Handbook of
Experimental Pharmacology

Continuation of Handbuch der experimentellen Pharmakologie

Vol. 55/II

Psychotropic Agents

Part II: Anxiolytics,
Gerontopsychopharmacological Agents,
and Psychomotor Stimulants

Contributors

C. Braestrup · P.B. Dews · S. Garattini · C. Giurgea · G. Greindl
W. Haefely · H. Hauth · L.R. Hines · F. Hoffmeister · S. Hoyer
M.L. Jack · S.A. Kaplan · S. Kazda · D.M. Loew · L. Pieri · P. Polc
S. Preat · L.A. Salazar · R. Samanin · R. Schaffner · C.R. Schuster
F. Seuter · L.H. Sternbach · J.M. Vigouret · J.E. Villarreal · T. Yanagita

Editors

F. Hoffmeister · G. Stille

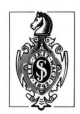

Springer-Verlag Berlin Heidelberg New York 1981

Professor Dr. F. HOFFMEISTER
Bayer AG, Institut für Pharmakologie, Aprather Weg 18a, D-5600 Wuppertal 1

Professor Dr. G. STILLE
Institut für Arzneimittel des Bundesgesundheitsamtes
Stauffenbergstraße 13, D-1000 Berlin 30

With 77 Figures

ISBN 3-540-10300-7 Springer-Verlag Berlin Heidelberg New York
ISBN 0-387-10300-7 Springer-Verlag New York Heidelberg Berlin

Library of Congress Cataloging in Publication Data. Main entry under title: Anxiolytics, gerontopsychopharmacological agents, and psychomotor stimulants. (Psychotropic agents; pt. 2) (Handbook of experimental pharmacology; v. 55/II). Includes bibliographies and index. 1. Tranquilizing drugs. 2. Geriatric psychopharmacology. 3. Stimulants. I. Braestrup, C. II. Hoffmeister, Friedrich. III. Stille, Günther, 1923–. IV. Series. V. Series: Handbook of experimental pharmacology; v. 55/II. QP905.H3 vol. 55/II [RM333] 615'.1s 80-28013 [615'.7882].

Printed in Germany

The use of registered names, trademarks, etc. in this publication does not imply, even in the absence of a specific statement, that such names are exempt from the relevant protective laws and regulations and therefore free for general use.

Typesetting, printing, and bookbinding: Brühlsche Universitätsdruckerei Giessen. 2122/3130-543210

Preface

This second volume continues the description of the psychotropic agents and discusses anxiolytics, gerontopsychopharmacological agents, and psychomotor stimulants.

Of these groups of substances, most of this volume has been devoted to anxiolytics as the authors have endeavored to convey as complete a picture as possible. The editors are of the opinion that particular attention should be given to anxiolytics with regard to their range of administration as this is the most frequently prescribed group of psychotropic drugs. In contrast to neuroleptics and thymoleptics, anxiolytics are a class of psychotropic drugs whose therapeutic effect can be recognized in animal experiments to some extent. This, together with the analysis of the biochemical mechanisms of their actions, permits a better understanding of material processes in the brain accompanying the emotions: anxiety and tension.

For the first time in the history of the Handbook the editors have devoted a whole chapter to gerontopsychopharmacological agents. In doing so they are also aware of the risk they are taking, at least from a pharmacological point of view, as gerontopsychopharmacological agents are an insufficiently defined and extremely heterogeneous group of substances. The only denominator the various subgroups of these agents have in common is that they are given in cases of dysfunctions, disorders, and diseases of the brain occurring mainly in the elderly. Here the question has been raised whether the therapeutic effects of all the substances in use are beyond doubt, or whether they are, at least in part, given because there is a pressing need for therapeutic intervention in these diseases of the elderly. Scientific psycho-pharmacology has long neglected research in this field with the result that, at present, little is known about relevant basic pharmacological mechanisms. As a result, the individual contributions are heterogeneous and should serve as a challenge to motivate further studies in this field rather than seeing the information contained in these chapters as being a complete description of this particular discipline.

Psychomotor stimulants in our day play a limited role in therapy. The social aspects of such stimulants, however, are enormous. With this in mind, the reader's attention is drawn to the volume on drug dependence edited by MARTIN (45/II). Independent of this knowledge of the effects of psychomotor stimulants, it is an absolute must for the pharmacologist to be able to understand the cerebral consequences of adrenergic, dopaminergic, and serotonergic stimulation.

Wherever possible and available, clinical pharmacology and therapeutic results are included to insure a better understanding and to describe the therapeutic relevance of pharmacological actions.

It was not the editor's intention to compile a textbook but rather to publish the views and convictions of the individual scientist. The reader, therefore, should not be surprised when he finds redundant or even contradictory opinions on one and the same theme in different chapters.

We believe that, in keeping with the tradition of the first volume, this second volume on psychotropic agents should not only be used as a reference book, but should also help to stimulate further research.

Wuppertal/Berlin   F. HOFFMEISTER · G. STILLE

List of Contributors

Dr. C. BRAESTRUP, Sct. Hans Mental Hospital, Dept. E, Psychopharmacological Research Laboratory, DK-4000 Roskilde

Dr. P. B. DEWS, Department of Psychiatry, Laboratory of Psychobiology, Harvard Medical School, 25 Shattuck Street, Boston, MA 02115/USA

Professor Dr. S. GARATTINI, Istitudo di Ricerche Farmacologiche "Mario Negri", Via Eritrea, 62, I-20157 Milano

Professor Dr. C. GIURGEA, University of Louvain, Neuropharmacological Department, UCB, Pharmaceutical Division, Rue Berkendael 68, B-1060 Bruxelles

Dr. G. GREINDL, University of Louvain, Neuropharmacological Department, UCB, Pharmaceutical Division, Rue Berkendael 68, B-1060 Bruxelles

Dr. W. HAEFELY, Pharma Research Department, F. Hoffmann-La Roche & Co AG, Grenzacherstraße 124, CH-4002 Basel

Dr. H. HAUTH, Sandoz AG, Pharmazeutisches Department, CH-4002 Basel

Dr. L. R. HINES, Hoffmann-La Roche, Inc., Research Division, Nutley, NJ 07110/USA

Professor Dr. F. HOFFMEISTER, Bayer AG, Institut für Pharmakologie, Postfach 101709, D-5600 Wuppertal 1

Professor Dr. S. HOYER, Institut für Pathochemie und Allgemeine Neurochemie im Zentrum Pathologie der Universität Heidelberg, Im Neuenheimer Feld 220–221, D-6900 Heidelberg

Dr. M. L. JACK, Department of Pharmacokinetics and Biopharmaceutics, Hoffmann-La Roche, Inc., Nutley, NJ 07110/USA

Dr. S. A. KAPLAN, Department of Pharmacokinetics and Biopharmaceutics, Hoffmann-La Roche, Inc., Nutley, NJ 07110/USA

Dr. S. KAZDA, Bayer AG, Institut für Pharmakologie, Postfach 101709, D-5600 Wuppertal 1

Dr. D. M. LOEW, Clinical Research, Sandoz, Inc., Hanover, NJ 07936/USA

Dr. L. PIERI, Pharma Research Department, F. Hoffmann-La Roche & Co AG, Grenzacherstraße 124, CH-4002 Basel

Dr. P. POLC, Pharma Research Department, F. Hoffmann-La Roche & Co AG Grenzacherstraße 124, CH-4002 Basel

Dr. S. PREAT, University of Louvain, Neuropharmacological Department, UCB, Pharmaceutical Division, Rue Berkendael 68, B-1060 Bruxelles

Dr. L.A. SALAZAR, Instituto Miles de Terapeutica Experimental, Apdo Postal 22026, MEX-México 22, D.F.

Dr. R. SAMANIN, Istituto di Ricerche Farmacologiche "Mario Negri", Via Eritrea, 62, I-20157 Milano

Dr. R. SCHAFFNER, Pharma Research Department, F. Hoffmann-La Roche & Co AG, Grenzacherstraße 124, CH-4002 Basel

Professor Dr. C.R. SCHUSTER, Department of Psychiatry, The University of Chicago, 950 East 59th Street, Chicago, IL 60637/USA

Dr. F. SEUTER, Bayer AG, Institut für Pharmakologie, Postfach 101709, D-5600 Wuppertal 1

Dr. L. H. STERNBACH, Hoffmann-La Roche Inc., Research Division, Nutley, NJ 07110/USA

Dr. J. M. VIGOURET, Preclinical Research, Pharmaceutical Division, Sandoz Ltd., CH-4002 Basel

Dr. J.E. VILLARREAL, Instituto Miles de Terapeutica Experimental, Apdo Postal 22026, MEX-México 22, D.F.

Dr. T. YANAGITA, Preclinical Research Laboratories, Central Institute for Experimental Animals, 1433 Nogawa, J-213 Kawasaki

Contents

Anxiolytics

CHAPTER 3

General Pharmacology and Neuropharmacology of Propanediol Carbamates.
W. HAEFELY, R. SCHAFFNER, P. POLC, and L. PIERI. With 1 Figure

CHAPTER 4

Behavioral Pharmacology of Anxiolytics. P. B. DEWS

CHAPTER 5

Biochemical Effects of Anxiolytics. C. BRAESTRUP. With 4 Figures

CHAPTER 8

Dependence-Producing Effects of Anxiolytics. T. YANAGITA. With 1 Figure

Gerontopsychopharmacological Agents

CHAPTER 9

Chemistry of Gerontopsychopharmacological Agents. H. HAUTH.
With 14 Figures

Contents

CHAPTER 10

Pharmacologic Approaches to Gerontopsychiatry. D. M. LOEW and
J. M. VIGOURET. With 2 Figures

CHAPTER 11

**Experimental Behavioral Pharmacology of Gerontopsychopharmacological
Agents.** C. GIURGEA, G. GREINDL, and S. PREAT. With 12 Figures

CHAPTER 12

Cerebrovascular Agents in Gerontopsychopharmacotherapy. F. HOFFMEISTER,
S. KAZDA, and F. SEUTER. With 4 Figures

CHAPTER 13

Biochemical Effects of Gerontopsychopharmacological Agents. S. HOYER

Psychomotor Stimulants

CHAPTER 14

The Pharmacological Profile of Some Psychomotor Stimulant Drugs Including Chemical, Neurophysiological, Biochemical, and Toxicological Aspects.
S. GARATTINI and R. SAMANIN. With 3 Figures

CHAPTER 15

The Behavioral Pharmacology of Psychomotor Stimulant Drugs. C. R. SCHUSTER

CHAPTER 16

The Dependence-Producing Properties of Psychomotor Stimulants.
J. E. VILLARREAL and L. A. SALAZAR. With 2 Figures

Contents

Part I: Antipsychotics and Antidepressants

Antipsychotics: Chemistry (Structure and Effectiveness)

Contents

Part III: Alcohol and Psychotomimetics, Psychotropic Effects of Central Acting Drugs

Alcohol

Psychotropic Effects of Central Acting Drugs

Anxiolytics

CHAPTER 1

The Chemistry of Anxiolytics

L. H. STERNBACH

A. Introduction

The anxiolytics are a group of CNS-active agents which in the last 25 years have played an ever-increasing role in the physician's armamentarium. They are mild sedatives with pronounced activity in anxiety, tension, and neuroses, including psychosomatic disorders. They generally do not act in psychoses, but are sometimes used in combination with neuroleptics to relieve anxiety in depressed psychotics. Several chemically completely unrelated classes of compounds are known to possess antianxiety properties and are discussed below. Although this chapter deals mainly with anxiolytics used in the United States, the sections on benzodiazepines (B.IV and B.V) include drugs used solely in other countries.

B. Classes of Antianxiety Agents

I. Barbiturates

Long before the terms anxiolytics or tranquilizers had been coined, barbiturates were used to achieve a calming effect in neurotic patients. Even now small doses of barbiturates are prescribed in some cases as antianxiety agents, e.g., phenobarbital, butabarbital, and amobarbital (1, 2, 3)[1], which are some of the most widely used representatives of a class of compounds which has yielded a host of useful drugs. They

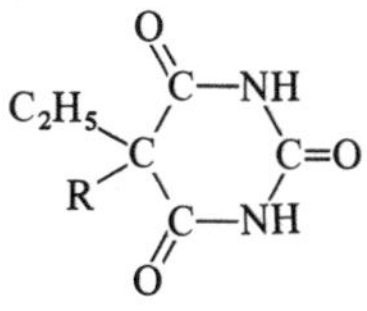

(1) R = C$_6$H$_5$

(2) R = CHCH$_2$CH$_3$
        |
        CH$_3$

(3) R = CH$_2$CH$_2$CH $<$ CH$_3$ / CH$_3$

---

[1] The drugs discussed in this chapter will be identified by their structural formulas, by their generic names, and in many cases by their trade names. The often cumbersome chemical names will be mentioned only exceptionally.

are disubstituted (at carbon 5) derivatives of barbituric acid and have been used since the beginning of the century, when the biologic activity of the diethyl derivative, barbital (Veronal), was discovered (FISCHER and v. MERING, 1903). Many hundreds of more or less potent, longer- or shorter-acting barbiturates have been prepared in the course of the last 75 years. They have found broad use as reliable hypnotics and in smaller doses as sedatives, anxiolytics, and antiepileptics.

II. Propanediols

A sweeping change in the treatment of neurotic patients took place when the first "tranquilizer", meprobamate, was discovered. It was synthesized by LUDWIG and PIECH (1951) in the course of synthetic studies concerned with modifications of the molecule of mephenesin (4), a glycerol derivative with short-acting muscle relaxant and anticonvulsant properties.

$$\text{benzene ring with } CH_3 \text{ and } OCH_2\overset{OH}{CH}CH_2OH$$

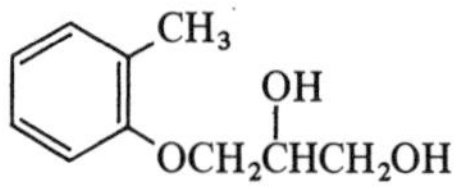

(4)

In the course of this work, it was found that simple 2-disubstituted propanediol (5) derivatives possessed superior, but very short-lasting anticonvulsant properties (LUDWIG and PIECH, 1951; BERGER, 1949).

$$HOCH_2-\underset{R_2}{\overset{R_1}{C}}-CH_2OH$$

(5)

A logical approach to longer-acting compounds was the blocking of the hydroxylic groups (LUDWIG and PIECH, 1951) to retard their metabolic degradation and elimination. One of these compounds, 2-methyl-2-propyl-1,3-propanediol dicarbamate (6) (BERGER, 1954) indeed possessed a superior spectrum of activity, received the

$$NH_2COOCH_2-\underset{CH_2CH_2CH_3}{\overset{CH_3}{C}}-CH_2OCONH_2$$

(6)

generic name meprobamate, and was introduced in 1955 under the trade name Miltown and in 1957 as Equanil. (For an excellent review see BERGER and LUDWIG, 1964).

This product was followed in 1965 by a close relative, tybamate (7), which possesses a similar pharmacologic and clinical spectrum of activity.

$$H_2NCOOCH_2-\underset{CH_2CH_2CH_3}{\overset{CH_3}{C}}-CH_2OCONHCH_2CH_2CH_2CH_3$$

(7)

Its synthesis was reported by BERGER and LUDWIG (1960) and its pharmacologic properties by BERGER et al. (1964). However, it never gained the broad acceptance of the first member of this series and was withdrawn from the market in 1977.

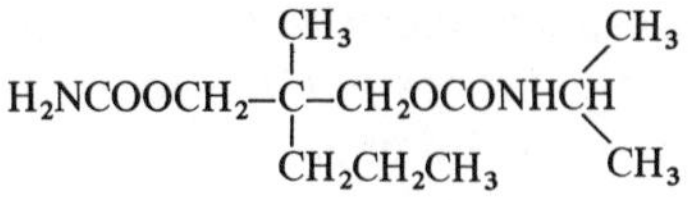

$$
\underset{\underset{\text{CH}_2\text{CH}_2\text{CH}_3}{|}}{\overset{\overset{\text{CH}_3}{|}}{\text{H}_2\text{NCOOCH}_2-\text{C}-\text{CH}_2\text{OCONHCH}}}\underset{\text{CH}_3}{\overset{\text{CH}_3}{\diagup}}
$$

(8)

Another member of this group is carisoprodol (8, Soma), which is used as a muscle relaxant relaxant but also has some sedative properties.

III. Compounds Belonging to Various Chemically Unrelated Classes

Some compounds belonging to other classes of drugs which were known to possess effects on the CNS were also used as anxiolytics. The centrally acting anticholinergic agent benactyzine (9) (for an exhaustive review see JACOBSON, 1964) found application in combination with meprobamate as Deprol.

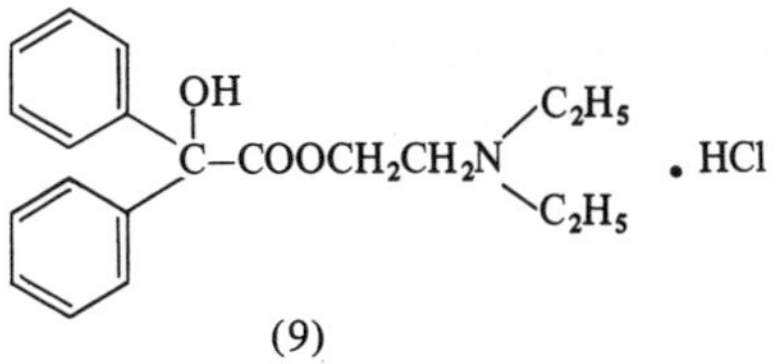

$$
\underset{\overset{|}{\text{C}}-\text{COOCH}_2\text{CH}_2\text{N}\diagup^{\text{C}_2\text{H}_5}_{\diagdown\text{C}_2\text{H}_5}}{\overset{\text{OH}}{|}} \quad \cdot \text{HCl}
$$

(9)

More widely used is hydroxyzine hydrochloride (10), a piperazine derivative closely related to the antihistamines which are known to have more or less pronounced sedative properties. It is the active ingredient of Atarax and Vistaril.

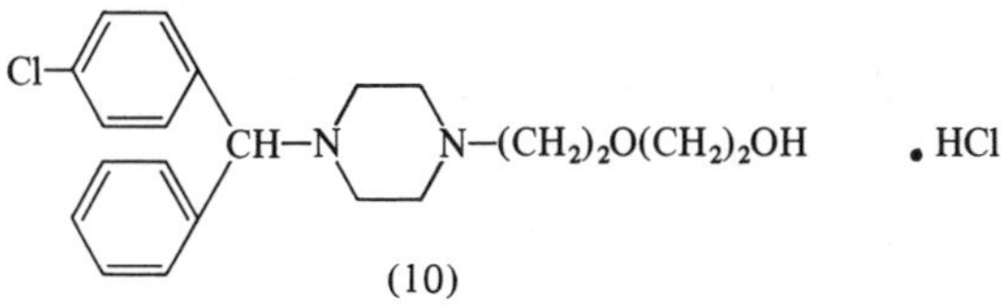

$$
\text{Cl}\text{---}\underset{\text{CH}-\text{N}}{\diagdown}\text{N}-(\text{CH}_2)_2\text{O}(\text{CH}_2)_2\text{OH} \quad \cdot \text{HCl}
$$

(10)

The synthesis of the product was first published by MORREN et al. in 1954, and in 1956, a description of the production method appeared in Chemical Week. A review article by MORREN et al. (1964) contains a detailed discussion of hydroxyzine and related compounds.

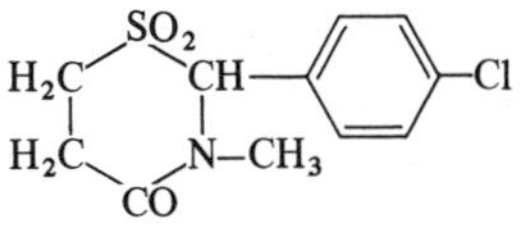

$$
\underset{\underset{\text{CO}}{\overset{|}{\text{H}_2\text{C}}}}{\overset{\overset{\text{SO}_2}{\diagup}}{\text{H}_2\text{C}}}\diagdown\underset{\text{N}-\text{CH}_3}{\overset{\text{CH}-}{|}}\text{---}\text{Cl}
$$

(11)

Completely unrelated chemically to the other products is the aryl-thiazanone derivative, chlormezanone (Trancopal, 11), which is a less frequently used anxiolytic. Its synthesis was published by SURREY et al. in 1958.

IV. 1,4-Benzodiazepines*

The most dramatic change in the physician's prescription pattern took place after the discovery of the anxiolytics of the 1,4-benzodiazepine type. The first member of this series was obtained by STERNBACH and REEDER (1961 a) in the course of a program aimed at the discovery of novel groups of CNS-active drugs. The chemical study of heterocyclic compounds led to the finding that the biologically inactive quinazoline N-oxide (12), on treatment with methylamine, underwent a ring enlargement to form

(12)   (13)

7-chloro − 2-methylamino-5-phenyl-3H-1,4-benzodiazepine 4-oxide (13), a compound containing a seven-membered heterocyclic ring system. The pharmacologic evaluation (RANDALL, 1961) showed that the product had interesting "tranquilizing" properties combined with a very low toxicity. This resulted in its clinical study and in the introduction in 1960 of its water-soluble hydrochloride under the trade name Librium. The product first had the generic name methaminodiazepoxide, which was later changed to chlordiazepoxide. Within a very short time it found general acceptance and by 1962 it was the most prescribed antianxiety agent.

Experiments concerned with transformations of this product led to the finding that chlordiazepoxide hydrochloride had a relatively short half-life in aqueous solution. After prolonged standing, it underwent hydrolysis with the loss of a molecule of methylamine and the formation of the pharmacologically equipotent lactam N-oxide 14 (STERNBACH and REEDER, 1961 b). An additional simplification of the molecular structure was the removal of the N-oxide oxygen in position 4 by reducing agents, which led to the highly active benzodiazepinone 15 (STERNBACH and REEDER, 1961 b).

Another transformation of the lactam N-oxide 14 is the so-called Polonovski rearrangement which occurs by treatment with acetic anhydride or acetyl chloride to yield the acetoxy derivative 16. This in turn is readily hydrolyzed to yield compound 17 (oxazepam), which possesses valuable antianxiety properties (BELL and CHILDRESS, 1962).

These transformations and additional studies showed that only the following relatively simple structural features were essential for the biologic activity of this new group of compounds:
1) The 1,4-benzodiazepine ring system
2) The substituent in the 7-position
3) The phenyl substituent in the 5-position.

These findings led to the synthesis and pharmacologic evaluation of thousands of experimental compounds possessing the above structural characteristics. Most of

---

* For the latest review article see STERNBACH, 1978

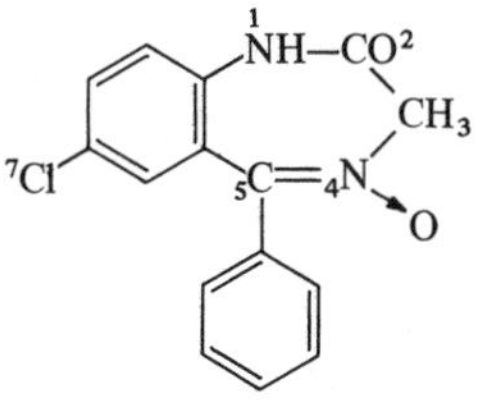

(14) 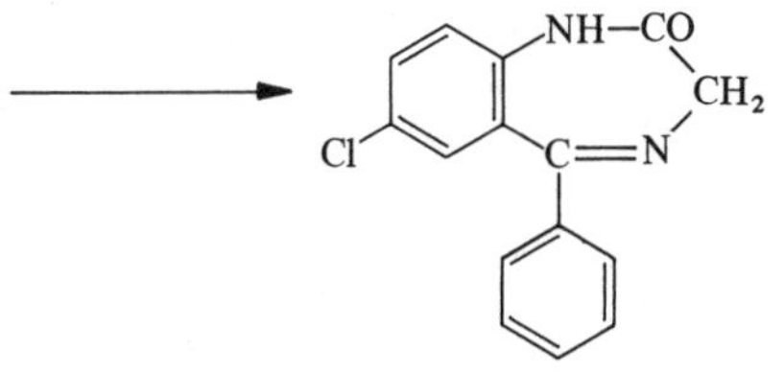   (15)

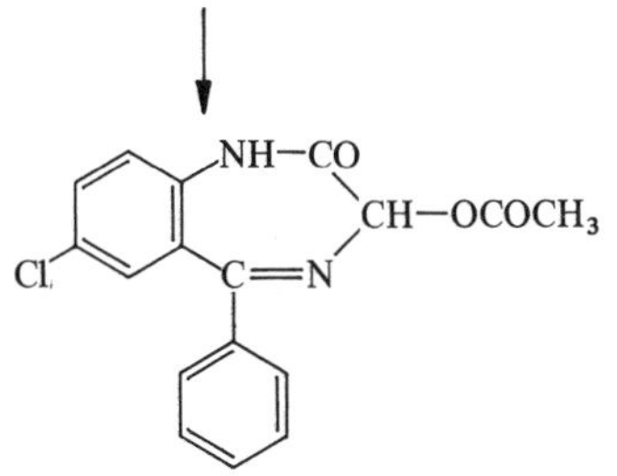

(16) 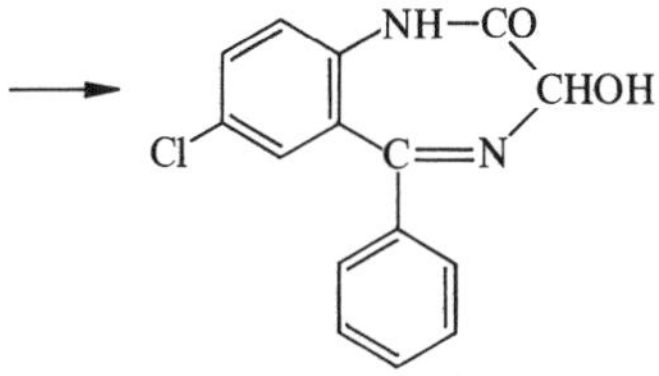   (17)

them showed pronounced muscle relaxant and sedative properties in animals. The monographs by STERNBACH et al. (1964, 1968) contain chemical and biologic data and the pertinent references. The first product to be introduced after Librium was the considerably more potent diazepam, which became available in 1963 under the trade name Valium. This compound 7-chloro-1,3-dihydro-1-methyl-5-phenyl-2H-1,4-benzodiazepinone (18) (STERNBACH and REEDER, 1961 b) gained general acceptance, surpassed Librium in popularity and, since 1969, is the antianxiety agent of choice.

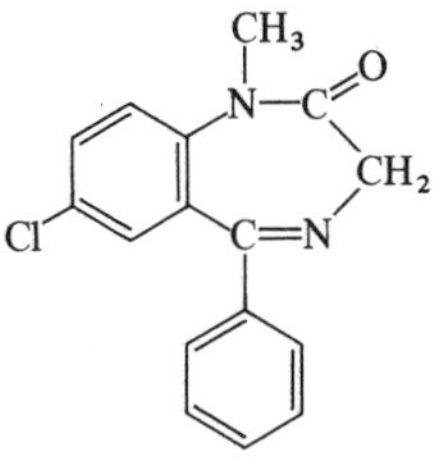

(18)

This product was followed in 1965 by oxazepam (17) which is marketed under various tradenames, e.g., in the United States as Serax, in Germany as Adumbran and Praxiten, and in Switzerland as Seresta.

An ever increasing number of 1,4-benzodiazepine derivatives followed; presently in the Unites States there are six 1,4-benzodiazepine anxiolytics at the physician's disposition. These are the three products shown below which are available in addition to chlordiazepoxide, diazepam, and oxazepam. The generic names, trade names, and dates of introduction are also listed.

Clorazepate (19) (SCHMITT et al., 1967, 1969) works essentially in the form of desmethyldiazepam (15) since it loses on ingestion the carboxylic substituent in the 3-position. Lorazepam (20) (BELL et al., 1968) is a close relative of oxazepam; prazepam (21) (WUEST, 1965; McMILLAN and PATTISON, 1965) is obtainable from desmethyldiazepam (15) by introduction of the cyclopropylmethyl substituent in position 1. A similarly simple derivative of 15 is pinazepam (31) (BENCONI et al., 1973), which contains a propargyl chain in the 1-position.

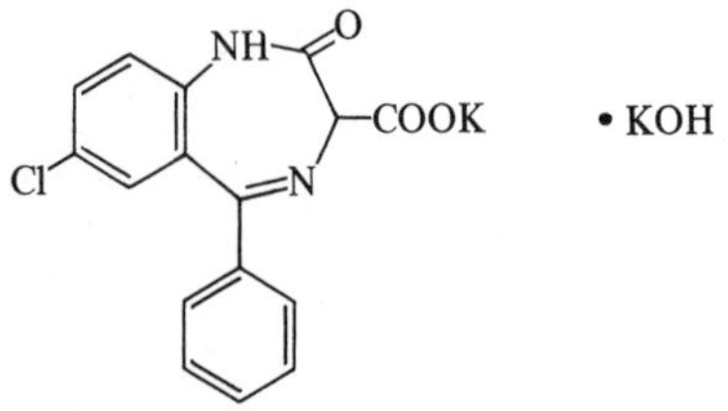

(19) *Clorazepate*
(Tranxene, 1972)

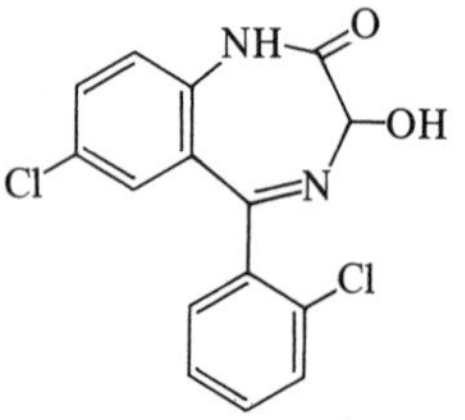

(20) *Lorazepam*
(Ativan, 1977)

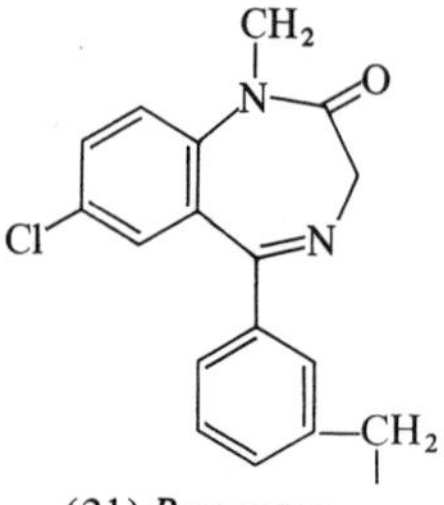

(21) *Prazepam*
(Verstran, 1977)

In addition to these anxiolytics, there are two more 1,4-benzodiazepine derivatives available in the United States. One is the hypnotic flurazepam (Dalmane, 22) (STERN-BACH et al., 1965), the other, clonazepam (Clonopin, 23) (STERNBACH et al., 1963), which is marketed as an anticonvulsant.

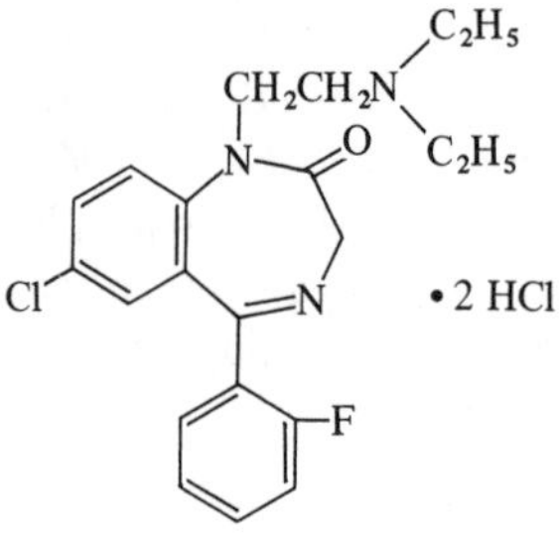

(22)

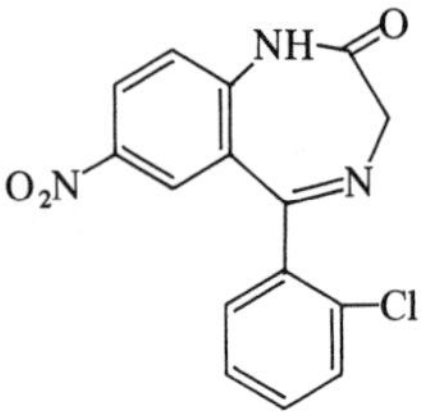

(23)

In other parts of the world there are other 1,4-benzodiazepine anxiolytics at the physician's disposition. Many of then are marketed worldwide, others only in a limited number of countries or in one country only.

The following shows, in chronological order, the formulas, generic names, and one of the trade names (many are marketed under various proprietary names) of benzodiazepines marketed in countries other than the United States.

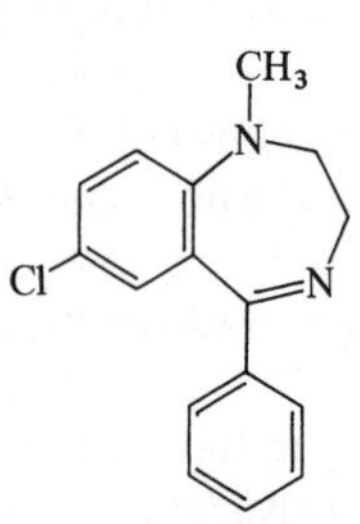

(24) Medazepam
(Nobrium, 1968)

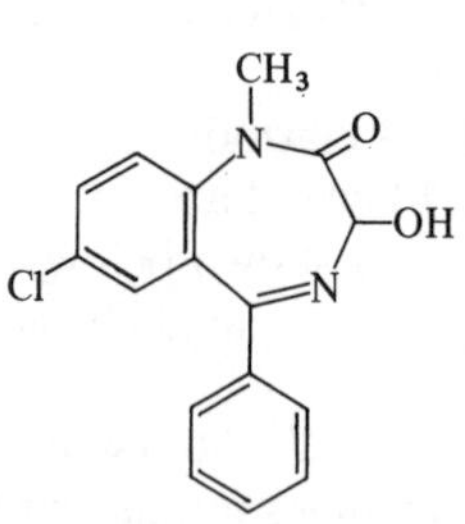

(25) Temazepam
(Levanxol, 1970)

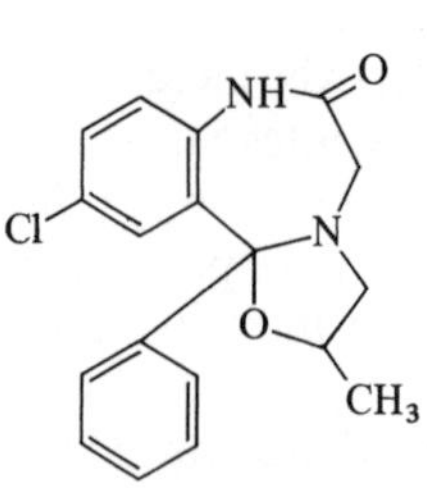

(26) Oxazolam
(Serenal, 1971)

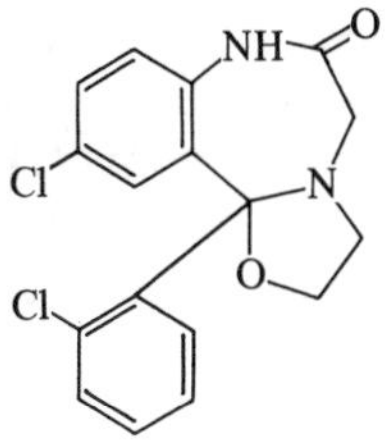

(27) Cloxazolam
(Sepazon, 1974)

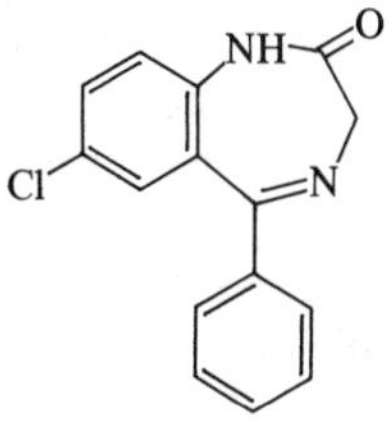

(15) Desmethyldiazepam
(Madar, 1973)

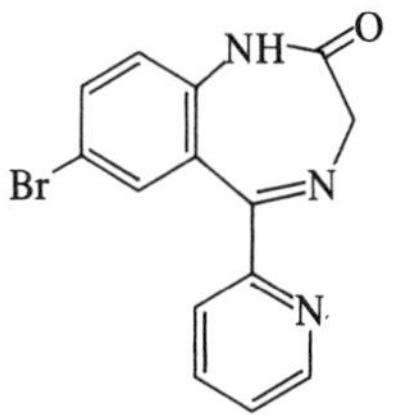

(28) Bromazepam
(Lexotanil, 1974)

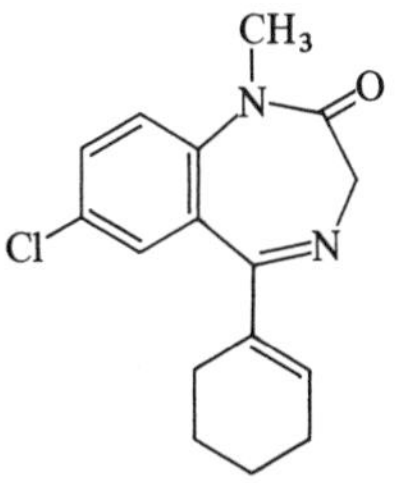

(29) Tetrazepam
(Myolastan, 1974)

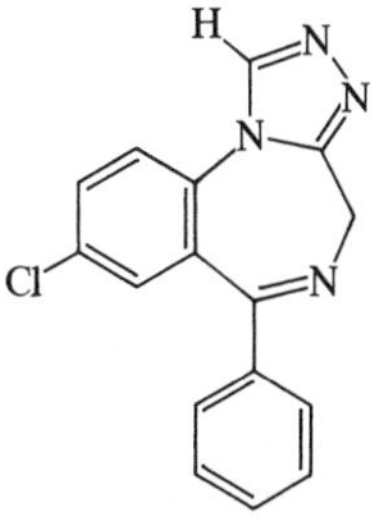

(30) Estazolam
(Eurodin, 1975)

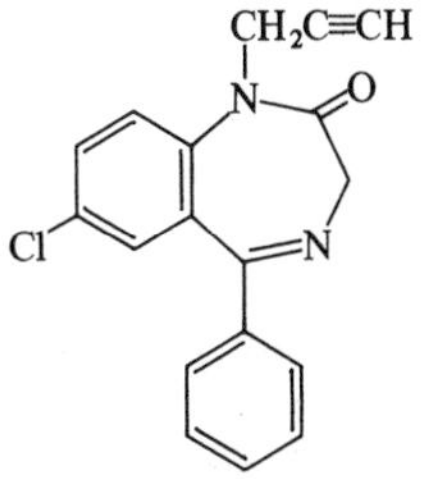

(31) Pinazepam
(Domar, 1975)

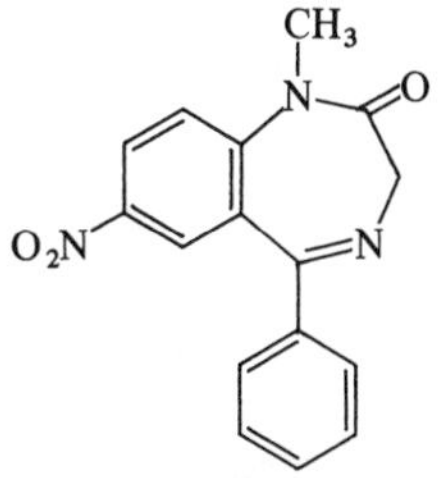

(32) Nimetazepam
(Erimin, 1977)

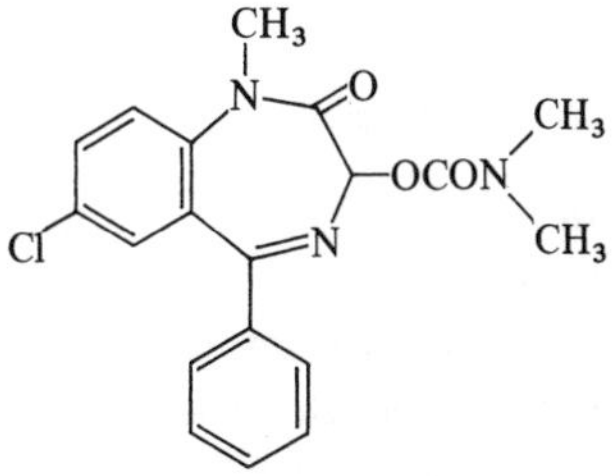

(33) Camazepam
(Albego, 1977)

All the commercially available products possess a pharmacophoric substituent in the 7-position which, as mentioned above, is of prime importance for the biologic activity. It is in most cases a chlorine atom, in some of the more potent compounds (23, 32, 34, 35) a nitro group (STERNBACH et al., 1963). The phenyl group in the 5-position is also present in all of these compounds; only bromazepam (28) (FRYER et al., 1964) has an α-pyridyl substituent in 5 (in addition to the bromine in 7), and tetrazepam (29) (SCHMITT et al., 1967, 1969) a cyclohexenyl group. Many of the most potent compounds, such as 20, 22, 23, 27, 35, and 36, bear an additional pharmacophore, a halogen in the 2′-position. Most of them have a carbonyl group in the 2-position and are thus related to diazepam. Three products, 20, 25 (BELL and CHILDRESS, 1962), and 33 (FERRARI and CASAGRANDE, 1974), are related to oxazepam (17) as they have an oxygen in the 3-position. Only one product (24) (ARCHER and STERNBACH, 1964; KAEGI, 1968) is currently on the market in which the benzodiazepine nucleus has a methylene group in the 2-position. It is metabolically converted into a benzodiazepinone having a carbonyl group in the 2-position (RIEDER and RENTSCH, 1968; SCHWARTZ and CARBONE, 1970).

Lately, 1,4-benzodiazepine derivatives have been introduced that have an additional ring attached to the heterocyclic part of the molecule as can be seen in the so-called oxazolobenzodiazepines oxazolam (26) and cloxazolam (27) (MIYADERA et al., 1971) and also in the biologically very potent "triazolobenzodiazepines" 30 (MEGURO and KUWADA, 1970) and 36 (HESTER et al., 1971). In two of these compounds (27 and 36) there is again a chlorine in the 2′-position which increases the pharmacologic activity.

Three more potent 1,4-benzodiazepine derivatives, shown below, are used as hypnotics.

(34) Nitrazepam (Mogadon, 1965)	(35) Flunitrazepam (Rohypnol, 1975)	(36) Triazolam (Halcion, 1977)

V. 1,5-Benzodiazepines

In view of their structural relationship to 1,4-benzodiazepines, 1,5-benzodiazepines have also lately evoked the interest of chemists and pharmacologists. Extended synthetic and pharmacologic studies have led to the discovery of pharmacologically active compounds (ROUSSEL UCLAF, 1968; HAUPTMANN et al., 1969; ROSSI et al., 1969; WEBER et al., 1972). Some of these also underwent clinical evaluation, which resulted in the introduction of clobazam (37) (Urbanyl), available in some European countries.

(37) Clobazam
(Urbanyl, 1975)

Acknowledgments. I would like to express my thanks to Dr. P. Sorter, head of the Scientific Literature Department and to his staff for literature searches, to the library staff for valuable help, to Dr. A. Rachlin for reviewing the manuscript, and to Mrs. Claudette Czachowski for excellent clerical work.

References

Anonymous: Tranquilizer's five-week scale-up. Chemical Week 70–71 (1956)

Archer, G.A., Sternbach, L.H.: Quinazolines and 1,4-benzodiazepines. XVI. Synthesis and transformations of 5-phenyl-1,4-benzodiazepine-2-thiones. J. Org. Chem. *29*, 231–233 (1964)

Bell, S.C., Childress, S.J.: A rearrangement of 5-aryl-1,3-dihydro-2H-1,4-benzodiazepine-2-one 4-oxides. J. Org. Chem. *27*, 1691–1695 (1962)

Bell, S.C., McCaully, R.J., Gochman, C., Childress, S.J., Gluckman, M.I.: 3-Substituted 1,4-benzodiazepin-2-ones. J. Med. Chem. *11*, 457–461 (1968)

Benconi, F., Tagliabue, R., Molteni, L.: 1-Propargyl 1,4-benzodiazepin-2-ones. Belgian Pat. 803315, assigned to Dr. L. Zambeletti S.P.A. (1973)

Berger, F.M.: Anticonvulsant action of 2-substituted-1,3-propanediols. Proc. Soc. Exp. Biol. Med. *71*, 270–271 (1949)

Berger, F.M.: The pharmacological properties of 2-methyl-2-n-propyl-1,3-propanediol dicarbamate (Miltown), a new interneuronal blocking agent. J. Pharmacol. Exp. Ther. *112*, 412–423 (1954)

Berger, F.M., Ludwig, B.J.: N-Monosubstituted-2,2-dialkyl-1,3-propanediols dicarbamates. U.S. Pat. 2937119 (1960)

Berger, F.M., Ludwig, B.J.: Meprobamate and related compounds. Psychopharmacological Agents, vol. 1, pp. 103–135. (Ed. M. Gordon) New York: Academic Press 1964

Berger, F.M., Kletzkin, M., Margolin, S.: Pharmacologic properties of a new tranquilizing agent 2-methyl-2-propyl-trimethylenebutylcarbamate carbamate (Tybamate). Med. Exp. *10*, 327–344 (1964)

Ferrari, G., Casagrande, C.: 1,4-Benzodiazepine derivatives. U.S. Pat. 3799920 (1974)

Fischer, E., Mering, v.: Über eine neue Klasse von Schlafmitteln, Ther. Ggw. *44*, 97 (1903); Chem. Zentralbl. *74*, I, 1155 (1903)

Fryer, R.I., Schmidt, R.A., Sternbach, L.H.: Quinazolines and benzodiazepines. XVII. Synthesis of 1,3-dihydro-5-pyridyl-2H-1,4-benzodiazepine derivatives. J. Pharm. Sci. *53*, 264–268 (1964)

Hauptmann, K.H., Weber, K.H., Zeile, K., Danneberg, P., Giesemann, K.: 1,5-Benzodiazepine derivatives. South African Pat. 6800803 (1968); Chem. Abstr. *70*, 106579 (1969)

Hester, J.B., Jr., Duchamp, D.J., Chidester, C.G.: A synthetic approach to new 1,4-benzodiazepine derivatives. Tetrahedron Letters *20*, 1609–1612 (1971)

Jacobson, E.: Benactyzine. Psychopharmacological Agents, Vol. 1, pp. 287–300. (Ed. M. Gordon) New York-London: Academic Press 1964

Kaegi, H.H.: Synthesis of 7-chloro-2,3-dihydro-1-methyl-5-phenyl-1H-1,4-benzodiazepine-5^{14}C hydrochloride. J. Labelled Comp. *4*, 363–367 (1968)

Ludwig, B.J., Piech, E.C.: Some anticonsulvant agents derived from 1,3-propanediols. J. Am. Chem. Soc. *73*, 5779–5781 (1951)

McMillan, F.H., Pattison, I.: Process for the production of 1-cycloalkyl derivatives of 1,4-benzodiazepine. U.S. Pat. 3192199 (1965)

Meguro, K., Kuwada, Y.: Syntheses and structures of 7-chloro-2-hydrazino-5-phenyl-3H-1,4-benzodiazepine and some isomeric 1,4,5-benzotriazocines. Tetrahedron Letters 4039–4042 (1970)

Miyadera, T., Terada, A., Fukunaga, M., Kawano, Y., Kamioa, T., Tamura, C., Takagi, H., Tachikawa, R.: Anxiolytic sedatives. 1. Synthesis and pharmacology of benzo[6,7]-1,4-diazepino[5,4-b]oxazole derivatives and analogs. J. Med. Chem. *14*, 520–526 (1971)

Morren, H., Denayer, R., Trolin, S., Grivsky, E., Linz, R., Strubbe, H., Dony, G., Marico, J.: Nouveaux derives 1,4-disubstitués de la piperazine. Etude de leurs propriétés antihistaminiques. Ind. Chim. Belg. *19*, 1176–1196 (1954)

Morren, H.G., Bienfet, V., Reyntjens, A.M.: Piperazine derivatives (except phenothiazines), Psychopharmacological Agents, Vol. 1, pp. 251–285. (Ed. M. Gordon) New York: Academic Press 1964

Randall, L.O.: Pharmacology of methaminodiazepoxide. Dis. Nerv. Syst. 21, 7–10 (1960); Pharmacology of chlordiazepoxide. Dis. Nerv. Syst. 22, 7–15 (1962)

Rieder, J., Rentsch, G.: Metabolismus und Pharmakokinetik des neuen Psychopharmakons 7-Chlor-2,3-dihydro-1-methyl-5-phenyl-1H-1,4-benzodiazepin (Ro 5-4556) beim Menschen. Arzneim. Forsch. *18*, 1545–1556 (1968)

Rossi, S., Pirola, O., Maggi, R.: 1,2,4,5-Tetrahydro-2,4-dioxo-3H-1,5-benzodiazepines. Chim. industria *51*, 479–483 (1969)

Roussel Uclaf. Benzo-1,5-diazepines C.N.S. depressants. Belg. Pat. 707667 (1968)

Schmitt, J., Comoy, P., Suquet, M., Boitard, J., Le Meur, J., Basselier, J.-J., Brunaud, M., Salle, J.: Sur un noveau myorelaxant de la classe des benzodiazépines: Le tetrazepam. Chim. Ther. *2*, 254–259 (1967)

Schmitt, J., Comoy, P., Suquet, M., Callet, G., Le Meur, J., Clim, T., Brunaud, M., Mercier, J., Salle, J., Siou, G.: Sur le nouvelles benzodiazépines hydrosolubles douées d'une puissante activité sur le syste'me nerveux central. Chim. Ther. *4*, 239–245 (1969)

Schwartz, M.A., Carbone, J.J.: Metabolism of ^{14}C-medazepam hydrochloride in dog, rat and man. Biochem. Pharmacol. *19*, 343–361 (1970)

Sternbach, L.H.: The benzodiazepine story. Progress in Drug Research. Vol. 22, pp. 229–267. (Ed. E. Jucker) Basel-Stuttgart: Birkhäuser 1978

Sternbach, L.H., Reeder, E.: Quinazolines and 1,4-benzodiazepines. II. The rearrangement of 6-chloro-2-chloromethyl-4-phenylquinazoline 3-oxide into 2-amino derivatives of 7-chloro-5-phenyl-3H-1,4-benzodiazepine 4-oxide. J. Org. Chem. *26*, 1111–1118 (1961a)

Sternbach, L.H., Reeder, E.: Quinazolines and 1,4-benzodiazepines. IV. Transformations of 7-chloro-2-methyl-amino-5-phenyl-3H-1,4-benzodiazepine 4-oxide. J. Org. Chem. *26*, 4936–4941 (1961b)

Sternbach, L.H., Fryer, R.I., Keller, O., Metlesics, W., Sach, G., Steiger, N.: Quinazolines and 1,4-benzodiazepines. X. Nitro-substituted 5-phenyl-1,4-benzodiazepine derivatives. J. Med. Chem. *6*, 261–265 (1963)

Sternbach, L.H., Randall, L.O., Gustafson, S.: 1,4-Benzodiazepines (chlordiazepoxide and related compounds). Psychopharmacol. Agents *1*, 137–224 (1964)

Sternbach, L.H., Archer, G.A., Earley, J.V., Fryer, R.I., Reeder, E., Wasyliw, N., Randall, L.O., Banziger, R.: Quinazolines and 1,4-benzodiazepines. XXV. Structure-activity relationships of aminoalkyl-substituted 1,4-benzodiazepin-2-ones. J. Med. Chem. *8*, 815–821 (1965)

Sternbach, L.H., Randall, L.O., Banziger, R., Lehr, H.: Structure-activity relationships in the 1,4-benzodiazepine series. Med. Res. Ser. *2*, 237–264 (1968)

Surrey, A.R., Webb, W.G., Gesler, R.M.: Central nervous system depressants. The preparation of some 2-aryl-4-metathiazanones. J. Am. Chem. Soc. *80*, 3469–3471 (1958)

Weber, K.H., Bauer, A., Hauptmann, H.H.: N-Aryl- and N-Heteroaryl-1H-1,5-benzodiazepin-2,4-[3H,5H]-dione. Liebigs Ann. Chem. *756*, 128–138 (1972)

Wuest, H.M.: 1-Cycloalkylmethyl derivatives of 1,4-benzodiazepine. U.S. Pat. 3192220 (1965)

CHAPTER 2

General Pharmacology and Neuropharmacology of Benzodiazepine Derivatives

W. Haefely, L. Pieri, P. Polc, and R. Schaffner

Introduction

This chapter deals with all pharmacologic effects of benzodiazepine-like compounds on neuronal and nonneuronal cells and tissues reported in the literature. In other words, we shall discuss all somatic effects of benzodiazepines investigated in experimental pharmacology and exclude effects on psychological functions which, in the animal, are identical with behavioral effects, since observation of free and scheduled behavior is the only means to obtain indirect information on drug-induced changes in the psychological activity of the laboratory animal. Behavioral effects of benzodiazepines are the subject of a special chapter in this volume (DEWS, 1981). We shall mention effects of benzodiazepines in man only on exceptional occasions.

Twenty years after the introduction of the first representative of the benzodiazepine class into therapy, the time has come to make a step beyond purely descriptive pharmacology and to consider the effects of these drugs in the light of a possible mechanism of action on the synaptic, cellular and molecular level. Research efforts of the past 7 years resulted in three important discoveries, namely (a) that benzodiazepines enhance GABAergic [γ-aminobutyric acid (GABA)] transmission throughout the mammalian central nervous system (HAEFELY et al., 1975b; COSTA et al., 1975b); (b) that they produce this effect by combining with receptor sites that are highly specific for this class of drugs (BRAESTRUP and SQUIRES, 1977; MÖHLER and OKADA, 1977a, b); and (c) that all the effects of benzodiazepines which are mediated by these receptors can be prevented or reversed by drugs that act as selective benzodiazepine antagonists, e.g., Ro 15–1788 (HUNKELER et al., 1981). We have attempted to make logical connections between individual pharmacologic observations and a single specific synaptic mechanism of action and yet to avoid too hypothetical speculations. We hope that this way of presenting the already enormous amount of available data will convince the sceptic reader of the value of the unifying notion of GABA-mediated effects of benzodiazepines and provoke relevant experiments to test this concept.

The term benzodiazepine, as it will be used throughout this chapter for the sake of brevity, should be understood in a broad sense and includes structural derivatives of benzodiazepines with similar pharmacologic activity. The benzol ring may be replaced by an aromatic heterocycle, the diazepine ring may contain the two nitrogen atoms in the 1,4-, the 1,5- or in the 2,4-position, or be replaced by an azepine ring.

A number of review articles and books, concerned entirely or in part with somatic effects of benzodiazepines, have appeared (ZBINDEN and RANDALL, 1967; RANDALL and SCHALLEK, 1968; GARATTINI et al., 1973; COSTA and GREENGARD, 1975; VAN DER KLEIJN et al., 1977; SCHALLEK, 1978; HAEFELY, 1978a; SCHALLEK and SCHLOSSER, 1979; SCHALLEK et al., 1979; FIELDING and LAL, 1979).

A. Acute Toxicity

I. Acute Toxicity in Man

From reports of accidental or suicidal ingestion of excessive amounts of drugs their approximative lethal doses can be estimated. A list of values of single oral lethal doses in man (Reggiani et al., 1968) for a few centrally active nonbenzodiazepine drugs is given in Table 1. In this Table, the drugs are listed according to the number of tablets that have to be taken in order to reach the approximate lethal dose. For benzodiazepines, uneventful recovery has been reported after ingestion of 500 mg (100 tablets) nitrazepam (Ridley, 1971), 500 mg (50 tablets) diazepam (Gilbert and Benson, 1972), 2,400 mg (80 tablets) flurazepam (Aderjan and Mattern, 1979), and 2,800 mg chlordiazepoxide (Malizia et al., 1965). No fatal outcome has been documented so far as a result of the ingestion of an overdose of these drugs when taken alone. Thus, acute lethal doses of these substances in man remain speculative. An extrapolated figure of 50–500 $mg \cdot kg^{-1}$ was presumed as the lethal dose of diazepam (Velvart, 1973). For chlordiazepoxide, the acute lethal dose in man was suggested to range between 200 and 300 $mg \cdot kg^{-1}$ (Malizia et al., 1965), which would require swallowing between 560 and 4,200 tablets or capsules.

II. Acute Toxicity in Animals

Acute toxicity in animals is usually indicated by the LD_{50}, which is the dose calculated to cause the death of half the animals administered a single dose of the substance. LD_{50} values as reported for diazepam from different laboratories are listed in Table 2. This is a representative example of the variability of results obtained in LD_{50} determinations, a field where methodologic standardization has not yet been universally adopted. For the substances listed in Table 3 and Table 4, minimal and maximal LD_{50} values were chosen from those reported in the literature, when possible. The acute intravenous doses as reported in the literature are not indicative of the acute toxic potency of benzodiazepines but, in fact, represent the toxicity of the vehicles used to solubilize the mostly very poorly water soluble active drugs.

III. General Comments on Acute Toxicity

Twenty years of extensive use of benzodiazepines have shown that acute lethal effects or irreversible somatic lesions or psychic disturbances do not occur in man with even tremendous overdoses, except under particular conditions such as, e.g., when combined with certain other drugs or on exposure to low ambient temperature (Aderjan and Mattern, 1979).

The high degree of safety is only in part due to the fact that benzodiazepines as a class belong to those drugs whose absolute lethal doses are high; a comparison of Tables 3 and 4 shows that a number of benzodiazepines have LD_{50} values similar to, e.g., meprobamate and barbiturates. More important for the high safety of benzodiazepines in practical terms is their high pharmacologic potency and, hence, their large therapeutic index. Because of their high potencies, the quantities of active ingredients in pharmaceutical formulations are very small, and the number of tablets or capsules that would contain sublethal or even lethal doses is simply too great to be swallowed (Aderjan and Mattern, 1979).

Table 1. Approximate oral lethal doses in man of several representative centrally active agents. (From REGGIANI et al., 1968, slightly modified and completed)

Drug with maximum content per tablet or capsule (mg)	Approximate lethal dose (LD) (mg)	Approximate therapeutic dose (ED) (mg)	Ratio LD/ED	Number of tablets containing LD	Ref.
Morphine (20)	60– 200	10– 20	3– 20	3– 10	DRILL (1958)
Chlorpromazine (100)	2,000	50– 100	20– 40	20	ALGERI et al. (1959)
Hexobarbitone (250)	2,000–10,000	250– 500	4– 40	8– 40	GLEASON et al. (1963)
Phenobarbitone (100)	2,000–10,000	100– 200	10– 100	20– 100	GLEASON et al. (1963)
Meprobamate (400)	20,000–40,000	400–1,200	20– 100	50– 100	CLEMMESEN (1965)
Glutethimide (250)	10,000–40,000	250– 500	20– 160	40– 160	RENNER (1965)
Chlordiazepoxide (25)	14,000–21,000	5– 50	280– 420	840–2,800	MALIZIA et al. (1965)
Diazepam (10)	3,500–35,000	2– 20	350–3,500	350–3,500	VELVART (1973)

Table 2. Intraperitoneal and oral LD$_{50}$ values for diazepam in mice and rats as reported from different laboratories

Mouse

Intraperitoneal		Per os		Ref.
LD$_{50}$ mg · kg^{-1}	95% Confidence limits	LD$_{50}$ mg · kg^{-1}	95% Confidence limits	
220				[1]
185	(294–382)			[2]
355				[3]
650				[4]
220		620	(560– 680)	[5]
332			(838–1,102)	[6]
		940	(642– 732)	[7]
			(550–1,610)	[8]
410			(560– 976)	[9]
270		930	(804–1,071)	[10]
		1,950	(1,300–2,923)	[11]

Rat

Intraperitoneal		Per os		Ref.
LD$_{50}$ mg · kg^{-1}	95% Confidence limits	LD$_{50}$ mg · kg^{-1}	95% confidence limits	
499	(416–599)			[12]
		710		[13]
663	(622–707)	2,075	(1,760–2,445)	[7]
		1,800		[14]

[1] SCHMITT et al. (1967)
[2] TAMAGNONE et al. (1974)
[3] MARCUCCI et al. (1971)
[4] HESTER et al. (1970)
[5] BANZIGER (1965)
[6] RANDALL et al. (1970)
[7] SHIBATA et al. (1967)
[8] ASAMI et al. (1975)
[9] NAKANISHI et al. (1972)
[10] KAMIOKA et al. (1972)
[11] HEILMAN et al. (1974)
[12] BABBINI et al. (1974)
[13] RANDALL and KAPPELL (1973)
[14] FERRINI et al. (1974)

Table 3. LD$_{50}$ values (mg·kg^{-1}) reported from different laboratories for various benzodiazepines. (Where two figures are given, they are the lowest and the highest reported)

Substance	Mouse		Rat	
	Intraperitoneal	Oral	Intraperitoneal	Oral
1,4-Benzodiazepines (7-chloro)				
Diazepam	185 [1] 650 [2]	620 [3] 1,950 [4]	499 [5] 663 [6]	710 [7] 2,075 [6]
Chlordiazepoxide	220 [8] 380 [9]	530 [7] 950 [9]		1,080 [8] 1,315 [7]
Flurazepam	260 [10] 290 [11]	660 [7] 870 [11]	200 [11]	1,232 [11] 2,400 [10]
Flurazepam	360 [12]	910 [12]		
Medazepam	360 [13] 550 [11]	475 [14] 1,070 [3]	220 [15]	900 [7] 1,650 [14]
Pinazepam	266 [6]	1,355 [6]	622 [6]	5,819 [6]
Tetrazepam	415 [16]	2,000 [16]		
Lorazepam (7-chloro, 3-OH)	986 [17]	3,170 [17]	1,730 [17]	>5,000 [17]
Oxazepam	3,270 [6]	12,000 [18]	1,535 [19] 5,000 [6]	>5,190 [6]
Clorazepate (7-chloro, 3-COOH)	290 [20]	700 [20]		3,050 [7]
Bromazepam (7-bromo, 5'pyridyl)		2,350 [3]		>3,000 [7]
Clonazepam (7-NO$_2$)		>4,000 [3]		
Flunitrazepam		1,980 [3]		485 [7]
Nitrazepam		1,550 [3] 2,300 [7]		825 [7]
Nimetazepam	970 [21]	910 [21]	970 [21]	1,150 [21]
Triazolam (triazolo)	>800 [22]			
Thiadipone (thio)	630 [23]	980 [23]		av. 2,000 [23]
"Y-7131" (thienotriazolo)	829 [24]	4,358 [24]	865 [24]	3,619 [24]
Brotizolam		>2,800 [25]		>3,546 [25]
Cloxazolam (oxazolidinotetrahydrol)	>2,000 [26]	3,300 [26]		
1,5-Benzodiazepines				
Clobazam	510 [9]	840 [9]		2,000 [9]

[1] Tamagnone et al. (1974)
[2] Hester et al. (1970)
[3] Banziger (1965)
[4] Heilman et al. (1974)
[5] Asami et al. (1974)
[6] Scrollini et al. (1975)
[7] Randall and Kappell (1973)

[8] Barzaghi et al. (1973)
[9] Nakanishi et al. (1972)
[10] Ikeda (1975)
[11] Randall et al. (1969)
[12] Asami et al. (1974)
[13] Randall et al. (1970)
[14] Ferrini et al. (1974)

[15] Gilbert and Benson (1972)
[16] Schmitt et al. (1967)
[17] Owen et al. (1971)
[18] Klupp and Kähling (1965)
[19] Babbini et al. (1973)
[20] Brunaud et al. (1970)
[21] Sakai et al. (1972)

[22] Rudzik et al. (1973)
[23] Fernandez-Tomé et al. (1975)
[24] Edanaca et al. (1978)
[25] Koch (1979)
[26] Kamioka et al. (1972)

Table 4. LD_{50} values ($mg \cdot kg^{-1}$) reported from different laboratories for tranquilizers other than benzodiazepines, as compared with phenobarbitone. Where two figures are given, they are the lowest and the highest reported

Substance	Mouse		Rat	
	Intraperitoneal	Oral	Intraperitoneal	Oral
Meprobamate	736 [1] 800 [2]	1,000 [3] 1,720 [4]	545 [2]	1,600 [2]
Methaqualone	555 [5]	1,130 [5]		
Methylpentynol		525 [6]		300–900 [6]
Phenobarbitone	340 [7]	325 [8]	190 [7]	660 [9]

[1] RANDALL et al. (1960)
[2] BERGER et al. (1964)
[3] ROBICHAUD et al. (1970)
[4] SHIBATA et al. (1967)
[5] SAITO et al. (1969)

[6] USDIN and AMAI (1963)
[7] GRUBER et al. (1944)
[8] REINHARD et al. (1952)
[9] SCHAFFARZICK and BROWN (1952)

A further point, which immediately emerges from a rapid inspection of Table 3, is the fact that not the slightest correlation exists between the pharmacologic potencies of benzodiazepines and their lethal doses. This clearly indicates that the lethal effects of benzodiazepines cannot be considered as the endpoint of an exaggeration of their main pharmacologic activity, but it strongly suggests that the lethal effects must be due to biologic actions that are completely unrelated to those underlying the main pharmacologic effects. This assumption is strongly supported by recent findings that specific benzodiazepine antagonists are unable to increase the LD_{50} of benzodiazepines; hence benzodiazepine receptors do not seem to mediate the lethal effects. Anticipating the evidence that will be offered in the subsequent paragraphs for a specific interaction of benzodiazepines with GABAergic synaptic transmission to produce their characteristic effects, we are on firm ground in assuming that sublethal and lethal effects are not due to their interaction with GABAergic mechanisms, but rather to relatively nonspecific membrane effects which can be observed with high concentrations of benzodiazepines (as with most other drugs).

B. Cardiovascular Effects

As will be shown below, benzodiazepines in therapeutic doses seem to have little, if any, direct effects on heart and blood vessels. However, these drugs have profound effects on brain structures involved in the control of emotional behavior and autonomic functions. The increasing awareness of the influence of emotional factors on autonomic functions and the extensive use of benzodiazepines have stimulated the interest in potential desired and undesired effects of this class of drugs on the cardiovascular system. In particular, benzodiazepines used as preanesthetics and induction agents, such as diazepam, flunitrazepam, lorazepam, and midazolam, have been studied in clinical conditions. They were reported to lower arterial blood pressure in patients undergoing surgery (DALEN et al., 1969; RAO et al., 1972; COLEMAN et al., 1973; COMER et al., 1973; JENKINSON et al., 1974; CÔTÉ et al., 1974; KORTTILA, 1975;

RIFAT and BOLOMAY, 1976; CÔTÉ et al., 1976; CONNER et al., 1978) and to either increase (RAO et al., 1972; COLEMAN et al., 1973; JENKINSON et al., 1974) or to fail to affect heart rate (DALEN et al., 1969; CÔTÉ et al., 1974; KORTTILA, 1975; CÔTÉ et al., 1976; RIFAT and BOLOMEY, 1976). Cardiac output and stroke volume were found to be reduced (DALEN et al., 1969; RAO et al., 1972; JENKINSON et al., 1974; CÔTÉ et al., 1974, 1976; RIFAT and BOLOMEY, 1976). An increase (RAO et al., 1972; JENKINSON et al., 1974) and a decrease (COLEMAN et al., 1973; RIFAT and BOLOMEY, 1976; FALK et al., 1978), as well as the absence of an effect (DALEN et al., 1969; COMER et al., 1973; CÔTÉ et al., 1974, 1976) on peripheral vascular resistance were observed. Diazepam was reported to decrease left ventricular end-diastolic pressure, rate of systolic pressure increase (dp/dt), and myocardial O_2 consumption in volunteers and patients (CÔTÉ et al., 1974, 1976). As an example of investigations in arterial hypertension, we mention the study of POZENEL et al. (1977) which showed that bromazepam reduced systolic and diastolic blood pressure in hypertensive patients after a single dose of 10 mg i.v. or after oral administration of 6–9 mg per day for 3 weeks. Most recently, MASSO and PEREZ (1979) performed a double-blind trial with bromazepam in hypertensive patients; the drug, 6 mg daily for 30 days, reduced both systolic and diastolic blood pressure to a similar extent as α-methyldopa.

I. Blood Pressure, Heart Rate, and Other Hemodynamic Parameters

1. Chlordiazepoxide

RANDALL et al. (1960) and MOE et al. (1962) observed transient hypotension and bradycardia in anesthetized dogs and cats after intravenous doses of chlordiazepoxide (1–16 mg · kg^{-1}). The effect on blood pressure was dose-dependent and long-lasting after higher doses (RANDALL et al., 1960; STERNBACH et al., 1964; RANDALL and SCHALLEK, 1968). Intraperitoneal administration to anesthetized cats (10 mg · kg^{-1}) and open-chest dogs (5 mg · kg^{-1}) resulted in a short-lasting decrease of blood pressure and heart rate and a reduction of myocardial contractile force (GLUCKMAN, 1965). A fall of blood pressure and biphasic effects on heart rate and myocardial contractile force were found after 5–15 mg · kg^{-1} i.v. in open-chest dogs by MADAN et al. (1963). A myocardial depressant effect after 10–20 mg · kg^{-1} i.v. was also found in the open-chest dog by HITCH and NOLAN (1971). CARROLL et al. (1961) observed a transient lowering of blood pressure and heart rate after chlordiazepoxide (10–20 mg · kg^{-1}) in cats, whereas no effect was found by SCHALLEK and ZABRANSKY (1966) in doses which depressed the hypothalamic-induced pressor response (20 mg · kg^{-1} i.v.). GLUCKMAN (1965) found no effect with 10 mg · kg^{-1} p.o. in conscious dogs. A decrease in blood pressure and an increase in heart rate with reduced rate of left ventricular pressure increase (dp/dt) was reported by MERLO et al. (1974) with 1 and 5 mg · kg^{-1} i.v. MCHUGH et al. (1978) reported a hypotensive effect in the normotensive as well as in the carotid sinus denervated hypertensive dog after an intravenous administration of 10 mg · kg^{-1}. The same authors also reported a hypotensive effect of chlordiazepoxide in genetically hypertensive rats (0.63–10 mg · kg^{-1} daily p.o. for 7 days) and in carotid sinus denervated dogs anesthetized with pentobarbitone or α-chloralose. The effects in hypertensive animals were more marked than in normotensives. In addition, a stronger hypotensive effect was observed under pentobarbitone anesthesia than under α-chloralose. In squirrel monkeys with elevated mean arterial blood pressures due to scheduling environmental stimuli, chlordiazepoxide (10 and 30 mg·kg⁻¹ i.m.) reduced blood pressure during time-out as well as time-on periods (BENSON et al., 1970).

2. Diazepam

A weak hypotensive and bradycardic effect after intravenous injections of diazepam in anesthetized dogs was reported by RANDALL et al. (1961). These effects were transient in moderate doses (1–8 mg·kg⁻¹ i.v.), but long-lasting after a higher dose (RANDALL et al., 1963). BRASSIER et al. (1966) found a dose dependency of this effect after intravenous bolus injections (1–10 mg·kg⁻¹) but no change of either blood pressure or heart rate after slow intravenous infusion. A very similar observation was made by TAYLOR et al. (1970). In the same preparation a transient decrease in blood pressure and heart rate occurred after 5–10 mg·kg⁻¹ i.p. (GLUCKMAN, 1965, 1971). In anesthetized cats transient hypotension and bradycardia were found by RANDALL et al. (1963) and GLUCKMAN (1965) with 4 mg·kg⁻¹ i.v. and 10 mg·kg⁻¹ i.p., respectively. CHAI and WANG (1966) observed in addition a decrease of the myocardial contractile force after 0.1 mg·kg⁻¹ i.v. Intraarterial injections (0.3 mg) of diazepam produced an immediate but transient increase of the femoral artery blood flow in the denervated limb which was unaffected by atropine (CHAI and WANG, 1966). After cumulative intravenous doses (0.125–16 mg·kg⁻¹), a biphasic effect on blood pressure, i.e., lowering with low doses and gradual recovery to predrug values with higher doses, was observed by HUDSON and WOLPERT (1970). Rapid intravenous injection of fairly high doses (2–15 mg·kg⁻¹) resulted in hypotension, bradycardia, and arrhythmias, with rapid recovery (SHARER and KUTT, 1971). This effect was also obtained with the diazepam solvent. Much weaker effects on blood pressure and heart rate were reported by the same authors after slow intravenous infusion (0.5 mg·kg⁻¹·min⁻¹) for up to 50 min. ANTONACCIO and HALLEY (1975) reported a decrease in blood pressure and heart rate in doses which inhibit hypothalamic-evoked pressor responses (0.1, 0.3 mg·kg⁻¹ i.v.). SCROLLINI et al. (1975) found a similar blood pressure lowering effect with comparable doses. No effect on blood pressure and heart rate with 0.3–10 mg·kg⁻¹ i.v. was observed in intact curarized cats (SCHALLEK and ZABRANSKY, 1966; SIGG and SIGG, 1969), whereas an increase in heart rate was reported in the spinal cat (KEIM and SIGG, 1973).

In the anesthetized rabbit diazepam produced a brief hypotension with tachycardia which was due to the constituents of the ampoule solution (PARKES, 1968). No effect on blood pressure and heart rate was found by SCROLLINI et al. (1975) with 20 mg·kg⁻¹ i.p. In the conscious rabbit a stabilizing effect on blood pressure and some bradycardia were observed with 2.5 mg·kg⁻¹ i.v. (PARKES, 1968). Systemic (0.1–1 mg·kg⁻¹) or intracerebro-ventricular (100 μg/20 μl) injection into anesthetized rats lowered blood pressure, an effect which was antagonized by the GABA-antagonist, picrotoxin (BOLME and FUXE, 1977). No effect on blood pressure was observed in spontaneously hypertensive rats (SHR) after 5 mg·kg⁻¹ i.v. (VAN ZWIETEN, 1977).

The development of a persistent hypertension was delayed in offspring of SHR injected daily with diazepam 1 mg·kg⁻¹ s.c. from the 1st day of life to the 12th week (SCHIEKEN, 1979). The mean arterial blood pressure reached by these rats after 8 weeks was significantly higher than the one of the corresponding Wistar Kyoto control rats, but was lower than the one of SHR injected with diazepam vehicle. No effect was observed on the mean arterial blood pressure of Wistar Kyoto rats injected daily with 1 mg·kg^{-1} s.c. diazepam (SCHIEKEN, 1979). The arterial hypertension, which gradually developed in rats exposed daily to stressful light and auditory stimuli, was prevented by daily administration of diazepam as a food admix; the drug also reduced the already established stress-induced hypertension (SEGAL, 1980). Diazepam 7.5 mg·kg^{-1} i.v. produced anesthesia in rats with loss of reaction to sound, pain, and corneal stimulation; cerebral blood flow, but not cerebral oxygen uptake, was decreased (CARLSSON et al., 1976). However, when combined with nitrous oxide, diazepam reduced cerebral oxygen uptake to a similar degree as observed under surgical anesthesia with barbiturates.

Several *hemodynamic studies* were performed with benzodiazepines in conscious or open-chest dogs. In a series of studies in the anesthetized dog with a cardiopulmonary bypass, ABEL et al. (1969, 1970a, b, c) studied the effect of diazepam (0.1, 0.2 mg·kg^{-1}), injected into the extracorporal circulation, on left ventricular dynamics and coronary and peripheral vascular resistance. In dogs with paced hearts and constant aortic pressure (ABEL et al., 1969, 1970c) an increase in left ventricular pressure and dp/dt_{max} was found, force-velocity and length-tension relations were improved, and coronary and peripheral vascular resistance decreased. At the same time myocardial O$_2$ consumption increased. By keeping coronary blood flow constant, left ventricular contractility was unchanged. Coronary vascular resistance and systemic vascular resistance decreased (ABEL et al., 1969, 1970a, b). Injections of diazepam into the coronary (0.25 mg·kg^{-1}) and systemic (0.5 mg·kg^{-1}) circulation, respectively, in animals with a separation of these circulations resulted in decreases of vascular resistances of the respective vascular beds (ABEL et al., 1969, 1970a, b). α- and β-adrenolytics, reserpine, atropine, or ganglionic blocking agents, but not vagotomy, partially inhibited or markedly reduced the effect of diazepam on coronary vascular resistance and systemic vascular resistance (ABEL et al., 1970a). Systemic injection of 5 and 10 mg·kg^{-1} diazepam was shown to decrease myocardial contractile force, blood pressure, and heart rate (GLUCKMAN, 1965, 1971) without affecting coronary or aortic flow (TAYLOR et al., 1970). Infusion of comparable amounts resulted in a decrease of myocardial contractile force, blood pressure and heart rate, but coronary and aortic flow were increased and myocardial O$_2$ consumption was reduced (TAYLOR et al., 1970). In dogs with a right-heart bypass, BIANCO et al. (1971) reported decreased mean arterial blood pressures and maximal rate of left ventricular pressure development dp/dt_{max} while left ventricular end-diastolic pressure was elevated. Coronary blood flow increased and the arterial-venous oxygen difference was reduced. This effect occurred after high cumulative intraarterial doses (6 × 2.5 mg). In dogs equipped additionally with a balloon catheter in the left ventricle, bolus injections of 10 mg diazepam produced a moderate lowering of aortic pressure and left ventricular dp/dt_{max}, whereas left ventricular end diastolic pressure remained unchanged. Again an increased coronary blood flow and a narrowing of the arterial-venous oxygen difference were observed (BIANCO et al., 1971). Comparable volumes of vehicle produced the same hemodynamic effects. FIELD et al. (1971) reported that 0.25 and 0.5 mg·kg^{-1} i.v. had no effect on left ventricular dynamics, whereas DANIELL (1975) found a decrease in myocardial contractile force and myocardial oxygen consumption and an increased coronary blood flow and cardiac output after diazepam (2 mg·kg^{-1} i.v.) and chlordiazepoxide (16 mg·kg⁻¹ i.v.). The effects on the coronary blood flow were abolished by either hexamethonium, phentolamine, or practolol. JONES et al. (1978) observed an increase in coronary blood flow after diazepam (0.5 and 2.5 mg·kg⁻¹ i.v.) in the absence of changes in the left ventricular dynamics. Finally, CLANACHAN and MARSHALL (1980 b) reported a transient fall in blood pressure and a more sustained increase of coronary blood flow in anesthetized dogs after diazepam 1–4 mg·kg⁻¹ i.v. Doses of diazepam which clearly increased coronary flow consistently potentiated and prolonged the vasodilator effect of adenosine.

STARLEY and MICHIE (1969) injected cumulative doses of diazepam (0.1, 0.4, 0.5 mg·kg⁻¹ i.v.) into conscious dogs. Right ventricular systolic pressure was reduced and left heart hemodynamics remained unchanged. In contrast, BLOOR et al. (1973) observed an increase of heart rate and coronary blood flow with reduced coronary vascular resistance and stroke volume after intravenous (0.5–1 mg·kg⁻¹) or intraarterial (0.05–0.1 mg·kg⁻¹) diazepam. Again the solvent was reported to produce essentially the same effects. KOROL and BROWN (1968) observed an increase in blood pressure and heart rate after 0.3 mg·kg⁻¹ i.v. in conscious unrestrained dogs, whereas SCROLLINI et al. (1975) described a slight hypotension and bradycardia (10 mg·kg⁻¹ i.v.). JONES et al. (1979) observed no change in heart rate and mean arterial blood pressure after 1.0 and 2.5 mg·kg⁻¹ i.v., however, a decrease of left ventricular dp/dt_{max} and an increase of cardiac output with unaltered coronary flow, systemic and coronary vascular resistance, stroke volume or stroke work was seen. A slight reduction of heart rate and of methylatropine-induced tachycardia was found by CHASSAING and DUCHÊNE-MARULLAZ (1973) in untrained restrained dogs (0.5–4 mg·kg⁻¹ i.v.), whereas tachycardia was observed in dogs equipped with a telemetric system (1–4 mg·kg⁻¹ i.v.). Tachycardia was also found by GEROLD et al. (1976) after diazepam in trained dogs. In doses of 1, 3, and 10 mg·kg⁻¹ u.o. the drug induced a dose-dependent, moderate, and long-lasting tachycardia without changes in systolic blood pressure. The increased heart rate initially coincided with behavioral stimulation, which is a typical benzodiazepine effect in dogs, and later with sedation. By pharmacologically eliminating the sympathetic and/or parasympathetic control on the heart with a β-adrenoceptor blocking agent and with the antimuscarinic, methylatropine, the authors were able to show that the chronotropic effect of diazepam was caused by a central reduction of the vagal tone to the cardiac pacemaker. No significant effect on the cardiac sympathetic tone was observed. In addition to a centrally elicited withdrawal of the cardiac vagal tone, diazepam had a negative chronotropic action of moderate intensity on the cardiac pacemaker, which became apparent only after the elimination of sympathetic and parasympathetic influences.

3. Other Benzodiazepines

A long-lasting hypotensive effect was reported by STERNBACH et al. (1964) for intravenous doses of nitrazepam (4 mg·kg⁻¹) in anesthetized dogs; moderate transient effects were seen after oxazepam (1 and 10 mg·kg⁻¹ i.p., GLUCKMAN, 1965), flurazepam (1–8 mg·kg⁻¹ i.v., RANDALL et al., 1969), lorazepam (1 and 5 mg·kg⁻¹ i.p., GLUCKMANN, 1971), triflubazam (0.5–8 mg·kg⁻¹ i.v., HEILMAN et al., 1974), temazepan (1–5 mg·kg⁻¹ i.v., MERLO et al., 1974), chlorazepate (up to 30 mg·kg⁻¹ i.v.,

BRUNAUD et al., 1970), triazolam (10 mg·kg^{-1} i.v., FURUKAWA et al., 1976) and midazolam (0.25–10 mg·kg^{-1} i.v., JONES et al., 1978), whereas medazepam (15 mg·kg^{-1} i.v., RANDALL et al., 1968), pinazepam (10 mg·kg^{-1} i.v., SCROLLINI et al., 1975), pyrazapon (2–32 mg·kg^{-1} i.v., POSCHEL et al., 1974), clobazam (10–50 mg·kg^{-1} i.p. and p.o., FIELDING and HOFFMANN, 1979) and camazepam (1–5 mg·kg^{-1} i.v., MERLO et al., 1974) were found to be inactive. Lorazepam (1 and 5 mg·kg^{-1} i.p.) was reported to reduce myocardial contractile force (GLUCKMAN, 1971). A decreased left ventricular dp/dt_{max}, and coronary flow with unchanged systemic vascular resistance and stroke volume were reported for midazolam (1 and 10 mg·kg^{-1} i.v., JONES et al., 1978). Midazolam (1–10 mg·kg^{-1} i.v.) increased cardiac output and decreased left ventricular dp/dt_{max} in conscious dogs without affecting coronary blood flow, systemic or coronary vascular resistance, stroke volume or stroke work (JONES et al., 1979). Bromazepam (1 mg·kg^{-1} i.v.) produced tachycardia in chloralose-urethane anesthetized dogs with intact cardiac innervation, and a slight bradycardia in dogs with acute cardiac denervation (GEROLD et al., 1976). In anesthetized cats a dose-dependent increase in blood pressure was reported for medazepam after intravenous doses of 4–16 mg·kg^{-1} i.v. (RANDALL et al., 1968); a short-lasting hypotension was observed after flurazepam (1–8 mg·kg^{-1} i.v., RANDALL et al., 1969) and oxazepam (10 mg·kg^{-1} i.p., GLUCKMAN, 1965). Also observed was a longer-lasting hypotension with bradycardia after clobazam 20 mg·kg^{-1} i.p. by BARZAGHI et al. (1973), but not by FIELDING and HOFFMANN (1979, 25–100 mg·kg^{-1} i.p.), some hypotension and bradycardia with lorazepam (1 and 5 mg·kg^{-1} i.p., GLUCKMAN, 1971) and no effect after pinazepam (cumulative doses up to 8 mg·kg^{-1} i.v.; SCROLLINI et al., 1975). Estazolam caused a marked and prolonged hypotension at 1 mg·kg^{-1} i.v., which was not modified by vagotomy or peripheral autonomic blocking agents but was abolished by spinal transection (SAJI et al., 1972); heart rate transiently increased and thereafter decreased for more than 2 h. Blood flow in the femoral and carotid artery was increased by up to 100% for a long time. Chlorazepate (10 mg·kg^{-1} i.v.) was reported to induce some bradycardia (BRUNAUD et al., 1970). In unrestrained conscious cats an intravenous infusion of medazepam up to a final dose of 15 mg produced a short-lasting fall in blood pressure and heart rate (HEINEMANN et al., 1969), but when injected into curarized cats a dose-dependent increase in blood pressure was reported (5–20 mg·kg^{-1} i.v., SCHALLEK et al., 1968, 1970). Flurazepam (20 mg·kg^{-1} i.v.) was also reported to increase blood pressure in curarized cats (SCHALLEK et al., 1968), whereas a short-lasting hypotension was observed with estazolam (SAJI et al., 1972). In anesthetized rabbits, flurazepam (20 mg·kg^{-1} i.p., BABBINI et al., 1975) and chlorazepate (10 mg·kg^{-1} i.v.; BRUNAUD et al., 1970) decreased the blood pressure, whereas doxefazepam (BABBINI et al., 1975), triazolam (FURUKAWA et al., 1976), and pinazepam (SCROLLINI et al., 1975) were ineffective. Estazolam injected in a high dose (10 mg·kg^{-1} i.v.) to conscious rabbits caused only a weak and transient hypotension and bradycardia; the same dose injected intraperitoneally produced a slight bradycardia (SAJI et al., 1972). In DOCA-saline hypertensive rats both medazepam (RANDALL et al., 1968) and flurazepam (RANDALL et al., 1969) were reported to have a hypotensive effect in sedative doses. Clonazepam had no effect in spontaneous hypertensive rats (BLUM et al., 1973). No change of blood pressure was observed with pyrazapon (2 × 50 mg·kg^{-1} p.o.) in perinephritic encapsulated hypertensive rats (POSCHEL et al., 1974).

In conscious dogs oxazepam (1–10 mg·kg^{-1} p.o.; Gluckman, 1965) did not change blood pressure or heart rate, whereas a slight decrease in blood pressure and some tachycardia was found with 10 mg·kg^{-1} pinazepam i.v. (Scrollini et al., 1975). Bromazepam in doses of 1, 3, and 10 mg·kg^{-1} p.o. had no effect on blood pressure but produced tachycardia and inhibited methylatropine-induced tachycardia in a study by Gerold et al. (1976) and produced a significant rise in arterial blood pressure with increased heart rate in a dose of 0.3 mg·kg^{-1} i.v. in experiments by Korol and Brown (1968). As shown for diazepam, the tachycardia induced by bromazepam (Gerold et al., 1976) was mainly due to a central reduction of the vagal tone to the heart. Clonazepam (0.3–10 mg·kg^{-1} p.o.) produced a non-dose-related hypotension (Blum et al., 1973). Wilson et al. (1974) reported that U-31,889 (0.5–2 mg·kg^{-1} i.v.), a triazolobenzodiazepine, decreased blood pressure and increased heart rate in a dose-dependent manner. Central venous pressure and pulmonary artery pressure were reduced. Slight bradycardia and hypotension were observed with 10 and 100 mg·kg^{-1} pyrazapon p.o. (Poschel et al., 1974).

II. Arrhythmias

Van Loon (1968) reported a case of reversion of ventricular arrhythmias to sinus rhythm with high intravenous doses of diazepam. The reversion occurred within minutes. However, in a study on patients who were injected with diazepam before attempting electrical cardioversion (atrial fibrillation, atrial flutter, atrial tachycardia, ventricular tachycardia) no beneficial effect was observed (Spracklen et al., 1970).

An increase in the threshold for electrically induced ventricular tachycardia was reported in anesthetized dogs after 1–2 mg·kg^{-1} diazepam i.v. (Spracklen et al., 1970), but the amount of K-strophanthin needed to induce arrhythmias was unaltered. In line with the failure of diazepam (0.5–1 mg·kg^{-1} i.v.) to restore K-strophantidin-induced arrhythmias was the lack of effect on ventricular tachycardia induced by ouabain as reported by Nevins et al. (1969). In contrast, Baum et al. (1971) reported a certain degree of reversal of ouabain-induced ventricular ectopic beats after 20 mg·kg^{-1} i.v. diazepam and lorazepam. Baum et al. (1971) also found that in anesthetized dogs 20 mg·kg^{-1} i.v. lorazepam and diazepam slightly reduced the maximal atrial following frequency, had no effect on aconitine-induced arrhythmias, slightly increased the threshold for ventricular fibrillation, and weakly affected epinephrine- and methylchloroform-induced arrhythmias. Acetylcholine-induced atrial arrhythmias in anesthetized dogs were not influenced up to high intravenous doses of chlordiazepoxide (Madan et al., 1963). Some reversion to sinus rhythm was observed with diazepam (1 mg·kg^{-1} i.v.) and chlordiazepoxide (10–30 mg·kg^{-1} i.v.) in conscious dogs with ligated ventral intraventricular branch of the left coronary artery (Madan et al., 1963; Gillis et al., 1974; Muir et al., 1975), whereas 50 mg·kg^{-1} i.v. pyrazapon had no effect at all (Poschel et al., 1974). Chlordiazepoxide was also reported to potentiate the antiarrhythmic effect and to prevent the neurotoxic effect of lidocaine in the same experimental situation (Gillis et al., 1974). In the anesthetized cat Gillis et al. (1974) reported that chlordiazepoxide (3–40 mg·kg^{-1} i.v.) reduced the number of ventricular ectopic beats induced by deslanoside and increased the sinus beats. This effect was no longer observed in spinalized animals. They also reported that the antiarrhythmic effect paralleled the reduction of an increased sympathetic discharge. PEARL et al. (1978 a) observed that diazepam (repeated injection of 10 mg bolus) tested on deslanoside arrhythmias was poorly active and in fact occasionally worsened the alterations of the rhythm. Essentially the same effects were seen with the solvent. In another paper the same authors (1978 b) reported that, when chlordiazepoxide was injected dissolved in polyethyleneglycol 400 instead of saline, no antiarrhythmic effect was obtained. DE JONG and HEAVNER (1973) described some activity of diazepam (0.25 mg$\cdot$kg^{-1} i.m.) against ventricular arrhythmias induced by high doses of lidocaine in anesthetized cats. Arrhythmias induced in unanesthetized rabbits with $BaCl_2$, ouabain or a combination of chloroform and isoprenaline were reduced by diazepam (5 mg$\cdot$kg^{-1} i.v.) and chlordiazepoxide (10 mg$\cdot$kg^{-1} i.v.) (ANDO et al., 1979).

In highly artificial conditions, chlordiazepoxide was found to facilitate the occurrence of arrhythmia (GASCON, 1977). Rats were treated on 5 consecutive days with the tremendous dose of 150 mg$\cdot$kg^{-1}. Acute stress induced by a 3-min period of electric shocks to the hindlegs resulted in a more marked tachycardia and in a higher incidence of ventricular extrasystoles than in untreated rats. Furthermore, ouabain 2.5 mg$\cdot$kg^{-1} injected intravenously every 15 min during 1 h, produced a higher incidence of ventricular arrhythmias in rats pretreated with the high dose of chlordiazepoxide than in untreated controls. The higher cardiotoxicity of stress and ouabain was ascribed to the marked increase of adrenaline in the adrenal glands produced by chlordiazepoxide (see Sect. X/IV.) and to the considerably greater absolute amount of adrenaline that was released by stress and ouabain from the adrenals.

III. Isolated Myocardium

In experiments in isolated cat papillary muscle, PRINDLE et al. (1970) described some reduction of peak isometric tension (T) and dT/dt with no change in the time to peak for chlordiazepoxide ($> 2 \times 10^{-5}$ mol$\cdot$l^{-1}) and no effect of diazepam ($\sim 10^{-5}$ mol$\cdot$l^{-1}), whereas SUGIMOTO et al. (1976) reported a depression of contractile tension of the rat papillary muscle with diazepam in a concentration of 2×10^{-6} mol$\cdot$l^{-1}. The same authors observed an increased refractory period and decreased maximal following frequency. In the guinea-pig papillary muscle flurazepam (2.5×10^{-5}–2×10^{-4} mol$\cdot$l^{-1}) reduced amplitude and maximum rate of rise (MRR) and increased the duration of the action potential; the transmembrane potential was unchanged (LIEBESWAR, 1972). As with quinidine or quinidine-like compounds, a recovery – even in the presence of flurazepam – of the decreased MRR was observed after switching off the stimulation. LIEBESWAR (1972) concluded that flurazepam interfered with the activated sodium channel. In canine heart Purkinje fibers and ventricular muscle, chlordiazepoxide ($\geq 10^{-4}$ mol$\cdot$l^{-1}) reduced the maximum rate of rise of the action potential and shortened its half-life with little change of the resting membrane potential (WANG and JAMES, 1979). A reduction of the refractory period and a shortening of the duration of the action potential was observed only in Purkinje fibers. The same authors reported that chlordiazepoxide depressed the enhanced repetitive discharge of subendocardial Purkinje fibers which survived acute myocardial infarction. A prolongation of repolarization and an increased refractory period was observed in rabbit auricular fibers with diazepam ($\sim 2 \times 10^{-5}$ mol$\cdot$l^{-1}) by TUGANOWSKI and WOLANSKI (1970). The depolarization velocity was decreased, but the action potential and the transmembrane potential were unchanged. In isolated rabbit auricles chlordiazepoxide (10^{-6}–3×10^{-4} mol·l^{-1}) had a negative inotropic (Moe et al., 1962) and negative chronotropic effect (Madan et al., 1963). No effect on adrenaline- or acetylcholine-induced tachycardia or bradycardia, respectively, was observed (3×10^{-4} mol·l^{-1}, Madan et al., 1963), but 10^{-5} mol·l^{-1} reduced the positive inotropic effect of adrenaline (Moe et al., 1962). Ando et al. (1979) reported that diazepam and chlordiazepoxide reduced the positive chronotropic effect of isoprenaline, adrenaline, and noradrenaline. A negative inotropic effect of chlordiazepoxide ($\sim 10^{-5}$ mol·l^{-1}) was described in isolated auricles of cats (Moe et al., 1962) and guinea pigs (Ferrini and Miragoli, 1973). Diazepam ($> 2 \times 10^{-5}$ mol·l^{-1}) was shown to depress contractile tension in electrically stimulated atria and papillary muscles, to increase refractory period and to decrease maximal following rate in rat atria (Sugimoto et al., 1976, 1978). In concentrations below 2×10^{-5} mol·l^{-1}, however, the contractile force of spontaneously beating right atria or electrically stimulated left atria and papillary muscles was increased. Stimulation-induced arrhythmias of rat or rabbit atria were prevented by diazepam (Sugimoto et al., 1976, 1978; Ando et al., 1979). In isolated guinea-pig auricles diazepam, temazepam and medazepam produced a negative ino- and chronotropic effect and SB 5,833 only a negative chronotropic effect (10^{-5} mol · l^{-1}, Ferrini and Miragoli, 1973). High concentrations of estazolam (3×10^{-4} mol·l^{-1}) had a negative inotropic and chronotropic effect (Saji et al., 1972), whereas clobazam (10^{-5} mol·l^{-1}) had no effect at all (Fielding and Hoffmann, 1979). In electrically driven guinea-pig left atria diazepam (10^{-6} and 10^{-5} mol·l^{-1}) significantly potentiated the negative inotropic effect of adenosine, but not that of 2-chloroadenosine (Clanachan and Marshall, 1980a). In primary cultures of rat myocardial cells exposed to diazepam (10^{-5}–10^{-4} mol·l^{-1}), tachycardia, arrhythmias, and cell death within 24 h were reported (Acosta and Chappel, 1977). In chick embryo hearts, diazepam produced a concentration-dependent negative inotropic and chronotropic effect. Cardiac standstill in diastole occurred with 2×10^{-4} mol·l^{-1} (Berry, 1975). Atropine did not influence the diazepam-induced depression but l-noradrenaline reversed the negative inotropic effect. The vehicle of diazepam was ineffective. Essentially the same, namely negative inotropic and chronotropic effects and standstill in diastole were observed with 3×10^{-4} mol·l^{-1} chlordiazepoxide in the perfused frog heart (Madan et al., 1963).

IV. Cardiovascular Responses to Central Nervous System Stimulation

Stimulation of various structures in the central nervous system is known to produce behavioral, cardiovascular, and a number of other autonomic responses.

A widely used structure to demonstrate the effect of benzodiazepines on centrally evoked blood pressure responses is the posterior hypothalamus. A decrease of the hypothalamic-evoked pressor response by chlordiazepoxide (10–20 mg·kg^{-1} i.v.) in curarized cats was found by Carroll et al. (1961), Schallek et al. (1964), Sternbach et al. (1964), Schallek and Zabransky (1966), and Randall et al. (1969). The same effect occurred in anesthetized and conscious dogs (5 mg·kg^{-1} i.v., Bolme et al., 1967); in the latter, tachycardia as well as behavioral responses in the conscious animal were reduced. An inhibitory effect was also found with diazepam (0.1–10 mg·kg^{-1} i.v.) in curarized or anesthetized cats (Randall et al., 1963; Schallek et al., 1964;

CHAI and WANG, 1966; SCHALLEK and ZABRANSKY, 1966; SIGG and SIGG, 1969; SIGG et al., 1971; ANTONACCIO and HALLEY, 1975; ANTONACCIO et al., 1978), but not in spinal cats (KEIM and SIGG, 1973), where in fact the stimulation-induced tachycardia was enhanced. The decrease of pressor responses after diazepam was prevented by bicuculline (ANTONACCIO et al., 1978). Diazepam (1–5 mg·kg^{-1} i.p.) diminished the evoked pressor response in anesthetized (MORPURGO, 1968) and unrestrained, unanesthetized rats (MORPURGO, 1968; KAWASAKI et al., 1979). Nitrazepam (0.1–10 mg·kg^{-1} i.v.; SCHALLEK et al., 1964; STERNBACH et al., 1964; SCHALLEK et al., 1966; FUKUDA et al., 1974), medazepam (10 mg·kg^{-1} i.v., RANDALL et al., 1968), flurazepam (10 mg·kg^{-1} i.v., RANDALL et al., 1969), chlorazepate (15 mg·kg^{-1} i.v., MERCIER et al., 1970) and estazolam (0.5–2 mg·kg^{-1} i.v., FUKUDA et al., 1974), were also reported to inhibit hypothalamic-evoked pressor responses.

Stimulation of the septum and of the amygdala evoked, depending on the exact locus of stimulation, pressor or depressor responses which were antagonized by benzodiazepines (CARROLL et al., 1961; CHOU and WANG, 1975; STOCK et al., 1976). The cardiac arrhythmias evoked by stimulation of limbic structures were completely blocked by chlordiazepoxide (10–20 mg·kg^{-1} i.v.; CARROLL et al., 1961).

Pressor responses evoked in cats by stimulation of mesencephalic structures such as central gray, reticular formation, dorsal and ventral tegmental structures were inhibited by 10–20 mg·kg^{-1} chlordiazepoxide i.v. (CARROLL et al., 1961), nitrazepam (2 mg·kg^{-1} i.v.; FUKUDA et al., 1974), and diazepam (0.1 and 0.3 mg·kg^{-1} i.v.; ANTONACCIO and HALLEY, 1975), but not by estazolam (FUKUDA et al., 1974).

Medullary evoked pressor or depressor responses were reported to be antagonized or unchanged by chlordiazepoxide (CARROLL et al., 1961; SCHALLEK and ZABRANSKY, 1966) and diazepam (CHAI and WANG, 1966; SCHALLEK and ZABRANSKY, 1966; ANTONACCIO and HALLEY, 1975; KAWASAKI et al., 1979) at a dose described as inhibiting the hypothalamic pressor response.

Cortically evoked pressor responses were also inhibited by chlordiazepoxide (CARROLL et al., 1961).

V. Cardiovascular Responses to Behavioral Experiments

Sustained blood pressure rises and other hemodynamic changes can be provoked by operant conditioning in laboratory animals. Chlordiazepoxide (3–30 mg·kg^{-1} i.m.) reduced the rates of responding as well as the mean arterial blood pressure in squirrel monkeys which had developed marked persistent elevations of mean arterial blood pressure during the behavioral experiments (BENSON et al., 1970). The effect of temazepam (10 mg·kg^{-1} p.o.) on emotional changes in coronary and systemic hemodynamics were studied in conscious dogs in which anxiety was induced by the classical conditioning procedure (BERGAMASCHI and LONGONI, 1973). The increases in heart rate, cardiac output, left ventricular work, and total peripheral vascular resistance were significantly reduced by temazepam. The conditioning-induced changes in coronary vascular bed were not altered significantly. Rats under a differential conditioning schedule had an increased heart rate and respiratory rate. Both parameters were markedly depressed after 20 mg·kg^{-1} chlordiazepoxide i.p. (YAMAGUCHI and IWAHARA, 1974).

VI. Cardiovascular Responses to Peripheral Stimulation

Pressor responses evoked by stimulation of the central stump of the cut sciatic nerve in intact anesthetized or curarized cats were antagonized by 2 mg·kg^{-1} diazepam i.v. (Chai and Wang, 1966; Pórszász and Gibiszer, 1970) and estazolam (2 mg·kg^{-1} i.v., Fukuda et al., 1974). In the *encéphale isolé* preparation, however, the pressor response was unchanged after estazolam. Hypertension evoked by noxious stimuli was decreased after 15 mg·kg^{-1} chlorazepate i.v. (Mercier et al., 1970), in curarized cats.

The effects of benzodiazepines on blood pressure changes and bradycardia evoked by stimulation of the central end of the vagal nerve have been studied by various authors. Unchanged responses after chlordiazepoxide (1–32 mg·kg^{-1} i.v., Randall et al., 1960; Sternbach et al., 1964), diazepam (1–8 mg·kg^{-1} i.v.; Randall et al., 1961; Randall et al., 1963; Sternbach et al., 1964), and triazolam (10 mg·kg^{-1} i.v., Furukawa et al., 1976) were reported in anesthetized dogs and a decreased pressor response was found after 4 mg·kg^{-1} i.v. of nitrazepam (Sternbach et al., 1964). The phenylephrine-induced reflex vagal bradycardia was dose-dependently inhibited by chlordiazepoxide (3, 10, and 20 mg·kg^{-1} i.v.) in anesthetized cats with an eliminated sympathetic component of the reflex by either pretreatment with propranolol or spinal cord transection (Quest et al., 1977). A depression of the reflex bradycardia and the biphasic pressor effect after stimulation of the afferent abdominal n. vagus were observed with 0.4 mg·kg^{-1} diazepam i.v. in anesthetized rats (Schumpelick, 1973). Reflex bradycardia evoked by stimulating the sinus nerve was inhibited by diazepam (0.2–3 mg·kg^{-1} i.v.) in the intact cat (Hockman and Livingston, 1971), whereas no inhibition was observed after decerebration or in the thalamic animal. After spinalization, diazepam (cumulative doses of 0.3–3 mg·kg^{-1} i.v.) had no effect on the reflex bradycardia induced by either stimulation of the sinus nerve, the central end of nervus vagus, the aortic depressor nerve, or by raising the intrasinal pressure (Keim and Sigg, 1973).

The pressor response occurring after bilateral occlusion of the carotid arteries was usually unchanged or somewhat attenuated after chlordiazepoxide (0.2–16 mg·kg^{-1} i.v., Randall et al., 1960; Moe et al., 1962; Sternbach et al., 1964; Varagic et al., 1964; Theobald et al., 1965), clobazam (20 mg·kg^{-1} i.p., Barzaghi et al., 1973), diazepam (0.1–8 mg·kg^{-1} i.v., Randall et al., 1961, 1963; Sternbach et al., 1964; Chai and Wang, 1966; Korol and Brown, 1968; Antonaccio and Halley, 1975), flurazepam (1–8 mg·kg^{-1} i.v., Randall et al., 1969), estazolam (1 mg·kg^{-1} i.v., Saji et al., 1972), pinazepam (20 mg·kg^{-1} i.p., Scrollini et al., 1975), and triazolam (10 mg·kg^{-1} i.v., Furukawa et al., 1976) in the various species studied. An increased hypertensive response was reported for bromazepam (0.3 mg·kg^{-1} i.v., Korol and Brown, 1968) and for medazepam (>4 mg·kg^{-1} i.v., Randall et al., 1968) and a decreased hypertensive response occurred after 4 mg · kg^{-1} nitrazepam i.v. (Sternbach et al., 1964) in the dog.

VII. Cardiac and Vasoconstrictor Responses to Various Agents

The vasoconstrictor response induced by hypoxia in isolated blood-perfused rat lungs was unaffected by diazepam ($\sim 2 \times 10^{-6}$ mol·l^{-1}, Bjertnaes, 1977). Using the perfused rat mesenteric artery preparation, Ally et al. (1978) found that diazepam

(55 µmol·l^{-1}) and chlordiazepoxide (890 µmol·l^{-1}) inhibited constrictor responses to noradrenaline and angiotensin II but not those to potassium and vasopressin. Since thromboxane A$_2$ supports vasoconstriction by noradrenaline and angiotensin II, but not by potassium and vasopressin, the authors postulated that the benzodiazepines acted as antagonists of thromboxane A$_2$. A reduced vasoconstrictor response to noradrenaline, angiotensin II, BaCl$_2$ and to lumbar sympathetic stimulation was observed in hindquarter perfusion experiments in spontaneous hypertensive rats (SHR) after a 12-week daily treatment with 1 mg·kg^{-1} diazepam (s.c., starting at day 1 of life) compared to diazepam-vehicle injected SHR (SCHIEKEN, 1979). The vascular reactivity of Wistar Kyoto rats treated according to the same schedule was unchanged (SCHIEKEN, 1979). In the anesthetized dog, bromazepam (1 mg·kg^{-1} i.v.) did not alter cardiac chronotropic responses to electrical stimulation of vagal or cardiac sympathetic preganglionic and postganglionic nerves (GEROLD et al., 1976).

A series of papers deal with the effects of benzodiazepines on blood pressure or heart rate changes after the systemic injection of noradrenaline, adrenaline, phenylephrine, tyramine, isoproterenol, serotonin, histamine, angiotensin, acetylcholine, eserine, and DMPP. No effect at all or inconsistent effects were reported with a large number of benzodiazepines (RANDALL et al., 1960, 1961, 1963, 1968, 1969; MOE et al., 1962; STERNBACH et al., 1964; VARAGIC et al., 1964; SCHALLEK et al., 1965; THEOBALD et al., 1965; BRASSIER et al., 1966; CHAI and WANG, 1966; SCHALLEK and ZABRANSKY, 1966; KOROL and BROWN, 1968; MORPURGO, 1968; MERCIER et al., 1970; SAJI et al., 1972; BARZAGHI et al., 1973; BERGAMASCHI and LONGONI, 1973; HEILMAN et al., 1974; ANTONACCIO and HALLEY, 1975; BABBINI et al., 1975; SCROLLINI et al., 1975; FURUKAWA et al., 1976; QUEST et al., 1977).

VIII. Conclusions

The very heterogeneous material presented in this section does not allow detailed conclusions to be made about the cardiovascular effects of benzodiazepines. A cautionary note on two methodological aspects is indicated. First, since most benzodiazepines are poorly water soluble, organic solvents were often used to administer these drugs; in many studies the effect of the vehicle alone was not investigated. Moreover, even if the solvent alone was found to be ineffective, it cannot be excluded that it altered the distribution of the active drug into tissues. Second, results obtained in anesthetized animals should be interpreted with great reservation. Since benzodiazepines potentiate the effects of anesthetics, many of the observed cardiovascular effects may be the result of a deeper state of general anesthesia.

Studies on isolated heart preparations and vessels show that benzodiazepines in concentrations below 10 µmol·l^{-1} do not produce significant effects, suggesting that a direct effect on heart and blood vessels is highly unlikely with therapeutic doses or corresponding pharmacologic doses (plasma levels were around 1 µmol·l^{-1} and brain levels about 3 times higher in rats 20 min after 5 mg·kg^{-1} diazepam i.v.; KLOTZ, 1979). However, such doses undoubtedly may produce hemodynamic changes in the intact animal, depending to a large extent on the conditions of the animal. The potent effect of benzodiazepines on many kinds of hemodynamic responses to peripheral and central stimuli strongly suggests that their effects on the cardiovascular system, when present, are caused by a central site of action. A representative example for such an action is the cardio-accelerating effect of diazepam and bromazepam in trained conscious dogs (GEROLD et al., 1976) and the inhibition of reflex bradycardia elicited by sinus nerve stimulation (HOCKMAN and LIVINGSTON, 1971). Although the exact site of action of these drugs which is responsible for the central depression of cardiac vagal tone remains to be elucidated, it is very tempting to speculate that it may be connected with the GABAergic synapses which have been proposed by BARMAN and GEBBER (1979), DI MICCO et al. (1979), DI MICCO and GILLIS (1979), and WIL-LIFORD et al. (1980a,b,c) to mediate a tonic inhibitory influence from forebrain and medullary structures onto cardiac vagal neurons in the nucleus tractus solitarii and/or nucleus ambiguus. A GABAergically mediated reduction of the activity of vascular sympathetic fibers (DI MICCO and GILLIS, 1979; SWEET et al., 1979) and a potentiating effect of benzodiazepines on this GABAergic activity have been suggested by BOLME and FUXE (1977) and ANTONACCIO et al. (1978). The great number of GABAergic neurons (MASSARI et al., 1976), their arrangement in series and in parallel in the central nervous system, and their probable involvement in the inhibitory control of both parasympathetic and sympathetic outflow from the medulla may explain why cardiovascular effects of benzodiazepines vary in function of the dose and the central state of the organism.

Since benzodiazepines in high concentrations have been found to inhibit the uptake of adenosine (see Sect. X/XI.), and in view of the part played by adenosine in the local regulation of blood flow and, possibly, in the noradrenergic transmission, part of their cardiovascular effects might be produced by their interaction with adenosine inactivation.

C. Effects on Respiration

I. Respiratory Control

Benzodiazepines are widely used as preanesthetics or induction agents. Their effects on the respiratory system were, as a consequence of its clinical use, extensively studied in humans. Therefore we also include, besides the animal data, some relevant clinical studies performed with benzodiazepines on respiration.

A series of papers deal with the effects of diazepam on the respiratory system in various animal species. RANDALL et al. (1961, 1963) and HEILMANN et al. (1974) observed no effect at all on the respiratory rate or amplitude in anaesthetized dogs up to 8 mg·kg^{-1} i.v. In contrast, STEPANEK (1973b, c) described with 1 and 3 mg·kg^{-1} i.v. a decrease of respiratory rate and minute volume together with reduced PaO_2, pH, O_2 saturation and increased $PaCO_2$, which corresponds to a picture of uncompensated, mixed respiratory and metabolic acidosis. At the same time an initial apnea and a deepening of the anesthesia were observed after the higher intravenous dose (3 mg·kg^{-1}). No effect on the respiration was observed after 0.3 mg·kg^{-1} i.v. in the conscious dog (KOROL and BROWN, 1968), but after single and repeated doses of 10 or 30 mg·kg^{-1} p.o. progressive uncompensated metabolic acidosis developed (STEPANEK, 1972, 1973a). In anesthetized cats, diazepam was reported by RANDALL et al. (1963) to have no effect on the respiration in high intravenous doses, whereas an increased respiratory rate was observed by CHOU and WANG (1975) after intravenous (0.28 mg·kg^{-1}) or intra-arterial (0.016 mg·kg^{-1}) injections in lightly anesthetized cats. ROSENSTEIN (1970) reported, with a dose of 0.1 mg·kg^{-1} i.v., a decrease in respiratory rate, tidal volume and minute volume and an increase in end-expiratory CO_2. A decrease of the slope of the CO_2 response curves ($V_T/\log [CO_2]$) and an elevation of the CO_2 threshold were reported by the same authors. In decerebrate cats, respiratory rate increased (ROSENSTEIN, 1970; CHOU and WANG, 1975) after very small intra-arterial or intravenous doses up to high intravenous doses (0.016 mg·kg^{-1} and 0.1–2 mg·kg^{-1}, respectively), the tidal volume was reduced (ROSENSTEIN, 1970; FLOREZ, 1971), but the minute volume increased (ROSENSTEIN, 1970). End-expiratory CO_2 was unchanged over a broad range of doses. FLOREZ (1971) reported both a decreased slope of the CO_2 response curves and an unchanged CO_2 threshold after 0.1–0.5 mg·kg^{-1}. The inspiratory response to stimulation of the inspiratory center was depressed to the same extent as the respiratory responsiveness to CO_2 (FLOREZ, 1971).

The results obtained with diazepam in the conscious rabbit are rather conflicting. PARKES (1968) reported that the brief rise in minute volume obtained with 2 mg·kg^{-1} i.v. was due to the constituents of the ampoule solution, but BRADSHAW and PLEUVRY (1971) observed some diminution of the respiratory volume and respiratory minute volume and respiratory rate with 8 mg·kg^{-1} i.v. Whereas essentially the same effects on respiratory rate were found after a comparable volume of solvent, no solvent effect was observed on minute volume in amounts contained in respiratory depressant doses of diazepam (BRADSHAW and PLEUVRY, 1971). The fall in respiratory minute volume and respiratory rate was accompanied by a small but significant rise of $PaCO_2$, pH, and standard bicarbonate (BRADSHAW et al., 1973). The respiratory depression observed with morphine was prolonged after 1 and 2 mg·kg^{-1} diazepam i.v. (BRADSHAW et al., 1973). An unaltered responsiveness of the respiratory system to CO_2 was found with 2.5 mg·kg^{-1} i.v. by PARKES (1968). A weak depression of respiratory rate in anesthetized rabbits was reported after 20 mg·kg^{-1} i.p. by SCROLLINI et al. (1975). In conscious, restrained rhesus monkeys, an inconsistent metabolic and respiratory acidosis was observed (MUNSON and WAGMAN, 1972) after an intravenous dose, which was shown to terminate local anesthetic-induced electrical seizure activity (0.1 mg·kg^{-1}). In anesthetized rats, SCHUMPELICK (1973) observed a slowing of spontaneous respiratory rate after diazepam 0.4 mg·kg^{-1} i.v., as well as a less pronounced inspiratory apnea in response to afferent abdominal vagus stimulation. BOLME and FUXE (1977) also described a reduction of respiratory rate after intraperitoneal (0.1–1 mg·kg^{-1}) or intracerebroventricular (100 µg/20 µl) injection of diazepam. In contrast, ISHIDA et al. (1974, 1979) reported a minimal elevation of respiratory rate. The same authors observed in the phrenic nerve a dose-dependent (0.33–10 mg·kg^{-1} i.v.) increase of interspike interval together with a decrease of the number of spikes for each inspiration in spontaneously breathing or artificially ventilated rats. These effects were not altered by midcollicular decerebration or after denervation of the carotid sinus. The increase of spike number and the decrease of the interspike intervals induced by ventilating the rats with hypoxic or hypercapnic gas mixtures were not altered by diazepam (ISHIDA et al., 1979). The intravenous injection of diazepam 7.5 mg·kg^{-1} to otherwise undrugged rats produced full surgical anesthesia; respiration, arterial oxygen, and CO_2 tensions were not significantly altered (CARLSSON et al., 1976). In conscious mice (1–80 mg·kg^{-1} i.p.), no effect (BRADSHAW et al., 1973) or a depression of respiratory rate, which could be ascribed to the solvent (BRADSHAW and PLEUVRY, 1971), was reported. Nevertheless, some potentiation of the respiratory depression by morphine was observed (BRADSHAW et al., 1973).

FLOREZ (1971) studied the respiratory effects of nitrazepam (0.1, 0.5 mg·kg^{-1} i.v.) and clonazepam (0.1 mg·kg^{-1} i.v.) in decerebrate cats. After both drugs, an increased respiratory rate, a reduced tidal volume, and an increased $PaCO_2$ were observed. The respiratory responsitivity to CO_2 inhalation and to stimulation of inspiratory neurons was consistently reduced.

No effects on respiration were reported for doxefazepam (BABBINI et al., 1975) and triazolam (FURUKAWA et al., 1976), weak or transient depression for estazolam (0.5–1 mg·kg^{-1} i.v., SAJI et al., 1972), clobazam (20 mg·kg^{-1} i.p., BABBINI et al., 1973), flurazepam (20 mg·kg^{-1} i.p., 40 mg·kg^{-1} p.o., BABBINI et al., 1975), and pinazepam (20 mg·kg^{-1} i.p., SCROLLINI et al., 1975) in anesthetized rabbits or cats. In curarized cats estazolam increased the discharge rate of the phrenic nerve (SAJI et al., 1972). In anesthetized dogs flurazepam was shown to inconsistently reduce the respiratory amplitude (RANDALL et al., 1969), whereas a reduction in amplitude together with an increased respiratory rate was reported for chlorazepate (1–10 mg·kg^{-1} i.v., BRUNAUD et al., 1970). After medazepam a weak increase in respiratory rate with unchanged respiratory amplitude was observed (RANDALL et al., 1968). In the conscious dog neither bromazepam (0.3 mg·kg^{-1} i.v., KOROL and BROWN, 1968) nor triflubazam (HEILMAN et al., 1974) influenced the respiratory system.

BILLINGSLEY et al. (1979) observed a respiratory depression in anesthetized rats and cats after tremendously high doses of chlordiazepoxide (120 mg·kg^{-1} i.v.), which was prevented in rats by intravenous picrotoxin and naloxone. This protective effect was absent in vagotomized animals. In cats, respiratory depression, but not hypotension and reflex bradycardia, was antagonized by naloxone. Stimulation of central nervous system structures, such as the areas dorsolateral to the trigeminal tract or the trigeminal nucleus (CHOU and WANG, 1975) or the nucleus amygdaloideus corticalis (KITO et al., 1977) in cats, elicits spasmodic respiratory reactions. CHOU and WANG (1975) found a depression of such responses after minute intraarterial or intravenous doses of clonazepam or diazepam in lightly anesthetized or midcollicular decerebrated cats. The spasmodic expiratory response evoked in anesthetized cats by stimulation of the amygdala was also depressed by 0.1 or 0.5 mg·kg^{-1} diazepam and chlordiazepoxide (i.v., KITO et al., 1977). They also showed that the emotional reactions occurring in conscious cats were reduced by diazepam (5 mg·kg^{-1} i.p.).

A weak to moderate, but still transient, respiratory depression with anesthetic doses of benzodiazepines was reported in most of the clinical studies. Signs of respiratory depression such as reduced tidal volume and respiratory minute volume together with an increased $PaCO_2$ or alveolar CO_2 and a slightly reduced PaO_2 were reported for diazepam (MASPOLI, 1967; DALEN et al., 1969; CATCHLOVE and KAFER, 1971; CÔTÉ et al., 1974). The respiratory rate tended to be increased (MASPOLI, 1967; CATCHLOVE and KAFER, 1971). A decrease in pH was found by MASPOLI (1967) and CÔTÉ et al. (1974). Essentially the same respiratory changes were reported for flunitrazepam (COLEMAN et al., 1973; BENKE et al., 1975; DIECKMANN et al., 1976). A pattern of cyclic hypo- and hyperventilation was seen after flunitrazepam (BENKE et al., 1975). Changes in respiratory pattern, i.e., periodic breathing, occurred after lorazepam, but not after diazepam (ADEOSHUN et al., 1978).

An impressive series of papers deals with the effects of benzodiazepines on the responsivity of the respiratory system to hypercapnic or hypoxic ventilatory drive. A reduction of slope of the V_T/log [CO_2] curves was usually observed with 5–10 mg p.o.

or 5–20 mg i.m. diazepam (GEISLER and HERBERG, 1967; HERBERG et al., 1968; CEGLA, 1973; UTTING and PLEUVRY, 1975; GASSER and BELLVILLE, 1976; PATRICK and SEMPIK, 1978). Inconsistent or no effects on the CO_2 response were also observed in comparable intravenous or intramuscular doses (SADOVE et al., 1965; STEEN et al., 1966; COHEN et al., 1969; CATCHLOVE and KAFER, 1971; LAKSHMINARAYAN et al., 1976). A potentiation of the depression of respiratory responses induced by either meperidine or morphine was reported by SADOVE et al. (1965) and UTTING and PLEUVRY, (1975). CEGLA (1973) observed, in addition, a reduction of the slope of the f/log [CO_2] curves. The threshold for the ventilatory response was either unchanged (COHEN et al., 1969) or increased (PATRICK and SEMPIK, 1978). The hypoxic ventilatory response was also reduced by diazepam (HUDSON, et al., 1974; LAKSHMINARAYAN et al., 1976). In contrast to diazepam neither lorazepam (COMER et al., 1973, 5 mg i.v. or i.m.; GASSER et al., 1975, 4 mg i.m.; CORMACK et al., 1977, 4 mg i.m.) nor chlordiazepoxide (SADOVE et al., 1965, 100 mg i.m.; STEEN et al., 1967, 1 mg·kg^{-1} i.v.) produced consistent effects on the ventilatory response to CO_2. The effects of meperidine and pethidine on the responsivity to hypercapnic ventilatory drive were potentiated by chlordiazepoxide (SADOVE et al., 1965; STEEN et al., 1967).

II. Cough

A cough response evoked in cats by electrical stimulation of a region dorsomedial to the trigeminal tract or to the corresponding nucleus was shown to be antagonized by very small intravenous or intraarterial doses of clonazepam (20 µg·kg^{-1} i.a., 40 µg·kg^{-1} i.v.) and diazepam (0.016 mg·kg^{-1} i.a., 0.3 mg·kg^{-1} i.v., CHOU and WANG, 1975). Peripherally evoked cough in cats after stimulating the laryngeal nerve or the tracheal mucosa was only minimally affected after 0.1 and 0.5 mg·kg^{-1} chlordiazepoxide or diazepam i.v. (KITO et al., 1977). Cough evoked in cats by ammonia insufflation or in dogs by stimulation of the tracheal mucosa was not inhibited by medazepam (16 and 32 mg·kg^{-1} i.v., RANDALL et al., 1968).

III. Bronchospasm

Bronchospasms induced in guinea pigs by either acetylcholine, serotonin (5-HT), histamine, or bradykinin were reported to be antagonized by 1–5 mg·kg^{-1} chlordiazepoxide (GLUCKMAN, 1965; THEOBALD et al., 1965; KOVÁCS and GÖRÖG, 1968) but not by diazepam or oxazepam up to 50 mg·kg^{-1} i.p. (GLUCKMAN, 1965). The antagonistic effect of chlordiazepoxide against acetylcholine and 5-HT, but not histamine, was prevented by the β-blocker dichloroisoproterenol (KOVÁCS and GÖRÖG, 1968). Chlordiazepoxide (100 µg) antagonized the anaphylactoid bronchospasm and the adenosine triphosphate (ATP)-induced bronchospasm in isolated perfused guinea-pig lungs. Bronchospasms provoked in cats by either 5-HT or histamine were inhibited by medazepam without altering basal bronchial resistance (RANDALL et al., 1968). Chlordiazepoxide ($\sim 10^{-3}$ mol·l^{-1}) antagonized contractions of the dog trachea induced by acetylcholine (MADAN et al., 1963). In the guinea-pig bronchi, triazolam (3×10^{-6} mol·l^{-1}) had no effect on the tone or on the contractions or relaxations induced by either acetylcholine, histamine, barium chloride, or 5-HT, whereas the effects of noradrenaline and adrenaline were slightly potentiated (FURUKAWA et al.,

1976). Estazolam caused a concentration-dependent (10^{-6}–10^{-4} mol·l^{-1}) reduction of contractions induced by both histamine and potassium (SAJI et al., 1972).

IV. Conclusions

Very conflicting results were obtained in the numerous studies on benzodiazepine effects on spontaneous respiration in animals and man. The best agreement seems to exist with regard to a respiratory depressant effect of intravenous injections of various benzodiazepines in anesthetized animals; the active doses were in most cases rather high. It seems reasonable to assume that this effect, at least in part, is due to a potentiation of anesthesia. In the absence of anesthesia, respiratory depressant doses of benzodiazepines are well above therapeutic ones or those required to obtain a pre-anesthetic state. Respiratory depressions may occur with therapeutic doses of benzodiazepines if medullary respiratory neurons are already depressed by other drugs or pathologic processes. The site of respiratory depressant action of benzodiazepines is most probably the medulla. In view of the well-documented potentiation of GABAergic synaptic transmission by benzodiazepines, it is of interest that systemic injections of GABA and other GABA mimetics have been shown to produce transient apnea in rats (HOLZER and HAGMUELLER, 1979) and that inspiratory and expiratory neurons of anesthetized rabbits and cats were depressed by iontophoresed GABA (FALLERT et al., 1979; TOLEIKIS et al., 1979).

D. Effects on the Gastrointestinal System

I. Stomach

1. Gastric Ulcers

A variety of experimental situations induce erosions of the gastric mucosa in experimental animals. The most commonly used method is restrained stress (sometimes combined with partial immersion in water). Unescapable electroshock, forced exertion, or reserpine also produce gastric erosions.

Benzodiazepines have been reported to prevent or, at least to reduce, the rate of occurrence or the severity of gastric mucosal erosions. Chlordiazepoxide was shown to reduce the number of ulcerations produced either by restrained stress in rats (50 mg·kg^{-1} i.p., HAOT et al., 1964), by restrained stress combined with immersion and forced exertion in mice (5–20 mg·kg^{-1} p.o., DAIRMAN and JUHASZ, 1978) or by unescapable electroshock in rabbits (50 mg·kg^{-1} i.p., DASGUPTA and MUKHERJEE, 1967a). Nitrazepam (15 and 20 mg·kg^{-1} s.c.) was shown by MERCIER and LUMBROSO (1967) to reduce the number of ulcerations occurring after restrained stress in both rats and mice. As already observed for chlordiazepoxide, diazepam at doses of 0.3–10 mg·kg^{-1} p.o. effectively diminished the incidence of gastric mucosal erosions in mice under restrained stress or forced exercise (DAIRMAN and JUHASZ, 1978). The same authors also found that a combined injection of either diazepam or chlordiazepoxide with anticholinergics resulted in an additive or supraadditive effect. An additive protective effect was also reported when 0.4 mg·kg^{-1} diazepam i.p. was combined with vagotomy in rats subjected to restrained stress (SCHUMPELICK and PASCHEN, 1974). In contrast to the already mentioned protective effects of the above benzodiazepines on stress-induced ulcers, no effect was reported for flurazepam (60 mg·kg^{-1} i.p.) on reserpine-induced ulcerations (RANDALL et al., 1969). Another approach to induce gastric ulcerations in rats is to ligate the pylorus. After such a procedure, chlordiazepoxide (125 mg·kg^{-1} s.c.) was shown to decrease the severity of ulcerations but not the number of ulcers (BORNMANN, 1961).

2. Gastric Secretion

Gastric acid secretion is in part controlled by central mechanisms. Since benzodiazepines were proposed for use in peptic ulcer therapy, we will include some clinical data on experimentally induced gastric acid secretion.

The most commonly used method to determine the influence of drugs on gastric acid secretion in rats is to ligate the pylorus and to measure, after a certain time, the volume and acidity of gastric juice which accumulated during that time. With this method it was demonstrated that diazepam inhibited the rate of volume secretion over a wide dose range, but affected acid secretion only at 2 mg·kg^{-1} i.v. or 2 mg intragastrically (BIRNBAUM, 1968). Somewhat contrasting results were reported by YAMAGUCHI et al. (1973), who observed only weak effects on the gastric juice secretion after prazepam (115 mg·kg^{-1} s.c.) and no effect after diazepam and chlordiazepoxide (>250 mg·kg^{-1} s.c.). Intraduodenal administration of bromazepam, chlordiazepoxide, diazepam, medazepam and midazolam reduced output of volume and acid (MÜLLER, personal communication). The changes in either acid secretion or juice volume were obtained with doses producing strong central nervous system effects (BIRNBAUM, 1968; YAMAGUCHI et al., 1973). In contrast to the clear-cut effects in the Shay rat, neither bromazepam, chlordiazepoxide, diazepam, medazepam, nor midazolam inhibited gastric acid secretion stimulated with either histamine or 4-methylhistamine in rats and dogs, respectively (MÜLLER, personal communication).

Results on the effect of benzodiazepines on basal as well as stimulated gastric acid secretion are also available from human studies. Diazepam decreased basal gastric secretion in volunteers and ulcer patients (10 mg p.o., BIRNBAUM et al., 1971; 0.14 mg·kg^{-1} i.v., BENNETT et al., 1975), but pentagastrin-stimulated gastric acid secretion was unchanged. Oxazepam (10 mg p.o.) was reported to influence basal acid secretion only marginally (SCHERBERGER et al., 1975; KUTZ et al., 1976). Pentagastrin-stimulated secretion was either unchanged (SCHERBERGER et al., 1975) or somewhat enhanced (KUTZ et al., 1976). No effect on insulin-stimulated gastric secretion was observed (KUTZ et al., 1976). A reduction of basal as well as betazole-stimulated gastric secretion was reported for bromazepam (0.1 mg·kg^{-1} i.v., STACHER and STÄRKER, 1974). This effect was much more pronounced in subjects who fell asleep and was reversed when the subjects were awakened. Natural sleep caused the same depression. Essentially the same effects were observed on the gastric acid response to hypoglycemia (STACHER and STÄRKER, 1975).

II. Liver and Pancreas

An important pathway for the elimination of benzodiazepines is the bile. The possibility that benzodiazepines could alter the excretion of other chemicals, especially of sulfobromophthaleine (BSP) or its glucuronide conjugate, will therefore be discussed.

In isolated perfused rat liver, KVETINA et al. (1969) showed that diazepam in high concentrations (2×10^{-4} mol $\cdot$ l^{-1}) moderately increased the bile flow and considerably decreased the excretion of BSP in the bile. The amount of excreted bilirubin was slightly increased. These effects were not due to the solvent and occurred without altering gross biochemical parameters of the liver. Chlordiazepoxide (5×10^{-4} mol $\cdot$ l^{-1}) also reduced BSP excretion and bile flow (ABERNATHY et al., 1975). The latter investigators also observed a decreased hepatic uptake of BSP.

A reduction of BSP excretion without significant alteration of bile flow after diazepam (5 mg $\cdot$ kg^{-1} i.v.) was observed in anesthetized rats (KVETINA et al., 1969). The effect on BSP excretion was dose-dependent (PLAA et al., 1975). Peak biliary BSP concentrations were markedly reduced, biliary T_m for BSP decreased, and a plasma BSP retention was observed. BSP glutathione excretion, however, was not influenced by diazepam. After a high oral dose of diazepam (150 mg $\cdot$ kg^{-1}) a decrease in peak BSP elimination rate, associated with a decrease of the proportions of conjugated to nonconjugated BSP in the bile was observed (HANASONO et al., 1976). Bile flow and hepatic uptake or storage of BSP were unaffected, but BSP conjugating activity decreased. After 5 days treatment with diazepam (150 mg $\cdot$ kg^{-1} p.o.), BSP elimination rate was unchanged but bile flow was enhanced. This choleretic response persisted for at least 24 h (HANASONO et al., 1976). VAILLE et al. (1979) showed that 16 mg $\cdot$ kg^{-1} diazepam i.v. slightly increased bile flow and considerably enhanced bilirubin excretion. These effects were not obtained after intraperitoneal administration of 32 mg $\cdot$ kg^{-1}, but were mimicked by the solvent used in the commercially available ampoule. Bile flow was reported to be unchanged after 125 mg $\cdot$ kg^{-1} p.o. chlordiazepoxide (BORNMANN, 1961). In conscious cholecystectomized dogs STEFKO and ZBINDEN (1963) observed a decreased bile flow and an increased intrabiliary pressure with high intravenous doses of diazepam (16 mg $\cdot$ kg^{-1}) and chlordiazepoxide (32 mg $\cdot$ kg^{-1}). Flurazepam (8 mg $\cdot$ kg^{-1} i.v.) increased bile flow under the same experimental conditions (RANDALL et al., 1969).

Taking into account that all these effects were obtained with doses of benzodiazepines well above the therapeutic range, the clinic relevance is questionable.

Benzodiazepines are sometimes used during insertion of the endoscope for retrograde cannulation of the pancreatic duct to measure pancreatic function by collecting pancreatic juice during stimulation with hormones. In a study in patients it was shown that diazepam (10 mg i.v.) did not significantly affect the trypsin or bilirubin output from pancreas or bile after stimulation with either secretin or cholecystokinin-pancreozymin (SAUNDERS et al., 1976), but that there was a delay in peak rates of secretion after injection of diazepam together with hyoscine.

III. Gastrointestinal Motility

The effects of benzodiazepines on the intestine were mainly studied under in vitro conditions with isolated organ preparations.

In reports on in vivo gastrointestinal motility it was shown that neither flurazepam nor medazepam or midazolam had effects in the charcoal-meal test (16 mg $\cdot$ kg^{-1} s.c.) or in dogs (4–8 mg $\cdot$ kg^{-1} i.v.) with gastric fistulae or "Thiry-Vella loop" (RANDALL et al., 1968, 1969; PIERI et al., 1981). Weak effects on the rabbit colon (0.5 mg $\cdot$ kg^{-1}

i.v. or i.d.) and in the Heidenhain dog (50 µg·kg^{-1} i.v.) are reported with diazepam (NIADA et al., 1978). The combination of diazepam with octatropine was shown to produce a synergistic inhibitory effect on stimulated (rabbit colon) as well as spontaneous (Heidenhain dog) gastrointestinal motility. Estazolam was reported to depress charcoal propulsion in mice at the dose of 45 mg·kg^{-1} p.o., whereas a weak but clear-cut increase in contractions of the stomach antrum was observed after 5 mg·kg^{-1} p.o. in dogs; intestinal motility was virtually unaffected in dogs (SAJI et al., 1972). Clobazam had no effect on intestinal motility in mice (FIELDING and HOFFMAN, 1979). Electrical stimulation of some areas of the cat brain such as the anterior sigmoid gyrus, limbic lobe and hypothalamus, produces inhibition of intestinal motility together with the blood pressure increase described above. This inhibition was antagonized by diazepam, nitrazepam, and lorazepam at doses that inhibited the pressure response as well (0.1–5 mg·kg^{-1} i.v., SCHALLEK et al., 1964), whereas chlordiazepoxide (10–20 mg·kg^{-1} i.v.) only marginally affected gastrointestinal inhibition (CARROLL et al., 1961; SCHALLEK et al., 1964).

Spontaneous contractions of the isolated rabbit intestine and its tone were reduced dose-dependently and the acetylcholine response was decreased by chlordiazepoxide (10^{-4}–3×10^{-4} mol·l^{-1}, MADAN et al., 1963). In the rabbit jejunum diazepam (10^{-5} mol·l^{-1}) potentiated the inhibitory effect of octatropine on the spontaneous pendular movements (NIADA et al., 1978). Chlorazepate (10^{-4} mol·l^{-1}) was reported to decrease the tone of the rat duodenum in vitro (BRUNAUD et al., 1970). In the rat intestine triazolam (3×10^{-5} mol·l^{-1}) affected neither the tone nor the response of the organ to acetylcholine, histamine, 5-HT, or barium chloride, but slightly enhanced the effects of noradrenaline and adrenaline (FURUKAWA et al., 1976).

A series of studies dealt with the effects of various benzodiazepines on isolated guinea-pig ileum. They showed that the inhibitory effects of benzodiazepines in high concentration (10^{-5}–10^{-3} mol·l^{-1}) on contractions induced by bradykinin, histamine, acetylcholine, carbachol, barium chloride, and coaxial electric stimulation as well as on relaxations induced by 5-HT were of the noncompetitive type (GARCIA LEME and ROCHA E SILVA, 1965; CAMPESE et al., 1972; SAJI et al., 1972; HUCK et al., 1975; PIERI et al., 1981, STUMPF, personal communication). Whereas the benzodiazepines were equally potent against acetylcholine, barium chloride, and carbachol, chlordiazepoxide was the most potent against histamine-induced contractions (LEEUWIN et al., 1975). The observed direct effects of benzodiazepines on intestinal smooth muscles are unlikely to occur with therapeutic doses.

IV. Conclusions

A relevant direct effect of benzodiazepines on the gastrointestinal system is unlikely to occur in doses or concentrations corresponding to even the highest doses used in therapy. However, through a central action, these drugs are able to influence gastric mucosa and gastrointestinal motility. The effects observed with high concentrations of benzodiazepines on intestinal smooth muscle in vitro are due to an unspecific membrane stabilizing action and are not mediated by benzodiazepine receptors, since they are not antagonized by a selective benzodiazepine antagonist (unpublished).

E. Effects on Other Autonomic Functions

Contractions of the nictitating membrane of anesthetized cats in response to adrenaline and noradrenaline were unaffected by chlordiazepoxide 0.6 mg · kg^{-1} i.v. (THEOBALD et al., 1965). The same authors also reported the virtual failure of this drug to antagonize adrenaline-induced contractions of guinea-pig seminal vesicles. Blood pressure increase and cardio-acceleration in response to stellate ganglion stimulation in spinal cats and in response to intravenous noradrenaline in anesthetized and acutely adrenalectomized cats were unaffected by diazepam up to a cumulative dose of 6 mg · kg^{-1} i.v. (CHAI and WANG, 1966); no change in nictitating membrane responses to postganglionic cervical sympathetic nerve stimulation was found. SCHALLEK and ZABRANSKY (1966) also reported that neither chlordiazepoxide (20 mg · kg^{-1} i.v.) nor diazepam (1–10 mg · kg^{-1} i.v.) affect the blood pressure increase due to stellate ganglion stimulation. In contrast, FURUKAWA et al. (1976) observed in anesthetized dogs a potentiation of the cardiovascular response to pre- or postganglionic stimulation of the cardiac sympathetic by triazolam (10 mg · kg^{-1} i.v.). No or inconsistent effects were reported with a variety of benzodiazepines on the blood pressure or heart rate changes in response to various drugs (see Sect. B/VII). Again, triazolam was an exception in that it potentiated the effects of noradrenaline and adrenaline at high intravenous doses in anesthetized dogs (FURUKAWA et al., 1976).

The hypotension or bradycardia in response to stimulation of the peripheral vagal nerve were reported to be unaffected by chlordiazepoxide (1–20 mg · kg^{-1} i.v., MOE et al., 1962; THEOBALD et al., 1965; QUEST et al., 1977) and diazepam (HOCKMAN and LIVINGSTON, 1971, 0.2–3 mg · kg^{-1} i.v.; SCROLLINI et al., 1975, 20 mg · kg^{-1} i.p.) in anesthetized cats or rabbits, whereas in the anesthetized dog flurazepam (1–8 mg · kg^{-1} i.v.) was found to attenuate stimulation-induced hypotension (RANDALL et al., 1969) and medazepam (4 mg · kg^{-1} i.v.) to prevent the asystole occurring after vagus stimulation (RANDALL et al., 1968). The release of acetylcholine in the chicken heart induced by vagal nerve stimulation was unaltered by diazepam 10^{-5} mol · l^{-1} (LINDMAR et al., 1979).

Salivation induced by pilocarpine was unaltered in anesthetized rabbit by chlordiazepoxide (6 mg · kg^{-1} i.v., THEOBALD et al., 1965) or in cats by clonazepam (1–10 mg · kg^{-1} i.v., OHNO, personal communication). In mice, bromazepam, chlordiazepoxide, diazepam, medazepam and midazolam were also ineffective up to high oral doses (MÜLLER, personal communication). Chlordiazepoxide (10–20 mg · kg^{-1} i.v., CARROLL et al., 1961) and clonazepam (1–10 mg · kg^{-1} i.v., OHNO, personal communication) did not affect salivation induced in cats by electrical stimulation of the hypothalamus and nucleus reticularis pontis. Salivation induced by stimulation of hypothalamic areas and the chorda tympani or by PGF$_{2\alpha}$ in dogs was unaffected by 1–10 mg · kg^{-1} i.v. clonazepam (OHNO, personal communication); the drug also failed to increase or decrease the spontaneous flow of saliva.

No antagonism of oxotremorine-induced peripheral effects was observed with chlordiazepoxide, diazepam and oxazepam (FROMMEL et al., 1960 b, 20 mg · kg^{-1} s.c.; GLUCKMAN, 1965, up to 40 mg · kg^{-1} i.p.). Oxotremorine-induced tremor in the mouse was inhibited by chlordiazepoxide, probably through its muscle relaxant effect (FROMMEL et al., 1960 a; THEOBALD et al., 1965; RANDALL et al., 1969).

Triazolam produced mydriasis in rabbits and slightly potentiated the mydriatic alarm response, but did not affect the mydriatic response to light (FURUKAWA et al., 1976).

In the isolated rat uterus, chlordiazepoxide (10^{-5}–3×10^{-4} mol·1^{-1}) antagonized the effects of histamine, 5-HT, and acetylcholine (RANDALL et al., 1960; MADAN et al., 1963). Chlorazepate had no effect after high intraduodenal or intravenous doses on the spontaneous contractility or on barium chloride-induced spasm under in vivo conditions (BRUNAUD et al., 1970). An inconsistent depression of rhythmic contractions and a very weak reduction of acetylcholine-induced spasms of the rat isolated uterus after a high concentration of estazolam (3×10^{-4} mol·1^{-1}) were reported (SAJI et al., 1972); in anesthetized rabbits the uterine tone was lowered in parallel with the arterial blood pressure after 2–5 mg·kg^{-1} i.v. In the guinea-pig uterus, triazolam (3×10^{-5} mol·1^{-1}) affected neither spontaneous contractions nor acetylcholine-, histamine-, 5-HT, or barium chloride-induced effects but slightly potentiated those of noradrenaline or adrenaline (FURUKAWA et al., 1976). Rabbit uterine segments exposed to 3×10^{-5} mol·1^{-1} chlordiazepoxide lost their resting tone and spontaneous contractility (CAVANAGH et al., 1966). In human myometrium strips both chlordiazepoxide (10^{-4} mol·1^{-1}) and diazepam (3×10^{-5} mol·1^{-1}) decreased tone and arrested spontaneous contractions (BERGER and NEUWEILER, 1961; CAVANAGH et al., 1966). The effects were reversible by washing. As in the uterus, triazolam did not affect the guinea-pig vas deferens, but slightly potentiated the effects of noradrenaline and adrenaline (FURUKAWA et al., 1976). A potentiation by diazepam (10^{-6} and 10^{-5} mol·1^{-1}) of adenosine-induced inhibition of isometric contraction of the rat vas deferens was reported by CLANACHAN and MARSHALL (1980a). In isolated guinea-pig seminal vesicles the adrenaline response was unaffected by chlordiazepoxide (THEOBALD et al., 1965). Diazepam, in very high concentrations, slightly diminished the noradrenaline response in rat seminal vesicles (RANDALL et al., 1963).

SILLÉN et al. (1980) reported that contractions of the m. detrusor vesicae induced in anesthetized rats by L-DOPA after peripheral decarboxylase inhibition were inhibited by intravenous diazepam (10 mg·kg^{-1}) as well as by systemic and intracerebroventricular muscimol, intracerebroventricular GABA and glycine. The inhibitory effect of diazepam, muscimol, and GABA, but not the effect of glycine, were antagonized by bicuculline, suggesting a GABAergic mechanism involved in the effect of diazepam on the urinary bladder function.

In the isolated portal vein of the rat, diazepam ($> 10^{-4}$ mol·1^{-1}) decreased the amplitude of the spontaneous myogenic activity as well as the contractions evoked by either KCl, field stimulation, or noradrenaline (BRADSHAW, 1976). This effect was mainly due to the constituents of the ampoule solution.

The increase of palmar skin conductivity in mice evoked by photostimulation was dose-dependently inhibited by chlordiazepoxide, chlorazepate, clonazepam, diazepam, lorazepam, medazepam, etc. (MARCY and QUERMONNE, 1974, 1975). The habituation of the skin conductance increase occurring during iterative photostimulation was speeded up by clonazepam (1 mg·kg^{-1} i.p., MARCY and QUERMONNE, 1976).

In conclusion, benzodiazepines had no consistent direct effects on smooth muscles and exocrine cells of various organs or on the response of the heart to various mediators.

F. Effects on Motor End Plate and Skeletal Muscle

Most of the muscle relaxant effects of benzodiazepines can be attributed to an effect on spinal and supraspinal mechanisms. However, benzodiazepines have been claimed to also exert some direct effects on the skeletal muscles and influence neuromuscular transmission to some extent. This section, therefore, will deal with direct effects of benzodiazepines on the peripheral motor system.

I. Neuromuscular Transmission In Vivo

The effects of benzodiazepines (in fact, almost exclusively diazepam) have been studied in situ in human, rabbit, cat, and rat neuromuscular preparations.

In humans the twitch response evoked in the adductor pollicis muscle by stimulation of the ulnar nerve was found to be unaffected after 0.15–0.2 mg·kg^{-1} diazepam i.v. by FELDMAN and CRAWLEY (1970) and BRADSHAW and MADDISON (1979) and reduced at an oral dose of 0.4 mg·kg^{-1} by LUDIN and ROBERT (1974). The contractile force after tetanic stimulation and the electromyographically recorded muscle evoked potentials were unaffected (LUDIN and ROBERT, 1974). In spastic patients with total or incomplete spinal lesions, action potential and twitch tension of the soleus muscle after popliteal nerve stimulation were reduced, whereas the latencies or the half-time of contraction or relaxation were unchanged (15–20 mg, VERRIER et al., 1976). In contrast, HOPF and BILLMAN (1973) found increased half-time of contraction or relaxation and an increased delay between the electrical and mechanical response in the hypothenar muscle after 15–30 mg p.o. The same authors also found that the conduction velocity in the motoneuron (n. ulnaris) was slowed down, that the negativity of the action potential was increased, and that the force of contraction was reduced, especially after repetitive activation. The elbow flexor (biceps brachii) developed a greater voltage for a corresponding tension (0.4 mg·kg^{-1} i.m., LUDIN and DUBACH, 1971), but again the conduction velocity in the corresponding motor nerve or in the muscle was decreased (40 mg p.o., HOPF, 1973). The authors concluded that the most likely explanation for these effects was a direct effect on contractile elements or on the electromechanical coupling.

In in situ preparations of anesthetized cats or rats most authors found no effect at all on the contractions of the anterior tibialis muscle (HAMILTON, 1967, 0.8 mg·kg^{-1} i.v.; CRANKSHAW and RAPER, 1968, 0.1 mg·kg^{-1} i.v.; HUDSON and WOLPERT, 1970, 1–16 mg·kg^{-1} i.v.; JOHNSON and LOWNDES, 1974, 2 mg·kg^{-1} i.v.), or on the twitch response in soleus muscle or in flexor hallucis longus (WEBB and BRADSHAW, 1973, 0.25–5 mg·kg^{-1} i.v.), elicited by single shock stimulation of either peroneal or sciatic nerve. Posttetanic potentiation of the twitch response was unaffected (CRANKSHAW and RAPER, 1968; WEBB and BRADSHAW, 1973; JOHNSON and LOWNDES, 1974). Soman-induced twitch potentiation was antagonized with 2 mg·kg^{-1} i.v., but the depression of posttetanic potentiation by soman was not (JOHNSON and LOWNDES, 1974). The twitch response of the anterior tibial muscle elicited by either sciatic nerve stimulation or by direct stimulation of the muscle in anesthetized rabbits was enhanced after 5 and 10 mg·kg^{-1} i.v. (CHEYMOL et al., 1967). Some inconsistent reduction of the twitches of the triceps surae in response to sciatic nerve stimulation was reported by BRAUSCH et al. (1973) in decerebrate cats (> 2 mg·kg^{-1} i.v.). The dynamic peak and the static discharge of the Ia afferents from muscle spindles in response to ramp stretch were unaltered (BRAUSCH et al., 1973).

II. In Vitro Neuromuscular Preparations

The effects reported in the literature with diazepam and chlordiazepoxide on the isolated phrenic nerve-hemidiaphragm preparation in rats are conflicting. Diazepam was demonstrated to have a depressant effect on the indirectly evoked twitch with or without effect on the direct muscle response ($\sim 3 \times 10^{-4}$ mol·l^{-1}, HAMILTON, 1967; DASGUPTA et al., 1969), or to increase the twitch amplitude in a dose-dependent manner (2×10^{-5}–2×10^{-4} mol·l^{-1}, MOUDGIL and PLEUVRY, 1970). CRANKSHAW and RAPER (1968) reported that diazepam, up to 3×10^{-4} mol·l^{-1}, did not influence the twitch response. VYSKOČIL (1977) found no effect on single action potentials but a blockade of trains of action potentials (10^{-6} and 10^{-5} mol·l^{-1}) occurred, which was dependent on the presence of Cl$^-$ in the medium. Cl$^-$ permeability was enhanced. Diazepam (3×10^{-5} mol·l^{-1}) inhibited the soman-induced twitch potentiation and drastically reduced the soman-induced repetitive activity in phrenic nerve, but did not affect orthodromic transmission (JOHNSON and LOWNDES, 1974). Miniature end-plate currents measured in the isolated mouse diaphragm were reduced and had shorter decay times at concentrations of 10^{-5}–10^{-4} mol·l^{-1}. The rising phase was unaffected. As a consequence, the postjunctional potential was reduced (TORDA and GAGE, 1977). Chlordiazepoxide was reported both to leave unaffected the indirectly or directly evoked response in the hemidiaphragm (3×10^{-4} mol·l^{-1}, DASGUPTA et al., 1969) and to inhibit both types of responses ($> 10^{-4}$ mol·l^{-1}, HAMILTON, 1967).

In the frog neuromuscular junction, especially the sciatic nerve-gastrocnemius muscle preparation, DASGUPTA et al. (1969) reported an abolition of the twitch response with an extremely high concentration of diazepam (10^{-2} mol·l^{-1}), whereas others found an increase of the twitch amplitude (VERGANO et al., 1969). VYSKOČIL (1978 a, b) reported that diazepam (10^{-5} mol·l^{-1}) did not at all influence the action potential. Neither the amplitude of the end-plate potentials nor the amplitude or the frequency of miniature end-plate potentials or the quantal release were changed. He also reported that the development of desensitization, occurring after acetylcholine pulses applied at a frequency of $1 \cdot s^{-1}$, was more rapid after 10^{-6} mol·l^{-1} diazepam, but that the recovery to normal sensitivity of the postjunctional membrane was unchanged.

In the frog sartorius neuromuscular preparation, diazepam was reported to reduce twitch height (5×10^{-5} mol·l^{-1}) and to slow the rate of fall of the negative afterpotential, without altering the membrane potential (1×10^{-4} mol·l^{-1}). The rate of Ca^{2+} efflux was reduced (BIANCHI and DE GROOF, 1977). In a similar preparation VYSKOČIL (1977) showed that comparable concentrations of diazepam did not at all influence single action potentials but blocked trains of action potentials. This effect was chloride dependent. In addition he observed an increase of the Cl$^-$ permeability, and he concluded that Cl$^-$ might counteract the effects of K$^+$ and therefore diminish the sustained depolarization occurring during repetitive activity. After chlordiazepoxide (5×10^{-5} mol·l^{-1}) the twitch tension was found to be increased, whereas the tension during tetanus decreased (OETLIKER, 1970). Contracture in response to high K$^+$ was normal but showed a slower recovery. OETLIKER (1970) concluded that the principal mechanism underlying these effects might be a blockade of a mechanism pumping Ca^{2+} back into the sarcoplasmic reticulum. An inhibitory effect of chlordiazepoxide $(10^{-4} \text{ mol} \cdot l^{-1})$ on the transport of Ca^{2+} through membranes has been shown by Mulé (1969). Lopez et al. (1979) recently found an increased twitch force and a de-layed decay of the twitch of frog skeletal muscle fibers under chlordiazepoxide $(10^{-5}-5 \times 10^{-4} \text{ mol} \cdot l^{-1})$; after injection of the Ca^{2+}-sensitive photoprotein aequorin into single muscle fibers an increased total light emission and a delayed light decay occurred parallel to the effect on the twitch force.

Contractions of either frog rectus by acetylcholine or of chick biventer cervicis by either acetylcholine or nicotine were blocked by chlordiazepoxide (Madan et al., 1963) and diazepam (Dretchen et al., 1971) in high concentrations $(10^{-4}-10^{-3} \text{ mol} \cdot l^{-1})$.

Untenable conclusions would be drawn from the results reported in the literature under in vitro conditions with benzodiazepines if it were not considered (a) that the concentrations used were well above those obtained with therapeutic doses and (b) that data are lacking with regard to the organic solvent used to solubilize diazepam. Nevertheless, the postulated inhibition of the sarcoplasmic Ca^{2+} uptake or an in-creased Cl^- permeability and counteraction of the effect of K^+ may to some extent account for the relaxant effect under conditions of tetanic stimulation.

III. Effects on Invertebrate Musculature

Ro 11–3128 (3-methyl clonazepam), a benzodiazepine with very potent central ner-vous system effects, has recently been shown to have schistosomicidal effects (Stoh-ler, 1978). Ro 11–3128 $(10^{-6} \text{ mol} \cdot l^{-1})$ produced a spastic paralysis of the muscula-ture of S. mansoni, an effect which was dependent on extracellular Ca^{2+} (Pax et al., 1978). They also showed that Ro 11–3128 decreased the efflux of K^+ and stimulated the influx of Na^+ and Ca^{2+}. With $10^{-5} \text{ mol} \cdot l^{-1}$ clonazepam, which produced the same effects as Ro 11–3128 on the musculature of S. mansoni, sustained depolariz-ation of the muscle cells was shown, which was strongly dependent on extracellular Na^+ and Ca^{2+} (Fetterer and Bennett, 1978). Drugs which are known to relax the musculature of schistosomes did not antagonize the effect of the two benzodiazepines.

On lobster muscle fibers flurazepam was found to inhibit dose-dependently depo-larizations in response to bath-applied or iontophoresed glutamate. The GABA re-sponse was unaffected. Higher concentrations of flurazepam $(> 200 \text{ } \mu\text{mol} \cdot l^{-1})$ some-times increased resting membrane conductance; this effect was insensitive to picrotox-in (Nistri and Constanti, 1978 a).

IV. Effects on Embryonic Muscles

Cultures of embryonic breast muscles of chicks exposed to exceedingly high concen-trations of diazepam $(5 \times 10^{-5}-10^{-4} \text{ mol} \cdot l^{-1})$ showed a reversibly inhibited cell dif-ferentiation and cell fusion (Bandman et al., 1978; Walker et al., 1979). An inhibition of the synthesis and accumulation of muscle specific protein (myosin heavy chain) was observed. This effect of diazepam was not due to the solvent and was specific for muscle cells.

V. Interaction with Neuromuscular Blockers

The coadministration of diazepam with various nondepolarizing or depolarizing neuromuscular blockers has produced conflicting results in human as well as in animal studies.

1. Tubocurarine

A potentiation by diazepam (5–10 mg·kg^{-1} i.v.) of an ineffective dose of tubocurarine was reported on sciatic nerve-anterior tibial muscle preparation in the anesthetized rabbit (CHEYMOL et al., 1967). The same authors showed in addition that when diazepam was injected during the recovery phase of the neuromuscular block, a reinstatement of that block occurred, even at a dose which enhanced by itself the twitch response evoked by either indirect or direct stimulation. A potentiation of tubocurarine block was also found in frog isolated sciatic nerve-gastrocnemius muscle preparation (VERGANO et al., 1969). A shortening of the tubocurarine block was observed in sciatic nerve-tibialis anterior preparation in anesthetized cats (3 mg·kg^{-1} i.v., FERNANDEZ and MARTINEZ, 1973), but no effect was seen on the sciatic nerve-flexor hallucis longus (0.2–5 mg·kg^{-1} i.v., WEBB and BRADSHAW, 1973) and sciatic nerve-gastrocnemius (1 mg·kg^{-1} i.v., DRETCHEN et al., 1971). No effect was found in the superfused chick biventer cervicis nerve-muscle preparation or in the human ulnar nerve-adductor pollicis muscle (0.5–0.6 mg·kg^{-1} i.v., DRETCHEN et al., 1971; 0.16 mg·kg^{-1} i.v., BRADSHAW and MADDISON 1979). In the isolated rat phrenic nerve-hemidiaphragm neuromuscular block was not influenced at all, but the twitch contraction of the curarized muscle was enhanced ($\sim 10^{-4}$ mol·l^{-1}, MOUDGIL and PLEUVRY, 1970).

2. Succinylcholine

A longer duration of neuromuscular block was observed after diazepam in sciatic nerve-anterior tibial muscle preparation in anesthetized cats (FERNANDEZ and MARTINEZ, 1973) and in the anesthetized dog in sciatic nerve-gastrocnemius muscle after 2–3 mg·kg^{-1} diazepam i.v. (SHARMA and SHARMA, 1978). Neuromuscular block was found unchanged after diazepam in the anesthetized rabbit sciatic nerve-anterior tibial preparation (5 and 10 mg·kg^{-1} i.v., CHEYMOL et al., 1967) and in the sciatic nerve-gastrocnemius preparation in decerebrate cats after 0.5–3 mg·kg^{-1} of either diazepam or lorazepam i.v. (SOUTHGATE and WILSON, 1971). In frog neuromuscular preparation the effect of succinylcholine was unchanged after diazepam (VERGANO et al., 1969). A reduction of the effect of succinylcholine was reported in humans (0.15 mg·kg^{-1} i.v., FELDMAN and CRAWLEY, 1970).

3. Gallamine

The combination of diazepam (5 and 10 mg·kg^{-1} i.v.) with gallamine produced effects that were opposite to those seen with succinylcholine. A faster recovery was observed in the isolated frog sciatic-gastrocnemius preparation (VERGANO et al., 1969), on the sciatic-anterior tibial muscle in anesthetized rabbits (CHEYMOL et al., 1967), and on the dog gastrocnemius neuromuscular preparation (2.5 mg·kg^{-1} i.v., SHARMA and SHARMA, 1978). On the human ulnar nerve-adductor pollicis muscle preparation,

Feldman and Crawley (1970) reported a potentiation and a slower recovery of the neuromuscular block after 0.2 mg·kg^{-1} i.v., an effect not found with a somewhat higher dose by Dretchen et al. (1971). No effect on neuromuscular blocking effect of gallamine was found in the anesthetized cat gastrocnemius preparation (0.5–1 mg·kg^{-1} i.v., Webb and Bradshaw, 1973; Dretchen et al., 1971) or in the superfused chick biventer cervicis nerve-muscle preparation (10^{-4} mol·l^{-1}, Dretchen et al., 1971).

Whether the described discrepancies are simply due to methodological differences or are accounted for by the neuromuscular system used cannot be conclusively answered. At least some differences may be explained by the use of high amounts of solvent, which was shown by Dretchen et al. (1971) to be responsible for the blockade of the tubocurarine and decamethonium effect on the indirectly evoked twitch response in anterior tibial muscle preparation of the dog and for the more rapid recovery after tubocurarine and gallamine in cat sciatic nerve-flexor hallucis longus preparation (Webb and Bradshaw, 1973).

VI. Conclusions

Very conflicting findings were reported on the direct effect of benzodiazepines on neuromuscular transmission. It seems that when an effect was observed, the doses or concentrations used were clearly above those that could be relevant for therapy.

G. Effects on the Kidney and Body Fluid Electrolytes

I. Urine

There are only few reports dealing with the effects of benzodiazepines on urine and electrolyte excretion by the kidneys.

Boris and Stevenson (1967) reported that neither diazepam nor chlordiazepoxide up to 160 mg·kg^{-1} s.c. had an effect on urine excretion in hydrated or dehydrated rats after an acute water load. Flurazepam (Randall et al., 1969), chlorazepate (Brunaud et al., 1970), clobazam (Fielding and Hoffmann, 1979), clonazepam (Blum et al., 1973), estazolam (Saji et al., 1972), and pyrazapon (Poschel et al., 1974) also failed to alter urinary output in rats. Chlorazepate (25 and 50 mg·kg^{-1} p.o.) increased Na$^+$ excretion and consequently the Na$^+$/K$^+$ ratio, but neither estazolam nor flurazepam changed electrolyte excretion. Clonazepam (3 and 10 mg·kg^{-1} p.o.) was reported to slightly diminish Na$^+$ excretion. Zamboni et al. (1972) observed an increased urine excretion in rats after 1 mg·kg^{-1} diazepam and bromazepam i.m., which was the consequence of an enhanced water intake. In rats deprived of water during urine collection, diazepam produced a weak diuretic effect (Zamboni et al., 1972).

In trained episiotomized dogs clonazepam (1 mg·kg^{-1} p.o.) did not influence urinary fluid or electrolyte excretion (Blum et al., 1973), whereas after flunitrazepam (0.2 and 0.4 mg·kg^{-1} p.o.) and nitrazepam (0.5 and 1 mg·kg^{-1} p.o.) an increased excretion of urine, Na$^+$ and Cl$^-$ was found (Daum, personal communication). K$^+$ excretion was unchanged after nitrazepam and decreased after flunitrazepam.

The effect of diazepam on glomerular filtration rate and on the effective renal plasma flow was studied in anesthetized rabbits (Guignard et al., 1975). Both glomerular filtration rate and effective renal plasma flow dropped transiently after a bolus injection of 2 mg·kg⁻¹. A concomitant drop in arterial blood pressure was observed. Renal function, however, was unaffected after slow intravenous infusion (5 mg·kg⁻¹·h⁻¹).

II. Blood Electrolytes

Serum levels of electrolytes in dogs (0.5 mg·kg⁻¹ i.v.) and humans (10–30 mg per day for 1 month) were reported to vary after diazepam within the normal physiologic range (SOLIMAN et al., 1965; CAHN, 1966).

III. Sodium Current in Frog Skin

The frog's skin provides a unique system for studying the effect of drugs on the active transport of sodium through epithelia by measuring the sodium short circuiting current. Addition of oxazepam (10^{-5} mol·l⁻¹) and chlordiazepoxide ($> 10^{-4}$ mol·l⁻¹) to the corial side resulted in a decreased sodium short circuiting current and a drop in membrane potential. The same effects occurred after adding oxazepam to the epidermal side (RÜBERG-SCHWEER and KARGER, 1970, 1974).

IV. Calcium Content of Synaptic Vesicles

PEYTON and BOROWITH (1979) injected rats with chlordiazepoxide 20 mg·kg⁻¹ i.p. The animals were decapitated 40 min later, and the cerebral cortex was separated into different subcellular fractions by differential and sucrose gradient density centrifugation. The fractions containing synaptic vesicles and synaptosomal ghosts contained significantly more (20%–40%) Ca^{2+} than the material from saline-injected rats. The Ca^{2+} content was unaltered in the fractions containing mainly synaptosomal and cell body mitochondria, damaged synaptosomes, and microsomes or in the synaptosomal supernatant. No significant changes in the Ca^{2+} content of synaptosomal subfractions were observed after chlorpromazine in the strongly sedative dose of 50 mg·kg⁻¹, whereas theophylline at 150 mg·kg⁻¹ markedly reduced the Ca^{2+} content of the fractions containing synaptic vesicles, synaptosomal ghosts, or synaptosomal mitochondria.

H. Effects on the Endocrine System

I. Male and Female Sexual Hormones

Chlordiazepoxide and diazepam administered subcutaneously for 100 days at daily doses ranging from 5 to 50 mg·kg⁻¹ to growing male and female albino rats had no influence on the weights of testes, penis, seminal vesicles, or prostates, on testicular descent, or on the weights of ovaries and uteri, on vaginal opening and cycling; no significant changes in luteinizing hormone (HL), luteotropic hormone (LTH), and lactation were observed (SUPERSTINE and SULMAN, 1966). In an early study (BORIS et al., 1961) chlordiazepoxide administered from 5 to 14 days had no effect on the pituitary-gonadal axis in rats. In contrast, in a study by ARGÜELLES and ROSNER (1975) on 35- to 55-year-old men with minor complaints of nervousness or mental tension, who took oral daily doses of 10–20 mg of diazepam for 2 weeks, plasma testosterone levels were significantly increased; the possible mechanism (altered activity of liver enzymes, changes in the clearance or synthesis of the hormone) was not investigated.

Female mice fed a diet containing either diazepam, chlordiazepoxide, oxazepam, prazepam, flurazepam, or nitrazepam showed significant decreases in the frequency of vaginal estrus (GUERRIERO and FOX, 1975). Mice exposed to the above-mentioned benzodiazepines prenatally and postnatally had delays in the age of vaginal perforation and first estrus concomitantly with reduced postnatal growth (FOX and GUERRIERO, 1978). Prenatal exposure alone did not produce postnatal growth deficit, but delayed vaginal opening.

II. Thyroid Hormones

The conflicting reports on possible interactions of benzodiazepines with thyroid function or thyroid hormone action have been discussed by EL-HAZMI (1975). Diazepam and chlordiazepoxide seem to compete for the thyroxine-binding site on serum proteins in vitro. However, in vivo, the two drugs did not consistently affect protein binding of thyroid hormones or their concentration in the circulating blood of man and rabbit. Chlordiazepoxide did not prevent thiouracil-induced thyroid enlargement in rats (BORIS et al., 1961).

III. Pituitary Hormones

1. Growth Hormone

KOULU et al. (1979) found that a single dose of diazepam (10 mg p.o.) increased serum growth hormone (GH) to about 300% for less than 2 h in healthy human volunteers, an effect which was prevented by pimozide and sodium valproate. Since dopamine is generally accepted to have a stimulant effect on GH release, the authors suggested that the effect of diazepam was due to an activation of tuberoinfundibular dopaminergic neurons (FUXE et al., 1975). No effect of diazepam at a daily dose of 40 mg on the release of GH was seen in patients (HAVARD et al., 1971). No clear-cut change in the level of GH was observed in healthy volunteers who took flurazepam 30 mg daily for 3 weeks (BIXLER et al., 1976). Diazepam abolished GH secretion of human volunteers in response to L-dopa and apomorphine (KOULU et al., 1980).

2. Prolactin

Various benzodiazepines were found to reduce the plasma prolactin level in rats after rather high oral doses and to partially or totally prevent the stimulation of prolactin release by sulpiride and haloperidol (LOTZ, personal communication); the most potent compounds were clonazepam and flunitrazepam (active at $1 \text{ mg} \cdot \text{kg}^{-1}$). In similar experiments by CHIELI et al. (1980), the decrease of basal plasma prolactin after diazepam ($10 \text{ mg} \cdot \text{kg}^{-1}$ i.p.) failed to reach statistical significance; however, the same dose of diazepam almost completely prevented the increase of prolactin produced by haloperidol $0.5 \text{ mg} \cdot \text{kg}^{-1}$. KOE (1979) observed a 60% decrease of plasma prolactin 1 h after a subcutaneous injection of diazepam ($9 \text{ mg} \cdot \text{kg}^{-1}$) in rats. No consistent change of plasma prolactin occurred in healthy men who took 30 mg flurazepam at bedtime over 3 weeks (BIXLER et al., 1976). Diazepam 15 mg per day in anxious patients failed to affect basal prolactin levels and the prolactin-stimulant effect of metoclopramide (WILSON et al., 1979).

3. Adrenocortical Steroids

High doses of benzodiazepines caused an elevation of plasma corticosteroids in rats (MARC and MORSELLI, 1969; LAHTI and BARSUHN, 1975; KEIM and SIGG, 1977; BARLOW et al., 1979), suggesting that some effect of acute high doses may be stressful to animals. Tolerance to the sedative and corticosteroid-elevating effect occurred on repeated administration (LAHTI and BARSUHN, 1975). A decrease of basal corticosteroid levels was, however, reported by KRULÍK and ČERNÝ (1971). The increase of plasma corticosteroids induced by the relatively mild stress of moving rats into a novel environment was blocked by diazepam, chlordiazepoxide, nitrazepam, and two triazolobenzodiazepines (LAHTI and BARSUHN, 1974). Diazepam reduced the rise of corticosteroids induced by restraint stress (KEIM and SIGG, 1977) and forced swimming (LE FUR et al., 1979); this effect was shown to be centrally mediated, since the drug did not alter the effect of adrenocorticotrophic hormone (ACTH) on isolated adrenals. BARLOW et al. (1979) could prevent the rise of corticosteroids induced by a mild noise stress with diazepam; the drug was, however, ineffective against severe stressors, such as electric foot shock and immobilization. A partial prevention of foot shock-induced elevation of corticosteroids was obtained by KRULÍK and ČERNÝ (1971) with both chlordiazepoxide and diazepam. Plasma corticosterone elevation in rats stressed by irregularly signaled foot shock was reduced by diazepam (BASSETT and CAIRNCROSS, 1974). In rabbits, chlordiazepoxide prevented the eosinopenia induced by electric shocks (DASGUPTA and MUKHERJEE, 1967 b); the drug also reduced eosinopenia induced by ACTH, but not that induced by cortisone.

IV. Conclusions

The effects of benzodiazepines on neuroendocrine functions are more subtle than, e.g., those of neuroleptics. It seems that low and moderate doses (producing distinct behavioral effects) do not or only very slightly affect the basal values of the hormones studied so far in physiologic conditions. However, neuroendocrine responses to various forms of emotional stress and to some drugs can be attenuated by benzodiazepines. This is clearly demonstrated for the stress-induced stimulation of the pituitary-adrenal axis. The antagonism of neuroleptic-induced hyperprolactinemia by benzodiazepines is likely to involve the tuberoinfundibular dopamine system, which is activated by these drugs, most probably indirectly via a direct action on GABA mechanisms that have been shown to be part of the prolactin control system (MÜLLER et al., 1979; LOCATELLI et al., 1979).

I. Effects on Cell Metabolism

I. Carbohydrates

RUTISHAUSER (1963) reported that chlordiazepoxide (30 mg·kg^{-1} i.p.) increased blood and brain glucose levels and the brain/blood glucose ratio in rats. Pyruvate and lactate also increased in the blood but not in the brain. Similar effects were obtained with chlorpromazine, reserpine, Ro 4-1284, and morphine, although changes in blood and brain glucose were less marked after phenobarbitone and methyprylone. No clear connection between hyperglycemia and hypothermia was seen. Since adrenalectomy prevented the hyperglycemia induced by chlordiazepoxide, it was assumed to be caused by some effect of the benzodiazepine on the adrenal gland. A 50% increase of glucose and lactate in the blood of rats was observed by Satoh and Iwamoto (1966) after 20 mg·kg^{-1} chlordiazepoxide i.p.; both effects were greatly reduced by removal of the adrenal medulla. In hooded-lister rats, chlordiazepoxide (10 mg·kg^{-1} i.p.) increased blood levels by about 30% (Nahorski, 1972). Brain glucose rose to a similar extent, resulting in an unaltered brain/blood glucose ratio. Evidence for a decreased glycolytic flux was found, since the levels of fructose-6-phosphate and of fructose-1,6-diphosphate were decreased. The levels of the tricarboxylate cycle intermediates, citrate, α-oxoglutarate, malate, and fumarate, were also reduced, whereas those of alanine, glutamine, GABA, and free ammonia were unaltered. These indexes of a depressed metabolic rate were similar to those described for general anesthetics and, therefore, believed to be the result, rather than the cause, of reduced neuronal activity. In contrast to chlordiazepoxide, trimethadione and ethosuximide increased the brain/blood glucose ratio, suggesting a facilitated glucose influx. Gey (1973) found a small (about 20%), rapid and transient increase of blood glucose in rats after single intraperitoneal doses of chlordiazepoxide (20 mg·kg^{-1}) and diazepam (4 mg·kg^{-1}). Pyruvate, lactate and maleate were decreased. More impressive than the elevation of blood glucose was the increase of the calculated intracellular glucose content in the brain tissue; little change was seen in the phosphorylated intermediates of glycolysis and in ATP. In contrast to Nahorski (1972), Gey (1973) suggested that glucose uptake into the brain was enhanced by the benzodiazepines. Gilbert et al. (1971) postulated that the increased brain glucose concentration observed after many anticonvulsant drugs was somehow involved in the anticonvulsant activity, possibly through membrane stabilization. Hyperglycemia was not observed in anxious patients after an oral dose of 25 mg chlordiazepoxide (Gottschalk et al., 1973); however, the drug appeared to reduce the hypoglycemic effect of insulin as judged from the glucose/insulin ratio.

The effect of benzodiazepines on the transport of sugars and ions in isolated rat skeletal muscle was studied by Bihler and Sawh (1978). The transport of ^{14}C-3-methylglucose into hemidiaphragms was depressed by diazepam in a concentration around 0.3 mmol·l^{-1} and markedly enhanced at concentrations of 1 mmol·l^{-1} and higher. This biphasic effect of diazepam was more pronounced in the presence of insulin. With 0.35 mmol·l^{-1} diazepam there was a small increase of the Na$^+$ and K$^+$ gradients; at 1 mmol·l^{-1} these ion gradients were markedly decreased. The influx of ^{45}Ca^{2+} was significantly depressed at concentrations that reduced sugar transport, but increased at higher concentrations. Chlordiazepoxide had essentially the same effects on glucose transport, intracellular concentrations of Na$^+$ and K$^+$, and Ca^{2+} influx. The effects of benzodiazepines on skeletal muscle were discussed on the basis of a hypothetical role of Ca^{2+} in sugar transport; "lower" concentrations of the drugs were assumed to stabilize, the highest concentrations to destabilize the membrane. The concentrations of benzodiazepines found to affect glucose and cations in skeletal muscle are, of course, much higher than those occurring after even massive overdoses.

II. Energy-Rich Phosphates

Chlordiazepoxide (60 mg·kg^{-1} i.p.) and meprobamate (200 mg·kg^{-1} i.p.) did not affect the levels of adenosine monophosphate (AMP), inorganic phosphate, phosphocreatinine, or the total adenine nucleotides (AMP+ADP+ATP) in the rat brain; chlordiazepoxide, but not meprobamate, decreased ATP and increased ADP and, hence, the ratio ATP/ADP (KAUL and LEWIS, 1963). Also in rats, 0.25 mg·kg^{-1} diazepam i.v. did not change the levels of cerebral high-energy phosphates or energy charge potential (MAEKAWA et al., 1980). In isolated mitochondria from rat brain, chlordiazepoxide and diazepam in a range of concentrations between 0.1 and 5 mmol·l^{-1} decreased respiration and oxidative phosphorylation, diazepam being seven times more potent than chlordiazepoxide (DAVIS et al., 1971). Part of the decreased oxidative phosphorylation was ascribed to an increase of ATPase activity. The possibility was also considered that the drugs were forming a permeability blocking monolayer on the mitochondrial membrane.

Na$^+$, K$^+$-ATPase from the microsomal fraction of beef brain homogenates was exposed to diazepam at various cation concentrations (UEDA et al., 1971). No stimulation of the enzyme activity was observed over a large range of concentrations of the drug. Diazepam, however, inhibited the enzyme noncompetitively at higher concentrations (apparent inhibitor constant 0.2 mmol·l^{-1}). Na$^+$, K$^+$-ATPase, but not Mg^{2+}-ATPase from rat brain synaptosomal preparations was inhibited by 55% in the presence of diazepam 0.2 mmol·l^{-1} (GILBERT and WYLLIE, 1976). Further fractionation of the synaptosomes showed that diazepam inhibited only the Na$^+$, K$^+$-ATPase associated with cell membranes but not that associated with mitochondria. The Mg^{2+}-ATPase of synaptic vesicles, however, was inhibited 60% by diazepam 0.25 mmol·l^{-1}, as by the other anticonvulsants, diphenylhydantoin and ethosuximide.

III. Lipids

Chlordiazepoxide (40 mg·kg^{-1} i.p.) was found to produce a sustained elevation of plasma-free fatty acids in rats similarly to theophylline (ARRIGONI-MARTELLI and CORSICO, 1969). The lipomobilizing effect of noradrenaline was potentiated by pretreatment with chlordiazepoxide or with theophylline. cAMP, which by itself (10 mg·kg^{-1}) had no effect on the plasma free fatty acid level, produced a threefold elevation of these lipids in rats pretreated with chlordiazepoxide. The lipomobilizing effect of chlordiazepoxide was almost doubled in rats pretreated with theophylline. The authors concluded that chlordiazepoxide, like theophylline, potentiated the lipomobilizing action of noradrenaline by inhibiting phosphodiesterase activity. In sharp contrast to the findings of ARRIGONI-MARTELLI and CORSICO (1969), KHAN et al. (1964) reported the lack of effect of 20 mg·kg^{-1} chlordiazepoxide (i.p.) on plasma free fatty acids in normal rats and on adrenaline-induced stimulation of free fatty acid release from fat pads. However, chlordiazepoxide completely prevented the increase of plasma free fatty acids in rat exposed to prolonged intermittent electric foot shocks.

In anxious patients, a single dose of chlordiazepoxide (25 mg) increased plasma free fatty acids and triglycerides (GOTTSCHALK et al., 1973).

Chlordiazepoxide was reported to inhibit the development of atherosclerosis in rabbits fed a cholesterol-rich atherogenic diet (CUPARENCU et al., 1969). Rabbits fed a cholesterol-rich diet for 2 months had elevated plasma levels of nonesterified fatty acids (NEFA) and reduced plasma lipoprotein lipase activity. Chlordiazepoxide, 10 mg·kg^{-1} p.o. daily for 2 months, doubled the levels of NEFA and plasma lipoprotein lipase activity in animals fed a normal diet. Rabbits fed the atherogenic diet and treated simultaneously with chlordiazepoxide had similar plasma NEFA levels and plasma lipoprotein lipase activity as those given a normal diet and the drug. Aortic lipolytic activity was doubled by the atherogenic diet alone, increased about 20-fold by chlordiazepoxide alone and increased about sevenfold in animals given the atherogenic diet together with chlordiazepoxide. The elevation of plasma lipoprotein lipase activity and aortic lipolytic activity by chlordiazepoxide was considered to account, at least in part, for the protective effect of the drug in experimental atherosclerosis. The same group of workers later found (Horák et al., 1976) that chlordiazepoxide, chlorazepate, diazepam, and lorazepam markedly reduced the hyperlipidemia (total lipids, total cholesterol, triglycerides) induced in rats by Triton WR-1339. No correlation was found between the lipid-lowering activity of these drugs and their effects on plasma viscosity (Cuparencu et al., 1970, 1979). The optimal dose for these compounds was 5 mg·kg^{-1}. Oxazepam, medazepam, nitrazepam, and tofisopam were weak or inactive. Chlordiazepoxide, chlorazepate, diazepam and lorazepam, after four consecutive daily doses of 5 mg·kg^{-1}, decreased serum cholesterol, triglyceride, and free fatty acids, but not phosphatides, in rabbits made hyperlipidemic by a diet rich in butter and cholesterol administered for 2 weeks (Feszt et al., 1977).

IV. Protein Synthesis

Diazepam (10 mg·kg^{-1} i.p.) increased the incorporation of ^{3}H-leucine into neuronal cell bodies in the ventral horn of the spinal cord, in the locus coeruleus, and in the trigeminal nucleus of rats (Jakoubek and Petrovický, 1976). In *E. coli* chlordiazepoxide at 3×10^{-3} mol·l^{-1}, but not diazepam, inhibited protein synthesis (Khafagy et al., 1977).

V. Miscellaneous

Javors and Erwin (1978, 1980) studied the inhibitory effect of several benzodiazepines on mouse brain aldehyde reductase in vitro to test the hypothesis that the anticonvulsant activity could be linked with the accumulation of aldehyde intermediates of biogenic amine metabolism. A good correlation was found between the inhibitory potencies of eight benzodiazepine derivatives on aldehyde reductase and the relative protective potencies in maximal electroshock convulsions in mice pretreated with 25 mg·kg^{-1} proadifen to reduce the metabolism of benzodiazepines. However, active concentrations of the drugs for enzyme inhibition were in the millimolar range and, hence, probably irrelevant. Chlordiazepoxide at 3×10^{-3} mol·l^{-1} but not diazepam inhibited RNA and DNA synthesis in *E. coli* (Khafagy et al., 1977). Chlordiazepoxide (0.6 mmol·l^{-1}) inhibited by 17% the transport of ^{45}Ca^{2+} between an aqueous phase and a lipid solvent phase mediated by phosphatidic acid (Mulé, 1969); similar effects were observed with various opiates, chlorpromazine, imipramine, and amphetamine, but not with barbiturates.

VI. Conclusions

Rather high doses of benzodiazepines produced an increase of blood glucose and plasma-free fatty acids. Therapeutic doses in man are apparently insufficient to affect these parameters. The nature of the hyperglycemic and lipomobilizing effect of benzodiazepines in animals has not been clearly established. Its partial or total prevention by adrenalectomy suggests that catecholamines may be involved and that benzodiazepines perhaps increase the effects of amines by inhibiting phosphodiesterase. The high concentrations of chlordiazepoxide and diazepam required to affect glucose transport in isolated skeletal muscle exclude any relevance of these effects for therapeutic doses. Experimental atherosclerosis and hyperlipidemia were found to be reduced by prolonged treatment with benzodiazepines.

Extremely high doses and concentrations of benzodiazepines depressed cell respiration and oxidative phosphorylation. A contribution of this unspecific effect to pharmacologic effects can be dismissed.

J. Miscellaneous Effects

I. Nociception

The demonstration of a true analgesic effect of drugs known to depress the central nervous system is an almost impossible task, since most tests available are based on behavioral responses to noxious stimuli.

Most of the benzodiazepines reported in the literature reduce responses to noxious stimuli at doses known to decrease motor activity. In the writhing test (phenylquinone or acetic acid; in mice), chlordiazepoxide, clobazam, clonazepam, estazolam, flurazepam, and medazepam were active in muscle-relaxant or sedating doses (RANDALL et al., 1968, 1969; SAJI et al., 1972; BARZAGHI et al., 1973; FENNESSY and SAWYNOK, 1973; FIELDING and HOFFMANN, 1979). At doses which effectively disturb the performance of mice in the horizontal wire test or on the rotating bar, chlordiazepoxide, chlorazepate, diazepam, flurazepam, medazepam, nitrazepam, and SAS 643 enhanced the reaction time on the hot plate (BRUNAUD et al., 1970; RANDALL and KAPPELL, 1973; BABBINI et al., 1975), whereas no elevation of pain threshold was reported after ataxic doses of either estazolam or nitrazepam (SAJI et al., 1972) and after diazepam (WELLER et al., 1968). Vocalization as a reaction to electrical stimulation of the mouse tail was reduced by pinazepam and diazepam at doses depressing the righting reflex (SCROLLINI et al., 1975). Intravenous injection of $2.5 \text{ mg} \cdot \text{kg}^{-1}$ diazepam produced a moderate increase of the stimulation threshold for vocalization; when bacitracin, which is believed to inhibit enzymatic degradation of enkephalins, was injected into a lateral cerebral ventricle a few minutes before, diazepam produced a marked antinociceptive effect (WÜSTER et al., 1980b). Naloxone ($10 \text{ mg} \cdot \text{kg}^{-1}$ i.p.) only partially reversed the threshold elevating effect of diazepam; these findings were taken as indirect evidence that diazepam was able to release endogenous opioids in some parts of the CNS (WÜSTER et al., 1980b). Only partial analgesia was observed in mice with high doses of diazepam ($> 100 \text{ mg} \cdot \text{kg}^{-1}$ i.p.) in tail-immersion, tail-pinch, and tail-shock procedures in mice (WELLER et al., 1968). Pain threshold elevation in the inflamed or noninflamed paw of rats was reported to be enhanced after $25–100 \text{ mg} \cdot \text{kg}^{-1}$ chlordiazepoxide s.c. (RANDALL et al., 1960) but unaffected after high doses of diazepam, flurazepam, medazepam, or nitrazepam (STERNBACH et al., 1964; RANDALL et al., 1968, 1969). An increase of pain threshold in the carrageenin-inflamed tail but not in the intact tail of mice was found with 10 mg·kg^{-1} estazolam and nitrazepam p.o., while 20 mg·kg^{-1} increased pain threshold under both conditions (SAJI et al., 1972). In contrast to the above-reported effects, neither chlordiazepoxide, diazepam, lorazepam, nor oxazepam were active in the rat tail-flick test (FROMMEL et al., 1960b; GUPTA and GAITONDE, 1964; GLUCKMAN, 1965, 1971). No antinociceptive effect was observed in the mouse tail-flick test with high oral doses of diazepam, medazepam, temazepam, or oxazepam (RANDALL et al., 1970). Chlordiazepoxide (25 and 50 mg·kg^{-1} i.m.) did not inhibit the licking response in rats or the jaw-opening reflex in rabbits to tooth pulp stimulation whereas the vocalization after-discharge was inhibited after 10–25 mg·kg^{-1} p.o. (HOFFMEISTER, 1968). With clobazam (20 mg·kg^{-1} i.p.) FIELDING and HOFFMANN (1979) observed a slight antinociceptive effect to electrical stimulation of the dental pulp. Measuring the flinch-jump threshold (electric shocks through grid floor) in rats, BODNAR et al. (1980) found chlordiazepoxide to be antinociceptive at 15 mg·kg^{-1} i.p. Tolerance to this action developed after daily administration for 14 days. There was a one-way cross tolerance between chlordiazepoxide and morphine and cold water swim, i.e., morphine-tolerant and cold-swim-adapted rats did not respond to chlordiazepoxide; however, chlordiazepoxide-tolerant animals had an attenuated cold swim analgesia but still reacted to morphine.

Using instrumental behavioral methods indication was obtained that chlordiazepoxide (5–20 mg·kg^{-1} i.p.) and diazepam (0.25 mg·kg^{-1} i.p.) reduced the motivation of rats and monkeys to escape a noxious stimulus (HOUSER and PARÉ, 1973; LINEBERRY and KULICS, 1978). The aversive threshold in rats as measured by an operant liminal escape procedure was enhanced by chlordiazepoxide (3–15 mg·kg^{-1} i.p.) but not by diazepam (0.5–5 mg·kg^{-1} i.p.); naloxone (20 mg·kg^{-1} s.c.) reversed the threshold elevation produced by chlordiazepoxide (KELLY et al., 1978a, b).

A well-controlled study in man suggests that diazepam 10 mg p.o. affects the emotional-motivational component of the pain experience, but not the sensory discriminative component or the central control of pain (CHAPMAN and FEATHER, 1973).

In drug interaction studies in the tail-flick test chlordiazepoxide was found to antagonize the analgesic effect of morphine in mice (0.1–50 mg·kg^{-1} s.c., WEIS, 1969) and guinea pigs (10 mg·kg^{-1} s.c., FROMMEL et al., 1960b), but to potentiate morphine analgesia in rats with 10 mg·kg^{-1} i.p. (GUPTA and GAITONDE, 1964). An antagonism of morphine in the mouse tail-flick was also demonstrated for diazepam (ED$_{50}$:3 mg·kg^{-1} s.c.), whereas oxazepam was inactive (RANDALL et al., 1970). With somewhat lower doses (1 mg·kg^{-1} i.p.) of diazepam and oxazepam, SHANNON et al. (1976) observed no antagonism of the analgesic effect of morphine or methadone in the mouse tail flick and hot plate test. CARABATEAS and HARRIS (1966) described a series of atypical benzodiazepines, which antagonized the analgesic effect of meperidine in the tail flick. A potentiation of the antinociceptive effect of morphine in the hot-plate test together with a potentiation of morphine's respiratory depressant effect was reported to occur after 2.5 mg·kg^{-1} diazepam i.p. (BRADSHAW et al., 1973). FENNESSY and SAWYNOK (1973) described a biphasic effect of chlordiazepoxide, clonazepam, diazepam, flurazepam, medazepam, and nitrazepam on the morphine analgesia in the phenylquinone writhing test; they all potentiated, at the dose of

10 mg·kg⁻¹ p.o., the effect of morphine after a short pretreatment interval but reduced morphine analgesia at longer pretreatment times. Chlordiazepoxide and clonazepam were shown to enhance and nitrazepam to reduce the analgesic action of sodium salicylate, whereas diazepam, flurazepam, and medazepam only potentiated the activity of sodium salicylate at a time when the sodium salicylate effect had disappeared completely (FENNESSY and SAWYNOK, 1973). BERGER et al. (1978) and ELLIS et al. (1977) potentiated the analgesic effects of D-propoxyphen in the mouse hotplate and rat tail-flick tests as well as in ischemic pain in humans by combining it with a variety of benzodiazepines. GROTTO and SULMAN (1967) report an antagonistic effect of chlordiazepoxide on paracetamol-induced analgesia in mice, but their results, in fact, show an enhancement.

II. Inflammation

Antiinflammatory activities of chlordiazepoxide, diazepam, flurazepam, nitrazepam, and pinazepam have been described in the carrageenin edema test or with the yeast inflammation method. Weak effects were achieved only with doses that had marked central nervous system effects (RANDALL et al., 1960, 1969; STERNBACH et al., 1964; BARZAGHI et al., 1973). Medazepam had no antiinflammatory effect in the carrageenin edema test or in the rat adjuvant arthritis model (RANDALL et al., 1968).

III. Food and Fluid Intake

A great number of papers deals with the effects of benzodiazepines on food and water consumption under free or instrumental behavioral conditions (COOPER, 1980b). Since a whole chapter in this handbook deals with the effects of benzodiazepines on instrumental behavior (DEWS, 1981), only effects in free behavioral situations will be considered in the following.

Already in very early papers benzodiazepines were described to enhance food intake in man (AYD, 1962; TOBIN and LEWIS, 1960) and in a variety of laboratory animals. RANDALL et al. (1960) reported that chlordiazepoxide 12.5–50 mg·kg⁻¹ s.c. enhanced food intake by 20%–60% in starved rats. A similar effect was also found in starved dogs with chlordiazepoxide in doses of 2.5–20 mg·kg⁻¹ p.o. (RANDALL and KAPPELL, 1961; STERNBACH et al., 1964) and later with diazepam 2 mg·kg⁻¹ p.o., but not with triflubazam (HEILMAN et al., 1974). Dogs treated with chlordiazepoxide for 13 weeks and rats treated for 14 days or 37 weeks showed an increased food consumption (ZBINDEN et al., 1961; STERNBACH et al., 1964). This effect was absent in chicks (ZBINDEN et al., 1961), but chlordiazepoxide (10 mg·kg⁻¹ i.m.) doubled the mean amount of food intake in nondeprived pigeons without affecting water intake (COOPER and POSADAS-ANDREWS, 1979). OPITZ and AKINLAJA (1966) found that chlordiazepoxide and oxazepam enhanced food consumption in rats during a long-term treatment. The effect of chlordiazepoxide acutely and chronically on several feeding parameters (e.g., rate and number of episodes) of rats was analyzed by COOPER and FRANCIS (1979b). A dose-dependent increase of food and water intake in starved rats was seen with diazepam and nitrazepam (STERNBACH et al., 1964), but not with flurazepam (RANDALL et al., 1969). NIKI (1965) found chlordiazepoxide to enhance food consumption even in satiated rats. In starved cats oxazepam, desmethyllorazepam, diazepam, chlordiazepoxide, medazepam, and pinazepam induced voraciousness, and satiated cats resumed voracious eating after benzodiazepines (0.3 mg·kg^{-1} i.p.; Fratta et al., 1976; Mereu et al., 1976). Della-Fera et al. (1980) studied the enhancing effect on food intake of several benzodiazepines in cats and puppies fed ad libitum; the triazolobenzodiazepines U 31,889 and U 37,576 were the most potent, but the increase of food intake was greater with elfazepam. Except for elfazepam, the effect on food intake occurred at doses that clearly produced ataxia or excitement. Diazepam also enhanced food intake in horses (Brown et al., 1976).

That the stimulant effect on food intake was not dependent on the environment or the time of feeding was shown by Wise and Dawson (1974), who found similar effects with diazepam in rats in their home cage, in the test box, during daytime and during nighttime. Cooper (1980a) provided evidence that increased food intake in rats after chlordiazepoxide and diazepam was induced by mechanisms independent of food neophobia. Presentation of novel food in a novel environment to rats under chlordiazepoxide, diazepam, or nitrazepam also resulted in a dose-dependent increase in food intake (Stephens, 1973). Chlordiazepoxide (5 and 10 mg·kg^{-1} i.p.) and diazepam (2.5 mg·kg^{-1} i.p.) increased eating of familiar food in food-deprived rats in a food preference test situation (Burton et al., 1980; Cooper, 1980a; Cooper and Crummy, 1978; Cooper and McClelland, 1980); higher doses of the compounds were required to enhance eating of novel food (Cooper, 1980a; Cooper and McClelland, 1980). Grouping or isolation of rats did not change the stimulant effect of chlordiazepoxide (Bainbridge, 1968). Soubrié et al., (1975b) showed that various benzodiazepines increased food intake in rats and mice irrespective of the environment or the degree of food deprivation. In addition it was shown that eating evoked in rats by tail pinching was enhanced by 5 mg·kg^{-1} chlordiazepoxide i.p. (Robbins et al., 1977). Eating can also be evoked, at least in some rats, by stimulation of the lateral hypothalamus. After 5 mg·kg^{-1} diazepam i.p. the threshold for evoking eating in "eater" rats was lowered, and stimulation in "noneater" rats now induced food consumption (Soper and Wise, 1971). Watson et al. (1980) found that 2.5 and 5 mg·kg^{-1} diazepam i.p. reduced the threshold for stimulation-bound eating but not for drinking. Bilateral injection of diazepam (20 µg/0.2 µl) into the ventromedial hypothalamus, but not into the lateral hypothalamus, led to an at least fourfold increase of food intake in non-starved rats (Anderson-Baker et al., 1979).

The stimulation of food intake by subcutaneous diazepam in rats was antagonized by small doses of naloxone (Gylys et al., 1979; Stapleton et al., 1979; Britton and Thatcher-Britton, 1980; Soubrié et al., 1980) and picrotoxin (Fletcher et al., 1980). An interaction of benzodiazepines with anorexigenic drugs was also reported. Indeed, amphetamine antagonized increased food intake after chlordiazepoxide in starved dogs (Sternbach et al., 1964). In rats, chlordiazepoxide (4–20 mg·kg^{-1} i.p.) at least partially antagonized the anorexigenic effect of amphetamine, fenfluramine, and fluoxetine (Borella et al., 1969; Iwahara, 1970; Cooper and Francis, 1978; Feldman and Smith, 1978). In cats, the anorexigenic effect of amphetamine, but not the hyperactivity and the stereotyped behavior, was antagonized by 3 mg·kg^{-1} i.p. oxazepam (Fratta et al., 1976).

Benzodiazepines were also shown to enhance the intake of water or other fluids. Sternbach et al. (1964) reported that 6–25 mg·kg^{-1} s.c. chlordiazepoxide, diazepam, and nitrazepam increased water intake in deprived rats. Enhanced water intake was also observed after bromazepam 1 mg·kg^{-1} s.c. (ZAMBONI et al., 1972). A dipsogenic effect in fluid-deprived rats was shown for 3–10 mg·kg^{-1} chlordiazepoxide and diazepam i.p., irrespective of whether water, water and tartaric acid, or sweetened water was offered (MAICKEL and MALONEY, 1973, 1974). An increased water intake was observed by SOUBRIÉ et al. (1976 a) in fluid-deprived rats or mice after diazepam (1–4 mg·kg^{-1} i.p.), chlordiazepoxide (8–16 mg · kg^{-1} i.p.), lorazepam (0.125–1 mg · kg^{-1} i.p.), nitrazepam (1–2 mg · kg^{-1} i.p.), and prazepam (8 mg · kg^{-1} i.p.) in a novel or familiar situation. Rats injected daily for 9 days with chlordiazepoxide (5–15 mg · kg^{-1} i.p.) and tested on the 9th day showed an enhanced water intake comparable to that observed after a single injection of the same doses of chlordiazepoxide (COOPER and FRANCIS, 1979 a). On the other hand FALK and BURNIDGE (1970) reported that in fluid-deprived rats 15 or 30 mg·kg^{-1} chlordiazepoxide s.c. did not enhance water intake but stimulated the intake of hypertonic saline. KURIBARA and TADOKORO (1978) found no effect of diazepam (4 mg·kg^{-1} i.p.), injected at the beginning of the dark period, on water consumption. PATEL and MALICK (1980) reported that chlordiazepoxide increased water consumption in satiated rats. The licking rate of rats tended to be increased during a 5-day treatment with chlordiazepoxide (8 mg·kg^{-1} i.p.), irrespective of whether familiar 32% or unfamiliar 4% sucrose was offered (FLAHERTY et al., 1980). Adjunctive drinking that developed in starved rats which had water spouts available during feeding sessions was enhanced with low doses of diazepam and ripazepam (SANGER and BLACKMAN, 1976). When sweetened or adulterated milk instead of water was offered to rats which were either naive or familiar, deprived or satiated, in the home cage or in a test box, increased drinking occurred after chlordiazepoxide, diazepam, lorazepam, medazepam, nitrazepam, and oxazepam or pyrazapon (GLUCKMAN, 1965, 1971; MARGULES and STEIN, 1967; POSCHEL, 1971; POSCHEL et al., 1974; JOHNSON, 1978).

Most authors concluded that the effects observed with benzodiazepines on food and water intake could not be explained by an effect on appetite (BURTON et al., 1980), but rather by a change of motivation for the offered food. However, recent findings point to an important role of GABAergic neurons in the hypothalamic control of feeding (KELLY and GROSSMAN, 1979; GRANDISON and GUIDOTTI, 1977). From studies of the effect of GABAmimetic muscimol, injected into discrete areas of the rat hypothalamus, KELLY et al. (1979) and OLGIATI et al. (1980) proposed that GABAergic neurons inhibited satiety mechanisms in the medial hypothalamus and inhibited feeding mechanisms in the lateral hypothalamus. If benzodiazepines enhanced GABAergic synaptic activity preferentially in the medial hypothalamus, as supposed by ANDERSON-BAKER et al. (1979), increased feeding would ensue as after local injection of muscimol. Another GABAergic synapse where benzodiazepines could act to produce their effect on food intake is the dorsal raphé nucleus; indeed, PRZEWLOCKA et al. (1979) found that local injection of GABA and muscimol into this nucleus reduced 5-HT and 5-HIAA in the hypothalamus, increased locomotor activity, and stimulated eating in satiated rats.

IV. Emesis

A few reports describe the effects of chlordiazepoxide, diazepam, flurazepam, and triflubazam on apomorphine-induced emesis in dogs. A weak antiemetic effect was

observed with 40 mg·kg⁻¹ chlordiazepoxide p.o. (RANDALL et al., 1960) and triflubazam (HEILMAN et al., 1974), whereas diazepam (40 mg·kg⁻¹ p.o.) and flurazepam
(0.1 mg·kg⁻¹ p.o.) were found inactive (STERNBACH et al., 1964; RANDALL et al.,
1969).

V. Body Temperature

No systematic studies of the hypothermic effects of benzodiazepines exist to our
knowledge. The following gives a few examples of the reported effects of chlordiazepoxide on body temperature in various species.

Chlordiazepoxide (12.5 and 50 mg·kg⁻¹ i.p.) lowered body temperature dose-dependently in mice (LOCKER and KOFFER, 1962). In rats body temperature was not
changed after chlordiazepoxide 20 mg·kg⁻¹ i.p. (THEOBALD et al., 1965), whereas
high doses lowered the body temperature in guinea pigs (FROMMEL et al., 1960 b). An
antipyretic effect was reported in guinea pigs (100 mg·kg⁻¹ s.c., FROMMEL et al.,
1960 b). A decreased body temperature was found in dogs, especially under low ambient temperature (10 mg·kg⁻¹ p.o., SCHMIDT et al., 1961); shivering occurring in animals exposed to low temperature was abolished. Hyperthermia induced by the combination of L-tryptophan and tranylcypromine was dose-dependently reduced in conscious cats by chlordiazepoxide, diazepam, and flurazepam (LIPPA et al., 1979); diazepam (0.3–1.5 mg·kg⁻¹ i.p.) did not significantly lower rectal temperature.

VI. Conclusions

The effect of benzodiazepines on pain perception and pain experience is still a matter
of controversy. A true antinociceptive activity in the usual animal tests could not be
observed in doses that had no marked effects on behavior and muscle tone and coordination. Interaction experiments with analgesics rather increased the confusion
about the effects of benzodiazepines on pain mechanisms. As will be shown in later
sections, benzodiazepines enhance presynaptic inhibition of signals from sensory
neurons; however, an increased primary afferent depolarization has so far been described only in I a afferents. It would be most interesting to study the effect of these
compounds on the presynaptic control of small-diameter afferents which are considered to conduct nociceptive messages. High-dose therapy of schizophrenics with
diazepam was found to produce very marked hypalgesia (BECKMANN and HAAS,
1980).

A consistent finding with benzodiazepines is their stimulant effect on food intake.
This effect on feeding is seen with familiar as well as with novel food. Accordingly,
these drugs may act directly on feeding mechanisms as well as increase food intake
indirectly through an anxiolytic effect. Evidence has been presented for a part played
by GABAergic mechanisms in feeding behavior, whereby several pathways may be involved (GRANDISON and GUIDOTTI, 1977; KELLY et al., 1977; KIMURA and KURIYAMA,
1975; PRZEWLOCKA et al., 1979; TAPPAZ and BROWNSTEIN, 1977). Since many instrumental behavioral tests are based on food as reinforcer, a more in-depth investigation
of the appetite stimulant effect of benzodiazepines is clearly indicated.

Benzodiazepines share a hypothermic effect with many other centrally active
drugs. It remains to be shown whether GABAergic mechanisms are also involved in

this activity of benzodiazepines, as results with GABA mimetics and GABA trans-aminase inhibitors tend to suggest.

K. Anticonvulsant Activity

Of all the somatic effects that benzodiazepines produce in the laboratory animal, the protection from epileptic seizures induced by various means, in particular by chemical convulsants, is the most impressive and the one that can be measured very reliably and simply. Although benzodiazepine derivatives reveal distinct differences in their neuropsychopharmacologic profile of action as assessed by the various laboratory methods available at present, the antagonistic action on pentetrazole-induced seizures predicts surprisingly well the overall psychotropic potency of these drugs in man (TALLMAN et al., 1980). This correlation is probably not the result of anticonvulsant action per se, because not all drugs active on pentetrazole-induced seizures exhibit benzodiazepine-like anxiolytic, sleep-inducing, and muscle relaxant activity in man. It seems rather that the synaptic effects which underlie the anticonvulsant activity of benzodiazepines are also the essential basis for their other effects and that, once we know the mechanism of the anticonvulsant activity, we may also begin to understand the molecular and cellular basis of their psychotropic effects.

The literature on the anticonvulsant actions of benzodiazepines is considerable. It does not seem meaningful to consider in this section the very many quantitative data obtained with a large number of benzodiazepines in all modifications of tests for an-ticonvulsant activity. We shall classify the essential findings according to whether they were elaborated in acute or chronic models of epilepsy and according to the means used to induce epileptiform activity.

I. Acute Models of Epilepsy

1. Chemical Convulsants

Pentetrazole (Pentylenetetrazole, Metrazole). The symptoms occurring after pente-trazole depend inter alia on the dose and the route and speed of administration. Among the various seizure components those most frequently used as experimental parameters are clonic and tonic convulsions (of the head, forelimbs, and hindlimbs) and death. There are two essentially different ways of assessing the protective effect of drugs on chemically induced convulsions. One consists in administering a fixed dose of the convulsant to a control and drug-treated group of animals, usually a dose found to produce the selected seizure component(s) in all or nearly all animals within a given time. The calculated effective or protective dose is that which prevents the ap-pearance of the selected symptoms in a definite percentage of animals. The other ap-proach is to determine the drug-induced change of the threshold dose of the convul-sant. In most experiments this is done by slow intravenous infusion of the convulsant until the occurrence of the seizure component. Both principles have their advantages and drawbacks. One advantage of the second approach is, e.g., the possibility to de-termine both potency and efficacy of an anticonvulsant. It is important to realize that the protective capacity of a drug will depend inter alia on the speed at which the epilep-tiform activities develop, viz. in a more protracted way after intraperitoneal or sub-

Table 5. ED_{50} values (mg · kg^{-1} p.o.) for some benzodiazepines in four routine screening tests used in the authors' laboratories. Rotarod and antipentetrazole activity were evaluated as described by BLUM et al. (1973)

Drug	Rotarod	Chimney	Pentetrazole	3-Mercaptopropionic acid
Diazepam	2.9	2.6	2.2	1.4
Bromazepam	0.37	0.34	0.49	0.78
Flunitrazepam	0.07	0.09	0.05	0.05
Medazepam	9	8	6.1	12.7
Triazolam	0.08	0.12	0.13	0.06
Estazolam	1.2	1.1	0.57	0.36
Midazolam	0.43	0.57	2.1	2.2

cutaneous administration, and very quickly after intravenous infusion. We prefer the latter method, in the modification described by BLUM et al. (1973), because it gave reproducible results over many years.

The early results reported by RANDALL et al. (1960, 1961, 1965a) in mice challenged with 125 mg · kg^{-1} pentetrazole s.c. clearly demonstrated the high potency of chlordiazepoxide, diazepam, and nitrazepam compared with other clinically used antiepileptics and meprobamate. In an extensive study SWINYARD and CASTELLION (1966) compared a series of benzodiazepines for their protective effect against a fixed dose of pentetrazole (85 mg · kg^{-1} s.c.) as well as for their ability to increase the intravenous threshold dose of the convulsant. Clonazepam was found by SWINYARD and CASTELLION (1966) to be particularly potent as an anticonvulsant, an observation which was essentially confirmed by other investigators (LECHAT et al., 1970; D'ARMAGNAC et al., 1971; BLUM et al., 1973). Oxazepam was found by GLUCKMAN (1965) to be virtually as potent as diazepam. COUTINHO et al. (1969, 1970) and MARCUCCI et al. (1968a, b, 1970, 1971, 1973) were mainly interested in relating anticonvulsant activity with the rate of metabolic degradation of benzodiazepines; differences in the duration of the antipentetrazole activity were observed by these authors and by BANZIGER (1965) and BANERJEE and YEOH (1977) in various animal species. The water-soluble oxazepam hemisuccinate was studied by BABBINI et al. (1969) and BABBINI and TORRIELLI (1972), and various triazolobenzodiazepines were investigated by NAKAJIMA et al. (1971a) and HESTER et al. (1971). MARCY and QUERMONNE (1975) determined in mice the antipentetrazole activity of several benzodiazepines as well as their effect on the palmar skin response; from the calculated ratio of the potencies for these two parameters, the authors classified various benzodiazepines as either "specifically anticonvulsant" or "sedative." A very high potency against pentetrazole seizures was reported for lorazepam (BRUNAUD and ROCAND, 1972; GLUCKMAN and STEIN, 1978). Activities of a series of benzodiazepines and their metabolites were reported by TRAVERSA et al. (1977). In Table 5 are listed the potencies of several classical benzodiazepines in the intravenous pentetrazole test as used in our laboratories. Results from the literature are given in Table 6. Some thienotriazolodiazepines were investigated by JOHNSON and FUNDERBURK (1978). STONE and JAVID (1978) compared a few benzodiazepines as antagonists of pentetrazole, bicuculline, picrotoxin, and 3-mercaptopropionic acid. JUHASZ and DAIRMAN (1977) as well as LIPPA and REGAN (1977) administered 2 mg · kg^{-1} p.o. diazepam daily for 4 or 7 days, respectively, and found that no tolerance developed to the antipentetrazole activity of benzodiazepine. How-

Table 6. ED_{50} values (mg · kg^{-1}) for various benzodiazepines obtained in horizontal wire, rotarod, and antipentetrazole tests

Drug	Traction test[a]	Rotarod[a]	Antipentetrazole test[a]
Diazepam	1.6 [1]	4.4 [1]	1.7 [1]
	29 [2]	3.4 [2]	1.4 [2]
	2.3 [6]	15 [4]	1.2 [3]
	16.9 [10]	30 [11]	1.6 [11]
	25 [11]	2.1 [6]	0.76 [6]
	7 [12] i.p.	7 [7]	1.4 [7]
	4 [13] i.p.	5.3 [10]	0.8 [12] i.p.
Chlordiazepoxide	3 [1]	13 [1]	5 [1]
	14 [5]	95 [4]	16.5 [3]
	58.5 [10]	14.2 [10]	10 [11]
	75 [11]	200 [11]	
Oxazepam	8.5 [1]	9.5 [1]	1.7 [1]
	13 [13] i.p.		
Medazepam	25 [1]	5 [1]	4.5 [1]
	8 [6]	18.5 [6]	3.1 [6]
	250 [11]	400 [11]	5 [11]
Lorazepam	2.5 [1]	0.4 [1]	0.07 [1]
Clonazepam	16 [2]	0.3 [2]	0.15 [2]
Nimetazepam		1.4 [4]	0.18 [4]
Flurazepam	3 [8]	6 [9]	2 [9]
Temazepam	40 [11]	50 [11]	6.4 [11]
	4 [13] i.p.		
Triazolam	0.6 [12] i.p.		0.04 [12] i.p.

[a] The values were obtained after oral administration except those indicated. Antipentetrazole activity was examined in various modifications of pentetrazole-induced seizures (see Sect. K.)

[1] Brunaud and Rocand (1972)
[2] Blum et al. (1973)
[3] Robichaud et al. (1970)
[4] Sakai et al. (1972)
[5] Fernandez-Tomé et al. (1975)
[6] Asami et al. (1975)
[7] Kamioka et al. (1972)
[8] Babbini et al. (1975)
[9] Randall and Kappel (1973)
[10] Nakanishi et al. (1972)
[11] Ferrini et al. (1974)
[12] Rudzik et al. (1973)
[13] Gall et al. (1978)

ever, both groups of investigators reported that the antistrychnine and antibicuculline activity of diazepam declined after this subchronic treatment schedule. A comparison of the potencies of several benzodiazepines as inhibitors of ^{3}H-diazepam binding in rat brain synaptosomes and as antagonists of pentetrazole in mice was made by Malick and Enna (1979).

Antipentetrazole activities of various benzodiazepines in the rat were reported by Banziger (1965), Marcucci et al. (1968a), Banerjee and Yeoh (1977), Matthews and McCafferty (1979), in the rabbit by Banziger (1965), and in the guinea pig by Marcucci et al. (1971a). In rats, Kleinrok et al. (1977) found that the antipentetrazole action of chlordiazepoxide, diazepam, oxazepam, and nitrazepam was enhanced by 5-HTP, 5-methoxytryptamine (combined with pargyline), or fenfluramine.

An interesting comparative study of 14 different benzodiazepines in the rat and the mouse antipentetrazole was published by DESMEDT et al. (1976) and NIEMEGEERS and LEWI (1979); the ED_{50} values for the various seizure components of these tests were listed together with those for the maximal electroshock test as well as for some tests indicative of muscle relaxation, motor incoordination and sedation. Using these activity profiles a spectral map of 49 anticonvulsants was constructed. The benzodiazepines are clearly separated from four other classes of anticonvulsants and, among themselves, are divided into three groups. Unfortunately, it is difficult, in the absence of corresponding data from man, to evaluate the relevance of the interesting differences elaborated in this sophisticated analysis.

CLINCKE and WAUQUIER (1979) administered pentetrazole in a subconvulsive dose ($40 \ mg \cdot kg^{-1}$ s.c.) 30 min before retesting rats which had been trained 24 h before in a single session to remain on a platform located above an electrifiable grid to avoid an electric shock. Pentetrazole reduced the latency to step down in this passive avoidance situation. Clonazepam ($0.04-0.63 \ mg \cdot kg^{-1}$ i.p.), as well as ethosuximide and trimethadione, antagonized the retention impairment of passive avoidance, whereas other antiepileptics were ineffective. CLINCKE and WAUQUIER (1979) concluded that the impaired information processing occurring after subconvulsive doses of pentetrazole was similar to the retrograde amnesia in petit mal absence, and that this passive avoidance paradigm discriminated effective anti-absence compounds from other antiepileptics.

Bicuculline. The GABA antagonist, bicuculline, has been used in mice and rats with similar methods as described for pentetrazole. Bicuculline is a much more potent convulsant than pentetrazole; the symptoms induced by the two convulsants are very similar. The anti-bicuculline effect of various benzodiazepines was described by BLUM et al. (1973), SCHLOSSER et al. (1973), HAEFELY et al. (1975 b), DINGLEDINE et al. (1978), STONE and JAVID (1978), WORMS et al. (1979), BUCKETT (1980), and MATTHEWS and McCAFFERTY (1979). There is agreement among the investigators that higher doses of benzodiazepines are required to obtain a similar degree of protection (or shift of the convulsive dose-response curve, respectively) against bicuculline than against pentetrazole. This finding by itself cannot be used as an argument in favor or against the concept that GABAergic mechanisms are primarily involved in the anticonvulsant action of benzodiazepines; indeed, the mode of action of pentetrazole in producing seizures is still not clear in spite of much experimental efforts, although an interaction with GABA-mediated synaptic processes (GABA release?, chloride conductivity?) seems to be at least partially involved. It is quite possible that the processes of GABAergic inhibition, which are blocked by pentetrazole, are more easily overcome by benzodiazepines than the blockade of GABA receptors produced by bicuculline.

According to JUHASZ and DAIRMAN (1977) and LIPPA and REGAN (1977) the daily administration of diazepam ($2 \ mg \cdot kg^{-1}$ p.o.) to mice for 4 and 7 days, respectively, produced a tolerance to the antibicuculline (and antistrychnine) activity, but not to the antipentetrazole activity.

Picrotoxin. Picrotoxin, like bicuculline, inhibits the effects of GABA. However, whereas bicuculline most probably acts at or near the GABA recognition site of the GABA receptor-chloride ionophore complex, picrotoxin is more likely to affect the chloride channel directly (TICKU et al., 1978). Various benzodiazepines were found to protect mice, rats, and chicks from convulsions induced by picrotoxin in roughly the same doses as those found to be active against bicuculline (COSTA et al., 1975 a; MAO

Table 7. Protection from convulsions induced in mice by thiosemicarbazide. (From MARKOVICH and OSTROVSKAYA, 1977)

Drug	ED_{50}, mg $\cdot$ kg^{-1} p.o.
Clonazepam	0.009 (0.005–0.014)
Lorazepam	0.034 (0.026–0.044)
Diazepam	0.45 (0.37–0.54)
Medazepam	1.8 (1.24–2.6)
Phenobarbitone	15.5 (11.9–20.15)
Diphenylhydantoin	No effect below 100 mg $\cdot$ kg^{-1}

et al., 1975 a; HORTON et al., 1976; SOUBRIÉ and SIMON, 1978; STONE and JAVID, 1978). Intrastriatal injection of several benzodiazepines delayed and reduced the forelimb myoclonus induced in rats by the microinjection of picrotoxin into the anterior caudate nucleus (JENNER et al., 1979).

Naloxone. This "pure" opiate antagonist (in the sense that it has no opiate agonistic activity) produces convulsive seizures in very high doses. Diazepam protected mice from naloxone-induced convulsions (DINGLEDINE et al., 1978). This and the interference of naloxone with specific GABA binding was taken by the authors as an indication for a GABA receptor blocking activity of naloxone (in much higher concentrations than required to block opiate receptors).

Inhibitors of the Biosynthesis of GABA. Benzodiazepines were found to be quite effective against seizures induced in rats by isoniacid, which depletes endogenous GABA by inhibiting glutamic acid decarboxylase (GAD) (MAO et al., 1975a; COSTA et al., 1975b; WOOD et al., 1979).

The more selective action of benzodiazepines against seizures induced by isoniacid than by other convulsants as compared with phenobarbitone, which was claimed by MAO et al. (1975a) and COSTA et al. (1975b), was not confirmed by LEMBECK and BEUBLER (1977) in mice.

Convulsive seizures induced in mice by a related GAD inhibitor, thiosemicarbazide, were also potently antagonized by benzodiazepines (HAEFELY et al., 1975; MARKOVICH and OSTROVSKAYA, 1977). ED_{50} values reported by the latter authors for four benzodiazepines, phenobarbitone, and diphenylhydantoin, are listed in Table 7. THIÉBOT et al. (1979) reduced the convulsive threshold dose of picrotoxin in rats by the previous intraperitoneal administration of 64 mg $\cdot$ kg^{-1} thiosemicarbazide; diazepam (4 mg $\cdot$ kg^{-1} i.p.) elevated the threshold dose of picrotoxin in control rats as well as in thiosemicarbazide-primed rats.

Convulsions occur with a very short latency after 3-mercaptopropionic acid (3-MPA) as compared with the other GAD inhibitors (HORTON and MELDRUM, 1973; KARLSSON et al., 1974). Diazepam and flunitrazepam (HAEFELY et al., 1975b) and many other benzodiazepines (unpublished data from our laboratories, see Table 5) prevented seizures and mortality induced by 3-MPA in mice at almost identical doses as they were found active against pentetrazole. STONE and JAVID (1978), using a different method, found chlordiazepoxide, diazepam, and nitrazepam less effective on 3-MPA-induced seizures than on those induced by pentetrazole. On the other hand, LÖSCHER (1979), comparing diazepam with a number of conventional anticonvulsant drugs (phenobarbitone ethosuximide, trimethadione, carbamazepine, phenytoin) in mice, found that diazepam was most effective against 3-MPA, its ED_{50} being identical to that against pentetrazole.

Administration of another GAD inhibitor, allylglycine (200 mg·kg^{-1} i.v.) enhances photically-induced epileptic responses in baboons *(Papio papio)* for a period of 6–10 h. Diazepam (0.5–1.5 mg·kg^{-1} i.v.) was highly effective against these facilitated myoclonic responses (MELDRUM et al., 1975). ASHTON and WAUQUIER (1979 b) studied a large number of anticonvulsants in rats in which seizures were induced by the i.v. injection of D, L-allylglycine. Clonazepam was the most potent drug. Trimethadione, ethosuximide, and meprobamate were inactive.

Bemegride. In mice, convulsive seizures induced by bemegride (30 mg·kg^{-1} s.c.) were antagonized with about the same potency (ED_{50} at 1 h $\sim$ 0.3 mg·kg^{-1} p.o. – ED_{50} at 24 h $\sim$ 1.5–3 mg·kg^{-1} p.o.) by cloxazolam and diazepam (KAMIOKA et al., 1972). Bemegride injected intravenously (4–9 mg·kg^{-1}) elicited tonic-clonic convulsions in freely moving cats; diazepam (2 mg·kg^{-1} s.c.) raised the bemegride threshold by more than 250% in cats (VAN DUJIN and VISSER, 1972). Seizures induced in rats by this convulsant analeptic were prevented by diazepam (SOUBRIÉ and SIMON, 1978). In gerbils, bemegride antagonized diazepam-cued behavior (JOHANSSON and JAERBE, 1975).

Ouabain. Ouabain injected in a small volume into the cerebral ventricles of rats induces running and leaping fits (when the drug is mainly concentrated in the hippocampus) and generalized clonic-tonic convulsions after higher volumes (when the drug also reaches the cerebellum and brain stem). Clonazepam protected rats from generalized clonic-tonic seizures (DAVIDSON et al., 1978). PETSCHE and RAPPELSBERGER (1970) induced focal cortical epilepsy in the rabbit by local application of ouabain on the cortical surface and recorded the electrical activity of the cortex and movements of the head and the contralateral body side. They obtained a status epilepticus lasting about 5 h, characterized by periods of cortical wave activity and the irregular appearance of myoclonic and generalized clonic-tonic seizures. Clonazepam suppressed seizures and myocloni at the dose of 0.25 mg·kg^{-1} i.v. Doubling the dose resulted additionally in a reduction of paroxysmal cortical activity (reduction of the amplitude of waves, prolongation of interburst intervals, and marked suppression of lateral and perpendicular propagation, while the focal activity in the deeper cortical layer was least affected).

Local Anesthetics. High parenteral doses of local anesthetics are well known to induce seizures; the mechanism of action is uncertain. EIDELBERG et al. (1963, 1965) were able to protect rats from convulsions induced by 60 mg·kg^{-1} cocaine i.p. with chlordiazepoxide, diazepam, clonazepam, and flunitrazepam; interestingly, tonic-clonic seizures by cocaine could also be prevented by previous destruction of both amygdalae by electrocoagulation. Similar results were obtained by ALDRETE and DANIEL (1971) with diazepam against convulsions induced by procaine, tetracaine, or lidocaine. Diazepam was found to prevent muscular rigidity and convulsions induced in cats by procaine and lidocaine (FEINSTEIN et al., 1970). Clonazepam increased the threshold dose of lidocaine for induction of paroxysmal EEG activity in the amygdala, hippocampus, and cerebral cortex of rabbits (GOGOLAK et al., 1973).

In Rhesus monkeys, paroxysmal cortical and subcortical EEG activity induced by intravenous infusion of lidocaine, mepivacaine, and bupivacaine was rapidly terminated by intravenous bolus injection of 0.1 mg·kg^{-1} diazepam (MUNSON and WAG-MAN, 1972). Similar effects were obtained with diazepam in convulsions induced in cats and monkeys (DE JONG and HEAVNER, 1973, 1974a, b). MAEKAWA et al. (1974) found in the dog that diazepam, which by itself reduced cerebral metabolism, prevented the increase of cerebral metabolism and the changes in cerebral circulation induced by high doses of lidocaine.

Penicillin. Penicillin reduces inhibitory GABAergic synaptic transmission probably at a postsynaptic (MACON and KING, 1979; ANTONIADIS et al., 1980) as well as at a presynaptic (CUTLER and YOUNG, 1979) site. In hippocampal slices penicillin-induced disinhibition resulted in dendritic burst firing and associated membrane depolarization shifts of pyramidal cells, which may be a first step in epileptogenesis (WONG and PRINCE, 1979).

DI ROCCO et al. (1974) studied the effect of clonazepam in rabbits. Penicillin was injected stereotaxically in the anterior part of the amygdala; this elicited within 20–150 s paroxysmal EEG activity in the amygdala, which then spread to other structures. Clonazepam 0.1–0.25 mg·kg^{-1} i.v. markedly reduced the spread of primary epileptiform discharges but only slightly affected the focal activity in the amygdala.

In cats anesthetized with pentobarbitone, SHARER and KUTT (1971) elicited focal cortical seizures by placing aqueous penicillin G on the anterior ectosylvian gyrus; diazepam infused intravenously at 0.25 mg·kg^{-1} decreased or abolished the spread of seizure discharges and also peripheral jerking, except in cats with foci produced by large amounts of penicillin. The cortical spike activity was never abolished, but was reduced in some instances with large doses of diazepam (1–2.4 mg·kg^{-1}). In another type of acute preparation (cat anesthetized with halothane and then immobilized with gallamine), lower doses of diazepam were sufficient to counteract electrical afterdischarges induced by intracortical application of penicillin; these investigators concluded that their preparation was a very sensitive indicator of the anticonvulsant effects of diazepam (STARK et al., 1974).

WEIHRAUCH et al. (1976) recorded paroxysmal EEG changes and convulsive seizures occurring in rabbits after the intravenous infusion of 2.4 mg·kg^{-1} benzylpenicillin over 50 min. Neither diazepam nor diphenylhydantoin reduced the amplitude or frequency of cortical spike potentials; however, diazepam (but not diphenylhydantoin) prevented the development of generalized convulsions in all animals.

Acute short-lasting epileptiform foci were induced in urethane-anesthetized rats by the local injection of benzylpenicillin into the cortex; both diazepam and diphenylhydantoin reduced the amplitude of spikes within the focus and, even more markedly, the amplitude of propagated spikes (GARTSIDE, 1978).

EDMONDS et al. (1974) injected minute quantities of penicillin into discrete intracortical sites in freely moving rats, studying the time course and extent of the penicillin-induced cortical paroxysmal activity. Diazepam (15–30 mg·kg^{-1} p.o.) was virtually ineffective, though eliciting slight ataxia in some animals at the highest dose used. EDMONDS et al. (1974) concluded that the therapeutic index of diazepam against penicillin-induced seizures in freely moving rats was very low.

Strychnine. Strychnine, although the best glycine antagonist presently available, seems to induce convulsions primarily by an action unrelated to glycine. The epileptiform syndrome evoked by strychnine differs in several respects from that seen after most other convulsants.

Antistrychnine activity is considered by many neuropharmacologists to reflect a muscle relaxant rather than an antiepileptic property.

Convulsions induced by strychnine in mice are reduced or prevented by benzodiazepines. The results of all investigators (Randall et al., 1960; Mustala and Penttilä, 1962; Lechat et al., 1970; Blum et al., 1973; Lembeck and Beubler, 1977; Soubrié and Simon, 1978; Dingledine et al., 1978; Worms et al., 1979) indicate more or less clearly that protective doses of benzodiazepines for strychnine-induced convulsions are higher than for seizures induced by other agents. Moreover, in our hands, the antistrychnine effect of benzodiazepines is much less reproducible than its antagonism of other convulsants. In the rat, diazepam intravenously was only one-tenth as potent against strychnine as against pentetrazole-induced seizures (Matthews and McCafferty, 1979). Giunta et al. (1970) found clonazepam surprisingly potent in increasing the threshold dose of strychnine for the induction of cortical paroxysmal activity in rabbits and cats. EEG spiking and convulsions of the Jacksonian type were induced in rabbits by topical application of strychnine on the sensorimotor cortex (Scotti de Carolis and Longo, 1967) and were blocked by intravenous injections of chlordiazepoxide, diazepam, and oxazepam in doses from 2 to 10 mg $\cdot$ kg^{-1}. After daily administration of diazepam (2 mg $\cdot$ kg^{-1} p.o.) to mice for 4 and 7 days, respectively, tolerance was observed to occur for the antistrychnine (and antibicuculline) activity of diazepam, but not for its antipentetrazole activity (Juhasz and Dairman, 1977; Lippa and Regan, 1977).

Acetylcholine, Carbachol. Hernández-Peón et al. (1964) applied minute crystals of acetylcholine or carbachol together with physostigmine to the amygdala, the midbrain, or the nucleus habenularis lateralis of unanesthetized, unrestrained cats; the resulting generalized seizures were markedly attenuated by diazepam.

Anticholinesterases. Convulsive seizure activity induced in monkeys by the intramuscular injection of soman was terminated and the paroxysmal EEG activity suppressed by the intravenous injection of diazepam, clonazepam, or nitrazepam. When given prior to soman, these benzodiazepines prevented seizures (Lipp, 1972, 1973, 1974). Atropine had no protective activity, indicating that central nicotinic receptors must be involved in the initiation of seizures.

Nicotine. Topical application of nicotine on the sensorimotor cortex of rabbits induced Jacksonian-type convulsions which were blocked by chlordiazepoxide, diazepam, and oxazepam (Scotti de Carolis and Longo, 1967).

Morphine. Similar results as with nicotine-induced convulsions were obtained by Scotti de Carolis and Longo (1967) with chlordiazepoxide, diazepam, and oxazepam on seizures induced by topical application of morphine in rabbits.

Kainic Acid. Kainic acid injected locally into the brain destroys cell bodies but spares axons and axon endings in the injected area. Injection of 2 µg kainic acid into the rat hippocampus results, upon awakening from anesthesia, in a period of abnormal behavior consisting of dystonic posture, hyperactivity, and episodic clonic convulsions. Diazepam, like phenobarbitone and carbamazepine, prevented the appearance of generalized convulsions; however, it failed to affect kainic acid-induced hyperactivity (Zaczek et al., 1978).

γ-Hydroxybutyrate. The EEG and behavioral effects induced by γ-hydroxybutyrate in *Macaca mulatta* have been proposed by Snead (1978) as an animal model of petit mal epilepsy. Ethosuximide and clonazepam normalized and diazepam marginally improved the EEG changes, while phenobarbitone was ineffective. However, the myoclonic jerks induced by γ-hydroxybutyrate were abolished by ethosuximide, significantly improved by diazepam, and worsened by clonazepam. Clinically, clonazepam has occasionally been observed to exacerbate myoclonic activity in atypical absence seizures. The different profile of activity of the two benzodiazepines, clonazepam and diazepam, in this animal model indicates that small qualitative differences may be clinically quite relevant and that the various derivatives do not differ from one another merely by properties such as potency and pharmacokinetics but also by their pharmacologic profile.

Barbiturate Withdrawal. Rats made physically dependent on barbiturates develop upon withdrawal a syndrome consisting of weight loss, increased susceptibility to sound-induced convulsions, and the occasional appearance of spontaneous convulsive seizures. The withdrawal syndrome could be prevented by chlordiazepoxide, meprobamate, primidone, and diphenylhydantoin; ethosuximide reduced the severity of seizures (NORTON, 1970).

Imipramine. High doses of imipramine induce convulsions and death in male Wistar rats. The LD_{90} (112 mg·kg^{-1} i.p.) was used to study its prevention by drugs. Doses protecting 50% of the animals from convulsions were 0.32 mg·kg^{-1} diazepam and 17.6 mg·kg^{-1} phenobarbitone i.p.; diphenylhydantoin was ineffective (BEAUBIEN et al., 1976).

Convulsant Benzodiazepine, Ro 5-3663. This compound at the dose of 30 mg·kg^{-1} i.p. precipitated convulsions in all injected mice. Diazepam protected the animals with an ED_{50} of 1.5 mg·kg^{-1} p.o. (SCHLOSSER et al., 1973). The GABA antagonistic property of the compound suggested by FRANCO and SCHLOSSER (1978), GELLER (1979), SCHLOSSER and FRANCO (1979 b), O'BRIEN and SPRIT (1980) was shown to be of the mixed competitive-noncompetitive type (SCHAFFNER et al., 1979).

Hyperbaric Oxygen. Oxygen at high pressure induces convulsions. Diazepam reduced these convulsions in the rabbit (TÓTH et al., 1969) and in mice (LEMBECK and BEUBLER, 1977), where it was more potent than phenobarbitone and baclofen. Convulsions induced by high oxygen/helium pressure (90 ATA) in rats were prevented by diazepam, and the symptoms of "high pressure nervous syndrome" were reduced (GRAN et al., 1980).

DL-*m-Fluorotyrosine.* This amino acid induces convulsions and death in mice. It was originally suggested to act through changes in catecholamine metabolism, but it now seems more likely that its metabolite, fluoroacetate, is the convulsant agent. Chlordiazepoxide in high doses antagonized the seizures induced by DL-m-fluorotyrosine (WEISSMAN and KOE, 1967).

2,4-Dimethyl-5-Hydroxymethylpyrimidin (DHMP). DHMP, which shows some structural relationship to barbiturates, induces convulsions in mice at the dose of 10 mg·kg^{-1} i.p. The oral ED_{50} for protective activity was 0.73 mg·kg^{-1} for clonazepam, 3.4 mg·kg^{-1} for diazepam, and 27 mg·kg^{-1} for chlordiazepoxide, 63 mg·kg^{-1} for phenobarbitone, and 770 mg·kg^{-1} for trimethadione; diphenylhydantoin was ineffective at 800 mg·kg^{-1} (BANZIGER and HANE, 1967).

Flurothyl. Chlordiazepoxide (1.25 mg·kg^{-1} i.p.) and diazepam (0.125 mg·kg^{-1} i.p.) prevented tonic seizures in mice following an intravenous dose of 0.05 ml 1% flurothyl in polyethyleneglycol (BOISSIER et al., 1968).

Caffeine. Marangos et al. (1979 a, b) mentioned preliminary results showing that benzodiazepines antagonize caffeine-induced seizures in animals. These findings were considered to support the view that benzodiazepines act at a receptor for endogenous purine derivatives (see Sect. Z, XII).

DDT. The insecticide DDT [1,1,1,-trichloro-2,2-bis(p-chlorophenyl)ethane] produces stimulus-sensitive myoclonic movements in mice. Clonazepam reduced DDT-induced myoclonus by 50% with 2 mg·kg⁻¹ i.p. The 5-HT receptor blockers methysergide, metergoline, and cinanserin reduced and the inhibitors of 5-HT-uptake, fluoxetine and chlorimipramine, potentiated the antimyoclonic effect of clonazepam (Chung Hwang and Van Woert, 1979).

Tetanus Toxin. Diazepam was the most potent of a number of drugs in preventing seizures and increasing survival rate of mice injected subcutaneously with tetanus toxin (Huck, 1979).

2. Electroconvulsive Shock

Of the many modifications of electroshock-induced convulsions (Swinyard, 1972), the antagonism of maximal electroshock seizures (MES) in mice is used most frequently. A short train of high frequency a.c. or d.c. current pulses is applied, usually through corneal electrodes, at a supramaximal current strength for the induction of a tonic extensor spasm and loss of consciousness; a varying percentage of mice die within 10 min after the seizure. Modifications less frequently used are (a) the so-called minimum electroshock seizure test, in which a current is applied that induces clonic seizures of the head, movements of the vibrissae, but no loss of consciousness or tonic extension; (b) the so-called low-frequency electroshock test (described by Swinyard and Castellion, 1966); and (c) the determination of electroshock threshold in the cat (Blum et al., 1973).

Benzodiazepines were found to be active in the MES test on the mouse by various authors (Randall et al., 1960, 1961, 1965a; Banziger, 1965; Gluckman, 1965; Klupp and Kähling, 1965; Swinyard and Castellion, 1966; Fournadjev et al., 1968; D'Armagnac et al., 1971; Dobrescu and Coeugniet, 1971; Barzaghi et al., 1973; Blum et al., 1973; Jeppsson and Ljungberg, 1975; Johnson and Funderburk, 1978; Gluckman and Stein, 1978; Niemegeers and Lewi, 1979). The active doses determined by these investigators (Table 8) vary enormously, especially for clonazepam (Swinyard and Castellion, 1966; Banziger and Hane, 1967; Lechat et al., 1970; Blum et al., 1973). In view of these discrepancies, it did not seem reasonable to discuss the relative potencies of benzodiazepines in the MES test. However, the wealth of values reported in the literature clearly indicates that the doses required to prevent maximal electroshock seizures are substantially higher than the protective doses for convulsions induced by most of the chemical agents. Niemegeers and Lewi (1979) presented data of a comparative study in the mouse of 14 benzodiazepine derivatives, which clearly show that the ED_{50} in the MES test were without exception higher than the doses producing ataxia and 10–20 times higher than the ED_{50} for antipentetrazole activity. Similar conclusions can also be drawn from data of different investigators reviewed by Reinhard and Reinhard (1977).

Table 8. ED_{50} values (mg·kg^{-1} p.o.) for various benzodiazepines in the "inclined screen," "maximal electroshock seizure," and "foot shock-induced fighting" tests

Drug	Inclined screen	Maximal electroshock seizure	Foot shock-induced fighting
Nitrazepam	15 [1] 8.3 [8] 5.8 [9]	31 [1] 26 [8]	5 [1] 25 [8]
Chlordiazepoxide	100 [2] 40* [5] 82 [7] 92 [8] 220 [9] 250 [11] 32.3 [12]	10.7 [5] 29 [2] 49 [7] 30 [8] 32 [11]	40 [2] 20* [4] 17 [7] 50 [8] 12.5 [11]
Diazepam	25 [3] 10* [5] 39 [7] 50 [8] 44 [9] 10 [10] 120 [11]	21 [4] 3.1 [5] 6.4 [3] 14 [7] 11.5 [8] 6.5 [10]	10 [3] 4 [7] 30 [8] 2.8 [11]
Medazepam	125 [2]	37 [2]	40 [2]
Oxazepam	225 [3] 40* [5]	28.5 [3] 4.6 [5]	40 [3]
Flurazepam	200 [6] 400 [8]	75 [6] 85 [8]	20 [6] 50 [8]
Prazepam	74 [7]	24 [7]	13 [7]
Nimetazepam	6.3 [8]	15 [8]	5.2 [8]
Triflubazam (1,5 benzodiazepine)	50 [11]	12.5 [11]	9 [11]

The values are ED_{50} as reported in the quoted papers (the values marked with an asterisk are ED_{100}).

[1] RANDALL et al. (1965a)   [7] ROBICHAUD et al. (1970)
[2] RANDALL et al. (1968)   [8] SAKAI et al. (1972)
[3] RANDALL et al. (1965b)   [9] NAKAJIMA et al. (1971)
[4] RANDALL et al. (1970)   [10] KAMIOKA et al. (1972)
[5] KLUPP and KÄHLING (1965)   [11] HEILMAN et al. (1974)
[6] RANDALL et al. (1969)   [12] ROBICHAUD and GOLDBERG (1974)

BANZIGER (1965), investigating chlordiazepoxide and diazepam in the MES test in mice, rats, and cats, found both compounds to have the shortest duration of action in the rat. Chlordiazepoxide was more potent than diazepam in the rat.

Chlordiazepoxide was observed by SOFIA and BARRY (1977) to increase the electroshock seizure threshold by 20% in mice at 10 mg·kg^{-1}, which was an inactive dose in the MES test. The protective action of chlordiazepoxide against maximal electroshock seizures in mice was markedly reduced by reserpine and the benzoquinolizine Ro 4-1284, but not by α-methyltyrosine and α-methyldopa (MENNEAR and RUD-ZIK, 1966); D-amphetamine, α-methyldopa and 5-hydroxytryptophan reversed the effect of reserpine.

The dose of clonazepam which increased the electroshock seizure threshold in the cat by 50% was determined as $0.84 \text{ mg} \cdot \text{kg}^{-1}$ p.o.; equieffective doses were $21 \text{ mg} \cdot \text{kg}^{-1}$ for phenobarbitone, $10.6 \text{ mg} \cdot \text{kg}^{-1}$ for diphenylhydantoin, and $2 \text{ mg} \cdot \text{kg}^{-1}$ for carbamazepine (BLUM et al., 1973).

3. Sensory Epilepsy (Audiogenic Seizures)

In specially inbred strains of mice an auditory stimulus with a defined frequency and intensity elicits a sequence of seizures from clonic to tonic convulsions, culminating in death (LEHMANN, 1964). Different benzodiazepines have been tested in this model, such as chlordiazepoxide (ED_{50} $4.4 \text{ mg} \cdot \text{kg}^{-1}$ p.o.), diazepam ($ED_{50} \sim 1.5 \text{ mg} \cdot \text{kg}^{-1}$ p.o.), prazepam (ED_{50} $1.7 \text{ mg} \cdot \text{kg}^{-1}$ p.o.) (ROBICHAUD et al., 1970), and nitrazepam (ED_{50} $0.14 \text{ mg} \cdot \text{kg}^{-1}$ i.p.) (COLLINS and HORLINGTON, 1969). For sensory epilepsy see also under K, II.3).

4. Spiking Activity Induced by Cortical Freezing

Spiking activity was induced in gallamine-immobilized cats by application of a dichlorodifluoromethane spray to the pial surface of gyrus posterior lateralis until whitening of the underlying cortex. Diazepam suppressed spiking activity (frequency and amplitude) in a dose-related manner ($0.25–0.5 \text{ mg} \cdot \text{kg}^{-1}$ i.v.) (HORI et al., 1979).

II. Chronic Models of Epilepsy

In order to improve the relevance of animal tests for the prediction of efficacy in human forms of epilepsy, which are mostly chronic diseases, several techniques have been developed to produce chronically epileptic animals. Benzodiazepines have been studied in some of these models.

1. Rats

Repeated stimulation of discrete brain areas with electric pulses that are not sufficiently strong to induce seizures in naive animals, results after a certain time in the appearance of persistent or periodic paroxysmal activities. This progressive induction is called "kindling effect." RACINE et al. (1975) found that diazepam in doses of 0.5–1 mg·kg⁻¹ i.p. delayed or blocked the kindling effect when repeated stimulation was in the amygdala, and blocked the generalized component of seizures when the electrodes were in the anterior neocortex (RACINE et al., 1979). Onset of kindling was, however, reported to be delayed by diazepam ($6 \text{ mg} \cdot \text{kg}^{-1}$ p.o.) without effect on clonic convulsions, when the site of stimulation was in the frontal cortex (GOFF et al., 1978). In some contrast to these findings are those of BABINGTON and WEDEKING (1973), who found chlordiazepoxide, diazepam, and oxazepam equally active against seizures in amygdaloid and sensory motor cortex kindled rats; these benzodiazepines were the most potent drugs tested. ASHTON and WAUQUIER (1979 a) examined the effect of 15 anticonvulsants in amygdaloid kindled rats; clonazepam, diazepam, and chlordiazepoxide were by far the most potent compounds (ED_{50} between 0.28 and 0.86 mg·kg^{-1} i.p.). Similar results were obtained by ALBERTSON et al. (1980) in a systematic study of a large series of anticonvulsants. They found clonazepam to be not only more potent than diazepam, but also more selective in diminishing the spread of afterdischarges to the cortex.

2. Cats

GUERRERO-FIGUEROA et al. (1967, 1968, 1969 a, b) induced "chronic" epilepsy by local implantation of aluminum oxide, penicillin, or cobalt into different brain regions. They observed the clinical signs of epileptic activity, recorded EEG activity and studied locally evoked potentials in unaffected structures as well as in primary and secondary foci. Diazepam and clonazepam depressed the spread of primary epileptiform discharges without producing significant changes of the epileptiform activity generated by the chemical irritants. Diazepam suppressed centrencephalic types of epilepsy (at 2 mg·kg^{-1} i.v.), but this was associated with complete muscle relaxation and a gross behavior of sedation and sometimes sleep.

In chronically instrumented cats with seizures induced by application of cobalt to the anterior suprasylvian gyrus, diazepam (2 mg·kg^{-1} s.c.) not only failed to inhibit these seizures but also actually exacerbated them (VAN DUJIN and VISSER, 1972). Clonazepam (0.2 mg·kg^{-1} s.c.) in the same experimental conditions was markedly active (VAN DUJIN, 1973).

3. Monkeys

Chronic Implantation of a Chemical Irritant. In monkeys *(Macaca mulatta)* made chronically epileptic by application of alumina cream on the cerebral cortex, chlordiazepoxide in high doses (5–35 mg·kg^{-1} i.v.) prevented clinical and EEG convulsant effects of challenge doses of intramuscular pentetrazole; in normal monkeys the same protection was seen against higher doses of pentetrazole (CHUSID and KOPELOFF, 1962). In a similar model clonazepam effectively reduced focal motor seizures and secondarily generalized tonic-clonic seizures (LOCKARD et al., 1979). Diazepam at 0.05 mg·kg^{-1} protected 20% of epileptic monkeys; 0.20 mg·kg^{-1} protected 100% (KOPELOFF and CHUSID, 1967).

In two rhesus monkeys with chemically irritative lesions in the septal region, GUERRERO-FIGUEROA et al. (1969 a) observed no effect or only a slight reduction of spontaneous epileptiform activity recorded from the primary focus, but a suppression of propagated activity after 2–5 mg·kg^{-1} clonazepam or diazepam i.v.

Sensory Epilepsy (Photosensitive Epilepsy). In man the most common and accepted form of "reflex" epilepsy is photosensitive epilepsy (NAQUET and MELDRUM, 1972). The baboon, *Papio papio*, obtained from the Casamance region of Senegal, has been shown to be a good model of human photosensitive epilepsy, since about 60% exhibit paroxysmal EEG and motor responses to flashing light pulsed at frequencies of 20–30 s^{-1} (KILLAM et al., 1967; KILLAM, 1979). In a series of investigations (STARK et al., 1970; KILLAM et al., 1973) with different anticonvulsants, it was observed that diazepam, clonazepam, and other benzodiazepines blocked seizures at doses below those effective in muscle relaxation. However, benzodiazepines seemed unable to maintain control of seizures with chronic administration of a constant dose; doubling the dose usually restored control of seizures, at least temporarily, whereas in some animals further increase of dose was required later, indicating development of tolerance.

4. Dogs

In beagles implanted stereotaxically with electrodes in the right basolateral amygdala, kindling seizures began with facial clonus, head nodding, salivation followed by opisthotonus, tonic extension of the forelegs and hindlegs, and running seizures, and terminated with wet shaking. Diazepam (2.5 mg·kg^{-1} p.o.) and phenobarbitone (10 mg·kg^{-1} p.o.) inhibited all phenomena in each of the three animals tested. Clonazepam (0.63 mg·kg^{-1} p.o.) protected two of the three animals against tonic and clonic seizures, but was ineffective against facial clonus. Kindling in dogs occurred rapidly and, when kindled, animals were susceptible to the development of spontaneous seizures and status epilepticus, which in three dogs could not be ameliorated by diazepam (WAUQUIER et al., 1979).

5. Domestic Fowl

Autosomal recessive mutation was reported to result in high seizure susceptibility in domestic fowl (CRAWFORD, 1970). Intermittent photic stimulation, muscular exertion, and heat stress induce grossly abnormal EEG activity (slow-wave, high-voltage activity and appearance of spiking) and a motor seizure pattern described as grand mal. Benzodiazepines were found to be the most potent drugs in reducing susceptibility to seizures (JOHNSON et al., 1979); the model was considered by these authors to have great predictability for human grand mal epilepsy.

III. Conclusions

Benzodiazepines are the most potent drugs in preventing or interrupting experimental epileptiform activity in animals and various forms of epilepsy in man. They are considerably more potent than barbiturates and tranquilizers of the meprobamate type, but also more potent than the "pure" antiepileptics such as hydantoins and carbamazepine. This potent anticonvulsant property is most pronounced on seizures induced by chemical agents; higher doses are required for the depression of convulsions induced by electroconvulsive shock.

The predictive potential of the numerous experimental animal models for the various forms of human epilepsy is not simple (MILLICHAP, 1969). Although benzodiazepines are generally considered to be the drugs of first choice in the treatment of status epilepticus, their therapeutic value in the chronic treatment of grand mal, Jacksonian, and temporal lobe epilepsies is less obvious. Most forms of petit mal epilepsy seem to be favorably affected by benzodiazepines. As with other antiepileptics, tolerance to the effect of benzodiazepines tends to develop and may induce or facilitate some forms of epilepsy while suppressing other forms. Compared to most other antiepileptics, the unwanted side effects of benzodiazepines (drowsiness and ataxia) are harmless.

The primary mechanism by which chemical convulsants induce paroxysmal neuronal activity are only partially understood. With few exceptions, they obviously affect synaptic inhibition rather than synaptic excitation. In contrast to the action of established GABA antagonists (e.g., bicuculline) and inhibitors of glutamic acid decarboxylase (e.g., various hydrazines), that of pentetrazole and penicillin is still a matter of controversy, although they certainly affect GABA mechanisms to some degree. The differing potencies of benzodiazepines in convulsions produced by the various chemical agents have been taken as evidence for or against a GABA-linked pharmacologic action of benzodiazepines. For example, the greater protective potency of these drugs against convulsions induced by GABA antagonists than against those elicited by strychnine, was inferred to reflect a primary interaction of benzodiazepines with GABAergic but not with glycinergic transmission (CURTIS et al., 1976a). The development of tolerance to the antibicuculline, but not to the antipentetrazole activity of diazepam, was considered to indicate that the latter effect (and the anticonflict activity) was unrelated to a facilitation of GABAergic transmission (JUHASZ and DAIRMAN, 1977; LIPPA and REGAN, 1977). Such a simple inference is not well founded. It should be realized that apparently similar paroxysmal activities may be generated by different attacks on neuronal circuits and that agents interfering with the same neurotransmitter system may produce different clinical seizure symptoms depending, e.g., on the speed of action (GABA receptor blockade versus inhibition of glutamate decarboxylase) and, hence, different susceptibility to anticonvulsant drug effects.

The crucial role of synaptic inhibition in epileptogenesis and anticonvulsant activity is becoming increasingly evident. Most straightforward is the situation in which epileptiform activity is induced with agents or procedures that depress GABAergic synaptic function. Attenuation or abolition of recurrent inhibition is a highly probable factor in initiating paroxysmal epileptiform activity in single neurons; in cortical foci induced by alumina gel a highly significant numerical decrease of GABAergic (GAD positive) nerve terminals was described (RIBAK et al., 1979). In pyramidal cells of hippocampal slices, penicillin, by reducing recurrent inhibition, changed the response to a single orthodromic stimulus from the normal EPSP (plus single spike) – IPSP sequence to dendritic burst firing and a depolarization shift which are typical events in "epileptic" neurons (WONG and PRINCE, 1979). Once epileptic activity has been generated in a pool of neurons by one mechanism or another, the spread to other regions and generalization of paroxysmal activity is normally prevented by the powerful synaptic inhibitory mechanisms in normal neurons ("surround inhibition," PRINCE and WILDER, 1967).

On the one hand, this well-documented role of synaptic inhibitory (mostly GABAergic) mechanisms in preventing epileptiform activity in single neurons and neuronal networks and, on the other hand, the evidence that benzodiazepines facilitate GABAergic synaptic transmission (see Sect. X), readily explain the anticonvulsant activity of these drugs. Most investigators found benzodiazepines (and other antiepileptics) to have no or little effect on paroxysmal activity in primary epileptic foci, probably because of morphological or functional lesions in the inhibitory circuits within the focus; however, these drugs potently prevent spreading and generalization, most probably by enhancing normal inhibitory mechanisms in structures that are not primarily affected. In accordance with this reasoning is the anticonvulsant activity of agents which increase the GABA content of the brain by inhibition of GABA trans-

Table 9. Minimum muscle relaxant doses of several benzodiazepines and phenobarbitone in the cat

Drug	Minimum effective dose (MED)[a], $mg \cdot kg^{-1}$ p.o.
Chlordiazepoxide	2
Diazepam	0.2
Medazepam	4
Flurazepam	2
Nitrazepam	0.1
Clonazepam	0.05
Flunitrazepam	0.02
Bromazepam	0.2
Phenobarbitone	50

[a] The minimum effective dose (MED) was the lowest dose at which muscle relaxation was observed. Muscle relaxation was identified by limpness in the legs when the cat was held by the scruff of the neck (Randall et al., 1960). At least three cats per dose at three dose levels were used. Data taken from Randall and Kappel (1973)

aminase. Maximal electroconvulsive shock, which results from a strong direct excitation of neurons throughout the brain, is less easily depressed by agents that act through improved synaptic inhibition.

L. Effects on Muscle Tone and Coordination

Most neuropharmacologists would probably agree that one of the most problematic tasks in the evaluation of psychotropic agents is the estimation of pure central muscle relaxant activity, i.e., the specific reduction of skeletal muscle tone which is not the consequence of a reduced vigilance. In states of natural drowsiness, such as orthodoxical and paradoxical sleep, muscle tone is physiologically reduced and it is, therefore, not surprising that drug-induced changes in the degree of arousal will also affect muscle tone. A further problem is that muscle relaxation is the therapeutic goal in situations of pathologically increased muscle tone and that it may be more difficult to reduce a normal muscle tone to below normal than to reduce an increased tone toward normal. Ataxia is often considered a logical consequence of reduced muscle tone and, therefore, a measurable index of muscle relaxation; this viewpoint may be correct. However, it should also be considered that a disturbance of muscle coordination may result from a drug action totally independent of changes in muscle tone.

I. Subjective Methods of Evaluating Muscle Tone and Coordination

It is possible to assess a reduction of normal muscle tone in a simple way. An experienced observer easily recognizes a muscle-relaxed mouse by the reduced resistance of the limbs when the animal is held gently in one hand. The relaxed animal is felt as an object of less consistency or firmness (i.e., its body is limp). The reduced muscle tone can be assessed by the resistance experienced by a finger or another object pressed into the abdomen. These simple measures entirely depend on subjective parameters; when routinely performed by the same highly experienced person, these tests yield reproducible results and are very helpful in the preliminary screening of compounds. Because of the lack of objective criteria and the impossibility of obtaining identical scores with different experimenters, values obtained in this way are absent in the literature except for a modification of the method in the cat. RANDALL and KAPPEL (1973) reported on the minimum effective doses of various benzodiazepines in a test (Table 9) in which cats are gently held by the neck and muscle relaxation is scored according to the degree to which the hindlegs hang down passively instead of being adduced toward the belly and also according to the degree of passive protrusion of the lower abdomen. The cat appears to be particularly sensitive to the muscle relaxant (and muscle incoordinating) action of benzodiazepines. Objective procedures have been described for the evaluation of ataxia, e.g., the observation of the printed traces of a walking animal (GAMBA, 1966) or of a cat forced to jump down an elevated frame. However, quantitative data on benzodiazepines, to our knowledge, have not been published. The doses producing ataxic gait in the mouse (subjective scores) have been evaluated for 14 benzodiazepines (NIEMEGEERS and LEWI, 1979).

II. Objective Tests Believed to Record Muscle Tone

1. Inclined Screen (or Plane) Tests

Many modifications (material of the plane, inclination, etc.) of the procedure originally described by PRADHAN and DE (1953) are routinely used and, all too often, believed to reveal muscle relaxation. The time is measured until an animal placed on an inclined plane slips off the screen. In Table 8 a number of ED_{50} values in inclined screen tests (and for comparison in maximal electroconvulsive shock and foot-shock-induced fighting tests) from the literature are given. The tremendous differences in the results obtained in various laboratories illustrate the importance of even small variations in the methods. Obviously, if the inclined screen test is considered to measure muscle relaxant activity, then the most divergent conclusions can be drawn.

2. Traction Test (Horizontal Wire Test)

This procedure, described by COURVOISIER (1956), measures the ability of mice hung with their forelegs on a horizontal wire or bar to heave themselves so as to grasp the wire also with their hindlegs within a limited time. Table 6 gives ED_{50} values from the literature as determined in traction tests and, for comparison, in rotarod and antipentetrazole tests. Differences by a factor of 20 in the ED_{50} values obtained in various laboratories are not exceptional and reflect modifications of the method.

3. Grip Strength Test

This test as described by VAN RIEZEN and BOERSMA (1969) is based on the ability of the mouse to grip a horizontal bar with its forepaws when pulled backwards by the tail; a system of weights and counterweights measures the force exerted on the bar. Using this method SOUBRIÉ and SIMON (1978) found that diazepam, at $2 \, mg \cdot kg^{-1}$, caused a marked decrease in the grip strength. TILSON and CABE (1978) have described a more selective measure of forelimb muscular strength using a precise strain gauge grip meter in the rat, which provides graded or continuous data. With this method the lowest effective dose required to produce a significant decrease in grip meter scores by chlorpromazine, chlordiazepoxide, and phenobarbitone were 5, 9, and 20 mg · kg^{-1}, respectively. By analogy with what will be pointed out for the rotarod test, it is questionable whether the procedure really assesses the muscular resistive force or some motivational factors.

4. Rotarod Test

In the various modifications of the rotarod test (DUNHAM and MIYA, 1957), the capacity of animals to retain their equilibrium on a slowly rotating horizontal bar is measured. Variations in training procedures, speed of rotating bar, type of material used for rotating bar, animal strain and way of handling, fixed time of measurement after injection or measurement at time of peak activity, criteria of test performance (number of doses, number of animals per dose, type of statistical evaluation) are some of the many variables that may influence the results (Table 6); therefore, only comparisons of data obtained in the same laboratory under the same experimental conditions are meaningful. In Table 5 the ED$_{50}$ values for some benzodiazepines determined in our laboratories are given together with values in the chimney test, antipentetrazole test and anti-3MPA test. The depressant effect of chlordiazepoxide on rotarod performance was antagonized by picrotoxin, but not by bicuculline in experiments of LIPPA et al. (1979). The potencies of several benzodiazepines in a rotarod test in mice were compared with their affinity for ^{3}H-diazepam binding sites in rat brain synaptosomes (MALICK and ENNA, 1979). A positive result in the rotarod test is given highly contradictory interpretations by various authors. For some of them, the test is believed to measure muscle relaxation or motor incoordination; some investigators used it for the determination of the dose producing "neurotoxicity" or "neuronal deficit" (two extremely misleading terms). For other authors, activity in this test is believed to reveal a sedative effect. Only a few of them have considered the possibility that drugs may reduce the performance of animals on the rotating bar by affecting motivation in some way. We believe that a reduced performance in the test may reflect quite different (muscle relaxant and incoordinating, sedative, stimulant) effects depending on technical variables and classes of drugs. In the modification used in our laboratories, the test does not seem to determine motor performance incapacitating effects of benzodiazepines, because the ED$_{50}$ values (see Table 5) are well below those at which a reduction of muscle tone or ataxia can be observed or spontaneous locomotor activity is altered.

5. Equilibrium Board

MOLINENGO (1964) described the equilibrium board test, which was used by SCROLLINI et al. (1975) for comparing pinazepam with diazepam. In this test, rats fasting from the previous evening are trained to reach their food by walking on a horizontal rod 10 mm in diameter and 1 m long placed 50 cm from the floor; ataxic rats are unable to reach the food and fall to the floor. In the equilibrium board test using rats, pinazepam was about $^1/_{10}$–$^1/_{12}$ as potent as diazepam. SOUBRIÉ and SIMON (1978) utilized a similar method to study the antagonism by bemegride and picrotoxin of the motor incoordination induced in the rat by a fixed dose of diazepam.

6. Chimney Test

This test, proposed by BOISSIER et al. (1960), is based on the escape reaction of the mouse which has to climb backwards in a glass tube (chimney) of appropriate diameter and length within a given time. It is complementary to the rotarod test and gives virtually identical results (see Table 5).

7. Aerial righting reflex

Rats held in an inverted position and then dropped require only a short distance in order to land on all four feet; this distance is increased by drugs that disturb motor coordination. Chlordiazepoxide at the dose of 8 mg $\cdot$ kg^{-1} i.p., which was active in a conflict test, had no effect on the aerial righting reflex, in contrast to ethanol (VOGEL et al., 1980).

8. Drug-Induced Rigidity

Several drugs have been used to increase the basal muscle tone, allowing an assessment of a muscle relaxant activity.

Etonitazene. BARNETT et al. (1974) measured the reduction by diazepam and flurazepam of rigidity induced by the narcotic analgesic etonitazene.

Reserpine. Reserpine (and Ro 4-1284) injected intravenously into rats produces a marked rigidity which can be measured by quantifying the spontaneous EMG activity of the extended hindlimbs (MORRISON and WEBSTER, 1973). Although the test was proposed for the evaluation of anti-Parkinson's disease agents, benzodiazepines were rather potent in reducing the increased neurogenic muscle tone (unpublished observations from our laboratories).

Fentanyl plus Droperidol. This combination is routinely used in anesthesiology for neuroleptanalgesia. The narcotic analgesic, fentanyl, is responsible for the Straub tail phenomenon which is induced in mice by the above combination. Prevention of this phenomenon was tested by NIEMEGEERS and LEWI (1979) in order to obtain some indication of muscle relaxant activity of benzodiazepines.

9. γ-Rigidity

Muscular rigidity induced in the cat by decerebration at the intercollicular level is considered to be due to an increased sensitivity of the tonic stretch reflex caused by the release of γ-motoneurons from a precollicular inhibitory influence. According to RANDALL et al. (1963) and HAEFELY et al. (1975), diazepam reduced γ-rigidity at the dose of 1 mg $\cdot$ kg^{-1} i.v. HUDSON and WOLPERT (1970) found even smaller doses of diazepam (0.125 mg $\cdot$ kg^{-1} i.v.) to be effective and MAXWELL et al. (1974) observed that in the rat, too, the intercollicular decerebrate rigidity was markedly affected by diazepam (1.2 mg $\cdot$ kg^{-1}). The effect of benzodiazepines in this model of muscular rigidity may be caused by one or several of the spinal and supraspinal actions to be described in Sect. R. It may be relevant that the inhibitor of GABA transaminase, aminooxyacetic acid, also reduced rigidity in intercollicularly decerebrate cats (HAEFELY et al., 1975).

10. α-Rigidity

The rigidity obtained by the anemic method in the cat (for references see MAXWELL and READ, 1972) is thought to be due primarily to the overactivity of the α-motoneuron system. SCHALLEK et al. (1964) found that chlordiazepoxide and diazepam inhibited α-rigidity with ED_{50} values of 26 mg·kg^{-1} and 2.5 mg·kg^{-1} i.v. Nitrazepam has been reported to almost completely abolish α-rigidity at the dose of 13 mg·kg^{-1} i.v. (RANDALL et al., 1965a). In comparing diazepam in the two types of rigidity (γ and α), MAXWELL and READ (1972) concluded that diazepam was more effective in reducing rigidity in the intercollicular, decerebrate cats than in the anemic, decerebrate cats.

11. Supraspinal and Spinal Cord Activities Related to Muscle Relaxation

This will be treated in the section on spinal cord functions (R).

III. Conclusions

In man, benzodiazepines, like all the other known centrally acting muscle relaxants, are effective as muscle relaxants at doses that produce some degree of drowsiness. Since muscle tension and pain are often associated with anxiety and other emotional disorders, it is difficult to clinically separate a "pure" muscle relaxant effect from one caused by emotional stabilization.

M. Effects on Spontaneous and Induced Motor Activity

Motor behavior is a complex of several activities including, for example, locomotion, exploration, and grooming. Although it is quite difficult, technically and conceptually, to separate all these components, a number of tests have been proposed to measure predominantly locomotor activity or exploratory behavior.

I. Locomotor Activity

1. Decrease in Mice

In mice tested in the Animex apparatus, only high doses of pinazepam (ED_{50} 77 mg·kg^{-1} p.o.) and diazepam (ED_{50} 44 mg·kg^{-1} p.o.) reduced locomotor activity (SCROLLINI et al., 1975). Measured with the same apparatus, clonazepam significantly decreased the activity phase of the first 5 night hours only in doses of 100 mg·kg^{-1} p.o. (BLUM et al., 1973). Considering the much lower ED_{50} values for diazepam and clonazepam in rotarod and chimney tests, it appears that the decrease of locomotor activity in mice is not a sensitive indication of the central effect of benzodiazepines.

   Using photocell activity cages, chlordiazepoxide produced a decrease of locomotor activity with an approximate ED_{50} of 100 mg·kg^{-1} p.o. Chronic administration of 100 mg·kg^{-1} twice daily for 14 days followed by the same dose of drug on the 15th day resulted in a marked decrease of drug effect as compared with acute administration (GOLDBERG et al., 1967). SANSONE (1979) also observed a tolerance to the depressant action of 20 and 30 mg·kg^{-1} chlordiazepoxide intraperitoneally after 5 consecutive days of administration. Also using photocell activity cages, Asami et al. (1975) found a decrease of locomotor activity after diazepam (ED_{50} 16.4 mg·kg^{-1} p.o.) and medazepam (ED_{50} 58 mg·kg^{-1} p.o.), whereas a new benzodiazepine derivative, 1-(β-methylsulfonylethyl)-5-(o-fluorophenyl)-7-chloro-1,3-dihydro-2H-1,4-benzodiazepin-2-one, was devoid of effect up to 256 mg·kg^{-1} p.o. Kamioka et al. (1972) reported ED_{50} values of 38 mg·kg^{-1} and 100 mg·kg^{-1} p.o. for diazepam and cloxazolam. According to Poschel et al. (1974) chlordiazepoxide decreased locomotor activity by 65% at 25 mg·kg^{-1} p.o., and diazepam by 39% at 12.5 mg·kg^{-1} p.o. Clobazam in doses ranging from 5 to 10 mg·kg^{-1} i.p. was more effective than chlordiazepoxide in reducing locomotor activity (Barzaghi et al., 1973). With another method, i.e., counting the number of revolutions in a revolving cage, Jindal et al. (1968) found that chlordiazepoxide and diazepam administered intraperitoneally in the mouse had no appreciable effect at 25 mg·kg^{-1} and 7 mg·kg^{-1} respectively, whereas Nakajima et al. (1971 b) observed a variable decrease from 27% to 50% with diazepam and nitrazepam 5–30 mg·kg^{-1} p.o. and ED_{50} for estazolam and alprazolam of 10.5 mg·kg^{-1} and 6.2 mg·kg^{-1}, respectively.

2. Increase in Mice

Comparing lorazepam, diazepam, chlordiazepoxide, and oxazepam and recording locomotion for 2 h by means of photocell activity cages, Gluckman (1971) concluded that these benzodiazepines were remarkably free of depressant effects in a wide dose range, both orally and intraperitoneally administered; stimulation was frequently seen particularly during the 2nd hour, most notably with lorazepam and diazepam, but also with chlordiazepoxide, while oxazepam was free of stimulant properties. An increased locomotor activity at 25 and 50 mg·kg^{-1} p.o. was also reported for cloxazolam (Kamioka et al., 1972) still using photocell activity cages. With a modified photocell method Klupp and Kähling (1965) found a biphasic effect of chlordiazepoxide and oxazepam: an increase of locomotor activity in the range of 5–40 mg·kg^{-1} p.o. and 5–20 mg·kg^{-1} p.o., respectively, and a decrease with higher doses. Sansone (1979) found that doses of 5 and 10 mg·kg^{-1} chlordiazepoxide intraperitoneally increased activity in mice. This stimulant effect was more marked after 5 consecutive days of administration. Higher doses of chlordiazepoxide decreased locomotor activity.

3. Decrease in Rats

Chlordiazepoxide was found to be ten times (ED_{50} 60 mg·kg^{-1} p.o.) more potent than meprobamate, but much less potent than chlorpromazine, in depressing the locomotor activity as measured during the night in "jiggle cages" (Randall et al., 1960; Randall, 1960). With a modification of the protocol, i.e., a duration of recording of only 10 min to utilize the first phase of orientational hypermotility in a novel environment (Borsy et al., 1960), flurazepam was found to be very potent in depressing locomotor activity (ED_{50} 4.5 mg·kg^{-1} i.p.) (Babbini et al., 1975). Borbély et al. (1975) found that chlordiazepoxide (i.p.) caused a dose-dependent reduction of motor activity in chronically thalamic rats, similar to its effect in the intact rat, and concluded that the presence of limbic structures was not necessary for the sedative effect of chlordiazepoxide.

II. Exploratory Behavior

1. Mice

AHTEE and SHILLITO (1970) used a "tunnel board," a wooden board onto which 12 plastic tunnels had been arranged in a symmetrical manner; the number of different tunnels entered by a mouse during the observation time was calculated and this gave the measure of exploration. Chlordiazepoxide, 25 or 50 mg·kg^{-1} i.p., and diazepam, 10 or 20 mg·kg^{-1} i.p., reduced exploratory behavior.

These authors also assessed motor activity of mice in an open metal box, where each mouse was placed individually after exploratory behavior had been assessed. Chlordiazepoxide and diazepam in similar doses, particularly in low ones, increased motor activity.

The hole-board method described by BOISSIER and SIMON (1962) offers a simple way of measuring exploratory activity by counting the number of head dips of the mouse in each of the 16 equally spaced holes, 3 cm in diameter, bored in the board. According to NOLAN and PARKES (1973), chlordiazepoxide, diazepam, nitrazepam, medazepam, oxazepam, and prazepam at low doses (BOISSIER et al., 1972) increased the number of head dips upon the first exposure to the hole-board, whereas flurazepam was ineffective at any dose tested (BOISSIER et al., 1972). BARZAGHI et al. (1973), using the hole-board method found that chlordiazepoxide and clobazam at doses of 5–10 mg·kg^{-1} i.p. always reduced exploratory behavior in mice, clobazam being more potent than chlordiazepoxide. Diazepam and pinazepam (ED$_{50}$ about 4–5 mg·kg^{-1} p.o. for both drugs) also reduced exploratory behavior evaluated with the hole-board test (SCROLLINI et al., 1975). A similar reduction was observed with orally administered diazepam and prazepam using a modified device (WEISCHER, 1976). Working with a simple box fitted with a floor consisting of four metal plates, MARRIOT and SMITH (1972) measured the number of plate crossings in unshocked mice, naive to the apparatus, as an indication of exploratory behavior (response to novelty). Chlordiazepoxide and diazepam, and also amylobarbitone and meprobamate, administered orally produced dose-dependent increases in plate-crossing; the effect was biphasic since higher doses, eliciting ataxia and general motor depression, decreased exploratory activity. In mice already familiar with the test situation, exploratory activity was not increased by chlordiazepoxide or amylobarbitone, whereas meprobamate still increased activity. An apparatus consisting of eight opaque Plexiglas toggle-floor boxes, divided into two compartments with an opening at the floor level, has also been used to measure the exploratory ambulation (crossings of the opening); in this experimental situation chlordiazepoxide (5 mg·kg^{-1} i.p.) produced stimulation of activity in naive mice, the effect being strongly pronounced at the commencement of the testing session and declining thereafter (VETULANI and SANSONE, 1978). Using the same apparatus, SANSONE (1979) found that repeated administration of chlordiazepoxide to mice enhanced the stimulant action of lower doses but reduced the depressant effect of higher doses. He concluded that tolerance developed to the depressant but not to the stimulant effects of chlordiazepoxide. A biphasic effect on exploratory activity in hole-board and open-field situations, i.e., an increase with lower doses and a decrease with higher doses, was observed in mice with demethyldiazepam and chlordemethyldiazepam (DE ANGELIS et al., 1979).

2. Rats

An open-field apparatus fitted with holes to study head-dipping behavior was used by NAKAMA et al. (1972), who found that diazepam (0.5–10 mg·kg⁻¹ i.p.) and particularly chlordiazepoxide (0.5–10 mg·kg⁻¹ i.p.) caused a marked increase in exploratory ambulation, but only slightly affected head-dipping behavior during the first 3 min; during the subsequent 3 min, however, the two compounds depressed both types of behavior. In a conventional open-field apparatus, IWAHARA and SAKAMA (1972) found with chlordiazepoxide (30 mg·kg⁻¹ p.o.) an increase of exploratory ambulation in the first few minutes of observation and a considerable reduction thereafter. The stimulant effect on exploratory locomotion completely disappeared on retesting on subsequent days. These results are in good agreement with those observed after chlordiazepoxide (6–50 mg·kg⁻¹ s.c.) on the exploratory behavior of rats placed in a Y-box, in the sense that increased exploration elicited by chlordiazepoxide was completely inhibited by a single previous exposure to the Y-box (MARRIOT and SPENCER, 1965). In a symmetrical Y-shaped box with a start door, ITOH and TAKAORI (1968) found with diazepam (0.5–2 mg·kg⁻¹ i.p.) a significant shortening in the start latency and a significant increase in the exploration of unexperienced rats, whereas the same doses in experienced rats resulted in a prolongation of the start latency and a decrease of locomotion and rearing frequencies. In rats placed for 8 min in a Y-maze the effect of chlordiazepoxide, oxazepam, diazepam, lorazepam, and nitrazepam (intraperitoneally, at three dose levels) was studied on exploratory behavior and intrasession habituation (SOUBRIÉ et al., 1977). Exploration (number of entries into the arms) was found to be increased by all these benzodiazepines (at low doses, whereas the highest dose reduced exploratory locomotion) only during the first 3 min of the test; no effect (or a weak reduction) was found during the last 5 min. Habituation (ratio between the number of entries made during the first 3 min and during the total time) was markedly enhanced by benzodiazepines.

It has been postulated that the benzodiazepines might remove a factor (fear?) that depresses exploratory activity of the animals in a novel situation and, therefore, that the increase in exploratory activity seen in the first few minutes after benzodiazepines was the consequence of their antianxiety effect. On subsequent experience sedation may then prevail. This suggestion does not seem to be supported by the experiments of KUMAR (1971 b), which show that chlordiazepoxide, administered to rats previously shocked in one arm only of a Y-maze, or to unshocked naive rats, equally increased the number of entries into both arms by both groups of rats.

3. Pigs

The exploratory behavior of pigs has been studied in two successive daily 20 min sessions in a two-compartment box by counting the number of crossings from one compartment to the other and observing the activity pattern. Injection of diazepam 1 mg·kg⁻¹ i.m. before the first session increased the number of crossings; treated pigs did not attempt to escape and tended to be more perseverative in their activity patterns than control pigs. When injected before the second session, diazepam did not modify the exploratory behavior. A factorial crossover design showed no evidence of state-dependent learning (DANTZER, 1977a, b).

III. Effects on Drug-Induced Changes in Motor Activity

1. Stimulants of Motor Activity

Amphetamine, Methamphetamine, Dexamphetamine. Dexamphetamine (5 mg·kg⁻¹ i.p.) increased locomotor activity of mice placed individually in a revolving activity cage. Chlordiazepoxide (25 mg·kg⁻¹ i.p.) and diazepam (7 mg·kg⁻¹ i.p.) injected 45 min prior to dexamphetamine did not reduce the stimulant effect of the latter drug on locomotion (Jindal et al., 1968).

Dexamphetamine (3.5 mg·kg⁻¹ i.p.) increased locomotor activity in mice as measured in photocell activity cages. At the dose of 0.5 mg·kg⁻¹ s.c. diazepam increased the effect of dexamphetamine. At the dose of 1 mg·kg⁻¹ i.p. diazepam produced only a weak, statistically insignificant increase. At the dose of 4 mg·kg⁻¹ i.p., diazepam did not affect the hypermotility induced by dexamphetamine, although it decreased spontaneous motility when administered alone (Soubrié et al., 1975a). On the other hand, according to Babbini et al. (1969), the increased locomotor activity elicited in the rat by methamphetamine (4 mg·kg⁻¹ i.p.) and recorded with jiggle-cage actometers was markedly inhibited by benzodiazepine derivatives: oxazepam (100–200 mg·kg⁻¹ i.p.), the water-soluble oxazepam hemisuccinate (33–71 mg·kg⁻¹ i.p.), its dimethylaminoethanol salt (20–41 mg·kg⁻¹ i.p.), and diazepam (12–24 mg·kg⁻¹ i.p.). Other investigators did not observe a reduction of amphetamine-induced hyperactivity in mice by benzodiazepines: diazepam administered 1 h before methamphetamine (5 mg·kg⁻¹ s.c.) in doses of 10, 50, and 100 mg·kg⁻¹ p.o., in fact potentiated this hyperactivity (Kamioka et al., 1972); the same results were obtained with nimetazepam 3–30 mg·kg⁻¹ p.o. (activity cages, methamphetamine 2 mg·kg⁻¹ i.p.; Sakai et al., 1972) and chlordiazepoxide 1 mg·kg⁻¹ (photocell activity cages, amphetamine 1.5 mg·kg⁻¹ i.p.; Sethy et al., 1970). No effect of diazepam and oxazepam at 10 mg·kg⁻¹ i.p. was seen on the locomotor stimulant action of d-amphetamine (1–30 mg·kg⁻¹ i.p.) (Shannon et al., 1976).

The combination amphetamine-barbiturate had been shown to increase, at some particular doses (1.2 mg·kg⁻¹ dexamphetamine s.c., 7.5 mg·kg⁻¹ amylobarbitone s.c.), exploratory activity of rats in a Y-shaped runway, the doses of the individual substances being virtually inactive per se; this has been regarded as an example of true mutual potentiation (Rushton and Steinberg, 1963). With chlordiazepoxide (25 mg·kg⁻¹ s.c.) in combination with dexamphetamine (dose as above) a strong potentiation was observed in the same experimental situation (Rushton and Steinberg, 1966, 1967; Kumar, 1971a; Rushton et al., 1973).

Methylphenidate. Chlordiazepoxide (25 mg·kg⁻¹ i.p.) and diazepam (7 mg·kg⁻¹ i.p.) did not reduce the stimulant effect of methylphenidate (10 mg·kg⁻¹ i.p.) on the locomotor activity of mice placed individually in a revolving activity cage (Jindal et al., 1968).

Cocaine. The increased locomotor activity elicited by cocaine (10 mg·kg⁻¹ i.p.) in mice placed individually in a revolving activity cage was not affected by chlordiazepoxide (25 mg·kg⁻¹ i.p.) and diazepam (7 mg·kg⁻¹ i.p.) (Jindal et al., 1968). Locomotor activity induced in mice by cocaine (8 mg·kg⁻¹ i.p.) and measured with photocells was not reduced by diazepam in a dose of 4 mg·kg⁻¹ i.p., which decreased spontaneous locomotor activity, whereas a low dose of diazepam (1 mg·kg⁻¹ i.p.) enhanced hyperactivity induced by cocaine (Soubrié et al., 1975a).

Locomotor activity in mice placed in a rectangular chamber of black perspex was recorded after cocaine administered intraperitoneally; cocaine increased locomotor activity during 3- or 5-min trials in a dose-related manner. Intraperitoneally administered chlordiazepoxide had little effect on locomotor activity, except for a depression at very high doses. Mixtures containing 20 mg·kg^{-1} cocaine and 15 mg·kg^{-1} chlordiazepoxide increased locomotor activity to a much greater extent than cocaine alone (D'MELLO and STOLERMAN, 1977). This effect of cocaine was similar to that already described for amphetamine.

Bemegride. In the open-field test in the rat, bemegride administered alone at 4 or 8 mg·kg^{-1} i.p. did not modify the locomotor activity; however, these doses antagonized the almost complete suppression of locomotor activity induced by diazepam 8 mg·kg^{-1} i.p. (SOUBRIÉ and SIMON, 1978).

Trihexyphenidyl. This antimuscarinic compound (8 mg·kg^{-1} i.p.) elicits hypermotility in mice in photocell activity cages. Diazepam at 2 mg·kg^{-1} i.p., which alone does not modify spontaneous motility, reduced the hypermotility induced by trihexyphenidyl. Oxazepam (4 mg·kg^{-1} i.p.) had a similar effect (SOUBRIÉ et al., 1975a).

Reserpine After Monoamine Oxidase Inhibitor. Reserpine (16 mg·kg^{-1} s.c.) induces hypermotility in mice given pargyline (150 mg·kg^{-1}) 24 h before. Diazepam and chlordiazepoxide depressed this type of hypermotility in a dose-related manner (SOUBRIÉ et al., 1975a).

Caffeine. In a special apparatus for measuring the spontaneous activity, caffeine (50 mg·kg^{-1} p.o.) in rats elicited a strong increase of motility. The approximate doses, which reduced this increase to 50%, were 12 mg·kg^{-1} p.o. for diazepam, 100 mg·kg^{-1} p.o. for chlordiazepoxide, and 160 mg·kg^{-1} p.o. for oxazepam (KLUPP and KÄHLING, 1965).

Opiates. In photocell activity cages, morphine (64 mg·kg^{-1} i.p.) elicited hyperactivity in mice. Diazepam (1 mg·kg^{-1} i.p.) induced a further increase of morphine hyperactivity; this increase was much weaker after diazepam 2 mg·kg^{-1}. At 4 mg·kg^{-1}, which decreased spontaneous motility per se, morphine hyperactivity was decreased. There was therefore a biphasic effect of diazepam, depending on the dose. The same was observed with prazepam and chlordiazepoxide: both increased morphine-induced hyperactivity at 2 mg·kg^{-1} and reduced it at 16 mg·kg^{-1} i.p. (SOUBRIÉ et al., 1975a). Different results were obtained by SHANNON et al. (1976). Stimulation of locomotor activity of mice by morphine (10–300 mg·kg^{-1} i.p.) was reduced by diazepam (0.1–1 mg·kg^{-1} i.p.) and oxazepam (10 mg·kg^{-1} i.p.) at doses which alone had no effect on locomotor activity; surprisingly, only oxazepam antagonized the stimulant effect of methadone.

Muscimol Intranigrally. Bilateral injection of 3 ng muscimol into the substantia nigra in nonanesthetized rats elicited continuous sniffing and head movements and an increase of locomotor activity, recorded cumulatively over 60 min. Muscimol, 10 and 30 ng, further increased hyperactivity. Nitrazepam 1 mg·kg^{-1}, diazepam 3 mg·kg^{-1}, and chlordiazepoxide 5 mg·kg^{-1}, administered orally 30 min before the intranigral injection of muscimol, significantly potentiated the hyperactivity induced by 3 ng muscimol (MATSUI and KAMIOKA, 1979).

2. Depressants of Motor Activity

Reserpine. Locomotor activity was reduced in mice by 0.5–1 mg·kg^{-1} reserpine i.p. In these mice, chlordiazepoxide at three doses (2.5, 5, and 10 mg·kg^{-1} i.p.) increased locomotor activity in comparison to saline (SANSONE, 1978b).

Additionally, the combination of chlordiazepoxide with amphetamine was found to have more marked effect than the two drugs alone, both in normal and reserpinized mice (SANSONE, 1975, 1977). In another experiment, most mice injected with reserpine (0.5 mg·kg^{-1} daily for 3 days) displayed motor depression; in approximately 50% of these mice chlordiazepoxide (5 mg·kg^{-1} i.p.) produced a marked hypermotility, lasting for at least 1 h (VETULANI and SANSONE, 1978).

α-*Methyl-p-tyrosine*. In the same experimental situation as used above with reserpine, α-methyl-p-tyrosine (50 mg·kg^{-1} i.p. 2 h before test), depressed the total locomotor activity of mice measured over 1 h. Chlordiazepoxide (5 mg·kg^{-1} i.p.), which significantly increased locomotor activity in saline-pretreated mice during the whole 1-h session, was inactive after α-methyl-p-tyrosine. This antagonism toward chlordiazepoxide was less evident during the first 10-min period (VETULANI and SANSONE, 1978).

IV. Induced Head-Turning

Contralateral head-turning induced in rats by electrical stimulation of the neostriatum was slowed by 50% by chlordiazepoxide (10.8 mg·kg^{-1}), diazepam (3.7 mg·kg^{-1}), lorazepam (1.5 mg·kg^{-1}), and clonazepam (0.6 mg·kg^{-1}) intraperitoneally. Diazepam lost its effect after a few days of dosing. Benzodiazepines potentiated the depressant effect on head-turning produced by injections of muscimol into the globus pallidus (CROSSMANN et al., 1979). Diazepam, GABA, and muscimol injected into the globus pallidus reduced head-turning provoked by stimulation of the striatum (SLATER and LONGMAN, 1979); inosine and nicotinamide injected together with diazepam abolished the effect of the latter.

V. Conclusions

The effects of benzodiazepines on spontaneous and induced motor activity vary in a bewildering manner depending on the doses and the experimental situation. The doses required to significantly reduce motor activity are usually considerably larger than those producing marked anticonvulsant and anxiolytic effects. Depression of motor activity is clearly not a characteristic effect of benzodiazepines and not a sensitive parameter for detecting active representatives of this chemical class, in particular in mice. The increase of exploratory activity, which has been observed with benzodiazepines in certain conditions, may reflect their anxiolytic or behavioral disinhibiting property. Accordingly, drug interaction experiments have yielded complex actions of benzodiazepines.

N. Benzodiazepines and Aggression

The effect of benzodiazepines on aggressive behavior has been studied extensively during the past 2 decades. The taming effect of chlordiazepoxide on "spontaneously" aggressive monkeys was among the first animal observations made with this class of anxiolytic drugs (RANDALL, 1959; RANDALL et al., 1960; HEISE and BOFF, 1961) and played an important part in the decision to initiate clinical studies with this compound. It was soon recognized that the complex behavioral patterns accompanying different types of aggressiveness and the variety of experimental paradigms used by the various investigators precluded a unifying hypothesis on the action of benzodiazepines on animal aggression (VALZELLI, 1967; DiMASCIO, 1973; ESSMAN, 1978; VALZELLI, 1979, DELINI-STULA and VASSOUT, 1979). Depending on the stimuli or other environmental factors that lead to behavioral patterns described as aggression, at least seven categories of aggressive responses can be differentiated (MOYER, 1968): (a) predatory aggression, (b) intermale aggression, (c) fear-induced aggression, (d) irritative (pain-induced) aggression, (e) territorial aggression, (f) maternal aggression, and (g) sex-related aggression. Some of these aggressive manifestations can be evoked and/or modulated by more or less clearly controlled experimental procedures including (a) electrical or chemical brain stimulation; (b) aversive stimulation, such as that elicited in pairs of mice and rats by electrical foot-shocks; (c) isolation, induced in mice, rats, and rabbits by a prolonged exclusion from social interaction; and (d) treatment with drugs known to affect the dynamics of central neurotransmitters.

Since benzodiazepines induce other effects (sedation, muscle relaxation) that could interfere with the motor expression of aggressive behavior, it is difficult to assess the specific effects of anxiolytics on aggression. Adding the differences in dose schedules (acute or chronic administration) and routes of administration used in the various studies to the above-mentioned variables, it is not surprising to find divergent results and interpretations of this subject. With these cautionary remarks in mind, an analysis of the available data of the literature should outline the general trends in the action of benzodiazepines on aggressive behavior in animals.

I. Spontaneous Aggression

A very impressive behavioral effect of chlordiazepoxide in the early studies of RANDALL and associates was the taming effect observed in vicious cynomolgus and rhesus monkeys with doses of chlordiazepoxide (1 mg·kg^{-1} p.o., RANDALL, 1960; RANDALL et al., 1960; 5 mg·kg^{-1} p.o. given during a week, HEISE and BOFF, 1961), which are clearly below those affecting general behavior or inducing ataxia. Subsequent studies (RANDALL et al., 1961; SCHECKEL and BOFF, 1968) extended this observation to diazepam (taming dose in cynomolgus monkey, 1 mg·kg^{-1} p.o.), nitrazepam (0.125 mg·kg^{-1}), bromazepam (1 mg·kg^{-1}), clonazepam (2.5 mg·kg^{-1}), flunitrazepam (0.5 mg·kg^{-1}), medazepam (5 mg·kg^{-1}), and flurazepam (5 mg·kg^{-1}). For chlordiazepoxide, the antiaggressive effect was shown to be due predominantly to the drug itself and not to its main metabolites, since after a single oral dose of ^{14}C-chlordiazepoxide the decline of the level of unchanged drug in blood, brain, and muscle was associated with a return of aggressivity over a period of 24 h, whereas the levels of N-desmethylchlordiazepoxide and the lactam metabolite remained constant within the same period in the three tissues (COUTINHO et al., 1971).

In studies investigating the social behavior of rhesus monkeys, DELGADO (1973) and DELGADO et al. (1976) found that dominant animals in pairs exhibited less aggressive attacks against submissive partners when either chlordiazepoxide (5 mg·kg^{-1} i.m.) was given to dominant animals or diazepam (5 mg·kg^{-1} i.m.) administered to dominant and/or submissive monkeys. In both studies these doses of benzodiazepines did not change the social hierarchy and did not impair motor performance. In another study, however, the submissive monkey increased its attacks against the dominant member of the colony, which had received chlordiazepoxide (5 mg·kg^{-1}), presumably to "challenge the apparent loss of authority" of the dominant partner (Apfelbach and Delgado, 1974). Socially induced suppression of behavior, but not aggression, was diminished after low doses of chlordiazepoxide (2 mg·kg^{-1} p.o.), diazepam (0.2 mg·kg^{-1}), cloxazolam (0.2 mg·kg^{-1}), oxazolam (2 mg·kg^{-1}), and CS 386, an oxazolobenzodiazepine (0.2 mg·kg^{-1}) (Kamioka et al., 1977).

In addition to monkeys, the taming effect of chlordiazepoxide was also observed in various wild zoo animals (Heuschele, 1961). In farm animals (poultry and pigs), however, diazepam administered orally or intramuscularly either reduced aggressivity along with signs of sedation and muscular impairment (Drumev et al., 1972) or even increased aggressive behavior (Dantzer, 1975). In contrast, the aggressivity of pigeons induced by nonreward in a positive reinforcement schedule of operant training, was suppressed during repeated administration of chlordiazepoxide (5 mg·kg^{-1} i.m. per day, Moore et al., 1976).

Important findings indicating more selective effects of benzodiazepines on distinct behavioral manifestations of aggression were demonstrated in cats. Aggressive-defensive behavior, characterized by hissing and striking with the paws against the experimenter's gloves, was abolished after 10 mg·kg^{-1} chlordiazepoxide p.o. However, "pure" attack occurring in rival fights between male cats and culminating in biting of the neck was not affected even with doses of chlordiazepoxide that induced ataxia (20 mg·kg^{-1} p.o.; Hoffmeister and Wuttke, 1969). Marked depressant effects of nitrazepam and nimetazepam, but not of diazepam, on aggressive-defensive behavior elicited by blowing air or approaching the cat with a stick were observed by Otsuka et al. (1973). In an attempt to further differentiate the effects of diazepam on aggressivity, Langfeldt and Ursin (1971) used spontaneously aggressive cats forced either to flee or to display a defensive behavior on being approached by a stick. Since diazepam (1 mg·kg^{-1} i.p.) depressed the affective defense response, but not the flight, the authors suggested that diazepam acted selectively on brain structures that regulate defense behavior, in particular the limbic system. In another study (Langfeldt, 1974), a dose of diazepam (1 mg·kg^{-1} i.p.) that did not sedate animals, induced a prey-play behavior in cats which would immediately kill a mouse when not drugged. Langfeldt (1974), therefore, assumed that diazepam had a depressant effect on an activation system related to aggressive behavior. Leaf et al. (1979) found no inhibition of mouse-killing behavior of cats with doses up to 16 mg·kg^{-1} chlordiazepoxide i.p. and 4 mg·kg^{-1} diazepam i.p., unless the drugs produced marked side-effects including ataxia. The animals used in this study were domesticated cats.

The spontaneous aggressivity in other mammalian species was not consistently altered by benzodiazepines. Mouse-killing by rats was either unaffected by doses of benzodiazepines that induced general motor impairment (Karli, 1961; Horovitz et al., 1965, 1966; Sofia, 1969; Goldberg, 1970; Valzelli and Bernasconi, 1971; Vassout and Delini-Stula, 1977) or was even enhanced by low doses of chlordiazepoxide (2.5 mg·kg^{-1} i.p.) and diazepam (1.25 mg·kg^{-1}), this latter effect persisting after chronic administration of chlordiazepoxide (Leaf et al., 1975). Antimuricidal effects of high doses of chlordiazepoxide (50 mg·kg^{-1} i.p.) exhibited tolerance on repeated administration of the drug, indicating that the general behavioral depression was primarily responsible for the antimuricidal action of chlordiazepoxide (Quenzer and

FELDMAN, 1975 a). KAMEI et al. (1975) found antimuricidal activity of diazepam and chlordiazepoxide, the ED_{50} values being 4.95 and 34.4 mg·kg^{-1} i.p., respectively. An interesting observation was made by MICZEK (1974), who studied dose-related effects of chlordiazepoxide on intraspecies aggressiveness of rats. In pairs of dominant and submissive rats, low doses of chlordiazepoxide (2.5–5 mg·kg^{-1} i.m.) given to the dominant rats increased aggressive responses, while a higher dose of the benzodiazepine (20 mg·kg^{-1}) suppressed them without reversing the dominance-subordination relationship. In pairs of aggressive and non-aggressive mice, diazepam (10 mg·kg^{-1} p.o.) and chlordiazepoxide (50 mg·kg^{-1} p.o.), administered to aggressive mice, reduced aggressive activity and increased social activities (sniffing, climbing) without inhibiting walking across the cage or rearing in the aggressive mice (KRŠIAK, 1979). Similarly, in pairs of golden hamsters, a rather high dose of chlordiazepoxide (50 mg·kg^{-1} p.o.) reduced aggressivity and increased sociability (POOLE, 1973). Chlordiazepoxide (50 mg·kg^{-1}) markedly attenuated spontaneous aggressiveness in minks without producing motor deficits (BAUEN and POSSANZA, 1970). In contrast, the time needed by a ferret to catch and kill rats was shortened after chlordiazepoxide (1 mg·kg^{-1} i.m., APFELBACH, 1978). The intense and frequent attacks occurring between male mice when a resident animal was confronted in its home cage with an intruder, was not affected by chlordiazepoxide in nondebilitating doses (MICZEK and O'DONNELL, 1980); when confrontation occurred in a neutral cage, attacks were less frequent. In this latter situation chlordiazepoxide (and ethanol) increased aggressive behavior.

The fighting behavior of male siamese fighting fish was diminished by doses of chlordiazepoxide (15 µg·ml^{-1} added to the aquarium) which had no effect on swimming performance (FIGLER et al., 1975). Chlordiazepoxide either did not affect the aggressive behavior of ants (KOSTOWSKI, 1966) and scorpions (MERCIER and DESSAIGNE, 1970) or reduced aggressivity in praying mantis only with debilitating doses (MERCIER et al., 1966). Regarding this inability to affect aggressiveness in invertebrates, it may be relevant that specific high-affinity binding sites for benzodiazepines have not been found in the nervous system of invertebrates (NIELSEN et al., 1978), as will be discussed in Sect. Z.

II. Isolation-Induced Aggression in Mice

The early observation that a dose of chlordiazepoxide (10 mg·kg^{-1} i.p.), which was lower than that producing motor impairment (20 mg·kg^{-1}), reduced fighting in a pair of previously isolated mice (SCRIABINE and BLAKE, 1962), has subsequently been confirmed in most investigations and extended to some other benzodiazepines. Whereas chlordiazepoxide (5–7 mg·kg^{-1} i.p.), medazepam (10 mg·kg^{-1}), and oxazepam (15 mg·kg^{-1}) induced antiaggressive activity without signs of overt motor impairment (VALZELLI et al., 1967; VALZELLI and BERNASCONI, 1971), the antiaggressive actions of diazepam (7.5 mg·kg^{-1} i.p.), nitrazepam (3.75 mg·kg^{-1}), N-desmethyldiazepam (3.75 mg·kg^{-1}), and N-methyl-oxazepam (3.75 mg·kg^{-1}) seemed to be related to their muscle-relaxant properties (VALZELLI, 1973). DA VANZO et al. (1966) and HOFFMEISTER and WUTTKE (1969) obtained an antifighting effect with chlordiazepoxide only with doses producing overt neurologic effects, while COLE and WOLF (1970) observed increased aggressiveness in previously isolated grasshopper mice after chlordiazepoxide. In an attempt to resolve the discrepancy on the specificity of benzodiazepine effects on the isolation-induced aggressivity in mice, Malick (1978) used repeated administration of diazepam (1 mg·kg^{-1} i.p. for 5 days). On the first day of administration a reduction in fighting as well as ataxia were observed, while tolerance to the motor impairment developed on subsequent days and thus unmasked a rather selective antiaggressive effect of diazepam.

III. Aggression in Grouped Male Mice

In contrast to the predominant antiaggressive effect of benzodiazepines in isolation-induced aggression in mice, aggressivity was enhanced in grouped male mice chronically fed a diet containing diazepam (Fox and Snyder, 1969), chlordiazepoxide (Fox et al., 1970), N-desmethyldiazepam, and oxazepam (Guaitani et al., 1971), nitrazepam and flurazepam (Fox et al., 1972), and prazepam (Fox et al., 1974). In line with these findings, aggressive behavior developed by dominant members in two fighting groups of mice was increased after acute administration of 3 mg·kg^{-1} chlordiazepoxide p.o. (Zwirner et al., 1975).

IV. Foot-Shock-Induced Aggression in Mice

The aggressive behavior elicited in a pair of mice subjected to mild electric foot shocks (Tedeschi et al., 1959, 1969) is particularly susceptible to the effect of benzodiazepines. Chlordiazepoxide (10 mg·kg^{-1} p.o.; Hoffmeister and Wuttke, 1969), chlordiazepoxide and diazepam (4.2 and 0.9 mg·kg^{-1} i.p. respectively, Sofia, 1969), flurazepam (20 mg·kg^{-1} p.o., Randall et al., 1969), chlordiazepoxide, diazepam, oxazepam, and nitrazepam (4.7; 2.1; 4.5; and 1.2 mg·kg^{-1} p.o., respectively; Christmas and Maxwell, 1970), prazepam (13 mg·kg^{-1} p.o., Robichaud et al., 1970), and a novel thienodiazepine (2.9 mg·kg^{-1} p.o.; Nakanishi et al., 1972) markedly reduced fighting behavior in mice at doses far below doses exhibiting signs of sedation or motor impairment. Effective doses of the above-mentioned and most other benzodiazepines (doses always refer to ED$_{50}$ values) are cited in reviews by Sternbach et al. (1964), Randall and Kappell (1973), Rudzik et al. (1973), and Randall et al. (1974). In an attempt to explain the antiaggressive effect of benzodiazepines, Quenzer and Feldman (1975 b) were unable to correlate the action of chlordiazepoxide on foot shock-induced fighting with mechanisms involving either 5-hydroxytryptamine or cyclic 3'5'-adenosine monophosphate (cAMP), although in a previous study (Quenzer et al., 1974) chlordiazepoxide and caffeine, both potent cAMP phosphodiesterase inhibitors (Beer et al., 1972), were shown to have additive effects on shock-induced aggression.

V. Aggression Induced in Rats by Brain Lesions

Conflicting reports exist on the effects of benzodiazepines on aggressiveness produced in rats by lesions in different brain areas. In the most frequently used model, i.e., rats made hyperirritable by bilateral ablation of the septum, benzodiazepines either reduced aggressive behavior or had no effect. Chlordiazepoxide (10–20 mg·kg^{-1} i.p.) was found to markedly depress the vicious behavior of septal rats (Schallek et al.,

1962; HOROVITZ et al., 1963; STARK and HENDERSON, 1966; BEATTIE et al., 1969). However, chlordiazepoxide (SOFIA, 1969; GOLDBERG, 1970) and diazepam (SOFIA, 1969) were ineffective in intraperitoneal doses below or equivalent to those inducing a motor deficit. Similarly, in rats made aggressive by bilateral destruction of the olfactory bulbs, chlordiazepoxide (MALICK et al., 1969) and diazepam (MALICK et al., 1969; VASSOUT and DELINI-STULA, 1977) were without effect. In contrast, when injected directly into the mamillary body region of the hypothalamus, chlordiazepoxide (50 µg) suppressed the muricidal behavior of olfactory bulbectomized rats (HARA et al., 1975a), whereas injections into different areas of the limbic system were inactive (WATANABE et al., 1979). Reduction of aggressivity was also observed after chlordiazepoxide (ED_{50}, 9 mg·kg^{-1} i.p.) in rats with bilateral lesions of the anterior hypothalamus (BLYTHER and MARRIOTT, 1969) as well as after oral administration of chlordiazepoxide (ED_{50}, 20 mg·kg^{-1}), diazepam (20 mg·kg^{-1}), and nitrazepam (14.5 mg·kg^{-1}) in rats with midbrain lesions (CHRISTMAS and MAXWELL, 1970). No effect was found with benzodiazepines in rats exhibiting aggressivity after bilateral lesion of the ventromedial hypothalamus (MALICK et al., 1969).

VI. Brain Stimulation-Induced Aggression in Cats, Rats, and Monkeys

High-frequency electrical stimulation of the hypothalamus, septum, or periaqueductal gray matter in freely moving animals elicits affective rage reactions which can be assessed by measuring the threshold current for evoking different manifestations of this behavior, such as hissing, growling, or defensive attack with striking paws (HESS, 1957; HUNSPERGER and BUCHER, 1967; BROWN et al., 1969). The early study performed by BAXTER (1964) indicated that a subchronic administration of chlordiazepoxide to cats (10 mg·kg^{-1} i.p.) increased the threshold for the hissing response induced by stimulation of the perifornical hypothalamic area on the 2nd day of administration. In a subsequent study the same dose of chlordiazepoxide was shown to raise the threshold for the hissing response within 1–2 h after administration (FUNDERBURK et al., 1970). Similar effects with elevation of the "hiss threshold" were observed with diazepam (4 mg·kg^{-1} i.p.) and oxazepam (12 mg·kg^{-1} i.p.) as early as 30 min after administration (MALICK, 1970). Our own investigations with stimulation of the perifornical hypothalamus demonstrated that a dose of diazepam (0.5 mg·kg^{-1} i.p.), which did not induce ataxia or sedation of the cats, significantly elevated the threshold for both the hissing and attack response (POLC, unpublished). MURASAKI et al. (1976) found that diazepam (1 mg·kg^{-1} i.p.) raised the threshold for the attack response more than that for the hissing response. A rather high dose of nitrazepam (5 mg·kg^{-1} i.p.), which concurrently diminished muscle tone, inhibited the rage reaction elicited by stimulation of the posterior hypothalamus and the septal area in cats (HERNÁNDEZ-PEÓN and ROJAS-RAMÍREZ, 1966).

An interesting observation, related to the findings of HOFFMEISTER and WUTTKE (1969) on spontaneously aggressive cats, was made in rats in which hypothalamic stimulation induced either an affective rage response or a quiet mouse-killing attack. Chlordiazepoxide (10 mg·kg^{-1} i.p.) abolished the affective response, but increased the quiet muricidal behavior (PANKSEPP, 1971). Chlordiazepoxide (1–10 mg·kg^{-1} i.p.) selectively depressed the escape response in rats to aversive stimulation of the periaqueductal gray matter without producing noticeable sedation or ataxia (SCHEN-

BERG and GRAEFF, 1978). The authors suggested that inhibition by benzodiazepines of the fight-flight system in the periaqueductal gray matter might be responsible for the antianxiety effects of this group of compounds. The flight reaction induced by hypothalamic stimulation was only delayed, but not abolished by 5 mg·kg⁻¹ diazepam i.p., a dose which reduced basal locomotor activity (MORPURGO, 1968).

Findings obtained with telemetric stimulation of brain areas in monkeys led DELGADO (1973) to conclude that benzodiazepines selectively depressed aggressiveness by an action on the limbic system or on the nociceptive system in the thalamus and central gray matter. A dose of chlordiazepoxide, which did not impair locomotion (8 mg·kg⁻¹ i.m.), given to the dominant animal in a monkey colony, blocked the violent fighting between the dominant and submissive monkey induced by radio stimulation of the olfactory area in the dominant partner. In the same study, the stimulation of Forel's field elicited aggressive behavior in a submissive monkey, which remained responsive to the attitude of the dominant partner, although the induced aggressiveness was inhibited after the same dose of chlordiazepoxide.

VII. Drug-Induced Aggression

While an inhibition of the biting response in mice injected with a high dose of DL-Dopa (500 mg·kg⁻¹ i.v.) was observed after diazepam (2.5 mg·kg⁻¹ i.p.), chlordiazepoxide (13 mg·kg⁻¹), and oxazepam (8.8 mg·kg⁻¹) (YEN et al., 1970), diazepam failed to influence biting behavior elicited in mice by apomorphine (OLPE, 1978). In an attempt to find out the site of action for the tranquilizing effects of benzodiazepines, NAGY and DECSI (1973) injected small amounts of diazepam (10–20 µg) locally into different limbic areas of cats in which the affective rage reaction was elicited by direct injections of carbachol into the hypothalamus. Direct injections of diazepam into amygdala and hypothalamus, and particularly into the anterobasal amygdaloid region, suppressed rage reactions. Injections into the hippocampus were ineffective. The same effects as obtained after direct application of diazepam into the anterobasal amygdala were also observed after intraperitoneal injection (2.3 mg·kg⁻¹) of the benzodiazepine, a dose that induced slight ataxia in these cats.

VIII. Induction of Aggressive Behavior

In addition to paradoxically increase existing aggressivity of grouped male mice, daily intraperitoneal injections of diazepam (4 mg·kg⁻¹) and flunitrazepam (2 mg·kg⁻¹) to male rats over 28 days induced aggressive behavior (WÜSTER et al., 1980a). Induction of mouse-killing behavior in rats by chlordiazepoxide (LEAF et al., 1975) could be blocked by lesions of the amygdala (GAY et al., 1976).

IX. Conclusions

Benzodiazepines affect animal aggressive behavior in differing ways, depending on variables such as the affective background, different forms of innate aggressivity, housing conditions, and quality of aversive somatosensory and social stimulation. Benzodiazepines exert the most pronounced antiaggressive activity with little apparent relation to sedative and muscle-relaxant effects in (a) some spontaneously aggressive monkeys and other wild animals, (b) isolation- and foot-shock-induced aggressiveness in mice, and (c) in cats, monkeys and rats, in which affective defensive behavior is evoked by brain stimulation. In contrast, no consistent effects of benzodiazepines were observed on the muricidal and brain lesion-induced aggressive behavior of rats, and these drugs enhanced aggressiveness in grouped male mice. It can be tentatively assumed that a depressant effect of benzodiazepines on limbic areas and their connections to the hypothalamus is responsible for the particular sensitivity to these drugs of the affectively motivated behavior, such as the rage reactions elicited by brain stimulation, and possibly also innate aggressiveness of wild animals. It is even possible that the same suppressant action of benzodiazepines would relieve anxiety and diminish aggressive behavior.

The paradoxical increase of aggressivity in grouped male mice can be explained by an inhibitory effect of benzodiazepines on frustration, which in animals housed in groups results in impairment of important motivational behavior such as feeding, drinking, and territorial defense (VALZELLI, 1979). The mechanisms by which benzodiazepines reduce aggressivity induced by prolonged isolation and electrical foot shocks are not easily understood. Perhaps benzodiazepines attenuate the sudden increase in intensity of social and somatosensory stimulation in mice placed together after prolonged isolation and diminish the stress response elicited by foot shocks, respectively. Hence, in the last two situations the antiaggressive effect of benzodiazepines would be rather indirect.

O. Interaction with Other Centrally Active Agents

In this section we consider briefly some of the interactions of benzodiazepine derivatives with other centrally acting agents not dealt with in other sections.

I. Synergism with "Centrally Depressant" Agents

1. General Anesthetics

Some propanediols and chlordiazepoxide reduced the doses of mebubarbitone and pentobarbitone required to induce a loss of the righting reflex (BOISSIER and SIMON, 1964). In doses which did not depress the righting reflex, chlordiazepoxide reinduced the loss of this reflex when given at the time of recovery of the reflex following barbiturates. Prolongation of barbiturate-induced anesthesia has been observed with different benzodiazepines and several barbiturates in various animal species (DE REPENTIGNY et al., 1976; CHAMBERS and JEFFERSON, 1977). Halothane-induced "sleeping time" (loss of righting reflex) in the mouse was prolonged by the simultaneous administration of nitrazepam, diazepam, flunitrazepam, chlordiazepoxide, medazepam, and oxazepam, in this order of potency; the organic solvent used for diazepam and flunitrazepam contributed to the observed potentiation of halothane effects (STUMPF et al., 1976; CHAMBERS et al., 1978). General anesthesia of the rabbit induced by equithesin was improved by the administration of diazepam as a preanesthetic (HODESSON et al., 1965). Based on the synergistic action of chloralose and chlordiazepoxide, this combination has been proposed as capable of maintaining a sufficient anesthesia in cats and rabbits for 6–12 h in acute neurophysiologic experiments (Steiner, 1969). Diazepam, flurazepam, and chlordiazepoxide potentiated the anesthetic effect of various steroid anesthetics in mice and rats (Gyermek, 1974). Diazepam, nitrazepam, flunitrazepam, and midazolam showed a marked synergism with the general anesthetic action of nitrous oxide in mice (Stumpf et al., 1975, 1979). In rats, diazepam intravenously accentuated the decrease of cerebral blood flow and cerebral oxygen consumption induced by nitrous oxide (Carlsson et al., 1976).

2. Ethanol

Several studies have shown an additive or supraadditive influence of benzodiazepines on the central depressant effect of ethanol (Forney et al., 1962; Gebhart et al., 1969; Bourrinet, 1971; Chan et al., 1978; Začková et al., 1978). The relative contribution of pharmacodynamic and pharmacokinetic mechanisms to this synergism is not yet clear (Hoyumpa et al., 1980; Vesell, 1980). In man, evidence exists for a pharmacokinetic (Molander and Duvhoek, 1976) as well as for a pharmacodynamic interaction (Dundee and Isaac, 1970). The interaction between ethanol and benzodiazepines may be more complicated than commonly believed and depends on the doses of both alcohol and the benzodiazepine as well as on the kind of benzodiazepine derivative. Indeed, Dundee and Isaac (1970) surprisingly found that after 100–140 mg chlordiazepoxide, the blood level of ethanol at which sleep occurred was higher than in the absence of the drug. This antagonism for sleep induction was not present after 50 mg chlordiazepoxide and 10–30 mg diazepam.

3. Neuroleptics

Benzodiazepines have been found to produce a loss of righting reflex when combined with a subhypnotic dose of chlorprothixene, and this effect has been used as a screening procedure to detect central depressant activity (Randall et al., 1968; Straw, 1975). The capacity of 14 benzodiazepines to prolong the loss of righting reflex induced by droperidol in mice has been measured by Niemegeers and Lewi (1979).

Various benzodiazepines were reported to enhance the cataleptic effect of different neuroleptics (Keller et al., 1976). This potentiation was paralleled by a reduction of the neuroleptic-induced increase of dopamine turnover. This type of interaction is discussed in more detail in connection with the effect of benzodiazepines on GABAergic transmission in the substantia nigra (X, X, 1).

4. Δ^9-Tetrahydrocannabinol (Δ^9 THC)

The interaction of chlordiazepoxide, ethanol, and phenobarbitone with the effect of Δ^9-THC in rats was studied using conditioned avoidance responses, locomotor activity, heart rate, body temperature, and performance in a rotarod test (Pryor et al., 1977). Chlordiazepoxide, as well as ethanol and phenobarbitone, enhanced the depressant effect of Δ^9-THC on most of these parameters. Chlordiazepoxide was the only agent which failed to enhance the Δ^9-THC-induced impairment of conditioned avoidance performance.

5. Anticholinesterases

The potent antagonistic action of benzodiazepines on seizures induced by anticholinesterases has been reported in the section dealing with the anticonvulsant effects. One observation, however, was made of a potentiating effect of chlordiazepoxide. This drug (as well as phenobarbitone and reserpine) increased the toxicity of carbaryl (WEISS and ORZEL, 1967). Perhaps this may be explained by the muscle relaxant effect of chlordiazepoxide, which may be harmful when the main effect of the anticholinesterase is to produce a muscular paralysis.

6. Muscimol

Chlordiazepoxide, diazepam, and nitrazepam were found to potentiate the hyperactivity induced in the rat by the bilateral injection of 3 ng muscimol into the substantia nigra (MATSUI and KAMIOKA, 1979); this "excitatory" effect of the benzodiazepines was explained by a facilitation of GABA-receptor stimulation. Various benzodiazepines, when given together with muscimol, increased the compulsive gnawing activity of mice induced by methylphenidate more than the benzodiazepines or muscimol alone (ARNT et al., 1979).

7. Scopolamine

Chlordiazepoxide as well as scopolamine slightly improved avoidance responding in mice being trained for shuttle-box performance. The facilitation of avoidance was more marked when the two drugs were combined, especially during the initial phases of training (SANSONE, 1978 a).

8. Analgesics

The interaction of benzodiazepines with analgesics was treated in Sect. J.I.

II. Antagonism with Centrally Active Agents

1. Opiate Antagonism

VON LEDEBUR et al. (1962) observed that nalorphine reduced the time during which guinea pigs passively remained in a lateral or supine position after chlordiazepoxide, chlorpromazine, and meprobamate and suggested the use of nalorphine as an antidote after ingestion of overdoses of central depressant drugs. Controversial clinical observations have been reported on the reversal of benzodiazepine effects by naloxone in man (MOSS, 1973; BELL, 1975; CHRISTENSEN and HÜTTEL, 1979) and have stimulated experiments in animals.

In the rat, naloxone in the extremely high dose of 60 mg·kg^{-1} i.p. blocked the anticonflict effect of chlordiazepoxide; mice that had lost the righting reflex after high doses of chlordiazepoxide regained this reflex, although remaining ataxic, after doses of 50 and 100 mg·kg^{-1} naloxone i.p., while the loss of righting reflex induced by barbiturates or meprobamate was unaffected (BILLINGSLEY and KUBENA, 1978). Naloxone (5 mg·kg^{-1} i.p.) reduced the increase by chlordiazepoxide (4 mg·kg^{-1}) and ethanol of operant responding of rats for lateral hypothalamic self-stimulation (LORENS and SAINATI, 1978). A small dose of naloxone (0.25 mg · kg⁻¹) reduced the stimulant effect of diazepam on food intake in satiated rats (STAPLETON et al., 1979). SOUBRIÉ et al. (1980) found that naloxone blocked some, but not all disinhibitory effects of diazepam on behavior of rats under aversive situations. Naloxone in much higher doses than required to block the effect of opiates has been shown to act as a GABA antagonist (DINGLEDINE et al., 1978) and to induce convulsions (BREUKER et al., 1976).

2. Anticholinesterases

Anecdotal clinical reports suggest that physostigmine may quickly reverse unconsciousness induced by diazepam. This analeptic property of physostigmine is probably an unspecific one, since the drug also antagonized central depression by neuroleptics (ROSENBERG, 1974; DI LIBERTI et al., 1975; LARSON et al., 1977). Moreover, physostigmine failed to reverse diazepam-induced sedation in patients undergoing dental extraction (GARBER et al., 1980). Experiments in rabbits, cats, and rats, measuring EEG, gross behavior, and mortality rate after lethal doses of diazepam confirmed the clinical observations (NAGY and DECSI, 1978). Since the antidote effect of physostigmine was still present after methylatropine, only central effects seem to be involved both in the lethal effects of diazepam and the antagonistic effect of the anticholinesterase. Benzodiazepines are also antidotes of anticholinesterases: in the rabbit diazepam prevented or blocked epileptic cortical activity induced by fluostigmine and, when added to atropine and obidoxime raised the LD_{50} of fluostigmine in rats about 80-fold (RUMP et al., 1973; RUMP and GRUDZINSKA, 1974; GRUDZINSKA et al., 1979). As will be discussed in the section on the interaction of benzodiazepines with acetylcholine, the antidote action of these drugs cannot be due to an effect on the cholinesterase itself.

3. Antimuscarinic Agents

The increased locomotor activity of mice induced by benztropine, scopolamine, atropine, and trihexyphenidyl was reduced or suppressed by diazepam in doses which by themselves did not reduce spontaneous activity (SIMON et al., 1974). Interaction experiments with picrotoxin, thiosemicarbazide, and strychnine suggested that the antagonistic effect of diazepam may involve a GABAergic mechanism (SOUBRIÉ et al., 1976 b).

4. Nicotine

A high dose of nicotine (120 mg · kg⁻¹ i.p.) induced electrocardiographic changes, convulsions, and death in about 90% of guinea pigs; bromazepam and diazepam (5 mg · kg⁻¹ i.m.) protected the animals from convulsions, changes in atrioventricular conduction, and mortality (MARINO et al., 1974). A similar protective effect on extensor seizures and mortality was also observed with diazepam and chlordiazepoxide in mice (ACETO, 1975).

5. Imipramine

Diazepam was found to block bradycardia, but to increase hypotension and hypothermia induced by imipramine in rats (CARPENTER et al., 1977).

6. Dibutyryl cAMP

The N^6,O^2-dibutyryl analogue of cAMP, in a dose-dependent manner, shortened the duration of "narcosis" in the rat induced by eight structurally different agents, among them diazepam (COHN et al., 1975).

7. Bemegride

Bemegride (a convulsant analeptic) normalized the diazepam-induced alteration of behavior of gerbils in an open-field situation (JÄRBE and JOHANSSON, 1977).

8. Caffeine

Caffeine dose-dependently reversed the depressant effect of diazepam on the performance of mice in a horizontal wire test (BONETTI and POLC, 1980); the doses of caffeine did not by themselves induce central stimulation. In contrast, caffeine antagonized the effect of phenobarbitone in this test situation only at high, stimulant doses. Caffeine also partially antagonized the effect of diazepam on the amplitude and duration of segmental dorsal root potentials in spinal cats, but was inactive on the changes in this potential induced by phenobarbitone. It is unlikely that the diazepam-caffeine antagonism is due to an interaction at benzodiazepine receptors; a purinergic mechanism might be involved (POLC et al., 1981). An antagonism between chlordiazepoxide and caffeine was not found on the behavior of rats and gerbils in a schedule of differential reinforcement of low rate (SANGER, 1980).

9. Dopa

Chlordiazepoxide (10 and 32 mg·kg^{-1} i.p.), but not diazepam (1 and 3.2 mg·kg^{-1} i.p.) potentiated the behavioral response of rats to L-Dopa after pretreatment with a monoamine oxidase inhibitor (BERENDSON et al., 1976).

III. Conclusions

The well-known synergism between benzodiazepines and general anesthetics is not surprising. It is probably the result of a combination of different mechanisms in reducing central nervous system excitability; indeed, all the general anesthetics studied in this combination experiment depress excitatory synapses, an effect which benzodiazepines lack in pharmacologic doses.

The synergistic action of benzodiazepines and ethanol is of particular interest because the latter, in a yet unknown way, also enhances GABAergic inhibitory transmission.

The interaction of benzodiazepines and neuroleptics both on the behavioral and neurochemical level suggests that this combination should be investigated carefully in the treatment of schizophrenia.

The antagonism of at least certain effects of benzodiazepines by naloxone may be of a rather complex nature. In higher doses, this opiate antagonist also seems to block GABA receptors. Moreover, benzodiazepines have been shown to alter the content of met-enkephalin in certain brain areas; whether this is an epiphenomenon or whether it points to a causal involvement of endorphins in certain actions of benzodiazepines, remains to be elucidated.

P. Effects on Peripheral Nervous Structures

I. Axonal Conduction

In isolated preganglionic cervical sympathetic nerve preparation of rabbits, diazepam and chlordiazepoxide reduced the amplitude of the compound action potential of B-fibers in a concentration-dependent manner (Clubley, 1978); chlordiazepoxide and diazepam were approximately equipotent, the concentration producing a 50% block of the compound action potential being 2×10^{-4} and 10^{-4} mol·l^{-1}, respectively, and of the order of potency of procaine. Chlorpromazine was 10–30 times more potent than the benzodiazepines. When injected intravenously in the anesthetized rabbit in a dose of 8 mg·kg^{-1}, diazepam and chlordiazepoxide did not consistently reduce the amplitude of the compound action potential of the preganglionic cervical sympathetic trunk (Clubley and Elliott, 1977). On nodes of Ranvier of isolated frog sciatic nerve fibers, chlordiazepoxide reduced the amplitude of single action potentials to 50% at about 10^{-3} mol·l^{-1} (Mitolo-Chieppa and Marino, 1972); at this concentration, the duration of the action potential was prolonged by about 20% and the threshold for excitation elevated by about 60%. Repetitive activity evoked by short high-frequency trains was reduced by chlordiazepoxide at about 2×10^{-4} mol·l^{-1}; the potency of chlordiazepoxide in the single node of Ranvier was similar to that of phenobarbitone. In the isolated frog sciatic nerve trunk, chlordiazepoxide at 3.4×10^{-3} mol·l^{-1} reduced the conduction velocity by about 20% (Pruett and Williams, 1966). In the isolated rat sciatic nerve trunk, midazolam had about one-tenth the local anesthetic potency of procaine (Pieri et al., 1981). In high concentrations, chlordiazepoxide ($> 10^{-3}$ mol·l^{-1}) and diazepam (0.5×10^{-3} mol·l^{-1}) produced conduction failure in the isolated giant axon of the earth-worm ventral cord by elevating the threshold for spike initiation, decreasing the rate of rise of the extracellularly recorded action potential, while having little effect on spike amplitude (Toman and Sabelli, 1968). The elevation of threshold could be transiently restored in the presence of diazepam by repetitive high-voltage stimulation. Chlordiazepoxide (3×10^{-5}–10^{-4} mol·l^{-1}) increased the threshold for spike initiation in the crayfish giant axon also (Wang and James, 1979). Amplitude and maximum rate of rise of the action potential were reduced, whereas the resting membrane potential remained unaltered. In the squid giant axon, the same authors observed with diazepam a suppression of two components of the membrane current, the transient Na$^+$ current being more affected than the steady state K$^+$ current.

II. Spontaneous and Evoked Activity in Sympathetic and Parasympathetic Nerves

In curarized cats, Sigg and Sigg (1969) observed a decrease of the spontaneous firing rate in splanchnic nerves and some attenuation of the activity in the preganglionic cervical sympathetic and the vagus nerve after diazepam (0.3 and 3 mg·kg^{-1} i.v.). The spontaneous excitatory episodes recorded from the cervical sympathetic nerve were clearly reduced after estazolam (0.25 mg·kg^{-1} i.v.) and nitrazepam (2 mg·kg^{-1} i.v.), but less markedly after diazepam (4 mg·kg^{-1} i.v., FUKUDA et al., 1974). The spontaneous activity in the cervical sympathetic of anesthetized rabbits was reduced by 8 mg·kg^{-1} diazepam and chlordiazepoxide i.v. in about half of the experiments (CLUBLEY and ELLIOT, 1977); the effect, when present, developed slowly and reached a peak about 60 min after the injection. Diazepam (0.1 mg·kg^{-1} i.v.) only slightly depressed a somatovisceral reflex, consisting of discharges in the preganglionic splanchnic nerve fibers in response to stimulation of forelimb cutaneous afferents in the cat (SCHLOSSER et al., 1975 b).

Diazepam 0.3 mg·kg^{-1} i.v. markedly reduced the hypothalamically evoked discharge in the splanchnic nerve in curarized cats (SIGG and SIGG, 1969); a slight or moderate depression of discharges was observed in cervical sympathetic and vagal nerves. Nitrazepam and estazolam 2 mg·kg^{-1} i.v. elevated the stimulation threshold in the posterior hypothalamus, midbrain reticular formation, and sciatic nerve to evoke responses in the preganglionic cervical sympathetic nerve (FUKUDA et al., 1974). The same authors also found that estazolam inhibited discharges in the cervical sympathetic nerve in response to sciatic nerve stimulation in the *cerveau isolé* cat. Evoked activity in renal sympathetic nerves of anesthetized cats in response to stimulation of the sciatic or vagal nerve was inhibited by diazepam, when stimulation was at high frequency, but enhanced when low frequency stimulation was used (PÓRSZÁSZ and GIBISZER, 1970). Nictitating membrane contractions evoked in curarized cats by stimulation of the posterior hypothalamus or the midbrain reticular formation or in response to sciatic nerve stimulation were inhibited by 2 mg·kg^{-1} of estazolam and nitrazepam i.v. (FUKUDA et al., 1974). However, using a similar preparation, SIGG et al. (1971) and CARROLL et al. (1961) failed to observe any effect of diazepam (3 mg·kg^{-1} i.v.) and chlordiazepoxide (20 mg·kg^{-1} i.v.) on nictitating membrane contractions evoked by hypothalamic stimulation. An attenuation by 1 mg·kg^{-1} diazepam i.v. of such responses was found in anesthetized cats by CHINN and BARNES (1978). A correlate of the cat nictitating membrane in the rat is the eyelid, whose contraction is sympathetically mediated; the response to hypothalamic stimulation was reduced by 5 mg·kg^{-1} diazepam i.p. (MORPURGO, 1968).

An attenuation by benzodiazepines of the stress-induced activation of the sympathoadrenal system was also found by measuring plasma and urinary catecholamines. Chlordiazepoxide (20 mg·kg^{-1} p.o.) abolished the increase of urinary catecholamine excretion induced by electric foot shock stress in rats (MICHALOVÁ et al., 1966). Also in the rat, 5 mg·kg^{-1} midazolam i.v. almost completely prevented the tremendous increase in plasma noradrenaline and adrenaline produced by exposure of the animals to a 1-min period of inescapable electric foot shock (DA PRADA et al., 1980).

III. Synaptic Transmission in Sympathetic Ganglia

The eyelid contraction in the rat in response to preganglionic cervical stimulation was unaffected by 5 mg·kg^{-1} diazepam i.p. (MORPURGO, 1968). Nictitating membrane contractions in chloralose-urethane anesthetized cats induced by electrical stimulation of the preganglionic nerves at 15·s^{-1} were reduced dose-dependently by diazepam in doses higher than 1 mg·kg^{-1} i.v. (CHAI and WANG, 1966); responses to postganglionic stimulation were unaffected. THEOBALD et al. (1965) found no consistent effect of chlordiazepoxide up to 3 mg·kg^{-1} in intact anesthetized cats. Estazolam (5 mg·kg^{-1} i.v.) moderately depressed the contractile response of the nictitating membrane to preganglionic stimulation in spinal cats; the response to postganglionic stimulation was unaltered (SAJI et al., 1972). No effect of clobazam (10 mg·kg^{-1} i.p., BARZAGHI et al., 1973) or of medazepam (up to 16 mg·kg^{-1} i.v.; RANDALL et al., 1968) was seen on nictitating membrane contractions evoked by preganglionic stimulation.

Using ganglionic surface recording, SCHLOSSER et al. (1977) observed a depolarization and transmission block in the cat superior cervical ganglion after injection of flurazepam in high doses between 3×10^{-7} and 5×10^{-6} mol into the arterial supply of the ganglion. Transmission block, but not depolarization, was antagonized by the GABA antagonists, bicuculline and picrotoxin. In doses below 3×10^{-7} mol, flurazepam and midazolam increased the amplitude and duration of ganglionic depolarization induced by GABA (SCHLOSSER and FRANCO, 1979 a); higher doses decreased the amplitude but still prolonged the duration of GABA-induced depolarization (SCHLOSSER et al., 1977; SCHLOSSER and FRANCO, 1979 a). An inconsistent and extremely weak potentiation of GABA-induced depolarization of the superfused isolated rat superior cervical ganglion was observed with 10^{-6}–10^{-4} mol·l^{-1} chlordiazepoxide (STRAUGHAN, 1977; BOWERY and DRAY, 1978), diazepam, flurazepam, and nitrazepam (STRAUGHAN 1977). However, chlordiazepoxide and diazepam consistently, although slightly, attenuated the blocking effect of bicuculline on GABA-induced depolarization (STRAUGHAN, 1977; BOWERY and DRAY, 1978). The atypical, convulsant benzodiazepine Ro 5–3663 (1 μmol), antagonized ganglionic depolarization induced by GABA and muscimol in the in situ superior cervical ganglion of the cat (FRANCO and SCHLOSSER, 1978); this antagonism was of the mixed competitive-noncompetitive type in the isolated rat superior cervical ganglion (SCHAFFNER et al., 1979).

A series of studies were performed with diazepam ($\geq 10^{-8}$ mol·l^{-1}) on the isolated bullfrog paravertebral sympathetic ganglion. No effects on the resting membrane potential or acetylcholine-induced effects were observed (SURIA and COSTA, 1974 b). EPSPs and IPSPs evoked by isolated single preganglionic stimuli were unaffected (SURIA and COSTA, 1973; SURIA et al., 1975). However, posttetanic potentiation of EPSPs was inhibited by diazepam (10^{-8} mol · l^{-1}) and chlordiazepoxide (10^{-6} mol · l^{-1}), while posttetanic potentiation of IPSPs was enhanced. The effect of diazepam on posttetanic potentiation of IPSPs was mimicked by dibutyryl cyclic 3′,5′-adenosine monophosphate and that on EPSPs by prostaglandins E$_1$ and E$_2$, arachidonic acid, and cyclic 3′,5′-guanosine monophosphate and blocked by SC 19220, a prostaglandin receptor blocker (SURIA and COSTA, 1974a, 1974b). Diazepam 10^{-6} mol · l^{-1} as well as GABA and dibutyryl cyclic 3′,5′-guanosine monophosphate produced a depolarization of presynaptic nerve terminals within the ganglion (SURIA and COSTA, 1975; SURIA, 1976). During this depolarization the amplitude of antidromic spikes induced by stimulation of presynaptic nerve endings was reduced. The effects of diazepam and GABA an presynaptic nerve endings were blocked by picrotoxin. The inhibitors of glutamic acid decarboxylase, isoniazid and thiosemicarbazide, prevented the depolarization of the presynaptic terminals by diazepam, but not that produced by GABA (COSTA et al., 1975c). The authors suggested that the depression of posttetanic potentiation of EPSPs observed after diazepam could be due to a presynaptic effect on transmitter release.

IV. Dorsal Root Ganglia

Diazepam 10^{-5} mol·l^{-1}, applied by superfusion to rat dorsal root ganglia in situ, did not influence the resting membrane potential and membrane conductance, but reduced the amplitude and the time course of the depolarization of ganglion cells produced by short GABA pulses. The amplitude of the depolarization induced by longer pulses of GABA was only minimally affected, whereas the very prolonged depolarization, which is seen after longer GABA pulses, was diminished by diazepam (LAMOUR, 1979; DESARMENIEN et al., 1980).

V. Conclusions

Direct effects of benzodiazepines on peripheral neuronal elements were only observed in concentrations that are well above those occurring after therapeutic doses. It is not surprising that drugs with high liposolubility affect neuronal membrane properties, when incorporated in sufficient amounts in hydrophobic phases of the membrane. These effects may be called "nonspecific" because they occur at much higher concentrations than required to produce the characteristic pharmacologic effects. They may, however, still be somehow specific in the sense that they may differ from those of other agents at comparable high concentrations because of unique structural properties.

Centrally induced changes of the activity of autonomic nervous fibers are to be expected with drugs which, like benzodiazepines, act on diencephalic structures involved in the control and integration of autonomic functions.

Q. Effects on Invertebrate Neurons

The effects of benzodiazepines on spike generation and conduction in invertebrate axons were described in the preceding chapter. A series of papers dealing with the effects of benzodiazepines on neurons of the marine snail, *Aplysia californica* will be briefly discussed.

The R2-cell, the giant cell of the pleural ganglion which has a very stable membrane potential, developed transient membrane potential oscillations in the presence of chlordiazepoxide (MURPHY et al., 1976), flurazepam, and medazepam in concentrations between 10^{-4} and 10^{-3} mol·l^{-1} (HOYER et al., 1976, 1978; HOYER, 1977). This effect on the membrane potential was accompanied either by a facilitation of the synaptic input from the right connective nerve or a suppression of the input from the genital pericardial nerve (MURPHY et al., 1976), which resulted in a firing pattern reminiscent of a bursting pacemaker cell (HOYER et al., 1976, 1978). In the bursting pacemaker cell (R15), chlordiazepoxide induced interburst hyperpolarization, an increased interburst interval, and a recruitment of an inhibitory input. A slight depolarization and a subsequent increase in firing rate, followed later by the appearance of inhibitory periods, was observed in the beating pacemaker cell, R14 (MURPHY et al., 1976). In L3 cells flurazepam (5×10^{-4} mol·l^{-1}) increased the duration and amplitude of the normal membrane potential oscillations. As a consequence of the increased duration of the depolarizing waves more action potentials were triggered per burst (HOYER et al., 1978). 10^{-4}–5×10^{-4} mol·l^{-1} reduced the firing rate, induced oscillations of the resting membrane potential, and sometimes induced double discharges

(HOYER et al., 1976). Regular cells (e.g., R3) became irregular in their firing pattern, whereas irregular cells (e.g., L7) showed a tendency to form bursts or multiple discharges (HOYER et al., 1978). The antidromic spike in R2 or R15 cells was markedly influenced by 10^{-4} mol·1^{-1}–10^{-3} mol·1^{-1} chlordiazepoxide, diazepam, flurazepam, medazepam, and oxazepam (HOYER et al., 1976; HOYER, 1977; MURPHY and KREISMAN, 1977). Overshoot and rate of rise were reduced and the rate of fall was decreased, which resulted in a prolonged action potential of reduced amplitude (HOYER et al., 1976; HOYER, 1977). In the R2 cell, MURPHY and KREISMAN (1977) found these effects of diazepam 10^{-4} mol·1^{-1} to be restricted to the soma spike; Ro 5–4864, a benzodiazepine with no central nervous system effects, was ineffective. The conduction velocity along the axon was reduced under diazepam (10^{-4} mol·1^{-1}) and flurazepam (5×10^{-4} mol·1^{-1}), which led to a conduction block after protracted exposure to flurazepam (HOYER, 1977; MURPHY and KREISMAN, 1977).

The EPSP of R15 cells, evoked by stimulation of the right connective (cholinergic) input, was reduced after 5×10^{-4} mol·1^{-1} flurazepam (HOYER et al., 1976; TREMBLAY and GRENON, 1977). Both benzodiazepines reduced the initial synaptic depression in a train of impulses at 1 Hz; the frequency-dependent facilitation was increased (TREMBLAY and GRENON, 1977; HOYER, personal communication). Posttetanic potentiation (PTP) was reduced, according to TREMBLAY and GRENON (1977). HOYER (personal communication) reported an enhancement and prolongation of posttetanic potentiation after 5×10^{-4} mol·1^{-1} flurazepam. In the same cell (R15) TREMBLAY and GRENON (1977) observed a weak depolarization and a slight reduction of the membrane resistance after flurazepam. IPSPs evoked in L5 or L12 cells after activation of the interneuron L8 were abolished within 10 min after 10^{-4} mol·1^{-1} flurazepam. This effect was irreversible after prolonged exposure (HOYER et al., 1976).

Iontophoretic application of acetylcholine to cells of the abdominal or pleural ganglion evokes a depolarization or hyperpolarization of the cell, which is accompanied by an increased or reduced activity in spontaneously active cells. The facilitation of cell firing was usually inhibited by benzodiazepines, whereas the reduction of spontaneous activity was only slightly affected (HOYER et al., 1976; HOYER, 1977). Some cells show a hyperpolarization in response to acetylcholine, consisting of two components: one with a short latency and a reversal potential corresponding to the equilibrium potential of Cl^- (~ -60 mV) and the other with a longer latency and a reversal potential corresponding to that of K^+ (~ -80 mV). Flurazepam, medazepam, oxazepam, and chlordiazepoxide at 2.5×10^{-4}–5×10^{-4} mol·1^{-1} blocked the short latency Cl^--dependent acetylcholine hyperpolarization but left the longer latency response virtually unaffected (HOYER et al., 1976; HOYER, 1977).

Aplysia neurons show different types of responses to iontophoretic GABA. The most common response is a fast hyperpolarization produced by a Cl^--conductance increase which is sensitive to bicuculline or picrotoxin (YAROWSKY and CARPENTER, 1978). This Cl^--dependent hyperpolarization was reversibly antagonized by 5×10^{-4} mol·1^{-1} flurazepam, whereas Na^+-dependent GABA depolarization was unaffected (HOYER, personal communication).

HOYER et al. (1976, 1978) studied the effects of flurazepam (2.5×10^{-4} and 5×10^{-4} mol·1^{-1}) under voltage clamp conditions on the current-voltage relationship of slow currents determining the resting membrane potential and of the more transient and much larger currents that flow during the action potential or during the depolarization. In R2 cells, a negative slope of the I-V curve for the slow current was observed under flurazepam. In cells with this negative slope under control conditions, such as R15, this property was accentuated under flurazepam. The much larger inward and outward currents flowing during an action potential or a membrane depolarization were reduced during the exposure to flurazepam, the Ca^{2+}-dependent K^+-outward current being more depressed. The inward current was shifted to more positive voltages. A fast inactivation of the outward current occurred in the presence of flurazepam.

Exposure of leeches to $1 \text{ mmol} \cdot l^{-1}$ flurazepam or $5 \text{ mmol} \cdot l^{-1}$ chlorazepate induced initial agitation followed by reduced activity, unresponsiveness to tactile stimuli, and complete anesthesia; all effects were easily reversible in drug-free solution (CORRADETTI et al., 1980). No specific ^{3}H-diazepam binding could be found in leech ganglia.

The relatively simple nervous systems of invertebrates are favoured models for the study of drug effects on neuronal membranes. Indeed, they have provided a great deal of useful detailed information on drug actions on passive and active properties of membranes and on the interaction of agents with specific neurotransmitters. In the case of benzodiazepines, however, the results obtained in invertebrate systems should be extrapolated with great caution to central neurons of higher animals and man. First, the concentrations that affected invertrebrate neurons were 10–1,000 times higher than the concentration of benzodiazepines determined in the brain of animals after pharmacologic doses. Second, the specific receptors, to which benzodiazepines bind with high affinity to induce their characteristic effects, are absent in invertebrates (NIELSEN et al., 1978). It seems, therefore, that the effects observed on invertebrate neurons are related rather to the effects of sublethal and lethal doses of benzodiazepines and not to their pharmacologic effects.

R. Effects of Spinal Cord Functions

The effects of benzodiazepines on spinal cord functions have been studied intensively for several reasons. One was to compare the effects of benzodiazepines with those of older muscle relaxant anxiolytics represented by meprobamate, which had been claimed to be an "interneuron blocking agent" (BERGER, 1954). The spinal cord is a favorite object of neuropharmacologists, because the rather advanced knowledge of its neuronal circuitry, the relative ease with which defined excitatory and inhibitory pathways can be stimulated and input-output relations studied, permit one to characterize a drug with respect to its actions on certain types of synapses or certain types of neuronal activity. A further advantage of spinal cord pharmacology is the possibility of isolating the cord at will from peripheral and/or central influences, which helps considerably in defining the site of action of a compound. It is not surprising, therefore, that the first evidence for a selective action of benzodiazepines on GABAergic synapses was obtained in spinal cord preparations. Whereas a great number of data are available on the effects of these drugs on motor functions of the spinal cord, little is known about their possible effects on sensory functions in the cord.

Early studies on benzodiazepines had already revealed their potent actions on spinal cord activities. In chloralose-anesthetized cats, polysynaptic flexor reflex contractions of the tibialis anterior muscle evoked by stimulation of the sciatic nerve were blocked by 2–3 mg·kg^{-1} chlordiazepoxide i.v. (Randall, 1960; Randall et al., 1961) and diazepam (0.4 mg·kg^{-1}) (Randall et al., 1961). These early findings were confirmed and extended in many laboratories. A drug may modulate synaptic transmission in the spinal cord of intact animals either by a primary action on supraspinal structures controlling spinal cord activities, or by a primary action within the spinal cord, or by a combination of both. We first discuss results which suggest or demonstrate a supraspinal site of action of benzodiazepines in modulating spinal cord activities.

I. Effects on Spinal Cord Activities Through a Supraspinal Site of Action

The finding that diazepam and nitrazepam (1–10 mg·kg^{-1} p.o., i.p. or i.v.) clearly diminished muscle tone in unrestrained freely moving cats without inducing somnolence or sleep (Hernández-Peón et al., 1964; Hernández-Peón and Rojas-Ramírez, 1966; Ghelarducci et al., 1966) led to the hypothesis that benzodiazepines depress spinal cord activities by reducing a tonic facilitatory influence exerted by the brain stem on spinal γ-motoneurons (Ghelarducci et al., 1966). These authors found in freely moving as well as in unanesthetized decerebrate and spinal cats that neither monosynaptic reflexes nor dorsal root potentials (DRPs) were affected by 1 mg·kg^{-1} nitrazepam i.v., a dose inducing marked hypotonia. Furthermore, the same dose of nitrazepam abolished the so-called γ-rigidity following precollicular decerebration, while leaving unaffected the α-rigidity produced by ablation of the cerebellum. The suggested supraspinal site of action received strong support from the study of Ngai et al. (1966). In decerebrate unanesthetized cats, they consistently observed that the marked depressant effect of low doses of diazepam (0.05 mg·kg^{-1} i.v.) on polysynaptic crossed extensor reflexes disappeared after subsequent spinal cord transection and that further injections of the drug had little additional effect on this reflex. The monosynaptic knee jerk was unaffected in decerebrate as well as in spinal cats (Ngai et al., 1966). On the other hand, facilitation and inhibition of the knee jerk induced by stimulation of the mesencephalic and bulbar reticular formation, respectively, were markedly reduced by diazepam (0.1 mg·kg^{-1} i.v.). The same dose of diazepam also depressed polysynaptic segmental reflexes and spontaneous activity of mesencephalic reticular neurons in decerebrate cats (Przybyla and Wang, 1968), but was much less effective on polysynaptic reflexes and spontaneous firing of spinal interneurons in spinal animals (Tseng and Wang, 1971 b). Depressant effects on the polysynaptic reflexes similar to those found after diazepam were observed in decerebrate cats with other benzodiazepines. In this respect clonazepam was the most potent compound (0.05 mg·kg^{-1} i.v.), followed by nitrazepam (0.1 mg·kg^{-1}), bromazepam (0.2 mg·kg^{-1}), and flurazepam (1 mg·kg^{-1}, Tseng and Wang, 1971 a). Additional evidence for a site of action of benzodiazepines in the brain stem was provided by studies in the rat. Diazepam (0.3 mg·kg^{-1} i.v.) diminished monosynaptic and polysynaptic spinal reflexes in intact anesthetized and decerebrate rats, but not in spinal rats (Nakanishi and Norris, 1971). Similarly, mono- and polysynaptic reflexes were reduced by oral administration of diazepam (10 mg·kg^{-1}), chlordiazepoxide (50 mg·kg^{-1}), and medazepam (50 mg·kg^{-1}) in decerebrate, but not in spinal rats (Kido et al., 1972). Schlosser et al. (1975 a, b) studied long latency spino-bulbospinal reflexes recorded in the ventral roots, elicited in chloralose-anesthetized cats by stimulation of the hind- and forelimb muscle as well as cutaneous afferents. These reflexes were depressed by diazepam in extremely small doses (0.01 mg·kg^{-1} i.v.), whereas a higher dose (0.1 mg·kg^{-1}) was required to reduce segmental mono- and polysynaptic ventral root reflexes in the same cat. A reflex response of the efferent nerve fibres to the posterior biceps muscle to stimulation of preganglionic fibres in the splanchnic nerve afferents ("viscerosomatic" reflex) was also very sensitive to the depressant effect of diazepam (0.001 mg·kg^{-1}). Conversely, diazepam (0.1 mg·kg^{-1} i.v.) was less potent in depressing efferent discharges of the preganglionic splanchnic nerve elicited by stimulation of the forelimb cutaneous afferents in the same intact anesthetized cats ("somatovisceral" reflex).

II. Effects Within the Spinal Cord

1. Mono- and Polysynaptic Reflexes

More recent studies have shown that in addition to a supraspinal site, benzodiazepines undoubtedly have a direct action on the spinal cord. HUDSON and WOLPERT (1970) used intact anesthetized, decerebrate, and spinal cats. While confirming the resistance to these drugs of the knee jerk in spinal as opposed to decerebrate animals, they found a depression of the facilitatory and inhibitory reticular effect on the knee jerk to be exerted by the same doses of diazepam (0.125–0.25 mg·kg^{-1} i.v.) which reduced facilitation of the knee jerk induced by sciatic nerve stimulation in spinal cats. Since facilitation of the knee jerk induced by stimulation of cervical spinal cord segments in spinal cats was also depressed by diazepam, the authors assumed that the drug was acting within the spinal cord, possibly in the region where supraspinal descending pathways impinge on the spinal cord neurons.

The finding that the knee jerk was not affected by benzodiazepines in intact anesthetized cats but that the monosynaptic reflex responses recorded in the ventral roots were depressed led CRANKSHAW and RAPER (1970) to propose that the mechanically evoked and recorded knee jerk with its asynchronous afferent input was more resistant to diazepam than the electrically evoked monosynaptic ventral root potentials, which are caused by synchronous volleys in afferents induced by single electrical shocks. Interestingly, SWINYARD and CASTELLION (1966) found monosynaptic ventral root reflexes elicited by single shocks applied to the dorsal roots to be unaltered in spinal cats after clonazepam. In contrast, small doses of this drug (0.05 mg·kg^{-1} i.v.) markedly reduced monosynaptic ventral root reflexes evoked by repetitive dorsal root stimulation.

Apart from this study, however, most investigators observed a depression by benzodiazepines of monosynaptic and polysynaptic ventral root reflexes induced by single shock afferent stimuli in spinal cats (SCHMIDT et al., 1967; CHANELET and LONCHAMPT, 1971; BLUM et al., 1973; POLC et al., 1974; MURAYAMA et al., 1972; POLC, unpublished observations).

2. γ-Motoneuron Activity

γ-Motoneurons, which discharge tonically in decerebrate and, to a smaller extent, in spinal cats, were markedly depressed by benzodiazepines in decerebrate cats (diazepam 1 mg·kg^{-1} i.v. in BALTZER and BEIN, 1973; doses of 0.2 mg·kg^{-1} of nitrazepam,

diazepam, and estazolam i.v. in Chiba and Nagawa, 1973; 0.1 mg·kg⁻¹ diazepam
i.v. in Polc et al., 1974; 0.01–0.05 mg·kg⁻¹ diazepam i.v. in Takano and Student,
1978). Similar doses of diazepam (0.1 mg·kg⁻¹ i.v.) were necessary to reduce the γ-
activity in spinal cats (Polc et al., 1974). This remarkably strong action of benzodiazepines on the γ-system, which is probably overactive in spasticity, would in part
explain the alleviation by diazepam of spastic symptoms in patients with complete
spinal cord transection (Cook and Nathan, 1967). Indirect (Polc et al., 1974) and
more direct evidence (Takano and Student, 1978) suggests that diazepam reduces
the activity of both dynamic and static γ-motoneurons.

3. Posttetanic Potentiation, Reciprocal and Recurrent Inhibition and Excitability of Motoneurons and Primary Afferents

Investigations including tests for posttetanic potentiation of monosynaptic ventral
root reflexes, disynaptic reciprocal and recurrent inhibition as well as direct excitability of motoneurons and primary afferent endings, failed to demonstrate any effects
of benzodiazepines on these parameters (Swinyard and Castellion, 1966; Schmidt
et al., 1967; Schlosser, 1971; Stratten and Barnes, 1971; Chanelet and Long-
champt, 1971; Polc, 1978; Nistri et al., 1980).

4. Presynaptic Inhibition

Schmidt et al. (1967) were the first to show that diazepam increased presynaptic inhibition of monosynaptic ventral root reflexes and enhanced depolarization of primary afferents recorded as dorsal root potentials (DRPs) in lightly anesthetized spinal
cats (Fig. 1). Doses of diazepam as small as 0.05 mg·kg⁻¹ increased the two presynaptic inhibitory phenomena, while larger doses (up to 0.5 mg·kg⁻¹ i.v.) were ineffective in postsynaptic inhibition, suggesting a selective action of diazepam on presynaptic inhibition in the spinal cord. This observation was later confirmed by all investigators and extended to other benzodiazepines as well as to other mammalian species
(Schlosser and Zavatski, 1969; Schlosser, 1971; Stratten and Barnes, 1971;
Chanelet and Lonchampt, 1971; Chiba and Nagawa, 1973; Menétrey et al., 1973;
Blum et al., 1973; Polc et al., 1974; Polc, unpublished observations; Chin et al., 1974;
Banna et al., 1974; Haefely et al., 1975b; 1978; Murayama et al., 1972; Murayama
and Suzuki, 1975; Suzuki and Murayama, 1976; Polzin and Barnes, 1976; Nicot
et al., 1976; Naftchi and Lowman, 1977; Naftchi et al., 1979). It is clear that the
spinal cord itself is the primary site of action for this effect of benzodiazepines on presynaptic inhibition, and some authors even believe that enhancement of presynaptic
inhibition may be the only direct action of benzodiazepines on the spinal cord (Stratten and Barnes, 1971; Chiba and Nagawa, 1973).

In several studies, presynaptic inhibition in the spinal cord evoked by stimulation
of supraspinal structures was also found to be affected by benzodiazepines. DRPs induced by stimulation of the brain stem reticular formation were enhanced by doses
of diazepam which were somewhat larger than those required to increase presynaptic
inhibition evoked by peripheral stimulation (0.3 mg·kg⁻¹ diazepam i.v. in Polc et al.,
1974; 1 mg·kg⁻¹ diazepam i.v. in Polzin and Barnes, 1976). In contrast, DRPs
evoked by cortical stimulation or heterosensory (optic and acoustic) stimuli were depressed by diazepam (Menétrey et al., 1973), and it is reasonable to suggest that this

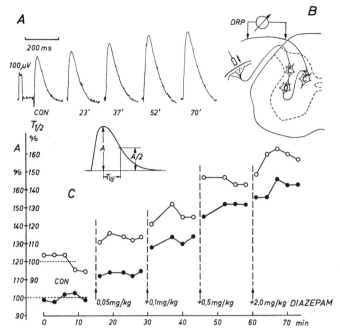

Fig. 1 A–C. Effect of diazepam on dorsal root potentials (DRP) in a cat under light pentobarbitone anesthesia. **A** shows averaged DRP at different times corresponding to the graphic presentation in **C**. DRP were elicited by mechanical deformation of the palmar skin of a hindleg (700 μm for 5 ms) and recorded from a L_7 dorsal rootlet as indicated schematically in **B**. In **C** are plotted the amplitude *(filled circles)* and the time for half-life *(open circles)* of DRP at times indicated on the *abscissa*. Diazepam was injected intravenously at the times indicated by *arrows*. The *ordinate* has a left-hand scale for the amplitude and a right-hand scale for the time to half-life of the DRP. (From SCHMIDT et al., 1967)

reduction was due to an effect of diazepam on supraspinal structures, and not at the axo-axonal synapses in the spinal cord. With accumulating evidence in the early 1970s that presynaptic inhibition in the spinal cord was mediated by a GABAergic interneuron (see CURTIS and JOHNSTON, 1974; LEVY, 1977), the early finding of a potentiating effect of benzodiazepines on this inhibition by SCHMIDT et al. (1967) and subsequent investigators appeared in a new light. Indeed, the possibility had to be considered that the action of benzodiazepines was closely related with GABAergic function. POLC et al. (1974) showed that the GABA antagonist, bicuculline, and benzodiazepines behaved as mutual surmountable antagonists in their effect on presynaptic inhibition, i.e. depression by bicuculline of presynaptic inhibition could be overcome by benzodiazepines and the benzodiazepine-induced potentiation reversed by the convulsant. Inhibition of GABA synthesis by thiosemicarbazide (POLC et al., 1974) or semicarbazide (BANNA et al., 1974) depressed presynaptic inhibition, but this depression could not be overcome with diazepam. These findings clearly indicated that the effect of benzodiazepines depended on the availability of GABA for release onto primary afferent endings but, of course, could not specify the exact locus of action of this drug in the pathway mediating presynaptic inhibition.

Attempts to answer the question of whether enhancement of presynaptic inhibition could account for all direct effects of benzodiazepines on the spinal cord went along two lines. Chanelet and Lonchampt (1971) studied the effect of local microinjection of diazepam (0.2–0.8 µl, 3.5×10^{-3} mol·l^{-1}) into different regions of the lumbosacral spinal cord of the cat. Diazepam reduced mono- and polysynaptic ventral root reflexes when injected into the ventral horn (lamina VII), but augmented DRP only if applied to the dorsal part of the dorsal horn (laminae I, II, and III). These findings are, however, no proof that reflex depression and enhancement of primary afferent depolarization are caused by two different effects of diazepam. Indeed, the concentration of the drug was rather high and might have affected ventral root reflexes in a nonspecific way; moreover, benzodiazepines might potentiate presynaptic inhibition at a site remote from the axo-axonal synapses on primary afferent endings, e.g., on GABergic cell bodies. A different approach for analyzing a possible causal connection between enhanced presynaptic inhibition and depression of reflex activity and γ-motoneuron discharge rates was used by Polc et al. (1974). They studied the effects of diazepam on various spinal cord activities after pharmacologically manipulating GABA synthesis and catabolism as well as receptor functions. On the one hand, thiosemicarbazide-induced augmentation of mono- and polysynaptic reflexes and depression of presynaptic inhibition were not antagonized by diazepam, indicating that the effectiveness of presynaptic inhibition could be responsible for the effect of diazepam on spinal reflexes. On the other hand, reflexes and γ-motoneuron activity were unaffected by aminooxyacetic acid (AOAA), a GABA-transaminase inhibitor. Hence, the important question of whether benzodiazepines have different, unrelated actions in the spinal cord, remains open. However, there is little doubt that presynaptic inhibition plays an important part in the central muscle relaxant action of benzodiazepines; in conditions of reduced presynaptic inhibition, such as in chronic spinal dogs and cats (Naftchi and Lowman, 1977; Naftchi et al., 1979), as well as in patients with incomplete cord transections (Verrier et al., 1975) and multiple sclerosis (Delwaide, 1970) diazepam (10–20 mg i.v.) concurrently increased presynaptic inhibition and reduced spasticity. In contrast, in cats made spastic by a temporary occlusion of the thoracic aorta, which preferentially destroys spinal interneurons, the virtually abolished DRPs were no longer enhanced by diazepam (Murayama and Suzuki, 1974).

5. Positive Dorsal Root Potentials

A more complex phenomenon, the so-called positive or hyperpolarizing DRPs, which is believed to represent disinhibition of primary afferent endings from a tonic depolarization (Mendell and Wall, 1964) and which can be elicited by stimulation of the bulbar and/or pontine reticular formation, was found to be inconsistently enhanced or depressed by diazepam (Polzin and Barnes, 1976).

6. Isolated Hemisected Frog Spinal Cord

While ventral root potentials evoked by dorsal root stimulation were slightly depressed (Pixner, 1966; Padjen and Bloom, 1975) or abolished (Evans et al., 1977) after addition of diazepam (0.5 mmol·l^{-1}) or chlordiazepoxide (1 mmol·l^{-1}) to the bath, DR-DRPs were either unaffected (Padjen and Bloom, 1975) or prolonged after diazepam (PIXNER, 1966) and flurazepam ($2.5 \, \mu mol \cdot l^{-1}$, NISTRI and CONSTANTI, 1978 a, b). If tetrodotoxin (TTX) was given before benzodiazepines to block the propagated impulse activity, diazepam ($0.5 \, mmol \cdot l^{-1}$) had no direct effect on motoneurons, but antagonized motoneuronal depolarization induced by the excitatory amino acid analogue, N-methyl-d-aspartate, without influencing depolarizations by glutamic and quiscalic acid (EVANS et al., 1977). Also in the isolated hemisected spinal cord of the frog exposed to TTX, flurazepam ($2.5–5 \, \mu mol \cdot l^{-1}$) had no consistent direct action on primary afferent endings, but depressed glutamate-induced depolarization of primary afferents. Flurazepam enhanced primary afferent depolarization induced by GABA at $2.5 \, \mu mol \cdot l^{-1}$; however, it depressed the effect of GABA with $5 \, \mu mol \cdot l^{-1}$ (NISTRI and CONSTANTI, 1978 a, b). In the frog hemisected spinal cord bathed in a medium containing high magnesium to block indirect synaptic effects, chlordiazepoxide ($10^{-4} \, mol \cdot l^{-1}$) selectively enhanced GABA-induced hyperpolarization of motoneurons without affecting hyperpolarizing responses to β-alanine and depolarization by glutamate (NICOLL and WOJTOWICZ, 1980). The drug had no direct GABA-mimetic action in contrast to barbiturates, which had a direct hyperpolarizing effect on motoneurons and reduced glutamate depolarization.

7. Isolated Hemisected Spinal Cord of the Immature Rat

In this preparation, diazepam ($50 \, \mu mol \cdot l^{-1}$) potentiated the responses of motoneurons to l-homocysteate and to a lesser extent to l-glutamate, but depressed the GABA-induced primary afferent depolarization (EVANS, 1977).

8. Activity of Single Interneurons

In unanesthetized spinal cats, diazepam ($0.05–0.1 \, mg \cdot kg^{-1}$ i.v.) slightly depressed the spontaneous firing of unidentified interneurons (TSENG and WANG, 1971 b). In anesthetized intact cats, the iontophoretic application of the thienotriazolodiazepine derivative, Ro 11–7800, on unidentified interneurons slightly reduced the amplitude of extracellularly recorded action potentials, suggesting a local anesthetic activity of this drug (CURTIS et al., 1976 b). In anesthetized spinal cats, DAVIES and POLC (1978) observed no decrease of the spontaneous firing of Renshaw cells and other, unidentified interneurons after iontophoretic application of midazolam. However, midazolam reduced the excitation of Renshaw cells by iontophoretic acetylcholine more than excitation by kainic acid (a potent, rigid analogue of glutamate) and N-methyl-d-aspartate (a potent analogue of aspartate). After intravenous injection, midazolam ($1 \, mg \cdot kg^{-1}$) depressed the activation of Renshaw cells elicited by submaximal orthodromic stimuli in dorsal roots, but not the stimulation evoked by ventral root stimulation. In unanesthetized spinal cats, $0.1 \, mg \cdot kg^{-1}$ diazepam i.v. depressed Renshaw cell spontaneous activity and discharges in response to submaximal ventral root volleys (POLC, unpublished).

9. Intracellular Studies on Spinal Motoneurons

Lumbosacral motoneurons of dial-anesthetized cats were recorded with a KCl-containing microelectrode, which increased the intracellular Cl^- concentration and thereby reversed the usually hyperpolarizing effect of GABA and muscimol into a depolarizing one. Iontophoretic application of flurazepam had no GABA-mimetic depolarizing action but selectively potentiated the effect of GABA and muscimol, but not of glycine. Intracellularly injected flurazepam and midazolam failed to affect the weak hyperpolarizing effect of intracellularly injected GABA, which is thought to result from the electrogenic Na^+-coupled transport of GABA (CONSTANTI et al., 1980; NISTRI et al., 1980).

10. Cultured Spinal Cord

In neurons of chick spinal cord in culture the pressure ejection of chlordiazepoxide in concentrations up to 10^{-4} mol·l^{-1} did not alter membrane potential or membrane conductance (CHOI et al., 1977). In a smaller concentration (10^{-7} mol·l^{-1}) the drug selectively augmented the depolarization produced by iontophorized GABA without affecting the response to glycine. Inhibitory synaptic potentials elicited by electrical stimulation of the culture were enhanced by chlordiazepoxide (10^{-7} mol·l^{-1}) and blocked by bicuculline (10^{-4} mol·l^{-1}). Very similar results were obtained by MACDONALD and BARKER (1978) in spinal cord cultures of the mouse with small amounts of iontophorized chlordiazepoxide. However, higher amounts of the drug depressed GABA-induced depolarizations and occasionally produced depolarization and conductance increase by themselves. In a recent study on cultured mouse spinal neurons, MACDONALD et al. (1979) observed a depolarizing response to flurazepam and desensitization to this effect upon repeated iontophoretic application of the drug.

III. Conclusions

It is well documented that benzodiazepines affect various neuronal activities in the spinal cord by both a supraspinal and a spinal site of action. At the supraspinal level, descending reticulospinal pathways, in particular those with a facilitatory influence on γ-motoneurons, appear to be very sensitive to benzodiazepines. At the spinal level, the most prominent effect of benzodiazepines is their marked enhancement of primary afferent depolarization subserving presynaptic inhibition. Whether the drugs depress spontaneous γ-motoneuron activity and mono- and polysynaptic reflexes by an additional mechanism independent of supraspinal control systems and intraspinal presynaptic inhibition, remains to be clarified. Most important, benzodiazepines lack any direct action on the excitability of motoneurons and primary afferent endings, and they fail to affect postsynaptic inhibition and posttetanic potentiation of ventral root reflexes in the spinal cord. Benzodiazepines in low concentration selectively enhance the synaptic effects of GABA. In marked contrast to the mechanisms subserving motor functions in the spinal cord, those involved in sensory processing have so far not been studied under the effect of benzodiazepines.

S. Effects on Dorsal Column Nuclei

The results obtained by POLC and HAEFELY (1976) with benzodiazepines in the cat dorsal column nuclei were crucial for the proposal (HAEFELY et al., 1975b, 1978) that

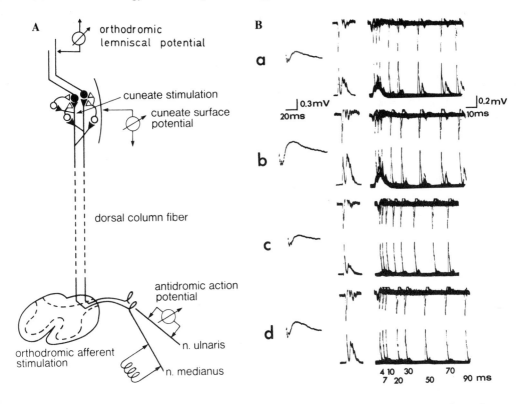

Fig. 2 A, B. Effect of diazepam on pre- and postsynaptic inhibition in the cuneate nucleus of a decerebrate cat and the interaction between diazepam and picrotoxin. **A** Schematic diagram of the pathways studied and of the sites of stimulation and recording. **B** Single cuneate surface potentials in *stabil left vertical row*; the N-wave (downward deflections) reflects monosynaptic excitation of cuneothalamic relay cells, the P-wave (upward wave) the depolarization of dorsal column fiber endings induced by orthodromic stimulation of the ipsilateral median nerve. The four pairs of potentials in the *second vertical row* are lemniscal potentials *(upper trace)* and the antidromic potential followed by the dorsal column reflex in the ulnar nerve *(lower trace)*; both potentials in each pair of traces were evoked by single shocks through an electrode within the nucleus ("cuneate stimulation" in **A**). The *third vertical row* shows the same potentials as the second row, but now elicited in intervals of 4, 7, 10, 20, 30, 50, 70, and 90 ms following a conditioning volley in the median nerve. The four horizontal rows are records in the control period a), after $0.3 \; mg \cdot kg^{-1}$ diazepam i.v. b), following $1 \; mg \cdot kg^{-1}$ picrotoxin i.v. after the first dose of diazepam c), and after a second dose of $1 \; mg \cdot kg^{-1}$ diazepam d). Diazepam did not alter the N-wave but increased the P-wave of the cuneate surface potential; it did not affect the excitability of cuneothalamic relay cells or of dorsal column fiber endings in the absence of conditioning stimuli *(second vertical row)*, but clearly enhanced the depression of cuneothalamic cells (due to postsynaptic inhibition) as well as the increase of excitability of primary afferents (due to depolarization of the endings of dorsal column fibers). Picrotoxin abolished the effect of the first dose of diazepam, but this blockade was overcome by a second, larger dose of diazepam. (From POLC and HAEFELY, 1976)

these drugs acted specifically as enhancers of GABAergic synaptic transmission. In fact, the clear-cut enhancement of presynaptic inhibition in the spinal cord and even the demonstration that this effect of benzodiazepines was entirely dependent on endogenous GABA (POLC et al., 1974; BANNA et al., 1974) did not permit one to decide whether these drugs selectively interacted with GABAergic synaptic transmission or with the special mechanism underlying primary afferent depolarization. POLC and HAEFELY (1976), therefore, decided to study the effect of benzodiazepines on a structure where GABA had been demonstrated to mediate both presynaptic and postsynaptic inhibition, and for this end the dorsal column nuclei offered themselves, with the additional advantage of relatively simple experimental accessibility. Impulses conducted in dorsal column fibers not only impinge on relay cells in the cuneate nucleus, which further project to the thalamus via the lemniscal pathway but, through collaterals, also excite GABA interneurons in this nucleus that produce primary afferent depolarization in much the same way as in the spinal cord, and, in addition, induce IPSPs in the relay cells, thus producing postsynaptic inhibition (CURTIS and JOHNSTON, 1974). Various benzodiazepines were found to simultaneously enhance presynaptic and postsynaptic inhibition in the cat cuneate nucleus (Fig. 2) and the same interactions of these drugs with GABA antagonists and inhibitors of GABA synthesis were found as were observed earlier in the spinal cord (POLC et al., 1974). These results made it clear that benzodiazepines were able to enhance the two types of synaptic inhibition which differ fundamentally in their mechanisms and functional consequences, but which in common had to be mediated by GABAergic interneurons. An important aspect of these interneurons is that they can be excited by inputs from both the periphery and higher forebrain structures. The functional consequence of enhanced presynaptic and postsynaptic inhibition after benzodiazepines in the dorsal column nuclei is not yet clear; it could depress overall sensory input and/or sharpen afferent signals from the periphery through increased lateral inhibition. The studies in the cuneate nucleus also showed that even high doses of benzodiazepines did not depress excitatory transmission in this structure, measured as the N-wave, according to ANDERSEN et al. (1964), in contrast to, e.g., barbiturates which dose-dependently depressed the synaptic excitatory transmission in the cuneate nucleus (POLC and HAEFELY, 1976). Unlike muscimol, the most potent GABA-mimetic drug, benzodiazepines did not affect the resting excitability of primary afferents and cuneo-thalamic relay cells (POLC and HAEFELY, 1978). Therefore, as in the spinal cord, enhancement of the GABAergic pre- and postsynaptic inhibition in the cuneate nucleus by benzodiazepines cannot be related to a direct activation of GABA receptors or a release of GABA from resting interneurons, but rather to some as yet unknown mechanism.

T. Benzodiazepines and Evoked Potentials in the Brain

A number of investigators have explored the action of benzodiazepines on potentials evoked in different brain regions by either sensory (visual, auditory) stimuli or electrical stimulation of the peripheral nerves or the brain itself. This technique, which contributed considerably to the identification of cerebral pathways, has also proved to be useful in studying sites of action of drugs.

I. Limbic Structures

In unanesthetized *cerveau isolé* cats, chlordiazepoxide (2–5 mg · kg^{-1} i.v.) reduced the amplitude of potentials evoked in the hippocampus by single shocks applied to the ipsilateral amygdala (MORILLO et al., 1962). Another study, using unanesthetized *cerveau isolé* and *encéphale isolé* cats, extended these observations to diazepam (2 mg · kg^{-1} i.v.), which clearly depressed the amygdalo-hippocampal evoked potentials and responses evoked in the amygdala by stimulation of the thalamic anteroventral nucleus, but failed to consistently affect the interhippocampal response evoked by contralateral hippocampal stimulation (MORILLO, 1962). Since the same dose of diazepam was ineffective on the cortical arousal response to high-frequency stimulation of the reticular formation, MORILLO (1962) concluded that benzodiazepines selectively depressed amygdalohippocampal connections, in particular in the amygdala. Similar results to those obtained by MORILLO et al. (1962) were later found by other investigators. In a systematic study in unanesthetized, immobilized cats, JALFRE et al. (1971) and HAEFELY (1978) observed a significant depression of the amplitude and, to a smaller extent, an increase in the latency of the amygdalo-hippocampal evoked potential after a dose as small as 0.003 mg · kg^{-1} flunitrazepam i.v. Diazepam (0.2 mg · kg^{-1}), chlordiazepoxide (0.8 mg · kg^{-1}), and medazepam (5.4 mg · kg^{-1}) were also effective, but less potent than flunitrazepam. In a series of experiments on unrestrained, freely moving cats and monkeys, GUERRERO-FIGUEROA et al. (1969 a) recorded local evoked potentials from several subcortical and cortical structures, which were elicited by stimuli applied by an electrode located at a distance of 0.2–0.5 mm from the recording electrodes. Clonazepam (1 mg · kg^{-1} i.p.) and diazepam depressed local evoked potentials not only in the septum, amygdala, and hippocampus, but also in the mesencephalic reticular formation, posterior and lateral hypothalamus, intralaminar thalamus, and preoptic area. In contrast, after oral administration of a much higher dose of clonazepam (15 mg · kg^{-1}), local evoked potentials in the subcortical substrates, assumed to be responsible for "anxiety" (posterior hypothalamus, reticular formation, amygdala), were depressed, whereas those in the intralaminar thalamus and cortex were unaffected. Local evoked potentials in septum, preoptic area, hippocampus, and lateral hypothalamus (substrates supposed to be responsible for "reward") were even enhanced (GUERRERO-FIGUEROA et al., 1969 b). Qualitatively similar effects were found with bromazepam and chlordiazepoxide (GUERRERO-FIGUEROA et al., 1973), triflubazam, a 1,5-benzodiazepine (GUERRERO-FIGUEROA and GALLANT, 1971) and lorazepam (GUERRERO-FIGUEROA et al., 1974). Since the same augmenting effects upon locally evoked potentials in the "reward" structures were observed after chronic administration of flurazepam as well as after oral administration of diazepam, bromazepam, chlordiazepoxide, and triflubazam, GUERRERO-FIGUEROA et al. (1973, 1974) postulated that a shift in the balance of activities from the "anxiety"-producing substrates to the "reward" system is relevant for the anxiolytic action of benzodiazepines.

Using multiple recording from different parts of the limbic system and diencephalon in unanesthetized immobilized cats, TSUCHIYA and KITAGAWA (1976) and TSUCHIYA (1977) observed a depression of hippocampal potentials evoked by stimulation of the amygdala, hypothalamus, and the central gray matter after several benzodiazepines (diazepam and fludiazepam).

The septohippocampal evoked potentials, however, were not affected by chlordi-azepoxide in curarized cats (SCHAFFNER et al., 1974). Rather high doses of nitrazepam ($7.5 \, \text{mg} \cdot \text{kg}^{-1}$ i.v.; $20\text{–}50 \, \text{mg} \cdot \text{kg}^{-1}$ p.o.) were used by VIETH et al. (1968) in their estimation of the threshold voltage needed to induce intracerebral evoked responses in unrestrained cats. Whereas interamygdaloid evoked potentials remained unaltered, nitrazepam markedly raised the stimulation threshold in the reticular formation and the hypothalamus for evoked responses in septum, amygdala, and hippocampus. In another study on immobilized *encéphale isolé* cats (HOLM, 1969), somewhat lower doses of nitrazepam ($3 \, \text{mg} \cdot \text{kg}^{-1}$ i.v.) elevated the stimulation threshold in the amygdala to evoke responses in all brain structures studied. However, only evoked potentials recorded in the hippocampus on stimulation of the reticular formation were clearly depressed after nitrazepam, while there was a slight elevation of the stimulus threshold in the reticular formation for evoked responses in the amygdala, centrum medianum thalami, ventroanterior thalamic nucleus, lateral hypothalamus, midbrain reticular formation, caudate nucleus, and pallidum. Opposite results to those obtained by HOLM (1969) were found by HEINEMANN et al. (1970) in unrestrained cats with slow intravenous infusion of medazepam. The stimulation thresholds for evoked responses in amygdaloid central nucleus to stimulation of septum and medial thalamus and vice versa, i.e., evoked responses in septum and medial thalamus to stimulation of the amygdala, were lowered during medazepam infusion. On the other hand, the connections between hippocampus and amygdala as well as between hippocampus and septum and thalamus were depressed, i.e., the thresholds for evoked potentials elicited and recorded within the amygdala, hippocampus, septum, and thalamus were elevated. In spite of marked divergence between the results of HOLM (1969) and HEINE-MANN et al. (1970) as well as the difficulty of interpretation because of the complexity of the results, the amygdala seemed to be the area most susceptible to the effect of benzodiazepines in both studies. In urethane-anesthetized rats, diazepam ($5 \, \text{mg} \cdot \text{kg}^{-1}$ i.v.) reduced posttetanic potentiation of the field potentials recorded from the pyramidal cells of the contralateral hippocampus upon stimulation of the dorsal hippocampal surface, but failed to affect the posttetanic potentiation of the granule cells or the responses to single stimuli (MATTHEWS and CONNOR, 1976). In contrast, evoked potentials in the hippocampal dentate area, elicited by single shocks applied to the ipsilateral entorhinal cortex and interpreted as synchronous excitation of granule cells, were markedly depressed by nitrazepam ($5 \, \text{mg} \cdot \text{kg}^{-1}$ i.p.) medazepam ($10 \, \text{mg} \cdot \text{kg}^{-1}$), and chlordiazepoxide ($30 \, \text{mg} \cdot \text{kg}^{-1}$) in unanesthetized rats (ANDREAS, 1978). KOBAYASHI et al. (1980) investigated the effect of benzodiazepines on amygdalo-cortical pathways. Short-latency negative responses in the gyrus proreus in response to stimulation of the magnocellular basal nucleus of the amygdala were depressed by $0.1\text{–}0.2 \, \text{mg} \cdot \text{kg}^{-1}$ physostigmine i.v., $10 \, \text{mg} \cdot \text{kg}^{-1}$ diazepam p.o., and $5\text{–}10 \, \text{mg} \cdot \text{kg}^{-1}$ chlordiazepoxide i.v. The authors suggested that benzodiazepines depressed the gyrus proreus responses by interacting with cholinergic inhibitory mechanisms.

II. Hypothalamus and Thalamus

The importance of the hypothalamus as a site of action of benzodiazepines was emphasized by MIYAKE (1965), who found a depression after chlordiazepoxide ($20 \, \text{mg} \cdot \text{kg}^{-1}$ i.p.) of the potential in the posterior hypothalamus evoked by single shocks in the sciatic nerve and of the facilitated hippocampal response to paired hypothalamic stimuli. In contrast, the same dose of chlordiazepoxide did not affect the evoked potentials elicited by sciatic nerve stimulation in the cortex, medial thalamus, reticular formation, hippocampus, and amygdala or the facilitation of the hypothalamic response evoked by paired stimuli in the limbic system. In anesthetized intact cats, diazepam (1 mg $\cdot$ kg^{-1} i.v.) depressed the excitability and elevated the threshold for evoked responses in the sensorimotor cortex induced by paired pulses applied to the ipsilateral ventrolateral thalamus (ENGLANDER et al., 1977). In unrestrained cats and unanesthetized *encéphale isolé* rabbits, chlordiazepoxide (10 mg $\cdot$ kg^{-1} i.v.), diazepam (2 mg $\cdot$ kg^{-1} i.v.) and the oxazolobenzodiazepine CS 370 (2 mg $\cdot$ kg^{-1} i.v.) reduced the evoked potentials in the central gray matter and, to a smaller degree, responses in the red nucleus and substantia nigra evoked by sciatic nerve stimuli. But even with much higher doses of the benzodiazepines the cortical recruiting response to thalamic stimuli was not affected (MORI et al., 1972). In unrestrained rabbits a high dose of chlordiazepoxide (30 mg $\cdot$ kg^{-1} i.v.) which was without effect on the recruiting cortical response to thalamic stimuli, increased the cortical responses evoked by hippocampal and reticular stimulation (MONNIER and GRABER, 1962). An enhancement of cortical evoked potentials in response to a stimulation of the unspecific thalamus and medial hypothalamus, and a diminution of the cortical response to a stimulation of the amygdala, was observed after chlordiazepoxide in unrestrained rabbits (SOLLERTINSKAYA and BALONOV, 1972).

III. Substantia Nigra

Single shocks in the caudate nucleus of the unanesthetized curarized cat evoke simple potentials in the ipsilateral substantia nigra pars compacta, which most probably represent the mass of IPSPs induced in nigral dopamine neurons mediated by the striatonigral GABAergic pathway, since the evoked response was dose-dependently depressed by picrotoxin and bicuculline, but resistant to strychnine (SCHAFFNER and HAEFELY, 1975; HAEFELY et al., 1975 b, 1978). Various benzodiazepines failed to affect the striatonigral evoked response, although they very potently prevented the depressant effect of bicuculline (HAEFELY et al., 1978).

IV. Brain Stem Reticular Formation

On the one hand, HERNÁNDEZ-PEÓN et al. (1964) and HERNÁNDEZ-PEÓN and ROJAS-RAMÍREZ (1966) found a clear-cut reduction by diazepam (5 mg $\cdot$ kg^{-1} i.p.) and nitrazepam (1 mg $\cdot$ kg^{-1} i.p.) of click-evoked potentials in the mesencephalic reticular formation in unrestrained cats, which showed no somnolence or sleep. On the other hand, chlordiazepoxide (2 mg $\cdot$ kg^{-1} i.v.) slightly enhanced the response evoked in the midbrain reticular formation by a stimulation of the sciatic nerve and the bulbopontine reticular formation in unanesthetized rabbits (WHITE et al., 1965).

V. Lateral Vestibular Nucleus

In the lateral vestibular nucleus of Deiters of unanesthetized curarized cats, single stimuli administered to Purkinje cell axons in the cerebellar white matter elicited a complex evoked field potential (HAEFELY et al., 1978). One component of this evoked potential was readily abolished by bicuculline and picrotoxin, but not by strychnine. As observed in the substantia nigra, various benzodiazepines prevented the depressant effect of bicuculline. Their order of potency was the same as in the usual pharmaco-logic screening tests for benzodiazepines.

VI. Visual System

Chlordiazepoxide produced a reversible diminution of the β-wave of the electroretino-gram of the isolated rabbit retina when applied in a very high concentration (10^{-3} mol $\cdot$ 1^{-1}) (HOMMER, 1968). A high dose of diazepam (4 mg $\cdot$ kg^{-1} i.v.) increased the latency of the visual cortical evoked potentials induced by light flashes (HEISS et al., 1969) in unanesthetized immobilized cats. In fact, much smaller doses of oxazepam (1–10 mg $\cdot$ kg^{-1} i.v. or i.p.) and clobazam (1.25 mg $\cdot$ kg^{-1} i.p.) reduced the amplitude of the late negative phase of the visual evoked responses in the retina, lateral genicu-late body and cortex to light flashes in unanesthetized cats and chronically implanted rabbits (DOLCE and KAEMMERER, 1967; GOLDBERG et al., 1974; GERHARDS, 1978). Within the same line of evidence, in midpontine pretrigeminal unanesthetized cats, BARNES and MOOLENAAR (1971) observed a depression by diazepam (1 mg $\cdot$ kg^{-1} i.v.) of the post-primary cortical evoked response to optic tract stimulation. In addition, these authors found a facilitation of the light-induced changes of the cortical response to the optic tract stimulation and an inhibition of the flash-produced enhancement of the cortical evoked potential in response to retinal stimulation after diazepam. Both picrotoxin-sensitive effects were attributed by BARNES and MOOLENAAR (1971) to an increase by diazepam of the presynaptic inhibition of neurons in the lateral geniculate body and the retina, respectively. A depression of cortical evoked responses to light flashes was also found by SHERWIN (1971) after diazepam (0.5 mg $\cdot$ kg^{-1} i.v.) in unan-esthetized immobilized cats. Similarly, the visual evoked responses to light flashes in the tectotegmental midbrain area of unrestrained rats were reduced by chlordiazepox-ide and diazepam (5 mg $\cdot$ kg^{-1} i.p.) (OLDS and BALDRIGHI, 1968).

VII. Cerebral Cortex

In addition to the cortical visual evoked potentials just discussed, rather recent evi-dence points to an action of benzodiazepines on nonvisually evoked responses at the cortical level. FRANK and JHAMANDAS (1970), using slabs of neuronally isolated cortex in decerebrate cats, observed a depression by diazepam (1–2 mg $\cdot$ kg^{-1} i.v.) of the sur-face-negative and surface-positive responses to a cortical surface stimulation. In un-anesthetized immobilized cats, transcallosal evoked potentials were not consistently altered by chlordiazepoxide (10–30 mg $\cdot$ kg^{-1} i.v.), whereas polysynaptic cortical evoked responses to sciatic nerve stimulation were reduced and their latency increased (GIURGEA and MOYERSOONS, 1972). On the other hand, potentials in the contralateral sensory-motor cortex elicited by tooth pulp stimulation were unaffected by chlordiaz-epoxide (10 mg $\cdot$ kg^{-1} i.p.), nitrazepam (10 mg $\cdot$ kg^{-1}), or clonazepam (1 mg $\cdot$ kg^{-1}). The same doses of the benzodiazepines, however, markedly diminished posttetanic potentiation of the tooth pulp-induced cortical evoked potentials in unanesthetized rabbits (BANSI et al., 1976). A discrete reduction of the amplitude and of the peak in the secondary complex of the somesthetic potential in the cortex evoked by sciatic nerve stimulation was found after diazepam and medazepam (5 mg·kg^{-1} s.c.) in the unanesthetized rat (LEHMANN and SCHMIDT, 1979). Further direct evidence for the cortical site of action of benzodiazepines was provided by ZAKUSOV et al. (1975, 1977). In the functionally isolated cortex of unanesthetized cats, diazepam (0.5 mg·kg^{-1} i.v.) depressed the early facilitation of the intracortical test response to paired cortical stimuli. In intact unanesthetized cats and rats diazepam also increased the early depression of the primary cortical test response to stimulation of the forepaw skin, induced by conditioning stimulation of the somatosensory cortex. All these effects of diazepam were reversibly antagonized by bicuculline, pentetrazole, and thiosemicarbazide. Since the dose of diazepam (0.5 mg·kg^{-1}), which increased the inhibition of the primary cortical response was virtually ineffective on the hippocampal evoked response to forepaw stimulation as well as on the interhippocampal potential, ZAKUSOV et al. (1975) assumed that benzodiazepines influenced neuronal circuitry in the neocortex more readily than in the hippocampus. Another investigation in unanesthetized immobilized cats confirmed and extended these observations to other benzodiazepines (ZAKUSOV et al., 1977). Clonazepam and lorazepam (0.1 mg·kg^{-1} i.v.) were more potent than diazepam (0.5 mg·kg^{-1} i.v.) and medazepam (20 mg·kg^{-1} i.v.) in depressing the early facilitation of the intracortical test response to paired stimuli applied to the somatosensory cortex.

VIII. Conclusions

From the numerous studies of evoked potentials in the brain no very clear picture of the effects of benzodiazepines emerges. The reasons for this are manifold. Few of the studies were systematic enough with respect to, e.g., the doses used. Dose-effect relations were only rarely examined; in many cases, the unique dose deliberately chosen was well above the therapeutic range. Moreover, an assessment of the significance of a given alteration of a distinct evoked potential by benzodiazepines requires that the effect of other centrally active agents in the same experimental situation be known. The interpretation of drug-induced changes in evoked potentials is not as simple as is often believed. Theoretically, drugs can affect an evoked potential by altering the excitability of the neuronal structures that are stimulated; such an alteration may result from a direct effect of drugs on the stimulated structures although this excitability may also be changed by influences from other structures that are primarily affected by a drug. Drugs may affect the neuronal pathway connecting the site of stimulation to the site of recording either directly or indirectly through other structures controlling the pathway. In evoked potential studies performed with benzodiazepines, constant (and deliberately chosen) intensities of stimulation were used; in only a few studies was the threshold of stimulation for a defined response measured. But even in the latter case, the exact site of a drug-induced alteration of the threshold cannot be deduced with certainty. In conclusion, considering the complex nature of evoked potentials in the brain and the many ways by which drugs may alter these responses, the available literature suggests that benzodiazepines affect many central structures. It seems, nevertheless, that certain brain areas are particularly sensitive to the effect of benzodiazepines, among them limbic cortical and subcortical structures; indeed, afferent and efferent connections of limbic areas were generally affected by smaller doses than were other pathways. However, the neocortex also appears to be an important target structure for benzodiazepines. It is probably more than mere coincidence that limbic structures and neocortex are among the brain areas containing the highest density of GABAergic synapses and of high-affinity binding sites for benzodiazepines. Future studies of evoked potentials with benzodiazepines should attempt to establish the role of GABAergic mechanisms in these responses.

U. Effects on Cortical and Subcortical Electroencephalogram (EEG)

Under this heading we discuss the effects of benzodiazepines on the animal EEG in the widest sense, i.e., on the electrical brain activity as it is recorded with macroelectrodes from the surface of the cerebral cortex (electrocorticogram, ECoG) as well as from subcortical structures considering drug-induced changes (a) in the composition of the spontaneous EEG in qualitative and quantitative terms; (b) in the EEG response to various natural or artificial stimuli (arousal reaction, recruiting and augmenting response, caudate spindles); (c) in the paroxysmal EEG pattern that is induced by and outlasts the repetitive stimulation within the same or other brain structures. Not included in this paragraph is the effect of benzodiazepines on the amount and organization of sleep, although these studies, of course, are based on the recording of EEG (see next section).

I. Spontaneous EEG

Studies in the early 1960s, performed by visual analysis in unanesthetized and unrestrained freely moving animals revealed a characteristic increase after benzodiazepines of a fast burst of spindle-like activity in the β-range, i.e., a pattern with high-frequency waves of high amplitude in the EEG.

In unanesthetized immobilized cats, chlordiazepoxide ($1.5 \, \text{mg} \cdot \text{kg}^{-1}$ i.v.) and diazepam ($0.5 \, \text{mg} \cdot \text{kg}^{-1}$ i.v.) induced rapid waves in the neocortex and hippocampus, which were grouped as spindle-like bursts (REQUIN et al., 1963). Virtually the same effects as after diazepam were found with nitrazepam ($0.5 \, \text{mg} \cdot \text{kg}^{-1}$ i.v.) in unanesthetized curarized cats (LANOIR et al., 1965); in freely moving cats with chronically implanted cortical and subcortical electrodes, nitrazepam ($0.5 \, \text{mg} \cdot \text{kg}^{-1}$ i.m.) led to the appearance of rapid high voltage waves in the neocortex, hippocampus, and amygdala, the latter structure exhibiting paroxysmal bursts of fast EEG-activity (LANOIR et al., 1965). A shift to higher frequencies in the spontaneous EEG was also observed in the neocortex of unrestrained freely moving cats after oral administration of chlordiazepoxide ($10 \, \text{mg} \cdot \text{kg}^{-1}$) and diazepam ($5 \, \text{mg} \cdot \text{kg}^{-1}$) (SCHALLEK and KUEHN, 1965). WINTERS and KOTT (1979) studied the effect of various doses of diazepam on EEG and behavior of freely moving cats with chronically implanted cortical and subcortical electrodes. Low doses of diazepam ($0.2\text{–}0.6 \, \text{mg} \cdot \text{kg}^{-1}$ i.p.) induced a so-called relaxed behavior characterized by an oscillation between wakefulness and sedation and predominance of 12–13 Hz waves in the EEG. Higher doses ($1\text{–}5 \, \text{mg} \cdot \text{kg}^{-1}$ i.p.) produced a transient period of sedation followed by activation and ataxia for 20–30 min. The EEG was dominated by high-frequency low-amplitude activity. About 30 min after the injection the phase of activation was followed by a phase of oscillation between activation and a prehypnotic state characterized by the cat's lying on one side and being unresponsive to noise (but responsive to noxious stimuli); the EEG had a mixed pattern of slow 7–9 Hz waves intermingled with high-frequency low-amplitude activity. The highest doses of diazepam used (10–15 mg · kg^{-1} i.p.) produced brief periods of sedation and activation, and, within 15 min after the injection, a hypnotic state behaviorally similar to the prehypnotic state but with reduced responsiveness to noxious stimuli. The EEG had a mixed pattern of 12–13 Hz bursts on a background of 3–4 Hz waves. Multiunit activity in the reticular formation was unaffected after the lowest doses of diazepam but depressed during the prehypnotic and hypnotic states. Rather high doses of chlordiazepoxide (30–40 mg · kg^{-1} i.v.) elicited in unanesthetized restrained rabbits slow waves and spindles in the neocortex, hippocampus, caudate nucleus, and medial thalamus for 30–60 min; this activity was then replaced by an EEG of small amplitude with the exception of the hippocampus, where both the frequency and amplitude of EEG-waves were increased (MONNIER and GRABER, 1962). In the same animal preparation, similar high intravenous doses of chlordiazepoxide (20–40 mg · kg^{-1}) and diazepam (5–10 mg · kg^{-1}) induced a mixed pattern of slow EEG waves intermingled with fast activity in the neocortex, whereas a general slowing of the EEG was found in subcortical structures (ARRIGO et al., 1965). In freely moving rabbits, the EEG during sleep induced by chlordiazepoxide (50 mg · kg^{-1} p.o.) was characterized by regular periodic bursts of fast activity (14–15 Hz) superimposed on slow waves in the motor cortex and caudate nucleus, an effect which was even more pronounced after nitrazepam (20 mg · kg^{-1} p.o.) (SOULAIRAC et al., 1965). Very similar effects were observed in more recent studies with diazepam, a new 1,4-benzodiazepine (1D 690; WATANABE et al., 1974) and flurazepam (OHMORI, 1977). Triazolam (0.2–0.5 mg · kg^{-1} i.v.) altered the EEG to a "drowsy pattern" (UEKI et al., 1978).

An interesting phenomenon appeared in a drug interaction study in freely moving rabbits (SCOTTI DE CAROLIS et al., 1969): the potent GABA agonist, muscimol (2 mg · kg^{-1} i.v.) produced tremor and ataxia, along with an EEG pattern consisting of slow (1–2 Hz) high amplitude waves intermingled with spikes in the cortex. Additional injection of diazepam (0.5–1 mg · kg^{-1} i.v.) dramatically changed the EEG, which became isoelectric with some interspersed spikes. This peculiar EEG effect, accompanied by a flaccid paralysis of the animal's musculature, was also observed to a smaller extent with pentobarbitone (10 mg · kg^{-1} i.v.) given after muscimol. In unrestrained rats, nitrazepam (10 mg · kg^{-1} p.o.) evoked a mixed pattern with fast waves superimposed on slow EEG activity in the neocortex and hippocampus during behavioral sleep, whereas EEG activity in the reticular formation and the olfactory bulb was virtually unaltered (SOULAIRAC et al., 1965). An intraperitoneal injection of chlordiazepoxide (10 mg · kg^{-1}) induced two types of fast spindle-like activity, one at 12–15 Hz and the other, burst-like, at 25–30 Hz in the neocortex of unrestrained rats. The simultaneous appearance of large slow waves characterized the EEG of subcortical structures (SZEKELY et al., 1974). In curarized rats, clonazepam (0.1 mg · kg^{-1} i.p.) induced slow high voltage waves (1–3 Hz) intermingled with spindle-like 10–13 Hz waves of high amplitude in the neocortex (HEIDLER et al., 1979). In baboons restrained in a chair, diazepam (2 mg · kg^{-1} i.p.) induced a fast electrocorticogram (ECoG) and attentive behavior; in the absence of drugs the monkeys were drowsy with an EEG pattern of synchronized 8–13 Hz rhythm (BOUYER et al., 1978). The authors ascribed the effect of diazepam to normalization of behavior altered by the stress of restraint, because the same pattern of fast activity (13–18 Hz) which was seen after diazepam in the restrained monkeys, also characterized the EEG of unrestrained, undrugged animals.

The first study of benzodiazepines using computer-assisted analysis of the EEG was done by EIDELBERG et al. (1965). By measuring the distribution of the spectral density of EEG, these authors observed in freely moving cats a clear-cut depression of the high-voltage spindling peak (40 Hz) in the amygdala without consistent changes in other subcortical and cortical structures after intraperitoneal injections of diazepam (5 mg·kg^{-1}), nitrazepam (2 mg·kg^{-1}), and flunitrazepam (1 mg·kg^{-1}). Power spectral analysis of the EEG in immobilized unanesthetized cats revealed an enhanced relative power in the frequency of 9–30 Hz in the cortex, hippocampus, and caudate nucleus after diazepam (10–20 mg·kg^{-1} i.v.), medazepam (20 mg·kg^{-1}), and chlordiazepoxide (10–20 mg·kg^{-1}), (SCHALLEK et al., 1968; SCHALLEK et al., 1970; SCHALLEK and THOMAS, 1971). In the squirrel monkey after diazepam (1 mg·kg^{-1} p.o.) and flurazepam (10–20 mg·kg^{-1} p.o.), two peaks in the power spectrum were observed in the ECoG, one in frequencies below 8 Hz and the other in the 20–50 Hz range, whereas the frequencies between 8 and 20 Hz were depressed (SCHALLEK and JOHNSON, 1976). JOY et al. (1971), using *Macaca nemestrina*, obtained results essentially similar to those obtained by SCHALLEK and JOHNSON (1976), although some subtle differences were apparent between various benzodiazepines. Low intramuscular doses of diazepam (0.1–1 mg·kg^{-1}), nitrazepam (1 mg·kg^{-1}), chlordiazepoxide (15 mg·kg^{-1}), clonazepam (0.1 mg·kg^{-1}), and flunitrazepam (0.1 mg·kg^{-1}) enhanced the spindle-like cortical activity in the β-frequency band (15–30 Hz) and at the same time reduced the aggressiveness without inducing sedation or ataxia. On the other hand, sedation occurred simultaneously with diminished aggressivity after a low intramuscular dose of medazepam (1 mg·kg^{-1}), which induced a slowing in the α-band and increased spindles. Finally, prazepam (up to 2 mg·kg^{-1} i.m.) did not increase spindle activity, even at doses producing ataxia. Higher doses of most benzodiazepines, however, decreased α-activity (8–13 Hz) and increased the activity in a low frequency band (< 5 Hz) in the neocortex and hippocampus, accompanied by sedation and ataxia. In *Macaca mulatta*, long-term ECoG recordings made it possible to evaluate the temporal changes in the spectral density after administration of various benzodiazepines and meprobamate. GEHRMANN and KILLAM (1978) observed interesting differences between meprobamate, which increased power and induced temporal stability at higher frequency bands (16–64 Hz) only with sedative doses (100 mg·kg^{-1} p.o.), benzodiazepine derivatives, which produced little sedation with doses (chlordiazepoxide, 20 mg·kg^{-1} p.o.; clonazepam, 0.04 mg·kg^{-1} i.m.) producing moderate energy increases at medium frequency (8–32 Hz) bands, and a benzodiazepine derivative with more sedative properties (chlorazepate, 7.5 mg·kg^{-1} p.o.) showing intermediate effects with more pronounced energy increases and a marked temporal fluctuation. In a study on unanesthetized restrained rabbits and decerebrate cats, diazepam and clobazam (3–10 mg·kg^{-1} i.p.) decreased the spectral density in the theta (5–8 Hz) and α-band, but increased power in the β-frequency band (> 15 Hz) (GERHARDS, 1978). Most recent experiments, performed on freely moving cats using telemetric EEG recording, revealed an enhanced fast activity (20–60 Hz) in the neocortex, midbrain reticular formation, medial amygdala and, especially, hippocampus after a low oral dose of diazepam ($0.5 \, \text{mg} \cdot \text{kg}^{-1}$). A simultaneous suppression of the hippocampal theta-rhythm as well as a decrease of the slower (5–20 Hz) and very fast frequencies (70–100 Hz) was noticed in all brain regions studied: cortex, hippocampus, amygdala, and mesencephalic reticular formation (HALLER, 1979).

In a few studies the effects of benzodiazepines on the spontaneous EEG activity of some particular structures were studied. In unanesthetized, immobilized, and chronically prepared rabbits, the spontaneous EEG of the red nucleus changed from predominant high frequency waves of small amplitude, observed also in adjacent brain regions of the alert rabbit, to a regular rhythm of 20–25 Hz after intravenous injections of high doses of chlordiazepoxide ($50 \, \text{mg} \cdot \text{kg}^{-1}$), diazepam ($8 \, \text{mg} \cdot \text{kg}^{-1}$), and oxazepam ($150 \, \text{mg} \cdot \text{kg}^{-1}$), but not nitrazepam ($8 \, \text{mg} \cdot \text{kg}^{-1}$) (GOGOLAK et al., 1969). A similar, but somewhat slower, regular EEG pattern (6–20 Hz) was found after medazepam ($50 \, \text{mg} \cdot \text{kg}^{-1}$ i.v.) and clonazepam ($2 \, \text{mg} \cdot \text{kg}^{-1}$ i.v.) in the anterior cerebellar lobe of unanesthetized curarized rabbits (GOGOLAK et al., 1972). The significance of this drug-induced rhythmic EEG activity in the cerebellorubral system remains unclear, although the abolition of this rhythm in the red nucleus after bilateral lesions of the brachium conjunctivum indicated that the rhythm originated in the cerebellum (GOGOLAK et al., 1970). In curarized rabbits, strychnine (0.1–$0.5 \, \text{mg} \cdot \text{kg}^{-1}$ i.v.) also induced a rhythmic activity in the cerebellorubral system, which was characterized by waves of higher amplitude than those seen with benzodiazepines. Interestingly, this strychnine effect was blocked by a rather low dose of clonazepam ($0.2 \, \text{mg} \cdot \text{kg}^{-1}$ i.v.; GOGOLAK et al., 1974). DE TRUJILLO et al. (1977) recorded the electrical activity of the cerebellar vermis and lumbar spinal cord in unanesthetized immobilized rabbits. Diazepam ($1 \, \text{mg} \cdot \text{kg}^{-1}$ i.v.) markedly augmented cerebellar 25 Hz waves without affecting the electrospinogram. The same dose of diazepam did not affect bursts of the high voltage spikes at 8–12 Hz induced by harmine ($2 \, \text{mg} \cdot \text{kg}^{-1}$ i.v.) in the cerebellum, although it abolished the same paroxysmal activity occurring after harmine in the spinal cord.

II. Arousal Reaction

Since the classic study of MORUZZI and MAGOUN (1949), demonstrating that high-frequency electrical stimulation of the brain stem reticular formation reproduced all electrocortical phenomena observed in the EEG arousal reaction associated with natural wakefulness, many studies have shown that the same pattern of low-voltage fast activity can be elicited in the cortex and hippocampus by stimulation of afferent pathways, posterior hypothalamus, and nonspecific thalamic nuclei (references in MAGOUN, 1963). In particular, changes of the electrical current or voltage required to induce EEG arousal by high frequency reticular stimulation were used to detect a drug effect on the ascending activating reticular system, assuming this to be a measure of drug effect on the excitability of the nonspecific reticular system and, hence, on vigilance.

The original finding of MORILLO (1962) that diazepam ($2 \, \text{mg} \cdot \text{kg}^{-1}$ i.v.) did not consistently affect the cortical arousal elicited by stimulation of the mesencephalic reticular formation in unanesthetized *encéphale isolé* cats at a dose that induced changes in the electrical activity of the limbic system, was later frequently observed in unanesthetized immobilized, and, unrestrained cats with various benzodiazepines. Chlordiazepoxide (1.5 mg·kg⁻¹ i.v.) and diazepam (0.5 mg·kg⁻¹ i.v.) did not alter the stimulus threshold for cortical EEG arousal in the reticular formation in unanesthetized immobilized cats (REQUIN et al., 1963). Similarly, nitrazepam up to a dose of 4 mg·kg⁻¹ i.v. did not alter the arousal threshold, although the EEG waves were higher and slower than during the control EEG arousal reaction (LANOIR et al., 1965) in unanesthetized curarized cats. In the same preparation, doses of clonazepam as low as 0.08–0.1 mg·kg⁻¹ i.v. markedly elevated the threshold for cortical arousal in the midbrain reticular formation, in contrast to chlordiazepoxide, diazepam, and nitrazepam (VUILLON-CACCIUTTOLO et al., 1970). In unrestrained cats, a depression of the EEG arousal reaction in the olfactory bulbs to hypothalamic stimuli was observed after nitrazepam (1 mg·kg⁻¹ i.p.; HERNÁNDEZ-PEÓN and ROJAS-RAMÍREZ, 1966). Also in unrestrained cats, KIDO et al. (1966) found an interesting difference in the action of chlordiazepoxide (20 mg·kg⁻¹ p.o.) on the EEG arousal reaction induced by stimulation of reticular formation and central gray matter. While chlordiazepoxide was without effect on the threshold in the reticular formation for cortical arousal, it markedly elevated the threshold in the central gray matter for hippocampal arousal. DOLCE and KAEMMERER (1967) observed a slight increase in the EEG arousal threshold in the reticular formation after oxazepam (1–10 mg·kg⁻¹ i.v., p.o., i.p., i.m.) in unanesthetized immobilized cats. In unanesthetized encéphale isolé cats, nitrazepam (0.5 mg·kg⁻¹ i.v.) did not clearly affect the threshold of stimulation in the pontine reticular formation for cortical arousal, but raised the threshold of hypothalamic stimulation for cortical arousal (VIETH et al., 1968). No change in the threshold stimulus in the reticular formation for cortical arousal was found in unrestrained as well as unanesthetized immobilized cats after flurazepam 1 mg·kg⁻¹ p.o. (RANDALL et al., 1969) and medazepam 12 mg·kg⁻¹ p.o. (SCHALLEK et al., 1970). The latter drug, however, elevated the threshold in the amygdala for cortical arousal (SCHALLEK et al., 1970). Similarly, chlordiazepoxide (10–40 mg·kg⁻¹ p.o.), diazepam (2–40 mg·kg⁻¹ p.o.), and a new 1,4-benzodiazepine (CS 370, 10–40 mg·kg⁻¹ p.o.) failed to affect the cortical arousal to reticular and hypothalamic stimuli in experiments of MORI et al. (1972) on unrestrained cats. Estazolam, which was ineffective on the cortical arousal response to reticular and sciatic nerve stimulation, raised the threshold of hypothalamic stimulation for cortical arousal in unanesthetized immobilized cats (FUKUDA et al., 1974). The same authors furthermore observed an elevated threshold in the hypothalamus and thalamus for hippocampal arousal in cerveau isolé cats after the same doses (0.25–0.5 mg · kg⁻¹ i.v.) of estazolam. In unanesthetized immobilized cats the cortical arousal response to sciatic nerve stimulation was depressed by diazepam (0.5 mg·kg⁻¹ i.v., ITO and SHIMIZU, 1976).

Rather inconsistent results were obtained in unanesthetized restrained, and, unrestrained rabbits with various benzodiazepines on the EEG arousal response in cortex and hippocampus to brain and/or peripheral afferent stimulation. High intravenous doses of chlordiazepoxide (30–40 mg · kg⁻¹) elevated the threshold in the reticular formation and posterior hypothalamus for cortical arousal (MONNIER and GRABER, 1962) in restrained unanesthetized rabbits. In the same preparation, lower intravenous doses of diazepam (1.25 mg·kg⁻¹) and nitrazepam (0.8 mg·kg⁻¹) also raised the threshold for cortical arousal in the midbrain reticular formation and proprioceptive afferents (GOGOLAK and PILLAT, 1965). However, as in cats, no effects of an oxazolobenzodiazepine (CS 370) (2 mg·kg⁻¹ i.v., 10–40 mg·kg⁻¹ p.o.), chlordiazepoxide

$(10–40 \text{ mg} \cdot \text{kg}^{-1}$ p.o.), or diazepam $(2–40 \text{ mg} \cdot \text{kg}^{-1}$ p.o.) were found in unanesthetized *encéphale isolé* rabbits upon the cortical arousal reaction to reticular and hypothalamic stimulation (MORI et al., 1972). In unrestrained rabbits, diazepam $(0.1–1 \text{ mg} \cdot \text{kg}^{-1}$ i.p.) and fludiazepam $(0.1–1 \text{ mg} \cdot \text{kg}^{-1})$ as well as flurazepam $(0.5 \text{ mg} \cdot \text{kg}^{-1}$ i.v.) elevated the threshold for hippocampal arousal in the hypothalamus (OTSUKA et al., 1975) and for cortical arousal in reticular formation, hypothalamus, and auditory system (OHMORI, 1977), respectively. Similarly, triazolam $(0.2–0.5 \text{ mg} \cdot \text{kg}^{-1}$ i.v.) suppressed the EEG arousal response to auditory stimuli and electrical stimulation of the mesencephalic reticular formation and posterior hypothalamus (UEKI et al., 1978).

In unanesthetized immobilized, and, unrestrained rats benzodiazepines did not seem to induce clear-cut changes in the EEG arousal reaction to stimulation of the reticular formation (TAKAGI et al. 1967, with chlordiazepoxide $40 \text{ mg} \cdot \text{kg}^{-1}$ i.p.; SOULAIRAC et al., 1965, with nitrazepam $20 \text{ mg} \cdot \text{kg}^{-1}$ p.o.). However, the threshold for hippocampal arousal in the reticular formation and, particularly, in the hypothalamus was elevated by chlordiazepoxide $(40 \text{ mg} \cdot \text{kg}^{-1}$ i.p., TAKAGI et al., 1967).

III. Hippocampal Theta-Rhythm

The regular rhythm of large amplitude slow EEG waves (5–7 Hz), the so-called theta-rhythm, was recognized by GREEN and ARDUINI (1954) to be a pattern of hippocampal activation, associated frequently with the low-voltage fast activity of the cortical EEG arousal described above. Most characteristically, benzodiazepines were found to depress the theta-activity of the hippocampus, both occurring spontaneously in attentive animals and during REM sleep and induced by brain stem stimulation, in unrestrained and restrained cats, rabbits and rats. Some of the effects of benzodiazepines on the spontaneous hippocampal theta-activity were described in the subheading under spontaneous EEG. Additional observations revealed a shift of the theta-rhythm to lower frequencies (3–4 Hz) during the REM sleep and wakefulness after diazepam $(2 \text{ mg} \cdot \text{kg}^{-1}$ p.o.), nitrazepam $(1 \text{ mg} \cdot \text{kg}^{-1}$ p.o.), and lorazepam $(1 \text{ mg} \cdot \text{kg}^{-1}$ p.o.) (BORENSTEIN et al., 1973), as well as after flunitrazepam $(0.1 \text{ mg} \cdot \text{kg}^{-1}$ i.p.) in unrestrained cats (POLC and HAEFELY, 1975) and with chlordiazepoxide $(20 \text{ mg} \cdot \text{kg}^{-1}$ i.p.) in unrestrained rats (IWAHARA et al., 1972). A reduction of hippocampal theta-activity was also found with flurazepam and a new 1,4-benzodiazepine (ID 690) in unrestrained rabbits (HASHIMOTO et al., 1973; OHMORI, 1977; WATANABE et al., 1974) as well as with diazepam and fludiazepam in unrestrained cats (OTSUKA et al., 1975) during wakefulness. Different benzodiazepines (diazepam, nitrazepam, flurazepam, and estazolam) diminished the frequency of the hippocampal theta-rhythm from 5 to 3 Hz during REM sleep as well as wakefulness in unrestrained cats (YAMAGUCHI et al., 1979).

The theta-rhythm occurring as the hippocampal arousal response to peripheral afferent and brain stimulation was depressed in unanesthetized rabbits by diazepam $(1.25 \text{ mg} \cdot \text{kg}^{-1}$ i.v.) and nitrazepam $(0.8 \text{ mg} \cdot \text{kg}^{-1}$ i.v.) (GOGOLAK and PILLAT, 1965). In unanesthetized *encéphale isolé* cats, a disappearance of the theta-rhythm induced by stimulation of pontine reticular formation was found after $0.5 \text{ mg} \cdot \text{kg}^{-1}$ nitrazepam i.v. (VIETH et al., 1968). Similarly, in unanesthetized immobilized cats clonazepam $(0.08–1 \text{ mg} \cdot \text{kg}^{-1}$ i.v.) reduced the theta-activity elicited by nociceptive stimulation (VUILLON-CACCIUTTOLO et al., 1970). The stimulation threshold for inducing hippocampal theta-rhythm in the thalamus and hypothalamus was elevated after estazolam (0.25–0.5 mg·kg⁻¹ i.v.) in unanesthetized *cerveau isolé* cats (FUKUDA et al., 1974) as well as with diazepam (0.1 mg·kg⁻¹ i.p.) and fludiazepam (0.1 mg·kg⁻¹) in unrestrained rabbits (OTSUKA et al., 1975), and with nitrazepam (1 mg·kg⁻¹ i.p.) and nimetazepam (1 mg·kg⁻¹) in unrestrained cats (OTSUKA et al., 1973). In an attempt to elucidate the mechanisms underlying the effects of benzodiazepines on the theta-rhythm, GRAY et al. (1975) found that chlordiazepoxide (4 mg·kg⁻¹ i.p.) elevated the threshold for driving the theta-frequency at 7.7 Hz in the hippocampus by septal stimulation in freely moving rats. Since similar effects were obtained after the suppression of activity in the noradrenergic neuronal system arising from the locus coeruleus, GRAY et al. (1975) proposed that an inhibition by benzodiazepines of noradrenergic tone in hippocampus may be the cause of their pronounced depressant effect on the theta-rhythm. In another study on freely moving rabbits, where an operant conditioning test was combined with the EEG recording, diazepam (2 mg·kg⁻¹ i.m.) shifted the hippocampal theta-rhythm to lower frequencies and simultaneously reduced the cortical arousal reaction during a conditioned avoidance response (BONFITTO et al., 1975).

IV. Cortical Recruiting and Augmenting Response

MORISON and DEMPSEY (1942) first described the progressively increasing wave-like response of the cortical EEG to low-frequency electrical stimulation of the medial thalamus. This cortical recruiting response resembles spontaneous spindle bursts, and both phenomena were thought to originate in the nonspecific thalamic nuclei which are involved in sleep mechanisms (references in MORUZZI, 1972). Effects of drugs on cortical recruiting were most frequently interpreted as alterations in thalamocortical mechanisms for internal inhibition and light sleep. A similar "waxing and waning" cortical response, the so-called augmenting response, can be elicited by low frequency stimulation of specific thalamic nuclei and is limited to the corresponding projection area of the cortex (MORISON and DEMPSEY, 1942).

The cortical recruiting response was not affected by high intravenous doses of chlordiazepoxide (30–40 mg·kg⁻¹) in restrained rabbits (MONNIER and GRABER, 1962) and by lower intravenous doses (2–5 mg·kg⁻¹) of the same compound in unanesthetized *cerveau isolé* cats (MORILLO et al., 1962). No consistent effect on the cortical recruiting was also observed after chlordiazepoxide (1.5 mg·kg⁻¹ i.v.), diazepam (0.5 mg·kg⁻¹), or clonazepam (0.8–1 mg·kg⁻¹) in unanesthetized curarized cats (REQUIN et al., 1963; VUILLON-CACCIUTTOLO et al., 1970). While diazepam (0.5–1 mg·kg⁻¹ i.v.) was without effect on the recruiting response to stimulation of the central medial thalamic nucleus, the same doses of the benzodiazepine markedly depressed the late negative component of the augmenting response elicited by stimulation of the ventrolateral thalamic nucleus in unanesthetized immobilized cats (SHERWIN, 1971). A similar differentiation of benzodiazepine effects was demonstrated in unrestrained rabbits, where flurazepam (0.5–5 mg·kg⁻¹ i.v.) reduced the augmenting response but slightly enhanced the recruiting response (OHMORI, 1977). However, in restrained rabbits diazepam (20 mg·kg⁻¹ p.o.) and an oxazolobenzodiazepine (CS 370) enhanced the augmenting response without influencing the recruiting response (MORI et al., 1972).

V. Caudate Spindles

Low-frequency stimulation of the caudate nucleus triggers spindle bursts in the ECoG, which seem to be mediated by the nonspecific thalamocortical system related to drowsiness and sleep (BUCHWALD et al., 1961). The only study dealing with the effect of benzodiazepines on this phenomenon showed an increased amplitude of the spindles recorded in the cortex upon stimulation of the head of the caudate nucleus after diazepam (0.5 mg·kg^{-1} i.v.) in unanesthetized immobilized cats (ITO and SHIMIZU, 1976).

VI. Ponto-geniculo-occipital (PGO) Waves

The effects of benzodiazepines on the PGO waves occurring during NREM and REM sleep as well as on the PGOs induced during wakefulness by pretreatment with reserpine, reserpine-like benzoquinolizine Ro 4–1284, or pCPA will be discussed in Sect. V/V.

VII. Afterdischarges

High frequency repetitive stimulation of diencephalic and limbic structures often produces discharges in the EEG of the same or adjacent brain regions, which can propagate to distant brain areas and, by inducing reverberating neuronal circuits, outlast the stimulation period (afterdischarges). A classic paper by HUNTER and JASPER (1949) described a behavioral arrest, accompanied by 3·s^{-1} spike and slow-wave pattern in the EEG induced by stimulation of the intralaminar thalamus in cats, a phenomenon bearing similarities to petit mal discharges in man. The current threshold for the induction of "afterdischarges" is a rather constant parameter in individual cats and rabbits and is frequently used as a sensitive measure of drug effects on what is believed to be the excitability of a particular brain area.

In several papers, SCHALLEK and associates described the marked depressant effects of various benzodiazepines on afterdischarges elicited in the cortex and limbic system upon stimulation of diencephalic and limbic brain structures. In unanesthetized immobilized cats, chlordiazepoxide (10 mg·kg^{-1} i.v.) decreased the duration of afterdischarges in the hippocampus and septum and reduced the amplitude of afterdischarges in the amygdala induced by stimulation of these limbic regions (SCHALLEK and KUEHN, 1960). In a later study on the same preparation, chlordiazepoxide (10 mg·kg^{-1} i.v.) was found to elevate the threshold and to diminish the duration and amplitude of afterdischarges in the central lateral thalamic nucleus, which were induced by stimulation of the medio-dorsal thalamus, cortex, or hippocampus. Higher doses of chlordiazepoxide (40 mg·kg^{-1} i.v.) also decreased the amplitude of the responses in cortex and hippocampus (SCHALLEK and KUEHN, 1963). The findings with chlordiazepoxide were confirmed and extended to other benzodiazepines in a study on unanesthetized, immobilized, and freely moving cats with chronically implanted electrodes (SCHALLEK et al., 1964). The threshold for the induction of afterdischarges induced in thalamus, cortex, and amygdala by stimulation of the same structures was significantly elevated with diazepam (10 mg·kg^{-1} i.v.), nitrazepam (10 mg·kg^{-1} i.v.), clonazepam (1 mg·kg^{-1} i.v.), and flunitrazepam (1 mg·kg^{-1} i.v.) in unanesthetized immobilized cats. On the other hand, afterdischarges in the neocortex were only slightly affected in freely moving cats. Stimulation of the amygdala and hippocampus in unrestrained cats induces staring, dilatation of pupils, and facial twitching resembling psychomotor seizures in man (Kaada et al., 1954). Morillo et al. (1962) observed an increase of the threshold for eliciting these behavioral manifestations of afterdischarges after chlordiazepoxide (10 mg·kg^{-1} i.m.). In freely moving cats Schallek et al. (1964) found an increase of the threshold for EEG afterdischarges in the amygdala and their behavioral correlates after chlordiazepoxide (10 mg·kg^{-1} p.o.), whereas diazepam (5 mg·kg^{-1} p.o.) and nitrazepam (1 mg·kg^{-1} p.o.) only shortened the duration of afterdischarges in amygdala and hippocampus. In other laboratories similar effects of benzodiazepines on afterdischarges in the limbic system were found. In unanesthetized curarized cats, chlordiazepoxide (3 mg·kg^{-1} i.v.) and diazepam (0.35 mg·kg^{-1} i.v.) depressed afterdischarges in the amygdala (Requin et al., 1963). In unrestrained cats, minute crystals of acetylcholine placed through a cannula into the amygdala evoked complex seizures which propagated to hippocampus, entorhinal cortex and brain stem, accompanied by clonic and clonic-tonic convulsions resembling status epilepticus. Nitrazepam (10 mg total dose, ca. 3.5 mg·kg^{-1} p.o. or i.p.) completely blocked electrographic and behavioral manifestations of seizures (Hernández-Peón and Rojas-Ramirez, 1966). In unanesthetized immobilized cats, diazepam (5 mg·kg^{-1} i.v.) reduced the amplitude and duration of afterdischarges in amygdala and isocortex (Dolce and Kaemmerer, 1967). The threshold for afterdischarges elicited by stimulation of amygdala and hippocampus was markedly raised after 20 mg·kg^{-1} chlordiazepoxide i.p. (Miyake, 1965). An interesting observation was made by Herink et al. (1976), who found that midbrain reticular lesions enhanced the depressant effect of diazepam (2.5 mg·kg^{-1} i.v.) on the afterdischarges in cortex, hippocampus, and midbrain elicited by stimulation of the septum in thiopentone-anesthetized rats. In restrained rabbits, the thienodiazepine, Y–6047, and diazepam did not affect the hippocampal afterdischarge in doses (40 mg·kg^{-1} i.p.) that significantly shortened the duration of amygdaloid afterdischarges (Nakanishi et al., 1972). In unrestrained rats, diazepam and chlordiazepoxide shortened the afterdischarges in the amygdala induced by local stimulation (Kamei et al., 1975).

In freely moving cats 1 mg·kg^{-1} nimetazepam and nitrazepam i.p. (Otsuka et al., 1973) as well as fludiazepam and diazepam (1 mg·kg^{-1} i.p.) shortened the duration of amygdaloid afterdischarges initially, but prolonged the afterdischarges 2–5 h after injection without clearly affecting the afterdischarges in the hippocampus (Otsuka et al., 1975). In the anesthetized rat the bicuculline- and pentetrazole-induced potentiation of the photically evoked afterdischarge in the visual cortex was suppressed by 15 mg·kg^{-1} diazepam i.p. (Bigler, 1977).

By using microinjections of diazepam in different limbic and diencephalic areas as well as systemic administration of diazepam, Nagy and Decsi (1973, 1979) attempted to localize the site of tranquilizing and anticonvulsant action of diazepam. In the first study with freely moving cats, intraperitoneal administration of diazepam (1 mg·kg^{-1}) produced a slow, high amplitude EEG pattern in cortical and subcortical leads. The injection of 50 μg diazepam mimicked this effect only if injected into the amygdaloid nucleus complex and particularly into its anterobasal portion, whereas the injections in the hippocampus were fully ineffective and those into the hypothalamus slightly effective (Nagy and Decsi, 1973). Similarly, pentetrazole-induced seizures and afterdischarges in the hippocampus provoked by stimulation of the amygdala were depressed in chronically implanted, slightly restrained rabbits only when diazepam (2×50 μg) was injected into the amygdala (anterior part), whereas injections into the dorsal hippocampus and the basal amygdaloid nucleus were ineffective (NAGY and DECSI, 1979). STOCK et al. (1976) could reverse several effects of intravenously infused medazepam (hypersynchronous EEG in septum and hippocampus, suppression of rage reaction) by stimulating electrically the basolateral amygdala in freely moving cats.

VIII. Conclusions

In spite of a large number of experimental studies, it is difficult to characterize in a few words the EEG changes induced by benzodiazepines. The main reason is the virtual lack of systematic dose-response studies (only exception: WINTERS and KOTT, 1979) and the greatly varying experimental conditions (immobilized and unrestrained animals, cable recording, telemetric techniques, route of administration, postdrug period, visual and computer-assisted analysis, statistical methods etc.).

On the one hand the spontaneous bioelectrical activity of cortical and subcortical structures seems to be affected by benzodiazepines in a distinct way. Most benzodiazepines have a tendency to shift the basal EEG pattern to waves of higher frequency and higher amplitude, particularly in neocortex, hippocampus, and amygdala. In addition, in pharmacologically relevant doses benzodiazepines depress the hippocampal theta-rhythm in the waking state and during REM sleep, as well as the theta-activity elicited by stimulation of subcortical areas. This depression is most frequently recognized as a shift of the theta-rhythm from the regular 5–7 Hz waves to slower waves in the delta range (3–4 Hz). Although the significance of benzodiazepine effects on spontaneous EEG is not known, it is tempting to speculate that at least the depression of the hippocampal theta-activity, which is frequently associated with attention and behavioral arousal, can be related to the sedative effects of benzodiazepines.

On the other hand, the arousal reaction in the neocortex, in most cases evoked by stimulation of the brain stem reticular formation, was not consistently found to be altered by benzodiazepines. This was often interpreted as being due to the absence of a pronounced direct action of benzodiazepines on the reticular formation, which would explain the absent or only slight sedation observed when benzodiazepines are given in the doses exhibiting selective antianxiety effects. The lack of marked effects of benzodiazepines on the cortical recruiting response, induced by stimulation of the nonspecific thalamic nuclei and associated with drowsiness, supports the above interpretation of a low sensitivity of structures directly involved in the regulation of vigilance states, i.e., reticular formation and thalamus, to the action of benzodiazepines.

In contrast, benzodiazepines are extremely potent in reducing the afterdischarges elicited in different limbic and diencephalic areas by repetitive stimulation of the same structures. From the available experimental data, the structure most susceptible to the depressant effect of benzodiazepines on this EEG phenomenon seems to be the amygdaloid complex. In this respect, the finding that diazepam selectively reduces rage reactions in unrestrained cats and simultaneously alters the EEG pattern as well as diminishes limbic afterdischarges in rabbits only when microinjected into the amygdala, supports a postulated "limbic site" of action of benzodiazepines for their antianxiety and, possibly, also anticonvulsant effects.

V. Benzodiazepines and Sleep

A number of different benzodiazepines were studied in unanesthetized, mostly freely moving animals with chronically implanted electrodes in an attempt to reproduce their well-known sleep-inducing effect in man. However, since sleep is a particularly fragile behavioral manifestation, susceptible to many influences from the animal itself and from the experimenter, it is not surprising that rather inconsistent results were obtained by various investigators who have used cats, rabbits, rats, and monkeys to determine the effects of benzodiazepines on the three basic vigilance states, i.e., wakefulness, nonrapid eye movement (NREM) sleep, and rapid eye movement (REM) sleep.

I. Cats

Because the physiology of sleep has been studied most intensively in cats, this species has also been the most frequently used in pharmacology. Almost all possible combinations of changes in REM sleep, NREM sleep and wakefulness have been reported.

A reduction of both REM and NREM sleep and an increase of wakefulness were found by Lanoir and Killam (1968) after nitrazepam and diazepam (0.25 mg·kg^{-1} i.p.). Very similar results were reported by Gogerty (1973) with flurazepam (10 mg·kg^{-1} i.p.) and by Schallek et al. (1972, 1973) with single oral doses of chlordiazepoxide (10 mg·kg^{-1}), clonazepam (4 mg·kg^{-1}), and flunitrazepam (4 mg·kg^{-1}).

A reduction of REM sleep and an increase of NREM sleep were observed by Dolce and Kaemmerer (1967) after oxazepam (1–10 mg·kg^{-1} p.o., i.p., or i.m.); frequent awakenings occurred accompanied by spindles (mixed sleep-wakefulness pattern). Clonazepam (0.08–1 mg·kg^{-1} i.p.) slightly augmented NREM sleep and markedly depressed REM sleep in the study by Vuillon-Cacciuttolo et al. (1970). A slight increase of REM sleep as the only effect was observed by Borenstein et al. (1973) with diazepam (2 mg·kg^{-1} p.o.).

No effect on the sleep-wakefulness cycle was reported by Borenstein et al. (1973) with nitrazepam (1 mg·kg^{-1} p.o.).

A selective increase of NREM sleep was found by Borenstein et al. (1973) with lorazepam (1 mg·kg^{-1} p.o.), by Straw (1975) with flurazepam (1 mg·kg^{-1} p.o.), and by Griauzde et al. (1979) with low doses of diazepam (0.3–0.9 mg·kg^{-1} i.p.).

A selective depression of NREM sleep occurred with intraperitoneal doses of diazepam above 1 mg·kg^{-1} (Griauzde et al., 1979) as well as after oral administration of diazepam (0.25 mg·kg^{-1} p.o.) and chlordiazepoxide (4 mg·kg^{-1} p.o.) (Straw, 1975).

An increase of both sleep stages and a decrease of wakefulness was seen by Schallek et al. (1973) when chlordiazepoxide (10 mg·kg^{-1} p.o.), clonazepam (4 mg·kg^{-1} p.o.), and flunitrazepam (4 mg·kg^{-1} p.o.) were administered on several consecutive days; the same doses of these benzodiazepines depressed both sleep stages after the first administration. The intravenous infusion of medazepam following a priming dose (total about 5 mg·kg^{-1}) and chlordiazepoxide (total about 0.2 mg·kg^{-1}) to achieve constant blood levels of the drugs over several hours, augmented both REM and NREM sleep and reduced the amount of wakefulness (Heinemann et al., 1968;

HEINEMANN and STOCK, 1973). A very small dose of flunitrazepam $(0.001 \text{ mg} \cdot \text{kg}^{-1}$ i.p.) enhanced REM sleep and, to a lesser extent, NREM sleep in cats prepared for telemetric recording (POLC and HAEFELY, 1975), whereas a higher dose $(0.1 \text{ mg} \cdot \text{kg}^{-1})$ had the opposite effect.

The effect of benzodiazepines on disturbed sleep of cats is of particular interest since many laboratory cats spend much of their time asleep (up to 70% of the recording time) and, hence, a hypnogenic effect of a drug cannot be easily demonstrated. When cats were made "insomniac" by small, otherwise behaviorally inactive doses of LSD or methylphenidate, flunitrazepam $(0.003 \text{ mg} \cdot \text{kg}^{-1} \text{ i.p.})$ partially reestablished normal sleep behavior (POLC and HAEFELY, 1975). Similar results were obtained on sleep depressed by small doses of morphine (SCHERSCHLICHT et al., 1979). Similarly, GOGERTY (1973) found an augmentation of both sleep stages with flurazepam $(10 \text{ mg} \cdot \text{kg}^{-1} \text{ i.p.})$ in cats whose sleep was disturbed by various arousing stimuli and electric foot shock. An attempt was undertaken in a recent study (GRIAUZDE et al., 1979) to elucidate the mechanism of the sleep-inducing action of diazepam. Lower doses of diazepam $(0.3–0.9 \text{ mg} \cdot \text{kg}^{-1} \text{ i.p.})$ increased, whereas higher doses of the drug depressed NREM sleep without affecting REM sleep. Since the simultaneously measured levels in the cerebrospinal fluid of 5-hydroxyindolacetic acid (5-HIAA) or homovanillic acid (HVA), respective metabolites of 5-hydroxytryptamine (5-HT) and dopamine were not altered by diazepam, GRIAUZDE et al. (1979) suggested that diazepam augmented NREM sleep by a mechanism unrelated to 5-HT, the monoamine implicated in the initiation of NREM sleep (JOUVET, 1972).

II. Rabbits

More consistent effects of benzodiazepines on the sleep-wakefulness cycle were observed in rabbits than in cats. The early report of an increased amount of sleep after oral administration of chlordiazepoxide $(50 \text{ mg} \cdot \text{kg}^{-1})$ and nitrazepam $(10 \text{ mg} \cdot \text{kg}^{-1})$ in partially restrained rabbits (SOULAIRAC et al., 1965) was confirmed by most investigators who have differentiated between NREM and REM sleep and who, in addition, administered smaller doses of benzodiazepines. KAWAKAMI et al. (1966) and GOLDSTEIN et al. (1967) found an augmentation of REM sleep in freely moving rabbits after oral administration of chlordiazepoxide $(3 \text{ mg} \cdot \text{kg}^{-1})$ or diazepam $(0.2 \text{ mg} \cdot \text{kg}^{-1})$ and after intravenous injection of chlordiazepoxide $(1 \text{ mg} \cdot \text{kg}^{-1})$, respectively. In another study, diazepam $(1 \text{ mg} \cdot \text{kg}^{-1} \text{ p.o.})$, but not nitrazepam $(1 \text{ mg} \cdot \text{kg}^{-1} \text{ p.o.})$, enhanced the amount of REM sleep, whereas NREM sleep was augmented by both benzodiazepines (HOFFMEISTER, 1972). Frequent awakenings characterized the sleep induced by both benzodiazepines in the latter study. In order to find an explanation for the discrepant effects of benzodiazepines in the various sleep studies, ZATTONI and ROSSI (1967) injected nitrazepam either systemically (intravenous) or into the carotid and vertebral artery of unanesthetized restrained rabbits. Administered intravenously or into the carotid artery, nitrazepam induced EEG synchronization with a sleep-like behavior, but when injected into the vertebral artery, the benzodiazepine elicited EEG arousal, accompanied by behavioral alertness. The authors suggested that nitrazepam depressed the neuronal structures responsible for wakefulness in the midbrain reticular formation and hypothalamus after the intracarotid administration, while depressing the sleep-promoting regions of the lower brain stem after intravertebral injection, thus eliciting arousal. The fact that intravenous injection produced the same effect as intracarotid application, i.e., a sleep-like state, indicated that the arousal system may be tonically more active than the hypnogenic system and, therefore, more susceptible to the depressant action of the benzodiazepine. Interestingly, Loizzo and Longo (1968) produced a REM sleep-like phenomenon by injection of diazepam ($0.2\ mg \cdot kg^{-1}$) into the vertebral artery in restrained rabbits, although an EEG synchronization without REM sleep was found after intravenous injection of diazepam ($0.5\ mg \cdot kg^{-1}$) in unrestrained rabbits.

III. Rats

Sleep-like behavior, accompanied by an unusual EEG pattern (fast spindles and high frequency waves), was induced by oral administration of nitrazepam ($10\ mg \cdot kg^{-1}$) in freely moving rats (Soulairac et al., 1965). In general agreement with this early report, nitrazepam augmented NREM sleep after acute administration ($1.1\ mg \cdot kg^{-1}$ p.o.; Gogerty, 1973) and enhanced both REM and NREM sleep after repeated dosing ($10\ mg \cdot kg^{-1} \cdot d^{-1}$ i.p.; Klygul et al., 1976); a rebound decrease of REM sleep was observed during withdrawal in the latter study. Low doses of nitrazepam ($0.3\ mg \cdot kg^{-1}$ i.p.), which did not produce side effects, reduced restlessness during sleep without significantly affecting different sleep states, whereas higher doses of the drug ($1\ mg \cdot kg^{-1}$) tended to reduce REM sleep along with the appearance of ataxia (Loew and Spiegel, 1976). A reduction of REM sleep and a slight increase of NREM sleep were observed after nitrazepam and temazepam in rats (Buonamici and Rossi, 1979). Estazolam ($5\ mg \cdot kg^{-1}$ i.p.) reduced NREM sleep in normal laboratory rats, but augmented NREM and REM sleep in rats rendered insomniac by pretreatment with an inhibitor of 5-HT synthesis, parachlorophenylalanine (Ikeda et al., 1973). If electric foot shock was used to induce insomnia, oral administration of flunitrazepam ($4\ mg \cdot kg^{-1}$) and of the imidazobenzodiazepine RU 31,158 ($8\ mg \cdot kg^{-1}$) enhanced the amount of NREM and REM sleep (Piper, 1977; James and Piper, 1978) in freely moving rats. An interesting observation was made by Monti et al., (1979a, b), who found that the combined administration of otherwise noneffective doses of diazepam ($1\ mg \cdot kg^{-1}$ i.p.) and gamma-hydroxybutyrate ($12.5\ mg \cdot kg^{-1}$ i.p.) enhanced NREM sleep (in particular, slow waves) in rats. Since this effect was prevented by pretreatment with a nonconvulsive dose of bicuculline ($2.5\ mg \cdot kg^{-1}$ i.p.), the authors suggested that an activation of GABA mechanisms could underlie the observed additive effect.

IV. Monkeys

Only few sleep studies with benzodiazepines were performed in monkeys. Moderate doses of clonazepam ($10\ mg \cdot kg^{-1}$ p.o.), flurazepam ($10–20\ mg \cdot kg^{-1}$ p.o.), and flunitrazepam ($2,5–5\ mg \cdot kg^{-1}$ p.o.) induced sedation without sleep in squirrel monkeys (Schallek et al., 1973). However, in *Cebus* monkeys flurazepam ($3.75\ mg \cdot kg^{-1}$) and temazepam ($3,75\ mg \cdot kg^{-1}$) increased the amount spent in NREM and REM sleep and correspondingly reduced the waking time (Gogerty, 1973). In rhesus monkeys diazepam (0.3 and $1\ mg \cdot kg^{-1}$ p.o.) and triazolam ($1\ mg \cdot kg^{-1}$ p.o.) augmented NREM sleep and reduced the amount of wakefulness without significantly affecting

REM sleep (STRAW, 1975). In contrast, a single high oral dose of nitrazepam (25 mg · kg^{-1}) markedly depressed REM sleep and reduced waking time while increasing the amount spent in NREM sleep in rhesus monkeys (DAVID et al., 1974). In the latter investigation the EEG recording was continued for some days after the acute administration; a strong rebound increase of REM sleep occurred after withdrawal of nitrazepam, an effect also found in man (OSWALD and PRIEST, 1965). Thus, monkeys would seem to be a good model for evaluating the effects of hypnotics in subhuman species. However, the necessity of restraining the monkey in a chair which creates an artificial situation, as well as high costs precluded a more extensive investigation of benzodiazepines on monkeys' sleep.

V. Ponto-geniculo-occipital (PGO) Waves

Ponto-geniculo-occipital waves are phasically occurring monophasic high amplitude waves, which characteristically have a burst-like appearance during REM sleep in cats, but which also occur as isolated waves during deeper periods of NREM sleep, in particular just preceding a REM sleep episode (JOUVET, 1972). In freely moving cats with electrodes chronically implanted in the lateral geniculate body, BORENSTEIN et al. (1973) and HARA et al. (1975b) found a marked increase of PGO waves occurring in bursts during REM sleep episodes as well as PGO waves elicited by pretreatment with reserpine after various benzodiazepines (nitrazepam and lorazepam, 1 mg · kg^{-1} p.o.; nitrazepam, 0.2 mg · kg^{-1} i.v., and diazepam, 0.4 mg · kg^{-1} i.v., respectively), whereas the same doses of the above benzodiazepines did not consistently alter the REM sleep itself.

These results were confirmed in investigations performed in unanesthetized immobilized cats, in which PGO waves were induced by the pretreatment either with *p*-chlorophenylalanine or with Ro 4-1284, a reserpine-like benzoquinolizine compound which depletes the monoaminergic nerve endings from monoamines (RUCH-MONACHON et al., 1976a). Since the facilitating effects of chlordiazepoxide (3 mg · kg^{-1} i.v.) on these pharmacologically produced PGO waves were abolished by lesions of the septum, medial forebrain bundle, amygdala, or by administration of atropine (MONACHON et al., 1973, RUCH-MONACHON et al., 1976b), it was assumed that a pathway descending from the forebrain, with an intercalated cholinergic synapse, would be responsible for the effects of benzodiazepines. On the other hand, in a more recent study on freely moving cats with electrodes implanted in the lateral geniculate body for recording the PGO waves, and in the midbrain reticular formation for recording the multiple unit activity, TSUCHIYA and FUKUSHIMA (1977) were unable to detect any clear-cut effects of diazepam (1 mg · kg^{-1} i.p.) or fludiazepam (0.5 mg · kg^{-1} i.p.) on PGO waves either during REM or NREM sleep, although the multiple unit activity in the midbrain reticular formation was markedly depressed during both sleep stages.

VI. Conclusions

The effects of benzodiazepines on the sleep-wakefulness cycle of animals are extremely complex. The interpretation of available data is made very difficult in the absence of systematic dose-response studies.

At first sight, the most striking and apparently paradoxical observation is the reduction of sleep, which occurred after single administrations of most doses of benzodiazepines in cats. This result of EEG studies is in line with gross behavioral observations showing that even high, ataxic doses produce a state of excitation, at least
initially, in cats and dogs. The reason for this behavioral stimulation is not fully
understood; the effect is, however, not unique for benzodiazepines, but is also consistently found with barbiturates in subanesthetic doses. It is also not known why the
stimulant effect is virtually absent in rodents and only rarely seen in man. An important similarity seems to exist, however, between man and cat, and this is the disturbing
effect of benzodiazepines on normal sleep patterns and their ability to normalize sleep
behavior disturbed by a variety of factors. In this respect, the sleep-reestablishing effect of benzodiazepines in cats made "insomniac" by small doses of LSD, methylphenidate, or morphine or by electric foot shock, may simulate more accurately the
sleep-inducing and -improving effect of benzodiazepines in insomniac patients.

More investigations are required before specific effects of benzodiazepines on sleep
mechanisms can be accepted or excluded. For the time being, it would appear safe to
assume that these drugs improve sleep primarily by attenuating emotional factors
which hinder the onset and maintained operation of normal sleep mechanisms. Taking into account the specific effect of benzodiazepines on GABAergic synapses, which
are widely distributed within the central nervous system, as well as the numerous brain
areas whose activity is affected by these drugs, one is inclined to suggest that benzodiazepines are able, in an essentially similar way, to affect various brain structures
with opposite effects on sleep. The overall effect of benzodiazepines on the amount and
organization of sleep may, then, depend primarily on the predrug level of activity in
these various structures.

W. Effects on Single- and Multiple-Unit Activity in the Brain

The analysis of drug effects on the "spontaneous" and evoked electrical activity of
single neurons as well as small neuronal populations in the central nervous system is
one of the most important recent achievements in neuropharmacology. The recording
of single neuron activity in different parts of the brain and spinal cord and the use of
iontophoretic and pressure ejection methods to administer the drugs into the immediate vicinity of neurons under study, provide information on possible direct effects
of drugs on the pattern of spontaneous as well as electrically and chemically induced
activity of identified neurons and on drug actions on the membrane properties of
neurons.

I. Limbic System

In chloralose-anesthetized cats, a small intravenous dose of nitrazepam ($0.15\,\mathrm{mg\cdot kg^{-1}}$)
did not induce any consistent changes in the spontaneous activity of neurons in the
hippocampus and lateral geniculate body (except for some bursting patterns), but
markedly depressed the increase of hippocampal neuronal discharge evoked by visual
stimuli (STEINER and HUMMEL, 1968). Since a visually evoked response of single
neurons in the lateral geniculate body was unaffected by nitrazepam, the authors sug-

gested a specific suppressant effect of the benzodiazepines on the visual afferent input to the hippocampus. However, in freely moving rats with chronically implanted semimicroelectrodes, OLDS and OLDS (1969) observed a strong depressant effect of intraperitoneal injections of chlordiazepoxide (10 mg · kg^{-1}) and diazepam (5 mg · kg^{-1}) on the spontaneous firing of hippocampal neurons, whereas meprobamate (80 mg · kg^{-}) was ineffective. In contrast, the same dose of meprobamate clearly reduced the spontaneous activity of midbrain reticular neurons, which were rather insensitive to diazepam (10 mg · kg^{-1}). Multiple unit activity in the preoptic area was slightly depressed by the above doses of both meprobamate and diazepam. In a later study in unrestrained rats, a conflict situation provoked an increase of neuronal discharges in the amygdala, and this effect was markedly diminished by chlordiazepoxide (5 mg · kg^{-1} i.p.) and diazepam (2.5 mg · kg^{-1} i.p.) (UMEMOTO and OLDS, 1975). In partial agreement with these observations, GUERRERO-FIGUEROA et al. (1973, 1974) found in unrestrained cats and rhesus monkeys a reduction of multi-unit activity after parenteral administration of diazepam, chlordiazepoxide, bromazepam, lorazepam, and triflubazam in the amygdala, posterior hypothalamus, intralaminar thalamus, and midbrain reticular formation (structures assumed by the authors to be responsible for aversive behavioral responses) as well as in hippocampus, septum, lateral hypothalamus, and preoptic area (structures considered to be parts of a "rewarding" system). Repeated oral administration of the benzodiazepines also depressed the neuronal activity of the aversive system while augmenting the spontaneous activity of neurons in the rewarding system. These rather complex results led GUERRERO-FIGUEROA et al. (1973) to postulate a shift in balance from the "anxiety-inducing" to the "rewarding part" of the limbic system after benzodiazepines. More recent investigations using small doses of systemic as well as iontophoretic injections of benzodiazepines from multibarreled micropipettes, confirmed these earlier observations on the marked sensitivity of the limbic structures to benzodiazepines. Doses as small as 0.05–0.1 mg · kg^{-1} diazepam i.v. clearly depressed the spontaneous neuronal activity in hippocampus, amygdala (CHOU and WANG, 1977), septum, cingulate gyrus, and lateral hypothalamus (ROBINSON and WANG, 1979) of unanesthetized immobilized cats. In the same studies a marked antagonism was observed between the excitatory action of morphine and the inhibitory effects of benzodiazepines on amygdala neurons. In another study with anesthetized rats, MATTHEWS and CONNOR (1977) found the spontaneous firing of pyramidal and granular cells in the hippocampus to be depressed by iontophoretically ejected medazepam, which also blocked the excitations of hippocampal neurons induced by acetylcholine and glutamate. Working with unanesthetized as well as anesthetized rats, WOLF and HAAS (1977) observed a clear-cut depression of spontaneously active pyramidal cells after diazepam (0.5 mg · kg^{-1} i.p.) and iontophoretically ejected Ro 11–7800 (a thieno-diazepine). Recurrent inhibition of pyramidal cells was prolonged by the two drugs. In urethane-anesthetized rats (MUNEKYIO and MESHI, 1979), 0.1–1 mg · kg^{-1} triazolam i.v. enhanced bicuculline-sensitive recurrent inhibition of hippocampal pyramidal cells. Triazolam depressed spontaneous activity of pyramidal cells in normal, but not in thiosemicarbazide-pretreated animals. The inhibition by iontophoretic GABA, but not glycine, was potentiated by triazolam. In unanesthetized immobilized cats, a similar enhancement of the bicuculline-sensitive recurrent inhibition of pyramidal cells was found by TSUCHIYA and FUKUSHIMA (1978) with small doses of diazepam and fludiazepam (0.3 mg · kg^{-1}

i.v.), whereas higher doses (1 mg·kg^{-1} i.v.) of both benzodiazepines were required to reduce the spontaneous firing of pyramidal cells. A depressant effect of iontophoresed chlordiazepoxide on the spontaneous activity of neurons in the corticomedial region of amygdala was reported by James et al. (1979).

Only two intracellular studies of the benzodiazepine effects in hippocampal cells have been published. Haas and Siegfried (1978), recording from pyramidal cells of slices of rat and human hippocampus, observed a hyperpolarization and, less frequently, an increase of membrane conductance, after adding diazepam, flurazepam, or the thienodiazepine, Ro 11–7800, to the bath. The amplitude of spontaneous and electrically induced action potentials was reduced, and the IPSPs elicited by alveus or fimbria stimulation were enhanced in some cells and reduced in others. In another paper, Haas et al. (1979) reported no change of the membrane potential of CA 1 pyramidal cells in the presence of diazepam 2×10^{-6} mol·l^{-1}.

Thus, it has been shown in different laboratories that benzodiazepines administered systematically or locally reduce the spontaneous and evoked activity of principal cells in amygdala and hippocampus. The most likely explanation for this effect is the potentiating action of benzodiazepines on GABA-mediated recurrent inhibition demonstrated in the hippocampus.

II. Cerebellum

It was an obvious step to investigate the effect of benzodiazepines on this structure because the neuronal circuitry of the cerebellum has been intensively studied, and the neurotransmitter released by inhibitory interneurons on the Purkinje cells has been identified as GABA (Curtis and Johnston, 1974). Moreover, motor side effects of benzodiazepines (ataxia, hypotonia) might be related to their action on the cerebellum. The early observation that diazepam (1 mg·kg^{-1} i.v.) augmented spontaneous Purkinje cell firing of decerebrate cats (Julien, 1972) seemed to find some support by Gähwiler (1976) and Ben-Neria and Lass (1977), both later studies using an in vitro technique. In one of these (Gähwiler, 1976) and in another investigation (Boakes et al., 1977), a bursting Purkinje cell activity with prolonged pauses was found, perhaps similar to that observed in the first single-unit study with benzodiazepines on hippocampal neurons (Steiner and Hummel, 1968). However, other investigators using continuous recording of spontaneous Purkinje cell activity found a consistent depression of Purkinje cell firing by various benzodiazepines (Pieri and Haefely, 1976; Lippa et al., 1977; Mariani and Delhaye-Bouchaud, 1978; Lippa et al., 1979). Depression of Purkinje cell firing in anesthetized rats by iontophoretically administered flurazepam was antagonized by picrotoxin, but not by bicuculline (Lippa et al., 1979). Both the reduction of spontaneous discharge and the tendency of Purkinje cells to built-up bursts separated by pauses can be accounted for by the increased GABAergic basket cell inhibition of Purkinje cells, which was observed after systemic or iontophoretic application of benzodiazepines in unanesthetized and anesthetized cats and rats (Curtis et al., 1976b; Geller et al., 1978; Montarolo et al., 1979). Basket cell inhibition of Purkinje cells seems to be extremely sensitive to the influence by benzodiazepines, since even in a dose which had no apparent effect on spontaneous Purkinje cell activity, diazepam (0.2 mg·kg^{-1} i.p.) augmented threshold basket cell inhibition (Geller et al., 1978). A depression of spontaneous Purkinje cell discharge as well as increased basket cell inhibition was induced by GABA, and the same dose of diazepam ($0.2 \ mg \cdot kg^{-1}$ i.p.), which did not affect the spontaneous discharge of Purkinje cells, potentiated the submaximal inhibition of Purkinje cell firing induced by iontophoresed GABA, but not that induced by noradrenaline. The effects of both GABA and benzodiazepines were suppressed in vivo and in vitro by GABA antagonists bicuculline and picrotoxin, but not by the glycine antagonist strychnine (LIPPA et al., 1977; GELLER et al., 1978; OKAMOTO and SAKAI, 1979). Furthermore, the dose-response curve for GABA-inhibition of the spontaneous cell activity in guinea-pig cerebellar slices was shifted to the left by chlordiazepoxide (OKAMOTO and SAKAI, 1979). Thus, earlier results showing an antagonism between GABA and benzodiazepines on the Purkinje cell activity (GÄHWILER, 1976; STEINER and FELIX, 1976 a, b) were not confirmed in recent investigations and could have been due either to a peculiarity of newborn rat cerebellar culture used by GÄHWILER (1976) or to inadequate methods (STEINER and FELIX, 1976a, b). In a recent study, diazepam ($0.1 - 1 \ mg \cdot kg^{-1}$ i.v.) potentiated the inhibition of Purkinje cell discharge induced by the stimulation of the raphé in chloralose-anesthetized cats (BARNES et al., 1979), an effect which was reversed by bicuculline.

Summarizing the effects of benzodiazepines on spontaneously active cerebellar Purkinje cells, it can be stated that the available evidence demonstrates a depressant effect of benzodiazepines on spontaneous activity and a potentiation of basket cell-mediated inhibition. The reduction of spontaneous activity is restricted to so-called simple spikes induced by mossy fiber activation, whereas the complex spikes produced by climbing fiber activation were unaffected by benzodiazepines (MARIANI and DE-LHAYE-BOUCHAUD, 1978; PIERI, 1978).

III. Cerebral Cortex

Spontaneous activity of cortical neurons in unanesthetized and anesthetized rabbits, cats, and rats was reduced after systemic injection of diazepam ($1 \ mg \cdot kg^{-1}$ i.v., ZAKUSOV et al., 1977; ZAKUSOV and KOZHECHKIN, 1978; PHILLIS, 1979), as well as by chlordiazepoxide, diazepam, and flurazepam applied iontophoretically (KOZHECHKIN and OSTROVSKAYA, 1977 b; PHILLIS, 1979; LIPPA et al., 1979). In addition, extremely small iontophoretic currents used to expel flurazepam from the micropipettes, which had no effect on ongoing activity of cortical neurons, clearly potentiated the small inhibition of neuronal firing elicited by a threshold stimulation of the nearby cortical surface (NESTOROS and NISTRI, 1978). Since pretreatment with the GABA synthesis inhibitor, thiosemicarbazide ($35 \ mg \cdot kg^{-1}$ i.v., 3 h before flurazepam) abolished the augmenting effect of flurazepam on cortical inhibition, but iontophoretically injected GABA still inhibited cortical neurons, NESTOROS and NISTRI (1978) suggested a presynaptic site of action of flurazepam, probably by increasing the release of GABA. A potentiating effect of diazepam ($1 \ mg \cdot kg^{-1}$ i.v.) and chlordiazepoxide on GABA- and adenosine-induced neuronal depression in the cortex was shown in rats and rabbits (KOZHECHKIN and OSTROVSKAYA, 1977a; ZAKUSOV et al., 1977; PHILLIS, 1979). Interestingly, both the adenosine- and flurazepam-evoked inhibition of neuronal activity in the sensorimotor cortex of anesthetized rats were abolished by $50–100 \ mg \cdot kg^{-1}$ theophylline i.v. (PHILLIS et al., 1979). In unanesthetized curarized rats clonazepam ($2 \ mg \cdot kg^{-1}$ i.m.) increased the inhibition of spontaneous firing of cells in the sensorimotor cortex produced by microiontophoretic application of GABA and reduced the activation on firing by iontophoresed acetylcholine and glutamate (SHMIDT et al., 1978). In urethane-anesthetized rats iontophoretically administered chlordiazepoxide reduced glutamate- and aspartate-induced excitation of spontaneously active, unidentified neurons in the sensorimotor cortex without consistently affecting acetylcholine-induced excitation or GABA-induced inhibition (ASSUMPÇÃO et al., 1979). Such a selective antagonism of excitatory amino acids by benzodiazepines was not observed in anesthetized cats by NESTOROS and NISTRI (1979), who found that iontophoretic flurazepam potentiated the inhibitory effects of GABA and antagonized those of 5-hydroxytryptamine on pericruciate cortical neurons driven by glutamate. The ejecting currents required to result in potentiation of GABA and inhibition of 5-hydrotryptamine were smaller than those required to reduce glutamate- and aspartate-induced excitation of the same neurons. Even higher currents were necessary to eject amounts of flurazepam that antagonized acetylcholine excitation, and these currents obviously interfered with the spike-generating mechanisms. KOZHECHKIN (1978) observed an augmenting effect of diazepam (1 mg·kg^{-1} i.v.) on the inhibition of spontaneously active cortical neurons evoked by direct cortical or sciatic nerve stimulation, as well as a depressant effect on the neuronal activation induced by sciatic nerve stimuli (KOZHECHKIN, 1978), effects which were reversibly antagonized by bicuculline (0.1 mg·kg^{-1} i.v., ZAKUSOV et al., 1977). In agreement with these observations, diazepam (0.5 mg·kg^{-} i.v.) was shown to prolong the postsynaptic recurrent inhibition of pyramidal tract cortical neurons in anesthetized and *encéphale isolé* cats (RAABE and GUMNIT, 1977). The finding of a decreased tonic and phasic multiple-unit activity of cortical pyramidal tract neurons after diazepam (3.5 mg·kg^{-1} i.m.) can probably be explained in the same way (VELASCO et al., 1977).

IV. Brain Stem and Diencephalic Structures

The effects of benzodiazepines on single neuronal activity in some brain stem and diencephalic regions have already been mentioned when discussing the descending reticular influence on the spinal cord (PRZYBYLA and WANG, 1968; TSENG and WANG, 1971 b) and the multiple-unit activity of the limbic midbrain area (OLDS and OLDS, 1969; GUERRERO-FIGUEROA et al., 1973).

The spontaneous activity of single unidentified medullar brainstem neurons was studied by DRAY and STRAUGHAN (1976) and by BOWERY and DRAY (1978). In intact anesthetized rats, iontophoretically ejected chlordiazepoxide and flurazepam reduced spontaneous as well as acetylcholine- and glutamate-induced firing, but had no effect on GABA- or glycine-produced depressions of spontaneous activity. On the other hand, iontophoretically ejected bicuculline antagonized the reduction of neuronal firing induced by flurazepam and GABA, but not that produced by glycine. Accordingly, strychnine selectively abolished the glycine effect without affecting GABA- or flurazepam-evoked depressions (DRAY and STRAUGHAN, 1976). Clonazepam (0.1 mg·kg^{-1} i.v.) reduced the spontaneous discharge of medullary neurons and partially reversed the blockade by iontophoretic bicuculline of GABA-induced depressions of spontaneous activity (BOWERY and DRAY, 1978).

A diminished spontaneous activity of identified neurons of the vestibular nucleus was observed after diazepam (0.2 mg·kg^{-1} i.v.) in decerebrate unanesthetized cats

(KIRSTEN and SCHOENER, 1972). In the same study diazepam prevented the short duration increase of vestibular neuronal firing produced by pentetrazole (5 mg·kg⁻¹ i.v.). Similar findings were obtained in a recent investigation by DEPOORTERE et al. (1978), who found a dose-dependent decrease of multi-unit activity in the lateral vestibular nucleus of Deiters after chlordiazepoxide and diazepam (0.1–3 mg·kg⁻¹ i.v.) in unanesthetized curarized cats. Enhancement of the neuronal activity evoked by picrotoxin (0.1 mg·kg⁻¹ i.v.) was suppressed by chlordiazepoxide. In contrast, STEINER and FELIX (1976a, b) observed in anesthetized cats a reduction by diazepam (0.5 mg·kg⁻¹ i.v.) of the Purkinje cell-evoked inhibition of antidromically activated Deiters' neurons. Since in this study diazepam blocked also the inhibition of antidromic potentials induced by iontophoretic GABA, these findings are in obvious contradiction with the wealth of studies dealing with the effect of benzodiazepines in postsynaptic inhibition. BARMACK and PETTOROSSI (1980) reported that small intravenous doses of diazepam (0.02–0.1 mg·kg⁻¹) reduced the sensitivity of secondary vestibular neurons of different vestibular nuclei to sinusoidal angular acceleration along vertical and longitudinal axes in unanesthetized, immobilized rabbits.

In the dorsal raphé nucleus of anesthetized and unanesthetized rats iontophoretically ejected flurazepam and chlordiazepoxide as well as intravenously administered diazepam (up to 8 mg·kg⁻¹) had no effect upon spontaneous neuronal activity, but depressed the firing rate after pretreatment with the GABA-transaminase inhibitor, aminooxyacetic acid (AOAA, 50 mg·kg⁻¹ i.v., 1 h before benzodiazepines, GALLAGER, 1978). In the same study, the three benzodiazepines also selectively potentiated the inhibitory effect of iontophoretically ejected GABA, whereas they were ineffective on depressions of the raphé cell activities produced by glycine and 5-hydroxytryptamine. In a later study in chloralhydrate anesthetized rats, GALLAGER et al. (1980) found no effect of 100 mg·kg⁻¹ diphenylhydantoin i.p. on the spontaneous activity of dorsal raphé neurons, but after diphenylhydantoin a depressant effect of diazepam (0.5 mg·kg⁻¹ i.v.) appeared. This finding was related to the observation that diphenylhydantoin enhanced specific ³H-diazepam binding in the brain in vitro and in vivo.

BUNNEY and AGHAJANIAN (1976) studied the effect of diazepam (0.8–20 mg·kg⁻¹ i.v.) on the assumed dopamine neuron activity in the zona compacta of the substantia nigra and the ventral tegmental area in anesthetized rats. Diazepam reversed the depression of dopamine neurons induced by amphetamine. On the other hand, WOLF and HAAS (1977) observed a depressant effect by benzodiazepines on the spontaneous firing of nigral neurons. The neuronal inhibition of the pars reticulata of the substantia nigra elicited in chloralose-anesthetized cats by stimuli applied to the nucleus accumbens was depressed by bicuculline (0.01–0.1 mg·kg⁻¹ i.v.), and this effect of bicuculline was reversed by diazepam 0.5 mg·kg⁻¹ i.v. (FUNG et al., 1979).

Additional evidence for an enhancement of inhibitory phenomena in the brain by benzodiazepines was provided by GELLER (1978) and GELLER et al. (1978) in experiments on cell cultures of tuberal hypothalamus. Bath application of diazepam (2×10^{-6} mol·l⁻¹) prolonged the inhibition of spontaneous single cell discharge evoked by electrical stimulation and iontophoretic GABA, but not depressions produced by iontophoretic glycine. Picrotoxin (10^{-5} mol·l⁻¹) blocked inhibitions elicited by electrical stimuli and GABA, glycine inhibitions being unaffected. In the same preparation flurazepam (10^{-5} mol·l⁻¹) potentiated GABA-induced submaximal inhibition of spontaneously active cells without affecting the depression induced by glycine. The convulsant benzodiazepine derivative Ro 5–3663 (10^{-4} mol·l^{-1}) antagonized GABA-induced inhibition (Geller, 1979).

Two studies demonstrated a depression by benzodiazepines of spontaneous and evoked activity of neurons intercalated in the visual pathway. While Heiss et al. (1969) observed a reduction of spontaneous and photically elicited firing of retinal neurons after diazepam (2–5 mg·kg^{-1} i.v.) in cats, Bigler (1976) noted a depression by diazepam (2–5 mg·kg^{-1} i.v.) of spontaneous and photically induced discharge of geniculocortical relay neurons as well as of spontaneous but not of evoked activity of inhibitory interneurons in the lateral geniculate body of anesthetized rats. Interestingly, in both studies a bursting oscillatory pattern of neuronal activity was sometimes observed after these rather high doses of diazepam, thus confirming the observations in the hippocampus and cerebellum mentioned previously.

In a most recent study in the cuneate nucleus of decerebrate cats, Polzin and Barnes (1979) found a reduction of spontaneously active and glutamate-excited cuneate neurons by iontophoretically applied diazepam and GABA. Both diazepam- and GABA-evoked depressions were antagonized by iontophoretically administered bicuculline or picrotoxin.

V. Conclusions

Benzodiazepines have been shown to depress the spontaneous and evoked activity of single principal neurons in various brain areas after both systemic and local administration. Although no direct comparison was made, it appears that the sensitivity of these neurons, which certainly subserve very dissimilar functions, was not essentially different in the cerebral and cerebellar cortex, in hippocampus and amygdala, in diencephalic structures, or in the lower brain stem. Convincing evidence supports the view that the effect of benzodiazepines on the neurons studied is due to an enhanced inhibitory control by local GABAergic interneurons.

X. Effects on Specific Neurotransmitter and Mediator Systems

In this section we discuss the effects of benzodiazepines on the functions of specific neurotransmitter and neuromediator (modulator) systems. We consider the available data on presynaptic and postsynaptic mechanisms obtained both with biochemical and neurophysiological methods. Some findings reported in this section have, of course, already been mentioned in other sections or will be commented on in Sect. Z.

I. Acetylcholine (ACh)

Several observations made over the past 2 decades suggest some kind of interaction of benzodiazepines with cholinergic mechanisms, e.g., the marked protective activity of these drugs against convulsions, muscular hyperactivity, and mortality produced by anticholinesterases (Gatti et al., 1973; Johnson and Lowndes, 1974; Lipp, 1973; Rump et al., 1973) or the finding that pentetrazole profoundly affects the dynamics of brain ACh (Giarman and Pepeu, 1962; Longoni et al., 1974; Mitchell, 1963; Beleslin et al., 1965; Gardner and Webster, 1973; Hemsworth and Neal, 1968;

GREEN, 1964). Furthermore, anecdotal clinical reports indicate that cholinesterase inhibitors are able to almost immediately restitute full consciousness in comatose patients after overdoses of benzodiazepines and in postoperative patients anesthetized with intravenous benzodiazepines. NAGY and DECSI (1978) described the use of physostigmine as an antidote against sublethal or lethal doses of diazepam in rats, rabbits, and cats. This interaction between benzodiazepines and anticholinesterases cannot be localized at the benzodiazepine receptors, since physostigmine failed to significantly inhibit ^{3}H-diazepam binding in concentrations up to 10^{-4} mol·l^{-1} [MÖHLER and OKADA, 1977a; BRAESTRUP and SQUIRES, 1978a; SPETH et al., 1978; see, however, SPEEG et al. (1979) for the effect of a commercially available injectable form of physostigmine].

1. Choline Acetyltransferase and Cholinesterases

Diazepam up to high concentrations did not affect choline acetyltransferase or cholinesterase activity in the mouse whole brain and rat striatum in vitro or mouse whole brain choline acetyltransferase in vivo (CONSOLO et al., 1972, 1974, 1975). HOLMES et al. (1978) studied a number of benzodiazepines for their effect on human plasma and red cell cholinesterase activity in vitro. At 1 mmol·l^{-1} concentration, compounds with an alkyl substituent on N1 were active on cholinesterase in plasma and, although to a much lesser degree, in red cells. Lower concentrations were not examined. Treatment of rats with diazepam, nitrazepam, clonazepam, chlordiazepoxide, and medazepam daily with 5 and 10 mg·kg^{-1} s.c. on 5 consecutive days did not alter cholinesterase activity in plasma and red cells (WIEZOREK et al., 1977).

2. ACh Content

The elevation of brain ACh levels by benzodiazepines is well documented. CONSOLO et al. (1972, 1974) and LADINSKI et al. (1973) reported that diazepam in doses between 5 and 40 mg·kg^{-1} i.p., as well as pentobarbitone (55 mg·kg^{-1}), increased ACh levels in the whole brain, the diencephalon, and the hemispheres of mice, but not in the cerebellum or mesencephalon. Choline levels were unaltered. After 5 mg·kg^{-1} i.v., the effect of diazepam lasted only for 4 h in the hemispheres and for 30 min in the diencephalon, whereas the protective effect against pentetrazole-induced seizures was longer-lasting. A similar increase of hemispheric ACh was found in rats and guinea pigs (CONSOLO et al., 1975). Diazepam had no effect on the level of ACh or choline in rat atria (CONSOLO et al., 1975). The same authors excluded hypothermia as a possible cause of the increased level of brain ACh after benzodiazepines. CHENEY et al. (1973) observed a 25% to 30% increase of whole brain ACh in the mouse after 2 mg·kg^{-1} diazepam; the steady-state concentrations of choline were unaltered. An increased ACh content of the synaptic vesicle fraction of the cerebral cortex of guinea pigs was found after various intraperitoneal doses of chlordiazepoxide and the benzodiazepine SCH 12,041 (ESSMAN, 1973). No change in the level of brain ACh after 5 mg·kg^{-1} chlordiazepoxide i.p. was found by DOMINO and OLDS (1972) in rats implanted with intracerebral electrodes for electrical self-stimulation; chlordiazepoxide also did not prevent the reduction of ACh produced by self-stimulation. A comparison of general anesthetics and benzodiazepines was made by SETHY (1978). Pentobarbitone

(30 mg·kg^{-1} and 60 mg·kg^{-1} i.p.) increased the ACh level in all rat brain areas studied, namely the cerebral cortex, the striatum, the hippocampus, and the brain stem. In contrast, diazepam and flurazepam at 100 mg·kg^{-1} and triazolam at 30 mg·kg^{-1} increased ACh only in cerebral cortex and striatum. Alprazolam and ketazolam at 100 mg·kg^{-1} had no significant effect on brain ACh. There was a good correlation, on the one hand, between sedation and loss of righting reflex and, on the other hand, the increase in ACh level. In another study, diazepam (5 mg·kg^{-1} i.p.) did not alter the ACh content of the striatum in rats, but prevented the increase of striatal ACh induced by picrotoxin (JAVOY et al., 1977). The increase of striatal ACh was shown by these authors to be caused by an enhanced dopaminergic activity in the striatum consequent to a release of nigral dopaminergic neurons from GABAergic inhibitory control. Another drug-induced change of brain ACh could be prevented by a benzodiazepine: As shown by CONSOLO et al. (1975), pentetrazole selectively decreased the ACh content in the hippocampus of rats; when the convulsant was administered together with diazepam, the hippocampal ACh level was not significantly different from that in vehicle-treated control animals.

3. ACh Turnover

Diazepam 7 µmol·kg^{-1} ($\sim$2 mg·kg^{-1} i.p.) and muscimol 8.8 µmol·kg^{-1} ($\sim$1 mg·kg^{-1} i.v.) decreased the rate of ACh turnover in the midbrain and cortex of the brain, but not in striatum and hippocampus (ZSILLA et al., 1976). In the mouse, diazepam, chlordiazepoxide, and another benzodiazepine, Ro 5-5807, reduced the specific activity of ACh in the brain following intravenous injection of phosphoryl (Me-^{14}C) choline (CHENEY et al., 1973).

4. ACh Release

Potassium-induced release of ACh from rat midbrain slices was not affected by chlordiazepoxide up to concentrations of 10^{-4} mol·l^{-1}, in marked contrast to the concentration-dependent inhibition of release observed with various barbiturates (RICHTER and WERLING, 1979).

5. Firing Rate of Central Cholinergic Neurons

So far no studies on identified central cholinergic neurones under the effect of benzodiazepines have been published.

6. Conclusions

The available data indicate that benzodiazepines, in pharmacologically relevant doses, produce an elevation of the ACh content of the brain, at least in some areas. These drugs do not affect the biosynthetic and catabolic enzymes and do not seem to inhibit the release of ACh at cholinergic nerve endings. The reduced turnover of ACh observed after benzodiazepines is therefore most likely due to a reduction of cholinergic neuron activity. There is no evidence that benzodiazepines affect cholinergic neurons directly; it is more probable that their primary action is on structures that control cholinergic neurons. This would also explain why the various cholinergic pathways in the brain do not seem to be uniformly affected by the drugs. It is not yet possible to correlate the changes in cholinergic systems with the pharmacologic effects of benzodiazepines. One hypothesis that can be tested is that the reduction of cholinergic neuron activity in the hippocampus observed after high doses might be involved in the amnesic effect of benzodiazepines (GHONEIM and MEWALDT, 1977; JONES et al., 1979a).

II. Dopamine (DA)

1. Dopamine Receptors

Diazepam did not inhibit the specific binding of ^{3}H-haloperidol and ^{3}H-DA in calf brain membranes (BURT et al., 1976).

2. Dopamine Uptake

Uptake of ^{3}H-DA into slices of the tuberculum olfactorium was moderately inhibited by diazepam in concentrations of 10^{-7}–10^{-5} mol·l^{-1} (FUXE et al., 1975).

3. Dopamine Release

Release of ^{3}H-DA, previously taken up by pieces of rat striatum, in response to KCl (15 mmol·l^{-1}) was enhanced by about 50% by diazepam (10^{-5} mol·l^{-1}), while the basal, unstimulated release was unaffected (MARTIN and MITCHELL, 1979). GABA did not enhance stimulated ^{3}H-DA release. Although this finding made an involvement of GABA in the effect of diazepam unlikely, bicuculline (10^{-5} mol·l^{-1}), but not picrotoxin (10^{-5} mol·l^{-1}), was able to partially antagonize the effect of diazepam on the stimulated DA release.

4. Brain Level of Dopamine

The DA level in the rat whole brain or in distinct brain areas was found to be either unaffected by benzodiazepines (CONSOLO et al., 1975; FENESSY and LEE, 1972; TAYLOR, 1969; TAYLOR and LAVERTY, 1973; PUGSLEY and LIPPMANN, 1975, 1976), slightly elevated (CORRODI et al., 1967; FENESSY and LEE, 1972; RASTOGI et al., 1976), or reduced (RASTOGI et al., 1977).

5. Turnover of Dopamine

Changes in the turnover of DA under the effect of benzodiazepines were studied by various methodological approaches. Measuring the decline of DA after inhibition of tyrosine hydroxylase (usually with α-methyltyrosine) either biochemically or by fluorescence microscopy, CORRODI et al. (1971) and LIDBRINK (1972) observed a small but significant decrease of DA turnover in the neostriatum and the limbic forebrain of rats after chlordiazepoxide and diazepam. The drugs potentiated the retardation of DA decline induced by immobilization stress. In contrast, both compounds slightly increased DA turnover in the median eminence of the hypothalamus and counteracted the stress-induced decrease of turnover (LIDBRINK, 1972). Effects similar to those of benzodiazepines were observed with three barbiturates and meprobamate (LIDBRINK, 1972; LIDBRINK et al., 1973); meprobamate (200 mg·kg⁻¹) enhanced the decrease of DA induced by immobilization stress in the striatum and accelerated the increase of DA turnover in the median eminence. An alteration of α-methyltyrosine-induced decrease of DA in various rat brain areas was also found by SHIBUYA et al. (1976) after diazepam, triazolam, and prazepam at 10 mg·kg⁻¹ i.p. Diazepam, desmethyldiazepam, and chlordiazepoxide partially counteracted the acceleration of DA turnover induced in the rat striatum by exposure to an ambient temperature of 4 °C (DOTEUCHI and COSTA, 1973); no effect was seen with these drugs in the brain of animals kept at an ambient temperature of 22 °C. The decline of dopamine fluorescence intensity induced by H 44/68 in the nucleus caudatus, nucleus accumbens, tuberculum olfactorium, and entorhinal cortex was attenuated by diazepam and chlordiazepoxide 10 mg·kg⁻¹ (FUXE et al., 1975). In contrast, the decline of DA fluororescence was enhanced by diazepam in the lateral external layer of the median eminence. The drug also partially counteracted the increase of DA turnover induced by pimozide. The effect of diazepam on DA turnover in striatum and limbic structures was not affected by maximal tolerated doses of strychnine, but by high doses of bicuculline. PUGSLEY and LIPPMANN (1975, 1976) observed that the α-methyltyrosine-induced decline of DA was attenuated by immobilization stress; chlordiazepoxide did not alter this effect of stress, but reduced the turnover in nonstressed rats.

Another way to assess DA turnover is to study the fate of ³H-DA in brain areas after its intracerebroventricular injection. Chlordiazepoxide (10 mg·kg⁻¹) retarded the disappearance of ³H-DA in cerebellum and striatum and increased the level of ³H-DA in the cerebellum already elevated by stress (PUGSLEY and LIPPMANN, 1975, 1976). Similar results in unstressed rats had been described by TAYLOR and LAVERTY (1969, 1973) in the striatum. Decrease or increase of the DA level may indicate an enhanced or reduced utilization of the transmitter. Electroshock stress decreased DA level in the striatum of rats, and diazepam and nitrazepam, but not chlordiazepoxide, all given in two doses of 10 mg·kg⁻¹ s.c., 2 and 4 h before death, prevented this decrease (TAYLOR and LAVERTY, 1969, 1973).

CHERAMY et al. (1977) measured the spontaneous release of ³H-DA in the caudate of encéphale isolé cats after biosynthesis from ³H-L-tyrosine using a push-pull cannula. Picrotoxin 2.5 mg·kg⁻¹ increased the spontaneous release of ³H-DA; diazepam (10 mg·kg⁻¹), which by itself did not affect the release, blocked the stimulating effect of picrotoxin.

Homovanillic acid (HVA) and 3,4-dihydroxyphenylacetic acid (DOPAC) as metabolites of DA were used to study the effect of benzodiazepines on DA turnover. The earliest indication for a reduced turnover of DA after benzodiazepines was the finding by DA PRADA and PLETSCHER (1966) that diazepam (10 mg·kg⁻¹ i.p.) significantly reduced HVA in the whole brain of rats. BARTHOLINI et al. (1973) confirmed this effect in rats kept at a room temperature of 22 °C; this dose also produced consistent hypothermia. When diazepam was given to rats kept at an ambient temperature of 32 °C, hypothermia was absent and the whole brain HVA level was not significantly different from those of untreated rats kept at 22 °C room temperature. Since exposure of rats to 32 °C ambient temperature induced a slight increase in body temperature and in

HVA, benzodiazepines under these conditions did not fail to affect DA turnover, but rather inhibited the increase caused by hyperthermia. No change of whole brain HVA in rats was observed by CONSOLO et al. (1975) 30 min after an intravenous injection of diazepam 5 mg · kg^{-1}. Administration of diazepam and bromazepam for 22 days at a daily dose of 10 mg · kg^{-1} s.c. to rats decreased locomotor activity to 39% and 51%, respectively, and decreased the level of HVA in the striatum, cerebral cortex, hypothalamus, pons-medulla, and midbrain by 5%–35% (RASTOGI et al., 1976). After a withdrawal period of 48 h, the DA levels were decreased by 20%–40% and striatal HVA tended to increase. A single dose of diazepam and bromazepam (10 mg · kg^{-1} s.c.) decreased spontaneous locomotor activity by about 70% and reduced striatal HVA by 28%, whereas striatal DOPAC was increased by 32% (RASTOGI et al., 1977, 1978). Clobazam, a 1,5-benzodiazepine, did not alter DA, HVA, or DOPAC, but decreased locomotor activity by 22%. HVA and DOPAC were found unaltered after diazepam and the thienodiazepine, Y-7131 (SETOGUCHI et al., 1978). KELLER et al. (1976) observed a 15% decrease in rat whole brain HVA after diazepam, chlordiazepoxide, flunitrazepam, and clonazepam (10 mg · kg^{-1} i.p.). The most marked effects of benzodiazepines on DA turnover were, however, found when DA turnover was accelerated by neuroleptics. The neuroleptic-induced increase of HVA in the rat brain was markedly attenuated by the administration of benzodiazepines prior to the neuroleptics (KELLER et al., 1976). Picrotoxin, at a dose which did not affect the HVA level by itself, reduced the effect of diazepam on haloperidol-induced elevation of HVA. The partial reversal of neuroleptic-induced rise of HVA by diazepam was seen in limbic structures as well as in the striatum. Various benzodiazepines potentiated the cataleptic effect of neuroleptics. The interactions of benzodiazepines with neuroleptics were mimicked by aminooxyacetic acid (AOAA), an inhibitor of GABA catabolism. FADDA et al. (1978) reported that diazepam at 2 mg · kg^{-1}, a dose which by itself did not affect rat brain DOPAC levels, prevented the increase of DOPAC induced in frontal cortex and nucleus accumbens by electric footshock stress; pentobarbitone (25 mg · kg^{-1}) was ineffective. Surprisingly, diazepam enhanced the increase of HVA in the striatum on the side of cortical spreading depression induced in rats with chronically implanted cannulas by the unilateral application of KCl on the surface of the cerebral cortex (BARTHOLINI et al., 1973). The complex and poorly understood interactions of neuronal pathways in cortical spreading depression do not permit a simple explanation of the effect of diazepam in this particular functional state.

   In cats with a permanent cannula in the cisterna magna, diazepam (0.3–1.5 mg · kg^{-1} i.p.) failed to alter the concentration of HVA in the cisternal cerebrospinal fluid (GRIAUZDE et al., 1979).

   The allosteric activation of striatal tyrosine hydroxylase occurring after administration of haloperidol to rats was reduced by diazepam and muscimol, but enhanced by picrotoxin and isoniazid (GALE et al., 1978).

   BISWAS and CARLSSON (1978) used the accumulation of endogenous L-DOPA after inhibition of aromatic L-aminoacid decarboxylase with 3-hydroxybenzylhydrazine (NSD 1015) to measure the effect of diazepam on the synthesis rate of catecholamines at the tyrosine hydroxylase step. Diazepam injected in doses of 1–10 mg · kg^{-1} i.p. to rats caused a decrease in DOPA accumulation. With 1 mg · kg^{-1} this decrease was significant only in the limbic forebrain; 3 and 10 mg · kg^{-1} caused a significant inhibition in both DA-rich limbic and striatal brain regions as well as in the portions of the hemisphere containing preferential noradrenaline nerve endings, whereas $3 \, \text{mg} \cdot \text{kg}^{-1}$ tended to be more effective than $10 \, \text{mg} \cdot \text{kg}^{-1}$ in reducing DOPA formation in DA-rich limbic areas and striatum. Doses higher than $10 \, \text{mg} \cdot \text{kg}^{-1}$ were not tested, although the difference in the effect of 3 and $10 \, \text{mg} \cdot \text{kg}^{-1}$ indicated the possibility that the effect of higher doses might reverse, i.e., lead to an increase of DOPA accumulation, as did GABA at $100 \, \text{mg} \cdot \text{kg}^{-1}$. Diazepam $3 \, \text{mg} \cdot \text{kg}^{-1}$ reduced the accelerating effect of GABA on DOPA formation, which was interpreted by the authors as a GABA antagonistic effect. Taking the DOPAC/DA ratio in discrete areas of the rat brain as an index of DA turnovers, LAVIELLE et al. (1978) found that mild electric foot shock produced a marked increase of the ratio selectively in frontal and cingulate cortex, two areas innervated by the mesocortical DA neuron system that originates in the ventrotegmental area of the midbrain (A 10-cell group), but not in areas innervated by mesolimbic and nigro-striatal dopaminergic pathways. The doubling of this ratio by stress was completely suppressed by pretreatment with diazepam ($5 \, \text{mg} \cdot \text{kg}^{-1}$ i.p.) and chlordiazepoxide ($10 \, \text{mg} \cdot \text{kg}^{-1}$ i.p.), which did not significantly alter the DOPAC/DA ratio in nonstressed rats.

6. Firing Rate of DA Neurons

The rather casual observations published so far contain conflicting data on the effect of benzodiazepines on single dopamine neurons in the mesencephalon. In rats anesthetized with urethane, diazepam in doses of $0.5-1.5 \, \text{mg} \cdot \text{kg}^{-1}$ i.p. reduced the firing rate of the three substantia nigra pars compacta cells studied (WOLF and HAAS, 1977). In rats anesthetized with chloral hydrate, diazepam in doses up to $8 \, \text{mg} \cdot \text{kg}^{-1}$ i.v. did not significantly alter the spontaneous firing rate of six substantia nigra cells, whereas in three other cells the firing rate was doubled after $1 \, \text{mg} \cdot \text{kg}^{-1}$ (GALLAGER, 1978). BUNNEY and AGHAJANIAN (1976) did not study the effect of diazepam alone on dopaminergic cells; however, in doses between 0.8 and $1.6 \, \text{mg} \cdot \text{kg}^{-1}$ i.v. the drug partially reversed the reduction of firing rate of zona compacta and ventral tegmental area cells produced by dexamphetamine in gallamine-immobilized rats. Pentobarbitone in a cumulative dose of $20 \, \text{mg} \cdot \text{kg}^{-1}$ had a similar effect, however, depressed the firing rate in the absence of dexamphetamine. Since the effect of diazepam on dexamphetamine-induced depression of firing resembled that obtained with the noncataleptic neuroleptic, clozapine, the authors suggested that diazepam might be active as an antipsychotic agent. LAURENT (personal communication) observed a dose-dependent decrease after midazolam of the spontaneous multiunit activity in the substantia nigra pars compacta of unanaesthetized *encéphale isolé* rats; a 50% decrease was achieved between 0.3 and $0.75 \, \text{mg} \cdot \text{kg}^{-1}$ i.v.

7. Conclusions

There is strong evidence that benzodiazepines reduce the turnover of DA in the nigro-striatal and mesolimbic system, whereas the reverse was found in the tuberoinfundibular system. Since benzodiazepines do not interfere directly with DA receptors or the biosynthesis and metabolism of DA and since the various DA systems are affected differently by these drugs, there is good reason to believe that the site of action is at synapses that modulate the activity of DA cells. The most likely candidate is a GABAergic synapse. The electrophysiologic correlate to the decreased turnover of DA after benzodiazepines, i.e., a reduction of the firing rate of dopaminergic neurons, requires further systematic investigation. How important the reduced activity of DA turnover is for the pharmacologic effects of benzodiazepines cannot be assessed at present. It is also not known whether tolerance to the effect of these drugs on DA neurons develops. While the effect of benzodiazepines on DA turnover was very small in animals kept under normal laboratory conditions, the depression of DA neuron activity was very pronounced under conditions of increased dopaminergic activity, such as in stress and after neuroleptic drugs. The increase of activity in the tuberoinfundibular DA system may explain, at least in part, the depressant effect of benzodiazepines on prolactin secretion (see Sect. H).

III. Noradrenaline (NA)

1. Noradrenaline Uptake

Chlordiazepoxide and diazepam did not inhibit the uptake of ^{3}H-NA into synaptosomal fractions of rat brain (CORRODI et al., 1971). A lack of uptake inhibition was also found by LIDBRINK and FARNEBO (1973) in cerebral cortex slices of rats with chlordiazepoxide, phenobarbitone, and pentobarbitone in a wide range of concentrations. Diazepam 1 mg·kg^{-1} failed to significantly alter the uptake of intracerebroventricularly injected ^{3}H-NA (NAKAMURA and THOENEN, 1972). Benzodiazepines were very weak inhibitors of the uptake of ^{14}C-NA by isolated membranes of bovine adrenal medulla (PLETSCHER, 1977); the IC$_{50}$ were 7×10^{-5} mol·l^{-1} and 5×10^{-4} mol·l^{-1} for diazepam and chlordiazepoxide, respectively. TAYLOR and LAVERTY (1969, 1973) found the uptake or ^{3}H-NA into synaptosomes of rat hypothalamus hardly affected by even high concentrations of benzodiazepines.

2. Noradrenaline Release

The spontaneous release and the field stimulation-induced release of NA from cerebral cortex slices of the rat were not affected by chlordiazepoxide (LIDBRINK and FARNEBO, 1973). The release of NA in the rat forebrain in response to electrical stimulation of ascending NA pathways was not decreased by chlordiazepoxide and diazepam.

3. Noradrenaline Levels

In the earliest report on the effect of benzodiazepines on endogenous NA levels, MOE et al. (1962) found no significant changes of the NA content of the brain of rabbits given a single intraperitoneal injection of chlordiazepoxide 100 mg·kg^{-1} or daily injections of 25 mg·kg^{-1} for 5 days; a small increase of cardiac NA was, however, observed 1 and 3 h after injection. TAYLOR (1969) and TAYLOR and LAVERTY (1969, 1973) also failed to find significant changes of the NA content in different brain areas of the rat after chlordiazepoxide and diazepam 10 mg·kg^{-1} s.c. However, the drugs counteracted the reduction of endogenous NA level induced by electroshock (TAYLOR and LAVERTY, 1969, 1973). Brain NA was unaltered in rats after 5 mg·kg^{-1} diazepam i.v. (CONSOLO et al., 1975). Of six benzodiazepines administered in doses corresponding to the ED_{50} in a rotarod test, only clonazepam, nitrazepam, and diazepam increased the NA level in the whole brain of mice (FENESSY and LEE, 1972), whereas chlordiazepoxide, medazepam, and flurazepam produced no significant effect. A 5-day treatment of rats with daily doses of 150 mg·kg^{-1} diazepam or a 7-day treatment with 25 mg·kg^{-1} or 50 mg·kg^{-1} did not result in any significant change of the NA level in the brain and heart (GASCON and LELORIER, 1975). A slight increase of the NA content in the brain stem of rats was reported by NAKAMURA and THOENEN (1972) after diazepam 1 mg·kg^{-1} i.p. Chlordiazepoxide 20 mg·kg^{-1} i.p. did not alter the NA content of the whole brain of stressed and unstressed rats (PUGSLEY and LIPPMANN, 1975, 1976). Diazepam and the thienodiazepine, Y-7131 at 10 mg·kg^{-1} i.p. retarded the depletion of NA in the diencephalon induced by foot shock stress (SETOGUCHI et al., 1978). An increase of the NA content of the hippocampus, hypothalamus, and pons-medulla was observed by RASTOGI et al. (1977) with a single dose of diazepam 10 mg·kg^{-1} s.c. in rats; this dose depressed spontaneous locomotor activity by 71%. At the same dose, the 1,5-benzodiazepine, clobazam, which depressed locomotor activity only by 22%, had no effect on NA levels. Bromazepam 10 mg·kg^{-1} s.c. also increased the NA content (RASTOGI et al., 1978a). Daily administration to rats of diazepam and bromazepam for 22 days with 10 mg·kg^{-1} s.c. decreased spontaneous locomotor activity to 39% and 51%, respectively, and elevated the NA content in the cerebral cortex, hypothalamus, pons-medulla, and midbrain by 20% to 50% (RASTOGI et al., 1976); a withdrawal period of 48 h increased spontaneous locomotor activity and reduced NA levels by 10%–40%. Diazepam (1 mg·kg^{-1} i.p.) prevented the decrease of brain NA level in rats submitted to craniocervical surgery (whiplash) (BOISMARE et al., 1978).

4. Noradrenaline Turnover

The decline of NA levels after inhibition of tyrosine hydroxylase with α-methyl-tyrosine or its methylester (H 44/68) was used by several workers to assess NA turnover after benzodiazepines. Measuring NA biochemically and by fluorescence microscopy in several brain regions of rats, CORRODI et al. (1971) and LIDBRINK (1972) found that chlordiazepoxide and diazepam retarded the decline of NA in the cerebral and cerebellar cortex as well as in the hippocampus, but not in the hypothalamus and lower brain stem, suggesting a decrease of NA turnover in locus coeruleus neurons, most probably by a decreased neuronal activity. Even more marked was the blockade of immobilization stress-induced increase of NA turnover. Similar results were obtained by SHIBUYA et al. (1976) after chlordiazepoxide, diazepam, triazolam, and prazepam at a dose of 10 mg·kg^{-1} i.p. Diazepam (10 mg·kg^{-1}) attenuated the increase of NA turnover induced by piperoxane, which is thought to block NA autoreceptors (FUXE et al., 1975). The same dose decreased the time course of NA depletion by H 44/68, as measured by the fluorescence of smear preparations of the cerebral cortex and counteracted the stimulation of turnover produced by yohimbine. PUGSLEY and LIPPMANN (1975, 1976) failed to find an attenuation of α-methyl-tyrosine-induced decline of NA in the whole brain of unstressed rats by chlordiazepoxide (20 mg·kg^{-1} i.p.); the drug, however, prevented the accelerated depletion of noradrenaline in stressed animals. The increased turnover rate of NA in the cerebellum and hypothalamus of rats and mice exposed to cold was reduced by diazepam, desmethyldiazepam, and chlordiazepoxide (DOTEUCHI and COSTA, 1973); no such effect was seen in animals kept at an ambient temperature of 22 °C. In mice, chlordiazepoxide (10 mg·kg^{-1}), diazepam (5 mg·kg^{-1}), but not flurazepam (10 mg·kg^{-1}) significantly attenuated the decrease of NA induced by α-methyl-tyrosine in the whole brain (DOMINIC et al., 1975). Three different barbiturates decreased the turnover of NA in the cerebral cortex of rats, but not in the hypothalamus (LIDBRINK, 1972; LIDBRINK et al., 1973). Meprobamate (200 mg · kg^{-1}) under the same conditions was ineffective. Both barbiturates and meprobamate, however, counteracted the increase of NA turnover in all brain parts induced by immobilization.

The fate of ^{3}H-NA injected intracerebroventricularly was also used to study the effect of benzodiazepines on NA turnover. The disappearance rate of ^{3}H-NA from various brain regions except the pons-medulla was slowed down by chlordiazepoxide, diazepam and nitrazepam (TAYLOR and LAVERTY, 1969, 1973). These compounds also attenuated the accelerated disappearance of ^{3}H-NA induced by electroconvulsive shock. Diazepam (1 mg·kg^{-1} i.p.) prolonged the half-life of injected ^{3}H-NA in the brain stem of rats (NAKAMURA and THOENEN, 1972). Chlordiazepoxide (10 mg·kg^{-1}) increased the level of ^{3}H-NA in cerebellum, thalamus-midbrain, and cerebral cortex (PUGSLEY and LIPPMANN, 1975, 1976); the stress-induced accelerated decline of ^{3}H-NA in these regions was prevented by the drug. WISE et al. (1972) and STEIN et al. (1973, 1975, 1977) proposed that the depressant effect of benzodiazepines on NA turnover was subject to tolerance upon repetitive administration. Indeed, they found that the fate of labeled NA and normetanephrine was clearly prolonged by a single dose of oxazepam (20 mg·kg^{-1} i.p.), but no longer after six daily consecutive doses. Results opposite to these were obtained by COOK and SEPINWALL (1975), who found no effect of a single dose of chlordiazepoxide (10 mg · kg^{-1} p.o.) on the fate of intracisternally injected ^{3}H-NA in the whole brain of rats. However, two or three identical doses, given either on consecutive days or at intervals of several days, markedly increased the ^{3}H-NA levels, suggesting a reduced utilization of this amine.

3-Methoxy-4-hydroxyphenylethylglycol sulphate (MOPEG) is a metabolite of NA in the rat brain and changes of its content allow conclusions to be drawn on the utilization of the amine. No changes in the content of MOPEG were found by CONSOLO et al. (1975) in the brain of rats injected intravenously with diazepam 5 mg·kg^{-1}. RASTOGI et al. (1978a) reported a decrease of the MOPEG level after bromazepam (10 mg·kg^{-1}). Similar results were obtained by SETOGUCHI et al. (1978) with the thienodiazepine, Y-7131, but not with diazepam (25 mg·kg^{-1} i.p.).

The accumulation of DOPA in NA-rich brain areas after inhibition of the decarboxylase of aromatic amino acids is an indication of the rate of NA synthesis at the step of tyrosine hydroxylase. BISWAS and CARLSSON (1978) found that diazepam in doses of 1,3, and 10 mg·kg^{-1} i.p. dose dependently depressed the rate of DOPA accumulation in the rat brain hemispheres induced by the inhibitor of decarboxylase, 3-hydroxybenzylhydrazine (NSD 1015).

5. Firing Rate of Noradrenaline Neurons

Based on indirect evidence, MONACHON et al. (1973) and HAEFELY et al. (1975a, 1976) arrived at the conclusion that benzodiazepines reduced the activity of noradrenergic locus coeruleus neurons. The increase of the density of ponto-geniculo-occipital

(PGO) waves in the lateral geniculate body of cats treated with the benzoquinolizine, Ro 4-1284, was assumed to be due to a reduced tonic activity of noradrenergic neurons that normally depress the activity of pontine generator cells for PGO waves. At present only preliminary data is available on the effect of benzodiazepines on the firing rate of individual noradrenergic neurons in the locus coeruleus. Gallager (1978) failed to find a significant change of the discharge rate of neurons in the locus coeruleus of rats after intravenous doses of diazepam up to 20 mg · kg^{-1}. Whether this was due to the anesthetic state of the animals studied and whether physiologic activation of these neurons, e.g., by noxious stimuli, can be reduced by benzodiazepines, remains to be studied. Laurent (personal communication) observed a dose-dependent decrease of spontaneous multiunit activity in the locus coeruleus of *encéphale isolé* rats after i.v. injections of midazolam and chlordiazepoxide; locus coeruleus neurons were less sensitive to these benzodiazepines than neurons in the substantia nigra and the dorsal raphé nucleus.

6. Benzodiazepine Actions and Destruction of Noradrenaline Neurons

The depressant effect of benzodiazepines on central NA systems and the obvious hypothesis that this may underly some of the actions of these drugs are in accord with the following two observations. Chlordiazepoxide raised the threshold for septal driving of the hippocampal theta-rhythm selectively at 7.7 Hz (Gray et al., 1975); a hippocampal theta-rhythm of this frequency is seen in rats exposed to nonreward after training in a rewarded runway task. An effect similar to that of chlordiazepoxide was obtained by inhibition of NA synthesis and selective chemical degeneration of the dorsal noradrenergic bundle. Chlordiazepoxide reversed the extinction of runway performance induced by nonreward in rats with intact noradrenergic systems, but not in animals with a lesioned dorsal noradrenergic bundle (Morris et al., 1979).

7. Conclusions

Although the literature on the interactions of benzodiazepines with central noradrenergic mechanisms is very heterogeneous in respect to drug, doses, methods, and species, the general conclusions may be drawn that benzodiazepines reduce the activity of central noradrenergic neurons. The effect is unequivocally shown for those neurons that originate in the locus coeruleus and project to the neocortex, limbic structures, and the cerebellum. The doses required to depress the turnover of NA were higher than those that produce clear-cut behavioral effects. This may indicate that benzodiazepines affect the normal activity of noradrenergic neurons very little and only in higher pharmacologic doses, but that they are very effective in counteracting the increased activity induced by stress. The concept that benzodiazepines lose their effect on the central noradrenergic tone upon repeated administration is based on experimental findings obtained in one laboratory and requires confirmation before it can be generally accepted. The problem is an important one because the reduction of activity or effectiveness of the ascending dorsal noradrenergic bundle is generally believed to account for sedation. Since the initial sedation seen with benzodiazepines both in man and in animals usually diminishes with repeated exposure to the drugs, it would be interesting to know whether the "tolerance" to the sedative effects is due to an "escape" of noradrenergic neurons from the depressant effect of benzo-diazepines or to a habituation of target structures to a persisting reduction in nor-adrenergic tone.

IV. Adrenaline

No data are available on the effect of anxiolytics on the dynamics of adrenaline in the central nervous system.

Treatment of rats for 5 days with daily doses of 150 mg·kg⁻¹ diazepam or for 7 days with daily doses of 25 or 50 mg·kg⁻¹ increased the adrenaline content of adrenals by about 30% (GASCON and LELORIER, 1975; GASCON, 1977). Perhaps this finding should be related to the enhanced induction of tyrosine hydroxylase in rat ad-renal medulla by multiple subcutaneous injections of isoprenaline or by intravenous injections of 6-hydroxydopamine, but not by reserpine or insulin after diazepam (SMITH et al., 1974). β-Adrenergic agonists release catecholamines from incubated rat adrenals, an effect which is accompanied by an increase of cAMP and enhanced by inhibitors of cAMP phosphodiesterase (GUTMAN and BOONYAVIROY, 1979). cAMP has also been postulated to be an essential step in the induction of tyrosine hy-droxylase (GUIDOTTI et al., 1976). Benzodiazepines have been found to inhibit phos-phodiesterase activity in various tissues (BEER et al., 1972; DALTON et al., 1974).

V. Phenylethylamine

Biosynthesis of ³H-phenylethylamine from ³H-L-phenylalanine in the brain of mice was markedly reduced by diazepam (75 mg·kg⁻¹) and chlordiazepoxide (75 mg·kg⁻¹) (HAVDALA et al., 1977).

VI. 5-Hydroxytryptamine (5-HT)

1. 5-HT-Receptors

Diazepam did not inhibit the stereospecific binding of D-LSD to brain membranes suggested to represent binding to central 5-HT receptors (BENNETT and SNYDER, 1975).

2. 5-HT Uptake

Diazepam did not affect the uptake of ¹⁴C-5-HT administered intracisternally in rats (CHASE et al., 1970). In synaptosomes from the brain of rats administered a daily dose of 10 mg·kg⁻¹ diazepam s.c. on 22 consecutive days, the uptake of ³H-5-HT was en-hanced by 31% (RASTOGI et al., 1978 b). After a 48-h withdrawal period, the synapto-somal uptake of ³H-5-HT was decreased by 30%. The uptake of ¹⁴C-5-HT by isolated human blood platelets was inhibited by 50% on exposure to chlordiazepoxide 10^{-3} mol·l⁻¹ and medazepam 10^{-4} mol·l⁻¹ (LINGJAERDE, 1973). Clonazepam in-hibited the uptake of ³H-5-HT by mouse brain synaptosomes by 23% at 10^{-5} and by 43% at 10^{-4} mol·l⁻¹, but at 8 mg·kg⁻¹ i.p. it did not affect ex vivo uptake (CHUNG HWANG and VAN WOERT, 1979).

3. 5-HT Release

Incubation of isolated rabbit blood platelets for 2 h with 1 mmol·l^{-1} chlordiazepoxide reduced their 5-HT content to nearly 50% (Pletscher et al., 1967). Spontaneous release of ^{14}C-5-HT from isolated human platelets was slightly inhibited by chlordiazepoxide 3×10^{-4} mol·l^{-1} and medazepam 10^{-5}–10^{-4} mol·l^{-1}. At 1 mmol·l^{-1} the drugs enhanced the spontaneous efflux of ^{14}C-5-HT (Lingjaerde, 1973).

The potassium-induced release of ^{3}H-5-HT from preloaded slices of rat amygdala, but not from hippocampal slices, was decreased by flurazepam 10^{-7}–10^{-5} mol·l^{-1} whereas the spontaneous efflux was enhanced (James et al., 1979). ACTH, although it did not affect the 5-HT release by itself, antagonized the modulating effect of flurazepam. These findings were believed to support the hypothesis that ACTH might be an endogenous anxiogenic compound and were taken as an indication that the interaction between ACTH and benzodiazepines in behavioral tests involved a 5-HT neuron system (File and Vellucci, 1978). Spontaneous release of ^{3}H-5-HT from preloaded mouse brain synaptosomes was increased by 24% and 50% with 10^{-5} and 10^{-4} mol·l^{-1} clonazepam, respectively (Chung Hwang and Van Woert, 1979).

4. 5-HT Levels

Most investigators observed an increase of 5-HT level in the brain after benzodiazepines. In the rat, chlordiazepoxide, diazepam, and oxazepam (20 mg·kg^{-1} i.p.) were found to significantly increase whole-brain 5-HT content (Bourgoin et al., 1975). Elevated levels of 5-HT in the rat brain and the spinal cord were also observed by Fernstrom et al. (1974) between 1 and 2 h after 5–20 mg·kg^{-1} diazepam i.p. A single dose of diazepam and clobazam (10 mg·kg^{-1} s.c.) increased the 5-HT content of rat hippocampus, hypothalamus, and midbrain (Rastogi et al., 1977, 1978 b). Six hours after the last of 22 daily injections of diazepam (10 mg·kg^{-1} s.c.) to rats the 5-HT content was elevated by 26–74% in all brain areas studied, i.e., cerebral cortex, hypothalamus, pons-medulla, midbrain, and striatum (Agarwal et al., 1977). An identical treatment increased the 5-HT content of whole-brain synaptosomes by 50% (Rastogi et al., 1978 b; Rastogi and Singhal, 1978); after 48 h of withdrawal the 5-HT content was reduced. In contrast to the above authors, Consolo et al. (1975) did not find any changes in the whole rat brain 5-HT after diazepam (5 mg·kg^{-1} i.v.), and clonazepam (4 mg·kg^{-1} i.p.) also failed to alter the 5-HT content (Jenner et al., 1978, Chung Hwang and Van Woert, 1979). Fenessey and Lee (1972) found only clonazepam out of six benzodiazepines active in elevating mouse whole-brain 5-HT at doses corresponding to ED$_{50}$ in a rotarod test. Jenner et al. (1975) and Chadwick et al. (1978), also working on the mouse, observed an elevation of whole-brain 5-HT by about 40% after acute administration of clonazepam (4 mg·kg^{-1}) and of diazepam (32 mg·kg^{-1}), whereas Chung Hwang and Van Woert (1979) found 5-HT unaffected after 4 mg·kg^{-1} diazepam i.p. After eight daily doses of 4 mg·kg^{-1} clonazepam i.p. the 5-HT level was normal (Jenner et al., 1975). In guinea pigs given clonazepam in doses between 5 and 20 mg·kg^{-1} i.p. the whole brain 5-HT content was almost doubled after 3 hours (Weiner et al., 1977). The effects of acute and subchronic treatment of hooded rats with chlordiazepoxide on brain 5-HT (File and Vellucci, 1978; Vellucci and File, 1979) is reported in the next section.

5. 5-HT Turnover

5-Hydroxyindoleacetic Acid (5-HIAA). A method frequently used to estimate 5-HT turnover is the measurement of the main metabolite of 5-HT, 5-HIAA.

An early study of DA PRADA and PLETSCHER (1966) showed that high intraperitoneal doses of diazepam (10 mg·kg^{-1}) and chlordiazepoxide (50 mg·kg^{-1}) elevated the whole brain level of 5-HIAA in rats by 24%–32%. Very similar results in the brain and spinal cord of rats were obtained by FERNSTROM et al. (1974) with diazepam. The effect of diazepam was influenced by prior food consumption. A protein-free carbohydrate and fat diet elevated brain 5-HT and 5-HIAA, and this effect was enhanced by diazepam. In contrast, a meal consisting of neutral amino acids plus carbohydrates prevented the rise of 5-HIAA otherwise induced by diazepam. An increase of rat brain 5-HIAA was also found by BOURGOIN et al. (1975) after 20 mg·kg^{-1} of chlordiazepoxide, diazepam, and oxazepam. AGARWAL et al. (1977) observed a marked rise of the 5-HIAA content in the cerebral cortex, hypothalamus, pons-medulla, midbrain, and striatum of rats 6 h after the last of 22 consecutive daily subcutaneous injections of diazepam and bromazepam (20 mg·kg^{-1}). The 5-HIAA levels were even higher after a withdrawal period of 3 days, although, at that time, the 5-HT content had fallen below control values. RASTOGI et al. (1977, 1978 b) reported on elevated 5-HIAA in the hippocampus, hypothalamus, and midbrain after single doses of diazepam (10 mg·kg^{-1} s.c.), clobazam and bromazepam. The same authors obtained similar increases in 5-HIAA in these three areas after 22 consecutive daily doses of diazepam (10 mg·kg^{-1} s.c.). An increase of rat brain 5-HIAA was obtained by JENNER et al. (1975, 1978) with 4 mg·kg^{-1} clonazepam i.p. acutely, but not after eight daily injections. In hooded rats, FILE and VELLUCCI (1978) assessed the turnover of brain 5-HT by measuring the 5-HIAA/5-HT ratio. A single dose of chlordiazepoxide (5 mg·kg^{-1} i.p.) did not significantly alter the 5-HT and 5-HIAA levels and, hence, the ratio in various brain regions. After five consecutive daily injections, however, the 5-HIAA/5-HT ratios were markedly decreased in hypothalamus, hippocampus, midbrain, and cerebral cortex due to an increase of 5-HT and a slight decrease of 5-HIAA. Since ACTH had an opposite effect, namely accelerated 5-HT turnover, the decrease of 5-HT turnover produced by chlordiazepoxide was proposed to be causally implicated in the anxiolytic action of benzodiazepines and the increase of 5-HT turnover in the anxiogenic action of ACTH (assessed in a social interaction model). The validity of the 5-HIAA/5-HT ratio as a measure of 5-HT turnover may be questioned in view of the effect of benzodiazepines on the efflux of 5-HIAA (see below). In a later study, the same authors (VELLUCCI and FILE, 1979) found no changes in the 5-HT and 5-HIAA levels after 25 days of treatment with 5 mg·kg^{-1} chlordiazepoxide i.p. Again, their conclusion that tolerance developed to the depressant effect of chlordiazepoxide on 5-HT turnover is not too convincing. Only two studies failed to find an increase of rat brain 5-HIAA after benzodiazepines, namely that of CONSOLO et al. (1975) using diazepam 5 mg·kg^{-1} and that of PUGSLEY and LIPPMANN (1975) using 20 mg·kg^{-1} chlordiazepoxide i.p.

SETOGUCHI et al. (1978) found that diazepam and the thienodiazepine, Y-7131, decreased the accumulation of 5-HIAA induced by probenecid in the rat brain, indicating a reduced formation of 5-HIAA. Both compounds suppressed the increase of 5-HIAA induced by foot shock stress.

In mice, chlordiazepoxide was found to decrease and nitrazepam to increase the brain level of 5-HIAA (FENNESSY and LEE, 1972); the doses corresponded to the ED_{50} in a rotarod test. CHADWICK et al. (1978) observed a dose-dependent rise of 5-HT and 5-HIAA after single doses of diazepam and clonazepam. The levels of the amine and of its acidic metabolite were normal 24 h after the last of eight daily injections of clonazepam (4 mg·kg^{-1}) and diazepam (32 mg·kg^{-1}). A further dose of either benzodiazepine, administered on the 9th day, produced a smaller increase of 5-HIAA than in drug-naive animals. Interestingly, diphenylhydantoin 20 mg·kg^{-1}, once or on 9 consecutive days, produced changes in 5-HT and 5-HIAA very similar to those seen after benzodiazepines. CHUNG HWANG and VAN WOERT (1979) found mouse brain 5-HT and 5-HIAA unaffected after clonazepam (4 mg·kg^{-1}), but significantly increased after diazepam (32 mg·kg^{-1} i.p.). In cats with a permanent cannula in the cisterna magna, diazepam (0.3–1.5 mg·kg^{-1} i.p.) did not change the concentration of 5-HIAA in the cisternal cerebrospinal fluid (GRIAUZDE et al., 1979).

Fate of Intracerebroventricularly Injected ^{14}C-*5-HT.* Using the fate of intracerebroventricularly injected labeled 5-HT, several authors obtained evidence for a reduced utilization of this amine after benzodiazepines. CHASE et al. (1970) reported that diazepam markedly retarded the decline of ^{14}C-5-HT and ^{14}C-5-HIAA in the rat brain; in addition the efflux of intracisternally injected ^{14}C-5-HIAA was retarded. Very similar results were obtained by LIPPMANN and PUGSLEY (1974) and PUGSLEY and LIPPMANN (1975, 1976) with 20 mg·kg^{-1} chlordiazepoxide i.p. STEIN et al. (1973) injected rats with chronically indwelling cannulas in the lateral ventricle once or daily on 6 consecutive days with 20 mg·kg^{-1} oxazepam i.p. ^{14}C-5-HT was injected intraventricularly 10 min before the single or the sixth dose of oxazepam; the animals were killed 3 h later. The concentrations of ^{14}C-5-HT and ^{14}C-5-HIAA in the midbrain-hindbrain were significantly higher in rats given oxazepam than in control animals, and there was no significant difference between single and repeated doses of oxazepam, suggesting the absence of tolerance to the depressant effect of benzodiazepines on 5-HT turnover.

COOK and SEPINWALL (1975) also studied the effect of a single dose and of multiple doses of chlordiazepoxide, given at various intervals, on the fate of intracisternally injected ^{14}C-5-HT in rats. Whereas a single oral dose of 10 mg·kg^{-1} chlordiazepoxide produced no significant effect, two and three identical doses, administered either on consecutive days or at intervals of several days consistently increased the ^{14}C-5-HT level in the whole brain, suggesting a reduced utilization of 5-HT. In mice, fludiazepam retarded the disappearance of intracerebrally injected ^{14}C-5-HT and ^{14}C-5-HIAA (NAKAMURA and FUKUSHIMA, 1977).

5-HT Depletion by H 75/12. α-Ethyl-3-hydroxy-4-methylphenethylamine (H 75/12) is an amine which is selectively taken up into 5-HT neurons and displaces 5-HT. Neither diazepam nor the thienodiazepine, Y-7131, prevented the 5-HT depletion induced by H 75/12 (LIPPMANN and PUGSLEY, 1974).

Time Course of 5-HT Depletion After Inhibition of Tryptophan Hydroxylase. p-Chlorophenylalanine blocks tryptophan hydroxylase; the time course of the depletion of 5-HT after this synthesis inhibitor depends on the rate of utilization of the amine. In rats, clonazepam (4 mg·kg^{-1} i.p.) reduced the 5-HT depletion induced by p-chlorophenylalanine (JENNER et al., 1978). Using another inhibitor of tryptophan hydroxylase, α-propyldopacetamide (H 22/54), LIDBRINK et al. (1973, 1974) found that chlordiazepoxide in doses above 10 mg · kg⁻¹ and diazepam in doses above 25 mg · kg⁻¹ reduced the 5-HT depletion in the cerebral cortex, but not in the rest of the brain. Chlordiazepoxide reduced the depletion of 5-HT induced by H 22/54 (LIPP-MANN and PUGSLEY, 1974).

Formation of ³H-5-HT and ³H-5-HIAA from ³H-Tryptophan. Chlordiazepoxide, diazepam, and flurazepam reduced the formation of ³H-5-HT and ³H-5-HIAA in the telencephalon of mice from intravenously injected ³H-tryptophan (DOMINIC, 1973; DOMINIC et al., 1975). Only diazepam significantly reduced 5-HT synthesis in the brain stem.

Accumulation of 5-HT and Decline of 5-HIAA After MAO Inhibition. Chlordiazep-oxide decreased the elevation of 5-HT in the thalamus-hypothalamus induced by the MAO inhibitor pargyline and further reduced the level of 5-HIAA already diminished by pargyline (PUGSLEY and LIPPMANN, 1975). ANTKIEWICZ-MICHALUK et al. (1975) studied the effect of chlordiazepoxide, oxazepam, temazepam, and nitrazepam (1 mg · kg⁻¹ p.o.) on the decline of 5-HIAA in the hypothalamus and brain stem of rats after inhibition of MAO by pargyline. All compounds reduced 5-HT turnover in both normal rats and in rats made aggressive by exposure in pairs to electric foot shock. Chlordiazepoxide was the most efficient drug. Interestingly, it reduced 5-HT turnover in the brain stem more markedly in unstressed than in stressed rats, while its depressant effect on hypothalamic 5-HT turnover was most marked in aggressive rats. CHUNG HWANG and VAN WOERT (1979) found the accumulation of 5-HT in mouse brain after pargyline unaffected by clonazepam, but reduced by diazepam.

Accumulation of 5-HTP after Inhibition of Decarboxylase. Accumulation of endog-enous 5-hydroxytryptophan (5-HTP) after inhibition of decarboxylase of aromatic amino acids is an index of the rate of synthesis of 5-HT at the step of tryptophan hy-droxylase. Clonazepam was found by JENNER et al. (1978) not to affect 5-HTP accu-mulation after the inhibitor NSD 1034. In contrast, BISWAS and CARLSSON (1978), us-ing 3-hydroxybenzyl-hydrazine (NSD 1015) as inhibitor, observed a significantly re-duced accumulation of 5-HTP in limbic areas, the striatum, and the "hemispheres" after diazepam in doses of 1, 3 and 10 mg · kg⁻¹ i.p. Very similar results were obtained by SANER and PLETSCHER (1979) with diazepam, but not with phenobarbitone (100 mg · kg⁻¹); the results were even more marked in reserpinized rats. The inhibitor of GABA transaminase, aminooxyacetic acid (AOAA, 25 mg · kg⁻¹ i.p.) produced a reduction of 5-HTP accumulation very similar to that seen after diazepam, 3 h after administration. AOAA and diazepam had an additive reducing effect on 5-HTP ac-cumulation. Picrotoxin (4 mg · kg⁻¹ i.p.) and bicuculline (1 mg · kg⁻¹ i.p.) had no sig-nificant effect by themselves on 5-HTP accumulation in reserpinized rats, but abol-ished the effect of diazepam and AOAA. These results were considered to be compati-ble with the view that benzodiazepines depressed 5-HT neuron activity by enhancing inhibitory GABAergic input. After reserpine, which increases 5-HT turnover, the in-hibitory GABAergic influence on 5-HT neurons and, hence, the facilitating effect of diazepam, was more marked than in nonreserpinized animals.

6. Effect on Brain and Plasma Tryptophan

Treatment of rats for 22 days with 10 mg · kg⁻¹ diazepam and bromazepam s.c. in-creased brain tryptophan concentration by 30% (AGARWAL et al., 1977); this modification disappeared after a withdrawal period of 2 days. A similar treatment with diazepam doubled the tryptophan content of rat brain synaptosomes (RASTOGI et al., 1978 b). A marked increase of brain tryptophan was also observed by BOURGOIN et al. (1975) after treatment of rats with single doses of diazepam, chlordiazepoxide, and oxazepam. Chlordiazepoxide decreased total tryptophan in serum by 20% and increased free tryptophan by 50%. Binding of ^{3}H-tryptophan to rat serum albumin was inhibited by chlordiazepoxide and diazepam and, to a lesser degree, by oxazepam. While DOMINIC et al. (1975) failed to find changes in brain tryptophan of mice after chlordiazepoxide, diazepam, and flurazepam, CHADWICK et al. (1978) found increased tryptophan levels after clonazepam and diazepam. CHUNG HWANG and VAN WOERT (1979) observed an increase of plasma tryptophan by both clonazepam and diazepam in mice, whereas brain tryptophan was only elevated after diazepam. This rise was of shorter duration than the changes in 5-HT and 5-HIAA. After nine daily doses, whole-brain tryptophan was increased by diazepam, but not by clonazepam. HÖCKEL et al. (1979) observed an increase of L-tryptophan uptake into slices of various rat brain regions in the presence of diazepam; a half-maximal effect was obtained at 10^{-4} mol·l^{-1}.

7. Efflux of 5-HIAA from the Brain

Diazepam inhibited the efflux from the brain of intracisternally injected ^{14}C-5-HIAA (CHASE et al., 1970). This indicates that this drug, and probably other benzodiazepines, inhibit the active process by which acidic amine metabolites are transported out of the brain and the cerebrospinal fluid. Results of JENNER et al. (1978) with probenecid blocking the active transport are consistent with this view. The demonstration of efflux inhibition by benzodiazepines casts doubts on the value of 5-HIAA determinations for estimating the turnover of brain 5-HT.

8. 5-HT Behavioral Syndrome

Stimulation of cerebral 5-HT receptors in mice with 5-hydroxytryptophan (5-HTP), tryptophan plus MAO inhibitors, with 5-HT intracerebrally, with lysergic acid diethylamide, mescaline, and 5-methoxytryptamine induces a characteristic syndrome with stereotyped head twitches. Similar head twitches were observed with low doses of fludiazepam, clonazepam, nitrazepam, and nimetazepam, whereas diazepam, chlordiazepoxide, flurazepam, oxazepam, and medazepam were ineffective up to 60 mg·kg^{-1} (NAKAMURA and FUKUSHIMA, 1976, 1977, 1978 a, b); cyproheptadine, a supposed 5-HT antagonist, blocked this syndrome. No tolerance to the induction of head twitches developed after repeated dosing. Fludiazepam-induced head twitches were reduced in mice in which 5-HT neurons had been previously destroyed by intracerebral 5,6-dihydroxytryptamine injections. On the other hand, fludiazepam enhanced the head twitching response to 5-methoxytryptamine. PUGSLEY and LIPPMANN (1976) could not increase the behavioral response to 5-HTP by 20 mg·kg^{-1} chlordiazepoxide i.p., but the drug inhibited the occurrence of head twitches with an ED_{50} of 36 mg·kg^{-1} s.c. (CORNE et al., 1963). CHADWICK et al. (1978) described abnormal head movements and a "wet-dog shake" response to pinna stimulation with clonazepam. In the presence of MAO inhibitors, pargyline or tranylcypromine, smaller doses

of clonazepam were required for these motor phenomena. In guinea pigs, 5-HTP produces a characteristic myoclonic bouncing stereotypy progressing to discontinuous
jerking movements of the entire body (WEINER et al., 1977). Clonazepam, in doses up
to 20 mg·kg^{-1}, did not modify the effect of 5-HTP.

9. Physicochemical Interaction Between 5-HT and Diazepam

GALZIGNA (1969) reported that diazepam could form a stable complex with 5-HT, in
which 5-HT must act as an electron donor. It is not known whether this test tube finding is of any relevance to the in vivo situation.

10. Electrical Activity of 5-HT Neurons

The spontaneous firing rate of single cells in the dorsal raphé nucleus, an important
site of origin for 5-HT neurons, was substantially decreased by doses of chlordiazepoxide below 1 mg·kg^{-1} i.v. in rats anesthetized with chloralhydrate (DALSASS and
STERN, 1976). Somewhat different results were obtained by GALLAGER (1978) under
apparently identical experimental conditions. Intravenous injections of diazepam (up
to 30 mg·kg^{-1}), chlordiazepoxide (up to 12 mg·kg^{-1}), and flurazepam (up to
30 mg·kg^{-1}), did not significantly affect the firing rate. However, diazepam
1 mg·kg^{-1} i.v. enhanced the depressant effect of iontophoretically administered GA-
BA without affecting the response to 5-HT. The potentiated response to iontophoresed GABA was specifically blocked by picrotoxin but unaffected by strychnine.
Diazepam did not affect the response to iontophoretically applied glycine. Iontophoretic application of chlordiazepoxide and flurazepam did not alter the spontaneous firing rate of raphé neurons, although the depressant effect of simultaneously
iontophoresed GABA was potentiated. In rats pretreated with the GABA transaminase inhibitor, aminooxyacetic acid (AOAA), the intravenous administration of
diazepam partially or totally inhibited spontaneous raphé unit activity, an effect
which was reversed by picrotoxin. In the dorsal raphé nucleus of unanaesthetized
encéphale isolé rats midazolam i.v. dose-dependently reduced the spontaneous multiunit activity (LAURENT, personal communication).

11. Conclusions

From the already large experimental evidence it would seem probable that benzodiazepines, at least at medium and high pharmacological doses, reduce the synthesis
and utilization of 5-HT in various central nervous structures. However, opposite conclusions were also drawn, e.g., by CHUNG HWANG and VAN WOERT (1979).

This effect cannot be explained by a direct action of benzodiazepines on biosynthetic or metabolizing steps or 5-HT receptors, on the uptake or on the release of
5-HT. All the evidence indicates that the activity of 5-HT neurons is reduced under
the effect of benzodiazepines, most probably by a modification of the input to 5-HT
cells. The high glutamic acid decarboxylase activity in the nucleus dorsalis raphé
(MASSARI et al., 1976) indicates the functional importance of GABAergic mechanism
in this area. One of the three studies, in which the firing rate of 5-HT neurons was
investigated, failed to demonstrate an effect of benzodiazepines on the spontaneous

firing rate. Perhaps this failure is due to the special situation of the immobilized animal. This tentative explanation gains support from Gallager's finding (1978) that GABA depressed the raphé neurons and that benzodiazepines, both after intravenous injection and iontophoretic application, selectively potentiated the inhibitory effect of GABA. However, diazepam markedly depressed the spontaneous firing in rats pretreated with AOAA, which may result in an increased release of accumulating GABA. Laurent (personal communication) found a dose-related depression of the spontaneous firing of raphé dorsalis neurons in *encéphale isolé* rats by midazolam. Besides reducing the activity of 5-HT neurons, benzodiazepines inhibit the active egress of 5-HIAA from the brain, which makes the measurement of brain 5-HIAA a questionable method for evaluating 5-HT turnover.

There is no indication that tolerance to the effect of benzodiazepines on 5-HT neuron activity occurs. Several observations are difficult to reconcile with the depressant effect of benzodiazepines on central 5-HT mechanisms. Indeed, higher doses of some benzodiazepines induced in mice a behavioral syndrome thought to be the result of 5-HT receptor stimulation. The nature of this phenomenon remains to be clarified.

Several authors (Stein et al., 1973, 1975, 1977; Warburton, 1974; Tye et al., 1977; File and Vellucci, 1978) postulated that the reduction of 5-HT activity induced by benzodiazepines is responsible for the behavioral disinhibition observed with these drugs in animal models believed to be relevant for the anxiolytic action. Recently, Thiébot et al. (1980 a, b) obtained a reduction of punishment-suppressed behavior by local injections of chlordiazepoxide and GABA, but not of muscimol into the nucleus raphé dorsalis of rats. Surprisingly, not even an additive effect was seen on simultaneous injection of chlordiazepoxide and GABA.

In the context of 5-HT mechanisms the specific interaction of benzodiazepines with the binding of L-tryptophan to plasma albumin has to be mentioned, although in quantitative terms it does not seem to be relevant.

VII. Histamine

Chlordiazepoxide and diazepam at $10 \text{ mg} \cdot \text{kg}^{-1}$ s.c. did not alter the levels of histamine and histidine or the activity of histidine decarboxylase and histamine methyltransferase in the hypothalamus of unstressed rats (Taylor and Laverty, 1973). However, exposure of rats to restraint boxes in a cold room at 4 °C for 2 h markedly reduced the histamine content, and this effect of stress was completely prevented by the two benzodiazepines.

VIII. Glutamate

Glutamate-induced depolarization of primary afferents in the hemisected frog spinal cord was noncompetitively antagonized by flurazepam in concentrations of 2.5–5 μmol·l^{-1} (Nistri and Constanti, 1978 a, b). Likewise, flurazepam (50–100 μmol·l^{-1}) noncompetitively antagonized glutamate-induced depolarization of muscle fibers of the lobster claw-opener muscle, and enhanced desensitization to glutamate. The authors proposed that flurazepam reduced the effect of glutamate by combining with the Na^+ channels regulated by glutamate receptors. Unfortunately, no other benzodiazepine has been examined in these studies; since flurazepam, due to its particular substitution (diethylaminoethyl on N_1), probably has more pronounced membrane stabilizing (Na^+ channel depressant) effects than congeners, its relatively potent glutamate-antagonistic action may not be representative of benzodiazepines in general. This view is supported by the failure of MACDONALD and BARKER (1978) to antagonize the depolarizing effect of glutamate in murine spinal cord neurons grown in dissociated cell culture with concentrations of diazepam and chlordiazepoxide that markedly potentiated the response to GABA, and by the absence of an effect of chlordiazepoxide 0.1 mmol·1^{-1} on glutamate-induced depolarization of motoneurons in the frog hemisected spinal cord (NICOLL and WOJTOWICZ, 1980). In this respect, benzodiazepines differed quite markedly from barbiturates, which depressed glutamate responses at the same concentrations as those required to enhance GABA responses.

IX. Glycine

1. Uptake and Release

Chlordiazepoxide and diazepam at 10^{-5} mol·1^{-1} did not affect uptake and K^+-induced release of ^{14}C-glycine in rat spinal cord synaptosomes (NELSON-KRAUSE and HOWARD, 1976).

2. Glycine Content

Ross et al. (1978) reported that diazepam (5 mg·kg^{-1} i.p.) produced highly significant differences in the diurnal changes of glycine concentrations in the pons and cerebellum of rats.

3. Glycine Receptor

Strychnine was proposed by YOUNG and SNYDER (1974) as a specific ligand for glycine receptor binding studies. These authors found that benzodiazepines were more potent than any other centrally active agent as inhibitors of ^3H-strychnine binding to rat spinal cord membrane fraction (YOUNG et al., 1974; SNYDER and ENNA, 1975; SNYDER et al., 1977). The most potent benzodiazepines tested, flunitrazepam and bromazepam, were active with a IC_{50} of 19 μmol·1^{-1}, which means that this affinity for the glycine receptor-like binding site is at best 1/10,000 of the affinity for benzodiazepine binding sites. The rank order of potency of benzodiazepines in displacing specific ^3H-strychnine binding was considered to correlate significantly with the rank order of pharmacologic potency in man and animals (SNYDER and ENNA, 1975; SNYDER et al., 1977), an opinion not shared by many pharmacologists. As an example, HUNT and RAYNAUD (1977) pointed to the small differences in the relative displacing potencies in the ^3H-strychnine binding assay of benzodiazepines as opposed to their marked differences in clinical potency. They also draw attention to the fact that displacement of ^3H-strychnine binding was rather well correlated with the liposolubility of the compounds and that nonanxiolytic tricyclic compounds existed with higher affinity for the ^3H-strychnine binding site than benzodiazepines. Concentrations of benzodiazepines required to displace ^{3}H-strychnine binding in vitro are well above those occurring in the animal central nervous system after reasonable pharmacologic doses.

CURTIS et al. (1976a) failed to find electrophysiologic support for the glycine hypothesis. Indeed, diazepam did not diminish the reduction by strychnine of the inhibitory action of glycine, both applied microiontophoretically on cat dorsal horn interneurons. CURTIS et al. (1976a) also found, like many other investigators, that benzodiazepines were weak as antagonists of strychnine-induced seizures in contrast to their high potency against seizures induced by the convulsant GABA antagonists or glutamate decarboxylase inhibitors. Studying single neurons in the dorsal raphé nucleus, GALLAGER (1978) found that diazepam, chlordiazepoxide, and flurazepam potentiated the depressant effect of iontophoretically applied GABA, but that these benzodiazepines neither mimicked nor enhanced the effect of iontophoresed glycine. Similarly, CHOI et al. (1977) observed in cultured chick spinal cord and MACDONALD and BARKER (1978) in cultured murine spinal cord cells that chlordiazepoxide potentiated the effect of GABA, but failed to alter the response to exogenous glycine. In cat motoneurons flurazepam enhanced the hyperpolarizing action of GABA, but not of glycine (NISTRI et al., 1980).

X. γ-Aminobutyric Acid (GABA)

The interaction of benzodiazepines with GABAergic mechanisms takes first place among recent studies on the mechanism of action of these drugs, since evidence from electrophysiologic (HAEFELY et al., 1975b) and biochemical (COSTA et al., 1975b) experiments for the potentiating effect on GABAergic synaptic transmission was presented at the first meeting concerned entirely with the mechanism of action of benzodiazepines (COSTA and GREENGARD, 1975). The explosive interest in benzodiazepines and GABA is the result of several concurrent developments, such as, e.g., the demonstration in the early 1970s of the neurotransmitter role of GABA in the mammalian central nervous system and the realization by pharmacologists of the role of GABAergic mechanisms for drug actions, as exemplified by the discovery that several potent convulsants were either GABA antagonists or inhibitors of GABA biosynthesis. Compared to the situation with monoamine transmitters, the electropharmacologic methods suited for the study of GABAergic inhibitory neurotransmission are simpler and biochemical indices of neuronal excitation and inhibition became available recently. It seems appropriate to start the discussion of benzodiazepine-GABA interaction with the findings on distinct GABAergic synapses.

1. GABAergic Synaptic Inhibition

Spinal Cord. SCHMIDT et al. (1967) were the first to describe a selective enhancement by diazepam of so-called presynaptic inhibition of spinal motoneurons in spinal cats; excitatory mechanisms and postsynaptic inhibition were found to be essentially unaffected.

These early findings were confirmed in many laboratories (SCHLOSSER and ZAVATSKI, 1969; SCHLOSSER, 1971; STRATTEN and BARNES, 1971; CHANELET and LONCHAMPT, 1971; PIXNER, 1966; NISTRI and CONSTANTI, 1978a, b; CHIBA and NAGAWA, 1973; MENETREY et al., 1973; BLUM et al., 1973; BANNA et al., 1974; MURAYAMA et al., 1972;

Suzuki and Murayama, 1976; Naftchi and Lowman, 1977; Naftchi et al., 1979; Chin et al., 1974; Polc et al., 1974; Nicot et al., 1976; Polzin and Barnes, 1976). Benzodiazepines seem to enhance presynaptic inhibition without significantly altering its time course, whereas barbiturates prolong presynaptic inhibition and have a moderate effect on the peak intensity of inhibition. As shown by Polc et al. (1974), there is a reversible antagonism between benzodiazepines and bicuculline in their effect on presynaptic inhibition. Bicuculline blocks the depolarization of Ia primary afferent endings induced by GABA (Sastry, 1979). Benzodiazepines lose their effect in animals in which GABA biosynthesis has been blocked (Polc et al., 1974; Banna et al., 1974). The effect of benzodiazepines on presynaptic inhibition is shared by inhibitors of GABA transaminase, and the combination of such inhibitors (particularly L-cycloserine) with benzodiazepines produces a pronounced enhancement of presynaptic inhibition. In cultures of embryonic chick spinal cord, chlordiazepoxide enhanced bicuculline-sensitive synaptic inhibition induced by stimulation of neighboring cells or axons (Choi et al., 1977). The recorded cells in this study were not identified, and GABAergic pathways mediating postsynaptic inhibition in the intact spinal cord are not known. In the frog hemisected spinal cord, flurazepam enhanced dorsal root potentials and increased the "noise" in primary afferent endings (Nistri and Constanti, 1978 a, b).

Dorsal Column Nuclei. The demonstration by Polc and Haefely (1976) that benzodiazepines enhanced both presynaptic and postsynaptic inhibition in the cat cuneate nucleus was of crucial importance for associating these drugs with GABAergic neurotransmission, because it showed that benzodiazepines did not specifically enhance the processes involved in primary afferent depolarization but also an essentially different type of inhibition in which GABA serves as mediator. In the cuneate nucleus, basically similar results were obtained as in the spinal cord with respect to interactions of benzodiazepines with GABA antagonists, inhibitors of GABA transaminase, and inhibitors of glutamic acid decarboxylase. Flurazepam enhanced the depolarizing effect of muscimol on primary afferents in slices of rat cuneate nucleus and markedly reduced the antagonistic effect of picrotoxin (Simmonds, 1980).

Cerebral Cortex. Recurrent (feedback) and collateral (feedforward) inhibition of principal neurons, mediated by GABAergic interneurons, was found to be enhanced by benzodiazepines (Raabe and Gumnit, 1977; Zakusov et al., 1977; Nestoros, 1979, Fig. 3), confirming previous results of Zakusov et al. (1975) on inhibitory mechanisms in isolated cortex slabs.

Hippocampus. Recurrent inhibition of hippocampal pyramidal cells, in which the GABAergic basket cells are involved, was intensified by diazepines in vivo (Wolf and Haas, 1977; Tsuchiya and Fukushima, 1978) and in tissue slices (Lee et al., 1979). In the latter case, an increased firing rate of GABAergic basket cells was found in the presence of diazepam.

Hypothalamus. In tissue culture, diazepam (10^{-6}–10^{-5} mol·1^{-1}) enhanced picrotoxin-sensitive recurrent inhibition of tuberal hypothalamic cells induced by focal electrical stimulation (Geller, 1978; Geller et al., 1978). This inhibition has been shown to be GABA-mediated (Geller and Woodward, 1979).

Cerebellar Cortex. Inhibition of cerebellar Purkinje cells by GABAergic basket cells was enhanced by diazepam in the studies reported so far (Curtis et al., 1976a; Geller et al., 1978; Montarolo et al., 1979). These findings are in excellent agree-

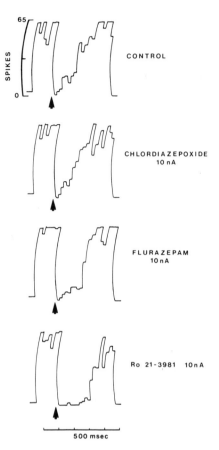

Fig. 3. Potentiation by three different benzodiazepines of electrically evoked cortical inhibition in a cat in fluothane anesthesia. Shown are peristimulus histograms from the same extracellularly recorded neuron in the postcruciate cerebral cortex. Each histogram shows the number of spikes *(ordinate)* occurring during each of 25 20-ms intervals for 128 consecutive 500-ms periods. Background firing of the neuron was maintained throughout at a steady submaximal rate by continuous release of Na L-glutamate (14 nA). In each record the sequence of events from left to right is *1* the prestimulus control firing; *2* at the arrow the electric stimulus (8.0 V, 2 Hz, 0.1 ms) to the surface of the cerebral cortex; *3* the reduced firing rate due to evoked inhibition; *4* the recovery of firing. The upper histogram is the predrug control. The three lower histograms were taken during the iontophoretic release of chlordiazepoxide, flurazepam, and midazolam (Ro 21-3981). Inhibition was allowed to return to control levels before each benzodiazepine was tested. (Courtesy of J. N. NESTOROS, unpublished)

ment with the depressant effect of benzodiazepines on the spontaneous and evoked firing rate of Purkinje cells (HAEFELY et al., 1975 b; PIERI and HAEFELY, 1976; MARIANI and DELHAYE-BOUCHAUD, 1978). They also explain why cGMP levels in the cerebellar cortex, which seem to be an index of the activity of Purkinje cells, are reduced by benzodiazepines (COSTA et al., 1975 b; GUIDOTTI, 1978).

Lateral Vestibular Nucleus of Deiters. The complex potential evoked in the nucleus of Deiters in response to single stimuli to cerebellar Purkinje cell axons in the parafastigial white matter contains a component that was easily blocked by bicuculline or picrotoxin, but not by strychnine (HAEFELY et al., 1978). This depressant effect of bicuculline was dose-dependently prevented by various benzodiazepines. The spontaneous multi-unit activity of Deiters' nucleus in cats was dose dependently reduced by chlordiazepoxide (ED_{50} 0.8 mg·kg^{-1} i.v.) (LLOYD et al., 1979).

Substantia Nigra. A GABAergic pathway is known to originate in the nucleus caudatus and to end in the substantia nigra on dopaminergic neurons projecting to the striatum. Electrical stimuli applied to the nucleus caudatus of immobilized cats evoked a potential in the substantia nigra. This simple evoked response was dose-dependently reduced and eventually abolished by bicuculline and picrotoxin, but not by strychnine and, therefore, considered to represent the summed GABAergic inhibitory postsynaptic potentials in nigral cells (SCHAFFNER and HAEFELY, 1975; HAEFELY et al., 1975b, 1978). While various benzodiazepines had no significant effect on the striatonigral evoked potential itself, they very potently prevented the depressant effect of GABA antagonists on this potential. These findings are probably related to the observation of WOLF and HAAS (1977) and LAURENT (personal communication) that diazepines reduced the spontaneous firing rate of nigral cells. Biochemical data on the effect of benzodiazepines on dopamine turnover agree well with the assumption that the drugs enhance an inhibitory GABAergic input to dopamine neurons in the mesencephalon (see Sect. X.II.5). The existence in the substantia nigra of GABAergic synapses that subserve other functions than inhibition of dopaminergic neurons is becoming increasingly evident. Intranigral injections of agents that affect GABAergic mechanisms produce effects that are unrelated to efferent DA neurons but rather involve different, yet unidentified, efferents. Benzodiazepines, injected into the pars reticulata of the substantia nigra, mimicked the effects of GABA mimetics and of compounds that elevate the nigral GABA content (WADDINGTON, 1976, 1977, 1978; WADDINGTON and LONGDEN, 1977; WADDINGTON and OWEN, 1978).

Noradrenergic Locus Coeruleus Cells. Although these neurons are known to receive GABAergic input, GALLAGER (1978) in preliminary studies failed to find a significant change in discharge rate of single locus coeruleus neurons of the rat with diazepam. Indirect evidence indicates that benzodiazepines might increase the tonic GABAergic input to locus coeruleus cells when these are in a state of hyperactivity due to amine depletion and, thereby, release the pontine generator cells for pontogeniculo-occipital waves from the inhibitory noradrenergic input (HAEFELY et al., 1975a, 1976; RUCH-MONACHON et al., 1976a, b, c).

Serotoninergic Dorsalis Raphé Cells. In agreement with the postulated GABAergic input to the dorsal raphé nucleus, GABA depressed the raphé neurons and benzodiazepines potentiated the GABA-mediated inhibition of these neurons (GALLAGER, 1978). The facilitation by benzodiazepines of the GABAergic inhibitory input to the serotoninergic raphé system is probably responsible for the reduction of 5-HT turnover being proposed to account for the anxiolytic action of benzodiazepines (STEIN et al., 1973, 1975, 1977).

In conclusion, benzodiazepines have been found to enhance transmission at all GABAergic synapses studied so far. However, this enhancement required different experimental procedures to become visible. In those experiments, in which afferents to a GABAergic interneuron were stimulated in order to activate a GABAergic synapse, an increased inhibition was immediately seen either as an increased amplitude of primary afferent depolarization (in presynaptic inhibition in the spinal cord or the cuneate nucleus) or an increased IPSP or silent period (e.g., in postsynaptic inhibition in the hippocampus). In those experiments, in which the axons of GABAergic neurons were stimulated, the ensuing field potential in the substantia nigra or vestibular nucleus was not increased by benzodiazepines, unless it had been depressed by a GABA antagonist. In the former group of experiments, a single stimulus applied to input neurons induced a burst of action potentials in GABAergic interneurons. Benzodiazepines theoretically might enhance either excitation of GABAergic interneurons, GABA release by a train of impulses, or the response to released GABA. In the latter case, a single stimulus applied to a GABAergic axon elicits a single action potential; the failure of benzodiazepines to increase the effect of such a single impulse in the axon might be due to a high safety factor of transmission, i.e., to the possibility that GABA released by a single pulse produced the maximum achievable hyperpolarization of the target neurons. The exact site of action of benzodiazepines (receptive part or axon terminal of the GABAergic neuron; subsynaptic membrane of GABAergic target cells) remains to be revealed.

2. GABA Release

In preloaded synaptosomes from mouse brain the release of ^{3}H-GABA in response to high potassium in the absence of calcium was enhanced by 10–100 μmol·l^{-1} diazepam; the same concentrations inhibited the Ca^{2+}-dependent K$^+$-induced release (OLSEN et al., 1977, 1978 b). Barbiturates were ineffective on both types of release. NELSON-KRAUSE and HOWARD (1976) did not observe any effect of 10^{-5} mol·l^{-1} diazepam on K$^+$-induced release of ^{14}C-GABA from rat cerebral cortex synaptosomes. MITCHELL and MARTIN (1978) used a rather low concentration of K$^+$ in the superfusing fluid (15 mmol·l^{-1}) to stimulate the release of ^{3}H-GABA from preloaded small pieces of rat frontal cortex. At 10^{-6} mol·l^{-1} diazepam and flurazepam enhanced the K$^+$-stimulated release by 31% and 38%, respectively; at 10^{-4} mol·l^{-1} both benzodiazepines markedly reduced the evoked release. Neither compound affected the resting release of ^{3}H-GABA. Surprisingly, the K$^+$-stimulated release of ^{3}H-GABA from striatal tissue was not affected by diazepam 10^{-5} mol·l^{-1} (MARTIN and MITCHELL, 1979). The high-potassium (24 mmol·l^{-1})-induced release of ^{3}H-GABA from preloaded slices of rat spinal cord was enhanced by diazepam in concentrations between 0.5 and 3 μmol·l^{-1}, unaffected by diazepam 10 μmol·l^{-1}, and depressed by diazepam 100 μmol·l^{-1} (MATSUMOTO et al., 1979). SCHACHT and BÄCKER (1979) studied the effect of diazepam and clobazam on the release of ^{3}H-GABA evoked by electric field stimulation from preloaded rat brain cortex slices. In the concentrations of 10^{-7} and 10^{-6} mol·l^{-1}, both benzodiazepines reduced the electrically induced overflow of ^{3}H-GABA. Interestingly, this depressant effect of the benzodiazepines was completely abolished by bicuculline. Hexobarbitone had a similar effect as the two benzodiazepines. The authors explained their results by assuming that benzodiazepines enhanced a hypothetical inhibitory effect of GABA on transmitter release through stimulation of terminal autoreceptors of GABAergic neurons.

The presently available data on GABA release do not allow a definitive conclusion to be drawn on a possible effect of benzodiazepines. Several drawbacks of the reported experiments should be eliminated in future work: labeling of GABA should be attempted by preloading with radioactive glucose, which may label a physiologically more relevant pool of the transmitter; several means of stimulation and various intensities of stimuli should be used, e.g., potassium, veratridine, electrical stimulation; and a wider range of benzodiazepines should be studied. As an example, stimulus parameters in the study of SCHACHT and BÄCKER (1979) were supramaximal, which might have masked a facilitating effect of benzodiazepines on submaximal release. Chemical and electrical stimulation of tissue slices may stimulate GABAergic neurons directly or indirectly, and other neurotransmitters released simultaneously may create situations that are too complex to be interpreted. Ideally, the effect of benzodiazepines should be examined on the release from a distinct GABAergic pathway in vivo.

3. GABA Uptake

Uptake of ^{3}H-GABA into slices and homogenates of rat cerebral cortex was not inhibited by chlordiazepoxide or diazepam at 0.3 mmol·l^{-1} (IVERSEN and JOHNSTON, 1971). Whereas NELSON-KRAUSE and HOWARD (1976) did not find an effect of diazepam 10^{-5} mol·l^{-1} on the uptake of ^{14}C-GABA by synaptosomes from rat cerebral cortex, a noncompetitive inhibition of uptake was observed by OLSEN et al. (1977, 1978a, b), who calculated that the concentration for 50% inhibition of GABA uptake accounted for the enhancement of GABAergic transmission by benzodiazepines. So far none of the more potent inhibitors of GABA uptake has been demonstrated to enhance GABAergic synaptic transmission after iontophoretic application.

4. GABA Content of the Central Nervous System

Diazepam at 5 and 10 mg·kg^{-1} i.p. increased the GABA content of the forebrain of mice by about 20% (SAAD, 1972). Similar results were obtained by HAEFELY et al. (1975b) in the whole brain of mice, although the dose necessary for a significant (17%) increase was 30 mg·kg^{-1}. In the rat whole brain, the same authors found a significant 4% increase after 30 mg·kg^{-1}. In the lumbosacral part of the spinal cord of spinal cats, the GABA content was elevated by 38% 2 h after an intravenous injection of 3 mg·kg^{-1} diazepam (HAEFELY et al., 1975b). PERIČIĆ et al. (1977) observed a significant increase in the GABA content of the substantia nigra, but not of the caudate nucleus or of the cingulate and pyriform cortex of rats after 5 or 10 mg·kg^{-1} diazepam; similar effects were seen with pentobarbitone. Diazepam at a dose of 15 mg·kg^{-1}, but not of 3.75 and 7.5 mg·kg^{-1} p.o., increased the GABA level in the whole brain of rats by about 10% without change in the activity of glutamic acid decarboxylase (TONG and EDMONDS, 1976).

5. GABA Turnover

The in vivo formation of GABA in mice was studied by HAEFELY et al. (1975b) using the ratio specific activity of ^{14}C-glutamate/specific activity of ^{14}C-GABA at different times after a single dose of 30 mg·kg^{-1} diazepam i.p. and 15 min after a subcutaneous injection of a tracer dose of 2-^{14}C-glucose. The ratio was significantly reduced 30 and 60 min after diazepam, indicating a reduced formation of ^{14}C-GABA. Similar findings were observed in the rat by SEMIGINOVOSKÝ et al. (1976). MAO et al. (1977) measured the formation of ^{13}C-GABA in the rat brain from ^{13}C-glucose infused intravenously. Diazepam 1 mg·kg^{-1} reduced the turnover rate in the caudate and nucleus accumbens, but not in the globus pallidus. A similar effect was seen after 1 mg·kg^{-1} muscimol i.v.

The reduction of the endogenous GABA level in the lumbosacral spinal cord of spinal cats induced by thiosemicarbazide was significantly attenuated by 3 mg·kg^{-1} diazepam (POLC et al., 1974). LÖSCHER and FREY (1977) found a reversal by 1.2 mg·kg^{-1} diazepam of the GABA-depleting effect of isoniazid in the mouse brain. Similar observations had been reported by SAAD (1972).

The increase of whole brain GABA in rats given aminooxyacetic acid was attenuated by 25 mg·kg^{-1} diazepam i.p. (FUXE et al., 1975). BERNASCONI and MARTIN (1978, 1979) used the rate of increase of endogenous GABA after irreversible inhibition of GABA transaminase with gabaculine as an index of GABA turnover in the mouse brain. Diazepam in doses from 0.01 to 10 mg·kg^{-1} i.p. produced a dose-dependent decrease of GABA turnover in the four brain regions studied (cerebellum, cerebral cortex, hippocampus, and corpus striatum). Similar findings were obtained with oxazepam, the enantiomer Ro 11-3129, which was active in the ^{3}H-diazepam binding assay, but not with the inactive enantiomer Ro 11-3625; other anticonvulsants, such as carbamazepine, sodium valproate, and phenobarbitone also reduced GABA turnover.

6. GABA Synthesizing and Metabolizing Enzymes

PERIČIĆ et al. (1977) found glutamic acid decarboxylase activity in the rat brain to be unaffected by diazepam. The inhibition of glutamic acid decarboxylase induced by isoniazid in the mouse brain was reversed by 1.2 mg·kg^{-1} diazepam (LÖSCHER and FREY, 1977).

In mouse brain homogenate, chlordiazepoxide at 0.1 μmol·l^{-1} inhibited the activity of GABA transaminase by 10%, whereas clonazepam and diazepam were inactive up to 5 μmol·l^{-1} (SAWAYA et al., 1975). CHAN-PALAY et al. (1979) obtained immunocytochemical evidence for an increase of GABA transaminase activity in the rat cerebellum after diazepam 25 mg·kg^{-1} i.p. The activity of succinic semialdehyde dehydrogenase was inhibited 30%–45% by diazepam in concentrations of 0.01–5 μmol·l^{-1}, unaffected by clonazepam, and slightly increased by chlordiazepoxide. According to LÖSCHER and FREY (1977) diazepam antagonized the inhibition of glutamate decarboxylase by isoniazid.

7. GABA Excretion in the Urine

A single dose of diazepam (5 mg) elevated the urinary GABA levels in two of four healthy volunteers, and similar changes were observed in surgical patients (TARVER et al., 1976). To determine the origin of the increased urinary GABA, rats were injected intracisternally with ^{3}H-GABA. Animals given 10 mg·kg^{-1} diazepam i.p. excreted 2–3 times more labeled GABA than controls. No effect on the excretion of intracisternally injected ^{3}H-glycine was found.

8. Interaction of Benzodiazepines with GABA

Absence of GABA mimetic Activity. Specific binding of ^{3}H (+)-bicuculline methiodide to synaptic membranes of rat cerebellum, proposed to represent interaction with GABA receptors, was unaffected by chlordiazepoxide and diazepam in concentrations up to 10^{-4} mol·l^{-1} (Möhler and Okada, 1977c). Inhibition of ^{3}H-muscimol binding by diazepam was also weak or absent (IC_{50}:10^{-5} mol·l^{-1}, Beaumont et al., 1978). Binding of ^{3}H-GABA to mouse brain synaptosomes was not significantly inhibited by diazepam 10^{-4} mol·l^{-1} (Olsen et al., 1978a, b; Hyttel, 1979). Thus, in GABA receptor binding assays, benzodiazepines in even extremely high concentrations, did not significantly displace specific ligands, demonstrating the absence of agonistic or antagonistic properties at GABA recognition sites.

When, in electrophysiologic experiments, physiological membrane effects were used as index of GABA mimetic action, which includes both stimulation of GABA recognition sites and subsequent molecular steps, most investigators failed to find unequivocal evidence for GABA mimetic properties of benzodiazepines. In the spinal cord of cats, high doses of GABA (100 mg·kg^{-1} i.v.) or low doses of muscimol (1 mg·kg^{-1} i.v.) induce depolarization of primary afferent endings (Levy, 1974; Polc and Haefely, 1977); no trace of a similar tonic depolarization was found with the highest doses of various benzodiazepines (Polc et al., 1974; Haefely et al., 1975b, 1979a; Polc, 1978). The same is true for primary afferent endings in the cat cuneate nucleus (Polc and Haefely, 1976). In the isolated hemisected frog spinal cord chlordiazepoxide failed to produce a hyperpolarization of motoneurons, in contrast to barbiturates (Nicoll and Wojtowicz, 1980). Intracellular recording from rat spinal ganglia cell bodies revealed no consistent effect of 10^{-6} and 10^{-5} mol·l^{-1} diazepam on resting membrane potential and conductance (Lamour, 1979, Desarmenien et al., 1980). In the isolated rat superior cervical ganglion, GABA and other GABA mimetics produce a depolarization; chlordiazepoxide up to 2 mmol·l^{-1} failed to depolarize the ganglion, while pentobarbitone had $^1/_{200}$ the potency of GABA (Bowery and Dray, 1978; Dray and Bowery, 1978). Somewhat different and more complex results were obtained in the cat superior cervical ganglion in situ. In this preparation, injections of flurazepam and midazolam in doses below 1 μmol into the arterial blood supply of the ganglion, enhanced and prolonged the depolarizing effect of GABA (Schlosser and Franco, 1979a). At higher doses, the effect of GABA was transiently reduced and, after a few minutes, prolonged. Flurazepam inconsistently produced ganglionic depolarization; this depolarization was not prevented in a reproducible manner by picrotoxin or bicuculline, which blocked the dose-dependent depolarizing effect of pentobarbitone.

Flurazepam and, less consistently, chlordiazepoxide depressed the spontaneous firing rate of single neurons in the rat medulla when applied by microiontophoresis (Dray and Straughan, 1976); the effect resembled that of GABA and glycine, but of course could not be ascribed to a direct stimulation of GABA receptors in spite of antagonism by bicuculline, because of the presence of endogenous GABA at the synapses.

In isolated single rat diaphragm muscle fibers diazepam in concentrations of 10^{-6} and 10^{-5} mol·l^{-1} increased the chloride conductance (Vyskočil, 1977). Since GABA did not produce such an effect, the membrane effect of diazepam cannot be mediated through GABA receptors.

OLSEN et al. (1978 b) measured the uptake of Cl^- by crayfish abdominal muscle in vitro; this uptake is stimulated by GABA mimetics. Diazepam did not mimic the effects of GABA in this preparation but inhibited the GABA-stimulated Cl^- uptake by 35% at 10^{-4} mol·l^{-1}.

Considering all the results reported, one may safely conclude that benzodiazepines do not act as agonists on GABA receptors. At high, probably pharmacologically irrelevant concentrations, they increase chloride conductance even in cells that lack GABA and specific benzodiazepine receptors. A modification of GABA-stimulated changes in the chloride conductance may be expected to occur, at least in high concentrations. The possibility of an antagonistic effect of benzodiazepines at the GABA recognition site (STEINER and FELIX, 1976 a, b; GÄHWILER, 1976) can be excluded with certainty.

Modification of GABA Effects by Benzodiazepines. Since benzodiazepines enhance GABAergic neurotransmission, the immediate question arises whether this may be caused by an increased effectiveness of GABA on its target cells. Therefore, a number of studies were conducted to examine the response to exogenous GABA under the effect of benzodiazepines.

Flurazepam and chlordiazepoxide, administered iontophoretically to single neurons in the rat medulla, did not consistently modify the depressant effect of iontophoresed GABA (DRAY and STRAUGHAN, 1976). In the isolated rat superior cervical ganglion, 90 μmol·l^{-1} chlordiazepoxide failed to alter the dose-response curve of GABA for depolarization (BOWERY und DRAY, 1978; DRAY and BOWERY, 1978); barbiturates usually had an extremely small potentiating effect on low doses of GABA and depressed the depolarizing response to doses of GABA above the ED_{50}. No potentiation of the depolarizing effect of GABA in isolated lobster muscle was observed with flurazepam (NISTRI and CONSTANTI, 1978 b). In rat spinal ganglion cells, 10^{-6} and 10^{-5} mol·l^{-1} diazepam never enhanced the depolarizing effect of GABA; in more than half of the cells studied with intracellular recording the peak of GABA-induced depolarization was reduced to varying degrees, the repolarization accelerated and the desensitization attenuated (LAMOUR, 1979, DESARMENIEN et al., 1980). Thus, in the medulla of intact cats as well as in three cell types in vitro, which contain both GABA receptors and GABAergic innervation (lobster skeletal muscle) or only GABA receptors (rat sympathetic and spinal ganglion cells), no consistent potentiation of GABA effects could be observed in the presence of benzodiazepines.

Other investigators have observed an enhancement of GABA effects by benzodiazepines in different neuron preparations. In 4- to 7-day-old cultures of embryonic chick spinal cords, chlordiazepoxide administered by pressure ejection enhanced the membrane conductance increase produced by pressure-ejected GABA without affecting the responses of single cells to glycine or altering the membrane conductance by itself (CHOI et al., 1977). The active concentrations of chlordiazepoxide were 10^{-7}–10^{-4} mol·l^{-1}; no antagonism of GABA effects was observed. The potentiating action of chlordiazepoxide was immediate and rapidly reversible upon termination of the pulses. No tolerance to the potentiating effect of the compound was observed with its continuous ejection. In cultures of fetal mouse spinal cord, MACDONALD and BARKER (1979) obtained similar results with iontophoresed diazepam and chlordiazepoxide. However, whereas an augmentation of GABA-mediated conductance increase was observed with low ejection currents, an antagonism occurred with higher currents. Occasionally, the benzodiazepines increased the conductance by themselves. The augmenting effect of diazepam was specific for GABA, since the responses to glycine remained unaffected. The time course of the GABA-induced conductance increase was not changed by the benzodiazepines. Effects on GABA responses similar to those seen with benzodiazepines were observed with barbiturates (MacDONALD and BARKER, 1979). In NB_{2a} neuroblastoma cells, which contain binding sites for GABA and benzodiazepines as well as "gabamodulin", diazepam (10^{-6} mol $\cdot$ l^{-1}) enhanced the increase in chloride flux elicited by threshold concentrations of GABA and muscimol (BARALDI et al., 1979a). Recording extracellularly from neurons in the sensorimotor cortex of anesthetized rabbits, chlordiazepoxide iontophoresed with a large range of ejecting currents regularly augmented the depressant effect of iontophoresed GABA (KOZHECHKIN and OSTROVSKAYA, 1977a). Similar results were obtained with systemically administered diazepam (KOZHECHKIN and OSTROVSKAYA, 1977b), and with iontophoresed flurazepam in cats (NESTOROS and NISTRI, 1979).

In the frog hemisected spinal cord, flurazepam in low concentration (2.5 μmol $\cdot$ l^{-1}) shifted the concentration-response curve of GABA for depolarization of dorsal roots to the left (NISTRI and CONSTANTI, 1978a, b). When doubling the concentration of flurazepam, the depolarizing effects of both GABA and, more markedly, glutamate were inhibited in a noncompetitive manner. The depression of GABA and glutamate responses by flurazepam were ascribed to a blockade of Na^+ channels and the evidence that glutamate acts entirely by opening Na^+ channels, while the GABA-induced depolarization of primary afferents is probably mediated by both Na^+ and Cl^- conductance increases. It should be recalled that flurazepam contains the same side chain on N_1 as procaine and may, therefore, not be totally representative for the benzodiazepine class. Also in the hemisected frog spinal cord NICOLL and WOJTOWICZ (1980) observed a selective enhancement of GABA-induced hyperpolarization of motoneurons by chlordiazepoxide 0.1 μmol $\cdot$ l^{-1}; no depression of GABA effects occurred. The effects of chlordiazepoxide in these experiments were not easily washed out. In the urethane-anesthetized rat, the depressant effect of iontophoresed GABA on the spontaneous firing rate of cerebellar Purkinje cells was markedly enhanced by 0.2 mg $\cdot$ kg^{-1} i.p. diazepam, while inhibitory responses to noradrenaline or glycine were unaffected (GELLER et al., 1978). The use of just threshold or just subthreshold test pulses of GABA in this study made the potentiating effect of diazepam particularly impressive. GABA-induced depressions of the spontaneous firing rate of rat tuberal hypothalamic cells in tissue culture were consistently enhanced during superfusion with 10^{-5} mol $\cdot$ l^{-1} diazepam and flurazepam, while the responses to glycine were unaffected (GELLER et al., 1978, 1979). The depressant effect of microiontophoresed GABA on the spontaneous firing rate of single units in the corticomedial regions of the amygdala in urethane-anesthetized rats was enhanced by chlordiazepoxide (JAMES et al., 1979).

Most investigators, who described the potentiating effect of benzodiazepines on responses to exogenous GABA, considered their findings as support for a postsynaptic site of action of benzodiazepines, i.e., a site in close connection with GABA receptors. Although this interpretation may be partially or totally correct, the possibility should not be overlooked that the drugs might potentiate ongoing GABAergic synaptic activity by a presynaptic site of action; an increased release of endogenous GABA would enhance the efficacy of exogenous GABA by simple additive synergism. This cautionary remark is particularly appropriate in view of the questionable GABA potentiating effects of benzodiazepines in isolated sympathetic ganglia, where GABAergic innervation is lacking, and in lobster skeletal muscle in vitro, where the GABAergic inhibitory neurons are not spontaneously active.

Ro 5-3663 is a simple benzodiazepine molecule with convulsant activities. This compound has been shown to be a rather specific, although not very potent antagonist of GABA (FRANCO and SCHLOSSER, 1978; SCHAFFNER et al., 1979; GELLER, 1979; SCHLOSSER and FRANCO, 1976b; O'BRIEN and SPIRT, 1980).

Interaction of Benzodiazepines with GABA Antagonists. The potent antagonism by benzodiazepines of the convulsant effect of GABA blocking agents and the prevention by GABA antagonists of some behavioral and neuropharmacologic effects of benzodiazepines fit very well into the view that these drugs affect GABAergic mechanisms, but they do not necessarily point to a direct molecular interaction between benzodiazepines and GABA antagonists at the GABA receptor. As examples, GABA antagonists reversibly abolished the potentiating effect of benzodiazepines on presynaptic inhibition in the spinal cord (POLC et al., 1974) and cuneate nucleus (POLC and HAEFELY, 1976), and benzodiazepines prevented the decrease of evoked potentials representing GABA inhibitory postsynaptic potentials in the substantia nigra (SCHAFFNER and HAEFELY, 1975; HAEFELY et al., 1975b, 1978) and Deiters' nucleus (HAEFELY et al., 1978). In the rat medulla, bicuculline antagonized the depressant effect of flurazepam and GABA on single cells (DRAY and STRAUGHAN, 1976) and chlordiazepoxide (but not flurazepam!) partially reversed the GABA antagonistic effect of bicuculline (BOWERY and DRAY, 1978). However, observations on the isolated rat superior cervical ganglion are rather suggestive of a direct interaction between benzodiazepines and bicuculline (at least in this preparation). Indeed, BOWERY and DRAY (1978) reported that chlordiazepoxide partially reversed the depression by bicuculline of the depolarizing effect of GABA. In this respect, chlordiazepoxide was more potent (threshold concentration $0.5 \ \mu mol \cdot l^{-1}$) than a series of barbiturates, although it differed from the latter by the failure to completely reverse the bicuculline effect. Interestingly, chlordiazepoxide reduced the GABA antagonistic effect of a subsequent exposure to bicuculline for over 40 min despite wash out. It should be recalled that chlordiazepoxide had no GABA mimetic effect in this preparation. BOWERY and DRAY (1978) suggested on the basis of their findings that GABA and GABA antagonists might act at different sites of GABA-receptor-ionophore complex, and that benzodiazepines could displace the GABA antagonist from a GABA-antagonist binding site to modulate the GABA recognizing part of the complex. Although this explanation is very tempting, it is difficult to reconcile with the failure of benzodiazepines to interact with the synaptosomal binding of ^3H (+) bicuculline methiodide in brain tissue (MÖHLER and OKADA, 1977c). In slices of rat cuneate nucleus, flurazepam more markedly reduced the GABA antagonist effect of picrotoxin than that of bicuculline (SIMMONDS, 1980). This effect was explained by an interaction of flurazepam with chloride channels or with the coupling between GABA receptors and chloride channels.

Benzodiazepines and GABA-Mediated Decrease of Cyclic Guanosine Monophosphate (cGMP). The effects of benzodiazepines on the GABA-mediated decline in cGMP content in the cerebellum are reported in Sect. Y.

Modulation by Benzodiazepines of Specific GABA Binding to Synaptosomal Membranes. A very interesting interaction of benzodiazepines with GABA receptor type binding sites in isolated membrane preparations has been reported which, if confirmed under less artificial conditions, will represent an important step toward an understanding of the molecular mechanisms by which benzodiazepines modulate GABA-mediated synaptic processes (COSTA et al., 1978; GUIDOTTI et al., 1978; TOFFANO et al., 1979, 1980; WILLOW and JOHNSTON, 1980).

The observations started from the well-documented fact that the characteristics of GABA receptor binding depend on the preparation of synaptic membranes (ENNA and SNYDER, 1977; OLSEN et al., 1978a; GUIDOTTI et al., 1978; HORNG and WONG, 1979; GREENLEE et al., 1978). ^{3}H-GABA binds to freshly prepared crude synaptic membrane preparations with a relatively low affinity (K_D around $0.2\ \mu\text{mol}\cdot\text{l}^{-1}$). Freeze-thawing and/or treatment with the detergent Triton X-100 alters the kinetic properties of ^{3}H-GABA binding; in addition to the low-affinity component, a second one with a higher affinity is unmasked (K_D around $0.02\ \mu\text{mol}\cdot\text{l}^{-1}$) and the density of specific binding sites increases (interestingly, detergents did not affect the binding characteristics of muscimol and other rigid analogues of GABA; WANG et al., 1979). A concept was proposed, according to which the receptor-ionophore complex is normally associated with an endogenous inhibitory factor ("gabamodulin") which reduces the affinity of the recognition site for GABA. Repeated freezing-thawing or treatment with detergents results in the separation of the receptor-inhibitor complex whereby the affinity of GABA is increased. Adding the supernatant of centrifuged membranes treated with Triton X-100 produces a concentration-dependent decrease of ^{3}H-GABA binding with the result that these treated membranes then behave like crude preparations in the ^{3}H-GABA binding assay. The inhibitory factor was subsequently purified and evidence found that it may be a relatively heat-stable, acidic protein with a molecular weight of about 15,000 (TOFFANO et al., 1979, 1980). Inhibition of high-affinity ^{3}H-GABA binding by the purified inhibitor was noncompetitive, suggesting a negative cooperative interaction between endogenous inhibitor and GABA recognition site.

Benzodiazepines added to fresh membranes were found to increase the Na$^+$-independent ^{3}H-GABA binding, although they were ineffective in membranes treated with Triton X-100. Thus, fresh membrane preparations preincubated with a benzodiazepine behaved like detergent-treated membranes and these drugs had an effect opposite to that of the endogenous inhibitor, which converted the functional state of detergent-treated membranes into one of fresh untreated membranes. There was a competitive antagonism between endogenous inhibitor and benzodiazepines for their effect on high-affinity binding of ^{3}H-GABA. To show this competition, membranes had to be incubated with benzodiazepines for some time prior to addition of the endogenous inhibitor. Not only were the binding characteristics of GABA modified by treatment of membranes, but also those of ^{3}H-diazepam binding. Indeed, both the maximal number of binding sites (B max) and the affinity (K_D) were greater in detergent-treated membranes. Addition of the purified endogenous inhibitor competitively inhibited ^{3}H-diazepam binding to Triton X-100-treated membranes. The hypothesis was thus formed that benzodiazepines competed with the endogenous inhibitor at a regulatory site of the GABA-binding macromolecule, occupation of this regulatory site by benzodiazepines increasing, and occupation by the endogenous inhibitor decreasing the specific binding of ^{3}H-GABA. Benzodiazepines, therefore, were proposed to modify GABAergic transmission by competitively interacting with an endogenous inhibitor protein that allosterically modulates the interaction of GABA with its receptor. In order to improve the evidence that inhibitor protein and GABA receptor occurred in the membranes of the same cells, fresh membranes prepared from neuroblastoma and glioma cell lines, which contain high-affinity binding sites for both ^{3}H-diazepam and ^{3}H-GABA were investigated (Baraldi et al., 1978). As in brain membranes, two populations of GABA receptors, differing in their K_D values, were obtained by extensive washing, freezing, and thawing or treatment with Triton X-100. Benzodiazepines increased the affinity of the untreated membranes for ^{3}H-GABA.

Although the concept of an interaction of benzodiazepines with an endogenous modulator of GABA affinity ("gabamodulin") would elegantly explain on a molecular level many of the benzodiazepine effects on GABAergic mechanisms, it has not remained uncontested. Maurer (1979 b) purified the "gabamodulin" according to Toffano et al. (1979, 1980) and arrived at the conclusion that this endogenous inhibitory factor was fully accounted for by endogenous GABA. GABA is released into the supernatant when synaptosomal membranes are exposed to osmotic shock or are frozen (Olsen et al., 1978 b). A clarification of the nature of "gabamodulin" is urgently needed. Moreover, the enhancement of GABA binding does not seem to be specific for benzodiazepines, since pentobarbitone was recently shown to produce a similar effect in crude preparations of rat brain membranes (Willow and Johnston, 1980). The effect of pentobarbitone was blocked by picrotoxin.

XI. Purine Nucleotides

Very low doses of diazepam (0.01–1 mg·kg^{-1} i.v.) markedly enhanced the depressant effect of iontophoretically administered adenosine-5′-monophosphate (AMP) on spontaneously firing neurons in the sensorimotor cortex of rats (Phillis, 1979). Similar potentiation was seen when diazepam was applied by microiontophoresis. A systemic or local doses of diazepam, which potentiated the effect of AMP, did not alter the spontaneous firing rate of cortical neurons. These electrophysiologic findings were explained by the inhibitory effect of diazepam on adenosine uptake in brain slices reported by Mah and Daly (1976). Perhaps this uptake inhibition also explains the enhanced adenosine-induced accumulation of cAMP in mouse cerebral cortex slices in the presence of clonazepam (Palmer et al., 1979). However, Skolnick et al. (1979 a) determined the concentration of radioactivity in the brain 10 min after intravenous injections of ^{3}H-diazepam in doses which were found to potentiate the neuronal depressant action of adenosine; they concluded that the approximate concentration (1–1.7 μmol·l^{-1}) after the injection of 1 mg·kg^{-1} were too small to inhibit adenosine uptake. In a subsequent study, Phillis et al. (1979) observed that theophylline (50–100 mg·kg^{-1} i.v.) antagonized the depressant effect of both adenosine and flurazepam (applied microiontophoretically) on single neurons in the rat cerebral cortex. Diazepam (10^{-6} and 10^{-5} mol·l^{-1}) potentiated the effect of adenosine on noradrenergic neuromuscular transmission in rat isolated vas deferens and guinea-pig atria in vitro (Clanachan and Marshall, 1980 a). More recently, Bender et al. (1980) and Phillis et al. (1980) reinvestigated the effect of diazepam and flurazepam on ^{3}H-adenosine uptake by synaptosomes of rat cerebral cortex. They found a 13% and 20%

inhibition by diazepam in concentrations of 10^{-8} and 10^{-7} mol·l^{-1}, respectively. The concentration-effect curve for this inhibition was very flat. Flurazepam was considerably less potent than diazepam as an inhibitor of ^{3}H-adenosine uptake.

These few observations on the interaction of benzodiazepines with purine nucleotides may be relevant in view of the proposed role of purine derivatives in synaptic functions of the central nervous system (BURNSTOCK, 1972; RIBEIRO, 1978; DAVIES and TAYLOR, 1979; OKADA, 1979) and the finding that endogenous brain purines have some affinity for the benzodiazepine binding sites. MACDONALD et al. (1979) observed that microiontophoretic application of inosine to mouse spinal neurons grown in tissue culture elicited two "transmitter-like" responses: a rapidly desensitizing excitatory and a nondesensitizing inhibitory response. Flurazepam imitated the excitatory response and blocked the inhibitory response to inosine. The authors, therefore, suggested that benzodiazepines might interact with purine receptors, which would, in fact, be identical with benzodiazepine receptors.

It would seem that at least some of the benzodiazepines might enhance postulated physiologic purinergic mechanisms in the CNS by inhibiting the cellular uptake of adenosine and, in addition, perhaps by inhibiting phosphodiesterase activity. This view receives some support by the rather selective partial reduction of some benzodiazepine effects by caffeine, an adenosine receptor blocking agent (POLC et al., 1981).

XII. Enkephalins

DUKA et al. (1979b) injected rats intravenously with doses of diazepam ranging from 0.1 to 2.5 mg·kg^{-1}. The level of met-enkephalin-like activity measured by a highly specific radioimmunoassay was increased by about 35% in the hypothalamus and decreased by about 25% in the striatum 5 min after the injection of the highest dose. Whereas the enkephalin level was no longer significantly different from controls after 20 min in the hypothalamus, it remained lowered for 60 min in the striatum and was normal again after 2 h. The enkephalin levels in medulla oblongata/pons and midbrain were unaltered by diazepam. The changes of leu-enkephalin levels seemed to parallel those of met-enkephalin. The concentrations of diazepam and active metabolites (measured by the receptor binding assay on isolated membranes) was highest 5 min after injection (about 0.5 μmol·l^{-1}) and declined rapidly within 60 min. The results were interpreted by the authors in the sense that benzodiazepines reduce the turnover of enkephalins in the hypothalamus, which is increased by stress, and increase the turnover of enkephalins in the striatum, possibly as a counterregulating mechanism which is switched on by the reduced turnover of GABA in the substantia nigra. The changes produced by diazepam in the striatal enkephalin level, but not in the hypothalamus, were mimicked by muscimol and aminooxyacetic acid and blocked by bicuculline and naloxone (DUKA et al., 1980). When diazepam (4 mg·kg^{-1} i.p.) and flunitrazepam (2 mg·kg^{-1} i.p.) were injected daily for 28 days, an increase of met-enkephalin occurred in the striatum, whereas met-enkephalin levels were unaltered in the hypothalamus and in the pons-medulla oblongata (WÜSTER et al., 1980a). The decrease of striatal met-enkephalin by a single dose of diazepam was blocked in animals treated for 28 days with morphine, but was enhanced in rats given ethanol for the same time. The changes in the met-enkephalin response observed after repeated treatment with benzodiazepines were explained by counterregulatory processes. It is interesting that the changes of striatal met-enkephalin observed after chronic benzodiazepines were similar to those seen after repeated treatment with haloperidol and chlorpromazine (Hong et al., 1978).

Preliminary experiments by Duka et al. (1979 b) suggested that diazepam (10^{-6} mol $\cdot$ l^{-1}) did not affect the basal release of met-enkephalin from striatal slices. The interaction of opiate antagonists with some effects of benzodiazepines was mentioned in Chap. J,I. Diazepam (2.5 mg $\cdot$ kg^{-1}) produced a moderate increase of pain threshold (vocalization) in rats (Wüster et al., 1980 b). This antinociceptive effect was greatly enhanced by the prior intracerebroventricular injection of bacitracin, believed to inhibit the enzymatic inactivation of enkephalins. Naloxone (10 mg $\cdot$ kg^{-1} i.p.) reduced the threshold elevation by the combination of diazepam and bacitracin.

XIII. Other Peptides

The interaction of benzodiazepines with ACTH has already been discussed in the section on 5-HT release (James et al., 1979) and 5-HT turnover (File and Vellucci, 1978).

XIV. Prostaglandins

Ally et al. (1978) observed that chlordiazepoxide and diazepam (IC$_{50}$, 890 and 55 µmol $\cdot$ l^{-1}) reduced and eventually abolished the vasoconstrictor effect of noradrenaline and angiotensin II in isolated perfused rat mesenteric artery preparation, but failed to block vasoconstriction produced by potassium and vasopressin. The concentration-response curve for the inhibitory effect of the benzodiazepines was shifted to the left by the addition of imidazole, an inhibitor of thromboxane A$_2$ formation. The authors postulated that the benzodiazepines acted as competitive antagonists of thromboxane A$_2$ and suggested that this prostaglandin could act as an endogenous ligand for benzodiazepine receptors in blood vessel and, possibly, also in the central nervous system. The problem is that no high affinity binding sites for benzodiazepines, corresponding to those present in the central nervous system, have been found in peripheral organs. The relevance of these findings in the isolated vessel preparation for the pharmacologic effects of benzodiazepines, therefore, remains uncertain.

Pentetrazole and picrotoxin in convulsive doses produced a dose-dependent increase of PGF$_{2\alpha}$, PGE$_2$ and TXB$_2$-like immunoreactive material in the brains of mice killed at the time of occurrence of seizures (Steinhauer et al., 1979). Diazepam, 10 mg $\cdot$ kg^{-1} i.p., injected 30 min before the convulsants prevented both the seizures and the rise in prostaglandins. A similar effect was obtained with trimethadione 500 mg $\cdot$ kg^{-1} i.p. Indomethacin blocked the increase in prostaglandins but was unable to prevent the seizures.

In contrast to diphenylhydantoin, 8.5 mg $\cdot$ kg^{-1} diazepam i.p. did not inhibit the decapitation-induced increase of unesterified free fatty acids, including arachidonic acid, in the brain of rats (Marion and Wolfe, 1978).

XV. Conclusions

Many of the presently established and putative neurotransmitter and mediator systems of the central nervous system have been reported to be affected by benzodiazepines. This is not at all surprising, but simply reflects the often neglected fact that even the most specific pharmacologic interaction with a single transmitter system within the complex neuronal machinery of the central nervous system must have consequences on the activity of a great number of other neuronal systems. The widespread effects of benzodiazepines on various electrical activities of many brain parts well illustrate this situation. The present knowledge suggests that benzodiazepines (a) modify the functions of some neurotransmitter systems indirectly by altering their neuronal input; (b) affect some other chemical synapses in a yet unknown way; (c) leave unaffected a few transmitter systems, and (d) specifically enhance transmission at GABAergic synapses.

1. Neurotransmitter Systems Indirectly Affected by Benzodiazepines

These systems comprise ACh, DA, NA, 5-HT and, possibly, histamine. Characteristically, benzodiazepines do not affect all central pathways using a given transmitter. Some pathways are either resistant to these drugs or are affected only at much higher doses than other neurons using the same transmitter. The direction of the changes induced by the drugs is usually a depression, although, in some cases, e.g., in the DA system, one pathway may be activated. The changes induced by benzodiazepines in the cholinergic and monoamine systems are below or at the limit of detection after low pharmacologic doses. Consistent changes are observed after high doses and in special conditions, in particular when these transmitter systems are abnormally activated, such as in stress or under the influence of other drugs (e.g., neuroleptics). A direct effect of benzodiazepines on presynaptic (transmitter synthesis, storage, release, uptake) or postsynaptic mechanisms (receptors and receptor-mediated events, inactivation) of these transmitter systems can be safely excluded. Therefore, the changes induced by benzodiazepines in the function of the ACh, DA, NA, 5-HT, and histamine system must result from a direct effect of these drugs on neuronal systems located upstream from the cholinergic and amine pathways. All the available data are consistent with the view that the changes occurring in these systems are secondary to modifications of GABAergic synapses.

2. Transmitter and Mediator Systems Affected in a Yet Unknown Way

The potentiation by benzodiazepines of synaptic effects of adenine nucleotides suggests the possibility that these drugs interact with a hypothetical physiological modulatory role on pre- and postsynaptic events of purine derivatives released from specific purinergic neurons or liberated concomitantly with other neurotransmitters. The relevance of these interactions with purines for the pharmacologic effects of benzodiazepines is yet obscure, as is the mechanism involved in this interaction.

The met-enkephalin levels in the hypothalamus and in the striatum of rats have been reported to be altered in the opposite direction by benzodiazepines. Whether the changes in this peptide are linked to certain specific effects of benzodiazepines, remains to be investigated. Some effects of benzodiazepines could be reduced by opiate antagonists. This, by itself, does not necessarily indicate a specific involvement of endogenous opiate-like compounds in certain effects of benzodiazepines, but may merely reflect the possibility that in complex behavioral functions the blockade of ongoing activity in endogenous opiate-like systems might interfere with the effects of benzodiazepines on other systems.

The possible interaction of benzodiazepines with other peptides (e.g., ACTH) and prostaglandins should be studied in the future.

3. Transmitter Systems Apparently Unaffected by Benzodiazepines

The present data fail to indicate changes in the dynamics of glutamate and glycine systems. The failure to detect changes in the turnover of these transmitters is most likely due to methodologic shortcomings.

4. Specific Enhancement of GABAergic Transmission

Data supporting the idea that benzodiazepines specifically enhance GABAergic transmission are increasing at a fast rate. At all GABAergic synapses investigated so far, the facilitating effect of benzodiazepines has been demonstrated. Consistent and marked facilitation was observed in studies of GABAergic synaptic inhibition induced by electrically stimulating the neuronal afferents to GABAergic interneurons (presynaptic inhibition in the spinal cord, pre- and postsynaptic inhibition in the dorsal column nuclei, recurrent inhibition in the hippocampus, hypothalamus, and cerebral and cerebellar cortex). Synaptic inhibition produced by directly stimulating axons of GABAergic projection neurons (striatonigral pathways, cerebellar Purkinje cell axons) was only enhanced by benzodiazepines when transmission had been reduced by depleting GABA or blocking GABA receptors. Attempts to explain the molecular mechanisms of action of benzodiazepines should take into account these differing findings on GABA interneurons and GABA projection neurons.

While the facilitating action of benzodiazepines on GABAergic transmission is no longer seriously in doubt, much effort is at present being made to understand the molecular mechanisms of action of these drugs. Theoretically, these drugs could affect GABAergic transmission by a presynaptic (on the GABA neuron itself) or by a postsynaptic (on GABA follower cells) site of action, and experimental support for both possibilities has been obtained. Presynaptically, benzodiazepines could enhance the response of GABAergic interneurons to their excitatory input, resulting in an increased firing of these cells; evidence for such an effect has been found in hippocampal slices (LEE et al., 1979). Another presynaptic site of action could be the GABAergic nerve terminal, where benzodiazepines might enhance excitation-secretion coupling; evidence for an enhanced potassium-induced release of GABA from brain has been provided (MITCHELL and MARTIN, 1978). Postsynaptically, benzodiazepines have been proposed to enhance the binding of GABA to its receptors by competing with an endogenous modulator of GABA receptor (gabamodulin), which physiologically decreases the affinity of GABA for binding sites in synaptic membranes (GUIDOTTI et al., 1979). An alternative postsynaptic mechanism of action is the suggested interaction with the coupling between GABA receptors and chloride channels or with the chloride channel itself (SIMMONDS, 1980).

Y. Benzodiazepines and Cyclic Nucleotides

I. Cyclic 3′,5′-Adenosine Monophosphate (cAMP)

Diazepam and clonazepam (7 mg·kg^{-1} i.p.) produced a slight increase of the cAMP level in the cerebellum, as did clonazepam in the cerebral cortex of mice. In the rat (GOVONI et al., 1976) and the mouse (LUST et al., 1978), cerebellar cAMP content was unaltered by various benzodiazepines in doses that markedly reduced the cerebellar cGMP level. However, the marked increase of cAMP produced in both structures by a convulsive dose of pentetrazole (100 mg·kg^{-1} s.c.) was completely prevented by the two benzodiazepines (PALMER et al., 1979). In isolated bullfrog sympathetic ganglion, diazepam (0.1 mmol·l^{-1}) markedly increased the basal content of cAMP; diazepam was more potent in this respect than theophylline and papaverine (SMITH et al., 1979). In in vitro studies with mouse cerebral cortex, diazepam and clonazepam (0.6 mmol·l^{-1}) increased the basal level of cAMP; clonazepam (and diazepam in tendency) augmented the elevation of cAMP by adenosine but reduced that evoked by ouabain (PALMER et al., 1979). In slices of guinea-pig cerebral cortex, diazepam, desmethyldiazepam, methyloxazepam, oxazepam, and chlordiazepoxide increased the basal level of cAMP at concentrations of 0.2 mmol·l^{-1} and 0.5 mmol·l^{-1} (SCHULTZ, 1974). All these compounds also enhanced the cAMP elevation induced by histamine and by the combination of histamine plus noradrenaline. The calculated EC$_{50}$ for diazepam was 50 μmol·l^{-1} in the case of histamine stimulation and 16 μmol·l^{-1} in the case of combined stimulation with histamine plus noradrenaline. Very similar results were obtained with chlordiazepoxide by HESS et al. (1975); however, these authors proposed that chlordiazepoxide affected cAMP by releasing adenosine. The adenosine-induced elevation of cAMP was only minimally enhanced by most benzodiazepines, probably because of the high level already achieved with adenosine alone. SCHULTZ (1974) interpreted these results as indicating an inhibitory effect of benzodiazepines on a low K$_m$ phosphodiesterase and suggested that active concentrations of these drugs could be reached by pharmacologically relevant doses. Different results were obtained in superfused slices of guinea-pig and rat cerebral cortex with the racemate and the enantiomers of oxazepam sodium hemisuccinate (TRAVERSA and NEWMAN, 1979). The pharmacologically more active d-isomer at 0.1 mmol·l^{-1} doubled the cAMP content in the absence of adenosine, whereas the l-isomer and the racemate were inactive. The racemate and the l-isomer, however, greatly reduced the cAMP increase induced by adenosine. The d-isomer was more potent than the l-isomer in inhibiting the uptake of adenosine by the slices. The accumulation of cAMP after oxazepam in the absence of exogenous adenosine was proposed to be mediated by adenosine, since theophylline, which blocks the stimulation of adenylate cyclase by adenosine, reduced the accumulation of cAMP induced by oxazepam.

In intact neuroblastoma cells, diazepam and, to a lesser degree, chlordiazepoxide at 0.5 mmol·l^{-1} enhanced the accumulation of cAMP induced by PGE$_1$ (SCHULTZ and HAMBRECHT, 1973). In the rat brain in vitro, BEER et al. (1972) found chlordiazepoxide and diazepam to be potent inhibitors of cAMP phosphodiesterase. In contrast to theophylline, these two drugs were more potent inhibitors in brain than in preparations from heart, fat cells, and adrenal glands. Comparing a number of agents for their inhibitory action on brain phosphodiesterase and their antipunishment effect in a conflict procedure (water licking test), the authors arrived at the conclusion that phosphodiesterase inhibition was the cause of the antianxiety effect of benzodiazepines. This view, however, is hardly supported by other evidence, and the apparent antianxiety effect of methylxanthines in the water licking test casts doubts on its predictive value for therapeutic anxiolytic activity. The inhibitory activity of benzodiazepines on brain phosphodiesterase was confirmed by DALTON et al. (1974). Medazepam, diazepam, chlordiazepoxide, N-desmethyldiazepam, oxazepam, and N-desmethyloxazepam inhibited cAMP phosphodiesterase activity in the supernatant of homogenates of rat brain and mouse neuroblastoma cells with potencies in the order of papaverine and dipyridamole and superior to that of thephylline. When diazepam 5 mg · kg^{-1} was administered to cats in vivo, no inhibition of phosphodiesterase activity could be detected in the brain ex vivo. The inhibitory effect on cAMP phosphodiesterase is therefore unlikely to be involved to a relevant degree in the pharmacologic actions of benzodiazepines; this view is also supported by the fact that medazepam, which is an inactive benzodiazepine prodrug requiring enzymatic transformation into an active metabolite, was as potent as diazepam on phosphodiesterase activity in the three brain regions.

In human blood platelets, chlordiazepoxide, diazepam, N-desmethyldiazepam, and oxazepam were weak inhibitors of phosphodiesterase or even inactive, as judged from potentiation of PGE$_1$-mediated inhibition of ADP-induced aggregation (HESS et al., 1975). At 1 mmol · l^{-1} they inhibited ADP-induced platelet aggregation, but obviously by a mechanism unrelated to phosphodiesterase inhibition. In vitro studies on inhibition of phosphodiesterase showed diazepam and chlordiazepoxide to be active in the rat brain (IC$_{50}$ of 33 and 110 µmol · l^{-1}, respectively), while on the cat heart enzyme 60 µmol · l^{-1} diazepam was required for 50% inhibition, and chlordiazepoxide proved inactive at 1 mmol · l^{-1} (WEINRYB et al., 1972). For comparison the IC$_{50}$ values for theophylline were 120 µmol · l^{-1} in the brain and 50 µmol · l^{-1} in the heart.

II. Cyclic 3′,5′-Guanosine Monophosphate (cGMP)

The study of cGMP in the cerebellum was an important biochemical approach in the discovery of benzodiazepine-GABA interactions. The starting point for this model was the finding that the cGMP content of the mouse cerebellum in vivo could be altered by stress, such as cold exposure (MAO et al., 1974) and by various drugs (COSTA et al., 1975a, b). In an attempt to define the neurotransmitters that regulate the cGMP content of the cerebellar cortex, it was most elegantly shown that increased activation of cerebellar Purkinje cells by either of the two excitatory afferent systems to the cerebellar cortex, the so-called climbing fibre system or the mossy fibre system, resulted in an increased cGMP content. A rather selective stimulation of climbing fibres can be obtained with the tremorigenic harmaline (COSTA et al., 1975a, b; BIGGIO et al., 1977b, c). An elevation of cerebellar cGMP is obtained by harmaline, by inhibiting the biosynthesis of GABA, e.g., with isoniazid, or by blocking GABA receptors with picrotoxin (SPANO et al., 1975; OPMEER et al., 1976; MAILMAN et al., 1978), but also after nonstressful locomotor activity (MEYERHOFF et al., 1979). Benzodiazepines alone were found to decrease the normal cGMP level in the cerebellar cortex and to prevent the rise of cGMP after harmaline, isoniazid, picrotoxin, pentetrazole, and electroshock, along with a reduction of convulsions (MAO et al., 1975a, b; COSTA et al., 1975a, b, 1976, 1978; SPANO et al., 1975; OPMEER et al., 1976; NAIK et al., 1976; GUI-

DOTTI, 1978; LUST et al., 1978; MAILMAN et al., 1978; CHAN-PALAY and PALAY, 1979; SZMIGIELSKI and GUIDOTTI, 1979).

The effects of systemic benzodiazepines could be mimicked by local injections of diazepam or the GABA mimetic, muscimol, into the cerebellar cortex. The difference between diazepam and muscimol was the dependence of the diazepam effect on the presence of endogenous GABA in the cerebellar cortex, whereas muscimol still reduced cGMP after depletion of endogenous GABA (BIGGIO et al., 1977a; COSTA et al., 1978). Diazepam was not able to further reduce the low level of cerebellar cGMP in "nervous" mutant mice, a genotype with a dramatic loss of Purkinje cells (MAO et al., 1975c). However, diazepam still reduced cerebellar cGMP in mice in which the climbing fibre system was eliminated by neurotoxic destruction of the olive by 3-acetyl-pyridine (BIGGIO et al., 1977b, c). Diazepam inhibited the rise of cerebellar cGMP induced by apomorphine (BIGGIO et al., 1976; BURKARD et al., 1976a, b) and amphetamine (GUMULKA et al., 1976), drugs that indirectly activate the excitatory input to the cerebellar cortex. An increase of the cGMP level in the medial forebrain and the cerebellum of mice occurred after stress induced by forced swimming in ice water for 30 s; pretreatment of the animals with $1 \ mg \cdot kg^{-1}$ diazepam markedly reduced the cGMP levels in both stressed and unstressed animals (DINNENDAHL and GUMULKA 1977). Pentobarbitone, chlorpromazine, haloperidol, reserpine, and aminooxyacetic acid (AOAA) had similar effects. In newborn rats, in which synaptic contacts on Purkinje cells are rudimentary, benzodiazepines failed to decrease cerebellar cGMP, while intracerebroventricularly injected GABA was active (SPANO et al., 1975; GOVONI et al., 1976). Diazepam also lowered the cGMP content of the deep cerebellar nuclei (BIGGIO et al., 1977b), whose neurons are strongly inhibited by the GABAergic cerebellar Purkinje cells. The increase of cerebellar cGMP induced by the intracerebroventricular injection of glutamate was inhibited by diazepam (COSTA et al., 1975a).

The relative potency of various benzodiazepines in reducing rat cerebellar cGMP level corresponded nicely with their potencies as sedatives and anxiolytics (GOVONI et al., 1976; BURKARD, personal communication).

The large number of data from experiments on cerebellar cGMP were interpreted as indications that benzodiazepines enhance in some way the GABAergic inhibitory input to cerebellar Purkinje cells and, by thus changing the balance between excitatory (glutamate) and inhibitory (GABAergic) inputs, decrease the formation of cGMP (COSTA et al., 1975a, b; GUIDOTTI, 1978). However, immunocytochemical studies in the cerebellum have shown a preferential localization of cGMP in neuroglial cells, and the relation between GABAergic transmission and cerebellar cGMP may, therefore, be more complicated (CHAN-PALAY and PALAY, 1979). Furthermore, it is still unknown whether the excitatory transmitter, presumably glutamate, excites Purkinje cells through the action of cGMP or whether the cGMP levels secondarily reflect the state of activity of these cells. It should also be mentioned that benzodiazepines were markedly more potent in reducing cGMP than barbiturates and that the anticonvulsant, diphenylhydantoin, was completely ineffective (COSTA et al., 1975b).

In tissue slices of rat substantia nigra, GABA ($0.5 \ mmol \cdot l^{-1}$) as well as chlordiazepoxide ($3 \ mmol \cdot l^{-1}$) reduced the level of cGMP (WADDINGTON and LONGDEN, 1977). In the isolated sympathetic ganglion, diazepam ($0.1 \ mmol \cdot l^{-1}$) elevated the basal content of cGMP (SMITH et al., 1979).

III. Conclusions

Several investigators have found an increase by benzodiazepines of resting or evoked cAMP levels in isolated tissues, which was ascribed to a release of adenosine or to an inhibition of phosphodiesterase. The high concentration of benzodiazepines required and their relative potencies make it very unlikely that these observations are relevant for the pharmacologic effects of these drugs.

The consistent decrease of cerebellar cGMP levels by benzodiazepines is not due to direct interactions with the cGMP generating and metabolizing mechanisms, but rather reflects the depressant effect of these drugs on the firing rate of neurons, whose synaptic excitation results in the increase of intracellular cGMP.

Z. Benzodiazepine Receptors

Using methods developed earlier for the demonstration of specific binding sites for neurotransmitters and their antagonists in cell-free systems, Squires and Braestrup (1977), Braestrup and Squires (1977), Möhler and Okada (1977a, b), and Bossmann et al. (1977) first demonstrated with ^{3}H-diazepam as ligand the presence of specific and saturable high-affinity binding sites for benzodiazepines in membrane preparations in rat and human central nervous system. The binding characteristics and the relative affinities of various representatives of this chemical class of compounds were compatible with the view that these binding sites, in part or entirely, are the receptors which mediate the specific pharmacologic effects of benzodiazepines. It is in this qualitative, rather than quantitative meaning, that the terms "benzodiazepine receptor" and "specific benzodiazepine binding site" will be used interchangeably in the following.

The early findings on benzodiazepine binding sites were rapidly confirmed and extended in many laboratories. Rat brain homogenates frozen for up to 1 month show little loss of ^{3}H-diazepam or ^{3}H-flunitrazepam binding capacity (Colello et al., 1978a), which greatly facilitates the investigation of these binding sites.

I. Main Characteristics of Benzodiazepine Receptors

1. Affinity

In in vitro benzodiazepine binding assays, the amount of ^{3}H-diazepam or ^{3}H-flunitrazepam of high specific activity bound to brain membrane is determined in the presence and absence of high concentrations of an unlabeled potent benzodiazepine (Fig. 4). The amount of radioactive ligand displaceable in the presence of the excess of unlabeled benzodiazepine is termed "specifically bound" and was found to be saturable with increasing concentrations of radioactive ligand, indicating that only a limited number of specific benzodiazepine binding sites are present in the tissue. In contrast, nondisplaceable binding ("nonspecific binding") increased linearly when the same concentrations of radioactive ligand were used.

The affinity of pharmacologically active benzodiazepines for these specific binding sites is very high, half-maximum saturation occurring, e.g., for diazepam at 2–

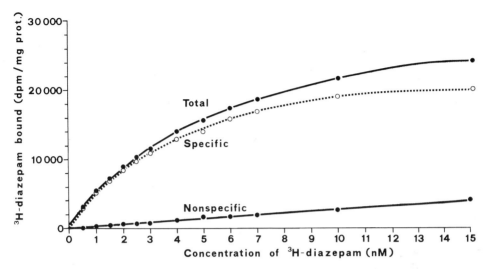

Fig. 4. Benzodiazepine receptor binding in rat cerebral cortex in vitro. Increasing concentrations of ³H-diazepam were incubated with crude synaptosomal preparations in the absence (total binding) and presence of 1 µM flunitrazepam (nonspecific binding). Specific binding is obtained by subtracting nonspecific from total binding. (Courtesy of Dr. H. Möhler)

8 nmol·l⁻¹. This high affinity permits a high degree of receptor occupation to be reached at the concentrations of benzodiazepines that occur in the brain after average pharmacological doses, even when taking into consideration that only an unknown part of free molecules is available for interaction with the receptors. All benzodiazepine derivatives investigated so far interacted in a purely competitive and reversible manner with specific binding of ³H-diazepam or ³H-flunitrazepam. A good correlation was found between their displacing potencies in the radioligand binding assay and their relative potencies in in vivo pharmacologic tests (and therapeutic activity). A large number of compounds structurally related to diazepam have been tested for their inhibitory effect on ³H-diazepam binding in many laboratories, and only a small part of these results have been published. Data available from the literature are, however, sufficient to demonstrate the correlation just mentioned (BRAESTRUP et al., 1977; MÖHLER and OKADA, 1977 a, 1978; BRAESTRUP and SQUIRES, 1978 a; MACKERER et al., 1978; MÜLLER et al., 1978 b; MALICK and ENNA, 1979). The few exceptions find a logical explanation in the fact that some compounds require biotransformation into pharmacologically active molecules and, therefore, are weakly active in the in vitro binding assay, or that some compounds are rapidly inactivated in vivo and, therefore, appear more potent in the in vitro binding assay than in in vivo tests.

Furthermore, enantiomers of benzodiazepines with a chirality center in position 3 differed in their potencies in displacing the radioligands from the specific binding sites, in agreement with the difference in pharmacologic activity of the stereoisomers (MÖHLER and OKADA, 1977 a, 1978; WADDINGTON and OWEN, 1978). Only the enantiomers of oxazepam were reported to lack stereospecific displacement of ³H-diazepam in membranes from rat spinal cord (MÜLLER et al., 1978 a).

2. Specificity

In the in vitro benzodiazepine binding assay using brain membrane preparations at $0\ ^\circ C$, nearly all of the radioactive ligand bound to the tissue is associated with the benzodiazepine specific binding sites (90%) at ligand concentrations that are of interest to pharmacologists $(1-1000\ nmol \cdot l^{-1}\ ^3H$-diazepam) (Möhler and Okada, 1977 a, b).

The ligand specificity of the receptor for molecules closely related to benzodiazepines is impressive. High affinities were found for compounds differing from the classical 1,4-benzodiazepines by substitution of ring A by aromatic heterocyclic rings (e.g., thiophene), by the position of the two nitrogens within ring B (e.g., 1,5-benzodiazepines), or by the lack of one nitrogen in ring B (e.g., 1-benzazepines). However, for hundreds of compounds not belonging to diazepines or azepines, no relevant affinity for the receptor was found apart from some triazolopyridazines, which show anticonvulsant and anxiolytic action and displace ^3H-diazepam and ^3H-flunitrazepam binding with K_i-values in the $10–1,000\ nmol \cdot l^{-1}$ range (Lippa et al., 1979; Squires et al., 1979 b, 1980; Klepner et al., 1979), the anxiolytic and hypnotic zopiclone (K_i $30\ nmol \cdot l^{-1}$ in ^3H-diazepam binding; Blanchard et al., 1979), and the inhibitor of adenosine uptake, dipyridamole (K_i $300\ nmol \cdot l^{-1}$) (Davies et al., 1980).

3. Irreversible Ligands

For several reasons, in particular for the isolation and purification of the presumed benzodiazepine receptor, for its autoradiographic localization in tissue slices, the availability of a highly specific irreversible ligand would be of immense utility. Two approaches were used to obtain a covalent binding of a ligand to the benzodiazepine recognition site. Rice et al. (1979) prepared a benzodiazepine with an isothiocyanate function in an ethane side chain attached to the nitrogen in position 1. This compound, coined "irazepine," was shown to inhibit benzodiazepine receptor binding in synaptosomal membranes in a noncompetitive fashion. Model experiments suggest that the presumably covalent binding of the ligand may occur through a thiourea or dithiocarbamate bridge to primary and secondary amine or mercaptan groups of the benzodiazepine binding molecule. The specificity of this ligand and, hence, its usefulness as a marker of the benzodiazepine receptor, remains to be demonstrated. In mice and rats, the systemic administration of irazepine did not result in a prolonged sedative effect (Bonetti, personal communication).

Another approach to the covalent labeling of the benzodiazepine receptors makes use of the photoaffinity labeling (Möhler et al., 1980 a). After incubating synaptosomal fractions of rat cerebral cortex with ^3H-flunitrazepam and illuminating with near UV light, followed by thorough washing, an apparently covalent binding of ^3H-flunitrazepam to the receptor was found. This irreversible binding could be prevented by simultaneous incubation with various active benzodiazepines with a potency corresponding to their affinity to the benzodiazepine receptor. Furthermore, there was an excellent inverse correlation between increase of irreversible ^3H-flunitrazepam binding and the reduction of reversible ^3H-diazepam binding sites. In addition to flunitrazepam, two other 7-nitrobenzodiazepines (clonazepam, nitrazepam) were found to interact irreversibly with benzodiazepine receptors in vitro (Johnson and Yamamura, 1979).

4. Solubilization

Solubilization of the specific benzodiazepine binding sites of brain membranes was achieved with digitonin (GAVISH et al., 1979), Lubrol (TALLMAN et al., 1980b; YOUSUFI et al., 1979) and Triton X-100 (CHIU and ROSENBERG, 1979) as detergents. Binding recovery in the former case was about 50% and the K_D value for flunitrazepam (1.5 nmol·l^{-1}) similar to that obtained with membrane bound receptors. A similar drug specificity was found with the solubilized and bound receptors using various active and inactive ligands. The temperature dependence of ^{3}H-diazepam binding was also present with the solubilized receptor preparation, however, GABA did not increase binding of ^{3}H-diazepam to the solubilized receptors (YOUSUFI et al., 1979).

II. Regional Distribution of Benzodiazepine Receptors

The density of specific benzodiazepine binding sites varies considerably (by a factor of 24) in various parts of the rat and human central nervous gray matter (BRAESTRUP and SQUIRES, 1977; BRAESTRUP et al., 1977; MÖHLER and OKADA, 1977a, 1978b; MACKERER et al., 1978; MÜLLER et al., 1978a; SPETH et al., 1978; PLACHETA and KAROBATH, 1979; YOUNG and KUHAR, 1980). Density is highest in the cerebral cortex, medium in the cerebellar cortex, limbic structures, thalamus and hypothalamus, and low in the lower brain stem and the spinal cord. The white matter (e.g., corpus callosum) contains virtually no binding sites. The apparent affinity constants did not differ significantly in the various structures. If a correlation between benzodiazepine receptor density and the density of neurotransmitter levels or receptors had to be done, it would be best, although not complete, with GABA (MÖHLER and OKADA, 1978). In all regions of the rat CNS, the number of ^{3}H-flunitrazepam binding sites was consistently smaller than that of GABA binding sites; the difference was most marked in the cerebellum (PLACHETA and KAROBATH, 1979). Using a newly developed light microscopic autoradiographic method, which circumvents the problems encountered with diffusible ligands, YOUNG and KUHAR (1979, 1980) studied the localization of benzodiazepine receptors in human, mouse and rat central nervous system labeled with ^{3}H-flunitrazepam. Specific binding sites were absent in the white matter, and there were interesting differences in the density of labeled binding sites in the various cell layers of cortical gray matter (Fig. 5). A very restricted distribution was also found in the dorsal horn of rat spinal cord. No simple correlation between the distribution of benzodiazepine and GABA receptors emerged from this investigation. Species differences in the distribution of benzodiazepine receptors in the cerebellar cortex call for caution in extrapolating animal data to the human nervous system.

Specific high-affinity binding sites for benzodiazepines, as they were characterized in the central nervous system, have not been detected in tissues outside the central nervous system except the retina (HOWELLS et al., 1979; OSBORNE, 1980; BORBE et al., 1980; PAUL et al., 1980). However, benzodiazepine binding sites with distinct characteristics were found in the kidney, lung, and liver cells, but not in skeletal muscle (BRAESTRUP and SQUIRES, 1977; MÖHLER and OKADA, 1977b). These "peripheral type" receptors differ from the central benzodiazepine receptors either in affinity or ligand specificity, or both. For instance, the centrally inactive benzodiazepine, Ro 5-4868, had a rather high affinity for binding sites in the kidney. Rat astrocytoma cells seem to contain benzodiazepine binding sites with similar characteristics to those

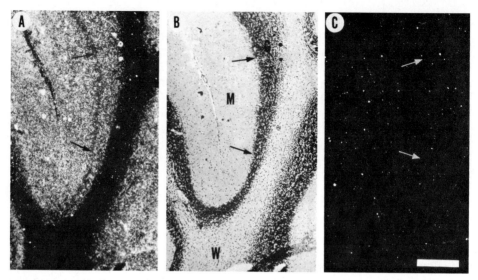

Fig. 5 A–C. Visualization of benzodiazepine receptors in human cerebellum using ^{3}H-fluni-trazepam binding. The dark-field photomicrograph in **A** shows the autoradiographic grain distribution over the tissue in **B**. The density of receptors is high in the molecular layer M and in the granule cell layer G, low in the Purkinje cell layer (indicated by *arrows*) and zero in the white matter W. The dark-field photomicrograph in **C** shows the blockade of receptor binding in an adjacent 4-µm section due to the addition of 1 µM clonazepam. Cryostat sections of tissue were thaw-mounted onto gelatin-coated slides and dipped into 1 µM ^{3}H-flunitrazepam of high specific activity. After 40 min incubation at 4 °C the sections were washed for 2 min and dried. Emulsion-coated coverslips were attached to the slide. After exposure for 2 weeks the coverslips were gently bent away from the tissue sections, the latent autoradiograms developed, and the tissues fixed and stained with pyronine Y. (From YOUNG and KUHAR, 1979)

found in the kidney (MALLORGA et al., 1979; STRITTMATTER et al., 1979 b). Of several cultured cell lines of neural origin, the rat C_6 glioma and mouse NB 41 A 3 neuroblastoma were found by SYAPIN and SKOLNICK (1979) to posses a large number of the "peripheral-type" benzodiazepine receptors. The authors discussed the possibility that an oncogenic mechanism was responsible for the transformation of the "central type" to the "peripheral type" benzodiazepine receptor.

Low affinity binding sites for benzodiazepines are found on plasma albumin. The K_D for chlordiazepoxide was determined to be 2.5×10^{-5} mol·l^{-1} by SOLLENNE and MEANS (1979). The sites are rather specific for benzodiazepines and L-tryptophan (MÜLLER and WOLLERT, 1975 a, b; BALL et al., 1979; FEHSKE et al., 1979). A high affinity of flunitrazepam for melanin-containing cells in the retina has been found (KUHN, 1980). These binding sites have not yet been characterized.

III. Multiplicity of Benzodiazepine Receptors

While early studies of the central benzodiazepine receptors in animal and human central nervous system appeared to indicate the presence of a uniform population of specific binding sites, SQUIRES et al. (1979 a, b, 1980), KLEPNER et al. (1979) and COUPET and SZUCS-MYERS (1979) first provided evidence for the heterogeneity of benzodiazepine receptors. Thermal inactivation of ^{3}H-flunitrazepam binding sites at 60 °C in 50 mmol·l^{-1} Na phosphate (but not in Tris buffer) suggested the presence of two components with half-lives of inactivation of about 8 and 70 min. Measurements of "off-rates" of the dissociation of radioligands in the presence of high concentrations of the respective unlabeled benzodiazepine (1 μmol·l^{-1}) showed a biphasic dissociation at 0 °C with components having half-lives of 2 and 9 min. Dissociation of ^{3}H-diazepam in the presence of a triazolopyridazine or cold diazepam was identical in respect to the fast component; however, the slow component of dissociation in the presence of the triazolopyridazine became even slower, the half-life being increased three-fold. The interpretation was that the triazolopyridazine compound had a significantly lower affinity for the "slow dissociating" binding site than for the "fast dissociating" one. Furthermore, in heat-pretreated membranes the interaction of triazolopyridazines with ^{3}H-diazepam and ^{3}H-flunitrazepam binding was indicative of two benzodiazepine binding sites. Further evidence for two populations of benzodiazepine receptors is derived from the finding that GABA and muscimol partially protected one population of binding sites from heat inactivation, but not the other one (SQUIRES et al., 1979 b). This protective property of GABA and muscimol is shared by the GABA mimetics, β-guanidino-propionic acid, β-alanine, and imidazole acetic acid. Surprisingly, however, the GABA mimetics, THIP and isoguvacine, failed to protect from heat inactivation. SQUIRES et al. (1979 c, 1980) proposed that a specific type of GABA receptors, stimulated by GABA mimetics of the GABA-muscimol type, but not by THIP and isoguvacine, cause conformational changes in the associated benzodiazepine receptors, making them more resistant to heat inactivation and increasing their affinities for diazepam and flunitrazepam. KLEPNER et al. (1979) proposed the presence of two distinct binding sites for benzodiazepines. Type I benzodiazepine receptors predominate in the cerebellum, have a high affinity for triazolopyrazines, and would not be coupled to GABA receptors and chloride channels; Type II benzodiazepine receptors predominate in the frontal cortex and hippocampus, have a low affinity for triazolopyridazines, and are coupled to GABA receptors and chloride conductance mechanisms. Whereas triazolopyridazines have a high affinity for Type I and a lower affinity for Type II receptors, benzodiazepines do not discriminate between the two. The suggestion that Type I receptors would mediate primarily anxiolytic activity, whereas Type II receptors would be responsible for sedative and ataxic effects, does not appear too convincing in view of the regional distribution of these binding sites. Evidence for the molecular heterogeneity of benzodiazepine binding sites ("isoreceptors") was provided by SIEGHART and KAROBATH (1980). After photoaffinity labeling of receptors with ^{3}H-flunitrazepam in membrane fractions of various rat brain regions, the membranes were dissolved in sodium dodecylsulphate (SDS) and subjected to SDS-polyacrylamide gel electrophoresis and fluorography. In the cerebellum irreversible binding of ^{3}H-flunitrazepam was restricted to a single protein band with an apparent molecular weight of 51,000 daltons. In other brain regions most of the radioactivity was associated with the same protein band (P_{51}), except in the spinal cord, where this band was very weakly labeled. The P_{51} benzodiazepine receptor seems to be identical with that described by MÖHLER et al. (1980a). Extracerebellar brain regions contain several other labeled protein bands in addition to P_{51} with apparent molecular weights of 53,000 (P_{53}), 55,000 (P_{55}), and 59,000 (P_{59}). The most prominent of these, P_{55}, was most highly labeled in hippocampal membranes.

Whereas diazepam inhibited irreversible binding of ^{3}H-flunitrazepam to P_{51} in cerebellum and to P_{51} and P_{55} in hippocampus to the same extent, the triazolopyridazine, CL 218,872, prevented irreversible binding to P_{51} more strongly than to P_{55}. SUPAVILAI and KAROBATH (1980) determined different K_D values for ^{3}H-flunitrazepam in hippocampal and cerebellar membrane preparations.

It appears likely, therefore, that at least two distinct populations of benzodiazepine receptors exist, which can be differentiated by their stability to heat, by the rate at which ligands dissociate from them, by their different affinities for triazolopyridazines, by their apparent association with two classes of GABA receptors, distinct by their different affinities for benzodiazepines, and by their apparent molecular weight. Whether these populations of receptors mediate different pharmacologic effects is yet unknown.

IV. Influence of Physical Factors on Benzodiazepine Binding

1. Temperature

Equilibrium of specific ^{3}H-diazepam binding is reached within 10–15 min at 0 °C and this time increases with temperature (BRAESTRUP and SQUIRES, 1977; MÖHLER and OKADA, 1977 b; BRILEY and LANGER, 1978; SPETH et al., 1979 a), whereas nonspecific binding is not temperature dependent (MÖHLER and OKADA, 1977 b). Arrhenius plots of the temperature dependence of ^{3}H-diazepam binding show a break in the curve which indicates that the binding site undergoes a conformational change at about 18 °C. At 37 °C the specific binding of ^{3}H-diazepam is only 2% of that occurring at 0 °C. The reason for this low binding of ^{3}H-diazepam at 37 °C, as opposed to that of ^{3}H-flunitrazepam, was investigated by BRAESTRUP and SQUIRES (1978 b), who found that the rate of dissociation of ^{3}H-diazepam was much more rapid than that of ^{3}H-flunitrazepam and that in centrifugation assays the binding of ^{3}H-diazepam was considerably less sensitive to temperature than in the usual filtration assays. The temperature dependence of ^{3}H-diazepam binding was also found with solubilized receptor proteins from cortical membranes (TALLMAN et al., 1980 b; YOUSUFI et al., 1979). When membrane preparations are stored at 37 °C in the presence or absence of a benzodiazepine, before equilibrium binding of a radiolabeled benzodiazepine is performed at 0 °C, the affinity is markedly enhanced (BRAESTRUP and SQUIRES, 1977; SPETH et al., 1979 b). It is not yet known whether this phenomenon is due to the postmortem degradation of factors that reduce the affinity of benzodiazepines for their binding sites or to the postmortem formation of GABA, which would enhance this affinity.

2. pH

The pH optimum of binding is rather broad, i.e., pH 6.5–9 in triphosphate buffer (MÖHLER and OKADA, 1977 b); in glycine-NaOH, pH optimum was 9.5 (BRAESTRUP and SQUIRES, 1977).

3. Ions

Early studies did not reveal significant effects of ionic changes on specific ^{3}H-diazepam binding (MÖHLER and OKADA, 1977 b). BOSMANN et al. (1977) observed that 10 mmol $\cdot$ l^{-1} EDTA lowered the binding of ^{3}H-diazepam to rat brain membranes by

20%, suggesting ionic requirements for optimal binding. Monovalent cations in high concentrations were all found to enhance the binding. Two more recent investigations gave somewhat discrepant results. MACKERER and KOCHMAN (1978), working with crude synaptic membrane preparations from the whole brain and spinal cord of rats found a very slight enhancement of ^{3}H-diazepam binding with various monovalent cations (except cesium) and a slight inhibition with monovalent anions. However, binding was markedly enhanced by divalent cations, Ni^{2+} being the most effective. This increased binding was due exclusively to an enhanced affinity. COSTA et al. (1979) observed that of 18 anions tested, only five produced a concentration-dependent enhancement of ^{3}H-diazepam binding at 0 °C, namely iodide, bromide, chloride, thiocyanate, and nitrate. This effect was absent at 37 °C. The enhanced binding at 0 °C was due to an increased affinity; only the dissociation rate constant, but not the association rate constant, was decreased. The correlation between the capacity of anions to enhance ^{3}H-diazepam binding and to serve as current carriers in the GABA-regulated chloride channel was not perfect. In spite of this and the absence of an anion effect at physiologic temperature, COSTA et al. (1979) and RODBARD et al. (1979) proposed that their results indicated an association between the benzodiazepine binding site and a chloride channel, possibly the same to which the GABA receptor is coupled, a view which has been questioned by CANDY and MARTIN (1979). In analogy to the opiate receptor, where agonist binding, but not antagonist binding is affected by the ion species in the presumed opiate-modulated conductance mechanism, COSTA et al. (1979) hypothetized that benzodiazepines acted as agonists at this receptor, while a potential endogenous ligand would behave as an antagonist.

V. Nature of the Benzodiazepine Binding Site

The destruction of the binding capacity of membrane fragment with trypsin and chymotrypsin (BRAESTRUP and SQUIRES, 1977; MÖHLER and OKADA, 1977b; LANG et al., 1979) indicated that the benzodiazepine receptor may be a protein. From enzymatic inactivation studies, BOSMANN et al. (1977) concluded that the binding site may be a complex involving protein, phospholipid, and N-acetylneuraminic acid. The membrane-bound benzodiazepine receptor appears to be rather stable; isolated membranes stored at −18 °C for 7 days showed no loss of activity (BRAESTRUP and SQUIRES, 1977). Incubating preparations at 50 °C–60 °C initially increased specific binding and then inactivated the receptor with a half-life of 3 h and 10 min, respectively (BRAESTRUP and SQUIRES, 1977). Incubation at pH 11 did not destroy specific binding, but at pH 2 specific activity completely disappeared within 20 min.

MÖHLER et al. (1980a) succeeded in covalently binding ^{3}H-flunitrazepam to the benzodiazepine receptor by photoaffinity labeling. P_2 fractions incubated with ^{3}H-flunitrazepam and brain tissue slices of rats injected intravenously with the radioligand were illuminated with near-UV light. The ^{3}H-flunitrazepam incorporated could not be washed out or separated from proteins or dialyzed after solubilization of the membranes, demonstrating its heat- and light-stable covalent binding to the receptor. Trypsin treatment of the photolabelled, solubilized P_2 fraction indicated that the binding site was a protein. By sodium-dodecyl-sulphate gel electrophoresis the molecular weight of the photolabelled receptor protein was calculated to be about 50,000 daltons. This protein may be part of a larger receptor complex solubilized in Lubrol by Tallman et al. (1980 b) and Lang et al. (1979). At present, it can only be speculated as to the part played by the protein identified by Möhler et al. (1980 a) in the supra-molecular complex which binds benzodiazepines and initiates the chain of events leading to the pharmacologic effects of these drugs.

VI. Cellular Localization of Benzodiazepine Receptors

The most important question which has to be answered before we may begin to understand the function of the benzodiazepine receptors in the synaptic pharmacology of benzodiazepines is that of the type of cells that bear the receptors. Mostly indirect approaches have been used so far for cellular localization.

Braestrup et al. (1978) did not detect specific high-affinity binding sites for ^{3}H-diazepam in primary cultures of mouse cerebral astrocytes and concluded that benzodiazepine receptors were probably confined to neurons and absent on glia. However, Baraldi et al. (1978, 1979 b) described high-affinity binding sites of diazepam in fresh membranes prepared from both NG_2 neuroblastoma and C_6 glioma cell lines; it is doubtful whether these benzodiazepine receptors are identical with those present in the central nervous system, since the relative potencies of various benzodiazepines as displacers of ^{3}H-diazepam binding differ considerably (Baraldi et al., 1979 a). Henn and Henke (1978) found more ^{3}H-diazepam binding in fractions from bovine cerebral cortex containing astroglial cells than in fractions enriched with nerve endings. Syapin and Skolnick (1979) compared ^{3}H-diazepam binding in a variety of cultured tumors cells lines of neural origin (gliomas, neuroblastomas, glioblastomas, astrocytomas, etc.). The number of binding sites was higher in a glioma and neuroblastoma cell line than in the rat cortex, but lower in other cell lines. The affinity was lower than in rat cortex and, most important, the order of potency of various benzodiazepines in displacing ^{3}H-diazepam was quite different from that found in rat cortex and similar to that found in membranes of rat kidney. Besides suggesting that benzodiazepine receptors may be present in different cell types, these studies also demonstrate that cultured cells, particularly from tumors, may not be representative for the binding sites in the intact normal central nervous system. Dudai and Yavin (1979) studied ^{3}H-flunitrazepam binding in neuronal-enriched and glia-enriched cultures of cells isolated from fetal rat brain and found similar binding characteristics in both types of cultures.

Another approach used for cellular localization of benzodiazepine receptors was the study of ^{3}H-diazepam binding sites in brains of animals with genetic and experimental degeneration of distinct neurons or neuronal pathways and in postmortem human brain affected by well-defined degenerative diseases. The number of ^{3}H-diazepam binding sites in the cerebellar cortex of mutant "nervous" mice was identical with that in normal littermates at an age of 15–21 days, when the Purkinje cells are still present in a normal number, but reduced by about 85% at the age of 60–70 days, when approximately 90% of the Purkinje cells in the cerebellar hemispheres had disappeared (Lippa et al., 1978 a). Similar findings in adult "nervous" mice were reported by Speth and Yamamura (1979), Skolnick et al. (1979 a), and Braestrup et al. (1979 b). An almost 50% reduction of ^{3}H-flunitrazepam binding sites in cerebellum was also found in "staggerer" mice, which are characterized by the absence of synaptic spines in Purkinje cell dendrites (Speth and Yamamura, 1979). In "reeler" and "weaver" mutant mice, which lack the excitatory granule cells in their cerebellar cortex, the number of ^{3}H-flunitrazepam binding sites was found to be normal (BRAES-TRUP et al., 1979 b) or higher by 44% and 25% than in normal control mice (SPETH and YAMAMURA, 1979). The K_D values for ^{3}H-flunitrazepam binding were identical in all mutant and normal mice. These findings support the view that most benzodiazepine binding sites in the cerebellar cortex are on Purkinje cells.

In the brain of patients with Huntington's chorea, ^{3}H-flunitrazepam and ^{3}H-diazepam binding was reduced by 50% in the putamen; however, it increased by 25% in the frontal cortex and cerebellum and was unchanged in the caudate nucleus (REISINE et al., 1978, 1979; MÖHLER and OKADA, 1978). K_D was increased about twofold and B_{max} decreased by 40% in putamen. K_D was unaltered in frontal cortex and cerebellum, but B_{max} increased by about 30%. The decreased affinity in the putamen was tentatively explained by the drastic depletion of GABA or by conformational changes of the receptor. Since it is known that basal ganglia in Huntington's chorea show a selective loss of small interneurons but rather a proliferation of glial elements, the moderate decrease of benzodiazepine receptor density was assumed to reflect the occurrence of part of them in glia cells. The increase of binding sites in the cortex and cerebellum was proposed to be a reaction to the loss of a "benzodiazepine-like" neurotransmitter. After local injection of the neurotoxic kainic acid into the striatum of rats, the number of striatal ^{3}H-flunitrazepam binding sites decreased dramatically, suggesting a preferential localization on neurons (SPERK and SCHLOEGEL, 1979). Kainic acid lesions of the rat cerebellar cortex, which spared only granule cells, drastically reduced the number of ^{3}H-diazepam binding sites and the content of gabamodulin; the specific ^{3}H-GABA binding sites were unaffected but the K_D for GABA decreased (BIGGIO et al., 1980a). Since granule cells are the only non-GABAergic neurons in the cerebellar cortex, these findings would suggest that benzodiazepine binding sites are mainly located on cerebellar GABAergic neurons.

A more direct approach to the localization of benzodiazepine receptors was used by BATTERSBY et al. (1979), MÖHLER and RICHARDS (1980) and MÖHLER et al. (1980a, b, 1981). It consists of covalently binding ^{3}H-flunitrazepam to the receptor by photoaffinity labeling and subsequent visualization of radioactivity by EM autoradiography. In the cerebral and cerebellar cortex of rats injected intravenously with ^{3}H-flunitrazepam and illuminated in vitro with near UV light, the radioactive ligand was selectively accumulated in the regions of "synaptic contacts", i.e., on nerve endings and adjacent synaptic and glial structures. In cerebellar slices radioactivity was found concentrated at synapses formed by Golgi cell axon endings on granule cells (but not at synapses between mossy fiber endings and granule cells) and by nerve endings on proximal dendrites of Purkinje cells. These findings clearly indicate the localization of benzodiazepine receptors at GABAergic synapses in the cerebellar cortex. It is, however, not yet possible to decide whether benzodiazepine receptors are presynaptic or postsynaptic to the GABAergic synapses. There was no indication for a general glial localization of benzodiazepine receptors.

VII. Subcellular Localization

Of the various subfractions of rat forebrain, the ones containing synaptosomal membranes and junctions had the highest number of binding sites for ^{3}H-diazepam and ^{3}H-flunitrazepam, whereas mitochondria and small and large synaptic vesicles were very poor in binding sites (Möhler and Okada, 1977a; Bosmann et al., 1978). The benzodiazepine receptor seems to follow the enzyme Na$^+$, K$^+$-ATP ase, a marker of outer cell membranes (Braestrup and Squires, 1978b). It is very likely, therefore, that the binding sites are localized mainly in synaptic membranes. Bosmann et al. (1980) described a saturable binding of ^{3}H-flunitrazepam to brain cell nuclei in vivo and in vitro. The K_D for this nuclear binding was, however, 25 times higher than for binding to synaptosomal membranes.

Specific low-affinity binding of ^{3}H-diazepam in kidney homogenates was associated with a fraction sedimenting with mitochondria (Braestrup and Squires, 1977).

VIII. Phylogenetic Development of Benzodiazepine Receptors

Nielsen et al. (1978) studied the presence of specific high-affinity binding sites of ^{3}H-diazepam in various species. In all vertebrate species studied (mammalia, birds, reptiles, amphibia, fishes) except the hagfish (*Myxine glutinosa*), which belongs to the genus *Cyclostomata*, specific ^{3}H-diazepam binding sites were found in the central nervous system. The K_D values varied at most by a factor of 3. Variations in the density of binding sites were greater. Benzodiazepine receptors could not be detected in invertebrates (earthworm, squid, wood louse, lobster, and locust). Specific ^{3}H-diazepam binding was also not detected in leech ganglia (Corradetti et al., 1980) It appears, therefore, that in the course of evolution benzodiazepine receptors (as defined in the central nervous system of man, calf, and rat) appeared in the brain with the development of higher bony fishes (Osteichthyes) from jawless fishes (Agnatha). There is some indication that the benzodiazepine receptors were somewhat modified with the evolution of higher vertebrates (tetrapoda). The absence of specific benzodiazepine receptors in invertebrates, in particular in crustacea and mollusca, is of uppermost importance, since these animals contain GABAergic neurons and are frequently used in electropharmacologic studies. Any effects that benzodiazepines may have in these species will, therefore, require very careful interpretation with regard to their specific character and the extrapolation to their mechanisms of action in the vertebrate central nervous system.

IX. Ontogenetic Development of Benzodiazepine Receptors

Braestrup and Nielsen (1978) studied the ontogenetic development of benzodiazepine receptors in the rat. At the earliest time investigated, 8 days before birth, specific binding of ^{3}H-diazepam in the whole brain amounted to 5.2% and the total number of binding sites to 2.5% of that in adults. Seven days after birth, an almost adult density of receptors was reached, and the total number increased steadily during the first 3 weeks to reach a plateau after about 4 weeks. There were no trends for age-dependent differences in K_D. Very similar findings on the ontogenetic development of benzodiazepine receptors were reported by Candy and Martin (1979) and Palacios et al. (1979). Interestingly, the enhancement of ^{3}H-flunitrazepam binding by anions and muscimol was the same at all ages (Palacios et al., 1979). Comparing ^{3}H-flunitrazepam binding to brain membranes of 2-month- and 14-month-old rats, Haefely et al. (1980) found no differences in K_D and B_{max}.

The ontogenetic development of benzodiazepine receptors was thus much more rapid than that of neurotransmitter receptors, e.g., muscarinic, dopamine, opiate, and GABA receptors.

X. In Vivo Demonstration of Benzodiazepine Receptors

The demonstration of a displaceable binding of benzodiazepines to specific brain sites in vivo has increased the confidence in findings obtained with isolated membrane preparations. It should be recalled that specific binding of ^{3}H-diazepam to isolated membranes is markedly dependent on the incubation temperature. Increasing the temperature increases both on and off rates of dissociation. The dissociation constant K_D is approximately 10 times higher at 37 °C than at 0 °C.

CHANG and SNYDER (1978) injected ^{3}H-diazepam or ^{3}H-flunitrazepam of high specific activity intravenously into mice. After various times, the animals were decapitated, the brain was rapidly homogenized and filtered, and total radioactivity (in the homogenate before filtering) was measured. Brain levels of unlabeled benzodiazepines were measured by the capacity of alcoholic brain extracts (containing the benzodiazepines) to inhibit specific ^{3}H-flunitrazepam binding in rat cortex membranes. Twenty minutes after the intravenous injection of a tracer dose of ^{3}H-flunitrazepam, total and bound radioactivity in the brain reached a peak. At this time 60% of the total tritium activity was particulate bound. Thereafter, both activities declined, particulate bound activity more rapidly than total activity, so that activity bound to the particulate fraction accounted for only 25% at 2 h and 13% at 24 h. Already after 1 h, only 30% of the total activity represented unmetabolized ^{3}H-flunitrazepam. The proportion of unmetabolized drug was greater in the particulate than in the soluble fraction. When various pharmacologic doses of four unlabelled benzodiazepines were administered 30 min before the injection of ^{3}H-flunitrazepam, the soluble radioactivity was unaltered; however, the bound activity was dose dependently reduced. ID_{50} (doses producing a 50% reduction of bound ^{3}H-flunitrazepam) were 0.7 μmol·kg^{-1} for clonazepam, approximately 1.8 μmol·kg^{-1} for flunitrazepam and diazepam, and 83 μmol·kg^{-1} for chlordiazepoxide. The concentrations of unlabelled benzodiazepines in the brain after pharmacologic doses were considerably higher than the concentrations producing 50% inhibition of ^{3}H-flunitrazepam binding in membrane preparations an 0 °C, namely 2.56 μmol·kg^{-1} brain after 3.5 μmol·kg^{-1} (0.9 mg·kg^{-1}) of diazepam i.p. However, doses of benzodiazepines which occupied 50% of the specific binding sites in vivo corresponded well with pharmacologically active doses in animals.

WILLIAMSON et al. (1978, 1979) found that binding of ^{3}H-diazepam to rat forebrain after intravenous injections remained constant up to 60 min after homogenization, whereas homogenization in 3 μmol·l^{-1} unlabelled diazepam reduced bound ^{3}H-diazepam to 50% within 1 min, providing good evidence that the observed binding had occurred in vivo and not during homogenization. When clonazepam or the two pharmacologically active enantiomers, Ro 11-3128 and Ro 11-6896, were injected simultaneously with the tracer dose of ^{3}H-diazepam, more than 75% of the specific binding of ^{3}H-diazepam was prevented in the rat forebrain, whereas the pharmacologically inactive enantiomers, Ro 11-3624 and Ro 11-6893, had no influence on ^{3}H-diazepam binding. Outside the central nervous system, ^{3}H-diazepam bound to liver, kidney, and abdominal skeletal muscle; however, no stereospecific displacement occurred in these peripheral tissues (Skolnick et al., 1979c). ^{3}H-Diazepam binding was always studied in tissues obtained 1 min after intravenous injection of the radioligand. An excellent correlation was found between the number of specific binding sites occupied and the protective effect of diazepam against pentetrazole-induced seizures (Skolnick et al., 1979c).

Lippa et al. (1978b) injected rats with various doses of diazepam and determined the amount of specifically bound ^{3}H-diazepam in crude P_2 synaptosomal fractions of the cerebral cortex of animals killed 30 min after intraperitoneal and 60 min after oral administration. The first doses to significantly inhibit ^{3}H-diazepam binding were 2–5 mg·kg^{-1} p.o.

Tallman et al. (1979) used ^{3}H-diazepam to study in vivo binding. Five minutes after the intravenous injection of a tracer dose of ^{3}H-diazepam to rats, about 15% of the total radioactivity in the brain was specifically bound, i.e., could be displaced within 20 min in vitro in the presence of 10^{-1} mol·l^{-1} chlordiazepoxide. Pretreatment with flurazepam and chlordiazepoxide, but not with the pharmacologically inactive Ro 5-5807, greatly reduced the amount of the specifically bound ^{3}H-diazepam without affecting the level of unspecifically bound tracer. Administration of aminooxyacetic acid or muscimol prior to the injection of tracer markedly increased the amount of total and specific binding of ^{3}H-diazepam.

Duka et al. (1979a) used ^{3}H-flunitrazepam for in vivo studies in the brain of mice. In contrast to Chang and Snyder (1978) they did not separately measure total and particulate-bound radioactivity, but only total radioactivity in some brain areas after combustion. Duka et al. (1979a) measured the highest radioactivity in hippocampus and cerebral cortex 5 min after the intravenous injection of a tracer dose of ^{3}H-flunitrazepam; the activity declined very rapidly within the next 40 min. The simultaneous injection of various benzodiazepines together with the radioligand resulted in a dose-dependent reduction of ^{3}H-flunitrazepam accumulation in the brain. This reduction was saturable; e.g., increasing the doses of cold flunitrazepam over 3 mg·kg^{-1} did not result in a more marked displacement (to about 25%) than after smaller doses. This value, therefore, most probably represents the nonspecifically bound or unbound ^{3}H-flunitrazepam. An excellent correlation between the ID_{50} for reduction of ^{3}H-flunitrazepam accumulation and ED_{50} for inhibition of pentetrazole-induced seizures was found for clonazepam, Ro 11-6896, flunitrazepam, diazepam, and chlordiazepoxide. The concentrations of ^{3}H-flunitrazepam after administration of receptor-saturating doses of nonlabeled flunitrazepam were very similar in various brain regions, suggesting a rather similar nonspecific benzodiazepine binding in these structures. However, there were marked differences in the amounts of displaceable ^{3}H-flunitrazepam in the various regions, reflecting the differences in the density of benzodiazepine receptors. The stereospecificity of inhibition of the ^{3}H-flunitrazepam binding was clearly demonstrated by the lack of displacement after the injection of the pharmacologically inactive *l*-enantiomer, Ro 11-6893, and the displacement with the pharmacologically active *d*-enantiomer, Ro 11-6896. Chlordiazepoxide was weak as a displacer of ^{3}H-flunitrazepam when given simultaneously with or shortly before the radioligand, but was quite potent when given 40–80 min before the ligand, in accordance with the biotransformation of the drug to active metabolites. Duka et al. (1979a) found, as did Chang and Snyder (1978), that the doses required to decrease the displaceable binding of ^{3}H-flunitrazepam resulted in concentrations in the brain of about 800 nmol·l^{-1} and, hence, considerably higher than required in vitro. The specific in vivo binding of ^{3}H-flunitrazepam in the striatum was reduced after intrastriatal injections of kainic acid in rats (SPERK and SCHLOEGL, 1979). PAUL et al. (1979) found an excellent correlation between receptor occupation by diazepam (measured in vivo) and its antipentetrazole activity at various times after an intraperitoneal injection of diazepam (4 mg·kg^{-1}) in mice. There was, however, no correlation between anticonvulsant effectiveness and the concentration of free or nonmembrane bound diazepam in the brain. Only about 30% of the specific binding sites were occupied at the time when diazepam protected all animals from seizures induced by the intraperitoneal dose of 80 mg·kg^{-1} of pentetrazole. The conclusions of PAUL et al. (1979) that a full anticonvulsant effect of diazepam requires only the occupation of 30% of the receptors is doubtful, because a higher dose of diazepam would have given a more marked anticonvulsant effect (tested against a higher dose of pentetrazole).

The demonstration of specific binding of benzodiazepines in the brain in vivo not only confirms the essential findings in isolated membrane preparations, but also provides a tool to measure the occupation of specific pharmacologic receptors by benzodiazepines (administered drug and active metabolites). This will enable one to correlate receptor occupation with pharmacologic effects in relation to dose and time. A "pharmacokinetics of drugs at the receptor site" is thus made possible and will provide extremely useful information for the understanding of the relations between drug concentrations in various body tissues and receptor occupation at any site of action.

Using ^{11}C-flunitrazepam and positron emission tomography, COMAR et al. (1979) could visualize the binding of the label in the brain of baboons under anesthesia and the displacement of ^{11}C-flunitrazepam by a subsequent injection of nonlabeled lorazepam. This is probably the first direct demonstration in a nontraumatic way of the distribution of a drug in the brain of a live animal and of its displacement by another agent acting on the same receptors.

XI. Plasticity of Benzodiazepine Receptors

Overstimulation and reduced stimulation of receptors for neurotransmitters are known to be capable of reducing and increasing, respectively, the number of these receptors ("down regulation," "up regulation"). It was therefore of interest to find out whether a similar regulation of the density of benzodiazepine receptors occurs under various conditions, such as acute and prolonged exposure to the drugs or extreme functional states of the central nervous system. Administration of 3 mg·kg^{-1} diazepam or 30 mg·kg^{-1} phenobarbitone in daily intraperitoneal injections over 30 days to rats did not result in significant changes in the number and affinity of benzodiazepine receptors as tested by specific ^{3}H-diazepam binding. However, a so far unexplained decrease of ^{3}H-GABA binding sites in the striatum and decrease of ^{3}H-quinuclidinylbenzilate (QNB) binding sites in the cerebellum was observed (MÖHLER et al., 1978a).

BRAESTRUP et al. (1979a) treated rats for 8 weeks with extremely high daily doses of diazepam (90 mg·kg^{-1}) and lorazepam (60 mg·kg^{-1}). There was no consistent change 5–11 days after withdrawal, in either the number of binding sites or the apparent affinity for ^{3}H-diazepam in membrane preparations of the forebrain. Daily ex-

posure of rats from 10 days before birth until 7 days after birth also failed to significantly affect brain benzodiazepine receptors. They concluded that tolerance to and
abstinence after withdrawal from prolonged administration of benzodiazepines could
not be attributed to changes in brain benzodiazepine receptors. Slightly different results were reported by Chiu and Rosenberg (1978) and Rosenberg and Chiu
(1979 a), who daily injected rats intraperitoneally with extremely high doses of flurazepam (60–150 mg·kg^{-1}) for 7–10 days; they found a 15% decrease of the maximal
binding capacity of the cerebral cortex for ^{3}H-diazepam without changes in the affinity constant.

DiStefano et al. (1979) administered male rats 170 mg·kg^{-1} diazepam in their
food for 35 days. On several days after withdrawal of diazepam specific binding of
^{3}H-diazepam and ^{3}H-flunitrazepam was markedly increased in brain synaptosomes.

Results very different from these were obtained by Speth et al. (1979 c) 1 h after
the injection of a single dose of diazepam (50 mg·kg^{-1} i.p.) in rats. The density of
[^{3}H]-flunitrazepam binding sites (B_{max}) was increased by about 140% in the total
brain homogenate.

Rats exposed to a standard conflict procedure for 5 min and decapitated immediately afterwards had a reduced (by 25%) binding capacity for ^{3}H-diazepam in membranes of the cerebral cortex (Lippa et al., 1978 b; 1979). A smaller effect on ^{3}H-diaze-
pam binding was produced by exposing rats during 5 min to 20 unavoidable electric
foot shocks. The authors proposed that conflict procedures and footshock stress
could release an endogenous ligand for the benzodiazepine receptor. Braestrup et al.
(1979 d) exposed rats and mice to several forms of stress for several days (electric foot
shock, immobilization, forced swimming, continuous amphetamine intoxication,
isolation) and found small increases, decreases and no changes of benzodiazepine
binding sites. No change in the K_D and B_{max} for ^{3}H-diazepam binding was found in
the brain of rats stressed by forced swimming (Le Fur et al., 1979). A very rapid
change in the number of benzodiazepine binding sites was observed to be induced by
generalized seizures evoked by electroshock or pentetrazole in rats (Paul and Skolnick, 1978; Skolnick et al., 1979 c). Fifteen to 30 min after maximal electroshock seizures, lasting for less than 1 min after a 1 s^{-1} stimulation with alternative current, the
number of ^{3}H-diazepam binding sites in crude synaptosomal fractions of the cerebral
cortex was increased by about 21%. The preseizure number was reached again 60 min
after the convulsions. A similar increase was found 30 min after convulsions induced
by pentetrazole; the affinity of ^{3}H-diazepam for binding sites was not affected. The
increase of binding sites depended on the occurrence of generalized seizures, because
subconvulsive electric pulses were ineffective. Cerebral hypoxia was made improbable
as the cause of these changes, since rats rendered hypoxic by inhalation of argon gas
did not show changes in their receptor number. Cross et al. (1979) observed no change
in ^{3}H-GABA binding to cerebral cortex membranes of rats given daily electroconvulsive shocks under halothane anesthesia. An increase of the number of ^{3}H-diazepam
binding sites was found in the hippocampal formation of rats in which kindling was
induced by repeated electrical stimulation of the amygdala (McNamara et al., 1980).

The number of ^{3}H-diazepam binding sites was found to be larger in Maudsley
nonreactive rats, particularly in the hypothalamus and hippocampus, than in Maudsley reactive rats (Robertson et al., 1978). These two strains of rats were selectively
bred for high and low levels of fearfulness. In a strain of inbred mice characterized

by high "emotionally" or "anxiety," the density of specific ^{3}H-diazepam binding sites was found to be significantly lower than in three other "nonemotional" strains (ROBERTSON, 1979).

Three weeks after deafferentation of the frontal cortex by coronal hemitransection in rats, ^{3}H-diazepam binding was significantly increased in the frontal cortex (LIPPA et al., 1979). This finding makes it unlikely that benzodiazepine receptors are located on terminals of afferents to or on cell bodies of afferents from the frontal cortex, but rather on intrinsic neurons (or glial elements). LIPPA et al. (1979) suggested that the increased binding might be a supersensitivity phenomenon. In the substantia nigra of rats in which the GABAergic striatonigral pathway had been lesioned 10 days previously by local injection of kainic acid into the caudate nucleus, the affinity constant (K_D) for ^{3}H-diazepam was decreased (from 3.1 to 8.7) without any change in the number of ^{3}H-diazepam binding sites (BIGGIO et al., 1979).

PODDAR et al. (1980) measured ^{3}H-diazepam binding in several brain areas of hamsters which were killed after various periods of sleep or wakefulness. Immediately after sleep, the binding of ^{3}H-diazepam in crude synaptosomal preparations was increased in all areas as compared to animals killed after corresponding periods of wakefulness. The increased binding was found to be due to an increased affinity and not to a change in the number of binding sites. The $30,000 \times g$ supernatant of the cerebral cortex of waking, but not sleeping hamsters was found to contain a benzodiazepine binding inhibitor, which was hypothetically considered to be either the gabamodulin, an endogenous benzodiazepine-like substance, or one of the postulated sleep peptides.

XII. Endogenous Ligands for Benzodiazepine Receptors

The most fascinating discovery of endogenous ligands for opiate-type receptors has led to an almost reflex-like search for brain constituents that could physiologically act as ligands for other drug receptors. The concept that drugs have to act as exogenous competitors for endogenous compounds at functional receptors in order to produce their pharmacologic effects is probably not valid in such a general form. Nevertheless, the very high specificity of benzodiazepine receptors led to the suspicion that these drugs are either substitutes for an endogenous molecule displaying "antianxiety" activity or competitors of endogenous "anxiogenic" agents.

Soon after the discovery of specific benzodiazepine receptors in the central nervous system the search for potential endogenous ligands in brain and other tissues started in several laboratories. MÖHLER et al. (1979) found three peaks in brain extracts which inhibited ^{3}H-diazepam binding. When the active material was identified as the purine derivatives inosine and hypoxanthine and as nicotinamide, their very weak affinities for the receptor (approximately $1/100,000$ the inhibitory potency of the most active benzodiazepines in ^{3}H-diazepam binding) made it appear unlikely that they would act as physiologic ligands. Perhaps more important than affinity, however, is the capability of a potential endogenous ligand to mimic or to antagonize the pharmacologic effects of benzodiazepines, provided they are administered in a way that permits their access to the receptor. A study of the effects of the three identified compounds in the whole animal after systemic administration of high doses and in the cat spinal cord after local infusion into the dorsal horn suggested that if any of them could be regarded as a potential endogenous ligand of physiologic relevance, nicotinamide would fulfill the requirements best (MÖHLER et al., 1979). SLATER and LONGMAN (1979) suggested that inosine and nicotinamide were rather antagonists of benzodiazepines than benzodiazepine-like agents. Inosine and hypoxanthine were also identified in the brain as endogenous inhibitors of benzodiazepine binding by SKOLNICK et al. (1978, 1979 b, c, d) and by MARANGOS et al. (1978, 1979 a). This group of investigators arrived at the conclusion that only purine derivatives, but not pyrimidines, interacted with ^{3}H-diazepam binding (MARANGOS et al., 1979 a). They also made preliminary structure-activity studies within the purine class. Inosine injected intracerebroventricularly delayed the onset of seizures induced by intraperitoneal injection of pentetrazole in mice (SKOLNICK et al., 1979 d). 7-Methyl-inosine was ineffective in inhibiting ^{3}H-diazepam binding in vitro and also did not protect mice from pentetrazole-induced seizures, whereas 2'-deoxyinosine, which was more potent than inosine in the ^{3}H-diazepam binding assay (see, however, TICKU and BURCH, 1980), was also more effective in increasing seizure latency. It is of interest that the concentrations of both inosine and hypoxanthine (metabolites of adenosine) were markedly increased in brain slices by electrical and chemical depolarization (PULL and MAC ILWAIN, 1972; SUN et al., 1977). ASANO and SPECTOR (1979) also identified inosine and hypoxanthine as brain constituents interacting with the benzodiazepine receptors. They used an antibody against diazepam as a surrogate receptor for the search of endogenous ligands in bovine brain extracts. The two purines competitively inhibited ^{3}H-diazepam binding with a K_i value of 1.3 mmol·l^{-1}. A number of other purine derivatives had similar (low) potencies, while the pyrimidines uracil and cytosine were inactive. The activity of methylxanthines in the ^{3}H-diazepam binding assay suggested that membrane-bound phosphodiesterase could act as the benzodiazepine receptor. However, this idea was invalidated by comparing phosphodiesterase inhibitory and ^{3}H-diazepam binding inhibitory potencies of various agents. DAMM et al. (1979) found a negative correlation between the potency of adenine derivatives for inhibition of ^{3}H-flunitrazepam binding in rat brain membranes and the depressant effect on the spontaneous firing rate of cerebellar Purkinje cells in situ; thus, adenosine was the most potent depressant of neuronal activity but the weakest ligand for the receptor. Guanine derivatives were even less potent than adenine derivatives and about equally potent as inosine and hypoxanthine. The most potent purine derivatives were the xanthines, theophylline, caffeine, and aminophylline (IC$_{50}$ 1 mmol·l^{-1}), theobromine being much less potent.

DAVIES et al. (1980), in a study of a series of purines in the ^{3}H-diazepam binding assay, found 1-methylisoguanosine to be the most potent in displacing ^{3}H-diazepam. This compound, which had been isolated from a marine sponge, produces some central nervous effects which resemble those of benzodiazepines. MACDONALD et al. (1979) compared the effects of inosine and flurazepam applied microiontophoretically on mouse spinal neurons grown in tissue culture and suggested that inosine had two distinct transmitter-like actions, one of which was mimicked and the other one blocked by flurazepam. They concluded that benzodiazepines might function as agonists at one putative purine receptor site and as antagonists at another and, hence, that benzodiazepine receptors were identical with the postulated purine receptors.

The presence of an unidentified endogenous factor in porcine and rat brain which inhibited ^{3}H-diazepam binding was reported by COLELLO et al. (1978 b). They separated an extract from porcine cerebral cortex on a sephadex G-75 column and tested the fractions for inhibitory activity on ^{3}H-diazepam and ^{3}H-flunitrazepam binding to rat brain homogenates. Competitive inhibitory activity was found in fractions containing entities between 1,000 and 2,000 ("benzodiazepine competitive factor II") and between 40,000 and 70,000 MW ("benzodiazepine competitive factor I"), the latter being 5 times more potent than the former. Factor I was heat stable but destroyed by trypsin digestion, suggesting a polypeptide nature. KAROBATH et al. (1978, 1979 a) described a "diazepam binding inhibitory factor" (DIF) in partially purified acetone extracts. The highest levels of DIF were found in skeletal muscle and myocardium of rats, while the brain of rats, mice, cows, and man contained less activity. Within the brain, cortical areas and hippocampus were richest in DIF.

Using an aqueous extraction method, MARANGOS et al. (1979) isolated two fractions which competitively inhibited ^{3}H-diazepam binding and which were heat stable and resistant to proteolytic degradation. Peak I (700–30,000 daltons) was only present in the brain and pituitary, whereas peak II (500–600 daltons) was also present in extracerebral porcine tissues.

BRAESTRUP and SQUIRES (1978 b) and BRAESTRUP and NIELSEN (1979, 1980) reported preliminary data suggesting the presence in the brain of a water-soluble protein with a molecular weight of approximately 70,000 which inhibited ^{3}H-diazepam binding. They also found unidentified inhibitory activity in the cerebrospinal fluid of a few patients without a history of benzodiazepine intake as well as in human urine. The urinary factor was initially characterized as highly lipophilic, inactivated by chymotrypsin and of a molecular weight of less than 500 (NIELSEN et al., 1979). Subsequent purification revealed the active component to be ethyl-β-carboline-3-carboxylate (NIELSEN et al., 1980). This β-carboline has a high affinity for the benzodiazepine binding sites (half maximal binding at about 1 nmol $\cdot$ l^{-1}). The isolated compound as such is most probably an artifact and not an endogenous component of the brain. Own preliminary results (unpublished) indicate that the β-carboline has no pharmacologic properties similar to diazepam; intravenously the compound has weak benzodiazepine antagonistic and convulsive actions.

Of all naturally occurring 20 amino acids, SQUIRES et al. (1979 b) found L-tryptophan to be the most potent inhibitor of ^{3}H-flunitrazepam binding, although the ID$_{50}$ of 5 mmol $\cdot$ l^{-1} is still very high. These authors also studied a number of tryptophan-containing dipeptides; L-tryptophanyl-glycine with an ID$_{50}$ of 80 μmol $\cdot$ l^{-1} was 10 times more potent than inosine. The problem of endogenous ligands for benzodiazepine receptors remains open, and much more work is needed before the concept of an endogenous "anxiogenic" or "anxiolytic" compound acting through benzodiazepine receptors can be accepted or refused.

PODDAR et al. (1980) found that the 30,000 $\times g$ supernatant of the cerebral cortex of waking, but not of sleeping hamsters contained an inhibitor of ^{3}H-diazepam binding. They considered the possibility that this inhibitor could be an endogenous benzodiazepine-like compound.

XIII. Modulation of Benzodiazepine Binding by GABA-Mimetic Compounds

A modulatory effect of GABA and other GABA mimetic agents on benzodiazepine binding to their receptors in vitro was reported almost simultaneously by several in-

dependent research groups (Briley and Langer, 1978; Gallager et al., 1978; Müller et al., 1978 a; Tallman et al., 1978; Wastek et al., 1978; Karobath and Sperk,
1979; Karobath et al., 1979 a, b; Williams and Risley, 1979). All these investigators
found that GABA increased in a concentration-dependent manner the binding of a
radiolabeled ligand to benzodiazepine binding sites in washed membranes. The increased binding was shown to be due to an increased affinity whereby only the association rate constant was changed, and there was no change in the number of binding
sites (Wastek et al., 1978). An EC_{50} of 1.6 $\mu mol \cdot l^{-1}$ was determined for GABA and
of 0.5 $\mu mol \cdot l^{-1}$ for muscimol. The degree of this enhancement depended on the previous treatment of membrane preparations; it was rather small in crude preparation
but amounted to more than 100% in extensively washed, frozen, and thawed membranes (Karobath and Sperk, 1979). It is interesting that GABA mimetics increased
the affinity of benzodiazepine binding from a low value in washed preparations to a
value usually found in crude preparations in the absence of exogenous GABA, suggesting that the reduction of affinity by washing is due to the removal of endogenous
GABA. This possibility has been proven to be correct by Martin and Candy (1978)
and Dudai (1979), who observed that supernatants from washes of crude membrane
preparations of the rat brain increased the binding of ^{3}H-diazepam and that this effect
of the supernatant was due to GABA. Several GABA mimetics had effects similar to
GABA, in particular muscimol, 4-trans-aminocrotonic acid, and DL-4-amino-2-hy-
droxybutyric acid (Karobath and Sperk, 1979). GABA and muscimol increased ^{3}H-
flunitrazepam binding also at 37 °C (Speth et al., 1979 a). Bicuculline, but not picrotoxin, inhibited the enhancing effect of GABA mimetic agents and slightly decreased
the basal affinity of membranes to the radiolabeled ligand. Compounds known to inhibit the uptake of GABA or its transamination were without effect on the benzodiazepine receptor interaction (Karobath and Sperk, 1979). The effect of muscimol
and bicuculline on ^{3}H-diazepam binding was absent in membranes prepared from 4-
day-old rats which, at this age, already contain a considerable density of benzodiazepine receptors, but only few GABA receptors (Briley and Langer, 1978).

A quantitative comparative study of various GABA mimetics led Karobath et al.
(1979 b) and Braestrup et al. (1979 c) to postulate that the GABA recognition site,
through which GABA mimetics modulate the affinity of the benzodiazepine receptor,
was different from the Na^+-independent high-affinity GABA binding site. Indeed,
there was no correlation between the relative potencies of GABA mimetics as stimulants of benzodiazepine binding and as inhibitors of ^{3}H-GABA binding (Karobath
et al., 1979 b; Maurer, 1979 a). Rigid molecules (e.g., muscimol, isoguvacine, THIP,
and imidazole-acetic acid) were less potent as stimulants of benzodiazepine binding
than more flexible analogues and, in part, even antagonized the effect of GABA
(Karobath and Lippitsch, 1979; Braestrup et al., 1979 c, 1980; Karobath et al.,
1980, 1981).

A modulation of benzodiazepine binding by GABAergic stimulation has also been
observed in vivo. Gallager et al. (1978) treated rats with aminooxyacetic acid
(AOAA) to increase the level of endogenous GABA; this treatment enhanced the
binding of ^{3}H-diazepam to membranes of the cerebral cortex by 20–25% as compared
with the binding to membranes of untreated animals. The effect was entirely due to
an increase of the affinity. The effect of pretreatment with AOAA or muscimol was
nullified by picrotoxin and bicuculline added to the membrane preparations, but not

by intraperitoneal injections of these compounds. GABA added to membranes from animals treated with AOAA did not further increase the enhanced binding of ^{3}H-diazepam. Surprisingly, baclofen and γ-butyrolactone, which lack direct GABA receptor-stimulating activity, mimicked the effect of AOAA and muscimol pretreatment. Inhibition of GABA biosynthesis by thiosemicarbazide had no significant effect on ^{3}H-diazepam binding in vitro. Pentobarbitone (25 mg·kg^{-1}) was also ineffective. ROSENBERG and CHIU (1979 b) obtained different results with AOAA. Acute elevation of GABA levels in rats by a single injection of 40 mg·kg^{-1} AOAA i.p. had no effect on the binding characteristics of ^{3}H-diazepam. Chronic elevation of brain GABA levels by two daily injections 10 mg·kg^{-1} AOAA i.p. for 7 days increased both nonspecific and specific binding of ^{3}H-diazepam. The authors concluded that the normal endogenous GABA levels were high enough to maximally enhance benzodiazepine binding.

The enhancing effect of GABA on ^{3}H-diazepam binding was absent in the retina (OSBORNE, 1980) and when a receptor complex solubilized from brain membranes was used (TALLMAN et al., 1980 b).

These findings suggest that GABA receptors are somehow coupled with benzodiazepine receptors, possibly forming a complex GABA receptor-ionophore-benzodiazepine receptor, and that GABA could act as an allosteric activator of the benzodiazepine receptor. The structure-activity relationship of GABA mimetics for stimulation of benzodiazepine binding provides evidence for the existence of a heterogeneous population of GABA receptors and indicates that only one type of GABA receptor is associated with benzodiazepine binding sites.

XIV. Enhancement of ^{3}H-Diazepam Binding by Other Compounds

BEER et al. (1978) and WILLIAMS and RISLEY (1979) described an enhancement of ^{3}H-diazepam binding in vitro by two pyrazolopyridine carboxylic acid compounds, SQ 20,009 (etazolate) and SQ 65,396, which had shown activity in animal models of anxiety. The increased binding was due exclusively to a decreased K_D for diazepam. Although these compounds are not GABA mimetics, their stimulant effect on ^{3}H-diazepam binding was blocked by (+)-bicuculline (WILLIAMS and RISLEY, 1979). The enhancement of ^{3}H-flunitrazepam binding by SQ 20,009 was entirely dependent on the presence of halide ions and blocked by picrotoxin (SUPAVILAI and KAROBATH, 1979, 1980), suggesting a functional interaction of benzodiazepine receptors with a chloride conductance mechanism. At concentrations higher than 10^{-5} mol·l^{-1} these compounds inhibited ^{3}H-diazepam binding. Since SQ 20,009 and SQ 65,396 are phosphodiesterase inhibitors, a few other inhibitors of this enzyme, as well as analogues of cAMP were also studied, but proved to be ineffective on ^{3}H-diazepam binding (WILLIAMS and RISLEY, 1979). Another nonbenzodiazepine anxiolytic, meprobamate, did not affect benzodiazepine binding. The meaning of the influence of pyrazolopyridines on benzodiazepine binding is at present obscure. The above-mentioned authors hypothesized that the pyrazolopyridines could interact with an endogenous inhibitor or modulator of benzodiazepine receptors.

Diphenylhydantoin was shown by GALLAGER et al. (1979) to enhance ^{3}H-diazepam binding by increasing its affinity for the receptor. The modification was assumed to be caused by an alteration of the membrane, since it could not be reversed by extensive washing. In contrast, Tunnicliff et al. (1979) reported that diphenylhydantoin inhibited ^{3}H-diazepam binding to specific membranes of rat cerebral cortex with a K_D of 0.9 μmol·l^{-1} and that the affinity of diphenylhydantoin for the benzodiazepine receptor was increased by GABA and muscimol. Similar results were found by Mimaki et al. (1980); in addition, chronic treatment of rats with daily doses of 200 mg·kg^{-1} diphenylhydantoin for 28 days resulted in a decrease of ^{3}H-flunitrazepam binding sites in cerebral and cerebellar cortex.

A novel macrocyclic lactone disaccharide anthelminthic, avermectin B_{1a}, was reported to enhance irreversibly ^{3}H-diazepam binding to rat brain membranes by increasing both affinity and the number of binding sites; the compound also potentiated the muscle relaxant and locomotor depressant effect of diazepam (Yarbrough, 1979; Williams and Yarbrough, 1979). Avermectin B_{1a} is reported to affect chloride channels in invertebrates.

The purine derivative, EMD 28,422 (N^6-2-(4-chlorophenyl)-bicyclo 2.2.2-octyl-(3)-adenosine) was reported to increase the binding of ^{3}H-diazepam both in vitro and when administered intraperitoneally (Skolnick et al., 1980a). The increased binding was due to an increase of binding sites (by 10–25%) rather than to a decrease of the apparent K_D. The compound depressed locomotor activity of mice, had a moderate protective effect on seizures induced by pentetrazole and caffeine, greatly enhanced the anticonvulsant activity of diazepam, and increased water drinking punished by electric current shocks applied to the drinking spout.

Skolnick et al. (1980b) reported that pentobarbitone in subanesthetic concentrations (10–50 μmol·l^{-1}) potentiated the enhanced ^{3}H-diazepam binding in vitro induced by GABA and, in anesthetic concentrations (100 μmol·l^{-1}), enhanced ^{3}H-diazepam binding in the absence of GABA. The effect of the combination of GABA and pentobarbitone was greater than the sum of the enhancement observed with either compound alone. Since both GABA and pentobarbitone activate Cl$^-$ conductance mechanisms in neuronal membranes, this effect was suggested to be important for the modification of benzodiazepine receptor affinity.

XV. Molecular Consequences of Benzodiazepine Receptor Stimulation

Quite an impressive amount of knowledge has been accumulated within a short time on the dynamics of benzodiazepine-receptor interaction; however, the crucial question in the context of benzodiazepine receptors has remained unresolved, namely the nature of the immediate molecular consequences in cell membranes that are triggered by the formation of benzodiazepine-receptor complexes to result eventually in enhanced GABAergic transmission.

A suggestion made by Costa's group (Costa and Guidotti, 1979) is that benzodiazepines prevent an endogenous inhibitor ("gabamodulin") from reducing the affinity of GABA for its receptors. According to this concept, benzodiazepines would prevent an endogenous compound from exerting its physiologic inhibitory function. "Gabamodulin", which is identical with the type II inhibitor of protein kinase, maintains the GABA receptor in a low-affinity state by inhibiting its phosphorylation into a high-affinity state (Toffano et al., 1980). Biggio et al. (1980a, b) suggested that benzodiazepine receptors and gabamodulin were located mainly on cerebellar Golgi cells and that gabamodulin was released together with GABA to act on the GABA receptors on granule cells. Benzodiazepines would inhibit the release of gabamodulin from Golgi cells and thereby enhance the effectiveness of GABA at the granule cell. TALL-MAN et al. (1980 b), MALLORGA et al. (1979), and STRITTMATTER et al. (1979 b) observed that the binding of benzodiazepines to specific binding sites in astrocytoma cells (which, however, show different ligand specificity as compared to those in mammalian brain) resulted in an enhancement of ^{3}H-methyl group incorporation into phosphati-dylcholine through stepwise addition of methyl groups to phosphatidylethanolamine. These investigators suggested, that in analogy to their interaction with "peripheral type" receptor, benzodiazepines might also trigger methylation of membrane lipids in the brain, thereby increasing the fluidity of the membranes, which would modulate the functioning of a GABA-receptor-ionophore complex. According to this hypo-thesis a direct effect of the binding of benzodiazepines to their receptors would be the activation of methyltransferase in synaptosomal membranes. In this context it is in-teresting that stimulation of phospholipid methylation in rat reticulocytes was found to unmask cryptic β-adrenergic receptors (STRITTMATTER et al., 1979 a). SIMMONDS (1980) arrived at a view similar to that of TALLMAN et al. (1980a, b) and hypotheti-cally located the benzodiazepine receptor either somewhat between the GABA recep-tor and the chloride channel or on the chloride ionophore itself in order to explain the reduction by flurazepam of the GABA antagonistic effect of picrotoxin on prima-ry afferent endings; according to his view the activated benzodiazepine receptor could increase the proportion of channel openings to GABA receptor activation or prolong the duration of channel opening induced by GABA receptor activation.

The above propositions for the functioning of benzodiazepine-receptor complexes assume a localization of these receptors in the postsynaptic membrane of the GA-BAergic synapse. LEE et al. (1979), as well as MITCHELL and MARTIN (1978), provided evidence for a presynaptic site of action of benzodiazepines either on the receptive parts or the terminals of the GABA neuron. A molecular mechanism by which ben-zodiazepines could either enhance the excitability of GABA neurons or increase stim-ulation-induced release of GABA has not yet been proposed.

AA. Benzodiazepine Antagonists

The characteristic profile of pharmacologic activity of benzodiazepines, which clearly distinguishes this class of drugs from other agents that also relieve anxiety, such as barbiturates and propanediole carbamates, can now be explained in part or entirely on the basis of specific enhancement of GABAergic neurotransmission (HAEFELY, 1977, 1978 a, b, c, 1979, 1980 a, b; HAEFELY et al., 1975 b, 1978, 1979 a, b). This action is initiated by the combination of benzodiazepines with specific receptors, and the af-finity of benzodiazepine derivatives for these receptors determines, together with pharmacokinetic properties and proneness to biotransformation, their pharmacologic potency in vivo.

In the case of receptors for endogenous ligands, such as neurotransmitters or hor-mones, molecules with sufficient affinity for the receptor can act either as agonists, antagonists, or partial agonists. Agonistic activity seems to depend on two properties; on the one hand, agonist molecules have a tridimensional shape and distribution of electric charges that permit a close attraction by short-distance forces between the sur-faces of the drugs and a small patch of the macromolecular receptor, the recognition and binding site; in addition to fitting to this site ("steric fit"), these molecules are apparently able to induce a change in the conformation of the receptor macromolecule which acts as a "pharmacologic stimulus", e.g., by causing an opening or closing of ion channels or by activating enzymes. Pure antagonists have a structure that enables binding to the recognition site or its immediate vicinity, they lack the structural requirements for the induction of the conformational change of the receptor. Partial agonists bind to the receptor, but their structure is not optimal for induction of the conformational change that underlies the "pharmacologic stimulus"; in the absence of a pure agonist, they produce a submaximal pharmacologic effect, while in the presence of an agonist they compete with its binding and block its effect.

Although it is at present not clear whether endogenous compounds interact with benzodiazepine receptors under physiologic or pathologic conditions, it is sensible to assume that, also for benzodiazepine receptors, agonists, antagonists, and partial agonists may exist or can be designed. For years we have occasionally tested benzodiazepine derivatives which were devoid of typical benzodiazepine activity in screening tests for possible benzodiazepine antagonistic activity, albeit without success.

Recently, we have found among derivatives of imidazobenzodiazepines bearing a carbonyl oxygen in place of the usual phenyl constituent, compounds with potent inhibitory activity on the specific binding of ^{3}H-diazepam in brain synaptosomal membranes without, however, any diazepam-like activity in vivo. These compounds prevented all typical central effects of diazepam when given prior to diazepam and immediately terminated the effects of diazepam when given at the peak of its action. One of them, Ro 15-1788, ethyl 8-fluoro-5,6-dihydro-5-methyl-6-oxo-4H-imidazo [1,5-a] [1,4] benzodiazepine-3-carboxylate (Hunkeler et al., 1981), is undergoing clinical trials. Briefly, this compound prevents or blocks characteristic benzodiazepine effects, such as muscle relaxation, anticonvulsant activity, decrease of locomotor activity, enhancement of presynaptic inhibition in the spinal cord, anticonflict activity, reduction of multiunit activity in raphé nuclei of the rat, decrease of cerebellar cGMP, and decrease of dopamine turnover. Ro 15-1788 does not block those benzodiazepine effects that are not mediated by specific benzodiazepine receptors, e.g., the schistosomicidal effect of some 7-nitrobenzodiazepines and the depression of contractile responses of the isolated guinea-pig ileum to transmural stimulation, which occurs at concentrations above 10^{-5} mol $\cdot$ l^{-1} and probably reflects a membrane stabilizing action. Ro 15-1788 does not prevent or block central effects of barbiturates, meprobamate, methaqualone, GABA agonists, GABA transaminase inhibitors, and ethanol. The compound has a very low toxicity and, up to very high doses, does not produce any behavioral or other pharmacologic effects and, in particular, is not convulsive. Ro 15-1788 is quite obviously a very selective and potent antagonist of specific benzodiazepine effects mediated by the high-affinity binding sites in brain membranes. This is a remarkable achievement in view of the considerable unsuccessful attempts to find selective antagonists of barbiturates and ethanol and may be compared with the discovery of opiate antagonists.

The availability of selective benzodiazepine antagonists has important theoretical and practical implications. Structure-activity studies with benzodiazepine agonists and antagonists should greatly augment our understanding of structural requirements for binding to and "activating" the receptor. Benzodiazepine antagonists will be useful tools in studying the possible existence and functional role of endogenous ligands for benzodiazepine receptors. They may help to clarify the question of multiplicity of benzodiazepine receptors and to distinguish between different receptors. A therapeutic use of selective benzodiazepine antagonists can be foreseen (1) in accidental and suicidal intoxications with benzodiazepines, where they would act as antidotes to reverse at least those components that are due to activation of benzodiazepine receptors; (2) in anesthesiology to terminate benzodiazepine effects when needed; and (3) in preventing central side effects of benzodiazepines action in the treatment of schistosomiasis.

AB. Concluding Remarks

The main pharmacologic actions of benzodiazepine anxiolytics may be grouped according to their therapeutic indications as shown in Table 10. In this chapter we have reviewed the literature on the somatic pharmacodynamics of these drugs; each section ended with a short summary. The present concluding remarks attempt to synthesize the available knowledge about the sites and mechanisms of action of benzodiazepines; in addition, some unresolved problems and directions of future research activities will be mentioned.

Organ Selectivity and General Tolerance

The active derivatives of the benzodiazepine class are characterized by a high affinity and selectivity for the central nervous system. In contrast to other neuropsychotropic agents used in therapy (antipsychotics, antidepressants, stimulants, etc.) they are devoid of any relevant direct action on organs and tissues outside the brain and the spinal cord, even at high pharmacologic doses. In fitting with this, high-affinity binding sites for benzodiazepines, as found in the central nervous system, are lacking in the periphery.

A further characteristic of benzodiazepines is the extraordinarily large safety margin; these drugs affect the central nervous system already in very low doses, whereas severe intoxication requires such high doses, that, in spite of the widespread use of these drugs, unequivocal proof is still lacking for the lethal outcome of accidental or suicidal overdosage of a benzodiazepine in the absence of other chemicals or additional harmful factors.

Table 10. Main pharmacologic actions of benzodiazepines and corresponding therapeutic uses

Pharmacological actions:	Therapeutic indications:
Antipunishment and antifrustration activity, behavioral disinhibition	Anxiety
	Anxious depression
Arousal reduction	Hyperemotional states
Antiaggressive activity	
Facilitation of sleep	Insomnia
Anticonvulsant action	Various forms of epileptiform activity
Attenuation of centrally mediated autonomic nervous and endocrine responses to emotions and to excessive afferent stimuli	Psychosomatic disorders (cardiovascular, gastrointestinal, hormonal)
Central muscle relaxation	Somatic and psychogenic muscle spasms, tetanus
Potentiation of the activity of centrally depressant agents, anterograde amnesia	Surgical anesthesia

Indirect Effects on Peripheral Functions

Changes induced by benzodiazepines in cardiovascular, respiratory, gastrointestinal, and hormonal functions are clearly of central origin. The normal activity of the autonomic nervous and endocrine system is hardly affected by these drugs; however, they potently attenuate excessive responses in these peripheral systems that are induced by stimulation of brain sites or afferent nerves or by emotional factors. The few mechanistic studies which were performed to analyze the effects of benzodiazepines on cardiovascular sympathetic and parasympathetic nerve activity as well as on pituitary function yielded results compatible with a primary involvement of hypothalamic and medullary GABAergic synapses.

Effects of Benzodiazepines on the Various Levels of the Neuraxis

Benzodiazepine effects have been studied on virtually all levels of the neuraxis with electrophysiologic and biochemical methods.

In the spinal cord, benzodiazepines consistently enhance segmental, heterosegmental, and descending presynaptic inhibition of Ia afferents, but seem to leave postsynaptic inhibition largely unaffected. The depression of mono- and polysynaptic reflexes and of spontaneous γ-motoneuron activity is, at least in part, due to the intensified presynaptic inhibitory control, though additional yet unknown mechanisms cannot be excluded. The effects of benzodiazepines on the intraspinal transmission of sensory influx seem to be negligible, but require more systematic investigation.

In the dorsal column nuclei of the caudal medulla both pre- and postsynaptic inhibitory mechanisms are enhanced.

Only limited studies were performed on the spontaneous and evoked activity in bulbopontine structures and in the mesencephalon. Although on the whole the lower brain stem does not seem to be particularly sensitive to the effect of benzodiazepines, part of their effects on cardiovascular and respiratory functions, on sleep behavior and skeletal muscle tone are undoubtedly induced in this part of the brain.

The cerebellum is consistently affected by benzodiazepines. An increasing number of central nervous functions are recognized to be modulated by cerebellar activity; this suggests that the cerebellum might also be involved in actions of benzodiazepines other than on muscle tone and coordination.

The effects of benzodiazepines on spontaneous and evoked neuronal activities in hypothalamus, thalamus, hippocampus, amygdala, and neocortex have been studied extensively in various experimental conditions; the drugs were found to be particularly potent in attenuating evoked potentials, afterdischarges, and other epileptoid activities in the neocortex and in limbic structures.

Effects on Distinct Neurotransmitter Systems

Of the several specific neurotransmitter systems that can be investigated with the presently available methods, most were found to be affected by benzodiazepines, albeit usually at rather high doses. Except for the tuberoinfundibular dopamine system, which is activated, cholinergic, noradrenergic, dopaminergic, and serotoninergic system are depressed by the drugs. This reduction is liminal in normal conditions, however quite marked in drug- or stress-induced situations which increase these pathways. Benzodiazepines fail to affect presynaptic and postsynaptic dynamics of these neurotransmitters directly; therefore, the drug-induced attenuation of the turnover of these neurotransmitters must be the result of a primary interaction with other neuronal systems.

Changes in the activity of pathways using excitatory amino acid transmitters cannot yet be assessed for technical reasons. Interactions of benzodiazepines with synaptic effects of purine derivatives have been found, but their relevance for the pharmacologic effect is yet uncertain. Benzodiazepines were found to alter the content of enkephalins in the hypothalamus and striatum, but the possible part played by these endogenous opiates in some actions of these drugs is at present very hypothetical.

Specific Effects of Benzodiazepines on GABAergic Synaptic Transmission

An increasing number of findings converges to support the view that benzodiazepines produce their effects by specifically enhancing GABAergic synaptic transmission (HAEFELY 1977, 1978a, b, c, 1979, 1980a, b; HAEFELY et al., 1975b, 1978, 1979a, b). The rather ubiquitous occurrence of GABA neurons in the central nervous system, in particular of GABAergic interneurons subserving feedforward and feedback inhibition of principal neurons, readily explains why electrophysiologic and biochemical studies have revealed benzodiazepine-induced changes in most of the brain structures examined. The recent finding of benzodiazepine receptor localization in these structures and the concurrent existence of high-affinity binding sites for benzodiazepines and GABAergic synapses are in perfect agreement with this specific synaptic activity. There is very strong evidence for the critical involvement of GABAergic mechanisms in most, if not all, major pharmacologic effects of benzodiazepines, e.g., their abolition by GABA antagonists and their partial imitation by inhibitors of GABA inactivation. The sequence of events leading to the pharmacologic effects of benzodiazepines according to the present state of knowledge is shown in the following schematic diagram:

Receptor	*Synapse (primary target)*	*Primary effector neurons*	*Secondary effector neurons*	*Whole organism*
				Psychic (behavioral) changes
Benzo-diazepine receptor activation →	Enhanced GABAergic neurotrans-mission →	Depression of spontaneous and evoked activity of various neurons with GABAergic input →	Changes in the activity of neurons dependent on primary effector neurons →	Changes in the neuronal activity of the CNS (e.g., in paroxysmal activity)
				Changes in autonomic functions (neurally or hormonally mediated)
Molecular	Synaptic	neuron pool (central)		Complex psychic and somatic domain

The formation of a benzodiazepine-receptor complex results in an enhancement of GABA-mediated synaptic inhibition. As a consequence, the activity of neurons with a GABAergic input ("primary effector neurons") is attenuated. Some of the pharmacologic effects, such as the anticonvulsant effect, may be fully or partially explained by the depression of "primary effector neurons" receiving GABAergic input. More complex effects may require alterations in "secondary effector neurons" in addition to the "primary effector pathways." The reason why benzodiazepines do not simply stop all neuronal activities at doses exerting their full enhancing effect on GABAergic transmission, is the dependence of the drug effect on ongoing activity in GABAergic neurons which, of course, varies enormously in the numerous circuits of the central nervous system; moreover, the maximum depression of neuronal activity which can be achieved through potentiated GABAergic transmission is limited because enhanced efficiency of GABAergic synapses, e.g. of those involved in local recurrent inhibiting pathways, does not only reduce the activity of GABAergically innervated target cells, but by this very effect in turn also decreases the excitatory input to GABAergic interneurons. In addition, the enhancement of GABAergic synaptic activity by benzodiazepines is of limited intensity at the single synapse. The obvious dependence of some benzodiazepine effects on various transmitter systems acting as secondary effectors explains the great number of possible interactions with other drugs.

Benzodiazepine Receptors

All or, at least, part of the saturable, high-affinity binding sites for radiolabeled benzodiazepines, at which active and antagonistic benzodiazepine derivatives compete to a relevant extent with the radioligand, are sites identical with the pharmacologic receptors for this class of drugs. Their distribution in the central nervous system corresponds to the sites where pharmacologic effects of benzodiazepines are found; their absence outside the central nervous system is consistent with the lack of direct peripheral effects of the drugs in pharmacologic doses.

The highly specific binding sites in brain membranes will be helpful in further defining the structural requirements for the activation of these receptors or of possible subgroups of them. The systematic use of the radio-receptor approach in combination with in vivo behavioral tests led to the discovery of molecules that have a high affinity for the benzodiazepine recognition site without being able to activate the receptor. Such pure benzodiazepine antagonists are likely to have an important therapeutic potential and be a most interesting scientific tool for a deeper understanding of the actions of benzodiazepines; partial agonists might reveal novel pharmacologic profiles.

The feasibility of measuring benzodiazepine receptor occupation in the animal brain in vivo opens the fascinating possibility of correlating receptor occupation in distinct central structures with certain pharmacologic effects as a function of dose and time. The recent discovery that flunitrazepam can be covalently coupled to the benzodiazepine receptor by photoaffinity labeling opens a most promising way for electron microscopic autoradiographic visualization and for isolation and identification of the receptor.

Many researchers are attracted by the idea that the benzodiazepine receptor should have a physiologically endogenous ligand; the endogenous brain constituents detected so far, however, do not seem to be "hot" candidates for the role of endogenous "benzodiazepines" with physiologic or pathological functions.

Benzodiazepine Receptor and Enhancement of GABAergic Synaptic Transmission

For some enthusiasts of receptor binding experiments the discovery of high-affinity binding sites for benzodiazepines appears as the answer to the question of how benzodiazepines act. Of course this is not true. There is at present no generally accepted view on the events which are triggered by the combination of a benzodiazepine with its receptor molecules and which result in enhanced GABAergic transmission. On the one hand, some evidence has been found for presynaptic sites of action of benzodiazepines at the GABAergic synapse. The possibility that the drugs increase the excitability of GABAergic interneurons merits testing. An enhanced release of GABA from GABAergic nerve terminals has been reported and requires confirmation. On the other hand, a number of results are compatible with a postsynaptic site of action. One attractive hypothesis proposes the existence of a supramolecular complex consisting of the GABA receptor, an inhibitory modulating protein ("gabamodulin"), the benzodiazepine receptor, and the chloride channel; the role of benzodiazepines would be to interact with or to displace gabamodulin and, thereby, to increase the affinity of the GABA receptor for GABA or to improve the coupling between the GABA receptor and chloride channel.

Benzodiazepines and Other Anxiolytics

Compounds from different chemical classes exist which have similar, although not identical pharmacologic profiles. The best-known are barbiturates, which produce neuropsychopharmacologic effects similar to those of benzodiazepines, although the two classes differ quite markedly in their dose-effect curves. The interesting fact in the present context is that barbiturates, too, enhance GABAergic transmission, albeit by a yet unsettled mechanism which differs from that of benzodiazepines. In contrast to the latter, barbiturates also strongly depress synaptic transmission at higher doses. Meprobamate and structurally related compounds have a pharmacologic profile which is very similar to that of benzodiazepines, though they differ quite markedly in their potencies. Surprisingly, however, meprobamate does not enhance GABAergic transmission. This comparison shows that similar neuropsychopharmacologic effects can be produced in the whole organism by different molecular and synaptic mechanisms of action.

Acknowledgments. We thank our colleagues Dr. E. P. Bonetti for assistance with the Section on acute toxicity and Drs. M. Da Prada, G. Häusler, H. Möhler and J.-P. Laurent for critical reading of parts of the manuscript.

References

Abel, R.M., Reis, R.L., Staroscik, R.N.: The pharmacological basis of coronary and systemic vasodilator actions of diazepam (valium). Br. J. Pharmacol. *39*, 261–274 (1970a)

Abel, R.M., Reis, R.L., Staroscik, R.N.: Coronary vasodilatation following diazepam (valium). Br. J. Pharmacol. *38*, 620–631 (1970b)

Abel, R.M., Staroscik, R.N., Reis, R.L.: The effects of diazepam on left ventricular contractility and coronary blood flow. Circulation *40*(3), 33 (1969)

Abel, R.M., Staroscik, R.N., Reis, R.L.: The effects of diazepam (valium) on left ventricular function and systemic vascular resistance. J. Pharmacol. Exp. Ther. *173*(2), 364–370 (1970c)

Abernathy, C.O., Smith, S., Zimmerman, H.J.: The effect of chlordiazepoxide hydrochloride on the isolated perfused rat liver. Proc. Soc. Exp. Biol. Med. *149*, 271–274 (1975)

Aceto, M.D.: The antinicotinic effects of drugs with clinically useful sedative-antianxiety properties. Pharmacology *13*, 458–464 (1975)

Acosta, D., Chappell, R.: Cardiotoxicity of diazepam in cultured heart cells. Toxicology *8*(3), 311–317 (1977)

Adeoshun, I.O., Healy, T.E.J., Patrick, J.M.: Ventilatory patterns in surgical patients premedicated with lorazepam or diazepam. Br. J. Pharmacol. *64*, 458P–459P (1978)

Aderjan, R., Mattern, R.: Eine tödlich verlaufene Monointoxikation mit Flurazepam (Dalmadorm). Probleme bei der toxikologischen Beurteilung. Arch. Toxicol. *43*, 69–75 (1979)

Agarwal, R.A., Lapierre, Y.D., Rastogi, R.B., Singhal, R.L.: Alterations in brain 5-hydroxytryptamine metabolism during the "withdrawal" phase after chronic treatment with diazepam and bromazepam. Br. J. Phamacol. *60*, 3–9 (1977)

Ahtee, L., Shillito, E.: The effect of benzodiazepines and atropine on exploratory behaviour and motor activity of mice. Br. J. Pharmacol. *40*, 361–371 (1970)

Albertson, T.E., Peterson, S.L., Stark, L.G.: Anticonvulsant drugs and their antagonism of kindled amygdaloid seizures in rats. Neuropharmacology *19*, 643–652 (1980)

Aldrete, J.A., Daniel, W.: Evaluation of premedicants as protective agents against convulsive (LD_{50}) doses of local anesthetic agents in rats. Anesth. Analg. (Cleve) *50*, 127–130 (1971)

Algeri, E.J., Katsas, G.G., McBay, A.: Toxicology of some new drugs, glutethimide, meprobamate and chlorpromazine. J. Forensic. Sci. *4*, 111 (1959)

Ally, A.I., Manku, M.S., Horrobin, D.F., Karmali, R.A., Morgan, R.O., Karmazyn, M.: Thromboxane A_2 as a possible natural ligand for benzodiazepine receptors. Neurosci. Letters *7*, 31–34 (1978)

Andersen, P., Eccles, J.C., Oshima, T., Schmidt, R.F.: Mechanisms of synaptic transmission in the cuneate nucleus. J. Neurophysiol. *27*, 1096–1116 (1964)

Anderson-Baker, W., McLaughlin, C.L., Baile, C.A.: Oral and hypothalamic injections of barbiturates, benzodiazepines and cannabinoids and food intake in rats. Pharmacol. Biochem. Behav. *11*, 487–491 (1979)

Ando, J., Akutagawa, M., Makino, M.: Antiarrhythmic effects of benzodiazepines. Japan J. Pharmacol. *29*, (Suppl.), P 15 (1979)

Andreas, K.: Der Einfluß von Benzodiazepinen auf durch Reizung des entorhinalen Kortex im Gyrus dentatus hippocampi der Ratte ausgelöste Potentiale. Acta biol. med. germ. *37*, 371–373 (1978)

Antkiewicz-Michaluk, L., Grabowska, M., Baran, L., Michaluk, J.: Influence of benzodiazepines on turnover of serotonin in cerebral structures in normal and aggressive rats. Arch. Immunol. Ther. Exp. (Warsz.) *23*, 763–767 (1975)

Antonaccio, M.J., Halley, J.: Inhibition of centrally-evoked pressor responses by diazepam: Evidence for an exclusively supramedullary action. Neuropharmacology *14*, 649–657 (1975)

Antonaccio, M.J., Kerwin, L., Taylor, D.G.: Effects of central GABA receptor agonism and antagonism on evoked diencephalic cardiovascular responses. Neuropharmacology *17*, 597–603 (1978)

Antoniadis, A., Müller, W.E., Wollert, U.: Inhibition of GABA and benzodiazepine receptor binding by penicillins. Neurosci. Letters *18*, 309–312 (1980)

Apfelbach, R.: Instinctive predatory behavior of the ferret (Putorius putorius furo L.) modified by chlordiazepoxide hydrochloride (librium). Psychopharmacology *59*, 179–182 (1978)

Apfelbach, R., Delgado, I.M.R.: Social hierarchy in monkeys (Macaca mulatta) modified by chlordiazepoxide hydrochloride. Neuropharmacology *13*, 11–20 (1974)

Argüelles, A.E., Rosner, J.: Diazepam and plasma-testerone levels. Lancet *1*, 607 (1975)

Arnt, J., Christensen, V., Scheel-Krüger, J.: Benzodiazepines potentiate GABA-dopamine stereotyped dependent gnawing in mice. J. Pharm. Pharmacol. *31*, 56–58 (1979)

Arrigo, A., Jann, G., Tonali, P.: Some aspects of the action of valium and of librium on the electrical activity of the rabbit brain. Arch. Int. Pharmacodyn. Ther. *154*(2), 364–373 (1965)

Arrigoni-Martelli, E., Corsico, N.: On the mechanism of lipomobilizing effect of chlordiazepoxide. J. Pharm. Pharmacol. *21*, 59–60 (1969)

Asami, Y., Otsuka, M., Hirohashi, T., Inaba, S., Yamamoto, H.: The synthesis and pharmacology of a novel benzodiazepine derivative, 1-methyl-5-/o-fluorophenyl/-7-chloro-1,3-dihydro-2H-1, 4-benzodiazepin-2-one/ID-540/. Arzneim. Forsch. *24*, 1563–1568 (1974)

Asami, Y., Otsuka, M., Akatsu, M., Kitagawa, S., Inaba, S., Yamamoto, H.: The synthesis and pharmacology of a novel benzodiazepine derivative, 1-(β-methylsulfonylethyl)-5-(o-fluorophenyl)-7-chloro-1,3-dihydro-2H-1,4-benzodiazepin-2-one (ID-622). Arzneim. Forsch. *25*, 534–539 (1975)

Asano, T., Spector, S.: Identification of inosine and hypoxanthine as endogenous ligands for the brain benzodiazepine-binding sites. Proc. Natl. Acad. Sci. USA *76*, 977–981 (1979)

Ashton, D., Wauquier, A.: Behavioral analysis of the effects of 15 anticonvulsants in the amygdaloid kindled rat. Psychopharmacology *65*, 7–13 (1979a)

Ashton, D., Wauquier, A.: Effects of some anti-epileptic, neuroleptic and gabaminergic drugs on convulsions induced by D,L-allylglycine. Pharmacol. Biochem. Behav. *11*, 221–226 (1979b)

Assumpção, J.A., Bernardi, N., Brown, J., Stone, T.W.: Selective antagonism by benzodiazepines of neuronal responses to excitatory amino acids in the cerebral cortex. Br. J. Pharmacol. *67*, 563–568 (1979)

Ayd, F.J.: A critical appraisal of chlordiazepoxide. J. Neuropsychiat. *3*, 117–180 (1962)

Babbini, M., Torrielli, M.V.: Investigation on pharmacological properties of hexadiphane, oxazepam hemisuccinate and of their combination. Curr. Ther. Res. *14*(6), 311–323 (1972)

Babbini, M., DeMarchi, F., Montanaro, N., Strocchi, P., Torrielli, M.V.: Chemistry and CNS-pharmacological properties of two hydrosoluble benzodiazepine derivatives. Arzneim. Forsch. *19*, 1931–1936 (1969)

Babbini, M., Torrielli, M.V., Gaiardi, M., Bartoletti, M., DeMarchi, F.: Influence of N 1,2-hydroxyethyl substitution on central activity of oxazepam and lorazepam. Pharmacology *10*, 345–353 (1973)

Babbini, M., Torrielli, M.V., Gaiardi, M., Bartoletti, M., DeMarchi, F.: Central effects of three fluorinated benzodiazepines in comparison with diazepam. Pharmacology *12*, 74–83 (1974)

Babbini, M., Torrielli, M.V., Strumia, E., Gaiardi, M., Bartoletti, M., DeMarchi, F.: Sedative-hypnotic properties of a new benzodiazepine in comparison with flurazepam. Arzneim. Forsch. *25*, 1294–1300 (1975)

Babington, R.G., Wedeking, P.W.: The pharmacology of seizures induced by sensitization with low intensity brain stimulation. Pharmacol. Biochem. Behav. *1*, 461–467 (1973)

Bainbridge, J.G.: The effect of psychotropic drugs on food reinforced behaviour and on food consumption. Psychopharmacologia *12*, 204–213 (1968)

Ball, H.A., Davies, J.A., Nicholson, A.N.: Effect of diazepam and its metabolites on the binding of L-tryptophan to human serum albumin. Br. J. Pharmacol. *66*, 92P–93P (1979)

Baltzer, V., Bein, H.J.: Pharmacological investigations with benzoctamine (Tacitin), a new psycho-active agent. Arch. Int. Pharmacodyn. Ther. *201*, 25–41 (1973)

Bandman, E., Walker, C.R., Strohman, R.C.: Diazepam inhibits myoblast fusion and expression of muscle specific protein synthesis. Science *200*, 559–561 (1978)

Banerjee, U., Yeoh, P.N.: The temporal dimensions of anticonvulsant action of some newer benzodiazepines against metrazol induced seizures in mice and rats. Med. Biol. *55*, 310–316 (1977)

Banna, N.R., Jabbur, S.J., Saadé, N.E.: Antagonism of the spinal action of diazepam by semicarbazide. Br. J. Pharmacol. *51*, 101–103 (1974)

Bansi, D., Krug, M., Schmidt, J.: Der Einfluß von Psychopharmaka auf durch Zahnpulpareizung ausgelöste kortikale Potentiale und langanhaltende posttetanische Erregbarkeitsänderungen. Acta Biol. Med. Germ. *35*, 613–625 (1976)

Banziger, R.F.: Anticonvulsant properties of chlordiazepoxide, diazepam and certain other 1,4-benzodiazepines. Arch. Int. Pharmacodyn. Ther. *154*(1), 131–136 (1965)

Banziger, R., Hane, D.: Evaluation of a new convulsant for anticonvulsant screening. Arch. Int. Pharmacodyn. Ther. *167*, 245–249 (1967)

Baraldi, M., Guidotti, A., Costa, E.: Benzodiazepine and GABA receptors in NB_{2a} neuroblastoma: Action on Cl^- fluxes. Soc. Neurosci., Abstr. 9th Ann. Meeting *5*, 301 (1979a)

Baraldi, M., Guidotti, A., Schwartz, J.P., Costa, E.: GABA receptors in clonal cell lines: A model for study of benzodiazepine action at molecular level. Science 205, 821–823 (1979 b)

Baraldi, M., Schwartz, J., Guidotti, A., Costa, E.: Regulation of the high affinity binding of diazepam and GABA to membranes of neuroblastoma and glioma cells. Pharmacologist 20, 373 (1978)

Barlow, S.M., Knight, A.F., Sullivan, F.M.: Plasma corticosterone responses to stress following chronic oral administration of diazepam in the rat. J. Pharm. Pharmacol. 31, 23–26 (1979)

Barmack, N.H., Pettorossi, V.E.: The influence of diazepam on the activity of secondary vestibular neurones in the rabbit. Neurosci. Letters 16, 339–344 (1980)

Barman, S.M., Gebber, G.L.: Picrotoxin- and bicuculline-sensitive inhibition of cardiac vagal reflexes. J. Pharmacol. Exp. Ther. 209, 67–72 (1979)

Barnes, C.D., Moolenaar, G.M.: Effects of diazepam and picrotoxin on the visual system. Neuropharmacology 10, 193–201 (1971)

Barnes, C.D., Strahlendorf, J.C., Strahlendorf, H.K.: Raphe stimulation modulates excitatory and inhibitory processes in the cerebellum. Soc. Neurosci., Abstr. 9th Ann. Meeting, 5, 98 (1979)

Barnett, A., Goldstein, J., Fiedler, E.P., Taber, R.I.: The pharmacology of fletazepam. A centrally-acting muscle relaxant. Arch. Int. Pharmacodyn. 212, 164–174 (1974)

Bartholini, G., Keller, H., Pieri, L., Pletscher, A.: The effect of diazepam on the turnover of cerebral dopamine. In: The Benzodiazepines; Garattini, S., Mussini, E., Randall, L.O. (eds.), pp. 235–239. New York: Raven Press 1973

Barzaghi, F., Fournex, R., Mantegazza, P.: Pharmacological and toxicological properties of clobazam (1-phenyl-5-methyl-8-chloro-1,2,4,5-tetrahydro-2,4-diketo-3H-1,5-benzodiazepine), a new psychotherapeutic agent. Arzneim. Forsch. 23, 683–686 (1973)

Basset, J.R., Cairncross, K.D.: Effects of psychoactive drugs on responses of the rat to aversive stimulation. Arch. Int. Pharmacodyn. 212, 221–229 (1974)

Battersby, M.K., Richards, J.G., Möhler, H.: Benzodiazepine receptor: photo affinity labeling and localization. Eur. J. Pharmacol. 57, 277–278 (1979)

Bauen, A., Possanza, G.J.: The mink as a psychopharmacological model. Arch. Int. Pharmacodyn. 186, 133–136 (1970)

Baum, T., Eckfeld, D.K., Shropshire, A.T., Rowles, G., Varner, L.L.: Observations on models used for the evaluation of antiarrhythmic drugs. Arch. Int. Pharmacodyn. 193, 149–170 (1971)

Baxter, B.L.: The effect of chlordiazepoxide on the hissing response elicited via hypothalamic stimulation. Life Sci. 3, 531–537 (1964)

Beattie, C.W., Chernov, H.I., Bernard, P.S., Glenny, F.H.: Pharmacological alteration of hyperreactivity in rats with septal and hypothalamic lesions. Int. J. Neuropharmacol. 8, 365–371 (1969)

Beaubien, A.R., Carpenter, D.C., Mathieu, L.F., MacConaill, M., Hrdina, P.D.: Antagonism of imipramine poisoning by anticonvulsants in the rat. Toxicol. Appl. Pharmacol. 38, 1–6 (1976)

Beaumont, K., Chilton, W.S., Yamamura, H.I., Enna, S.J.: Muscimol binding in rat brain: association with synaptic GABA receptors. Brain Res. 148, 153–162 (1978)

Beer, B., Klepner, C.A., Lippa, A.S., Squires, R.F.: Enhancement of ^{3}H-diazepam binding by SQ 65,396: a novel anti-anxiety agent. Pharmacol. Biochem. Behav. 9, 849–851 (1978)

Beer, B., Chasin, M., Clody, D.E., Vogel, J.R., Horovitz, Z.P.: Cyclic adenosine monophosphate phosphodiesterase in brain: effect on anxiety. Science 176, 428–430 (1972)

Beleslin, D., Polak, R.L., Sproul, O.H.: The effects of leptazol and strychnine on the acetylcholine release from the cat brain. J. Physiol. (Lond.) 181, 308–316 (1965)

Bell, E.F.: The use of naloxone in the treatment of diazepam poisoning. J. Pediatrics 87, 803–804 (1975)

Bender, A.S., Phillis, J.W., Wu, P.H.: Diazepam and flurazepam inhibit adenosine uptake by rat brain synaptosomes. J. Pharm. Pharmacol. 32, 293–294 (1980)

Benke, A., Balogh, A., Reich-Hilscher, B.: Der Einfluß von Flunitrazepam (Rohypnol) auf die Atmung. Wien. Klin. Wschr. 87(10), 656–658 (1975)

Ben-Neria, Y., Lass, Y.: Facilitation of synaptic transmission by diazepam in a perfused frog cerebellum. Experientia *33*(11), 1484 (1977)

Bennett, J.P., Snyder, S.H.: Stereospecific binding of D-lysergic acid diethylamide (LSD) to brain membranes: relationship to serotonin receptors. Brain Res. *94*, 523–544 (1975)

Bennett, P.N., Davies, P., Frigo, G.M., Weerasinghe, W.M.T., Lennard-Jones, J.E.: Effect of diazepam on unstimulated and on stimulated gastric secretion. Scand. J. Gastroenterol. *10*(1), 102–103 (1975)

Benson, H., Herd, J.A., Morse, W.H., Kelleher, R.T.: Hypotensive effects of chlordiazepoxide, amobarbital and chlorpromazine on behaviorally induced elevated arterial blood pressure in the squirrel monkey. J. Pharmacol. Exp. Ther. *173*(2), 399–406 (1970)

Berendson, H., Leonard, B.E., Rigter, H.: The action of psychotropic drugs on DOPA induced behavioural responses in mice. Drug. Res. *26*, 1686–1689 (1976)

Bergamaschi, M., Longoni, A.M.: Cardiovascular events in anxiety: Experimental studies in the conscious dog. Am. Heart J. *86*(3), 385–394 (1973)

Berger, F.M.: The pharmacological properties of 2-methyl-2-n-propyl-1,3-propandiol dicarbamate (Miltwon), a new interneuronal blocking agent. J. Pharmacol. Exp. Ther. *112*, 413–423 (1954)

Berger, F.M., Dille, J.M., Johnson, H.L.: The analgesic action of combinations of propoxyphene and benzodiazepines. Abstracts 7th Int. Congress Pharmacology, Part 1, p. 204. Paris: Pergamon 1978

Berger, F.M., Kletzkin, M., Margolin, S.: Pharmacologic properties of a new tranquillizing agent, 2-methyl-2-propyltrimethylene butylcarbamate carbamate (Tybamate). Med. Exp. *10*, 327–344 (1964)

Berger, M., Neuweiler, W.: Die medikamentöse Relaxation des menschlichen Uterus. Wissenschaftl. Ausstellung, 3. Weltkongreß der Int. Fed. f. Gynäkol., Wien, 1961

Bernasconi, R., Martin, P.: Effects of diazepam and baclofen on the GABA turnover rate in various brain regions. Naunyn-Schmiedebergs Arch. Pharmacol. *302* (Suppl.), R 58 (1978)

Bernasconi, R., Martin, P.: Effects of antiepileptic drugs on the GABA turnover rate. Naunyn-Schmiedebergs Arch. Pharmacol. *307* (Suppl.), R 63 (1979)

Berry, D.G.: Effects of diazepam on the isolated chick embryo heart. Proc. Soc. Exp. Biol. Med. *150*, 240–243 (1975)

Bianchi, C.P., de Groof, R.C.: Direct effect of diazepam on muscle contraction. Scientific Exhibit., Ann. Congr. Rehabil. Med., Miami (Florida), Oct 31th-Nov 3rd, 1977

Bianco, J.A., Shanahan, E.A., Ostheimer, G.W., Guyton, R.A., Powell, W.J., Jr., Daggett, W.M.: Cardiovascular effects of diazepam. J. Thorac. Cardiovasc. Surg. *62*, 125–130 (1971)

Biggio, G., Costa, E., Guidotti, A.: Different mechanisms mediating the decrease of cerebellar cGMP elicited by haloperidol and diazepam. Adv. Biochem. Psychopharmacol. *15*, 325–335 (1976)

Biggio, G., Costa, E., Guidotti, A.: Regulation of 3',5'-cyclic guanosine monophosphate content in deep cerebellar nuclei. Neurosciences 2, 49–52 (1977a)

Biggio, G., Costa, E., Guidotti, A.: Pharmacologically induced changes in the 3',5'-cyclic guanosine monophosphate content of rat cerebellar cortex: differences between apomorphine, haloperidol and harmaline. J. Pharmacol. Exp. Ther. *200*, 207–215 (1977b)

Biggio, G., Brodie, B.B., Costa, E., Guidotti, A.: Mechanisms by which diazepam, muscimol, and other drugs change the content of cGMP in cerebellar cortex. Proc. Natl. Acad. Sci. USA *74*, 3592–3596 (1977c)

Biggio, G., Corda, M.G., Lamberti, C., Gessa, G.L.: Changes in benzodiazepine receptors following GABAergic denervation of substantia nigra. Eur. J. Pharmacol. *58*, 215–216 (1979)

Biggio, G., Corda, M.G., De Montis, G., Gessa, G.L.: Differential effects of kainic acid on benzodiazepine receptors, GABA receptors, and GABA-modulin in the cerebellar cortex. In: Receptors for Neurotransmitters and Peptide Hormones. Pepeu, G., Kuhar, M.J., Enna, S.J. (eds.), pp. 265–270. New York: Raven Press 1980a

Biggio, G., Corda, M.G., De Montis, G., Stefanini, E., Gessa, G.L.: Kainic acid differentiates GABA receptors from benzodiazepine receptors in the rat cerebellum. Brain Res. *193*, 589–593 (1980b)

Bigler, E.D.: Diazepam modification of evoked and spontaneous lateral geniculate activity. Electroenceph. Clin. Neurophysiol. *41*, 429–433 (1976)

Bigler, E.D.: Comparison of effects of bicuculline, strychnine, and picrotoxin with those of pentylenetetrazol on photically evoked afterdischarges. Epilepsia 18, 465–470 (1977)

Bihler, I., Sawh, P.C.: Effects of benzodiazepines on the transport of sugars and ions in rat skeletal muscle in vitro. Molecular Pharmacol. 14, 879–883 (1978)

Billingsley, M.L., Kubena, R.K.: The effects of naloxone and picrotoxin on the sedative and anticonflict effects of benzodiazepines. Life Sci. 22, 897–906 (1978)

Billingsley, M., Suria, A., Williams, J.: Effects of picrotoxin, naloxone, and vagotomy on chlordiazepoxide-induced respiratory depression. Arch. Int. Pharmacodyn. Ther. 242, 95–103 (1979)

Birnbaum, D.: The effect of valium on basal gastric secretion in rats. Med. Psychosomatica 13(1), 1–4 (1968)

Birnbaum, D., Karmeli, F., Tefera, M.: The effect of diazepam on human gastric secretion. Gut 12, 616–618 (1971)

Biswas, B., Carlsson, A.: On the mode of action of diazepam on brain catecholamine metabolism. Naunyn-Schmiedebergs Arch. Pharmacol. 303, 73–78 (1978)

Bixler, E.O., Kales, A., Santen, R., Vela-Bueno, A., Soldatos, C.R., Kotas, K.M.: Effects of flurazepam (dalmane) on anterior pituitary secretion. Res. Commun. Chem. Pathol. Pharmacol. 14(3), 421–429 (1976)

Bjertnaes, L.J.: Hypoxia-induced vasoconstriction in isolated perfused lungs exposed to injectable or inhalation anesthetics. Acta Anaesthesiol. Scand. 21, 133–147 (1977)

Blanchard, J.C., Boireau, A., Garret, C., Julou, L.: In vitro and in vivo inhibition by zopiclone of benzodiazepine binding to rodent brain receptors. Life Sci. 24, 2417–2420 (1979)

Bloor, C.M., Leon, A.S., Walker, D.E.: Coronary and systemic hemodynamic effects of diazepam (valium) in the unanesthetized dog. Res. Commun. Chem. Pathol. Pharmacol. 6(3), 1043–1051 (1973)

Blum, J.E., Haefely, W., Jalfre, M., Polc, P., Schärer, K.: Pharmakologie und Toxikologie des Antiepileptikums Clonazepam. Arzneim. Forsch. 23, 377–400 (1973)

Blyther, S., Marriott, A.S.: The effects of drugs on the hyper-reactivity of rats with bilateral anterior hypothalamic lesions. Br. J. Pharmacol. 37, 507P–508P (1969)

Boakes, R.J., Martin, I.L., Mitchell, P.R.: Burst firing of cerebellar Purkinje neurones induced by benzodiazepines. Neuropharmacology 16, 711–713 (1977)

Bodnar, R.J., Kelly, D.D., Thomas, L.W., Mansour, A., Brutus, M., Glusman, M.: Chlordiazepoxide antinociception: cross-tolerance with opiates and with stress. Psychopharmacology 69, 107–110 (1980)

Boismare, F., Le Poncin-Lafitte, M., Boquet, J.: Traitement par le diazépam et la lévamépromazine des conséquences hémodynamiques d'un traumatisme cranio-cervical expérimental chez le rat. J. Pharmacol. (Paris) 9, 285–296 (1978)

Boissier, J.-R., Simon, P.: La réaction d'exploration chez la souris. Thérapie 17, 1225–1232 (1962)

Boissier, J.-R., Simon, P.: Tranquillisants et anesthésie: quelques aspects pharmacologiques. Anesth. Analgés 21, 455–463 (1964)

Boissier, J.-R., Tardy, J., Diverres, J.-C.: Une nouvelle méthode simple pour explorer l'action „tranquillisante": le test de la cheminée. Med. Exp. 3, 81–84 (1960)

Boissier, J.-R., Zebrowska-Lupina, I., Simon, P.: Profil psychopharmacologique du prazépam. Arch. Int. Pharmacodyn. 196, 330–344 (1972)

Boissier, J.-R., Simon, P., Villeneuve, A., Larousse, C.: Flurothyl in mice: seizure, post-convulsive behavior, and interactions with psychotropic drugs. Can. J. Physiol. Pharmacol. 46, 93–100 (1968)

Bolme, P., Fuxe, K.: Possible involvement of GABA mechanisms in central cardiovascular and respiratory control. Studies on the interaction between diazepam, picrotoxin and clonidine. Med. Biol. 55(5), 301–309 (1977)

Bolme, P., Ngai, S.H., Uvnäs, B., Wallenberg, L.R.: Circulatory and behavioural effects on electrical stimulation of the sympathetic vasodilator areas in the hypothalamus and the mesencephalon in unanesthetized dogs. Acta Physiol. Scand. 70, 334–346 (1967)

Bonetti, E.P., Polc, P.: Antagonism by caffeine of diazepam, phenobarbitone and 1-methylisoguanosine effects. Abstracts 12th CINP Congress, Göteborg, 22–26 June 1980, p.86

Bonfitto, M., Della Bella, D., Santini, V.: Study of the action of some centrally acting drugs on the EEG and on a conditioned avoidance reflex in the rabbit. Arch. Int. Pharmacodyn. Ther. *217*, 131–139 (1975)

Borbe, H.O., Müller, W.E., Wollert, V.: The identification of benzodiazepine receptors with brain-like specificity in bovine retina. Brain Res. *182*, 466–469 (1980)

Borbély, A.A., Jost, M., Huston, J.P., Waser, P.G. Caffeine and chlordiazepoxide: Effects on motor activity in the chronic thalamic rat. Arch. Pharmacol. *290*, 285–296 (1975)

Borella, L.E., Paquette, R., Herr, F.: The effect of some CNS depressants on the hypermotility and anorexia induced by amphetamine in rats. Can. J. Physiol. Pharmacol. *47*, 841–847 (1969)

Borenstein, P., Gekiere, F., Brindeau, F., Cleau, M., Allegre, G.: Etude comportementale et polygraphique de trois benzodiazépines et d'un barbiturique chez le chat implanté libre. Ann. Med. Psychol. (Paris) *131*, 13–43 (1973)

Boris, A., Stevenson, R.H.: The effects of some psychotropic drugs on dehydration induced antidiuretic hormone activity in the rat. Arch. Int. Pharmacodyn. Ther. *166*, 486–498 (1967)

Boris, A., Costello, J., Gower, M.M., Welsch, J.A.: Endocrine studies of chlordiazepoxide. Proc. Soc. Exp. Biol. Med. *106*, 708–710 (1961)

Bornmann, G.: Zum Einfluß einiger psychotroper Substanzen auf Magen und Gallefluß. Arzneim. Forsch. *11*, 89–90 (1961)

Borsy, J., Csanyi, E., Lazar, I.: A method of assaying tranquillizing drugs based on the inhibition of orientational hypermotility. Arch. Int. Pharmacodyn. *124*, 180–190 (1960)

Bosmann, H.B., Case, R., DiStefano, P.: Diazepam receptor characterization: specific binding of a benzodiazepine to macromolecules in various areas of rat brain. FEBS Lett. *82*, 368–372 (1977)

Bosmann, H.B., Penney, D.P., Case, K.R., DiStefano, P., Averill, K.: Diazepam receptor: specific binding of [^{3}H]diazepam and flunitrazepam to rat brain subfractions. FEBS Lett. *87*, 199–202 (1978)

Bosmann, H.B., Penney, D.P., Case, K.R., Averill, K.: Diazepam receptor: specific nuclear binding of [^{3}H]flunitrazepam. Proc. Natl. Acad. Sci. USA *77*, 1195–1198 (1980)

Bourgoin, S., Héry, F., Ternaux, J.P., Hamon, M.: Effects of benzodiazepines on the binding of tryptophan in serum. Consequences on 5-hydroxyindoles concentrations in the rat brain. Psychopharmacol. Commun. *1*, 209–216 (1975)

Bourrinet, P.: Influence de l'alcoolisation aiguë et chronique sur l'activité de quelques benzodiazépines chez la souris. Thérapie *26*, 687–700 (1971)

Bouyer, J.-J., Dedet, L., Debray, O., Rougeul, A.: Restraint in primate chair may cause unusual behavior in baboons; electrocorticographic correlates and corrective effects of diazepam. Electroenceph. Clin. Neurophysiol. *44*, 562–567 (1978)

Bowery, N.G., Dray, A.: Reversal of the action of amino acid antagonists by barbiturates and other hypnotic drugs. Br. J. Pharmacol. *63*, 197–215 (1978)

Bradshaw, E.G.: The vasodilator effects of diazepam in vitro. Br. J. Anaesth. *48*, 817–818 (1976)

Bradshaw, E.G., Maddison, S.: Effect of diazepam at the neuromuscular junction. Br. J. Anaesth. *51*, 955–960 (1979)

Bradshaw, E.G., Pleuvry, B.J.: Respiratory and hypnotic effects of nitrazepam, diazepam and pentobarbitone and their solvents in the rabbit and the mouse. Br. J. Anaesth. *43*, 637–643 (1971)

Bradshaw, E.G., Biswas, T.K., Pleuvry, B.J.: Some interactions between morphine and diazepam in the mouse and rabbit. Br. J. Anaesth. *45*, 1185–1190 (1973)

Braestrup, C., Nielsen, M. Ontogenetic development of benzodiazepine receptors in the rat brain. Brain Res. *147*, 170–173 (1978)

Braestrup, C., Nielsen, M.: Benzodiazepine receptors and their possible endogenous ligands. Acta Physiol. Scand. Suppl. *473*, 10 (1979)

Braestrup, C., Nielsen, M.: Benzodiazepine receptors. Drug Res. *30*, 852–857 (1980)

Braestrup, C., Squires, R.F.: Specific benzodiazepine receptors in rat brain characterized by high-affinity ^{3}H-diazepam binding. Proc. Nat. Acad. Sci. USA *74*, 3805–3809 (1977)

Braestrup, C., Squires, R.F., Pharmacological characterization of benzodiazepine receptors in the brain. Eur. J. Pharmacol. *48*, 263–270 (1978a)

Braestrup, C., Squires, R.F., Brain specific benzodiazepine receptors. Br. J. Psychiat. *133*, 249–260 (1978 b)

Braestrup, C., Albrechtsen, R., Squires, R.F.: High densities of benzodiazepine receptors in human cortical areas. Nature *269*, 702–704 (1977)

Braestrup, C., Nissen, C., Squires, R.F., Schousboe, A.: Lack of brain specific benzodiazepine receptors on mouse primary astroglial cultures, which specifically bind haloperidol. Neurosci. Letters *9*, 45–49 (1978)

Braestrup, C., Nielsen, M., Squires, R.F.: No changes in rat benzodiazepine receptors after withdrawal from continuous treatment with lorazepam and diazepam. Life Sci. *24*, 347–350 (1979 a)

Braestrup, C., Nielsen, M., Biggio, G., Squires, R.F.: Neuron localization of benzodiazepine receptors in cerebellum. Neurosci. Letters *13*, 219–224 (1979 b)

Braestrup, C., Nielsen, M., Krogsgaard-Larsen, P., Falch, E.: Partial agonists for brain GABA/benzodiazepine receptor complex. Nature *280*, 331–333 (1979 c)

Braestrup, C., Nielsen, M., Nielsen, E.B., Lyon, M.: Benzodiazepine receptors in the brain as affected by different experimental stresses: the changes are small and not unidirectional. Psychopharmacology *65*, 273–277 (1979 d)

Braestrup, C., Nielsen, M., Krogsgaard-Larsen, P., Falch, E.: Two or more conformations of benzodiazepine receptors depending on GABA receptors and other variables. In: Receptors for Neurotransmitters and Peptide Hormones. Pepeu, G., Kuhar, M.J., Enna, S.J. (eds.), pp. 301–312. New York: Raven Press (1980)

Brassier, J., Eben-Moussi, E., Allain, P., Van den Driessche, J.: Action du diazépam sur la pression sanguine et sur la réactivité cardio-vasculaire du chien à l'adrénaline et à la noradrénaline. Thérapie *21*, 379–385 (1966)

Brausch, U., Henatsch, H.-D., Student, C., Takano, K.: Effect of diazepam on development of stretch reflex tension. In: The Benzodiazepines. Garattini, S., Mussini, E., Randall, L.O. (eds.), pp. 531–543. New York: Raven Press 1973

Breuker, E., Dingledine, R., Iversen, L.L.: Evidence for naloxone and opiates as GABA antagonists. Br. J. Pharmacol. *58*, 458P (1976)

Briley, M.S., Langer, S.Z.: Influence of GABA receptor agonists and antagonists on the binding of ^{3}H-diazepam to the benzodiazepine receptor. Eur. J. Pharmacol. *52*, 129–132 (1978)

Britton, D.R., Thatcher-Britton, K.: Naloxone reversible and non-naloxone reversible behavioral effects of diazepam. Fed. Proc. *39*, Abstr. 2561 (1980)

Brown, J.L., Hunsperger, R.W., Rosvold, H.E.: Defense, attack, and flight elicited by electrical stimulation of the hypothalamus of the cat. Exp. Brain Res. *8*, 113–129 (1969)

Brown, R.F., Houpt, K.A., Schryver, H.F.: Stimulation of food intake in horses by diazepam and promazine. Pharmacol. Biochem. Behav. *5*, 495–497 (1976)

Brunaud, M., Rocand, J.: Une nouvelle benzodiazépine: le lorazépam. Mise au point pharmacologique. Agressologie *13*, 363–375 (1972)

Brunaud, M., Navarro, J., Salle, J., Siou, G.: Pharmacological, toxicological and teratological studies on dipotassium-7-chloro-3-carboxy-1,3-dihydro-2,2-dihydroxy-5-phenyl-2H-1,4-benzodiazepine-chloroazepate (dipotassium chlorazepate, 4306 CB), a new tranquillizer. Arzneim. Forsch. *20*(1), 123–125 (1970)

Buchwald, N.A., Wyers, E.J., Okuma, T., Heuser, G.: The caudate spindle. 1. Electrophysiological properties. Electroenceph. Clin. Neurophysiol. *13*, 509–518 (1961)

Buckett, W.R.: Intravenous bicuculline in mice facilitates in vivo evaluation of drugs affecting GABA-like mechanisms. Br. J. Pharmacol. *68*, 177P–178P (1980)

Bunney, B.S., Aghajanian, G.K.: The effect of antipsychotic drugs on the firing of dopaminergic neurons: A reappraisal. In: Antipsychotic drugs: Pharmacodynamic and Pharmacokinetics. Sedwall, G., Uvnäs, B., Zottermann, Y. (eds.), pp. 305–318. Oxford: Pergamon Press 1976

Buonamici, M., Rossi, A.C.: Acute effects of temazepam and nitrazepam on the sleep-wake cycle of the rat: An EEG study. 3rd Int. Congress Sleep Res. Abstracts, 168, Tokyo, 1979

Burkard, W.P., Pieri, L., Haefely, W.: In vivo changes of guanosine 3',5'-cyclic phosphate in rat cerebellum by dopaminergic mechanisms. J. Neurochem. *27*, 297–298 (1976 a)

Burkard, W.P., Pieri, L., Haefely, W.: Changes of rat cerebellar guanosine 3',5'-cyclic phosphate by dopaminergic mechanisms in vivo. Adv. Biochem. Psychopharmacol. *15*, 315–324 (1976 b)

Burnstock, G.: Purinergic nerves. Pharmacol. Rev. *24*, 509–581 (1972)

Burt, D.R., Creese, I., Snyder, S.H.: Properties of [^{3}H]haloperidol and [^{3}H]dopamine binding associated with dopamine receptors in calf brain membranes. Mol. Pharmacol. *12*, 800–812 (1976)

Burton, M.J., Cooper, S.J., Posadas-Andrews, A.: Interactions between chlordiazepoxide and food deprivation determining choice in a food-preference test. Br. J. Pharmacol. *68*, 157P–158P (1980)

Cahn, B.: Electrolyte and hormonal balance in human subjects following diazepam administration. Curr. Ther. Res. *8*(5), 256–260 (1966)

Campese, V.M., Russo, C.R., Marino, A.: Effetti di un nuovo benzodiazepinico (bromazepam) sull'intestino isolato di cavia. Boll. Soc. Ital. Biol. Sper. *48*, 807–809 (1972)

Candy, J.M., Martin, I.L.: The postnatal development of the benzodiazepine receptor in the cerebral cortex and cerebellum of the rat. J. Neurochem. *32*, 655–658 (1979)

Carabateas, P.M., Harris, L.S.: Analgesic antagonists. I. 4-Substituted 1-acyl-2,3,4,5-tetrahydro-1H-1,4-benzodiazepines. J. Med. Chem. *9*, 6–10 (1966)

Carlsson, C., Hägerdal, M., Kaasik, A.E., Siesjö, B.K.: The effects of diazepam on cerebral blood flow and oxygen consumption in rats and its synergistic interaction with nitrous oxide. Anaesthesiology *45*, 319–325 (1976)

Carpenter, D.C., Hrdina, P.D., Beaubien, A.R.: Effects of phenobarbital and diazepam on imipramine-induced changes in blood pressure, heart rate and rectal temperature of rats. Res. Commun. Chem. Pathol. Pharmacol. *18*, 613–625 (1977)

Carroll, M.N., Jr., Hoff, E.C., Kell, J.F., Jr., Suter, C.G.: The effects of ethanol and chlordiazepoxide in altering autonomic responses evoked by isocortical and paleocortical stimulation. Biochem. Pharmacol. *8*, 15 (1961)

Catchlove, R.F.H., Kafer, E.R.: The effects of diazepam on the ventilatory response to carbon dioxide and on steady-state gas exchange. Anesthesiology *34*(1), 9–13 (1971)

Cavanagh, D., Albores, E., Todd, J.: Comparative effects of two benzodiazepine compounds on isolated human myometrium. Am. J. Obstet. Gynecol. *94*(1), 6–13 (1966)

Cegla, U.H.: The use of CO_2 response curves to determine the respiration-depressant action of drugs with diazepam as an example. Pneumonologie *149*, 219–228 (1973)

Chadwick, D., Gorrod, J.W., Jenner, P., Marsden, C.D., Reynolds, E.H.: Functional changes in cerebral 5-hydroxytryptamine metabolism in the mouse induced by anticonvulsant drugs. Br. J. Pharmacol. *62*, 115–124 (1978)

Chai, C.Y., Wang, S.C.: Cardiovascular actions of diazepam in the cat. J. Pharmacol. Exp. Ther. *154*(2), 271–280 (1966)

Chambers, D.M., Jefferson, G.C.: Some observations on the mechanism of benzodiazepine-barbiturate interactions in the mouse. Br. J. Pharmacol. *60*, 393–399 (1977)

Chambers, D.M., Jefferson, G.C., Ruddick, C.A.: Halothane-induced sleeping time in the mouse: its modification by benzodiazepines. Eur. J. Pharmacol. *50*, 103–112 (1978)

Chan, A.W.K., Greizerstein, H.B., Strauss, W.: Interaction of chlordiazepoxide with ethanol. Pharmacologist *20*(3), 159 (1978)

Chanelet, J., Lonchampt, P.: Action du diazépam sur la moelle épinière du chat. J. Physiol. (Paris) *63*, 185A (1971)

Chang, R.S.L., Snyder, S.H.: Benzodiazepine receptors: labeling in intact animals with ^{3}H-flunitrazepam. Eur. J. Pharmacol. *48*, 213–218 (1978)

Chan-Palay, V., Palay, S.L.: Immunocytochemical localization of cyclic GMP: light and electron microscopic evidence for involvement of neuroglia. Proc. Natl. Acad. Sci. USA *76*, 1485–1488 (1979)

Chan-Palay, V., Wu, J.-Y., Palay, S.L.: Immunocytochemical localization of γ-aminobutyric acid transaminase at cellular and ultrastructural levels. Proc. Natl. Acad. Sci. USA *76*, 2067–2071 (1979)

Chapman, C.R., Feather, B.W.: Effects of diazepam on human pain tolerance and pain sensitivity. Psychosom. Med. *35*, 330–340 (1973)

Chase, T.N., Katz, R.I., Kopin, I.J.: Effect of diazepam on fate of intracisternally injected serotonin ^{14}C. Neuropharmacology *9*, 103–108 (1970)

Chassaing, C., Duchene-Marullaz, P.: Diazepam et fréquence cardiaque du chien non narcosé. J. Pharmacol. (Paris) *4*(4), 465–470 (1973)

Cheney, D.L., Trabucchi, M., Hanin, I., Costa, E.: Effect of several benzodiazepines on concentrations and specific activities of choline and acetylcholine in mouse brain. Pharmacologist *15*, 162 (1973)

Chéramy, A., Nieoullon, A., Glowinski, J.: Blockade of the picrotoxin-induced in vivo release of dopamine in the cat caudate nucleus by diazepam. Life Sci. *20*, 811–816 (1977)

Cheymol, J., Van den Driessche, J., Allain, P., Eben-Moussi, E.: Diazépam et curarisation. Anesth. Anal. (Paris) *24*, 329–336 (1967)

Chiba, S., Nagawa, Y.: Effects of new S-triazolobenzodiazepine (D-40TA) and other central muscle relaxants on spinal and supraspinal reflexes in cats. Japan. J. Pharmacol. *23*, 83–96 (1973)

Chieli, T., Cocchi, D., Fregnan, G.B., Müller, E.E.: Neuroleptic-induced prolactin rise: Influence of pharmacological alterations of different neurotransmitter systems. Experientia *36*, 463–465 (1980)

Chin, J.H., Crankshaw, D.P., Kendig, J.J.: Changes in the dorsal root potential with diazepam and with the analgesics aspirin, nitrous oxide, morphine and meperidine. Neuropharmacology *13*, 305–315 (1974)

Chinn, Ch., Barnes, Ch.D.: Comparative effects of propranolol and diazepam on hypothalamically-evoked sympathetic response. Pharmacologist *20*(3), 207 (1978)

Chiu, T.H., Rosenberg, H.C.: Reduced diazepam binding following chronic benzodiazepine treatment. Life Sci. *23*, 1153–1158 (1978)

Chiu, T.H., Rosenberg, H.C.: Differential effects of triton X-100 on benzodiazepine and GABA binding in a frozen-thawed synaptosomal fraction of rat brain. Eur. J. Pharmacol. *58*, 335–338 (1979)

Choi, D.W., Farb, D.H., Fischbach, G.D.: Chlordiazepoxide selectively augments GABA action in spinal cord cell cultures. Nature *269*, 342–344 (1977)

Chou, D.T., Wang, S.C.: Studies on the localization of central cough mechanism: Site of action of antitussive drugs. J. Pharmacol. Exp. Ther. *194*(3), 499–505 (1975)

Chou, D.T., Wang, S.C.: Unit activity of amygdala and hippocampal neurons: Effects of morphine and benzodiazepines. Brain Res. *126*(3), 427–440 (1977)

Christensen, K.N., Hüttel, M.: Naloxone does not antagonize diazepam-induced sedation. Anesthesiology *51*, 187 (1979)

Christmas, A.J., Maxwell, D.R.: A comparison of the effects of some benzodiazepines and other drugs on aggressive and exploratory behaviour in mice and rats. Neuropharmacology *9*, 17–29 (1970)

Chung Hwang, E., Van Woert, M.H.: Antimyoclonic action of clonazepam: the role of serotonin. Eur. J. Pharmacol. *60*, 31–40 (1979)

Chusid, J.G., Kopeloff, L.M.: Chlordiazepoxide as an anticonvulsant in monkeys. Proc. Soc. Exp. Biol. Med. *109*, 546–548 (1962)

Clanachan, A.S., Marshall, R.J.: Therapeutic concentrations of diazepam potentiate the effects of adenosine on isolated cardiac and smooth muscle. Br. J. Pharmacol. *68*, 148P–149P (1980a)

Clanachan, A.S., Marshall, R.J.: Diazepam potentiates the coronary vasodilator actions of adenosine in anaesthetized dogs. Br. J. Pharmacol. *70*, 66P–67P (1980b)

Clemmesen, C.: Behandlung von Vergiftungen mit Psychopharmaka. Ther. Umschau *22*, 170 (1965)

Clincke, G., Wauquier, A.: Metrazol-produced impairment of passive avoidance retention specifically antagonized by anti-petit mal drugs. Psychopharmacology *66*, 243–246 (1979)

Clubley, M.: The action of CNS drugs on an isolated sympathetic nerve preparation of rabbit. Eur. J. Pharmacol. *50*, 175–181 (1978)

Clubley, M., Elliott, R.C.: Centrally active drugs and the sympathetic nervous system of rabbits and cats. Neuropharmacology *16*, 609–616 (1977)

Cohen, R., Finn, H., Steen, S.N.: Effect of diazepam and meperidine, alone and in combination, on respiratory response to carbon dioxide. Anesth. Analg. *48*(3), 353–355 (1969)

Cohn, M.L., Cohn, M., Taylor, F.H., Scattaregia, F.: A direct effect of dibutyryl cyclic AMP on the duration of narcosis induced by sedative, hypnotic, tranquiliser and anaesthetic drugs in the rat. Neuropharmacology *14*, 483–487 (1975)

Cole, H.F., Wolf, H.H.: Laboratory evaluation of aggressive behavior of the grasshopper mouse. J. Pharmaceut. Sci. *59*, 969–971 (1970)

Colello, G.D., Case, K., Bosmann, H.B.: Benzodiazepine binding to specific rat brain fractions: assay parameters. Pharmacologist *20*, 273 (1978a)

Colello, G.D., Hockenbery, D.M., Bosmann, H.B., Fuchs, S., Folkers, K.: Competitive inhibition of benzodiazepine binding by fractions from porcine brain. Proc. Natl. Acad. Sci. USA *75*, 6319–6323 (1978b)

Coleman, A.J., Downing, J.W., Moyes, D.G., O'Brien, A.: Acute cardiovascular effects of Ro 5-4,200: A new anaesthetic induction agent. S. Afr. Med. J. *47*(9), 382–384 (1973)

Collins, A.J., Horlington, M.: A sequential screening test based on the running component of audiogenic seizures in mice, including reference compound PD50 values. Br. J. Pharmacol. *37*, 140–150 (1969)

Comar, D., Maziere, M., Godot, J.M., Berger, G., Soussaline, F., Menini, Ch., Arfel, G., Naquet, R.: Visualisation of ^{11}C-flunitrazepam displacement in the brain of the live baboon. Nature *280*, 329–331 (1979)

Comer, W.H., Elliott, H.W., Nomof, N., Navarro, G., Kokka, N., Ruelius, H.W., Knowles, J.A.: Pharmacology of parenterally administered lorazepam in man. J. Int. Med. Res. *1*, 216–225 (1973)

Conner, J.T., Katz, R.L., Pagano, R.R., Graham, C.W.: Ro 21-3981 for intravenous surgical premedication and induction of anesthesia. Anesth. Analg. (Cleve) *57*, 1–4 (1978)

Consolo, S., Garattini, S., Ladinsky, H.: Action of the benzodiazepines on the cholingergic system. Adv. Biochem. Psychopharmacol. *14*, 63–80 (1975)

Consolo, S., Ladinsky, H., Peri, G., Garattini, S.: Effect of central stimulants and depressants on mouse brain acetylcholine and choline levels. Eur. J. Pharmacol. *18*, 251–255 (1972)

Consolo, S., Ladinsky, H., Peri, G., Garattini, S.: Effect of diazepam on mouse whole brain and brain areas acetylcholine and choline levels. Eur. J. Pharmacol. *27*, 266–268 (1974)

Constanti, A., Krnjević, K., Nistri, A.: Intraneuronal effects of inhibitory amino acids. Can. J. Physiol. Pharmacol. *58*, 193–204 (1980)

Cook, J.B., Nathan, P.W.: On the site of action of diazepam in spasticity in man. J. Neurol. Sci. *5*, 33–37 (1967)

Cook, L., Sepinwall, J.: Behavioral analysis of the effects and mechanisms of action of benzodiazepines. Adv. in Biochem. Psychopharmacol. *14*, 1–28 (1975)

Cooper, S.J.: Effects of chlordiazepoxide and diazepam on feeding performance in a food-preference test. Psychopharmacology *69*, 73–78 (1980a)

Cooper, S.J.: Benzodiazepines as appetite-enhancing compounds. Appetite *1*, 7–19 (1980b)

Cooper, S.J., Crummy, Y.M.T.: Enhanced choice of familiar food in a food preference test after chlordiazepoxide administration. Psychopharmacology *59*, 51–56 (1978)

Cooper, S.J., Francis,, R.L.: Feeding parameters in the rat: Interactions of chlordiazepoxide with (+)-amphetamine or fenfluramine. Br. J. Pharmacol. *64*, 378P–379P (1978)

Cooper, S.J., Francis, R.L.: Water intake and time course of drinking after single or repeated chlordiazepoxide injections. Psychopharmacology *65*, 191–195 (1979a)

Cooper, S.J., Francis, R.L.: Effects of acute or chronic administration of chlordiazepoxide on feeding parameters using two food textures in the rat. J. Pharm. Pharmacol. *31*, 743–746 (1979b)

Cooper, S.J., Posadas-Andrews, A.: Food and water intake in the non-deprived pigeon after chlordiazepoxide administration. Psychopharmacology *65*, 99–101 (1979)

Cooper, S.J., McClelland, A.: Effects of chlordiazepoxide, food familiarization, and prior shock experience on food choice in rats. Pharmacol. Biochem. Behav. *12*, 23–28 (1980)

Cormack, R.S., Milledge, J.S., Hanning, C.D.: Respiratory effects and amnesia after premedication with morphine or lorazepam. Br. J. Anaesth. *49*, 351–360 (1977)

Corne, S.J., Pickering, R.W., Warner, B.T.: A method for assessing the effects of drugs on the central nervous actions of 5-hydroxytryptamine. Br. J. Pharmac. *20*, 106–120 (1963)

Corradetti, R., Moroni, F., Pepeu, G.: Pharmacological effects of benzodiazepines in the leech: benzodiazepine and GABA receptors and GABA level. Pharmacol. Res. Commun. *12*, 581–585 (1980)

Corrodi, H., Fuxe, K., Hökfelt, T.: The effect of some psychoactive drugs on central monoamine neurons. Eur. J. Pharmacol. *1*, 363–368 (1967)

Corrodi, H., Fuxe, K., Lidbrink, P., Olson, L.: Minor tranquillizers, stress and central catecholamine neurons. Brain Res. *29*, 1–16 (1971)

Costa, E., Greengard, P. (eds.): Mechanism of action of benzodiazepines. New York: Raven Press 1975

Costa, E., Guidotti, A.: Molecular mechanisms in the receptor action of benzodiazepines. Ann. Rev. Pharmacol. Toxicol. *19*, 531–545 (1979)

Costa, E., Guidotti, A., Mao, C.C.: Diazepam, cyclic nucleotides and amino acid neurotransmitters in rat cerebellum. In: Neuropsychopharmacology. Boissier, J.-R., Hippius, H., Pichot, P. (eds.), pp. 849–856. Amsterdam: Excerpta Medica 1975 a

Costa, E., Guidotti, A., Mao, C.C.: Evidence for involvement of GABA in the action of benzodiazepines: studies on rat cerebellum. Adv. Biochem. Psychopharmacology *14*, 113–130 (1975 b)

Costa, E., Guidotti, A., Mao, C.C.: A GABA hypothesis for the action of benzodiazepines. In: GABA in nervous system function. Roberts, E., Chase, T.N., Tower, D.B. (eds.), pp. 413–426. New York: Raven Press 1976

Costa, E., Guidotti, A., Toffano, G.: Molecular mechanisms mediating the action of diazepam on GABA receptors. Br. J. Psychiat. *133*, 239–248 (1978)

Costa, E., Guidotti, A., Mao, C.C., Suria, A.: New concepts on the mechanism of action of benzodiazepines. Life Sci. *17*, 167–186 (1975 c)

Costa, T., Rodbard, D., Pert, C.B.: Is the benzodiazepine receptor coupled to a chloride anion channel? Nature *277*, 315–317 (1979)

Côté, P., Campeau, L., Bourassa, M.G.: Therapeutic implications of diazepam in patients with elevated left ventricular filling pressure. Am. Heart J. *91*(6), 747–751 (1976)

Côté, P., Guéret, P., Bourassa, M.G.: Systemic and coronary hemodynamic effects of diazepam in patients with normal and diseased coronary arteries. Circulation *50*, 1210–1216 (1974)

Coupet, J., Szucs-Myers, V.A.: On the multiplicity of benzodiazepine receptors and their distribution in the rat brain. Abstracts 9th Ann. Meeting Soc. Neuroscience, Atlanta 1979, p. 552 (1979)

Courvoisier, S.: Pharmacodynamic basis for the use of chlorpromazine in psychiatry. J. Clin. Exp. Psychopath. *17*, 25–37 (1956)

Coutinho, C.B., Cheripko, J.A., Carbone, J.J.: Relationship between the duration of anticonvulsant activity of chlordiazepoxide and systemic levels of the parent compound and its major metabolites in mice. Biochem. Pharmacol. *18*, 303–316 (1969)

Coutinho, C.B., Cheripko, J.A., Carbone, J.J.: Correlation between the duration of the anticonvulsant activity of diazepam and its physiological disposition in mice. Biochem. Phamacol. *19*, 363–379 (1970)

Coutinho, C.B., King, M., Carbone, J.J., Manning, J.E., Boff, E., Crews, T.: Chlordiazepoxide metabolism as related to the reduction in the aggressive behaviour of cynomolgus primates. Xenbiotica *1*(3), 287–301 (1971)

Crankshaw, D.P., Raper, C.: Some studies on peripheral actions of mephenesin, methocarbamol and diazepam. Br. J. Pharmacol. Chemother. *34*(3), 579–590 (1968)

Crankshaw, D.P., Raper, C.: Mephenesin, methocarbamol, chlordiazepoxide and diazepam: action on spinal reflexes and ventral root potentials. Br. J. Pharmacol. *38*, 148–156 (1970)

Crawford, R.D.: Epileptiform seizures in domestic fowl. J. Hered. *61*, 185–188 (1970)

Cross, A.J., Deakin, J.F.W., Lofthouse, R., Longden, A., Owen, F., Poulter, M.: On the mechanism of action of electroconvulsive therapy: some behavioural and biochemical consequences of repeated electrically induced seizures in rats. Br. J. Pharmacol. *66*, 111P (1979)

Crossmann, A.R., Lee, L.A., Longman, D.A., Slater, P.: Effects of benzodiazepines and barbiturates in a GABA-dependent animal model: interactions with muscimol in the globus pallidus. Br. J. Pharmacol. *66*, 493P–494P (1979)

Cuparencu, B., Mocan, R., Safta, L.: The influence of chlordiazepoxide on the plasma lipoprotein lipase activity and on the lipolytic activity of the aorta in normal and cholesterol fed rabbits. Cor Vasa *12*, 248–251 (1970)

Cuparencu, B., Ticsa, I., Safta, L., Rosenberg, A., Mocan, R., Brief, G.: Influence of some psychotropic drugs on the development of experimental atherosclerosis. Cor Vasa *11*, 112–121 (1969)

Cuparencu, B., Vincze, J., Horak, J., Hancu, N.: Effects of the hypolipidaemic benzodiazepine derivatives on plasma viscosity in triton WR-1339-induced hyperlipidaemia in rats. Agressologie 20, 177–182 (1979)

Curtis, D.R., Johnston, G.A.R.: Amino acid transmitters in the mammalian central nervous system. Ergebn. Physiol. 69, 97–188 (1974)

Curtis, D.R., Game, C.J.A., Lodge, D.: Benzodiazepines and central glycine receptors. Br. J. Pharmacol. 56, 307–311 (1976a)

Curtis, D.R., Lodge, D., Johnston, G.A.R., Brand, S.J.: Central actions of benzodiazepines. Brain Res. 118, 344–347 (1976b)

Cutler, R.W.P., Young, J.: The effect of penicillin on the release of γ-aminobutyric acid from cerebral cortex slices. Brain Res. 170, 157–163 (1979)

Dairman, W.M., Juhasz, L.: A study in mice of benzodiazepine-anticholinergic interaction: Protection against restraint-immersion and forced exertion-induced gastric mucosal erosion. Pharmacology 17, 104–112 (1978)

Dalen, J.E., Evans, G.L., Banas, J.S., Jr., Brooks, H.L., Paraskos, J.A., Dexter, L.: The hemodynamic and respiratory effects of diazepam (valium). Anesthesiology 30(3), 259–263 (1969)

Dalsass, M., Stern, W.C.: Effects of chlordiazepoxide on spontaneous raphe unit activity in the anesthetized rat. Neurosci. Abstr. 2, 865 (1976)

Dalton, C., Crowley, H.J., Sheppard,, H., Schallek, W.: Regional cyclic nucleotide phosphodiesterase activity in cat central nervous system: effects of benzodiazepines. Proc. Soc. Exp. Biol. Med. 145, 407–410 (1974)

Damm, H.W., Müller, W.E., Wollert, U.: Is the benzodiazepine receptor purinergic? Eur. J. Pharmacol. 55, 331–333 (1979)

Daniell, H.B., Cardiovascular effects of diazepam and chlordiazepoxide. Eur. J. Pharmacol. 32, 58–65 (1975)

Dantzer, R.: Analyse séquentielle de l'action d'une benzodiazépine, chez le porc, suivant l'intensité de l'agression. Ann. Rech. Vétér. 6, 165–171 (1975)

Dantzer, R.: Etude des effets du diazépam sur le comportement explorateur du porc. Psychopharmacology 51, 317–321 (1977a)

Dantzer, R.: Behavioral effects of benzodiazepines: a review. Biobehavioral Rev. 1, 71–86 (1977b)

Da Prada, M., Pletscher, A.: On the mechanism of chlorpromazine-induced changes of cerebral homovanillic acid levels. J. Pharm. Pharmacol. 18, 628–630 (1966)

Da Prada, M., Pieri, L., Picotti, G.B.: Effect of midazolam (a water soluble benzodiazepine) on stress-induced increase of plasma catecholamines. In: Catecholamines and Stress: Recent Advances. Usdin, E., Kvetňanský, R., Kopin, I.J. (eds.), pp. 231–236. Amsterdam: Elsevier 1980

D'Armagnac, J., Boismarc, F., Streichenberger, G., Lechat, P.: Activité anticonvulsive comparée de huit benzodiazépines. Thérapie 26, 439–450 (1971)

Dasgupta, S.R., Mukherjee, B.P.: Effect of chlordiazepoxide on stomach ulcers in rabbit induced by stress. Nature 215, 1183 (1967a)

Dasgupta, S.R., Mukherjee, B.P.: Effect of chlordiazepoxide on eosinopenia of stress in rabbits. Nature 213, 199–200 (1967b)

Dasgupta, S.R., Ray, N.M., Mukherjee, B.P.: Studies on the effect of diazepam (valium) on neuromuscular transmission in skeletal muscles. Indian J. Physiol. Pharmacol. 13, 79–80 (1969)

DaVanzo, J.P., Daugherty, M., Ruckardt, R., Kang, L: Pharmacological and biochemical studies in isolation-induced fighting mice. Psychopharmacologia 9, 210–219 (1966)

David, J., Grewal, R.S., Wagle, G.P.: Persistent electroencephalographic changes in rhesus monkeys after single doses of pentobarbital, nitrazepam and imipramine. Psychopharmacology 35, 61–75 (1974)

Davidson, D.L.W., Tsukada, Y., Barbeau, A.: Ouabain induced seizures: Site of production and response to antivonvulsants. Can. J. Neurol. Sci. 5, 405–413 (1978)

Davies, J., Polc, P.: Effect of a water soluble benzodiazepine on the responses of spinal neurones to acetylcholine and excitatory amino acid analogues. Neuropharmacology 17, 217–220 (1978)

Davies, L.P., Taylor, K.M.: The role of adenosine in neural transmission. In: Muscle, nerve and brain degeneration, Kidman, A.D., Tomkins, J.K. (eds.) pp. 94–110. Amsterdam: Excerpta Medica 1979

Davies, L.P., Cook, A.F., Poonian, M., Taylor, K.M.: Displacement of [^{3}H]diazepam binding in rat brain by dipyridamole and by l-methylisoguanosine, a marine natural product with muscle relaxant activity. Life Sci. 26, 1089–1095, (1980)

Davis, L.F., Gatz, E.E., Jones, J.R.: Effects of chlordiazepoxide and diazepam on respiration and oxidative phosphorylation in rat brain mitochondria. Biochem. Pharmacol. 20, 1883–1887 (1971)

De Angelis, L., Traversa, V., Vertura, R.: Demethyldiazepam and chlordemethyldiazepam: comparison on behavioral tests. Curr. Ther. Res. 26, 920–930 (1979)

Delgado, J.M.R.: Antiaggressive effects of chlordiazepoxide. In. The Benzodiazepines. Garattini, S., Mussini, E., Randall, L.O. (eds.), pp. 419–432. New York: Raven Press 1973

Delgado, J.M.R., Grau, C., Delgado Garcia, J.M., Rodero, J.M.: Effects of diazepam related to social hierarchy in rhesus monkeys. Neuropharmacology 15, 409–414 (1976)

Delini-Stula, A., Vassout, A.: Differential effects of psychoactive drugs on aggressive responses in mice and rats. In: Psychopharmacology of Aggression. Sandler, M. (ed.), pp. 41–60. New York: Raven Press 1979

Della-Fera, M.A., Baile, C.A., McLaughlin, C.L.: Feeding elicited by benzodiazepine-like chemicals in puppies and cats: Structure-activity relationships. Pharmacol. Biochem. Behav. 12, 195–200 (1980)

Delwaide, P.J.: Etude expérimentale de l'hyperréflexie tendineuse en clinique neurologique. Thèse. Arscia, pp. 324. Bruxelles (1970)

Depoortere, H., Lourdelet, J., Lloyd, K.G., Bartholini, G.: Effect of psychoactive drugs on the activity of a GABA-mediated synapses. 7th Int. Congr. Pharmacol., 1978, Abstract, pp. 754. Paris: Pergamon Press 1978

De Repentigny, L., Hanasono, G.K., Plaa, G.L.: The influence of acute diazepam pretreatment on the action and disposition of 14 C-pentobarbital in rats. Can. J. Physiol. Pharmacol. 54, 671–674 (1976)

Desarmenien, M., Lamour, Y., Feltz, P.: Effects of diazepam on GABA-evoked depolarization in rat dorsal root ganglia in vivo. Prog. Neuro-Psychopharmacol. 4, 31–36 (1980)

Desmedt, L.K.C., Niemegeers, C.J.E., Lewi, P.J., Janssen, P.A.J.: Antagonism of maximal metrazol seizures in rats and its relevance to an experimental classification of antiepileptic drugs. Arzneim. Forsch. 26, 1592–1603 (1976)

Dews, P.B.: This volume

De Trujillo, G.C., de Carolis, A.S., Longo, V.G.: Influence of diazepam, L-dopa and dopamine on the cerebellar and spinal electrical patterns induced by harmine in the rabbit. Neuropharmacology 16, 31–36 (1977)

Dieckmann, W., Frank, W., Schlotter, C.: Der Einfluß von „Rohypnol" auf die Atmung. In: Bisherige Erfahrungen mit „Rohypnol" (Flunitrazepam) in der Anästhesiologie und Intensivtherapie. Hügin, W., Hossli, G., Gemperle, M. (eds.), pp. 64–71. Basel: Editiones Roche 1976

Di Liberti, J., O'Brien, M.L., Turner, T.: The use of physostigmine as an antidote in accidental diazepam intoxication. J. Pediatrics 86, 106–107 (1975)

DiMascio, A.: The effects of benzodiazepines on aggression: Reduced or increased? Psychopharmacologia 30, 95–102 (1973)

DiMicco, J.A., Gillis, R.A.: Neuro-cardiovascular effects produced by bicuculline in the cat. J. Pharmacol. Exp. Ther. 210, 1–6 (1979)

DiMicco, J.A., Gale, K., Hamilton, B., Gillis, R.: GABA receptor control of parasympathetic outflow to heart: Characterization and brainstem localization. Science 204, 1106–1109 (1979)

Dingledine, R., Iversen, L.L., Breuker, E.: Naloxone as a GABA antagonist: Evidence from iontophoretic, receptor binding and convulsant studies. Eur. J. Pharmacol. 47, 19–27 (1978)

Dinnendahl, V., Gumulka, S.W.: Stress-induced alterations of cyclic nucleotide levels in brain: effects of centrally acting drugs. Psychopharmacology 52, 243–249 (1977)

Di Rocco, C., Maira, G., Meglio, M., Rossi, G.F.: Studio sperimentale dell'azione antiepilettica del clonazepam sull'epilessia rinencefalica „acuta" del coniglio. Riv. Neurologia 44, 155–168 (1974)

Di Stefano, P., Case, K.R., Colello, G.D., Bosmann, H.B.: Increased specific binding of ^{3}H-diazepam in rat brain following chronic diazepam administration. Cell Biol., Intern. Reports *3*, 163–167 (1979)

D'Mello, G., Stolerman, I.P.: Interaction of cocaine with chlordiazepoxide assessed by motor activity in mice. Br. J. Pharmacol. *59*, 141–145 (1977)

Dobrescu, D., Coeugniet, E.: Recherches expérimentales sur l'action anticonvulsivante de certaines associations médicamenteuses. Ann. Pharm. Franç. 29(9–10), 501–506 (1971)

Dolce, G., Kaemmerer, E.: Neurophysiologische Untersuchungen mit 7-Chlor-1,3-dihydro-3-hydroxy-5-phenyl-2H-1,4-benzodiazepin-2-on im Tierexperiment. Arzneim. Forsch. *17*, 1057–1060 (1967)

Dominic, J.A.: Suppression of brain serotonin synthesis and metabolism by benzodiazepine minor tranquilizers. In: Serotonin and Behavior. Baschas, J., Usdin, E. (eds.) pp. 149–155, New York: Academic Press 1973

Dominic, J.A., Sinha, A.K., Barchas, J.D.: Effect of benzodiazepine compounds on brain amine metabolism. Eur. J. Pharmacol. *32*, 124–127 (1975)

Domino, E.F., Olds, M.E.: Effects of d-amphetamine, scopolamine, chlordiazepoxide and diphenylhydantoin on self-stimulation behaviour and brain acetylcholine. Psychopharmacologia *23*, 1–16 (1972)

Doteuchi, M., Costa, E.: Pentylenetetrazol convulsions and brain catecholamine turnover rate in rats and mice receiving diphenylhydantoin or benzodiazepines. Neuropharmacology *12*, 1059–1072 (1973)

Dray, A., Bowery, N.G.: GABA convulsants and their interactions with central depressant agents. In: GABA-neurotransmitters. Krogsgaard-Larsen, P., Scheel-Krüger, J., Kofod, H. (eds.), pp. 376–389. Copenhagen: Munksgaard 1978

Dray, A., Straughan, D.W.: Benzodiazepines: GABA and glycine receptors on single neurons in the rat medulla. J. Pharm. Pharmacol. *28*, 314–315 (1976)

Dretchen, K., Ghoneim, M.M., Long, J.P.: The interaction of diazepam with myoneural blocking agents. Anaesthesiology 34(5), 463–468 (1971)

Drill, V.A.: Pharmacology in medicine. New York: McGraw Hill 1958

Drumew, D., Georgiew, B., Koitschew, K., Dilow, P., Mendow, C.: Die Wirkung von Diazepam (Faustan) bei landwirtschaftlichen Nutztieren. Monatsh. Vet. Med. *27*, 615–621 (1972)

Dudai, Y.: Modulation of benzodiazepine binding sites in calf cortex by an endogenous factor and GABAergic ligands. Brain Res. *167*, 422–425 (1979)

Dudai, Y., Yavin, E.: Binding of [3H] flunitrazepam to differentiating rat cerebral cells in culture. Brain Res. *177*, 418–422 (1979)

Duka, T., Höllt, V., Herz, A.: In vivo receptor occupation by benzodiazepines and correlation with the parmacological effect. Brain Res. *179*, 147–156 (1979a)

Duka, T., Wüster, M., Herz, A.: Rapid changes in enkephalin levels in rat striatum and hypothalamus induced by diazepam. Naunyn-Schmiedebergs Arch. Pharmacol. *309*, 1–5 (1979b)

Duka, T., Wüster, M., Herz, A.: Benzodiazepines modulate striatal enkephalin levels via a GABAergic mechanism. Life Sci. *26*, 771–776 (1980)

Dundee, J.W., Isaak, M.: Interaction of alcohol with sedatives and tranquillisers (a study of blood levels at loss of consciousness following rapid infusion). Med. Sci. Law *10*, 220–224 (1970)

Dunham, N.W., Miya, T.S.: A note on a simple apparatus for detecting neurological deficit in rats and mice. J. Am. Pharm. Assoc. (Sci. Ed.) *46*, 208–209 (1957)

Edanaca, M., Horizone, H., Okuda, K., Kita, T.: Studies on psychotropic drugs. Acute, subacute, and chronic toxication of 6-/o-Chlorophenyl/8-ethyl-1-methyl-4H-s-triazolo(3,4-c)-thieno(2,3-c)(1,4) diazepine (Y-7131). Pharmacometrics *16*, 1021–1046 (1978)

Edmonds, H.L., Stark, L.G., Hollinger, M.A.: The effects of diphenylhydantoin, phenobarbital and diazepam on the penicillin-induced epileptogenic focus in the rat. Exp. Neurol. *45*, 377–386 (1974)

Eidelberg, E., Lesse, H., Gault, F.P.: An experimental model of temporal lobe epilepsy: Studies of the convulsant properties of cocaine. In: EEG and Behavior. Glaser, G.H. (ed.), pp. 272–283. New York: Basic Books 1963

Eidelberg, E., Neer, H.M., Miller, M.K.: Anticonvulsant properties of some benzodiazepine derivatives. Neurology *15*, 223–230 (1965)

El-Hazmi, M.A.F.: On the interaction between thyroid hormones and the tranquillisers librium and valium. Clin. Chim. Acta *63*(2), 211–221 (1975)

Ellis, M.E., Johnson, H.L., Berger, F.M.: Benzodiazepine enhancement of propoxyphene analgesia. Fed. Proc. *36*, 1024 (1977)

Englander, R.N., Johnson, R.N., Brickley, J.J., Hanna, G.R.: Effects of antiepileptic drugs on thalamocortical excitability. Neurology *27*, 1134–1139 (1977)

Enna, S.J., Snyder, S.H.: Influence of ions, enzymes and detergents on gamma-aminobutyric acid receptor binding in synaptic membranes of rat brain. Mol. Pharmacol. *13*, 442–453 (1977)

Essman, W.B.: Subcellular actions of benzodiazepines. In: The Benzodiazepines. Garattini, S., Mussini, E., Randall, L.O. (eds.), pp. 177–190. New York: Raven Press 1973

Essman, W.B.: Benzodiazepines and aggressive behavior. Mod. Probl. Pharmacopsychiatry *13*, 13–28 (1978)

Evans, R.H. Effects of central depressant drugs on the isolated hemisected spinal cord of the immature rat. Br. J. Pharmacol. *60*, 273P–274P (1977)

Evans, R.H., Francis, A.A., Watkins, J.C.: Differential antagonism by chlorpromazine and diazepam of frog motoneurone depolarization induced by glutamate-related amino acids. Eur. J. Pharmacol. *44*, 325–330 (1977)

Fadda, F., Argiolas, A., Melis, M.R., Tissari, A.H., Onali, P.L., Gessa, G.L.: Stress-induced increase in 3,4-dihydroxyphenylacetic acid (DOPAC) levels in the cerebral cortex and in n. accumbens: reversal by diazepam. Life Sci. *23*, 2219–2224 (1978)

Falk, R.B., Denlinger, J.K., Nahrwold, M.L., Todd, R.A.: Acute vasodilation following induction of anaesthesia with intravenous diazepam and nitrous oxide. Anesthesiology *49*, 149–150 (1978)

Falk, J.L., Burnidge, G.K.: Fluid intake and punishment-attenuating drugs. Physiol. Behav. *5*, 199–202 (1970)

Fallert, M., Böhmer, G., Dinse, H.R.O., Sommer, T.J., Bittner, A.: Microelectrophoretic application of putative neurotransmitters onto various types of bulbar respiratory neurons. Arch. Ital. Biol. *117*, 1–12 (1979)

Fehske, K.J., Müller, W.E., Wollert, U.: A highly reactive tyrosine residue as part of the indole and benzodiazepine binding site of human serum albumin. Biochim. Biophys. Acta *577*, 346–359 (1979)

Feinstein, M.B., Lenard, W., Mathias, J.: The antagonism of local anesthetic induced convulsions by the benzodiazepine derivative diazepam. Arch. Int. Pharmacodyn. *187*, 144–154 (1970)

Feldman, S.A., Crawley, B.E.: Interaction of diazepam with the muscle-relaxant drugs. Br. Med. J. *1970 II*, 336–338 (1970)

Feldman, R.S., Smith, W.C.: Chlordiazepoxide-fluoxetine interactions on food intake in free-feeding rats. Pharmacol. Biochem. Behav. *8*, 749–752 (1978)

Fennessy, M.R., Lee, J.R.: The effect of benzodiazepines on brain amines of the mouse. Arch. Int. Pharmacodyn. Ther. *197*, 37–44 (1972)

Fennessy, M.R., Sawynok, J.: The effect of benzodiazepines on the analgesic effet of morphine and sodium salicylate. Arch. Int. Pharmacodyn. Ther. *204*, 77–85 (1973)

Fernandez, P.L., Martinez, A.M.: The interaction of diazepam with neuromuscular blocking agents. J. Internat. Res. Commun. *1*(6), 14 (1973)

Fernandez-Tomé, M.P., Fuentes, J.A., Madronero, R., del Rio, J.: Pharmacological properties of 6,7-tetramethylene-5-phenyl-1,2-dihydro-3H-thieno(2,3-e)(1,4)-diazepin-2-one (QM-6008, Thiadipone), a new psychotropic drug. Arzneim. Forsch. *25*(6), 926–934 (1975)

Fernstrom, J.D., Shabshelowitz, H., Faller, D.V.: Diazepam increases 5-hydroxyindole concentrations in rat brain and spinal cord. Life Sci. *15*, 1577–1584 (1974)

Ferrini, R., Miragoli, G.: Effetti inotropi e cronotropi di alcune benzodiazepine sull'atrio isolato di cavia. Boll. Soc. Ital. Biol. Sper. *49*, 644–647 (1973)

Ferrini, R., Miragoli, G., Taccardi, B.: Neuropharmacological studies on SB 5833, a new psychotherapeutic agent of the benzodiazepin class. Arzneim. Forsch. *24*, 2029–2032 (1974)

Feszt, T., Buska, C., Cuparencu, B., Horak, J.: Influence of some benzodiazepines on serum lipids levels in hyperlipidaemic rabbits. Agressologie *18*, 265–267 (1977)

Fetterer, R.E., Bennett, J.L.: Clonazepam and praziquantel: Mode of antischistosomal action. Fed. Proc. *37*, 604 (1978)

Field, D.E., Malpass, C.A., Jr., Frank, M.J.: Hemodynamic and electrocardiographic effects following the acute administration of chlorpromazine and diazepam. Clin. Res. *19*(2), 313 (1971)

Fielding, S., Hoffmann, I.: Pharmacology of anti-anxiety drugs with special reference to clobazam. Br. J. Clin. Pharmacol. *7*, 7S–15S (1979)

Fielding, S., Lal, H. (eds.): Anxiolytics. New York: Futura Publishing Company, Inc. Mount Kisco 1979

Figler, M.H., Klein, R.M., Thompson, C.S.: Chlordiazepoxide (librium)-induced changes in intraspecific attack and selected non-agonistic behaviors in male Siamese fighting fish. Psychopharmacologia *42*, 139–145 (1975)

File, S.E., Vellucci, S.V.: Studies on the role of ACTH and of 5-HT in anxiety, using an animal model. J. Pharm. Pharmacol. *30*, 105–110 (1978)

Flaherty, C.F., Lombardi, B.R., Wrightson, J., Deptula, D.: Conditions under which chlordiazepoxide influences gustatory contrast. Psychopharmacology *67*, 269–277 (1980)

Fletcher, A., Green, S.E., Hodges, H.M., Summerfield, A.: Evidence for a role of Gaba in benzodiazepine effects on feeding in rats. Br. J. Pharmacol. *69*, 274P–275P (1980)

Florez, J.: The action of diazepam, nitrazepam, and clonazepam on the respiratory center of decerebrate cats. Eur. J. Pharmacol. *14*, 250–256 (1971)

Forney, R.B., Hulpieu, H.R., Hughes, F.W.: The comparative enhancement of the depressant action of alcohol by eight representative ataractic and analgesic drugs. Experientia *18*, 468–470 (1962)

Fournadjev, G., Boismare, F., Lechat, P.: Activité comparée de diverses associations d'anticonvulsivants vis-à-vis l'électrochoc chez la souris. Thérapie *23*, 1363–1370 (1968)

Fox, K.A., Guerriero, F.J.: Effect of benzodiazepines on age of vaginal perforation and first estrus in mice. Res. Commun. Chem. Pathol. Pharmacol. *21*, 181–184 (1978)

Fox, K.A., Snyder, R.L.: Effect of sustained low doses of diazepam on aggression and mortality in grouped male mice. J. Comp. Physiol. Psychol. *69*, 663–666 (1969)

Fox, K.A., Guerriero, F.J., Zanghi, D.C.: Oxazepam, prazepam, and aggression in mice. Pharmacol. Res. Commun. *6*, 301–306 (1974)

Fox, K.A., Tuckosh, J.R., Wilcox, A.H.: Increased aggression among grouped male mice fed chlordiazepoxide. Eur. J. Pharmacol. *11*, 119–121 (1970)

Fox, K.A., Webster, J.C., Guerriero, F.J.: Increased aggression among grouped male mice fed nitrazepam and flurazepam. Pharmacol. Res. Commun. *4*, 157–162 (1972)

Franco, S., Schlosser, W.: GABA antagonistic effect of a convulsant benzodiazepine. Fed. Proc. *37*, 613 (1978)

Frank, G.B., Jhamandas, K., Effects of general depressant drugs on the electrical responses of isolated slabs of cat's cerebral cortex. Br. J. Pharmacol. *39*, 707–715 (1970)

Fratta, W., Mereu, G., Chessa, P., Paglietti, E., Gessa, G.: Benzodiazepine-induced voraciousness in cats and inhibition of amphetamine-anorexia. Life Sci. *18*, 1157–1166 (1976)

Frommel, E., Fleury, C., Schmidt-Ginzkey, J., Béguin, M.: De la pharmacodynamie différentielle thymoanaleptiques et des substances „neuroleptiques" en expérimentation animale. Thérapie *15*, 1175–1198 (1960a)

Frommel, E., Fleury, C., Schmidt-Ginzkey, J., Béguin, M.: De l'action pharmacodynamique d'un nouveau tranquillisant: le méthaminodiazépoxide ou librium, étude expérimentale. Thérapie *15*, 1233–1244 (1960b)

Fukuda, N., Saji, Y., Nagawa, Y.: Neuropharmacological studies of effect of new central depressant, 8-chloro-6-phenyl-4H-S-triazolo (4,3-a)(1,4) benzodiazepine (D-40TA) on EEG and central sympathetic activating mechanism in cats. Japan. J. Pharmacol. *24*, 75–88 (1974)

Funderburk, W.H., Foxwell, M.H., Hakala, M.W.: Effects of psychotherapeutic drugs on hypothalamic-induced hissing in cats. Neuropharmacology *9*, 1–7 (1970)

Fung, S.J., Strahlendorf, H.K., Strahlendorf, J.C., Barnes, C.D.: Attenuation of nucleus accumbens induced inhibition of substantia nigra unit activity by bicuculline. 9th Ann. Meeting Soc. Neurosci., Abstr. *5*, 71 (1979)

Furukawa, T., Yamazaki, M., Hiraga, Y., Fukazawa, E., Kushiku, K., Nakano, U., Yoshihara, K., Ichimasa, S., Tokuda, M.: Potentiation of effects of catecholamines and sympathetic stimulation by a triazolobenzodiazepine. Japan. J. Pharmacol. *26*, Suppl., 52P (1976)

Fuxe, K., Agnati, L.F., Bolme, P., Hökfelt, T., Lidbrink, P., Ljungdahl, A., de la Mora, M.P., Ögren, S.-O.: The possible involvement of GABA mechanisms in the action of benzodiazepines on central catecholamine neurons. Adv. Biochem. Psychopharmacol. *14*, 45–61 (1975)

Gähwiler, B.H.: Diazepam and chlordiazepoxide: Powerful GABA antagonists in explants of rat cerebellum. Brain Res. *107*, 176–179 (1976)

Gale, K., Costa, E., Toffano, G., Hong, J.-S., Guidotti, A.: Evidence for a role of nigral γ-aminobutyric acid and substance P in the haloperidol-induced activation of striatal tyrosine hydroxylase. J. Pharmacol. *206*, 29–38 (1978)

Gall, M., Lahti, R.A., Rudzik, A.D., Duchamp, D.J., Chidester, C., Scahill, T.: Novel anxiolytic agents derived from α-amino-α-phenyl-o-tolyl-4H-triazoles and -imidazoles. J. Med. Chem. *21*, 542–548 (1978)

Gallager, D.W.: Benzodiazepines: Potentiation of a GABA inhibitory response in the dorsal raphé nucleus. Eur. J. Pharmacol. *49*, 133–143 (1978)

Gallager, D.W., Thomas, J.W., Tallman, J.F.: Effect of GABAergic drugs on benzodiazepine binding site sensitivity in rat cerebral cortex. Biochem. Pharmacol. *27*, 2745–2749 (1978)

Gallager, D.W., Mallorga, P., Tallman, J.F.: Diphenylhydantoin: Interaction with [^{3}H]diazepam binding site in brain and anticonvulsant activity. 9th Ann. Meeting Soc. Neurosci. Atlanta. Abstr. *5*, 193 (1979)

Gallager, D.W., Mallorga, P., Tallman, J.F.: Interaction of diphenylhydantoin and benzodiazepines in the CNS. Brain Res. *189*, 209–220 (1980)

Galzigna, L.: Interaction between diazepam and serotonin. FEBS Letters *3*, 97–98 (1969)

Gamba, A.: Un nuovo metodo per tests di coordinazione motoria sul topo. Boll. Chim. Farm. *105*, 148–153 (1966)

Garattini, S., Mussini, E., Randall, L.O. (Eds.): The Benzodiazepines. New York: Raven Press 1973

Garber, J.G., Ominsky, A.J., Orkin, F.K., Quinn, P.: Physostigmine-atropine solution fails to reverse diazepam sedation. Anesth. Analg. *54*, 58–60 (1980)

Garcia Leme, J., Rocha e Silva, M.: Competitive and non-competitive inhibition of bradykinin on the guinea-pig ileum. Br. J. Pharmacol. *25*, 50–58 (1965)

Gardner, C.R., Webster, R.A.: The effect of some anticonvulsant drugs on leptazol and bicuculline induced acetylcholine efflux from rat cerebral cortex. Br. J. Pharmacol. *47*, 652P (1973)

Gartside, I.B.: The actions of diazepam and phenytoin on a low dose penicillin epileptiform focus in the anaesthetized rat. Br. J. Pharmacol. *62*, 289–292 (1978)

Gascon, A.L.: Effect of acute stress and ouabain administration on adrenal catecholamine content and cardiac function of rats pretreated with diazepam. Can. J. Physiol. Pharmacol. *55*, 65–71 (1977)

Gascon, A.L., Lelorier, J.: Increase in catecholamine content of the rat adrenals after pretreatment with diazepam. Can. J. Physiol. Pharmacol. *53*, 1198–1199 (1975)

Gasser, J.C., Bellville, J.W.: The respiratory effects of hydroxyzine, diazepam and pentazocine in man. Anaesthesia *31*, 718–723 (1976)

Gasser, J.C., Kaufman, R.D., Bellville, J.W.: Respiratory effects of lorazepam, pentobarbital and pentazocine. Clin. Pharmacol. Ther. *18*, 170–174 (1975)

Gatti, G.L., Bonavoglia, F., Michalek, H.: Brain acetylcholine levels in diazepam attenuation of DFP toxicity in mice. Abstracts, 4th Int. Meeting Int. Soc. Neurochem., Tokyo, p. 492 (1973)

Gavish, M., Chang, R.S.L., Snyder, S.H.: Solubilization of histamine H-1, GABA and benzodiazepine receptors. Life Sci. *25*, 783–790 (1979)

Gay, P.E., Potter, L.S., Cole, S.O.: Interacting effects of amygdala lesions with chlordiazepoxide and pilocarpine on mouse killing by rats. Bull. Psychonomic Soc. *7*, 69–71 (1976)

Gebhart, G.F., Plaa, G.L., Mitchell, C.L.: The effects of ethanol alone and in combination with phenobarbital, chlorpromazine, or chlordiazepoxide. Toxicol. Appl. Pharmacol. *15*, 405–414 (1969)

Gehrmann, J.E., Killam, K.F., Jr.: Studies of central functional equivalence. I. Time-varying distribution of power in discrete frequency bands of the EEG as a function of drug exposure. Neuropharmacology *17*, 747–759 (1978)

Geisler, L., Herberg, D.: Untersuchungen über den Einfluß einiger häufig verwendeter Pharmaka auf die Erregbarkeit des Atemzentrums beim Menschen. Therapiewoche 47, 1941–1943 (1967)

Geller, H.M.: Transmitter mechanisms of basal hypothalamus in tissue culture. In: Iontophoresis and Transmitter Mechanisms in the Mammalian Central Nervous System. Ryall, R.W., Kelly, J.S. (eds.), pp. 212–214. Amsterdam: Elsevier 1978

Geller, H.M.: Water soluble benzodiazepines with agonistic and antagonistic actions on GABA-induced inhibition in cultured hypothalamus. Neurosci. Letters 15, 313–318 (1979)

Geller, H.M., Woodward, D.J.: Synaptic organization of tuberal hypothalamus in tissue culture: Effects of electrical stimulation and blockers of synaptic transmission. Exp. Neurol. 64, 535–552 (1979)

Geller, H.M., Taylor, D.A., Hoffer, B.J.: Benzodiazepines and central inhibitory mechanisms. Naunyn-Schmiedebergs Arch. Pharmacol. 304, 81–88 (1978)

Gerhards, H.J.: Neuropharmacological profile of clobazepam, a new 1',5'-benzodiazepine. Psychopharmacology 58, 27–33 (1978)

Gerold, M., Cavero, I., Riggenbach, H., Wall, M., Haeusler, G.: Analysis of cardiac chronotropic responses to diazepam and bromazepam in conscious dogs. Eur. J. Pharmacol. 35, 361–368 (1976)

Gey, K.F.: Effect of benzodiazepines on carbohydrate metabolism in rat brain. In: The Benzodiazepines. Garattini, S., Mussini, E., Randall, L.O. (eds.), pp. 243–255. New York: Raven Press 1973

Ghelarducci, B., Lenzi, G., Pompeiano, O.: A neurophysiological analysis of the postural effects of a benzodiazepine. Arch. int. Pharmacodyn. 163, 403–421 (1966)

Ghoneim, M.M., Mewaldt, S.P.: Studies on human memory: the interactions of diazepam, scopalamine, and physostigmine. Psychopharmacology 52, 1–6 (1977)

Giarman, N.J., Pepeu, G.: Drug-induced changes in brain acetylcholine. Br. J. Pharmacol. 19, 226–234 (1962)

Gilbert, J.J., Benson, D.F.: Transient global amnesia: report of two cases with definite etiologies. J. Nerv. Ment. Dis. 154, 461–464 (1972)

Gilbert, J.C., Wyllie, M.G.: Effects of anticonvulsants and convulsant drugs on the ATPase activities of synaptosomes and their components. Br. J. Pharmacol. 56, 49–57 (1976)

Gilbert, J.C., Gray, P., Heaton, G.W.: Anticonvulsant drugs and brain glucose. Biochem. Pharmacol. 20, 240–243 (1971)

Gillis, R.A., Thibodeaux, H., Barr, L.: Antiarrhythmic properties of chlordiazepoxide. Circulation 49, 272–282 (1974)

Giunta, F., Ottino, C.A., Rossi, G.F., Tercero, E.: Studio sperimentale dell'azione antiepilettica di un nuovo derivato benzodiazepinico (Ro 5-4023). Riv. Neurol. 11, 213–223 (1970)

Giurgea, C.E., Moyersoons, F.E.: On the pharmacology of cortical evoked potentials. Arch. Int. Pharmacodyn. Ther. 199, 67–68 (1972)

Gleason, N.M., Gosselin, R.E., Hodge, H.C. (eds.): Clinical Toxicology of Commercial Products. Baltimore, Md.: William and Wilkins 1963

Gluckman, M.I.: Pharmacology of oxazepam (serax), a new antianxiety agent. Curr. Ther. Res. 7, 721–740 (1965)

Gluckman, M.I.: Pharmacology of 7-chloro-5-(o-chlorophenyl)-1,3-dihydro-3-hydroxy-2H-1,4-benzodiazepin-2-one (lorazepam; Wy 4036). Arzneim. Forsch. 21, 1049–1055 (1971)

Gluckman, M.I.: Pharmacology of lorazepam. J. clin. Psychiatry 39, 3–10 (1978)

Goff, D., Miller, A.A., Webster, R.A.: Anticonvulsant drugs and folic acid on the development of epileptic kindling in rats. Br. J. Pharmacol. 64, 406P (1978)

Gogerty, J.H.: Pharmacological methods and prediction of the clinical value of hypnotic agents. In: Sleep: Physiology, Biochemistry, Psychology, Pharmacology, Clinical Implications. 1st Europ. Congr. Sleep Res., Basel, 1972, Koella, W.P., Levin, P. (eds.), pp. 69–83. Basel: Karger 1973

Gogolak, G., Pillat, B.: Effect of mogadon on the arousal reaction in rabbits. Prog. Brain Res. 18, 229–230 (1965)

Gogolak, G., Liebeswar, G., Stumpf, C.: Action of drugs on the electrical activity of the red nucleus. Electroenceph. clin. Neurophysiol. 27, 296–303 (1969)

Gogolak, G., Liebeswar, G., Stumpf, C., Williams, H.: The relationship between barbiturate-induced activities in the cerebellum and the red nucleus of the rabbit. Electroenceph. Clin. Neurophysiol. 29, 67–73 (1970)

Gogolak, G., Krijzer, F., Stumpf, C.: Action of central depressant drugs on the electrocerebellogram of the rabbit. Arch. Pharmacol. 272, 378–386 (1972)

Gogolak, G., Stumpf, C., Tschakaloff, C.: Antikonvulsive Wirkung von Clonazepam und Ro 8-4192 gegen Penicillin- und Lidocain-Krämpfe. Arzneim. Forsch. 23, 545–549 (1973)

Gogolak, G., Huck, S., Porges, P., Stumpf, C.: Action of strychnine and central depressants on the cerebello-rubral system. Arch. Int. Pharmacodyn. Ther. 207, 322–332 (1974)

Goldberg, H., Horvath, T.B., Meares, R.A.: Visual evoked potentials as a measure of drug effects on arousal in the rabbits. Clin. Exp. Pharmacol. Physiol. 1, 147–154 (1974)

Goldberg, M.E.: Pharmacologic activity of a new class of agents which selectively inhibit aggressive behavior in rats. Arch. Int. Pharmacodyn. Ther. 186, 287–297 (1970)

Goldberg, M.E., Manian, A.A., Efron, D.H.: A comparative study of certain pharmacologic responses following acute and chronic administrations of chlordiazepoxide. Life Sci. 6, 481–491 (1967)

Goldstein, L., Gardocki, J.F., Mundschenk, D.L., O'Brien, G.: The effect of psychotropic drugs on the occurrence of paradoxical sleep in rabbits and cats. Fed. Proc. 26, 506 (1967)

Gottschalk, L.A., Noble, E.P., Stolzoff, G.E., Bates, D.E., Cable, C.G., Uliana, R.L., Birch, H., Fleming, E.W.: Relationships of chlordiazepoxide blood levels to psychological and biochemical responses. In: The Benzodiazepines. Garattini, S., Mussini, E., Randall, L.O. (eds.), pp. 257–280. New York: Raven Press 1973

Govoni, S., Fresia, P., Spano, P.F., Trabucchi, M.: Effect of desmethyldiazepam and chlordesmethyldiazepam on 3',5'-cyclic guanosine monophosphate levels in rat cerebellum. Psychopharmacology 50, 241–244 (1976)

Gran, L., Coggin, R., Bennett, P.B.: Diazepam under hyperbaric conditions in rats. Acta Anaesth. Scand. 24, 404–411 (1980)

Grandison, L., Guidotti, A.: Stimulation of food intake by muscimol and beta endorphin. Neuropharmacology 16, 533–536 (1977)

Gray, J.A., McNaughton, N., James, D.T.D., Kelly, P.H.: Effect of minor tranquillisers on hippocampal theta rhythm mimicked by depletion of forebrain noradrenaline. Nature 258, 424–425 (1975)

Green, J.D., Arduini, A.: Hippocampal electrical activity in arousal. J. Neurophysiol. 17, 533–557 (1954)

Greenlee, D.V., Van Ness, P.C., Olsen, R.W.: Endogenous inhibitor of GABA binding in mammalian brain. Life Sci. 22, 1653–1662 (1978)

Griauzde, M.L., Chen, E.H., Radulovački, M.: Effects of diazepam on sleep, temperature, 5-hydroxyindoleacetic acid and homovanillic acid in cisternal cerebrospinal fluid of cats. Pharmacology 19, 149–155 (1979)

Grotto, M., Sulman, F.G.: Interaction of analgesic effects of psychopharmaca. Arch. Int. Pharmacodyn. Ther. 170, 257–263 (1967)

Gruber, C.M., Ellis, F.W., Freedman, G.: A toxicological and pharmacological investigation of sodium sec-butyl ethyl barbituric acid (butisol sodium). J. Pharmacol. Exp. Ther. 81, 254–268 (1944)

Grudzinska, E., Gidynska, T., Rump, S.: Therapeutic value of anticonvulsant drugs in poisonings with an organophosphate. Arch. Int. Pharmacodyn. 238, 344–350 (1979)

Guaitani, A., Marcucci, F., Garattini, S.: Increased aggression and toxicity in grouped male mice treated with tranquilizing benzodiazepines. Psychopharmacologia 19, 241–245 (1971)

Guerrero-Figueroa, R., Gallant, D.M.: Electrophysiological study of the action of a new benzodiazepine derivative (ORF-8063) on the central nervous system. Curr. Ther. Res. 13, 747–758 (1971)

Guerrero-Figueroa, R., Rye, M.M., Gallant, D.M.: Effects of diazepam on three per second spike and wave discharges. Curr. Ther. Res. 9, 522–535 (1967)

Guerrero-Figueroa, R., Rye, M.M., Guerrero-Figueroa, C.: Effects of diazepam on secondary subcortical epileptogenic tissues. Curr. Ther. Res. 10, 150–166 (1968)

Guerrero-Figueroa, R., Rye, M.M., Heath, R.G.: Effects of two benzodiazepine derivatives on cortical and subcortical epileptogenic tissues in the cat and monkey. I. Limbic system structures. Curr. Ther. Res. 11, 27–39 (1969 a)

Guerrero-Figueroa, R., Rye, M.M., Heath, R.G.: Effects of two benzodiazepine derivatives on cortical and subcortical epileptogenic tissues in the cat and monkey. II. Cortical and centrencephalic structures. Curr. Ther. Res. *11*, 40–50 (1969b)

Guerrero-Figueroa, R., Gallant, D.M., Guerrero-Figueroa, C., Gallant, J.: Electrophysiological analysis of the action of four benzodiazepines derivatives on the central nervous system. In: The Benzodiazepines. Garattini, S., Mussini, E., Randall, L.O. (eds.), pp. 489–512. New York: Raven Press 1973

Guerrero-Figueroa, R., Guerrero-Figueroa, E., Sneed, G.A., Kennedy, M.J.: Effects of lorazepam on CNS structures: Neurophysiological and behavioral correlations. Curr. Ther. Res. *16*, 137–146 (1974)

Guerriero, F.J., Fox, K.A.: Benzodiazepine-induced suppression of estrous cycles in C57 BL/6 J mice. Res. Commun. Chem. Pathol. Pharmacol. *11*, 155–158 (1975)

Guidotti, A.: Synaptic mechanisms in the action of benzodiazepines. In: Psychopharmacology: A generation of progress. Lipton, M.A., DiMascio, A., Killam, K.F. (eds.), pp. 1349–1357. New York: Raven Press 1978

Guidotti, A., Kurosawa, A., Costa, E.: Association between the increase of cAMP content and the trans-synaptic induction of tyrosine hydroxylase in rat adrenal medulla. Naunyn-Schmiedebergs Arch. Pharmacol. *295*, 135–140 (1976)

Guidotti, A., Toffano, G., Costa, E.: An endogenous protein modulates the affinity of GABA and benzodiazepine receptors in rat brain. Nature *275*, 553–555 (1978)

Guidotti, A., Toffano, G., Baraldi, M., Schwartz, J.P., Costa, E.: A molecular mechanism for the facilitation of GABA receptor function by benzodiazepines. In: GABA-Neurotransmitters. Krogsgaard-Larsen, P., Scheel-Krüger, J., Kofod, H. (eds.), pp. 406–415. Copenhagen: Munksgaard 1979

Guignard, J.P., Filloux, B., Lavoie, J., Pelet, J., Torrado, A.: Effect of intravenous diazepam on renal function. Clin. Pharmacol. Ther. *18*, 401–404 (1975)

Gumulka, S.W., Dinnendahl, V., Schönhöfer, P.S., Stock, K.: Dopaminergic stimulants and cyclic nucleotides in mouse brain. Effects of dopaminergic antagonists, cholinolytics, and GABA agonists. Naunyn-Schmiedebergs Arch. Pharmacol. *295*, 21–26 (1976)

Gupta, S.K., Gaitonde, B.B.: Analgesic activity of a new quinoline derivative Ro 4-1778. Indian J. Physiol. Pharmacol. *8*, 27–32 (1964)

Gutman, Y., Boonyaviroy, P.: Activation of adrenal medulla adenylate cyclase and catecholamine secretion. Naunyn-Schmiedebergs Arch. Pharmacol. *307*, 39–44 (1979)

Gyermek, L.: Benzodiazepines for supplementing steroid anesthesia. Life Sci. *14*, 1433–1436 (1974)

Gylys, J.A., Chamberlain, J.H., Wright, R.N., Doran, K.M.: Interaction between diazepam and naloxone in conflict, novel food intake and antimetrazol tests. Fed. Proc. *38*, 863 (1979)

Haas, H.L., Siegfried, J.: Intracellular recording from cortical slices of rat and man in vitro: Action of diazepines. Experientia *34*, 924 (1978)

Haas, H.L., Schaerer, B., Vosmansky, M.: A simple perfusion chamber for the study of nervous tissue slices in vitro. J. Neurosci. Meth. *1*, 323–325 (1979)

Haefely, W.E.: Synaptic pharmacology of barbiturates and benzodiazepines. Agents Actions *7*, 353–359 (1977)

Haefely, W.: Behavioral and neuropharmacological aspects of drugs used in anxiety and related states. In: Psychopharmacology: A Generation of Progress. Lipton, M.A., DiMascio, A., Killam, K.F. (eds.), pp. 1359–1374. New York: Raven Press 1978a

Haefely, W.E.: Central actions of benzodiazepines: General Introduction. Br. J. Psychiat. *133*, 231–238 (1978b)

Haefely, W.: GABA as a neurotransmitter and target for drugs. In: Dimensions in health research: Search for the medicine of tomorrow. Weissbach, H., Kunz, R.M. (eds.), pp. 195–208 New York: Academic Press 1978c

Haefely, W.: Involvement of GABA in the actions of neuropsychotropic agents. Int. J. Neurol. *13*, 53–66 (1979)

Haefely, W.: Biological basis of the therapeutic effects of benzodiazepines. In: First International Symposium. Benzodiazepines Today and Tomorrow. Priest, R.G., Vianna Filho, U., Amrein, R., Skreta, M. (eds.) pp. 19–45. Lancaster: MTP Press, 1980a

Haefely, W.: GABA and the anticonvulsant action of benzodiazepines and barbiturates. In: GABA and other inhibitory Neurotransmitters. Brain Research Bull. *5*, Suppl. 2., 873–878 (1980b)

Haefely, W., Jalfre, M., Ruch-Monachon, M.-A.: A pathway and neurotransmitters involved in the control of noradrenergic locus coeruleus neurons. In: Chemical Tools in Catecholamine Research. Almgren, O., Carlsson, A., Engel, J. (eds.), Vol. II, pp. 135–142. Amsterdam: North-Holland Publishing Company 1975a

Haefely, W., Kulcsár, A., Möhler, H., Pieri, L., Polc, P., Schaffner, R.: Possible involvement of GABA in the central actions of benzodiazepines. In: Mechanism of Action of Benzodiazepines. Costa, E., Greengard, P. (eds.), pp. 131–151. New York: Raven Press 1975b

Haefely, W., Ruch-Monachon, M.-A., Jalfre, M., Schaffner, R.: Interaction of psychotropic agents with central neurotransmitters as revealed by their effects on PGO-waves in the cat. Drug Res. *26*, 1036–1039 (1976)

Haefely, W., Keller, H.H., Pieri, L., Polc, P., Schaffner, R., Zihlmann, R.: Interaction of minor tranquillizers with synaptic processes mediated by GABA. In: Neuro-Psychopharmacology. Proc. 10th C.I.N.P. Congr., Québec, 1976. Deniker, P., Radouco-Thomas, C., Villeneuve, A. (eds.), pp. 907–916. Oxford: Pergamon Press 1978

Haefely, W., Polc, P., Schaffner, R., Keller, H.H., Pieri, L., Möhler, H.: Facilitation of GABAergic transmission by drugs. In: GABA-Neurotransmitters, Krogsgaard-Larsen, P., Scheel-Krüger, J., Kofod, H. (eds.), pp. 357–375. Copenhagen: Munksgaard 1979a

Haefely, W., Polc, P., Pieri, L., Schaffner, R.: Effects of benzodiazepines on the electrical activity of the central nervous system: correlation with synaptic pharmacology. In: Neuro-Psychopharmacology. Proc. 11th C.I.N.P. Congr., Wien 1978, Saletu, B., Berner, P., Hollister, L. (eds.), pp. 449–458. New York: Pergamon Press 1979b

Haefely, W., Bandle, E., Burkard, W.P., Da Prada, M., Keller, H.H., Kettler, R., Möhler, H., Richards, J.G.: Pharmacology of central neurotransmitters in advanced age. In: Etats déficitaires cérébraux liés à l'âge. Tissot, R. (ed.), pp. 329–353. Genève: Georg 1980

Haller, J.: Quantification of the psychotropic drug-induced changes in the feline EEG. Ph. D. thesis, pp. 1–266. Basel 1979

Hamilton, J.T.: Muscle relaxant activity of chlordiazepoxide and diazepam. Can. J. Physiol. Pharmacol. *45*, 191–199 (1967)

Hanasono, G.K., De Repentigny, L., Priestly, B.G., Plaa, G.L.: The effects of oral diazepam pretreatment on the biliary excretion of sulfobromophtalein in rats. Can. J. Physiol. Pharmacol. *54*, 603–612 (1976)

Haot, J., Djahanguiri, B., Richelle, M.: Action protectrice du chlordiazépoxide sur l'ulcère de contrainte chez le rat. Arch. Int. Pharmacodyn. Ther. *148*, 557–559 (1964)

Hara, C., Watanabe, S., Ueki, S.: Effects of drugs injected into the hypothalamus on muricide and EEG in the olfactory bulbectomized rats. Jpn. J. Pharmacol. *25*, Suppl., 45P (1975)

Hara, T., Masuda, K., Miyake, H.: Effects of psychotropic drugs on the PGO wave occuring in REM sleep and on the reserpine-induced PGO waves. Adv. Sleep Res. *2*, 131–154 (1975)

Hashimoto, T., Shuto, K., Ichikawa, S.: Studies on flurazepam. I. Effects of flurazepam on the central nervous system. Pharmacometrics *7*, 381–398 (1973)

Havard, C.W.H., Saldanha, V.F., Bird, R., Gardner, R.: Effects of centrally acting drugs on pituitary adrenal axis. Acta Endocrinol. (Kbh.) *155*, 31 (1971)

Havdala, H., Borison, R., Diamond, B.: Anesthetics and anesthetic premedicants upon biogenic amine turnover. Fed. Proc. *36*, 1004 (1977)

Heidler, I., Mares, J., Trojan, S.: Influence of rivotril (clonazepam) on the spontaneous EEG in rats. Activ. Nerv. Sup. (Praha) *21*, 13–14 (1979)

Heilman, R.D., Bauer, E.W., Da Vanzo, J.P.: Pharmacologic studies with triflubazam (ORF 8063): a new psychotherapeutic agent. Curr. Ther. Res. *16*, 1022–1032 (1974)

Heinemann, H., Stock, G.: Chlordiazepoxide and its effect on sleep wakefulness behavior in unrestrained cats. Arzneim. Forsch. *23*, 823–825 (1973)

Heinemann, H., Hartmann, A., Sturm V.: Der Einfluß von Medazepam auf die Schlaf-Wach-Regulation von wachen, unnarkotisierten Katzen. Arzneim. Forsch. *18*, 1557–1559 (1968)

Heinemann, H., Stosiek, U., Hartmann, A.: The effect of medazepam (Nobrium) on the sleep-wake regulation and on the blood pressure of alert, non-anesthetized cats. Arch. Exp. Pathol. Pharmacol. *203*, 220 (1969)

Heinemann, H., Hartmann, A., Stock, G., Sturm, V.: Die Wirkung von Medazepam auf Schwellen subcorticaler, limbischer Reizantworten, gemessen an unnarkotisierten, frei beweglichen Katzen. Arzneim. Forsch. *20*, 413–415 (1970)

Heise, G.A., Boff, E.: Taming action of chlordiazepoxide. Fed. Proc. *20*, 393 (1961)

Heiss, W.-D., Hoyer, J., Heilig, P.: Die Wirkung von Psychopharmaka auf visuell evozierte Potentiale der Katze. Vision Res. *9*, 507–513 (1969)

Henn, F.A., Henke, D.J.: Cellular localization of ^{3}H-diazepam receptors. Neuropharmacology *17*, 985–988 (1978)

Herberg, D., Geisler, L., Bohr, W., Utz, G.: Untersuchungen am Menschen über den Einfluß verschiedener Pharmaka auf die CO_2-sensible zentrale Atmungsregulation mittels CO_2-Antwortkurven. Pharmacol. Clin. *1*, 54–62 (1968)

Herink, J., Hrdina, V., Květina, J., Nemeček, S.: Facilitation of after-discharges in the limbic system after a mesencephalic lesion and effect of diazepam. Activ. Nerv. Sup. (Praha) *18*, 234–235 (1976)

Hernández-Peón, R., Rojas-Ramírez, J.A.: Central mechanisms of tranquilizing, anticonvulsant and relaxant actions of Ro 4-5360. Int. J. Neuropharmacol. *5*, 263–267 (1966)

Hernández-Peón, R., Rojas-Ramírez, J.A:, O'Flaherty, J.J., Mazzuchelli-O'Flaherty, A.L.: An experimental study of the anticonvulsive and relaxant actions of valium. Int. J. Neuropharmacol. *3*, 405–412 (1964)

Hess, W.R.: The functional organization of the diencephalon. New York: Grune and Stratton 1957

Hess, S.M., Chasin, M., Free, C.A., Harris, D.N.: Modulators of cyclic AMP systems. Adv. Biochem. Psychopharmacol. *14*, 153–167, 1975

Hester, J.B., Rudzik, A.D., Kamdar, B.V.: 6-phenyl-4H-s-triazolo (4,3-a)(1,4) benzodiazepines which have central nervous system depressant activity. J. Med. Chem. *14*, 1078–1081 (1971)

Hester, J.B., Rudzik, A.D., Veldkampf, W.: Pyrrolo (3,2,1.JK) (1,4)benzodiazepines and pyrrolo (1,2,3-EF) (1,5)benzodiazepines which have central nervous system activity. J. Med. Chem. *13*, 827–835 (1970)

Heuschele, W.P.: Chlordiazepoxide for calming Zoo animals. J. Am. Vet. Med. Assoc. *139*, 996–998 (1961)

Hitch, D.C., Nolan, S.P.: Changes in myocardial performance and total peripheral resistance produced by the administration of chlordiazepoxide. J. Thorac. Cardiovasc. Surg. *61*, 352–358 (1971)

Höckel, S.H.J., Müller, W.E., Wollert, U.: Diazepam increases L-tryptophan uptake into various regions of the rat brain. Res. Commun. Psychol. Psychiatr. and Behav. *4*, 467–475 (1979)

Hockman, C.H., Livingston, K.E.: Inhibition of reflex vagal bradycardia by diazepam. Neuropharmacology *10*, 307–314 (1971)

Hodesson, S., Rich, S.T., Washington, J.O., Apt, L.: Anesthesia of the rabbit with equi-thesin following the administration of preanesthetics. Lab. Animal Care *15*, 336–344 (1965)

Hoffmeister, F.: Effects of psychotropic drugs on pain. In: "Pain", Proc. of the Int. Symposium on Pain, Paris, 1967, Soulairac, A., Cahen, J., Charpentier, J. (eds.), pp. 309–319. London, New York: Academic Press 1968

Hoffmeister, F.: Elektroenzephalogramm und Verhalten von Kaninchen im physiologischen und medikamentösen Schlaf. 3. Mitt.: Einfluß von Hypnotika auf das Schlafverhalten des Kaninchens; Besprechung der Ergebnisse und Zusammenfassung. Arzneim. Forsch. *22*, 563–569 (1972)

Hoffmeister, F., Wuttke, W.: On the actions of psychotropic drugs on the attack- and aggressive-defensive behaviour of mice and cats. In: Aggressive Behaviour, Garattini, S., Sigg, E.B. (eds.), pp. 273–280. Amsterdam: Excerpta Medica Foundation 1969

Holm, E.: Schlafmittelwirkungen auf subkortikale Hirngebiete. In: Der Schlaf, Neurophysiologische Aspekte. Jovanović, U.J. (ed.), pp. 163–182. München: Johann Ambrosius Barth 1969

Holmes, J.H., Kanfer, I., Zwarenstein, H.: Effect of benzodiazepine derivatives on human blood cholinesterase in vitro. Res. Commun. Chem. Path. Pharmacol. *21*, 367–370 (1978)

Holzer, P., Hagmüller, K.: Transient apnoe after systemic injection of GABA in the rat. Naunyn-Schmiedebergs Arch. Pharmacol. *308*, 55–60 (1979)

Hommer, K.: Die Wirkung den Chinins, Chlorochins, Jodacetats und Chlordiazepoxids auf das ERG der isolierten Kaninchennetzhaut. Albrecht v. Graefes Arch. Klin. Exp. Ophthal. *175*, 111–120 (1968)

Hong, J.-S., Yang, H.-Y.T., Fratta, W., Costa, E.: Rat striatal methionine-enkephalin content after chronic treatment with cataleptogenic and noncataleptogenic antischizophrenic drugs. J. Pharmacol. Exp. Ther. *205*, 141–147 (1978)

Hopf, H.C.: Anticonvulsant drugs and spike propagation of motor nerves and skeletal muscle. J. Neurol. Neurosurg. Psychiatry *36*, 574–580 (1973)

Hopf, H.C., Billmann, F.: The effect of diazepam on motor nerves and skeletal muscle. Z. Neurol. *204*, 255–262 (1973)

Horak, J., Cuparencu, B., Cucuinanu, M., Opincaru, A., Seusan, E., Vincze, I.: Effects of some benzodiazepine derivatives on triton WR-1339-induced hyperlipidaemia in rats. Atherosclerosis *24*, 81–97 (1976)

Hori, M., Ito, T., Yoshida, K., Shimizu, M.: Effect of anticonvulsants on spiking activity induced by cortical freezing in cats. Epilepsia *20*, 25–36 (1979)

Horng, J.S., Wong, D.T.: γ-Aminobutyric acid receptors in cerebellar membranes of rat brain after a treatment with triton X-100. J. Neurochem. *32*, 1379–1386 (1979)

Horovitz, Z.P., Furgiuele, A.R., Brannick, L.J., Burke, J.C., Craver, B.N.: A new chemical structure with specific depressant effects on the amygdala and on the hyper-irritability of the "septal rat". Nature *200*, 369–370 (1963)

Horovitz, Z.P., Ragozzino, P.W., Leaf, R.C.: Selective block of rat mouse-killing by antidepressants. Life Sci. *4*, 1909–1912 (1965)

Horovitz, Z.P., Piala, J.J., High, J.P., Burke, J.C., Leaf, R.C.: Effects of drugs on the mouse-killing (muricide) test and its relationship to amygdaloid function. Int. J. Neuropharmacol. *5*, 405–411 (1966)

Horton, R.W., Meldrum, B.S.: Seizures induced by allylglycine, 3-mercapto-propionic acid and 4-deoxypyridoxine in mice and photosensitive baboons, and the different modes of inhibition of cerebral glutamic acid decarboxylase. Br. J. Pharmacol. *49*, 52–63 (1973)

Horton, R.W., Meldrum, B.S., Sawaya, M.C.B., Stephenson, J.D.: Picrotoxin convulsions and GABA metabolism after injection of anticonvulsants in chicks. Eur. J. Pharmacol. *40*, 101–106 (1976)

Houser, V.P., Paré, W.P.: Analgesic potency of sodium salicylate, indomethacin, and chlordiazepoxide as measured by the spatial preference technique in the rat. Psychopharmacologia *32*, 121–131 (1973)

Howells,R.D., Miller, J.M., Simon, E.J.: Benzodiazepine binding sites are present in retina. Life Sci. *25*, 2131–2136 (1979)

Hoyer, J.: Wirkungsmechanismen von Benzodiazepinen. Elektrophysiologische Untersuchungen an Nervenzellen der Meeresschnecke Aplysia Californica. Pharmakopsychiatr. Neuropsychopharmakol. *10*, 271–280 (1977)

Hoyer, J., Klee, M.R., Heiss, W.-D.: Voltage clamp analysis of the action of a benzodiazepine on aplysia ganglion cells. In: Neurobiology of Invertebrates, Gastropoda Brain, 3rd Int. Symp., Tihány/Hung., 1975, Salanki, J. (ed.): pp. 253–265. Budapest: Akad. Kiadó 1976

Hoyer, J., Park, M.R., Klee, M.R.: Changes in ionic currents associated with flurazepam-induced abnormal discharges in Aplysia neurons. In: Abnormal neuronal discharges. Chalazonitis, N., Boisson, M. (eds.), pp. 301–316. New York: Raven Press 1978

Hoyumpa, A.M., Desmond, P.V., Roberts, R.K., Nichols, S., Johnson, R.F., Schenker, S.: Effect of ethanol on benzodiazepine disposition in dogs. J. Lab. Clin. Med. *95*, 310–322 (1980)

Huck, S.: The estimation of the survival rate of tetanus-intoxicated mice. A model for screening anti-tetanus drugs. Naunyn-Schmiedebergs Arch. Pharmacol. *308*, 77–79 (1979)

Huck, S., Stacher, G., Gogolak, G., Stumpf, C.: Action of six commonly used benzodiazepines on isolated guinea pig ileum preparation. Arch. Int. Pharmacodyn. *218*, 77–83 (1975)

Hudson, R.D., Wolpert, M.K.: Central muscle relaxant effects of diazepam. Neuropharmacology *9*, 481–488 (1970)

Hudson, L.D., Lakshminarayan, S., Sahn, S.A., Weil, J.V.: Diminished hypoxic ventilatory drive following diazepam. Amer. Rev. Respir. Dis. *109*, 694 (1974)

Hunkeler, W., Möhler, H., Pieri, L., Polc, P., Bonetti, E.P., Cumin, R., Schaffner, R., Haefely, W.: Selective antagonists of benzodiazepines. Nature *290*, 514–516 (1981)

Hunsperger, R.W., Bucher, V.M.: Affective behaviour produced by electrical stimulation in the forebrain and brain stem of the cat. Prog. Brain Res. *27*, 103–127 (1967)

Hunt, P., Raynaud, J.-P.: Benzodiazepine activity: is interaction with the glycine receptor, as evidenced by displacement of strychnine binding, a useful criterion? J. Pharm. Pharmacol. *29*, 442–444 (1977)

Hunter, J., Jasper, H.H.: Effects of thalamic stimulation in unanesthetized animals. Electroenceph. Clin. Neurophysiol. *1*, 305–324 (1949)

Hyttel, J.: Characterization of ^{3}H-GABA receptor binding to rat brain synaptosomal membranes: Effect of non GABAergic compounds. Psychopharmacology *65*, 211–214 (1979)

Ikeda, M.: Cumulative LD 50 – Table No. 3. Pharmacometrics *9*, 601–614 (1975)

Ikeda, H., Take, Y., Itoh, Y., Nagawa, Y.: Hypnotic effect of 8-chloro-6-phenyl-4H-S-triazolo (4,3,-a) (1,4) benzodiazepine (D-4OTA) in experimentally induced insomnia and brain serotonin in rats. Jpn. J. Pharmacol. *23*, 77 (1973)

Ishida, Y., dal Ri, H., Schmidt, G.: Effects of diazepam on discharge pattern in single fibres of phrenic nerve. Arch. Pharmacol. *289*, Suppl., R 35 (1974)

Ishida, Y., dal Ri, H., Schmidt, G., Vetterlein, F.: Actions of diazepam on the discharge pattern of phrenic motoneurones in rats. Neuropharmacology *18*, 679–687 (1979)

Ito, T., Shimizu, M.: Effect of psychotropic drugs on caudate spindle in cats. Jpn. J. Pharmacol. *26*, 527–534 (1976)

Itoh, H., Takaori, S.: Effects of psychotropic agents on the exploratory behavior of rats in a Y-shaped box. Jpn. J. Pharmacol. *18*, 344–352 (1968)

Iversen, L.L., Johnston, G.A.R.: GABA uptake in rat central nervous system: Comparison of uptake in slices and homogenates and the effects of some inhibitors. J. Neurochem. *18*, 1939–1950 (1971)

Iwahara, S.: Interactions between the effects of chlordiazepoxide and amphetamine on food-intake and spontaneous motor activity in the rat. Jpn. Psychol. Res. *12*, 82–86 (1970)

Iwahara, S., Sakama, E.: Effects of chlordiazepoxide upon habituation of open-field behavior in white rats. Psychopharmacologia *27*, 285–292 (1972)

Iwahara, S., Oishi, H., Yamazaki, S., Sakai, K.: Effects of chlordiazepoxide upon spontaneous alternation and the hippocampal electrical activity in white rats. Psychopharmacologia *24*, 496–507 (1972)

Jakoubek, B., Petrovický, P.: Incorporation of 4,5-^{3}H leucine into the neurons of locus ceruleus and other nerve cells in stressed rats: effect of diazepam. Psychopharmacology *50*, 193–197 (1976)

Jalfre, M., Monachon, M.A., Haefely, W.: Effects on the amygdalo hippocampal evoked potential in the cat of four benzodiazepines and some other psychotropic drugs. Arch. Pharmakol. *270*, 180–191 (1971)

James, G.W.L., Piper, D.C.: A method for evaluating potential hypnotic compounds in rats. J. Pharmacol. Methods *1*, 145–154 (1978)

James, T.A., Macleod, N.K., Mayer, M.L.: A functional antagonism between benzodiazepines and ACTH? Br. J. Pharmacol. *66*, 115P–116P, 1979

Järbe, T.U.C., Johansson, J.O.: Pentobarbital, diazepam and bemegride: their effects on open-field behavior in the gerbil (meriones unguiculatus). Arch. Int. Pharmacodyn. *25*, 88–97 (1977)

Javors, M., Erwin, V.G.: Correlation between IC 50 for inhibition of aldehyde reductase and ED_{50} for protection against maximal electroshock by a series of benzodiazepines. Pharmacologist *20*, 184 (1978)

Javors, M., Erwin, V.G.: Effects of benzodiazepines and valproic acid on brain aldehyde reductase and a proposed mechanism of anti-convulsant action. Biochem. Pharmacol. *29*, 1703–1708 (1980)

Javoy, F., Euvrard, C., Herbert, A., Glowinski, J.: Involvement of the dopamine nigrostriatal system in the picrotoxin effect on striatal ACh levels. Brain Res. *126*, 382–386 (1977)

Jenkinson, J.L., MacRae, W.R., Scott, D.B., Gould, J.F.: Haemodynamic effects of diazepam used as a sedative for oral surgery. Br. J. Anaesth. *46*, 294–297 (1974)

Jenner, P., Chadwick, D., Reynolds, E.H., Marsden, C.D.: Altered 5-HT metabolism with clonazepam, diazepam and diphenylhydantoin. J. Pharm. Pharmacol. *27*, 707–710 (1975)

Jenner, P., Marsden, C.D., Pratt, J., Reynolds, E.H.: Altered serotoninergic activity in mouse brain induced by clonazepam. Br. J. Pharmacol. *64*, 432P (1978)

Jenner, P., Marsden, C.D., Pratt, J., Reynolds, E.H.: Modulation of picrotoxin-induced forepaw myoclonus in the rat by benzodiazepines. Br. J. Pharmacol. *67*, 440P (1979)

Jeppsson, R., Ljungberg, S.: Anticonvulsant activity in mice of diazepam in an emulsion formulation for intravenous administration. Acta Pharmacol. Toxicol. *36*, 312–320 (1975)

Jindal, M.N., Doctor, R.B., Kelkar, V.V., Chonsey, H.K.: Certain aspects of pharmacological profiles of chlordiazepoxide and diazepam. Indian J. Physiol. Pharmacol. *12*, 141–152 (1968)

Johansson, J.O., Järbe, T.U.C.: Diazepam as a discriminative cue: its antagonism by bemegride. Eur. J. Pharmacol. *30*, 372–375 (1975)

Johnson, D.D., Lowndes, H.E.: Reduction by diazepam of repetitive electrical activity and toxicity resulting from soman. Eur. J. Pharmacol. *28*, 245–250 (1974)

Johnson, D.D., Davis, H.L., Crawford, R.D.: Pharmacological and biochemical studies in epileptic fowl. Fed. Proc. *38*, 2417–1423 (1979)

Johnson, D.N.: Effect of diazepam on food consumption in rats. Psychopharmacology *56*, 111–112 (1978)

Johnson, D.N., Funderburk, W.H.: AHR-3219, a new antianxiety agent. Prog. Neuro-Psychopharmacol. *2*, 443–448 (1978)

Johnson, R.W., Yamamura, H.I.: Photoaffinity labeling of the benzodiazepine receptor in bovine cerebral cortex. Life Sci. *25*, 1613–1620 (1979)

Jones, D.J., Stehling, L.C., Zauder, H.L.: A comparison of the effects of Ro 21-3981 and diazepam on the cardiovascular system in dogs. Pharmacologist *20*, 254 (1978)

Jones, D.J., Stehling, L.C., Zauder, H.L.: Cardiovascular responses to diazepam and midazolam maleate in the dog. Anesthesiology *51*, 430–434 (1979)

Jones, D.M., Jones, M.E.L., Lewis, M.J., Spriggs, T.L.B.: Drugs and human memory: effects of low doses of nitrazepam and hyoscine on retention. Br. J. clin. Pharmac. *7*, 479–483 (1979)

de Jong, R.H., Heavner, J.E.: Diazepam and lidocaine-induced cardiovascular changes. Anesthesiology *39*, 633–638 (1973)

de Jong, R.H., Heavner, J.E.: Convulsions induced by local anaesthetic: time course of diazepam prophylaxis. Can. Anaesth. Soc. J. *21*, 153–158 (1974a)

de Jong, R.H., Heavner, J.E.: Diazepam prevents and aborts lidocaine convulsions in monkeys. Anesthesiology *41*, 226–230 (1974b)

Jouvet, M.: The role of monoamines and Acetylcholine-containing neurons in the regulation of the sleep-waking cycle. Ergebn. Physiol. *64*, 167–307 (1972)

Joy, R.M., Hance, A.J., Killam, K.F., Jr.: A quantitative electroencephalographic comparison of some benzodiazepines in the primate. Neuropharmacology *10*, 483–497 (1971)

Juhasz, L., Dairman, W.: Effect of sub-acute diazepam administration in mice on the subsequent ability of diazepam to protect against metrazol and bicuculline induced convulsions. Fed. Proc. *36*, 377 (1977)

Julien, R.M.: Cerebellar involvement in the antiepileptic action of diazepam. Neuropharmacology *11*, 683–691 (1972)

Kaada, B.R., Andersen, P., Jansen, J.: Stimulation of the amygdaloid nuclear complex in unanesthetized cats. Neurology *4*, 48–64 (1954)

Kamei, C., Masuda, Y., Oka, M., Shimizu, M.: Effects of antidepressant drugs on amygdaloid after-discharges in rats: Jpn. J. Pharmacol. *25*, 359–365 (1975)

Kamioka, T., Nakayama, I., Akiyama, S., Takagi, H.: Effects of oxazolam, cloxazolam, and CS-386, new anti-anxiety drugs, on socially induced suppression and aggression in pairs of monkeys. Psychopharmacology *52*, 17–23 (1977)

Kamioka, T., Takagi, H., Kobayashi, S., Suzuki, Y.: Pharmacological studies on 10-chloro-11b-(2-chlorophenyl)-2,3,5,6,7,11b-hexahydrobenzo-(6,7)-1,4-diazepino(5,4-b)-oxazol-6-one (CS-370), a new psychosedative agent. Arzneim. Forsch. *22*, 884–891 (1972)

Karli, P.: Action du méthaminodiazépoxide (librium) sur l'agressivité interspécifique rat-souris. C.R. Soc. Biol. *155*, 625–627 (1961)

Karlsson, A., Fonnum, F., Malthe-Sorenssen, D., Storm-Mathisen, J.: Effect of the convulsive agent 3-mercaptopropionic acid on the levels of GABA, other amino acids and glutamate decarboxylase in different regions of rat brain. Biochem. Pharmacol. *23*, 3053–3061 (1974)

Karobath, M., Lippitsch, M.: THIP and isoguvacine are partial agonists of GABA-stimulated benzodiazepine receptor binding. Eur. J. Pharmacol. *58*, 485–488 (1979)

Karobath, M., Sperk, G.: Stimulation of benzodiazepine receptor binding by γ-aminobutyric acid. Proc. Natl. Acad. Sci. USA *76*, 1004–1006 (1979)

Karobath, M., Sperk, G., Schönbeck, G.: Evidence for an endogenous factor interfering with ^{3}H-diazepam binding to rat brain membranes. Eur. J. Pharmacol. *49*, 232–236 (1978)

Karobath, M., Sperk, G., Schönberg, G.: Evidence for an endogenous compound interfering with ^{3}H-diazepam binding to rat brain membranes. In: Biological Psychiatry Today. Obiols, J., Bullús, C., Gonzáles Monclús, E., Pujol, J. (eds.), pp. 114–118. Amsterdam: Elsevier/North Holland Biomedical Press 1979 a

Karobath, M., Placheta, P., Lippitsch, M., Krogsgaard-Larsen, P.: Is stimulation of benzodiazepine receptor binding mediated by a novel GABA receptor? Nature *278*, 748–749 (1979 b)

Karobath, M., Placheta, P., Lippitsch, M., Krogsgaard-Larsen, P.: Characterization of GABA-stimulated benzodiazepine receptor binding. In: Receptors for Neurotransmitters and Peptide Hormones. Pepeu, G., Kuhar, M.J., Enna, S.J. (eds.), pp. 313–320. New York: Raven Press 1980

Karobath, M., Placheta, P., Lippitsch, M.: Different structural requirements of GABAergic drugs for stimulation of ^{3}H-diazepam binding and inhibition of NA$^+$-independent ^{3}H-GABA binding. Brain Res. (in press) 1981

Kaul, C.L., Lewis, J.J.: Effects of minor tranquillizers on brain phosphate levels in vivo. Biochem. Pharmacol. *12*, 1279–1282 (1963)

Kawakami, M., Negoro, H., Takahashi, T.: Neuropharmacological studies on the mechanisms of paradoxical sleep in the rabbit. Japan. J. Physiol. *16*, 667–683 (1966)

Kawasaki, H., Watanabe, S., Ueki, S.: Effects of psychotropic drugs on pressor and behavioral responses to brain stimulation in unrestrained, unanesthetized rats. Pharmacol. Biochem. Behav. *10*, 907–915 (1979)

Keim, K.L., Sigg, E.B.: Vagally mediated cardiac reflexes and their modulation by diazepam and pentobarbital. Neuropharmacology *12*, 319–325 (1973)

Keim, K.L., Sigg, E.B.: Plasma corticosterone and brain catecholamines in stress: effect of psychotropic drugs. Pharmacol. Biochem. Behav. *6*, 79–85 (1977)

Keller, H.H., Schaffner, R., Haefely, W.: Interaction of benzodiazepines with neuroleptics at central dopamine neurons. Naunyn-Schmiedebergs Arch. Pharmacol. *294*, 1–7 (1976)

Kelly, D.D., Bodnar, R.J., Brutus, M., Woods, C.F., Glusman, M.: Differential effects upon liminal-escape pain thresholds of neuroleptic, antidepressant and anxiolytic drugs. Fed. Proc. *37*, 470 (1978 a)

Kelly, D.D., Brutus, M., Bodnar, R.J.: Differential effects of naloxone upon elevations in liminal-escape pain thresholds induced by psychotropic drugs: reversal of chlordiazepoxide but enhancement of neuroleptic "analgesia". Abstracts 7th Int. Congr. of Pharmacol., Part 1, p. 119. Paris: Pergamon Press (1978 b)

Kelly, J., Grossman, S.P.: GABA and hypothalamic feeding systems. II. A comparison of GABA, glycine and acetylcholine, agonists and their antagonists. Pharmacol. Biochem. Behav. *11*, 647–652 (1979)

Kelly, J., Alheid, G.F., Newberg, A., Grossman, S.P.: GABA stimulation and blockade in the hypothalamus and midbrain: effects on feeding and locomotor activity. Pharmacol. Biochem. Behav. *7*, 537–541 (1977)

Kelly, J., Rothstein, J., Grossman, S.P.: GABA and hypothalamic feeding systems. I. Topographic analysis of the effects of microinjections of muscimol. Physiol. Behav. *23*, 1123–1134, (1979)

Khafagy, E.Z., El-Laithy, A.F., El-Makkawi, H.K., El-Darawy, Z.I.: New aspects concerning the mechanism of action of tranquilizers. The influence of some tranquilizers on protein and nucleic acid syntheses. Biochem. Pharmacol. *26*, 1205–1211 (1977)

Khan, A.A.: Preliminary in vitro study of diazepam and droperidol on oestrus rat uterus. Br. J. Anaesth. *52*, 349–354 (1980)

Khan, A.V., Forney, R.B., Hughes, F.W.: Plasma free fatty acids in rats after shock as modified by centrally active drugs. Arch. Int. Pharmacodyn. *151*, 466–474 (1964)

Kido, R., Matsushita, A., Takesue, H.: Effect of 7-chloro-2,3-dihydro-1-methyl-5-phenyl-1H-1,4-benzodiazepine (S 804, Ro 5-4556, medazepam) on spinal reflexes and decerebrate rigidity. Pharmacometrics (Tokyo) *6*, 243–249 (1972)

Kido, R., Yamamoto, K., Matsushita, A.: Analysis of central nervous system depressants in cats with permanently implanted electrodes. Progr. Brain Res. *213*, 130–141 (1966)

Killam, E.K.: Photomyoclonic seizures in the baboon, Papio papio. Fed. Proc. *38*, 2429–2433 (1979)

Killam, E.K., Matsuzaki, M., Killam, K.F.: Studies of anticonvulsant compounds in the Papio papio model of epilepsy. In: Chemical Modulation of brain function. Sabelli, H.C. (ed.), pp. 161–171. New York: Raven Press 1973

Killam, K.F., Killam, E.K., Naquet, R.: An animal model of light sensitive epilepsy. Electroenceph. Clin. Neurophysiol. 22, 497–513 (1967)

Kimura, H., Kuriyama, K.: Distribution of gamma-aminobutyric acid (GABA) on the rat hypothalamus: functional correlates of GABA with activities of appetite controlling mechanisms. J. Neurochem. 24, 903–907 (1975)

Kirsten, E.B., Schoener, E.P.: Antagonism of pentylenetetrazol excitation by anticonvulsants on single brain stem neurons. Neuropharmacology 11, 591–599 (1972)

Kito, G., Kasé, Y., Miyata, T.: A cough-like respiratory response induced by electrical stimulation of the amygdaloid complex in the cat. Arch. Int. Pharmacodyn. 227, 82–92 (1977)

Kleinrok, Z., Przegalinski, E., Sczuczwar, S., Participation of 5-hydroxytryptamine in anticonvulsive action of benzodiazepines. Pol. J. Pharmacol. Pharm. 29, 385–391 (1977)

Klepner, C.A., Lippa, A.S., Benson, D.I., Sano, M.C., Beer, B.: Resolution of two biochemically and pharmacologically distinct benzodiazepine receptors. Pharmacol. Biochem. Behav. 11, 457–462 (1979)

Klotz, U.: Effect of age on levels of diazepam in plasma and brain of rats. Naunyn-Schmiedebergs Arch. Pharmacol. 307, 167–169 (1979)

Klupp, H., Kähling, J.: Pharmakologische Wirkung von 7-Chlor-1,3-dihydroxy-5-phenyl-2H-1,4-benzodiazepin-2-on. Arzneim. Forsch. 15, 359–365 (1965)

Klygul, T.A., Kadlecova, O., Vikhlyaev, Y.I.: Effect of prolonged administration of nitrazepam on sleep cycles in rats. Byull. Éksp. Biol. Med. U.S.S.R. 81, 197–199 (1976)

Kobayashi, K., Hara, T., Iwata, N.: Effects of benzodiazepine compounds on amygdalofugal pathways. Japan. J. Pharmacol. 29, (Suppl) 32P (1980)

Koch, H.: Brotizolam, 2-Bromo-4-(2-chlorophenyl)-9-methyl-6H-thieno-/3,2-f/-1,2,4-triazolo-/4,3-a/-1,4-diazepine, WE-941. Drugs Future 4, 85–88 (1979)

Koe, B.K.: Biochemical effects of antianxiety drugs on brain monoamines. In: Anxiolytics. Fielding, S., Lal, H. (eds.): pp. 173–195. Mount Kisco, N.Y.: Futura Publ. Comp. 1979

Kopeloff, L.M., Chusid, J.G.: Diazepam as anticonvulsant in epileptic and normal monkeys. Int. J. Neuropsychiatry 3, 469–471 (1967)

Korol, B., Brown, M.L.: A behavioral and autonomic nervous system study of Ro 5-3350 and diazepam in conscious dogs. Pharmacology 1, 115–128 (1968)

Korttila, K.: The effect of diazepam, flunitrazepam and droperidol with an analgesic on blood pressure and heart rate in man. Arzneim. Forsch. 25, 1303–1306 (1975)

Kostowski, W.: A note on the effects of some psychotropic drugs on the aggressive behaviour in the ant, formica rufa. J. Pharm. Pharmacol. 18, 747–749 (1966)

Koulu, M., Lammintausta, R., Dahlström, S.: Effects of some γ-aminobutyric acid (GABA)-ergic drugs on the dopaminergic control of human growth hormone secretion. J. Clin. Endocr. Metab. 51, 124–129 (1980)

Koulu, M., Lammintausta, R., Kangas, L., Dahlström, S.: The effect of methysergide, pimozide, and sodium valproate on the diazepam-stimulated growth hormone secretion in man. J. Clin. Endocr. Metab. 48, 119–122 (1979)

Kovacs, I.B:, Görög, P.: Effect of chlordiazepoxide on bronchoconstriction. Arch. Int. Pharmacodyn. 173, 27–33 (1968)

Kozhechkin, S.N.: Changes in the electrical activity of the cerebral cortex neurons in the rabbit following intravenous diazepam injection. Byull. Éksp. Biol. Med. U.S.R.R. 85, 41–45 (1978)

Kozhechkin, S.N., Ostrovskaya, R.U.: Increased sensitivity of sensory-motor cortex neurons of rabbits to γ-aminobutyric acid under the effect of diazepam (microiontophoretic study). Byull. Éksp. Biol. Med. U.S.S.R. 82, 1448–1450 (1976)

Kozhechkin, S.N., Ostrovskaya, R.U.: Are benzodiazepines GABA antagonists? Nature 269, 72–73 (1977)

Krulik, R., Černý, M.: Effect of chlordiazepoxide on stress in rats. Life Sci. 10, 145–151 (1971)

Kršiak, K.: Effects of drugs on behavior of aggressive mice. Br. J. Pharmacol. 65, 525–533 (1979)

Kuhn, H.: Autoradiographic evidence for binding of [³H]-flunitrazepam (Rohypnol®) to melanin granules in the cat eye. Experientia 36, 863–865 (1980)

Kumar, R.: Extinction of fear. I. Effects of amylobarbitone and dexamphetamine given separately and in combination on fear and exploratory behavior in rats. Psychopharmacologia *19*, 163–187 (1971 a)

Kumar, R.: Extinction of fear. II. Effects of chlordiazepoxide and chlorpromazine on fear and exploratory behavior in rats. Psychopharmacologia *19*, 297–312 (1971 b)

Kuribara, H., Tadokoro, S.: Effects of psychotropic drugs on water drinking behavior in rats. Japan. J. Pharmacol. *28*, 51P (1978)

Kutz, K., Schuler, G., Brenner, U., Miederer, S.E.: Vergleichende Untersuchungen über die Wirkung von Anticholinergika auf die basale und die durch Pentagastrin und Hypoglykämie stimulierte Magensekretion. Klin. Wochenschr. *54*, 485–492 (1976)

Kvetina, J., Guaitani, A., Pugliatti, C., Veneroni, E.: Effect of diazepam on liver function of rats. Pharmacology *2*, 17–20 (1969)

Ladinski, H., Consolo, S., Peri, G., Garattini, S.: Increase in mouse and rat brain acetylcholine levels by diazepam. In: The Benzodiazepines. Garattini, S., Mussini, E., Randall, L.O. (eds.), pp. 241–242. New York: Raven Press, 1973

Lahti, R.A., Barsuhn, C.: The effect of minor tranquilizers on stress-induced increases in rat plasma corticosteroids. Psychopharmacologia *35*, 215–220 (1974)

Lahti, R.A., Barsuhn, C.: The effect of various doses of minor tranquilizers on plasma corticosteroids in stressed rats. Res. Commun. Chem. Pathol. Pharmacol. *11*, 595–603 (1975)

Lakshminarayan, S., Sahn, S.A., Hudson, L.D., Weil, J.V.: Effect of diazepam on ventilatory responses. Clin. Pharmacol. Ther. *20*, 178–183 (1976)

Lamour, Y.: Les propriétés depolarisantes du GABA au niveau des neurones du ganglion rachidien du rat: Application à la pharmacologie de l'inhibition présynaptique. PhD Thesis, Université Pierre et Marie Curie, Paris, 1979

Lang, B., Barnard, E.A., Chang, L.-R., Dolly, J.O.: Putative benzodiazepine receptor: A protein solubilized from brain. FEBS Lett. *104*, 149–153 (1979)

Langfeldt, T.: Diazepam-induced play behavior in cats during prey killing. Psychopharmacologia *36*, 181–184 (1974)

Langfeldt, T., Ursin, H.: Differential action of diazepam on flight and defense behavior in the cat. Psychopharmacologia *19*, 61–66 (1971)

Lanoir, J., Killam, E.K.: Alteration in the sleep-wakefulness patterns by benzodiazepines in the cat. Electroenceph. Clin. Neurophysiol. *25*, 530–542 (1968)

Lanoir, J., Dolce, G. Chirinos, E., Naquet, R.: Etude neurophysiologique du Ro 4-5360. C. R. Soc. Biol. *159*, 431–435 (1965)

Larson, G.F., Hurlbert, B.J., Wingard, D.W.: Physostigmine reversal of diazepam-induced depression. Anesth. Analg. *56*, 348–351 (1977)

Lavielle, S., Tassin, J.-P., Thierry, A.-M., Blanc, G., Herve, D., Barthelémy, L., Glowinski, J.: Blockade by benzodiazepines of the selective high increase in dopamine turnover induced by stress in mesocortical dopaminergic neurons of the rat. Brain Res. *168*, 585–594 (1978)

Leaf, R.C., Wnek, D.J., Gay, P., Corcia, R.M., Lamon, S.: Chlordiazepoxide and diazepam induced mouse killing by rats. Psychopharmacologia *44*, 23–28 (1975)

Leaf, R.C., Wnek, D.J., Lamon, S., Gay, P.: Despite various drugs, cats continue to kill mice. Pharmacol. Biochem. Behav. *9*, 445–452 (1979)

Lechat, P., Boismare, F., Streichenberger, G., D'Armagnac, J.: Evaluation expérimentale des propriétés antiépileptiques d'une nouvelle benzodiazépine: le Ro 5-4023. Thérapie *25*, 893–905 (1970)

Lee, H.K., Dunwiddie, T.V., Hoffer, B.J.: Interaction of diazepam with synaptic transmission in the in vitro rat hippocampus. Naunyn-Schmiedebergs Arch. Pharmacol. *309*, 131–136 (1979)

Leeuwin, R.S., Djojodibroto, R.D., Groenewoud, E.T.: The effects of three benzodiazepines and of meprobamate on the action of smooth muscle stimulants on the guinea pig ileum. Arch. Int. Pharmacodyn. *217*, 18–21 (1975)

Le Fur, G., Guilloux, F., Mitrani, N., Mizoule, J. Uzan, A.: Relationships between plasma corticosteroids and benzodiazepines in stress. J. Pharmacol. Exp. Ther. *211*, 305–308 (1979)

Lehmann, A.: Contribution à l'étude psychophysiologique et neuropharmacologique de l'épilepsie acoustique de la souris et du rat. Agressologie *5*, 311–351 (1964)

Lehmann, K., Schmidt, J.: Beeinflussung somatosensorisch ausgelöster Kortexpotentiale durch Psychopharmaka. Acta Biol. Med. Germ. *38*, 619–625 (1979)

Lembeck, F., Beubler, E.: Convulsions induced by hyperbaric oxygen: inhibition by phenobarbital, diazepam and baclofen. Arch. Pharmacol. *297*, 47–51 (1977)

Levy, R.A.: GABA: a direct depolarizing action at the mammalian primary afferent terminal. Brain Res. *76*, 155–160 (1974)

Levy, R.A.: The role of GABA in primary afferent depolarization. Prog. Neurobiol. *9*, 211–267 (1977)

Lidbrink, P.: Turnover changes in central monoamine neuron systems after minor tranquillizers and barbiturates. Acta Pharmacol. Toxicol. (Kbh.) *31*, Suppl. I, 5 (1972)

Lidbrink, P., Farnebo, L.-O.: Uptake and release of noradrenaline in rat cerebral cortex in vitro: no effect of benzodiazepines and barbiturates. Neuropharmacology *12*, 1087–1095 (1973)

Lidbrink, P., Corrodi, H., Fuxe, K., Olson, L.: The effect of benzodiazepines, meprobamate, and barbiturates on central monoamine neurons. In: The Benzodiazepines. Garattini, S., Mussini, E., Randall, L.O. (eds.), pp. 203–223. New York, Raven Press 1973

Lidbrink, P., Corrodi, H., Fuxe, K.: Benzodiazepines and barbiturates: Turnover changes in central 5-hydroxytryptamine pathways. Eur. J. Pharmacol. *26*, 35–40 (1974)

Liebeswar, G.: The depressant action of flurazepam on the maximum rate of rise of action potentials recorded from guinea pig papillary muscles. Arch. Pharmacol. *275*, 445–456 (1972)

Lineberry, C.G., Kulics, A.T.: The effects of diazepam, morphine and lidocaine on nociception in rhesus monkeys: a signal detection analysis. J. Pharmacol. Exp. Ther. *205*, 302–310 (1978)

Lindmar, R., Löffelholz, K., Weide, W.: Inhibition by pentobarbital of acetylcholine release from the postganglionic parasympathetic neuron of the heart. J. Pharmacol. Exp. Ther. *210*, 166–173 (1979)

Lingjaerde, O.: Effect of benzodiazepines on uptake and efflux of serotonin in human blood platelets in vitro. In: The Benzodiazepines. Garattini, S., Mussini, E., Randall, L.O. (eds.), pp. 225–233. New York: Raven Press 1973

Lipp, J.: Effect of diazepam upon soman-induced seizure activity and convulsions. Electroenceph. Clin. Neurophysiol. *32*, 557–560 (1972)

Lipp, J.: Effect of benzodiazepine derivatives on soman-induced seizure activity and convulsions in the monkey. Arch. Int. Pharmacodyn. Ther. *202*, 244–251 (1973)

Lipp, J.: Effect of small doses of clonazepam upon soman-induced seizure activity and convulsions. Arch. Int. Pharmacodyn. Ther. *210*, 49–54 (1974)

Lippa, A.S., Regan, B.: Additional studies on the importance of glycine and GABA in mediating the actions of benzodiazepines. Life. Sci. *21*, 1779–1784 (1977)

Lippa, A.S., Greenblatt, E.N., Pelham, R.W.: The use of animal models for delineating the mechanisms of action of anxiolytic agents. In: Animal models in psychiatry and neurology. Hanin, I., Usdin, E. (eds.), pp. 279–292. Oxford: Pergamon 1977

Lippa, A.S., Sano, M.C., Coupet, J., Klepner, C.A., Beer, B.: Evidence that benzodiazepine receptors reside on cerebellar Purkinje cells: studies with "nervous" mutant mice. Life Sci. *23*, 2213–2218 (1978 a)

Lippa, A.S., Klepner, C.A., Yunger, L., Sano, M.C., Smith, W.V., Beer, B.: Relationship between benzodiazepine receptors and experimental anxiety in rats. Pharmacol. Biochem. Behav. *9*, 853–856 (1978 b)

Lippa, A.S., Coupet, J., Greenblatt, E.N., Klepner, C.A., Beer, B.: A synthetic non-benzodiazepine ligand for benzodiazepine receptors: a probe for investigating neuronal substrates of anxiety. Pharmacol. Biochem. Behav. *11*, 99–106 (1979)

Lippmann, W., Pugsley, T.A.: Effects of benzoctamine and chlordiazepoxide on turnover and uptake of 5-hydroxytryptamine in the brain. Br. J. Pharmac. *51*, 571–575 (1974)

Lloyd, K.G., Worms, P., Depoortere, H., Bartholini, G.: Pharmacological profile of SL 76002, a new GABA-mimetic drug. In: GABA-Neurotransmitters. Krogsgaard-Larsen, P., Scheel-Krüger, J., Kofod, H. (Eds.), pp. 308–325. Copenhagen: Munksgaard 1979

Locatelli, V., Cocchi, D., Frigerio, D., Betti, R., Krogsgaard-Larsen, P., Racagni, G., Müller, E.E.: Dual γ-aminobutyric acid control of prolactin secretion in the rat. Endocrinology *105*, 778–785 (1979)

Lockard, J.S., Levy, R.H., Congdon, W.C., DuCharme, L.L., Salonen, L.D.: Clonazepam in a focal-motor monkey model: efficacy, tolerance, toxicity, withdrawal, and management. Epilepsia *20*, 683–695 (1979)

Locker, A., Koffer, E.: Senkung der Körpertemperatur bei Mäusen durch Librium. Experientia *18*, 28–29 (1962)

Loew, D.M., Spiegel, R.: Polygraphic sleep studies in rats and humans. Arzneim. Forsch. *26*, 1032–1035 (1976)

Loizzo, A., Longo, V.G.: A pharmacological approach to paradoxical sleep. Physiol. Behav. *3*, 91–97 (1968)

Longoni, R., Mulas, A., Pepeu, G.: Drug effect on acetylcholine level in discrete brain regions of rats killed by microwave irradiation. Br. J. Pharmacol. *52*, 429P–430P (1974)

Lopez, J.R., Helland, L.A., Wanek, L.A., Rudel, R., Taylor, S.R.: Calcium transients in skeletal muscle are not necessarily antagonized by muscle "relaxants". Biophys. J. *25*, 119a (1979)

Lorens, S.A., Sainati, M.: Naloxone blocks the excitatory effect of ethanol and chlordiazepoxide on lateral hypothalamic self-stimulation behavior. Life Sci. *23*, 1359–1364 (1978)

Löscher, W.: 3-Mercaptopropionic acid: Convulsant properties, effects on enzymes of the γ-aminobutyrate system in mouse brain and antagonism by certain anticonvulsant drugs, aminooxyacetic acid and gabaculine, Biochem. Pharmacol. *28*, 1397–1407 (1979)

Löscher, W., Frey, H.-H.: Effect of convulsant and anticonvulsant agents on level and metabolism of γ-aminobutyric acid in mouse brain. Naunyn-Schmiedebergs Arch. Pharmacol. *296*, 263–269 (1977)

Ludin, H.P., Dubach, K.: Action of diazepam on muscular contraction in man. J. Neurol. *199*, 30–38 (1971)

Ludin, H.P., Robert, F.: The action of diazepam on human skeletal muscle. Eur. Neurol. *11*, 345–352 (1974)

Lust, W.D., Kupferberg, H.J., Yonekawa, W.D., Penry, J.K., Passonneau, J.V., Wheaton, A.B.: Changes in brain metabolites induced by convulsants or electroshock: effects of anticonvulsant agents. Mol. Pharmacol. *14*, 347–356 (1978)

Macdonald, R.L., Barker, J.L.: Benzodiazepines specifically modulate GABA-mediated postsynaptic inhibition in cultured mammalian neurones. Nature *271*, 563–564 (1978)

Macdonald, R.L., Barker, J.L.: Enhancement of GABA-mediated postsynaptic inhibition in cultured mammalian spinal cord neurons: a common mode of anticonvulsant action. Brain Res. *167*, 323–336 (1979)

MacDonald, J.F., Barker, J.L., Paul, S.M., Marangos, P.J., Skolnick, P.: Inosine may be an endogenous ligand for benzodiazepine receptors on cultured spinal neurons. Science *205*, 715–717 (1979)

Mackerer, C.R., Kochman, R.L.: Effects of cations and anions on the binding of ^{3}H-diazepam to rat brain. Proc. Soc. Exp. Biol. Med. *158*, 393–397 (1978)

Mackerer, C.R., Kochman, R.L., Bierschenk, B.A., Bremner, S.S.: The binding of ^{3}H-diazepam to rat brain homogenates. J. Pharmacol. Exp. Ther. *206*, 405–413 (1978)

Macon, J.B., King, D.W.: Penicillin iontophoresis and the responses of somatosensory cortical neurons to amino acids. Electroenceph. Clin. Neurophysiol. *47*, 52–63 (1979)

Madan, B.R., Sharma, J.D., Vyas, D.S.: Action of methaminodiazepoxide on cardiac, smooth and skeletal muscles. Arch. Int. Pharmacodyn. *143*, 127–137 (1963)

Maekawa, T., Sakabe, T., Takeshita, H.: Diazepam blocks cerebral metabolic and circulatory responses to local anesthetic-induced seizures. Anesthesiology *41*, 381–391 (1974)

Maekawa, T., Oshibuchi, T., Imamura, A., Takeshita, H.: Effects of psychotropic drugs on the cerebral energy state and glycolytic metabolism in the rat: diazepam, clomipramine and chlorpromazine. Biochem. Pharmacol. *29*, 15–18 (1980)

Magoun, H.W.: The waking brain, 2nd Edition. Springfield, Ill.: C.C. Thomas 1963

Mah, H.D., Daly, J.W.: Adenosine-dependent formation of cyclic AMP in brain slices. Pharmacol. Res. Commun. *8*, 65–79 (1976)

Maickel, R.P., Maloney, G.J.: Effects of various depressant drugs on deprivation-induced water consumption. Neuropharmacology *12*, 777–782 (1973)

Maickel, R.P., Maloney, G.J.: Taste phenomena influences on stimulation of deprivation-induced fluid consumption of rats. Neuropharmacology *13*, 763–767 (1974)

Mailman, R.B., Mueller, R.A., Breese, G.R.: The effect of drugs which alter GABA-ergic function on cerebellar guanosine-3′,5′-monophosphate content. Life Sci. *23*, 623–628 (1978)

Malick, J.B.: Effects of selected drugs on stimulus-bound emotional behavior elicited by hypothalamic stimulation in the cat. Arch. Int. Pharmacodyn. *186*, 137–141 (1970)

Malick, J.B.: Selective antagonism of isolation-induced aggression in mice by diazepam following chronic administration. Pharmacol. Biochem. Behav. *8*, 497–499 (1978)

Malick, J.B., Enna, S.J.: Comparative effects of benzodiazepines and non-benzodiazepine anxiolytics on biochemical and behavioral tests predictive of anxiolytic activity. Commun. Psychopharmacol. *3*, 245–251 (1979)

Malick, J.B., Sofia, R.D., Goldberg, M.E.: A comparative study of the effects of selected psychoactive agents upon three lesion-induced models of aggression in the rat. Arch. Int. Pharmacodyn. *181*, 459–465 (1969)

Malizia, E., Bertolini, G., Venturi, V.M.: Comparison between experimental responses and clinical intoxications caused by central nervous system depressants and by antihistaminic drugs. Proc. Europ. Soc. Drug Toxicol. *6*, 179–184 (1965)

Mallorga, P., Strittmatter, W.J., Hirata, F., Tallman, J.F., Axelrod, J.: β-Adrenergic agonists and benzodiazepines stimulate membrane phospholipid methylation in rat astrocytoma cells. 9th Ann. Meeting Soc. Neurosci., Abstr. *5*, 654 (1979)

Mao, C.C., Guidotti, A., Costa, E.: Interactions between γ-aminobutyric acid and guanosine cyclic 3′,5′-monophosphate in rat cerebellum. Mol. Pharmacol. *10*, 736–745 (1974)

Mao, C.C., Guidotti, A., Costa, E.: Evidence for an involvement of GABA in the mediation of the cerebellar cGMP decrease and the anticonvulsant action of diazepam. Naunyn-Schmiedebergs Arch. Pharmacol. *289*, 369–378 (1975a)

Mao, C.C., Guidotti, A., Costa, E.: Inhibition by diazepam of the tremor and the increase of cerebellar cGMP content elicited by harmaline. Brain Res. *83*, 516–519 (1975b)

Mao, C.C., Guidotti, A., Landis, S.: Cyclic GMP: reduction of cerebellar concentrations in "nervous" mutant mice. Brain Res. *90*, 335–339 (1975c)

Mao, C.C., Marco, E., Revuelta, A., Bertilsson, L., Costa, E.: The turnover rate of γ-aminobutyric acid in the nuclei of telencephalon: Implications in the pharmacology of antipsychotics and of a minor tranquilizer. J. Biol. Psychiatry *12*, 359–371 (1977)

Marangos, P.J., Paul, S.M., Greenlaw, P., Goodwin, F.K., Skolnick, P.: Demonstration of an endogenous, competitive inhibitor(s) of [^{3}H]-diazepam binding in bovine brain. Life Sci. *22*, 1893–1900 (1978)

Marangos, P.J., Paul, S.M., Goodwin, F.K., Skolnick, P.: Putative endogenous ligands for the benzodiazepine receptor. Life Sci. *25*, 1093–1102 (1979a)

Marangos, P.J., Clark, R., Martino, A.M., Paul, S.M., Skolnick, P.: Demonstration of two new endogenous "benzodiazepine-like" compounds from brain. Psychiat. Res. *1*, 121–130 (1979b)

Marc, V., Morselli, P.L.: Effect of diazepam on plasma corticosterone levels in the rat. J. Pharm. Pharmacol. *21*, 784–786 (1969)

Marcucci, F., Guaitani, A., Kvetina I., Mussini, E., Garattini, S.: Species difference in diazepam metabolism and anticonvulsant effect. Eur. J. Pharmacol. *4*, 467–470 (1968)

Marcucci, F., Fanelli, R., Mussini, E., Garattini, S.: Further studies on the long lasting antimetrazol activity of diazepam in mice. Eur. J. Pharmacol. *11*, 115–116 (1970)

Marcucci, F., Guaitani, A., Fanelli, R., Mussini, E., Garattini, S.: Metabolism and anticonvulsant activity of diazepam in guinea pigs. Biochem. Pharmacol. *20*, 1711–1713 (1971a)

Marcucci, F., Mussini, E., Guaitani, A., Fanelli, R., Garattini, S.: Anticonvulsant activity and brain levels of diazepam and its metabolites in mice. Eur. J. Pharmacol. *16*, 311–314 (1971b)

Marcucci, F., Mussini, E., Martelli, P., Guaitani, A., Garattini, S.: Metabolism and anticonvulsant activity of deuterated N-demethyldiazepam. J. Pharm. Sci. *62*, 1900–1902 (1973)

Marcy, R., Quermonne, M.A.: Anhydrotic effect of benzodiazepines in mice. Experientia *30*, 783–784 (1974)

Marcy, R., Quermonne, M.A.: Benzodiazepines: a comparison of their effects in mice on the magnitude of the plantar skin conductivity response and on pentylenetetrazole-induced seizures. Experientia *31*, 954–955 (1975)

Marcy, R., Quermonne, M.A.: Decremental skin conductance response in mice, during iterative photostimulation; an attention-sustaining capacity model for psychopharmacological research. Br. J. Pharmacol. *58*, 437–438 (1976)

Margules, D.L., Stein, L.: Neuroleptics vs. Tranquilizers: Evidence from animal behavior studies of mode and site of action. In: Neuro-Psychopharmacology. Proc. 5th C.I.N.P. Congr. Brill, H. (ed.), pp. 108–120. Amsterdam: Excerpta Medica 1967

Mariani, J., Delhaye-Bouchaud, N.: Effect of diazepam on the spontaneous and harmaline-induced electrical activity of Purkinje cells in the cerebellum of the rat and rabbit. Neuropharmacology 17, 45–51 (1978)

Marino, A., Campese, V.M., Cuomo, V., Calabrese, P.: Influenza del bromazepam e del diazepam sulla tossicità acuta e sulle alterazioni ecgrafiche da nicotina nella cavia. Boll. Soc. Ital. Biol. Sper. 50, 769–774 (1974)

Marion, J., Wolfe, L.S.: Increases in vivo of unesterified fatty acids, prostaglandin $F_{2\alpha}$ but not thromboxane B_2 in rat brain during drug induced convulsions. Prostaglandins 16, 99–110 (1978)

Markovich, V.V., Ostrovskaya, R.U.: Cortical inhibition processes and the anticonvulsant action of benzodiazepine derivatives. Byull. Éksp. Biol. Med. U.S.S.R. 84(10), 1429–1432 (1977)

Marriott, A.S., Smith, E.F.: An analysis of drug effects in mice exposed to a simple novel environment. Psychopharmacologia 24, 397–406 (1972)

Marriott, A.S., Spencer, P.S.J.: Effects of centrally acting drugs on exploratory behavior in rats. Br. J. Pharmacol. 25, 432–441 (1965)

Martin, I.L., Candy, J.M.: Facilitation of benzodiazepine binding by sodium chloride and GABA. Neuropharmacology 17, 993–998 (1978)

Martin, I.L., Mitchell, P.R.: Diazepam facilitates the potassium stimulated release of [^{3}H]-dopamine from rat striatal tissue. Br. J. Pharmacol. 66, 107P (1979)

Maspoli, M.: Le Valium, son action sur la respiration. Schweiz. Med. Wschr. 97, (10) 320–324 (1967)

Massari, V.J., Gottesfeld, Z., Jacobowitz, D.M.: Distribution of glutamic acid decarboxylase in certain rhombencephalic and thalamic nuclei of the rat. Brain Res. 118, 147–151 (1976)

Masso, M., Pérez, H.: Double-blind clinical trial of bromazepam and α-methyldopa in arterial hypertension. Pharmatherapeutica 2(3), 195–204 (1979)

Matsumoto, K., Ono, H., Fukuda, H.: Effects of diazepam and baclofen on the release of GABA from slices of rat spinal cord. Jap. J. Pharmacol. 29, 48P (1979)

Matsui, Y., Kamioka, T.: Potentiation of muscimol-induced hyperactivity by benzodiazepines. J. Pharm. Pharmacol. 31, 427–428 (1979)

Matthews, W.D., Connor, J.D.: Effects of diphenylhydantoin and diazepam on hippocampal evoked responses. Neuropharmacology 15, 181–186 (1976)

Matthews, W.D., Connor, J.D.: Actions of iontophoretic phenytoin and medazepam on hippocampal neurons. J. Pharm. Exp. Ther. 201, (3) 613–621 (1977)

Matthews, W.D., McCafferty, G.P.: Anticonvulsant activity of muscimol against seizures induced by impairment of GABA-mediated neurotransmission. Neuropharmacology 18, 885–889 (1979)

Maurer, R.: The GABA agonist THIP, a muscimol analogue, does not interfere with the benzodiazepine binding site on rats cortical membranes. Neurosci. Letters 12, 65–68 (1979a)

Maurer, R.: Characterization of an endogenous inhibitor of ^{3}H-muscimol binding isolated from rat brain. Experientia 35, 939 (1979b)

Maxwell, D.R., Read, M.A., The effects of some drugs on the rigidity of the cat due to ischaemic or intercollicular decerebration. Neuropharmacology 11, 849–855 (1972)

Maxwell, D.R., Read, M.A., Sumpter, E.A.: Pharmacology of M&B 18.706, a drug which selectively reduced decerebrate rigidity. Br. J. Pharmacol. 50, 35–45 (1974)

McHugh, S.L. Ram, N., Gray, M.I., Rosenthale, M.E.: Effects of chlordiazepoxide in hypertensive animals. Fed. Proc. 37, 353 (1978)

McNamara, J.O., Peper, A., Patrone, V.: Repeated seizures induce long-term increase in hippocampal benzodiazepine receptors. Proc. Natl. Acad. Sci. USA 77, 3029–3033 (1980)

Meldrum, B.S., Horton, R.W., Toseland, P.A.: A primate model for testing anticonvulsant drugs. Arch. Neurol. 32, 289–294 (1975)

Mendell, L.M., Wall, P.D.: Presynaptic hyperpolarization: a role for fine afferent fibres. J. Physiol. (Lond.) 172, 274–294 (1964)

Menétrey, D., Decaud-Gasarabwe, J., Besson, J.M.: Effects of diazepam on dorsal root potentials induced by cortical paroxysmal activity. Eur. J. Pharmacol. 24, 158–163 (1973)

Mennear, J.H., Rudzik, A.D.: Mechanism of action of anticonvulsant drugs. 3. Chlordiazepoxide. J. Pharm. Sci. 55, 640–641 (1966)

Mercier, J., Dessaigne, S.: Influence exercée par quelques drogues psycholeptiques sur le comportement du scorpion. C. R. Soc. Biol. *164*, 341–344 (1970)

Mercier, J., Lumbroso, S.: Influence exercée par la 1,3 dihydro-7-nitro-5-phényl-2H,1,4 benzodiazépine-2-one (Mogadon) sur l'ulcère de contrainte du rat et de la souris albinos. Pharmacodyn. Ther. *167* (1), 35–38 (1967)

Mercier, J., Dessaigne, S., Etzensperger, P.: Influence exercée par la chlordiazépoxide sur le comportement de la mante religieuse. C. R. Soc. Biol. *160*, 133–136 (1966)

Mercier, J., Dessaigne, S., Manez, J.: Neurophysiological study of dipotassium chlorazepate (4306 CB). Arzneim. Forsch. *20*, (1) 125–127 (1970)

Mereu, G.P., Fratta, W., Chessa, P., Gessa, G.L.: Voraciousness induced in cats by benzodiazepines. Psychopharmacology *47*, 101–103 (1976)

Merlo, L., Noseda, V., Ferrini, R., Miragoli, G., Marchetti, G.: Effect of camazepam (SB-5833), a new antianxious drug, on cardiac contractility and coronary hemodynamics. Arzneim. Forsch. *24*(11), 1759–1762 (1974)

Meyerhoff, J.L, Lenox, R.H., Kant, G.J., Sessions, G.R., Mougey, E.H., Pennington, L.L.: The effect of locomotor activity on cerebellar levels of cGMP. Life Sci. *24*, 1125–1130 (1979)

Michalová, C., Hrubeš, V., Beneš, V.: The influence of chlordiazepoxide on biochemical reactions to experimental stress in rats. Activ. Nerv. Sup. (Praha) *8*, 458–459 (1966)

Miczek, K.A.: Intraspecies aggression in rats: Effects of d-amphetamine and chlordiazepoxide. Psychopharmacologia *39*, 275–301 (1974)

Miczek, K.A., O'Donnell, J.M.: Alcohol and chlordiazepoxide increase suppressed aggression in mice. Psychopharmacology *69*, 39–44 (1980)

Millichap, J.G.: Relation of laboratory evaluation to clinical effectiveness of antiepileptic drugs. Epilepsia *10*, 315–328 (1969)

Mimaki, T., Deshmukh, P.P., Yamamura, H.I.; An interaction of phenytoin (DPH) with benzodiazepine receptor in rat brain. Pharmacologist *22*, 185 (1980)

Mitchell, J.F.: The spontaneous and evoked release of acetylcholine from the cerebral cortex. J. Physiol. (Lond.) *165*, 98–116 (1963)

Mitchell, P.R., Martin, I.L.: The effects of benzodiazepines on K+-stimulated release of GABA. Neuropharmacology *17*, 317–320 (1978)

Mitolo-Chieppa, D., Marino, A.: Effetti di un tranquillante (il chlordiazepossido) e di un barbiturico (il luminal) sull' attività elettrica di fibre nervose isolate di rana. Boll. Soc. Ital. Biol. Sper. *48*(23), 1042–1044 (1972)

Miyake, H.: Electrophysiological studies on the action of chlordiazepoxide in cats. Psychiat. Neurol. Jap. *67*, 992–1004 (1965)

Moe, R., Bagdon, R.E., Zbinden, G.: The effects of tranquilizers on myocardial metabolism. Angiology *13*(1), 4–12 (1962)

Möhler, H., Okada, T.: Benzodiazepine receptors: demonstration in the central nervous system. Science *198*, 849–851 (1977a)

Möhler, H., Okada, T.: Properties of ^{3}H-diazepam binding to benzodiazepine receptors in rat cerebral cortex. Life Sci. *20*, 2101–2110 (1977b)

Möhler, H., Okada, T.: GABA receptor binding with ^{3}H (+)bicuculline-methiodide in rat CNS. Nature *267*, 65–67 (1977c)

Möhler, H., Okada, T.: The benzodiazepine receptor in normal and pathological human brain. Br. J. Psychiat. *133*, 261–268 (1978)

Möhler, H., Richards, J.G.: Benzodiazepine receptors: electronmicroscopic localization in the brain. In: Psychopharmacology and Biochemistry of Neurotransmitter Receptors. Olsen, R.W., Yamamura, N.I., Usdin, E. (eds.), pp. 649–654. Amsterdam: Elsevier 1980b

Möhler, H., Okada, T., Enna, S.J.: Benzodiazepine and neurotransmitter binding in rat brain after chronic administration of diazepam or phenobarbital. Brain Res. *156*, 391–395 (1978a)

Möhler, H., Okada, T., Heitz, P., Ulrich, J.: Biochemical identification of the site of action of benzodiazepines in human brain by ^{3}H-diazepam binding. Life Sci. *22*, 985–996 (1978b)

Möhler, H., Polc, P., Cumin, R., Pieri, L., Kettler, R.: Nicotinamide is a brain constituent with benzodiazepine-like actions. Nature *278*, 563–565 (1979)

Möhler, H., Battersby, M.K., Richards, J.G.: Benzodiazepine receptor protein identified and visualized in brain tissue by a photoaffinity label. Proc. Natl. Acad. Sci. USA 77, 1666–1670 (1980a)

Möhler, H., Wu, J.-Y., Richards, J.G.: Benzodiazepine receptors: autoradiographical and immunocytochemical evidence for their localization in regions of GABAergic synaptic contacts. In: GABA and Benzodiazepine receptors. Costa, E., Di Chiara, G., Gessa, G.L. (eds.), pp. 139–146. New York: Raven Press 1981

Möhler, H., Battersby, M.K., Richards, J.G., Polc, P., Cumin, R., Pieri, L., Kettler, R.: Benzodiazepine receptor: localization by photoaffinity labelling and isolation of a possible endogenous ligand. In: Receptors for neurotransmitters and peptide hormones. Pepeu, G., Kuhar, M.J., Enna, S.J. (eds.), pp. 295–299. New York: Raven Press 1980c

Molander, L., Duvhök, C.: Acute effects of oxazepam and methylperone, alone and in combination with alcohol on sedation, coordination and mood. Acta Pharmacol. Toxicol. 38, 145–160 (1976)

Molinengo, L.: Azione di alcuni depressivi del SNC sulla coordinazione motoria del ratto. Arch. Ital. Sci. Farmacol. 14, 288–291 (1964)

Monachon, M.A., Jalfre, M., Haefely, W.: A modulating effect of chlordiazepoxide on drug-induced PGO spikes in the cat. In: The Benzodiazepines. Garattini, S., Mussini, E., Randall, L.O. (eds.), pp. 513–529. New York: Raven Press 1973

Monnier, M., Graber, S.: Classification électrophysiologique des substances psycholeptiques. (Position du chlordiazépoxide „Librium"). Arch. Int. Pharmacodyn. 140(1–2), 206–216 (1962)

Montarolo, P.G., Raschi, F., Strata, P.: Interactions between benzodiazepines and GABA in the cerebellar cortex. Brain Res. 162, 358–362 (1979)

Monti, J.M., Altier, H., D'Angelo, L.: The effects of the combined administration of gamma-hydroxybutyrate and diazepam on sleep parameters in the rat. J. Neur. Trans. 45, 177–183 (1979a)

Monti, J.M., Altier, H., D'Angelo, L: Diazepam, GABA agonists and antagonists and the sleep wakefulness cycle. Adv. Biosci. 21, 65–73 (1979b)

Moore, M.S., Tychsen, R.L., Thompson, D.M.: Extinction-induced mirror responding as a baseline for studying drug effects on aggression. Pharmacol. Biochem. Behav. 4, 99–102 (1976)

Mori, M., Nishijima, Y., Iwata, N.: Neuropharmacologic studies on the effects of CS-370, a new psychotherapeutic agent, upon the central nervous system. Folia Pharmacol. Jap. 68(3), 314–329 (1972)

Morillo, A.: Effects of benzodiazepines upon amygdala and hippocampus of the cat. Int. J. Neuropharmacol. 1, 353–359 (1962)

Morillo, A., Revzin, A.M., Knauss, T.: Physiological mechanisms of action of chlordiazepoxide in cats. Psychopharmacologia 3, 386–394 (1962)

Morison, R.S., Dempsey, E.W.: A study of thalamo-cortical relations. Am. J. Physiol. 135, 281–292 (1942)

Morpurgo, C.: Pharmacological modifications of sympathetic responses elicited by hypothalamic stimulation in the rat. Br. J. Pharmacol. 34, 532–542 (1968)

Morris, M.D., Tremmel, F., Gebhart, G.F.: Forebrain noradrenaline depletion blocks the release by chlordiazepoxide of behavioural extinction in the rat. Neurosci. Letters 12, 343–348 (1979)

Morrison, A.B., Webster, R.A.: Reserpine rigidity and adrenergic neurones. Neuropharmacology 12, 725–733 (1973)

Moruzzi, G.: The sleep-waking cycle. Ergebn. Physiol. 64, 1–165 (1972)

Moruzzi, G., Magoun, H.W.: Brain stem reticular formation and activation of the EEG. Electroenceph. Clin. Neurophysiol. 1, 455–473 (1949)

Moss, L.M.: Naloxone reversal of non-narcotic induced apnea. J. Am. Coll. Emer. Phys. 1, 46–48 (1973)

Moudgil, G., Pleuvry, B.J.: Diazepam and neuromuscular transmission. Brit. Med. J. 1970II, 734–735 (1970)

Moyer, K.E.: Kinds of aggression and their physiological basis. Commun. Behav. Biol. 2, 65–87 (1968)

Muir, W.W., Werner, L.L., Hamlin, R.L.: Antiarrhythmic effects of diazepam during coronary artery occlusion in dogs. Am. J. Vet. Res. 36(8), 1203–1206 (1975)

Mulé, S.J.: Inhibition of phospholipid-facilitated calcium transport by central nervous system-acting drugs. Biochem. Pharmacol. 18, 339–346 (1969)

Müller, W.E., Wollert, U.: Benzodiazepines: Specific competition for the binding of L-trypto-phan to human serum albumin. Naunyn-Schmiedebergs Arch. Pharmacol. *288*, 17–27 (1975a)

Müller, W.E., Wollert, U.: High stereospecificity of the benzodiazepine binding site on human serum albumin. Studies with d- and l-oxazepam hemisuccinate. Mol. Pharmacol. *11*, 52–60 (1975b)

Müller, W.E., Schläfer, U., Wollert, U.: Benzodiazepine receptor binding in rat spinal membranes. Neurosci. Letters *9*, 239–243 (1978a)

Müller, W.E., Schläfer, U., Wollert, U.: Benzodiazepine receptor binding: The interactions of some non-benzodiazepine drugs with specific [³] diazepam binding to rat brain synaptosomal membranes. Naunyn-Schmiedebergs Arch. Pharmacol. *305*, 23–26 (1978b)

Müller, E.E., Cocchi, D., Locatelli, V., Krogsgaard-Larsen, P., Brund, F., Racagni, G.: GABAergic neurotransmission and the secretion of prolactin in the rat. In: GABA-neurotransmitter. Krogsgaard-Larsen, P., Scheel-Krüger, J., Kofod, H. (eds.), pp. 518–532. Copenhagen: Munksgaard 1979

Munekyio, K., Meshi, T.: Effect of triazolam on the activities of the hippocampal pyramidal cells in rats. Jap. J. Pharmacol. *29* (Suppl.) 47P (1979)

Munson, E.S., Wagman, I.H.: Diazepam treatment of local anesthetic-induced seizures. Anesthesiology *37*(5), 523–528 (1972)

Murasaki, M., Hara, T., Oguchi, T., Inami, M., Ikeda, Y.: Action of enpiprazole on emotional behavior induced by hypothalamic stimulation in rats and cats. Psychopharmacology *49*, 271–274 (1976)

Murayama, S., Suzuki, T.: Effects of benzodiazepines on spinal reflex potentials: experiments on ischemic spinal rigid cats. Japan. J. Pharmacol. *24*, Suppl., 105 (1974)

Murayama, S., Suzuki, T.: Spinal action of lorazepam. Chiba Med. J. *51*(4), 201–204 (1975)

Murayama, S., Uemura, H., Suzuki, T.: Effects of benzodiazepines on spinal reflexes in cats. Japan. J. Pharmacol. *22*, Suppl., 117 (1972)

Murphy, M.F., Kreisman, N.R.: Effects of 1,4-benzodiazepines on antidromic invasion in the giant neuron of aplysia californica. 7th Ann. Meeting Soc. Neurosci. Abstr. *3*, 143 (1977)

Murphy, M.F., King, W.M., Kreisman, N.R.: Effects of chlordiazepoxide on identified neurons in the abdominal ganglion of aplysia californica. Pharmacologist *18*(2), 137 (1976)

Mustala, O.O., Penttilä, O.I.: Anticonvulsant action of some new skeletal muscle relaxants in strychnine convulsions in mice. Acta Pharmacol. Toxicol. (Kbh.) *19*, 247–250 (1962)

Naftchi, N.E., Lowman, E.W.: The effect of diazepam on presynaptic inhibition. Scientific Exhibit at the Am. Acad. of Rehab. Med., pp. 1–15. Miami Beach, 1977

Naftchi, N.E., Schlosser, W., Horst, W.D.: Changes in the GABAsystem with development of spasticity in paraplegic cats. In: GABA-Biochemistry and CNS Functions. Mandel, P., De Feudis, F. (eds.), pp. 431–450. New York: Raven Press 1979

Nagy, J., Decsi, L.: Location of the site of the tranquilizing action of diazepam by intralimbic application. Neuropharmacology *12*, 757–768 (1973)

Nagy, J., Decsi, L.: Physostigmine, a highly potent antidote for acute experimental diazepam intoxication. Neuropharmacology *17*, 469–475 (1978)

Nagy, J., Decsi, L.: Further studies on the site of action of diazepam: Anticonvulsant effect in the rabbit. Neuropharmacology *18*, 39–45 (1979)

Nahorski, S.R.: Biochemical effects of the anticonvulsants trimethadione, ethosuximide and chlordiazepoxide in rat brain. J. Neurochem. *19*, 1937–1946 (1972)

Naik, S.R., Guidotti, A., Costa, E.: Central GABA receptor agonists: Comparison of muscimol and baclofen. Neuropharmacology *15*, 479–484 (1976)

Nakajima, R., Hattori, C., Nagawa, Y.: Structure-activity relationship of 5-triazolo-1,4-benzodiazepines in central nervous depressant action. Japan. J. Pharmacol. *21*, 489–495 (1971a)

Nakajima, R., Take, Y., Moriya, R., Saji, Y., Yui, T., Nagawa, Y., Pharmacological studies on new potent central depressants, 8-chloro-6-phenyl-4H-s-triazolo[4,3a][1,4] benzodiazepine (D-40TA) and its 1-methyl analogue (D-65MT). Japan. J. Pharmacol. *21*, 497–519 (1971b)

Nakama, M., Ochiai, T., Kowa, Y.: Effects of psychotropic drugs on emotional behaviour: Exploratory behaviour of naive rats in holed open field. Japan. J. Pharmacol. *22*, 767–775 (1972)

Nakamura, M., Fukushima, H.: Head twitches induced by benzodiazepines and the role of biogenic amines. Psychopharmacology 49, 259–261 (1976)

Nakamura, M., Fukushima, H.: Effect of fludiazepam on turnover of serotonin in mouse brain. Japn. J. Pharmacol. 27, 905–908 (1977)

Nakamura, M., Fukushima, H.: Effect of 5,6-dihydroxytryptamine on the head twitches induced by 5-HTP, 5-HT, mescaline and fludiazepam in mice. J. Pharm. Pharmacol. 30, 56–58 (1978 a)

Nakamura, M., Fukushima, H.: Effects of reserpine, para-chlorophenylalanine, 5,6-dihydroxytryptamine and fludiazepam on the head twitches induced by 5-hydroxytryptamine or 5-methoxytryptamine in mice. J. Pharm. Pharmacol. 30, 254–256 (1978 b)

Nakamura, K., Thoenen, H.: Increased irritability: a permanent behaviour change induced in the rat by intraventricular administration of 6-hydroxydopamine. Psychopharmacologia 24, 359–372 (1972)

Nakanishi, T., Norris, F.H., Jr.: Effect of diazepam on rat spinal reflexes. J. Neurol. Sci. 13, 189–195 (1971)

Nakanishi, M., Tsumagari, T., Takigawa, Y., Shuto, S., Kenjo, T., Fukuda, T.: Studies on psychotropic drugs. XIX. Psychopharmacological studies of 1-methyl-5-o-chlorophenyl-7-ethyl-1,2-dihydro-3H-thieno(2,3-e)(1,4)diazepine-2-one (Y-6047). Arzneim. Forsch. 22 (11), 1905–1914 (1972)

Naquet, R., Meldrum, B.S.: Photogenic Seizures in Baboon. In: Experimental Models of Epilepsy. Purpura, D.P., Penry, J.K., Tower, D.B., Woodbury, D.M., Walter, R.D. (eds.), pp. 373–406. New York: Raven Press 1972

Nelson-Krause, D.C., Howard, B.D.: Release of glycine and gamma aminobutyric acid from synaptosomes prepared from rat central nervous tissue. Fed. Proc. 35(3), 543 (1976)

Nestoros, J.N.: Benzodiazepine receptors and cortical inhibition. Abstr., CFBS Meeting, Vancouver, June 1979

Nestoros, J.N., Nistri, A.: A presynaptic component of the action of iontophoretically applied flurazepam on feline cortical neurones. Can. J. Physiol. Pharmacol. 56, 889–892 (1978)

Nestoros, J.N., Nistri, A.: Effects of microiontophoretically applied flurazepam on responses of cerebral cortical neurones to putative neurotransmitters. Can. J. Physiol. Pharmacol. 57, 1324–1329 (1979)

Nevins, M.A., Mattes, L.M., Spritzer, R.C., Weisenseel, A.C., Donoso, E., Friedberg, C.K., Ineffectiveness of diazepam as an antiarrhythmic agent. J. Mt. Sinai Hosp. 36, 408–414 (1969)

Ngai, S.H., Tseng, D.T.C., Wang, S.C.: Effect of diazepam and other central nervous system depressants on spinal reflexes in cats: a study of site of action. J. Pharmacol. Exp. Ther. 153, 344–351 (1966)

Niada, R., Omini, C., Prino, G., Folco, G.C., Milani, S., Berti, F.: Synergistic interaction between diazepam and octatropine-methylbromide at the gastrointestinal level. Pharmacol. Res. Commun. 10(10), 951–960 (1978)

Nicoll, R.A., Wojtowicz, J.M.: The effects of pentobarbital and related compounds on frog motoneurons. Brain. Res. 191, 225–237 (1980)

Nicot, G., Decaud-Gasarabwe, J., Besson, J.: Action du diazépam et du clonazépam sur les phénomènes d'inhibition présynaptique au niveau spinal chez le lapin. J. Pharmacol. (Paris) 7(1), 17–26 (1976)

Nielsen, M., Braestrup, C., Squires, R.F.: Evidence for a late evolutionary appearance of brain-specific benzodiazepine receptors: an investigation of 18 vertebrate and 5 invertebrate species. Brain Res. 141, 342–346 (1978)

Nielsen, M., Gredal, D., Braestrup, C.: Some properties of ^{3}H-diazepam displacing activity from human urine. Life Sci. 25, 679–686 (1979)

Nielsen, M., Schou, H., Braestrup, C.: ^{3}H-Propyl β-carboline-3-carboxylate binds specifically to brain benzodiazepine receptors. J. Neurochem. 36, 276–285 (1981)

Niemegeers, C.J.E., Lewi, P.J.: The anticonvulsant properties of anxiolytic agents. In: Industrial Pharmacology. Fielding, S., Lal, H., (eds.), Vol. III, pp. 141–158. New York: Futura Publishing Co., Mount Kisco, 1979

Niki, H.: Chlordiazepoxide and food intake in rat. Jap. Psychol. Res. 7, 80–85 (1965)

Nistri, A., Constanti, A.: Effects of flurazepam on amino acid-evoked responses recorded from the lobster muscle and the frog spinal cord. Neuropharmacology 17, 127–135 (1978 a)

Nistri, A., Constanti, A.: A quantitative study of benzodiazepine-aminoacid interactions on the lobster muscles and the frog spinal cord. In: Iontophoresis and transmitter mechanisms in the mammalian central nervous system. Ryall, R.W., Kelly, J.S. (eds.), pp. 273–275. Amsterdam: Elsevier 1978 b

Nistri, A., Constanti, A., Krnjević, K.: Electrophysiological studies on the mode of action of GABA on vertebrate central neurons. In: Receptors for Neurotransmitters and Peptide Hormones. Pepeu, G., Kuhar, M.J., Enna, S.J. (eds.), pp. 81–90. New York: Raven Press 1980

Nolan, N.A., Parkes, M.W.: The effects of benzodiazepines on the behaviour of mice on a hole-board. Psychopharmacologia 29, 277–288 (1978)

Norton, P.: The effects of drugs on barbiturate withdrawal convulsions in the rat. J. Pharm. Pharmacol. 22, 763–766 (1970)

O'Brien, R.A., Spirt, N.M.: The inhibition of GABA-stimulated benzodiazepine binding by a convulsant benzodiazepine. Life Sci. 26, 1441–1445 (1980)

Oetliker, H.: Action of chlordiazepoxide on contractile mechanism in single fibres of frog muscle. Experientia 26 (6), 682 (1970)

Ohmori, K.: Electroencephalographic effect of flurazepam in rabbits. Nippon Yakurigaku Zasshi 73, (8) 939–954 (1977)

Okada, Y.: Inhibitory action of adenosine and adenine nucleotides on the postsynaptic potential (PSP) of an olfactory cortex slice of the guinea pig. In: Neurobiology of chemical transmission. Otsuka, M., Hall, Z.W. (eds.), pp. 223–234. New York: John Wiley & Sons 1979

Okamoto, K., Sakai, Y.: Augmentation by chlordiazepoxide of the inhibitory effects of taurine, beta-alanine and GABA on spike discharges in guinea-pig cerebellar slices. Brit. J. Pharmacol. 65, 277–285 (1979)

Olds, M.E., Baldrighi, G.: Effects of meprobamate, chlordiazepoxide, diazepam and sodium pentobarbital on visually evoked responses in the tectotegmental area of the rat. Int. J. Neuropharmacol. 7, 231–239 (1968)

Olds, M.E., Olds, J.: Effects of anxiety-relieving drugs on unit discharges in hippocampus, reticular midbrain and pre-optic area in the freely moving rat. Int. J. Neuropharmacol. 8, 87–103 (1969)

Olgiati, V.R., Netti, C., Guidobono, F., Pecile, A.: The central GABAergic system and control of food intake under different experimental conditions. Psychopharmacology 68, 163–167 (1980)

Olpe, H.-R.: Pharmacological manipulations of the automatically recorded biting behavior evoked in rats by apomorphine. Eur. J. Pharmacol. 51, 441–448 (1978)

Olsen, R.W., Lamar, E.E., Byless, J.D.: Calcium-induced release of γ-aminobutyric acid from synaptosomes. Effects of tranquilizer drugs. J. Neurochem. 28, (2) 299–305 (1977)

Olsen, R.W., Ticku, M.K., Greenlee, D., Van Ness, P.: GABA receptor and ionophore binding sites: interaction with various drugs. In: GABA-Neurotransmitters. Krogsgaard-Larsen, P., Scheel-Krüger, J., Kofod, H. (eds.), pp. 165–178. Copenhagen: Munksgaard 1978 a

Olsen, R.W., Ticku, M.K., Van Ness, P., Greenlee, D.: Effects of drugs on γ-aminobutyric receptors, uptake, release and synthesis in vitro. Brain Res. 139, 277–294 (1978 b)

Opitz, K., Akinlaja, A.: Zur Beeinflussung der Nahrungsaufnahme durch Psychopharmaka. Psychopharmacologia 9, 307–319 (1966)

Opmeer, F.A., Gumulka, S.W., Dinnendahl, V., Schönhöfer, P.S.: Effects of stimulatory and depressant drugs on cyclic guanosine 3′,5′-monophosphate and adenosine 3′,5′-monophosphate levels in mouse brain. Naunyn-Schmiedebergs Arch. Pharmacol. 292, 259–265 (1976)

Osborne, N.N.: Benzodiazepine binding to bovine retina. Neuroscience Letters 16, 167–170 (1980)

Oswald, I., Priest, R.G.; Five weeks to escape the sleeping-pill habit. Br. Med. J. 165 II, 1093–1095 (1965)

Otsuka, M., Tsuchiya, T., Kitagawa, S.: Electroencephalographic and behavioral studies on the central action of nimetazepam (S-1530) in cats. Arzneim. Forsch. 23 (5), 645–652 (1973)

Otsuka, M., Tsuchiya, T., Kitagawa, S.: Electrophysiological and behavioral effects of 1-methyl-5-(o-fluorophenyl)-7-chloro-1,3-dihydro-2H-1,4-benzodiazepin-2-one (ID-540) in cats and rabbits. Arzneim. Forsch. 25 (5), 755–759 (1975)

Owen, G., Hatfield, G.K., Pollock, J.J., Steinberg, A.J., Tucker, W.E., Agersborg, H.P.K., Jr.: Toxicity studies of lorazepam, a new benzodiazepine, in animals. Arzneim. Forsch. *21*, 1065–1073 (1971)

Padjen, A., Bloom, F.: Problems in the electrophysiological analysis of the site of action of benzodiazepines. In: Advances in Biochemical Psychopharmacology. Costa, E., Greengard P. (eds), Vol. 14, pp. 93–102. New York: Raven Press 1975

Palacios, J.M., Niehoff, D.L., Kuhar, M.J.: Ontogeny of GABA and benzodiazepine receptors: effects of Triton-X-100, bromide and muscimol. Brain Res. *179*, 390–395 (1979)

Palmer, G.C., Jones, D.J., Medina, M.A., Stavinoha, W.B.: Anticonvulsant drug actions on in vitro and in vivo levels of cyclic AMP in the mouse brain. Epilepsia *20*, 95–104 (1979)

Panksepp, J.: Drugs and stimulus-bound attack. Physiol. Behavior *6*, 317–320 (1971)

Parkes, M.W.: The pharmacology of diazepam. In: Diazepam in anaesthesia. Knight, P.F., Burgess, C.C. (eds.), pp. 1–7. Bristol: John Wright and Sons Ltd. 1968

Patel, J.B., Malick, J.B.: Effects of isoproterenol and chlordiazepoxide on drinking and conflict behaviors in rats. Pharmacol. Biochem. Behav. *12*, 819–821 (1980)

Patrick, J.M., Sempik, A.K.: The effect of diazepam on the threshold of the ventilatory response to CO_2. Brit. J. Pharmacol. *64*, 454P–455P (1978)

Paul, S.M., Skolnick, P.: Rapid changes in brain benzodiazepine receptors after experimental seizures. Science *202*, 892–894 (1978)

Paul, S.M., Syapin, P.J., Paugh, B.A., Moncada, V., Skolnick, P.: Correlation between benzodiazepine receptor occupation and anticonvulsant effects of diazepam. Nature *281*, 688–689 (1979)

Paul, S.M., Zatz, M., Skolnick, P.: Demonstration of brain specific benzodiazepine receptors in rat retina. Brain Res. *187*, 243–246 (1980)

Pax, R., Bennett, J.L., Fetterer, R.: A benzodiazepine derivative and praziquantel: effects on musculature of schistosoma mansoni and schistosoma japonicum. Arch. Pharmacol. *304*(3), 309–315 (1978)

Pearl, D.S., Quest, J.A., Gillis, R.A.: Effect of diazepam on digitalis-induced ventricular arrhythmias in the cat.. Toxicol. Appl. Pharmacol. *44*, 643–652 (1978a)

Pearl, D.S., Quest, J.A., Gillis, R.A.: Use of various solvents to study the effect of diazepam on cardiac rhythm. Toxicol. Appl. Pharmacol. *44*, 653–656 (1978b)

Peričič, D., Walters, J.R., Chase, T.N.: Effect of diazepam and pentobarbital on aminooxyacetic acid-induced accumulation of GABA. J. Neurochem. *29*, 839–846 (1977)

Petsche, H., Rappelsberger, P.: Der Strophanthinstatus als Modell für Auswertung antikonvulsiver Medikamente. Pharmakopsychiat. Neuro-Psychopharm. *3*, 151–161 (1970)

Peyton, J.C., Borowitz, J.L.: Chlordiazepoxide and theophylline alter calcium levels in subcellular fractions of rat brain cortex. Proc. Soc. Exp. Biol. Med. *161*, 178–182 (1979)

Phillis, J.W.: Diazepam potentiation of purinergic depression of central neurons. Can. J. Physiol. Pharmacol. *57*, 432–435 (1979)

Phillis, J.W., Edstrom, J.P., Ellis, S.W., Kirkpatrick, J.R.: Theophylline antagonizes flurazepam-induced depression of cerebral cortical neurons. Can. J. Physiol. Pharmacol. *57*, 917–920 (1979)

Phillis, J.W., Bender, A.S., Wu, P.H.: Benzodiazepines inhibit adenosine uptake into rat brain synaptosomes. Brain Res. *195*, 494–498 (1980)

Pieri, L.: Effect of a new imidazobenzodiazepine and a thienotriazolodiazepine on spontaneous activity of cerebellar Purkinje neurons in the rat. Abstr. 11th C.I.N.P. Congr., p. 40, Wien, 1978

Pieri, L., Haefely, W.: The effect of diphenylhydantoin, diazepam and clonazepam on the activity of Purkinje cells in the rat cerebellum. Arch. Pharmacol. *296*, 1–4 (1976)

Pieri, L., Schaffner, R., Scherschlicht, R., Polc, P., Sepinwall, J., Davidson, A., Möhler, H., Cumin, R., Da Prada, M., Burkard, W.P., Keller, H.H., Müller, R.K.M., Gerold, M., Pieri, M., Cook, L., Haefely, W.: Pharmacology of midazolam. Arzneim. Forsch. (in press) 1981

Piper, D.C.: Stress-induced partial insomnia: a model for the evaluation of potential hypnotic compounds. Brit. J. Pharmacol. *59*, 509P (1977)

Pixner, D.B.: The effect of some drugs upon synaptic transmission in the isolated spinal cord of the frog. J. Physiol. (Lond.) *189*, 15P–17P (1966)

Plaa, G.L., Besner, J.-G., Caillé, G.: Effect of diazepam on sulfobromophthalein excretion. In: Clinical Pharmacology of Psychoactive Drugs. Sellers, E.M. (ed.), pp. 203–218, Toronto: Alcoholism and Drug Addiction Research Foundation 1975

Placheta, P., Karobath, M.: Regional distribution of Na⁺-independent GABA and benzodiazepine binding sites in rat CNS. Brain Res. *178*, 580–583 (1979)

Pletscher, A.: Effect of neuroleptics and other drugs on monoamine uptake by membranes of adrenal chromaffin granules. Brit. J. Pharmacol. *59*, 419–424 (1977)

Pletscher, A., Da Prada, M., Foglar, G.: Differences between neuroleptics and tranquilizers regarding metabolism and biochemical effects. Proc. Vth Int. Congr. C.I.N.P., Washington, 1966, pp. 101–107. Amsterdam: Excerpta Medica 1967

Poddar, M.K., Urquart, D., Sinha, A.K.: Diazepam binding in brain after sleep and wakefulness. Brain Res. *193*, 519–528 (1980)

Polc, P.: Intravenous GABA, muscimol, baclofen and diazepam: GABA-ergic transmission in the spinal cord and cuneate nucleus of cats. Abstr. 11th C.I.N.P. Congr., p. 40, Wien, 1978

Polc, P., Haefely, W.: Effects of flunitrazepam on the sleep of cats. In: Sleep 1974. Levin, P., Koella, W.P. (eds.), pp. 303–305. Basel: Karger 1975

Polc, P., Haefely, W.: Effects of two benzodiazepines, phenobarbitone and baclofen on synaptic transmission in the cat cuneate nucleus. Arch. Pharmacol. *294*, 121–131 (1976)

Polc, P., Haefely, W.: Effects of systemic muscimol and GABA in the spinal cord and superior cervical ganglion of the cat. Experientia *33*, 809 (1977)

Polc, P., Haefely, W.: Psychotropic drugs and GABAergic transmission in the cat cuneate nucleus. In: Iontophoresis and Transmitter Mechanisms in the mammalian central nervous system. Ryall, R.W., Kelly, J.S. (eds.), pp. 276–278. Amsterdam: Elsevier 1978

Polc, P., Möhler, H., Haefely, W.: The effect of diazepam on spinal cord activities: Possible sites and mechanisms of action. Arch. Pharmacol. *284*, 319–337 (1974)

Polc, P., Bonetti, E.P., Pieri, L., Cumin, R., Angioi, R.M., Haefely, W.E.: Caffeine antagonizes several central effects of diazepam. Life Sci. *28*, 2265–2275 (1981)

Polzin, R.L., Barnes, C.D.: The effect of diazepam and picrotoxin on brainstem evoked dorsal root potentials. Neuropharmacology *15*, 133–137 (1976)

Polzin, R.L., Barnes, C.D.: Effect of diazepam on GABAergic cuneate neurones. Neuropharmacology *18*, 431–434 (1979)

Poole, T.B.: Some studies on the influence of chlordiazepoxide on the social interaction of golden hamsters (mesocricetus auratus). Br. J. Pharmacol. *48*, 538–545 (1973)

Pórszász, J., Gibiszer, K.P.: Effect of somatic and vegetative afferent stimuli on efferent sympathetic activity. Acta Physiol. Acad. Sci. Hung. *37*, 353–354 (1970)

Poschel, B.P.H.: A simple and specific screen for benzodiazepine-like drugs. Psychopharmacologia *19*, 193–198 (1971)

Poschel, B.P.H., McCarthy, D.A., Chen, G., Ensor, C.R.: Pyrazapon (CI-683): a new antianxiety agent. Psychopharmacologia *35*, 257–271 (1974)

Pozenel, H., Bückert, A., Amrein, R.: The antihypertensive effect of lexotan (bromazepam) – a new benzodiazepine derivative. Int. J. Clin. Pharmacol. *15*(1), 31–39 (1977)

Pradhan, S.N., De, N.N., Hayatin Methiopide: A new curariform drug. Br. J. Pharmacol. *8*, 399–405 (1953)

Prince, D.A., Wilder, B.J.: Control mechanism in cortical epileptogenic foci. "Surround" inhibition. Arch. Neurol. *16*, 194–202 (1967)

Prindle, K.H., Jr., Gold, H.K., Cardon, PV., Epstein, S.E.: Effects of psychopharmacologic agents on myocardial contractility. J. Pharmacol. Exp. Ther. *173*(1), 133–137 (1970)

Pruett, J.K., Williams, B.B., Effects of some psychotropic agents on peripheral nerve conduction rate. J. Pharm. Sci. *55*(10), 1139–1141 (1966)

Pryor, G.T., Larsen, F.F., Carr, J.D., Braude, M.C.: Interactions of Δ9-tetrahydrocannabinol with phenobarbital, ethanol and chlordiazepoxide. Pharmacol. Biochem. Behav. *7*, 331–345 (1977)

Przewlocka, B., Stala, L., Scheel-Krüger, J.: Evidence that GABA in the nucleus dorsalis raphé induces stimulation of locomotor activity and eating behavior. Life Sci. *25*, 937–945 (1979)

Przybyla, A.C., Wang, S.C.: Locus of central depressant action of diazepam. J. Pharm. Exp. Ther. *163*(2), 439–447 (1968)

Pugsley, T.A., Lippmann, W.: Effects of taclamine (Ay-22,214), a new psychoactive agent, on catecholamine and serotonin metabolism. Arch. Int. Pharmacodyn. *213*, 73–87 (1975)

Pugsley, T.A., Lippmann, W.: Effects of pyrroxan and chlordiazepoxide on biogenic amine metabolism in the rat brain. Psychopharmacology *50*, 113–118 (1976)

Pull, I., McIlwain, H.: Metabolism of [^{14}C]adenine and derivatives by cerebral tissues, superfused and electrically stimulated. Biochem. J. *126*, 975–981 (1972)

Quenzer, L.F., Feldman, R.S.; The mechanism of anti-muricidal effects of chlordiazepoxide. Pharmacol. Biochem. Behav. *3*, 567–571 (1975 a)

Quenzer, L.F., Feldman, R.S.: Chlordiazepoxide effects on brain amines and cAMP in suppression of aggression. In: Neuropsychopharmacology. Boissier, J.R., Hippius, H., Pichot, P. (eds.), pp. 890–906. Amsterdam: Excerpta Medica 1975 b

Quenzer, L.F., Feldman, R.S., Moore, J.W.: Toward a mechanism of the anti-aggression effects of chlordiazepoxide in rats. Psychopharmacologia *34*, 81–94 (1974)

Quest, J.A., Freer, L.S., Kunec, J.R., Gillis, R.A.: Chlordiazepoxide inhibition of reflex vagal bradycardia in the cat. Life Sci. *21*, 659–666 (1977)

Raabe, W., Gumnit, R.J.: Anticonvulsant action of diazepam: Increase of cortical postsynaptic inhibition. Epilepsia *18*, 117–120 (1977)

Racine, R., Burnham, W.M., Livingston, K.: The effect of procaine hydrochloride and diazepam, separately or in combination, on cortico-generalized kindled seizures. Electroenceph. Clin. Neurophysiol. *47*, 204–214 (1979)

Racine, R., Livingstone, K., Joaquin, A.: Effects of procaine HCl, diazepam and diphenylhydantoin on seizure development in cortical and subcortical structures in rats. Electroenceph. Clin. Neurophysiol. *38*, 355–365 (1975)

Randall, L.O.: Pharmacology of methaminodiazepoxide. Dis. Nerv. System *21*, (Suppl. 3) 7–10 (1960)

Randall, L.O., Kappell, B.: Pharmacology of chlordiazepoxide (librium) and analogues. Biochem. Pharmacol. *8*(1), 15 (1961)

Randall, L.O., Kappell, B.: Pharmacological activity of some benzodiazepines and their metabolites. In: The Benzodiazepines. Garattini, S., Mussini, E., Randall, L.O. (eds.), pp. 27–51. New York: Raven Press 1973

Randall, L.O., Schallek, W.: Pharmacological activity of certain benzodiazepines. In: Psychopharmacology. A review of Progress 1957–1967. Efron, D.H. (ed.), pp. 153–184. Washington: U.S. Government Printing Office 1968

Randall, L.O., Scheckel, C.L., Banziger, R.F.: Pharmacology of the metabolites of chlordiazepoxide and diazepam. Curr. Ther. Res. *7*, 590–606 (1965 a)

Randall, L.O., Scheckel, C.L., Pool, W.: Pharmacology of medazepam and metabolites. Arch. Int. Pharmacodyn. *185*, 135–148 (1970)

Randall, L.O., Schallek, W., Sternbach, L.H., Ning, R.Y.: Chemistry and pharmacology of the 1,4-benzodiazepines. Psychopharmacol. Agents *3*, 175–281 (1974)

Randall, L.O., Schallek, W., Heise, G.A., Keith, E.F., Bagdon, R.E.: The psychosedative properties of methaminodiazepoxide. J. Pharmacol. Exp. Ther. *129*, 163–171 (1960)

Randall, L.O., Schallek, W., Scheckel, C., Bagdon, R.E., Rieder, J.: Zur Pharmakologie von Mogadon, einem Schlafmittel mit neuartigem Wirkungsmechanismus. Schweiz. Med. Wschr. *95*(10), 334–337 (1965 b)

Randall, L.O., Schallek, W., Scheckel, C., Banzinger, R., Moe, R.A.: Zur Pharmakologie des neuen Psychopharmakons 7-Chlor-2,3-dihydro-1-methyl-5-phenyl-1H-1,4-benzodiazepin (Ro 5-4556). Arzneim. Forsch. *18*, 1542–1545 (1968)

Randall, L.O., Schallek, W., Scheckel, C.L., Stefko, P.L., Banziger, R.F., Pool, W., Moe, R.A.: Pharmacological studies on flurazepam hydrochloride (Ro 5-6901), a new psychotropic agent of the benzodiazepine class. Arch. Int. Pharmacodyn. *178*, 216–241 (1969)

Randall, L.O., Heise, G.A., Schallek, W., Bagdon, R.E., Banziger, R., Boris, A., Moe, R.A., Abrams, W.B.: Pharmacological and chemical studies on valium, a new psychotherapeutic agent of the benzodiazepine class. Curr. Ther. Res. *3*, 405–425 (1961)

Randall, L.O., Schallek, W., Scheckel, C., Banziger, R., Boris, A., Moe, R.A., Bagdon, R.E., Schwartz, M.A., Zbinden, G.: Zur Pharmakologie von Valium, einem neuen Psychopharmakon der Benzodiazepinreihe. Schweiz. Med. Wschr. *93*(22), 794–797 (1963)

Rao, S., Sherbaniuk, R.W., Prasad, K., Lee, S.J.K., Sproule, B.J.: Cardiopulmonary effects of diazepam. Clin. Pharmacol. Ther. *14*(2), 182–189 (1972)

Rastogi, R.B., Singhal, R.L.: Brain 5-hydroxytryptamine metabolism: adaptive changes after long-term administration of psychotropic drugs. Gen. Pharmacol. *9*, 307–314 (1978)

Rastogi, R.B., Lapierre, Y.D., Shinghal, R.L.: Evidence for the role of brain norepinephrine and dopamine in "rebound" phenomenon seen during withdrawal after repeated exposure to benzodiazepines. J. Psychiatr. Res. *13*, 65–75 (1976)

Rastogi, R.B., Lapierre, Y.D., Singhal, R.L.: Effects of a new benzodiazepine bromazepam on locomotor performance and brain monoamine metabolism. J. Neural Transm. *42*, 251–261 (1978a)

Rastogi, R.B., Lapierre, Y.D., Singhal, R.L.: Synaptosomal uptake of norepinephrine and 5-hydroxytryptamine and synthesis of catecholamines during benzodiazepine treatment. Can. J. Physiol. Pharmacol. *56*, 777–778 (1978b)

Rastogi, R.B., Agarwal, R.A., Lapierre, Y.D., Singhal, R.L.: Effects of acute diazepam and clobazam on spontaneous locomotor activity and central amine metabolism in rats. Eur. J. Pharmacol. *43*, 91–98 (1977)

Reggiani, G., Hürlimann, A., Theiss, E.: Some aspects of the experimental and clinical toxicology of chlordiazepoxide. Proc. Eur. Soc. Study Drug Toxicol. *9*, 79–97 (1968)

Reinhard, J.F., Kimura, E.T., Scudi, J.V.: Pharmacologic characteristics of 1-(ortho-toluoxy)2,3-bis(2,2,2-trichloro-1-hydroxyethoxy)-propane. J. Pharmacol. Exp. Ther. *106*, 444–452 (1952)

Reinhard, J.F., Reinhard, J.F., Jr.: Experimental evaluation of anticonvulsants. In: Anticonvulsants. Vida, J.A. (ed.), pp. 57–111. New York: Academic Press 1977

Reisine, T.D., Wastek, G.J., Yamamura, H.I.: Alterations in benzodiazepine binding sites in Huntington's disease. Pharmacologist *20*(3), 240 (1978)

Reisine, T.D., Wastek, G.J., Speth, R.C., Bird, Ed.D., Yamamura, H.I.: Alterations in the benzodiazepine receptor of Huntington's diseased human brain. Brain Res. *165*, 183–187 (1979)

Renner, E.: Die Haemodialyse bei exogenen Vergiftungen und Stoffwechselkrankheiten. Internist (Berlin) *6*, 196 (1965)

Requin, S., Lanoir, J., Plas, R., Naquet, R.: Etude comparative des effets neurophysiologiques du Librium et du Valium. C.R. Soc. Biol. *157*, 2015–2019 (1963)

Ribak, C.E., Harris, A.B., Vaughin, J.E., Roberts, E.: Inhibitory GABAergic nerve terminals decrease at sites of local epilepsy. Science *205*, 211–241 (1979)

Ribeiro, J.A.: ATP; related nucleotides and adenosine on neurotransmission. Life Sci. *22*, 1373–1380 (1978)

Rice, K.C., Brossi, A., Tallmann, J., Paul, S.M., Skolnick, Ph.: Irazepine, a noncompetitive, irreversible inhibitor of ^{3}H-diazepam binding to benzodiazepine receptors. Nature *278*, 854–855 (1979)

Richter, J.A., Werling, L.L.: K-stimulated acetylcholine release: Inhibition by several barbiturates and chloral hydrate but not by ethanol, chlordiazepoxide or 11-OH-Δ^9-tetrahydrocannabinol. J. Neurochem. *32*, 935–941 (1979)

Ridley, C.M.: Bullous lesions in nitrazepam overdosage. Br. Med. J. *3*, (1971)

Rifat, K., Bolomey, M.: Les effets cardio-vasculaires du "Rohypnol" utilisé comme agent d'induction anesthésique. In: Bisherige Erfahrungen mit „Rohypnol" (Flunitrazepam) in der Anästhesiologie und Intensivtherapie. Hügin, W., Hossli, G., Gemperle, M. (eds.), pp. 84–97. Basel: Editiones Roche 1976

Robbins, T.W., Philipps, A.G., Sahakian, B.J.: Effects of chlordiazepoxide on tail pinch-induced eating in rats. Pharmacol. Biochem. Behav. *6*, 297–302 (1977)

Robertson, H.A., Benzodiazepine receptors in "emotional" and "non-emotional" mice: comparison of four strains. Eur. J. Pharmacol. *56*, 163–166 (1979)

Robertson, H.A., Martin, I.L., Candy, J.M., Differences in benzodiazepine receptor binding in Maudsley reactive and Maudsley non-reactive rats. Eur. J. Pharmacol. *50*, 455–457 (1978)

Robichaud, R.C., Goldberg, M.E.: Pharmacological properties of two chlordiazepoxide metabolites following microsomal enzyme inhibition. Arch. Int. Pharmacodyn. *211*, 165–173 (1974)

Robichaud, R.C., Gylys, J.A., Sledge, K.L., Hillyard, I.W.: The pharmacology of prazepam. A new benzodiazepine derivative. Arch. Int. Pharmacodyn. *185*, 231–227 (1970)

Robinson, J.H., Wang, S.C.: Unit activity of limbic system neurons: effect of morphine, diazepam and neuroleptic agents. Brain Res. *166*, 149–159 (1979)

Rodbard, D., Costa, T., Pert, C.B.: Is the benzodiazepine receptor coupled to a chloride channel? Nature *280*, 173–174 (1979)

Rosenberg, H.: Physosostigmine reversal of sedative drugs. J. Am. Med. Ass. *229*, 1168 (1974)

Rosenberg, H.C., Chiu, T.H.: Decreased ^{3}H-diazepam binding is a specific response to chronic benzodiazepine treatement. Life Sci. *24*, 803–808 (1979 a)

Rosenberg, H.C., Chiu, T.H.: Benzodiazepine binding after in vivo elevation of GABA. Neurosci. Letters *15*, 277–281 (1979 b)

Rosenstein, R.: Latent respiratory depression with diazepam in unanesthetized decerebrate cats. Pharmacologist *12*(2), 219 (1970)

Ross, F.H., Sermons, A.L., Walker, Ch.A.: The influence of diazepam on the circadian rhythm of glycine in the rodent brain. Pharmacologist *20*, 241 (1978)

Ruch-Monachon, M.A., Jalfre, W., Haefely, W.: Drugs and PGO waves in the lateral geniculate body of the curarized cat. I. PGO wave activity induced by Ro 4-1284 and by p-chlorophenylalanine (PCPA) as a basis for neuropharmacological studies. Arch. Int. Pharmacodyn. Ther. *219*, 251–268 (1976 a)

Ruch-Monachon, M.A., Jalfre, M., Haefely, W.: Drugs and PGO waves in the lateral geniculate body of the curarized cat. IV. The effect of acetylcholine, GABA and benzodiazepines on PGO wave activity. Arch. Int. Pharmacodyn. Ther. *219*, 308–325 (1976 b)

Ruch-Monachon, M.A., Jalfre, M., Haefely, W.: Drugs and PGO waves in the lateral geniculate body of the curarized cat. V. Miscellaneous compounds. Synopsis of the role of central neurotransmitters on PGO wave activity. Arch. Int. Pharmacodyn. Ther. *219*, 326–346 (1976 c)

Rudzik, A.D., Hester, J.B., Tang, A.H., Straw, R.N., Friis, W.: Triazolobenzodiazepines, a new class of central nervous system-depressant compounds. In: The Benzodiazepines. Garattini, S., Mussini, E., Randall, L.O. (eds.), pp. 285–298. New York: Raven Press 1973

Rüberg-Schweer, M., Karger, W.: Beeinflussung des Ionentransports an Membranen durch Tranquilizer. Eur. J. Physiol. *316*, R74 (1970)

Rüberg-Schweer, M., Karger, W.: Beeinflussung des Na$^+$-Transportes an der isolierten Froschhaut durch Meprobamate, Carisoprodol, Oxazepam und Phenobarbital. Arzneim. Forsch. *24*(10), 1568–1574 (1974)

Rump, S., Grudzinska, E.: Investigations on the effects of diazepam in acute experimental intoxication with fluostigmine. Arch. Toxikol. (Berl.) *31*, 223–232 (1974)

Rump, S., Grudzinska, E., Edelwejn, Z.: Effects of diazepam on epileptiform patterns of bioelectrical activity of the rabbit's brain induced by fluostigmine. Neuropharmacology *12*, 813–817 (1973)

Rushton, R., Steinberg, H.: Mutual potentiation of amphetamine and amylobarbitone measured by activity in rats. Br. J. Pharmacol. *21*, 295–305 (1963)

Rushton, R., Steinberg, H.: Combined effect of chlordiazepoxide and dexamphetamine on activity of rats in an unfamiliar environment. Nature *211*, 1312–1313 (1966)

Rushton, R., Steinberg, H.: Drug combinations and their analysis by means of exploratory activity in rats. In: Neuropharmacology. Bill, H., Cole, J.O., Deniker, P., Hippius, H., Bradley, P.B. (eds.), pp. 464–470. Amsterdam: Excerpta Medica 1967

Rushton, R., Steinberg, H., Tomkiewicz, M.: Effects of chlordiazepoxide alone and in combination with amphetamine on animal and human behaviour. In: The Benzodiazepines. Garattini, S., Mussini, E., Randall, L.O. (eds.), pp. 355–366. New York: Raven Press 1973

Rutishauser, M.: Beeinflussung des Kohlenhydratstoffwechsels des Rattenhirns durch Psychopharmaka mit sedativer Wirkung. Arch. Exp. Pathol. Pharmakol. *245*, 396–413 (1963)

Saad, F.S.: Effect of diazepam on γ-aminobutyric acid (GABA) content of mouse brain. J. Pharm. Pharmacol. *24*, 839–840 (1972)

Sadove, M.S., Balagot, R.C., McGrath, J.M.: Effects of chlordiazepoxide and diazepam on the influence of meperidine on the respiratory response to carbon dioxide. J. New Drugs *5*, 121–124 (1965)

Saito, C., Sakaim, S., Yukawa, Y., Yamamoto, H., Tagaki, H.: Pharmacological studies on 2-methyl-3(2′methyl-4′-chlorophenyl)-5-chloro-4(3H)-quinazolinone (SL-164). Arzneim. Forsch. *19*, 1945–1949 (1969)

Saji, Y., Mikoda, T., Ishi, H., Sato, H., Fukui, H., Koike, S., Fukuda, T., Nagawa, Y.: Pharmacodynamic effects of 8-chloro-6-phenyl-4H-5-triazolo(4,3a)(1,4)benzodiazepine (D-4OTA), a new central depressants. J. Takeda Res. Lab. *31*, 186–205 (1972)

Sakai, Sh., Kitagawa, S., Yamamoto, H.: Pharmacological studies on 1-methyl-7-nitro-5-phenyl-1,3-dihydro-2H-1,4-benzodiazepin-2-one (S-1530). Arzneim. Forsch. *22*, 534–539 (1972)

Saner, A., Pletscher, A.: Effect of diazepam on cerebral 5HT synthesis. Eur. J. Pharmacol. *55*, 315–318 (1979)

Sanger, D.J.: The effects of caffeine on timing behaviour in rodents: comparison with chlordiazepoxide. Psychopharmacology *68*, 305–309 (1980)

Sanger, D.J., Blackman, D.E.: Effects of diazepam and ripazepam on two measures of adjunctive drinking in rats. Pharmacol. Biochem. Behav. *5*, 139–152 (1976)

Sansone, M.: Facilitation of avoidance learning by chlordiazepoxide-amphetamine combinations in mice. Psychopharmacologia (Berl.) *41*, 117–121 (1975)

Sansone, M.: Effects of chlordiazepoxide, amphetamine and their combinations on avoidance behaviour of reserpinized mice. Pharmacol. Res. Commun. *9*, 879–884 (1977)

Sansone, M.: Effects of chlordiazepoxide-scopolamine combinations on shuttle-box avoidance performance of mice. Arch. Int. Pharmacodyn. *235*, 93–102 (1978 a)

Sansone, M.: Facilitating effects of chlordiazepoxide on locomotor activity and avoidance behaviour of reserpinized mice. Psychopharmacology *59*, 157–160 (1978 b)

Sansone, M.: Effects of repeated administration of chlordiazepoxide on spontaneous locomotor activity in mice. Psychopharmacology *66*, 109–110 (1979)

Sastry, B.R.: γ-Aminobutyric acid and primary afferent depolarization in feline spinal cord. Can. J. Physiol. Pharmacol. *57*, 1157–1167 (1979)

Satoh, T., Iwamoto, T.: Neurotropic drugs, electroshock, and carbohydrate metabolism in the rat. Biochem. Pharmacol. *15*, 323–331 (1966)

Saunders, J.H.B., Masoero, G., Wormsley, K.G.: Effect of diazepam and hyoscine butylbromide on response to secretin and cholecystokinin-pancreozym in man. Gut *17*, 351–353 (1976)

Sawaya, M.C.B., Horton, R.W., Meldrum, B.S.: Effects of anticonvulsant drugs on the cerebral enzymes metabolizing GABA. Epilepsia *16*, 649–655 (1975)

Schacht, U., Bäcker, G.: In vitro studies on GABA release. Br. J. Clin. Pharmacol. *7*, 25S–31S (1979)

Schaffarzick, R.W., Brown, B.J.: The anticonvulsant activity and toxicity of methylparafynol (Dormison) and some other alcohols. Science *116*, 663–665 (1952)

Schaffner, R., Haefely, W.: The effects of diazepam and bicuculline on the strio-nigral evoked potential. Experientia *31*, 732 (1975)

Schaffner, R., Jalfre, M., Haefely, W.: Effects of different pharmacological agents on the septohippocampal evoked potential (SHEP) in the cat. J. Pharmacol. (Paris) *5* (Suppl. 2), 89 (1974)

Schaffner, R., Polc, P., Möhler, H.: A convulsant benzodiazepine (RO 05-3663): Evidence for a mixed competitive/non-competitive GABA antagonism. Neurosci. Letters, Suppl. 3, 228 (1979)

Schallek, W., Preclinical pharmacology of anxiolytics. In: Principles of psychopharmacology. Clark, W.G., Del Giudice, J. (eds.), 2nd ed., pp. 325–342. New York: Academic Press 1978

Schallek, W., Kuehn, A.: Effects of psychotropic drugs on limbic system of cat. Proc. Soc. Exp. Biol. Med. *105*, 115–117 (1960)

Schallek, W., Kuehn, A.: Effects of trimethadione, diphenylhydantoin and chlordiazepoxide on after-discharge in brain of cat. Proc. Soc. Exp. Biol. Med. *112*, 813–816 (1963)

Schallek, W., Kuehn, A.: Effects of benzodiazepines on spontaneous EEG and arousal responses of cats. Prog. Brain Res. *18*, 231–238 (1965)

Schallek, W., Zabransky, F.: Effects of psychotropic drugs on pressor responses to central and peripheral stimulation in cat. Arch. Int. Pharmacodyn. Ther. *161* (1), 126–131 (1966)

Schallek, W., Thomas, J.: Effects of benzodiazepines on spontaneous electrical activity of subcortical areas in brain of cat. Arch. Int. Pharmacodyn. Ther. *192* (2), 321–337 (1971)

Schallek, W., Johnson, T.C.: Spectral density analysis of the effects of barbiturates and benzo-diazepines on the electrocorticogram of the squirrel monkey. Arch. Int. Pharmacodyn. Ther. *223*(2), 301–310 (1976)

Schallek, W., Schlosser, W.: Neuropharmacology of sedatives and anxiolytics. Mod. Probl. Pharmacopsychiatry *14*, 157–173 (1979)

Schallek, W., Kuehn, A., Jew, N.: Effects of chlordiazepoxide (librium) and other psychotropic agents on the limbic system of the brain. Ann. N.Y. Acad. Sci. *96*, 303–314 (1962)

Schallek, W., Zabransky, F., Kuehn, A.: Effects of benzodiazepines on central nervous system of cat. Arch. Int. Pharmacodyn. *149*(3–4), 467–483 (1964)

Schallek, W., Levinson, Th., Thomas, J.: Power spectrum analysis as a tool for statistical eval-uation of drug effects on electrical activity of brain. Int. J. Neuropharmacol. *7*, 35–46 (1968)

Schallek, W., Kuehn, A., Kovacs, J.: Effects of chlordiazepoxide hydrochloride on discrimina-tion responses and sleep cycles in cats. Neuropharmacology *11*, 69–79 (1972)

Schallek, W., Horst, W.D., Schlosser, W.: Mechanisms of action of benzodiazepines. Adv. Pharmacol. Chemother. *16*, 45–87 (1979)

Schallek, W., Thomas, J., Kuehn, A., Zabransky, F.: Effects of Mogadon on responses to stim-ulation of sciatic nerve, amygdala and hypothalamus of cat. Int. J. Neuropharmacol. *4*, 317–326 (1965)

Schallek, W., Kovacs, J., Kuehn, A., Thomas, J.: Some observations on the neuropharmacol-ogy of medazepam hydrochloride (Ro 5-4556). Arch. Int. Pharmacodyn. *185*, 149–158 (1970)

Schallek, W., Kovacs, J., Kuehn, A., Thomas, J.: Studies on clonazepam, flunitrazepam and related benzodiazepines in cat and monkey. Arch. Int. Pharmacodyn. *206*(1), 161–180 (1973)

Scheckel, L.L., Boff, E.: The effect of drugs on conditioned avoidance and aggressive be-haviour. in: Use of nonhuman primates in drug evaluation. Vagtborg, H. (ed.), pp. 301–312. Austin: Univ. of Texas Press 1968

Schenberg, L.C., Graeff, F.G.: Role of the periaqueductal gray substance in the antianxiety ac-tion of benzodiazepines. Pharmacol. Biochem. Behav. *9*, 287–295 (1978)

Scherberger, R.-R., Kaess, H., Brückner, S.: Untersuchungen über die Wirkung eines Anticho-linergikums in Verbindung mit einem Tranquilizer auf die Magensaftsekretion beim Men-schen. Arzneim. Forsch. *25*(9), 1460–1463 (1975)

Scherschlicht, R., Schneeberger, J., Steiner, M., Haefely, W.: Delta sleep inducing peptide (DISP) antagonizes morphine insomnia in cats. 3rd Int. Congress Sleep Res., Abstracts p. 14, Tokyo 1979

Schieken, R.M.: The effect of diazepam upon the development of hypertension in the spontane-ously hypertensive rat. Pediat. Res. *13*, 992–996 (1979)

Schlosser, W.: Action of diazepam on the spinal cord. Arch. Int. Pharmacodyn. *194*, 93–102 (1971)

Schlosser, W., Franco, S.: Modification of GABA-mediated depolarization of the cat ganglion by pentobarbital and two benzodiazepines. Neuropharmacology *18*, 377–381 (1979a)

Schlosser, W., Franco, S.: Reduction of γ-aminobutyric acid (GABA)-mediated transmission by a convulsant benzodiazepine. J. Pharmacol. Exp. Ther. *211*, 290–295 (1979b)

Schlosser, W., Zavatsky, E.: Pharmacological investigation of transmission and presynaptic in-hibition of the cells of the dorsal spinocerebellar tract of the cat. Pharmacologist *11*, 265 (1969)

Schlosser, W., Franco, S., Kuehn, A.: Modification of the cat ganglionic activity and GABA-induced depolarization by pentobarbital and flurazepam. 7th Ann. Meeting Soc. Neurosci. *3*, 1 (1977)

Schlosser, W., Franco, S., Sigg, E.B.: Differential attenuation of somatovisceral and visceroso-matic reflexes by diazepam, phenobarbital and diphenylhydantoin. Neuropharmacology *14*, 525–531 (1975b)

Schlosser, W., Zavatsky, E., Franco, S., Sigg, E.B.: Analysis of the action of CNS depressant drugs on somato-somatic reflexes in the cat. Neuropharmacology *14*, 517–523 (1975a)

Schlosser, W., Zavatsky, E., Kappell, B., Sigg, E.B.: Antagonism of bicuculline and Ro 5-3663 by diazepam. Pharmacologist *15*(2), 162 (1973)

Schmidt, R., Kappey, F., Albers, C.: Die Beeinflussung der Thermoregulation des Hundes durch Chlordiazepoxyd (Librium). Arch. Exp. Pathol. Pharmakol. *242*, 293–303 (1961)

Schmidt, R.F., Vogel, M.E., Zimmermann, M.: Die Wirkung von Diazepam auf die präsynaptische Hemmung und andere Rückenmarksreflexe. Arch. Exp. Pathol. Pharmakol. *258*, 69–82 (1967)

Schmitt, J., Comoy, P., Suquet M., Boitard, J., LeMeur, L., Basselier, J.J., Brunaud, M., Salle, J.: Sur un nouveau myorelaxant de la classe des benzodiazépines, le tétrazépam. Chim. Ther. *2*, 254–259 (1967)

Schultz, J.: Adenosine 3′,5′-monophosphate in guinea pig cerebral cortical slices. Effect of benzodiazepines. J. Neurochem. *22*, 685-690 (1974)

Schultz, J., Hamprecht, B.: Adenosine 3′,5′-monophospate in cultured neuroblastoma cells: Effect of adenosine, phosphodiesterase inhibitors and benzodiazepines. Arch. Pharmacol. *278*, 215–225 (1973)

Schumpelick, V.: Wirkung von Diazepam auf einige durch afferente abdominale Vagusreizung ausgelöste kardiovaskuläre und respiratorische Reflexe. Arzneim. Forsch. *23*(4), 514–519 (1973)

Schumpelick, V., Paschen, U.: Vergleich der protektiven Wirkung von Diazepam und Vagotomie auf das Stressulkus der Ratte. Arzneim. Forsch. *24*(2), 176–179 (1974)

Scotti de Carolis, A., Longo, V.G.: Studies on the anticonvulsant properties of some benzodiazepines (chlordiazepoxide, diazepam, oxazepam). Arzneim. Forsch. *17*, 1580–1582 (1967)

Scotti de Carolis, A., Lipparini, F., Longo, V.G.: Neuropharmacological investigations on muscimol, a psychotropic drug extracted from Amanita Muscaria. Psychopharmacologia *15*, 186–195 (1969)

Scriabine, A., Blake, A.: Evaluation of centrally acting drugs in mice with fighting behaviour induced by isolation. Psychopharmacologia *3*, 224–226 (1962)

Scrollini, F., Caliari, S., Romano, A., Torchio, P.: Toxicological and pharmacological investigations of pinazepam (7-chloro-1-propargyl-5-phenyl-3H-1,4-benzodiazepine-2-one) a new psychotherapeutic agent. Arzneim. Forsch. *25*, 934–940 (1975)

Segal, M.: Effect of diazepam (Valium) on chronic stress-induced hypertension in the rat. Experientia *37*, 298–299 (1981)

Semiginovský, B., Safanda, J., Sobotka, R., Jakoubek, B., Pavlík, A.: The cerebral GABA, β-alanine, lysine and ethanolamine content and conversion of ^{14}C from U ^{14}C-D-glucose into their molecule during emotional stress in rats. Effect of pyrithioxin and diazepam pretreatment. Activ. Nerv. Sup. (Praha) *18*, 218–220 (1976)

Sethy, V.H.: Effect of hypnotic and anxiolytic agents on regional concentration of acetylcholine in rat brain. Arch. Pharmacol. *301*, 157–161 (1978)

Sethy, V.H., Naik, P.Y., Sheth, U.K.: Effect of d-amphetamine sulphate in combination with CNS depressants on spontaneous motor activity of mice. Psychopharmacologia (Berl.) *18*, 19–25 (1970)

Setoguchi, M., Takehara, S., Nakajima, A., Tsumagari, T., Takigawa, Y.: Effects of 6-(o-chlorophenyl)-8-ethyl-1-methyl-4H-s-triazolo[3,4-c]thieno [2,3-e][1,4]diazepine (Y-7,131) on the metabolism of biogenic amines in brain. Drug. Res. *28*, 1165–1169 (1978)

Shannon, H.E., Holtzman, S.G., Davis, D.C.: Interaction between narcotic analgesics and benzodiazepine derivatives on behavior in the mouse. J. Pharmacol. Exp. Ther. *199*, 389–399 (1976)

Sharer, L., Kutt, H.: Intravenous administration of diazepam. Effects on penicillin-induced focal seizures in the cat. Arch. Neurol. *24*, 169–175 (1971)

Sharma, K.K., Sharma, U.C.: Influence of diazepam on the effect on neuromuscular blocking agents. J. Pharm. Pharmacol. *30*, 64 (1978)

Sherwin, I.: Differential action of diazepam on evoked cerebral responses. Electroencephalogr. Clin. Neurophysiol. *30*, 445–452 (1971)

Shibata, S., Sasakawa, S., Fujita, Y.: The central depressant profile of carbamate ester of glycerol ether: 3-(1,2,3,4-Tetrahydro-7-napthyloxy)-2-hydroxy-propyl carbamate. Toxicol. Appl. Pharmacol. *11*, 591–602 (1967)

Shibuya, T., Sato, K., Matsuda, H., Nishimori, T., Hayashi, M., Nomura, K., Chen, P.C.: Effects of benzodiazepines on brain monoamines. Japn. J. Pharmacol. *26*, Suppl., 102 (1976)

Shmidt, I., Eler, I., Fisenko, V.P.: Effect of clonazepam on neuronal activity in the senso-motor cortex in rabbit's brain. Russian Pharmacol. Toxicol. *41*, 231–234 (1978)

Sieghart, W., Karobath, M.: Molecular heterogeneity of benzodiazepine receptors. Nature *286*, 285–287 (1980)

Sigg, E.B., Sigg, T.D.: Hypothalamic stimulation of preganglionic autonomic activity and its modification by chlorpromazine, diazepam and pentobarbital. Int. J. Neuropharmacol. *8*, 567–572 (1969)

Sigg, E.B., Keim, K.L., Kepner, K.: Selective effect of diazepam on certain central sympathetic components. Neuropharmacology *10*, 621–629 (1971)

Sillén, U., Persson, B., Rubenson, A.: Involvement of central GABA receptors in the regulation of the urinary bladder function of anaesthetized rats. Naunyn-Schmiedebergs Arch. Pharmacol. *314*, 195–200 (1980)

Simmonds, M.A.: A site for the potentiation of GABA-mediated responses by benzodiazepines. Nature *284*, 558–560 (1980)

Simon, P., Soubrié, P., Boissier, J.R.: Hyperactivité motrice induite chez la souris par un anticholinergique central: antagonisme par les benzodiazépines. J. Pharmacol. (Paris) *5*, 93 (1974)

Skolnick, P., Marangos, P.J., Goodwin, F.K., Edwards, M., Paul, S.: Identification of inosine and hypoxanthine as endogenous inhibitors of ^{3}H-diazepam binding in the central nervous system. Life Sci. *23*, 1473–1480 (1978)

Skolnick, P., Paul, S.M., Marangos, P.J.: Brain benzodiazepine levels following intravenous administration of [^{3}H]-diazepam: relationship to the potentiation of purinergic depression of central nervous system neurons. Can. J. Physiol. Pharmacol. *57*, 1040–1042 (1979a)

Skolnick, P., Syapin, P.J., Paugh, B.A.: Reduction in benzodiazepine receptors associated with Purkinje cell degeneration in "nervous" mutant mice. Nature *277*, 397–399 (1979b)

Skolnick, P., Marangos, P.J., Syapin, P., Goodwin, F.K., Paul, S.: CNS benzodiazepine receptors: Physiological studies and putative endogenous ligands. Pharmacol. Biochem. Behav. *10*, 815–823 (1979c)

Skolnick, P., Syapin, J.P., Paugh, B.A., Moncada, V., Marangos, P.J., Paul, S.M.: Inosine, an endogenous ligand of the brain benzodiazepine receptor, antagonizes pentylenetetrazole-evoked seizures. Proc. Natl. Acad. Sci. USA *76*, 1515–1518 (1979d)

Skolnick, P., Lock, K.-L., Paugh, B., Marangos, R., Windsor, R., Paul, S.: Pharmacologic and behavioral effects of EMD 28422: a novel purine which enhances (^{3}H)diazepam binding to brain benzodiazepine receptors. Pharmacol. Biochem. Behav. *12*, 685–689 (1980a)

Skolnick, P., Paul, S.M., Barker, J.L.: Pentobarbital potentiates GABA-enhanced ^{3}H-diazepam binding to benzodiazepine receptors. Eur. J. Pharmacol. *65*, 125–127 (1980b)

Slater, P., Longman, D.A.: Effects of diazepam and muscimol on GABA-mediated neurotransmission: interactions with inosine and nicotinamide. Life Sci. *25*, 1963–1967 (1979)

Smith, R.D., Breese, G.R., Mueller, R.A.: Potentiation of drug initiated adrenal tyrosine hydroxylase induction by diazepam. Arch. Pharmacol. *284*, 195–206 (1974)

Smith, P.A., Weight, F.F., Lehne, R.A.: Potentiation of Ca^{2+}-dependent K^+ activation by theophylline is independent of cyclic nucleotide elevation. Nature *280*, 400–402 (1979)

Snead, O.C.: Gamma hydroxybuyrate in the monkey. III. Effect of intravenous anticonvulsant drugs. Neurology *28*, 1173–1179 (1978)

Snyder, S.H., Enna, S.J.: The role of central glycine receptors in the pharmacologic actions of benzodiazepines. Adv. Biochem. Psychopharmacol. *14*, 81–91 (1975)

Snyder, S.H., Enna, S.J., Young, A.B.: Brain mechanisms associated with therapeutic actions of benzodiazepines: focus on neurotransmitters. Am. J. Psychiatr. *134*, 662–665 (1977)

Sofia, R.D.: Effects of centrally active drugs on four models of experimentally-induced aggression in rodents. Life Sci. *8*(1), 705–716 (1969)

Sofia, R.D., Barry, H.: Comparative activity of Δ^9-tetrahydrocannabinol, diphenylhydantoin, phenobarbital and chlordiazepoxide on electroshock seizure threshold in mice. Arch. Int. Pharmacodyn. Ther. *228*, 73–78 (1977)

Soliman, M.K., El Amrousi, S., Khamis, M.Y.: The influence of tranquillizers and barbiturate anaesthesia on the blood picture and electrolytes of dogs. Vet. Rec. *77*, 1256–1259 (1965)

Sollenne, N.P., Means, G.E.: Characterization of a specific drug binding site of human serum albumin. Mol. Pharmacol. *15*, 754–757 (1979)

Sollertinskaya, T.N., Balonov, L.Y.: Electrophysiologic analysis of diencephalo amygdaloid interrelations. Fiziol Zh. Sechenov. *58*(7), 1050–1058 (1972)

Soper, W.Y., Wise, R.A.: Hypothalamically induced eating: Eating from "non-eaters" with diazepam. TIT J. Life Sci. *1*, 79–84 (1971)

Soubrié, P., Simon, P.: Comparative study of the antagonism of bemegride and picrotoxin on behavioural depressant effects of diazepam in rats and mice. Neuropharmacology *17*, 121–125 (1978)

Soubrié, P., Simon, P., Boissier, J.R.: Effets du diazépam sur six modèles d'hyperactivité chez la souris. Psychopharmacologia *45*, 197–201 (1975 a)

Soubrié, P., Simon, P., Boissier, J.R.: Antagonism of diazepam against central anticholinergic drug-induced hyperactivity in mice: involvement of a GABA mechanism. Neuropharmacology *15*(12), 773–776 (1976 b)

Soubrié, P., Jobert, A., Thiébot, M.H.: Differential effects of naloxone against the diazepam-induced release of behavior in rats in three aversive situations. Psychopharmacology *69*, 101–105 (1980)

Soubrié, P., Kulkarni, S., Simon, P., Boissier, J.R.: Effets des anxiolytiques sur la prise de nourriture de rats et de souris placés en situation nouvelle ou familière. Psychopharmacologia *45*, 203–210 (1975 b)

Soubrié, P., De Angelis, L., Simon, P., Boissier, J.R.: Effets des anxiolytiques sur la prise de boisson en situation nouvelle et familière. Psychopharmacol. *50*, 41–45 (1976 a)

Soubrié, P., Thiébot, M., Simon, P., Boissier, J.R.: Effets des benzodiazépines sur les phénomènes d'inhibition qui contrôlent les comportements exploratoires et le recueil de l'information chez le rat. J. Pharmacol. (Paris) *8*, 393–403 (1977)

Soulairac, A., Cahn, J., Gottesmann, C., Alano, J.: Neuropharmacological aspects of the action of hypogenic substances on the central nervous system. Progr. Brain Res. *18*, 194–220 (1965)

Southgate, P.J., Wilson, A.B.: Pharmacological interaction of lorazepam with thiopentone sodium and skeletal neuromuscular blocking drugs. Brit. J. Pharmacol. *43*, 434P-435P (1971)

Spano, P.F., Kumakura, K., Govoni, S., Trabucchi, M.: Postnatal development and regulation of cerebellar cyclic guanosine monophosphate system. Pharmacol. Res. Commun. *7*, 223–237 (1975)

Speg, K.V., Wang, S., Avant, G.R., Berman, M.L., Schenker, S.: Antagonism of benzodiazepine binding in rat and human brain by antilirium®. Life Sci. *24*, 1345–1350 (1979)

Sperk, G., Schlögl, E: Reduction of number of benzodiazepine binding sites in the caudate nucleus of the rat after kainic acid injections. Brain Res. *170*, 563–567 (1979)

Speth, R.C., Yamamura, H.I.: Benzodiazepine receptors: Alterations in mutant mouse cerebellum. Eur. J. Pharmacol. *54*, 397–399 (1979)

Speth, R.C., Bresolin, N., Yamamura, H.I.: Acute diazepam administration produces rapid increases in brain benzodiazepine receptor density. Eur. J. Pharmacol. *59*, 159–160 (1979 c)

Speth, R.C., Wastek, G.J., Yamamura, H.I.: Benzodiazepine receptors: temperature dependence of ^{3}H-flunitrazepam binding. Life Sci. *24*, 351–358 (1979 a)

Speth, R.C., Wastek, G.J., Johnson, P.C., Yamamura, H.I.: Benzodiazepine binding in human brain: characterization using [^{3}H-]flunitrazepam. Life Sci. *22*, 859–866 (1978)

Speth, R.C., Wastek, G.J., Reisine, T.D., Yamamura, H.I. Benzodiazepine receptors: effect of tissue preincubation at 37 °C. Neurosci. Letters *13*, 243–247 (1979 b)

Spracklen, F.H.N., Chambers, R.J., Schrire, V.: Value of diazepam (valium) in treatment of cardiac arrhythmias. Brit. Heart J. *32*, 827–832 (1970)

Squires, R.F., Braestrup, C.: Benzodiazepine receptors in rat brain. Nature *266*, 732–734 (1977)

Squires, R.F., Naquet, R., Riche, D., Braestrup, C.: Increased thermolability of benzodiazepine receptors in cerebral cortex of a baboon with spontaneous seizures. A case report. Epilepsia *20*, 215–221 (1979 a)

Squires, R.R., Benson, D.I., Braestrup, C., Coupet, J., Klepner, C.A., Myers, V., Beer, B: Some properties of brain specific benzodiazepine receptors: new evidence for multiple receptors. Pharmacol. Biochem. Behav. *10*, 825–830 (1979 b)

Squires, R.F., Klepner, C.A., Benson, D.I.: Multiple benzodiazepine receptor complexes: some benzodiazepine recognition sites are coupled to GABA receptors and ionophores. In: Receptors for Neurotransmitters and Peptide Hormones. Pepeu, G., Kuhar, M.J., Enna, S.J. (eds.) pp. 285–293 New York: Raven Press 1980

Stacher, G., Stärker, D.: Inhibitory effect of bromazepam on basal and betazole-stimulated gastric acid secretion in man. Gut *15*, 116–120 (1974)

Stacher, G., Stärker, D.: Inhibitory effect of bromazepam on insulin-stimulated gastric acid secretion in man. Am. J. Dig. Dis. *20*, 156–161 (1975)

Stapleton, J.M., Lind, M.D., Merriman, V.J., Reid, L.D.: Naloxone inhibits diazepam-induced feeding in rats. Life Sci. *24*, 2421–2426 (1979)

Stark, P., Henderson, J.K.: Differentiation of classes of neurosedatives using rats with septal lesions. Int. J. Neuropharmacol. *5*, 385–389 (1966)

Stark, L.G., Killam, K.F., Killam, E.K.: The anticonvulsant effects of phenobarbital, diphenylhydantoin and two benzodiazepines in the baboon. J. Pharmacol. Exp. Ther. *173*, 125–132 (1970)

Stark, L.G., Edmonds, H.L., Keesling, P.: Penicillin-induced epileptogenic foci. I. Time course and the anticonvulsant effects of diphenylhydantoin and diazepam. Neuropharmacology *13*, 261–267 (1974)

Starley, J.W., Michie, D.D.: Hemodynamic alterations produced by intravenous diazepam in conscious, unrestrained dogs. Curr. Ther. Res. *11*(12), 796–801 (1969)

Steen, S.N., Weitzner, S.W., Amaha, K., Martinez, L.R.: The effect of diazepam on the respiratory response to carbon dioxide. Can. Anaesth. Soc. J. *13*(4), 374–377 (1966)

Steen, S.N., Amaha, K., Weitzner, S.W., Martinez, L.R.: The effect of chlordiazepoxide and pethidine, alone and in combination, on the respiratory response to carbon dioxide. Br. J. Anaesth. *39*, 459–463 (1967)

Stefko, P.L., Zbinden, G.: Effect of chlorpromazine, chlordiazepoxide, diazepam and chlorprothixene on bile flow and intrabiliary pressure in cholecystectomized dogs. Am. J. Gastroenterol. *39*, 410–417 (1963)

Stein, L., Wise, C.D., Belluzzi, J.D.: Effects of benzodiazepines on central serotoninergic mechanisms. Adv. Biochem. Psychopharmacol. *14*, 29–44 (1975)

Stein, L., Wise, C.D., Berger, B.D.: Antianxiety action of benzodiazepines: decrease in activity of serotonin neurones in the punishment system. In: The Benzodiazepines. Garattini, S., Mussini, E., Randall, L.O. (eds.), pp. 299–326. New York: Raven Press 1973

Stein, L., Belluzzi, J.D., Wise, C.D.: Benzodiazepines: Behavioural and neurochemical mechanisms. Am. J. Psychiatry *134*, 665–669 (1977)

Steiner, F.A., Hummel, P.: Effects of nitrazepam and phenobarbital on hippocampal and lateral geniculate neurones in the cat. Int. J. Neuropharmacol. *7*, 61–69 (1968)

Steiner, F.A., Felix, D.: Antagonistic effects of GABA and benzodiazepines on vestibular and cerebellar neurones. Nature *260*, 346–347 (1976a)

Steiner, F.A., Felix, D.: GABA inhibition on central neurones: antagonistic effects of benzodiazepines. Experientia *32*, 763 (1976b)

Steiner, J.E.: A combination narcosis suitable for acute neurophysiological experiments. Electroenceph. Clin. Neurophysiol. *27*, 220 (1969)

Steinhauer, H.B., Anhut, H., Hertting, G.: The synthesis of prostaglandins and thromboxane in the mouse brain in vivo. Influence of drug induced convulsions, hypoxia and the anticonvulsants timethadione and diazepam. Naunyn-Schmiedebergs Arch. Pharmacol. *310*, 53–58 (1979)

Stepanek, J.: Effects of benzoctamine and diazepam on acid-base balance, respiration rate and heart rate in the dog. Arch. Pharmacol. *274* (Suppl.) R 111 (1972)

Stepanek, J.: Changes in acid-base balance, respiration rate and heart rate upon repeated oral administration of benzoctamine and diazepam to conscious dogs. Arch. Int. Pharmacodyn. Ther. *202*, 135–152 (1973a)

Stepanek, J.: Alterations in acid-base balance in the dog after intravenous administration of benzoctamine and diazepam, compared with those induced by thiopental. Arch. Int. Pharmacodyn. Ther. *204*, 350–360 (1973b)

Stepanek, J.: Beeinflussung der Atmung und der arteriellen O_2-Sättigung durch Benzoctamin oder Diazepam am Hund. Schweiz. Med. Wochenschr. *103*(4), 145–148 (1973c)

Stephens, R.J.: The influence of mild stress on food consumption in untrained mice and the effect of drugs. Br. J. Pharmacol. *49*, 146P (1973)

Sternbach, L.H., Randall, L.O., Gustafson, S.R.: 1,4-Benzodiazepines (Chlordiazepoxide and related compounds). Psychopharmacol. Agents *1*, 137–222 (1964)

Stock, G., Heinemann, H., Bergande, F.: Changes in excitability of amygdaloid and septal nuclei induced by medazepam hydrochloride. Psychopharmacologia 46(2), 197–203 (1976)
Stohler, H.R.: Ro 11-3128 – A novel schistosomicidal compound. In: Proc. 10th Int. Congr. Chemother., Zürich, 1977. Siegenthaler, W., Lüthy, R. (eds.). Washington: Am. Soc. Microbiol. 1978
Stone, W.E., Javid, M.J.: Benzodiazepines and phenobarbital as antagonists of dissimilar chemical convulsants. Epilepsia 19(4), 361–368 (1978)
Stratten, W.P., Barnes, C.D.: Diazepam and presynaptic inhibition. Neuropharmacology 10, 685–696 (1971)
Straughan, D.W.: Current views on the mechanisms of action of the benzodiazepines. Arch. Farmacol. y Toxicol. 3, 3–22 (1977)
Straw, R.N.: Pharmacological evaluation of hypnotic drugs in infrahuman species as related to clinical utility. In: Hypnotics – Methods of evaluation and development. Kagan, F., Harwood, T., Ridals, K., Rudzik, A.D., Sorer, H. (eds.), pp. 65–85. New York: Spectrum Publications 1975
Strittmatter, W.J., Hirata, F., Axelrod, J.: Phospholipid methylation unmasks cryptic β-adrenergic receptors in rat reticulocytes. Science 204, 1205–1207 (1979a)
Strittmatter, W.J., Hirata, F., Axelrod, J., Mallorga, P., Tallman, J.F., Henneberry, R.C.: Benzodiazepines and β-adrenergic receptor ligands independently stimulate phospholipid methylation. Nature 282, 857–859 (1979b)
Stumpf, C., Gogolak, G., Huck, S., Andics, A.: Wirkung zentral dämpfender Pharmaka auf die Stickoxydul-Narkose. Anaesthesist 24, 264–268 (1975)
Stumpf, C., Gogolak, G., Huck, S., Andics, A.: Beeinflussung der Halothannarkose durch zentral dämpfende Pharmaka. Anaesthesist 25, 579–584 (1976)
Stumpf, C., Jindra, R., Huck, S., Ewers, H.: Wechselwirkungen zwischen Stickoxydol und zentral dämpfend wirkenden Pharmaka. Anaesthesia 28, 3–8 (1979)
Sugimoto, J., Nagata, M., Ikeda, Y.: The effects of diazepam on rat isolated heart muscle. Clin. Exp. Pharmacol. Physiol. 5(6), 655–663 (1978)
Sugimoto, J., Ikeda, Y., Shimamoto, J., Morita, M.: Comparative studies on the actions of chlorpromazine and diazepam in isolated rat heart. Jap. J. Pharmacol. 26 (Supp.), 133P (1976)
Sun, M.C., McIlwain, H., Pull, I.: The metabolism, of adenine derivatives in different parts of the brain of the rat, and their release from hypothalamic preparations on excitation. J. Neurobiol. 7, 109–122 (1977)
Supavilai, P., Karobath, M.: Stimulation of benzodiazepine receptor binding by SQ 20,009 is chloride-dependent and picrotoxin-sensitive. Eur. J. Pharmacol. 60, 111–113 (1979)
Supavilai, P., Karobath, M.: Heterogeneity of benzodiazepine receptors in rat cerebellum and hippocampus. Eur. J. Pharmacol. 64, 91–93 (1980)
Superstine, E., Sulman, F.G.: The mechanism of the push and pull principle VIII. Endocrine effects of chlordiazepoxide, diazepam and guanethidine. Arch. Int. Pharmacodyn. 160(1), 133–146 (1966)
Suria, A.: Cyclic GMP modulates the intensity of post-tetanic potentiation in bullfrog sympathetic ganglia. Neuropharmacology 15, 11–16 (1976)
Suria, A., Costa, E.: Benzodiazepines and posttetanic potentiation in sympathetic ganglia of the bullfrog. Brain Res. 50, 235–239 (1973)
Suria, A., Costa, E.: Diazepam inhibition of post-tetanic potentiation in bullfrog sympathetic ganglia: Possible role of prostaglandins. J. Pharmacol. Exp. Ther. 189(3), 690–696 (1974a)
Suria, A., Costa, E.: Possible mechanisms of action of benzodiazepines. J. Pharmacol. (Paris) 5 (Suppl. 1), 94–95 (1974b)
Suria, A., Costa, E.: Action of diazepam, dibutyryl cGMP and GABA on presynaptic nerve terminals in bullfrog sympathetic ganglia. Brain Res. 87(1), 102–106 (1975)
Suria, A., Lehne, R., Costa, E.: Possible mechanisms of action of benzodiazepines. In: Neuropsychopharmacology. Boissier, J.R., Hippius, H., Pichot, R. (eds.), pp. 729–734. Amsterdam: Excerpta Medica 1975
Suzuki, T., Murayama, S.: Dorsal root reflex potential and diazepam: Relationship between GABA content and the effect. Japn. J. Pharmacol. 26, 99P (1976)

Sweet, C.S., Wenger, H.C., Gross, D.M.: Central antihypertensive properties of muscimol and related γ-aminobutyric acid agonists and the interaction of muscimol with baroreceptor reflexes. Can. J. Physiol. Pharmacol. *57*, 600–605 (1979)

Swinyard, E.A.: Electrically induced convulsions. In: Experimental Models of Epilepsy. Purpura, D.P., Penry, J.K., Tower, D.B., Woodbury, D.M., Walter, R.D. (eds.), pp. 433–458. New York: Raven Press 1972

Swinyard, E.A., Castellion, A.W.: Anticonvulsant properties of some benzodiazepines. J. Pharmacol. Exp. Ther. *151*(3), 369–375 (1966)

Syapin, P.J., Skolnick, P.: Characterization of benzodiazepine binding sites in cultured cells of neural origin. J. Neurochem. *32*, 1047–1059 (1979)

Székely, J.I., Borsy, J., Kiraly, I.: Chlordiazepoxide induced beta spindle activity in rats. Activ. Nerv. Sup. (Praha) *16*(1), 44–46 (1974)

Szmigielski, A., Guidotti, A.: Action of harmaline and diazepam on the cerebellar content of cyclic GMP and on the activities of two endogenous inhibitors of protein kinase. Neurochem. Res. *4*, 189–199 (1979)

Takagi, K., Kasuya, Y., Tachikawa, S.: The effect of certain psychotropic drugs on arousal responses in rats' EEG. Nippon Yakugaku Zasshi *87*(7), 781–787 (1967)

Takano, K., Student, J.C.: Effect of diazepam on the γ-motor system indicated by the responses of the muscle spindle of the triceps surae muscle of the decerebrate cat to the muscle stretch. Arch. Pharmacol. *302*, 91–101 (1978)

Tallman, J.F., Thomas, J.W., Gallager, D.W.: GABAergic modulation of benzodiazepine binding site sensitivity. Nature *274*, 384–385 (1978)

Tallman, J.F., Thomas, J.W., Gallager, D.W.: Identification of diazepam binding in intact animals. Life Sci. *24*, 873–880 (1979 a)

Tallman, J.F., Paul, S.M., Skolnick, P., Gallager, D.W.: Receptors for the age of anxiety: Pharmacology of the benzodiazepines. Science *207*, 274–281 (1980 a)

Tallman, J.F., Gallager, D.W., Mallorga, P., Thomas, J.W., Strittmatter, W., Hirata, F., Axelrod, J.: Studies on benzodiazepine receptors. In: Receptors for Neurotransmitters and Peptide Hormones. Pepeu, G., Kuhar, M.J., Enna, S.J. (eds.), pp. 277–283. New York: Raven Press 1980 b

Tamagnone, G.F., Torrielli, M.V., Demarchi, F.: A new benzodiazepine 1-(2-hydroyethyl)-3-hydroxy-7-chloro-1,3-dihydro-5-(o-fluorophenyl)-2H-1,4-benzodiazepine-2-one.   J. Pharm. Pharmacol. *26*, 566–567 (1974)

Tappaz, M.L., Brownstein, M.J.: Origin of glutamate-decarboxylase (GAD)-containing cells in discrete hypothalamic nuclei. Brain Res. *132*, 95–106 (1977)

Tarver, J., Bautz, G., Horst, W.D.: Effect of diazepam on urinary GABA levels. Pharmacologist *18*, 130 (1976)

Taylor, K.M.: The effect of minor tranquilizers on stress-induced noradrenaline turnover in the rat brain. Proc. Univ. Otago School *47*, 33–35 (1969)

Taylor, K.M., Laverty, R.: The effect of chlordiazepoxide, diazepam and nitrazepam on catecholamine metabolism in regions of the rat brain. Eur. J. Pharmacol. *8*, 296–301 (1969)

Taylor, K.M., Laverty, R.: The interaction of chlordiazepoxide, diazepam and nitrazepam with catecholamines and histamine in regions of the rat brain. In: The benzodiazepines. Garattini, S., Mussini, E., Randall, L.O. (eds.), pp. 191–202. New York: Raven Press 1973

Taylor, P.L., Daniell, H.B., Bagwell, E.E.: Studies on the myocardial hemodynamic and metabolic effects of diazepam in the dog. Pharmacologist *12*(2), 233 (1970)

Tedeschi, D.H., Fowler, P.J., Miller, R.B., Macko, E.: Pharmacological analysis of footshock-induced fighting behaviour. In: Aggressive Behaviour. Garattini, S., Sigg, E.B. (eds.), pp. 245–252. Amsterdam: Excerpta Medica 1969

Tedeschi, R.E., Tedeschi, D.H., Mucha, A., Cook, L., Mattic, P.A., Fellows, E.J.: Effecs of various centrally acting drugs on fighting behaviour of mice. J. Pharm. Exp. Ther. *125*, 28–34 (1959)

Theobald, W., Büch, O., Kunz, H.A.: Vergleichende Untersuchungen über die Beeinflussung vegetativer Funktionen durch Psychopharmaka im akuten Tierversuch. Arzneim. Forsch. *15*(2), 117–125 (1965)

Thiébot, M.-H., Jobert, A., Soubrié, P.: Nature des mécanismes gabaergiques impliqués dans l'effet protecteur des benzodiazépines vis-à-vis des crises convulsives induites chez le rat par la picrotoxine. J. Pharmacol. (Paris) *10*, 3–11 (1979)

Thiébot, M.-H., Jobert, A., Soubrié, P.: Conditioned suppression of behaviour: its reversal by intra raphe microinjection of chlordiazepoxide and GABA. Neurosci. Letters *16*, 213–217 (1980a)

Thiébot, M.-H., Jobert, A., Soubrié, P.: Chlordiazepoxide and GABA injected into raphé dorsalis release the conditioned behavioural suppression induced in rats by a conflict procedure without nociceptive component. Neuropharmacology *19*, 633–641 (1980b)

Ticku, M.K., Burch, T.: Purine inhibition of ^{3}H-γ-aminobutyric acid receptor binding to rat brain membranes. Biochem. Pharmacol. *29*, 1217–1220 (1980)

Ticku, M.K., Van Ness, P.C., Haycock, J.W., Levy, W.B., Olsen, R.W.: Dihydropicrotoxinin binding sites in rat brain: comparison to GABA receptors. Brain Res. *150*, 642–647 (1978)

Tilson, H.A., Cabe, P.A.: Assessment of chemically-induced changes in the neuromuscular function of rats using a new recording grip meter. Life Sci. *23*, 1365–1370 (1978)

Tobin, J.M., Lewis, N.D.C.: New psychotherapeutic agent, chlordiazepoxide. Use in treatment of anxiety states and related symptoms. J. Amer. Med. Ass. *174*, 1242–1249 (1960)

Toffano, G., Guidotti, A., Costa, E.: Un possibile meccanismo molecolare per l'azione del diazepam sui recettori del GABA. Riv. Farmacol. Ter. *10*, 72–83 (1979)

Toffano, G., Leon, A., Massotti, M., Guidotti, A., Costa, E.: GABA-Modulin: a regulatory protein for GABA receptors. In: Receptors for Neurotransmitters and Peptide Hormones. Pepeu, G., Kuhar, M.J., Enna, S.J. (eds.), pp. 133–142. New York: Raven Press 1980

Toleikis, J.R., Wang, L., Boyarsky, L.L.: Effects of excitatory and inhibitory amino acids on phasic respiratory neurons. J. Neurosci. Res. *4*, 225–235 (1979)

Toman, J.E.P., Sabelli, H.C.: Neuropharmacology of earthworm giant fibers. Int. J. Neuropharmacol. *7*, 543–566 (1968)

Tong, H.S., Edmonds, H.L.: The effects of diazepam on the central gabaminergic system. Proc. West. Pharmacol. Soc. *19*, 122–124 (1976)

Torda, T.A., Gage, P.W.: Postsynaptic effect of i.v. anaesthetic agents at the neuromuscular junction. Brit. J. Anaesth. *49*, 771–776 (1977)

Toth, S., Ungar, B., Szilagyi, T.: Data to the anticonvulsive effect of Valium® diazepam in experimental hyperoxia and guinea pig anaphylaxis. Int. J. Clin. Pharmacol. *2*, 139–141 (1969)

Traversa, U., Newman, M.: Stereospecific influence of oxazepam hemisuccinate on cyclic AMP accumulation elicited by adenosine in cerebral cortical slices. Biochem. Pharmacol. *28*, 2363–2365 (1979)

Traversa, U., De Angelis, L., Vertua, R.: On the hypnogenic and anticonvulsant activities of demethyldiazepam and chlordemethyldiazepam: time-effect relations. J. Pharm. Pharmacol. *29*, 504–506 (1977)

Tremblay, J.P., Grenon, G.: Benzodiazepines mimic the presynaptic action of GABA on a cholinergic synapse of Aplysia. 7th Annu. Meeting Soc. Neurosci., 1977. Abstr. *3*, 520 (1977)

Tseng, T.C., Wang, S.C.: Locus of central depressant action of some benzodiazepine analogues. Proc. Soc. Exp. Biol. Med. *137*, 526–30 (1971a)

Tseng, T.C., Wang, S.C.: Locus of action of centrally acting muscle relaxants, diazepam and tybamate. J. Pharmacol. Exp. Ther. *178*(2), 350–360 (1971b)

Tsuchiya, T.: Effects of 1,4 benzodiazepines with a long side chain in position 1 on the evoked potentials recorded in the limbic system and hypothalamus. Neuropharmacology *16*(4), 259–266 (1977)

Tsuchiya, T., Fukushima, H.: Effects of benzodiazepines on PGO firings and multiple unit activity in the midbrain reticular formation in cats. Electroenceph. Clin. Neurophysiol. *43*(5), 700–706 (1977)

Tsuchiya, T., Fukushima, H.: Effects of benzodiazepines and pentobarbitone on the GABAergic recurrent inhibition of hippocampal neurons. Eur. J. Pharmacol. *48*, 421–424 (1978)

Tsuchiya, T., Kitagawa, S.: Effects of benzodiazepines and pentobarbital on the evoked potentials in the cat brain. Jap. J. Pharmacol. *26*, 411–418 (1976)

Tuganowski, W., Wolanski, A.: The effect of diazepam on the electrical properties of auricular fibers. Diss. Pharm. Pharmacol. *22*, 369–372 (1970)

Tunnicliff, G., Smith, J.A., Ngo, T.T.: Competition for diazepam receptor binding by diphenyl-hydantoin and its enhancement by γ-aminobutyric acid. Biochem. Biophys. Res. Commun. *91*, 1018–1024 (1979)

Tye, N.C., Everitt, B.J., Iversen, S.D.: 5-Hydroxytryptamine and punishment. Nature *268*, 741–743 (1977)

Ueda, U., Wada, T., Ballinger, C.M.: Sodium- and potassium-activated ATPase of beef brain. Effects of some tranquilizers. Biochem. Pharmacol. *20*, 1697–1700 (1971)

Ueki, S., Watanabe, S., Fujiwara, M.: Behavioural and EEG effects of triazolam in comparison with those of diazepam. Folia Pharmacol. Jap. *74*, 597–614 (1978)

Umemoto, M., Olds, M.E.: Effects of chlordiazepoxide, diazepam and chlorpromazine on conditional emotional behaviour and conditioned neuronal activity in limbic, hypothalamic and geniculate regions. Neuropharmacology *14*, 413–425 (1975)

Usdin, E., Amai, R.L.S.: Psychopharmacol. Serv. Center Bull. *2*, 17–93 (1963)

Utting, H.J., Pleuvry, B.J.: Benzoctamine – a study of the respiratory effects of oral doses in human volunteers and interactions with morphine in mice. Br. J. Anaesth. *47*, 987–992 (1975)

Vaille, C., Souchard, M., Chariot, J.: Action du diazépam et de quelques alcools utilisés comme solvant sur la sécrétion biliaire du rat. Ann. Pharm. Franc. *37*, 5–12 (1979)

Valzelli, L.: Drugs and aggressiveness. Adv. Pharmacol. *5*, 79–108 (1967)

Valzelli, L.: Activity of benzodiazepines on aggressive behaviour in rats and mice. In: The benzodiazepines. Garattini, S., Mussini, E., Randall, L.O. (eds.), pp. 405–418. New York: Raven Press 1973

Valzelli, L.: Effect of sedatives and anxiolytics on aggressivity. Mod. Probl. Pharmacopsychiatry *14*, 143–156 (1979)

Valzelli, L., Bernasconi, S.: Differential activity of some psychotropic drugs as a function of emotional level in animals. Psychopharmacologia (Berl.) *20*, 91–96 (1971)

Valzelli, L., Giacalone, E., Garattini, S.: Pharmacological control of aggressive behaviour in mice. Eur. J. Pharmacol. *2*, 144–146 (1967)

Van der Kleijn, E., Vree, T.B., Guelen, P.J.M.: 7-Chloro-1,4-benzodiazepines: Diazepam, desmethyldiazepam, oxydiazepam, oxydesmethyl-diazepam (oxazepam), and chlordiazepoxide. In: Psychotherapeutic drugs. Usdin, E., Forrest, I.S. (eds.) Part II, pp. 997–1037. New York: Dekker 1977

Van Duijn, H.: Superiority of clonazepam over diazepam in experimental epilepsy. Epilepsia *14*, 195–202 (1973)

Van Duijn, H., Visser, S.L.: The action of some anticonvulsant drugs on cobalt-induced epilepsy and on the bemegride threshold in alert cats. Epilepsia *13*, 409–420 (1972)

Van Loon, G.R.: Ventricular arrhythmias treated by diazepam. Can. Med. Ass. J. *98*, 785–787 (1968)

Van Riezen, H., Boersma, L.: A new method for quantitative grip strength evaluation. Eur. J. Pharmacol. *6*, 353–356 (1969)

Van Zwieten, P.A.: The interaction between clonidine and various neuroleptic agents and some benzodiazepine tranquilizers. J. Pharm. Pharmacol. *29*, 229–234 (1977)

Varagić, V., Krstić, M., Mihajlović, L.: The effect of psychopharmacological agents on the hypertensive response to eserine in the rat. Int. J. Neuropharmacol. *3*, 273–277 (1964)

Vassout, A., Delini-Stula, A.: Effets de β-bloqueurs (propranolol et oxprénolol) et du diazépam sur différents modèles d'agressivité chez le rat. J. Pharmacol. (Paris) *8*, 5–14 (1977)

Velasco, M., Velasco, F., Cepeda, C., de Anda, A.M.: Effect of diazepam on pyramidal tract and electromyographic multiple unit activities of cats with chronic epileptogenic foci. Neuropharmacology *16*(4), 299–301 (1977)

Vellucci, S.V., File, S.E.: Chlordiazepoxide loses its anxiolytic action with long-term treatment. Psychopharmacology *62*, 61–65 (1979)

Velvart, J.: Medizinisch-toxikologische Probleme. Schweiz. Apoth. Ztg. *111*, 228–231, 1973

Vergano, F., Zaccagna, C.A., Zuccaro, G., Barile, C.: Proprietà miorilassanti del diazepam. Minerva Anest. *35*, 91–94 (1969)

Verrier, M., McLeod, S., Ashby, P.: The effect of diazepam on presynaptic inhibition in patients with complete and incomplete spinal cord lesions. Can. J. Neurol. Sci. *2*, 179–184 (1975)

Verrier, M., Ashby, P., McLeod, S.: Effects of diazepam on muscle contraction in spasticity. Am. J. Phys. Med. 55(4), 184–191 (1976)

Vesell, E.S.: Elucidation of the pharmacokinetic interaction between acutely administered ethanol and benzodiazepines. J. Lab. Clin. Med. 95, 305–309 (1980)

Vetulani, J., Sansone, M.: Stimulatory effect of chlordiazepoxide on locomotor activity in mice: importance of noradrenergic transmission. Pol. J. Pharmacol. Pharm. 30, 791–798 (1978)

Vieth, J.B., Holm, E., Knopp, P.R.: Electrophysiological studies on the action of mogadon on central nervous structures of the cat. A comparison with pentobarbital. Arch. Int. Pharmacodyn. 171(2), 323–338 (1968)

Von Ledebur, I., Frommel, E., Béguin, M.: Nalorphine antagonism to the narcotic action of chlorpromazine, meprobamate and metaminodiazepoxide (librium). Med. Exp. 7, 177–179 (1962)

Vuillon-Cacciuttolo, G., Issautier, G., Naquet, R.: Etude neurophysiologique du Ro 5-4023. C.R. Soc. Biol. 164, 572–576 (1970)

Vyskočil, F.: Diazepam blockade of repetitive action potentials in skeletal muscle fibres. A model of its membrane action. Brain Res. 133(2), 315–328 (1977)

Vyskočil, F.: Effects of some centrally acting drugs on neuromuscular transmission and desensitization. In: Iontophoresis and transmitter mechanisms in the mammalian central nervous system. Ryall, R.W., Kelly, J.S. (eds.), pp. 239–241. Amsterdam: Elsevier/North-Holland 1978a

Vyskočil, F.: Effect of diazepam on the frog neuromuscular junction. Eur. J. Pharmacol. 48, 117–124 (1978b)

Waddington, J.L.: A behavioural model of the GABA-facilitating action of benzodiazepines: Rotational behaviour after unilateral intranigral injection of chlordiazepoxide. Br. J. Pharmacol. 58, 453P (1976)

Waddington, J.L.: GABA-like properties of flurazepam and baclofen suggested by rotational behaviour following unilateral intranigral injection: a comparison with the GABA agonist muscimol. Brit. J. Pharmacol. 60, 263P–264P (1977)

Waddington, J.L.: Behavioural evidence for GABAergic activity of the benzodiazepine flurazepam. Eur. J. Pharmacol. 51, 417–421 (1978)

Waddington, J.L., Longden, A.: Rotational behaviour and cGMP responses following manipulation of nigral mechanisms with chlordiazepoxide. Naunyn-Schmiedebergs Arch. Pharmacol. 300, 233–237 (1977)

Waddington, J.L., Owen, F.: Stereospecific benzodiazepine receptor binding by the enantiomers of oxazepam sodium hemisuccinate. Neuropharmacology 17, 215–216 (1978)

Walker, C.R., Bandman, E., Strohman, R.C.: Diazepam induces relaxation of chick embryo muscle fibres in vitro and inhibits myosin synthesis. Exp. Cell. Res. 123, 285–291 (1979)

Wang, C.M., James, C.A.: An analysis of the direct effect of chlordiazepoxide on mammalian cardiac tissues and crayfish and squid giant axons: possible basis of antiarrhythmic activity. Life Sci. 24, 1357–1365 (1979)

Wang, Y.J., Salvaterra, P., Roberts, E.: Characterization of [^{3}H] muscimol binding to mouse brain membranes. Biochem. Pharmacol. 28, 1123–1128 (1979)

Warburton, D.M.: Modern biochemical concept of anxiety. Implications for psychopharmacological treatment. Int. Pharmacopsychiat. 9, 189–205 (1974)

Wastek, G.J., Speth, R.C. Reisine, T.D., Yamamura, H.I.: The effect of γ-aminobutyric acid on ^{3}H-flunitrazepam binding in rat brain. Eur. J. Pharmacol. 50, 445–447 (1978)

Watanabe, S., Inoue, M., Ueki, S.: Effects of psychotropic drugs injected into the limbic structures on mouse-killing behaviour in the rat with olfactory bulb ablations. Jap. J. Pharmacol. 29, 493–495 (1979)

Watanabe, S., Kawasaki, H., Nishi, H., Ueki, S.: Electroencephalographic effects of 5-(O-chlorophenyl)-1,3-dihydro-1-methyl-7-nitro-2H-1,4-benzodiazepine-2-one (ID-690) in rabbits with chronic electrode implants. Folia Pharmacol. Jap. 70(4), 531–542 (1974)

Watson, P.J., Short, M.A., Huenink, G.L., Hartman, D.F.: Diazepam effects on hypothalamically elicited drinking and eating. Physiol. Behav. 24, 39–44 (1980)

Wauquier, A., Ashton, D., Melis, W.: Behavioural analysis of amygdaloid kindling in beagle dogs and the effects of clonazepam, diazepam, phenobarbital, diphenylhydantoin and flunarizine on seizure manifestation. Exp. Neurol. 64, 579–586 (1979)

Webb, S.N., Bradshaw, E.G.: An investigation, in cats, into the activity of diazepam at the neuromuscular junction. Brit. J. Anaesth. *45*, 313–318 (1973)

Weihrauch, T.R., Rieger, H., Köhler, H., Voigt, R., Höffler, D., Krieglstein, J.: Einfluß von Diazepam und Phenytoin auf durch Penicillin induzierte zerebrale Krampfanfälle. Arzneim. Forsch. *26*(3), 379–382 (1976)

Weiner, W.J., Goetz, C., Nausieda, P.A., Klawans, H.L.: Clonazepam and 5-hydroxytryptophan-induced myoclonic stereotypy. Eur. J. Pharmacol. *46*, 21–24 (1977)

Weinryb, I., Chasin, M., Free, C.A., Harris, D.N., Goldenberg, H., Michel, I.M., Paik, V.S., Phillips, M., Samaniego, S., Hess, S.M.: Effects of therapeutic agents on cyclic AMP metabolism in vitro. J. Pharm. Sci. *61*, 1556–1567 (1972)

Weis, J.: Morphine antagonistic effect of chlordiazepoxide (librium). Experientia *25*(4), 381 (1969)

Weischer, M.L.: Eine einfache Versuchsanordnung zur quantitativen Beurteilung von Motilität und Neugierverhalten bei Mäusen. Psychopharmacology *50*, 275–279 (1976)

Weiss, L.R., Orzel, R.A.: Enhancement of toxicity of anticholinesterases by central depressant drugs in rats.. Toxicol. Appl. Pharmacol. *10*, 334–339 (1967)

Weissman, A., Koe, B.K.: m-Fluorotyrosine convulsions and mortality: relationship to catecholamine and citrate metabolism. J. Pharmacol. Exp. Ther. *155*, 135–144 (1967)

Weller, C.P., Ibrahim, I., Sulman, F.G.: Analgesic profile of tranquillizers in multiple screening tests in mice. Arch. Int. Pharmacodyn. Ther. *176*, 176–192 (1968)

White, R.P., Sewell, H.H., Rudolph, A.S.: Drug-induced dissociation between evoked reticular potentials and the EEG. Electroenceph. Clin. Neurophysiol. *19*, 16–24 (1965)

Wiezorek, W.D., Liebmann, H., Stremmel, D.: Wirkung von Benzodiazepinderivativen auf die Cholinesteraseaktivität im Blut von Ratten. Pharmazie *32*, 530–532 (1977)

Williams, M., Risley, E.A.: Enhancement of binding of ³H-diazepam to rat brain membranes in vitro by SQ 20,009, a novel anxiolytic, γ-aminobutyric acid (GABA) and muscimol. Life Sci. *24*, 833–842 (1979)

Williams, M., Yarbrough, G.G.: Enhancement of in vitro binding and some of the pharmacological properties of diazepam by a novel anthelmintic agent, avermectin B$_{1a}$. Eur. J. Pharmacol. *56*, 273–276 (1979)

Williamson, M.J., Paul, S.M., Skolnick, P.: Labelling of benzodiazepine receptors in vivo. Nature *275*, 551–553 (1978a)

Williamson, M.J., Paul, S.M., Skolnick, P.: Demonstration of [³H] diazepam binding to benzodiazepine receptors in vivo. Life Sci. *23*(19), 1935–1940 (1978b)

Williford, D.J., Hamilton, B.C., Gillis, R.A.: Evidence that a Gabaergic mechanism at nucleus ambiguus influences reflex-induced vagal activity. Brain Res. *193*, 584–588 (1980a)

Williford, D.J., DiMicco, J.A., Gillis, R.A.: Evidence for the presence of tonically active forebrain GABA system influencing central sympathetic outflow in the cat. Neuropharmacology *19*, 245–250 (1980b)

Williford, D.J., Hamilton, B.C., Souza, J.D., Williams, T.P., Di Micco, J.A., Gillis, R.A.: Central nervous system mechanisms involving GABA influence arterial pressure and heart rate in the cat. Circulation Res. *47*, 80–88 (1980c)

Willow, M., Johnston, G.A.R.: Enhancement of GABA binding pentobarbitone. Neurosci. Letters *18*, 323–327 (1980b)

Wilson, J.D., King, D.J., Sheridan, B.: Tranquilizers and plasma prolactin. Brit. Med. J. *1979I*, 123–124

Wilson, R.D., Phillips, C., Phillips, M.: Cardiorespiratory effects of U-31.889 a dose response evaluation. Pharmacologist *16*(2), 301 (1974)

Winters, W.D., Kott, K.S.: Continuum of sedation, activation and hypnosis or hallucinosis: a comparison of low dose effects of pentobarbital, diazepam or gamma-hydroxybutyrate in the cat. Neuropharmacology *18*, 877–884 (1979)

Wise, R.A., Dawson, V.: Diazepam-induced eating and lever pressing for food in sated rats. J. Comp. Physiol. Psychol. *86*, 930–941 (1974)

Wise, C.D., Berger, B.D., Stein, L.: Benzodiazepines: anxiety-reducing activity by reduction of serotonin turnover in the brain. Science *177*, 180–183 (1972)

Wolf, P., Haas, H.L.: Effects of diazepines and barbiturates on hippocampal recurrent inhibition. Naunyn-Schmiedebergs Arch. Pharmacol. *299*, 211–218 (1977)

Wong, R.K.S., Prince, D.A., Dendritic mechanisms underlying penicillin-induced epileptiform activity. Science *204*, 1228–1231 (1979)

Wood, J.D., Russel, M.P., Kyrylo, E., Newstead, J.D.: Stability of synaptosomal GABA levels and their use in determining the in vivo effects of drugs: convulsant agents. J. Neurochem. *33*, 61–68 (1979)

Worms, P., Depoortere, H., Lloyd, K.G., Neuropharmacological spectrum of muscimol. Life Sci. *25*, 607–614 (1979)

Wüster, M., Duka, T., Herz, A.: Diazepam effects on striatal met-enkephalin levels following long-term pharmacological manipulations. Neuropharmacology *19*, 501–505 (1980a)

Wüster, M., Duka, T., Herz, A.: Diazepam-induced release of opioid activity in the rat brain. Neurosci. Letters *16*, 335–337 (1980b)

Yamaguchi, K., Iwahara, S.: Effects of chlordiazepoxide upon differential heart rate conditioning in rats. Psychopharmacologia *39*(1), 71–79 (1974)

Yamaguchi, I., Katsuki, S., Ohashi, T., Kumada, S.: The relationship between gastric secretory inhibition and cerebral and gastric levels of monoamines in pylorus-ligated rats. Jap. J. Pharmacol. *23*, 523–534 (1973)

Yamaguchi, N., Makihara, M., Kubota, M., Ito, T., Yoshimoto, H., Nakamura, K.: Influence of the hypnotics on the hippocampal slow activity during sleep and wakefulness in cats. 3th Int. Congress Sleep Res., Abstracts, p. 44, Tokyo 1979

Yarbrough, G.G.: Enhancement of in vitro binding and some of the pharmacological properties of diazepam by a novel anthelmintic agent, avermectin B_{1a}. Eur. J. Pharmacol. *56*, 273–276 (1979)

Yarowsky, P.J., Carpenter, D.D.: Receptor for gamma-aminobutyric acid (GABA) on Aplysia neurons. Brain Res. *144*, 75–94 (1978)

Yen, H.C.Y., Katz, M.H., Krop, S.: Effects of various drugs on 3,4-dihydroxyphenyl-alanine (DL-Dopa)-induced excitation (aggressive behaviour) in mice. Toxicol. Appl. Pharmacol. *17*, 597–604 (1970)

Young, A.B., Snyder, S.H.: Strychnine binding in rat spinal cord membranes associated with the synaptic glycine receptor: cooperativity of glycine interactions. Mol. Pharmacol. *10*, 790–809 (1974)

Young, A.B., Zukin, S.R., Snyder, S.H.: Interaction of benzodiazepines with central nervous glycine receptors: Possible mechanism of action. Proc. Natl. Acad. Sci. USA *71*(6), 2246–2250 (1974)

Young, W.S., Kuhar, M.J.: Autoradiographic localization of benzodiazepine receptors in the brains of humans and animals. Nature *280*, 393–395 (1979)

Young, W.S., Kuhar, M.J.: Radiohistochemical localization of benzodiazepine receptors in rat brain. J. Pharmacol. Exp. Ther. *212*, 337–346 (1980)

Yousufi, M.A.K., Thomas, J.W., Tallman, J.F.: Solubilization of benzodiazepine binding site from rat cortex. Life Sci. *25*, 463–470 (1979)

Začková, P., Zamazalová, I., Lazniček, M.: Influence of ethylalcohol on the effect of benzodiazepines in rats and mice. Activ. Nerv. Sup. (Praha) *20*(4), 242–244 (1978)

Zaczek, R., Nelson, M.F., Coyle, J.T.: Effects of anaesthetics and anticonvulsants on the action of kainic acid in the rat hippocampus. Eur. J. Pharmacol. *52*, 323–327 (1978)

Zakusov, V.V., Kozhechkin, S.N.: Brain cortex neurons tolerance of repeat diazepam introduction. Farmakol. i Toksikol. *2*, 135–138 (1978)

Zakusov, V.V., Ostrovaskaya, R.U., Markovich, V.V., Molodavkin, G.M., Bulayev, V.M.: Electrophysiological evidence for an inhibitory action of diazepam upon cat brain cortex. Arch. Int. Pharmacodyn. Ther. *241*, 188–205 (1975)

Zakusov, V.V., Ostrovaskaya, R.U., Kozhechkin, S.N., Markovich, V.V., Molodavkin, G.M., Voronina, T.A.: Further evidence for GABAergic mechanisms in the action of benzodiazepines. Arch. Int. Pharmacodyn. Ther. *229*, 313–326 (1977)

Zamboni, P., Renna, G., Cortese, I.: Effetto delle benzodiazepine sulla sete e sulla diuresi del ratto. Boll. Soc. Ital. Biol. Sper. *48*(21), 711–713 (1972)

Zattoni, J., Rossi, G.F.: A study of the hypnogenic action of "mogadon" by selective injection into carotid and vertebral circulation. Physiol. Behav. *2*, 277–282 (1967)

Zbinden, G., Randall, L.O.: Pharmacology of benzodiazepines: Laboratory and clinical correlations. Adv. Pharmacol. *5*, 213–291 (1967)

Zbinden, G., Bagdon, R.E., Keith, E.F., Phillips, R.D., Randall, L.O.: Experimental and clinical toxicology of chlordiazepoxide (librium). Toxicol. Appl. Pharmacol. *3*, 619–637 (1961)
Zsilla, G., Cheney, D.L., Costa, E.: Regional changes in the rate of turnover of acetylcholine in rat brain following diazepam or muscimol. Naunyn-Schmiedebergs Arch. Pharmacol. *294*, 251–255 (1976)
Zwirner, P.P., Porsolt, R.D., Loew, D.M., Inter-group aggression in mice. A new method for testing the effects of centrally active drugs. Psychopharmacologia (Berl.) *45*, 133–138 (1975)

Addendum*

Section B

Brissette, Y., Gascon, A.L.: The cardiorespiratory toxicity of ouabain in benzodiazepine-treated rats. Toxicol. Appl. Pharmacol. *55*, 235–244 (1980)
Morishima, H.O., Sakuma, K., Bruce, S.L., Pedersen, H., Dyrenfurth, I., Daniel, S.H., Finster, M.: The effect of diazepam on maternal and fetal stress responses in the sheep. Dev. Pharmacol. Ther. *1*, 374–381 (1980)
Nugent, M., Artru, A.A., Michenfelder, J.D.: Cerebral effects of midazolam and diazepam. Anaesthesiology *53*, S 8 (1980)
Persson, B.: Cardiovascular effects of intracerebroventricular GABA, glycine and muscimol in rat. Arch. Pharmacol. *313*, 225–236 (1980)
Siemkowicz, E.: Improvement of restitution from cerebral ischemia in hyperglycemic rats by pentobarbital or diazepam. Acta Neurol. Scand. *61*, 368–376 (1980)

Section C

Jordan, C., Tech, B., Lehane, J.R., Jones, J.G.: Respiratory depression following diazepam: Reversal with high-dose naloxone. Anesthesiology *53*, 293–298 (1970)

Section G

Leslie, S.W., Friedman, M.B., Coleman, R.R.: Effects of chlordiazepoxide on depolarization-induced calcium influx into synaptosomes. Biochem. Pharmacol. *29*, 2439–2443 (1980)

Section H

Bruni, G., Dal Pra, P., Dotti, M.T., Segre, G.: Plasma ACTH and cortisol levels in benzodiazepine treated rats. Pharmacol. Res. Commun. *12*, 163–175 (1980)
Conklin, K.A., Graham, C.W., Murad, S., Dandall, F.M., Katz, R.L.: Midazolam and diazepam: maternal and fetal effects in the pregnant ewe. Obstet. Gynecol. *56*, 471–474 (1980)
Matthew, E., Engelhardt, D.L., Laskin, J.D., Zimmermann, E.A.: Melanotropic effects of benzodiazepines: correlation with a high-affinity receptor. Ann. Neurol. *81*, 92 (1980)
Morishima, H.O., Sakuma, K., Bruce, S.L., Pedersen, H., Dyrenfurth, I., Daniel, S.H., Finster, M.: The effect of diazepam on maternal and fetal stress responses in the sheep. Dev. Pharmacol. Ther. *1*, 374–381 (1980)
Vogel, R.A., Frye, G.D., Wilson, J.H., Kuhn, C.M., Koepke, K.M., Mailman, R.B., Mueller, R.A., Breese, G.R.: Attenuation of the effects of punishment by ethanol: comparison with chlordiazepoxide. Psychopharmacology *71*, 123–129 (1980)
Wilkinson, M., Moger, W.H., Grovestine, A.D.: Chronic treatment with Valium (diazepam) fails to affect the reproductive system of the male rat. Life Sci. *27*, 2285–2291 (1980)

Section I

Smith, D.W., Rehncrona, S.: Inhibitory effects of different barbiturates on lipid peroxidation in brain tissue in vitro: comparison with the effects of promethazine and chlorpromazine. Anaesthesiology *53*, 186–194 (1980)

---

* Additional papers which became available until December 1980.

Section J

Cooper, S.J.: Effects of enantiomers of oxazepam sodium hemisuccinate on water intake and antagonism of picrotoxin- or naloxone-induced suppression of drinking by chlordiazepoxide in the rat. Neuropharmacology *19*, 861–865 (1980)

Cooper, S.J., Francis, R.L.: Interaction of chlordiazepoxide and anorectic agents on rate and duration parameters of feeding in the rat. Psychopharmacology *69*, 261–265 (1980)

Vogel, R.A., Frye, G.D., Wilson, J.H., Kuhn, C.M., Koepke, K.M., Mailman, R.B., Mueller, R.A., Breese, G.R.: Attenuation of the effects of punishment by ethanol: comparison with chlordiazepoxide. Psychopharmacology *71*, 123–129 (1980)

Section K

Antoniadis, A., Müller, W.E., Wollert, U.: Benzodiazepine receptor interactions may be involved in the neurotoxicity of various penicillin derivatives. Ann. Neurol. *8*, 71–73 (1980)

Callaghan, D.A., Schwark, W.S.: Pharmacological modification of amygdaloid-kindled seizures. Neuropharmacology *19*, 1131–1136 (1980)

Ito, T., Hori, M., Yoshida, K., Shimizu, M.: Facilitation of tungistic acid gel-induced cortical epilepsy in rats by depression of the reticular formation. Arch. Int. Pharmacodyn. *245*, 271–282 (1980)

Lal, H., Shearman, G.T., Fielding, S., Dunn, R., Kruse, H., Theurer, K.: Evidence that GABA mechanisms mediate the anxiolytic action of benzodiazepines: a study with valproid acid. Neuropharmacology *19*, 785–789 (1980)

Nisticó, G., Sarro, G.B., Rotiroti, D., Silvestri, R., Marmo, E.: Antagonism by classical antiepileptics and sodium valproate of cefazolin induced experimental epilepsy in rats. Res. Commun. Chem. Path. Pharmacol. *29*, 429–444 (1980)

Robertson, H.A.: Audiogenic seizures: increased benzodiazepine receptor binding in a susceptible strain of mice. Eur. J. Pharmacol. *66*, 249–252 (1980)

Rommelspacher, H., Nanz, C.: Pharmacodynamic effects of harmane, a β-carboline formed in vivo. Arch. Pharmacol. *313*, R 34 (1980)

Sepinwall, J., Cook, L.: Mechanism of action of the benzodiazepines: behavioural aspect. Fed. Proc. *39*, 3024–3031 (1980)

Snead, D.C., Bearden, L.J.: Anticonvulsants specific for petit mal antagonize epileptogenic effect of leucine enkephalin. Science *210*, 1031–1033 (1980)

Snead, D.C., Bearden, L.J., Pegram, V.: Effect of acute and chronic anticonvulsant administration on endogenous γ-hydroxybutyrate in rat brain. Neuropharmacology *19*, 47–52 (1980)

Section L

Igarashi, M., Storey, V.O.: Locomotor body equilibrium after diazepam injection in the squirrel monkey. ORL *36*, 33–36 (1973)

Igarashi, M., Levy, J.K., O-Uchi, T., Homick, J.L.: Diazepam-induced ataxia in trotting squirrel monkeys. Agressologie *21*, 151–153 (1980)

McCabe, B.F., Sekitani, T., Ryu, J.H.: Drug effects on postlabyrinthectomy nystagmus. Arch. Otolaryngol. *98*, 310–313 (1973)

Rackham, A.: Opiate-induced muscle rigidity in the rat: effects of centrally acting agents. Neuropharmacology *19*, 855–859 (1980)

Rommelspacher, H., Nanz, C.: Pharmacodynamic effects of harmane, a β-carboline formed in vivo. Arch. Pharmacol. *313*, R 34 (1980)

Vogel, R.A., Frye, G.D., Wilson, J.H., Kuhn, C.M., Koepke, K.M., Mailman, R.B., Mueller, R.A., Breese, G.R.: Attenuation of the effects of punishment by ethanol: comparisons with chlordiazepoxide. Psychopharmacology *71*, 123–129 (1980)

Section M

Cuomo, V., Cortese, I.: Effects of bicuculline and chlordiazepoxide on locomotor activity and avoidance performance in rats. Experientia *36*, 1208–1210 (1980)

Martin, J.R., Oettinger, R., Driscoll, P., Baettig, K.: Effects of chlordiazepoxide and imipramine on maze exploration by rats. Neurosci. Letters Suppl. *5*, 262 (1980)

Sansone, M.: Influence of benzodiazepine tranquilizers on amphetamine-induced locomotor stimulation in mice. Psychopharmacology *71*, 63–65 (1980)

Sansone, M.: Influence of benzodiazepine tranquilizers on scopolamine-induced locomotor stimulation in mice. Psychopharmacology *71*, 243–245 (1980)

Sansone, M., Oliverio, A.: Effects of chlordiazepoxide-morphine combination on spontaneous locomotor activity in three inbred strains of mice. Arch. Int. Pharmacodyn. *247*, 71–75 (1980)

Section N

Poshivalov, V.P.: The integritiy of the social hierarchy in mice following administration of psychotropic drugs. Br. J. Pharmacol. *70*, 367–373 (1980)

Section O

Henrik, J., Fusek, J., Hrdina, V.: The effect of clonazepam on atropine spikes in the limbic system. Acta Nerv. Sup. (Praha) *22*, 209–210 (1980)

Kuruvilla, A., Uretsky, N.J.: Effects of sodium valproate on motor functions influenced by GABA. Pharmacologist *22*, 185 (1980)

Kusaka, M., Horikawa, A., Meshi, T., Maruyama, Y.: Interaction of triazolam with desimipramine. Effects of single and repeated treatment on certain pharmacologic responses and brain catecholamine levels. Psychopharmacology *70*, 255–261 (1980)

Menon, M.K., Clark, W.G., Vivonia, C.: Interaction between phencyclidine (PCP) and GABAergic drugs: clinical implications. Pharmacol. Biochem. Behav. *12*, 113–117 (1980)

Persson, B.: Cardiovascular effects of intracerebroventricular GABA, glycine and muscimol in rat. Arch. Pharmacol. *313*, 225–236 (1980)

Rackham, A.: Opiate-induced muscle rigidity in the rat: effects of centrally acting agents. Neuropharmacology *19*, 855–859 (1980)

Risch, C., Kripke, D., Janowsky, D.: Flurazepam effects on methylphenidate-induced stereotyped behaviour. Psychopharmacology *70*, 79–82 (1980)

Sansone, M.; Influence of benzodiazepine tranquilizers on amphetamine-induced locomotor stimulation in mice. Psychopharmacology *71*, 63–65 (1980)

Sansone, M.: Influence of benzodiazepine tranquilizers on scopolamine-induced locomotor stimulation in mice. Psychopharmacology *71*, 243–245 (1980)

Sansone, M., Oliverio, A.: Effects of chlordiazepoxide-induced combinations on spontaneous locomotor activity in three inbred strains of mice. Arch. Int. Pharmacodyn. *247*, 71–75 (1980)

Thiébot, M.-H., Kloczko, J., Chermat, R., Simon, P., Soubrié, P.: Oxolinic acid and diazepam: their reciprocal antagonism in rodents. Psychopharmacology *6*, 91–95 (1980)

Section Q

Trembley, J.P., Grenon, G.: Benzodiazepines modify synaptic depression, frequency facilitation and PTP of an identified cholinergic synapse of aplysia. Life Sci. *27*, 491–496 (1980)

Section U

Bouyer, J.-J., Rougeul, A.: Comparative anxiolytic and hypnotic effects of 3 benzodiazepines on baboons. Electroencephalogr. Clin. Neurophysiol. *49*, 401–405 (1980)

Fairchild, M.D., Jenden, D.J., Mickey, M.R., Yale, C.: The quantitative measurement of changes in EEG frequency spectra produced in the cat by sedative-hypnotics and neuroleptics. Electroencephalogr. Clin. Neurophysiol. *49*, 382–390 (1980)

Iwata, N., Mikuni, N.: EEG change in the conscious rat during immobility induced by psychological stress. Psychopharmacology *71*, 117–122 (1980)

Section W

Barmack, N.H., Pettorossi, V.E.: The influence of a GABA agonist, diazepam, on the vestibuloocular reflexes of the rabbit. Brain Res. Bull. *4*, 697 (1979)

Geller, H.M., Hoffer, B.J., Taylor, D.A.: Electrophysiological actions of benzodiazepines. Fed. Proc. *39*, 3016–3023 (1980)

Grant, S.J., Huang, Y.H., Redmont, D.E.: Benzodiazepines attenuate single unit activity in the locus coeruleus. Life Sci. *27*, 2231–2236 (1980)

Matsuoka, I., Chikamori, Y., Takaori, S., Morimoto, M.: Effects of chlorpromazine and diaze-pam on neuronal activities of the lateral vestibular nucleus in cats. Arch. Otorhinolaryngol. (N.Y.) *209*, 89–95 (1975)

Phillis, J.W., Wu, P.H.: Interactions between the benzodiazepines, methylxanthines and adenosine. J. Can. Sci. Neurol. *7*, 247–249 (1980)

Riley, M., Scholfield, C.N.: Diazepam produces a mild intensification of inhibition. J. Physiol. (Lond.) *305*, 102 P–103 P (1980)

Ryu, J.H., McCabe, B.F.: Effects of diazepam and dimenhydrinate on the resting activity of the vestibular neuron. Aerospace Med. *45*, 1177–1179 (1974)

Sekitani, T., McCabe, B.F., Ryu, J.H.: Drug effects on the medial vestibular nucleus. Arch. Otolaryng. *93*, 581–589 (1971)

Section X

Balfour, D.J.K.: Effects of GABA and diazepam on ^{3}H-serotonin release from hippocampal synaptosomes. Eur. J. Pharmacol. *68*, 11–16 (1980)

Cananzi, A.R., Costa, E., Guidotti, A.: Potentiation by intraventricular muscimol of the an-ticonflict effect of benzodiazepines. Brain Res. *196*, 447–453 (1980)

Gallager, D.W., Mallorga, P., Thomas, J.W., Tallman, J.F.: GABA-benzodiazepine inter-actions: physiological, pharmacological and developmental aspects. Fed. Proc. *39*, 3034–3049 (1980)

Gavish, M., Snyder, S.H.: Benzodiazepine recognition sites on GABA receptors. Nature *287*, 651–652 (1980)

Geller, H.M., Hoffer, B.J., Taylor, D.A.: Electrophysiological actions of benzodiazepines. Fed. Proc. *39*, 3016–3023 (1980)

Grant, S.J., Huang, Y.H., Redmont, D.E.: Benzodiazepines attenuate single unit activity in the locus coeruleus. Life Sci. *27*, 2231–2236 (1980)

Guidotti, A., Baraldi, M., Leon, A., Costa, E.: Benzodiazepines: a tool to explore the biochem-ical and neurophysiological basis of anxiety. Fed. Proc. *39*, 3039–3042 (1980)

Kennedy, B., Leonard, B.E.: Similarity between the action of nicotinamide and diazepam on neurotransmitter metabolism in the rat. Biochem. Soc. Trans. *8*, 59–60 (1980)

Mitchell, P.R., Martin, I.L.: Facilitation of striatal potassium-induced dopamine release – novel structural requirements for a presynaptic action of benzodiazepines. Neuropharma-cology *19*, 147–150 (1980)

Namima, M., Sakai, Y., Okamoto, K.: Effects of chlordiazepoxide on K^+-evoked release of labeled GABA, taurine and glycine from cerbellar and cerebral slices of guinea pigs. Jap. J. Pharmacol. *29*, Suppl., 192 P (1979)

Oka, M., Yamada, K., Yoshika, K., Shimizu, M.: Avoidance enhancement and discriminative response control by anxiolytics with drugs acting on the GABA system. Jap. J. Pharmacol. *30*, 325–336 (1980)

Persson, B.: Cardiovascular effects of intercerebroventricular GABA, glycine and muscimol in rat. Arch. Pharmacol. *313*, 225–236 (1980)

Phillis, J.W., Wu, P.H.: Interactions between the benzodiazepines, methylxanthines and adenosine. J. Can. Sci. Neurol. *7*, 247–249 (1980)

Phillis, J.W., Siemens, R.K., Wu, P.H.: Effects of diazepam on adenosine and acetylcholine re-lease from rat cerebral cortex: further evidence for a purinergic mechanism in action of diazepam. Br. J. Pharmacol. *70*, 341–348 (1980)

Porta, R., Camardella, M., Verruti, A., De Negri, P., Miele, L., Della Pietra, G.: The in vitro inhibition of indoleamine N-methyltransferase by antipsychotic drugs and benzo-diazepines. Res. Commun. Psychol. Psychiat. Behav. *5*, 177–184 (1980)

Riley, M., Scholfield, C.N.: Diazepam produces a mild intensification of inhibition. J. Physiol. (Lond.) *305*, 102 P–103 P (1980)

Suzuki, T., Fukumori, R., Yoshii, T., Yanaura, S., Satoh, T., Kitagawa, H.: Effect of p-chloro-phenylalanine on diazepam withdrawal signs in rats. Psychopharmacology *71*, 91–98 (1980)

Wu, P.H., Phillis, S.W., Bender, A.S.: Inhibition of [^{3}H]diazepam binding to rat brain cortical synaptosomal membranes by adenosine uptake blockers. Eur. J. Pharmacol. *65*, 459–460 (1980)

Section Y

Kageyama, H., Kurosawa, A.: A probable site of action of diazepam in rat cerebellar GABA system. Life Sci. *27*, 1783–1789 (1980)

Section Z

Airaksinen, M.M., Mikkonen, E.: Effects of some β-carbolines on rat brain benzodiazepine and opiate receptors. Arch. Pharmacol. *313*, R 34 (1980)

Antoniadis, A., Müller, W.E., Wollert, U.: Benzodiazepine receptor interactions may be involved in the neurotoxicity of various penicillin derivatives. Ann. Neurol. *8*, 71–73 (1980)

Antoniadis, A., Müller, W.E., Wollert, U.: Central system stimulating and depressing drugs as possible ligands of the benzodiazepine receptor. Neuropharmacology *19*, 121–124 (1980)

Bennett, J.L.: Characteristics of antischistosomal benzodiazepine binding sites in schistosoma mansoni. J. Parasitol. (in press)

Braestrup, C., Nielsen, M.: Searching for endogenous benzodiazepine receptor ligands. Trends Pharmacol. Sci. *1*, 424–427 (1980)

Braestrup, C., Nielsen, M.: Multiple benzodiazepine receptors. Trends Neurosci. *3*, 301–303 (1980)

Doble, A., Iversen, L.L.: Effect of temperature on GABA/benzodiazepine receptor coupling. Neurosci. Letters Suppl. *5*, 70 (1980)

Fehnske, K.J., Borbe, H.O., Müller, W.E., Rommelspacher, H., Wollert, U.: β-Carbolines, potent inhibitors of specific ^{3}H-flunitrazepam binding. Arch. Pharmacol. *313*, R 34 (1980)

Freund, G.: Benzodiazepine receptor loss in brains of mice after chronic alcohol consumption. Life Sci. *27*, 987–992 (1980)

Gallager, D.W., Mallorga, P., Thomas, J.W., Tallman, J.F.: GABA-benzodiazepine interactions: physiological, pharmacologigal and developmental aspects. Fed. Proc. *39*, 3043–3049 (1980)

Gavish, M., Snyder, S.H.: Benzodiazepine recognition sites on GABA receptors. Nature *287*, 651–652 (1980)

Guidotti, A., Baraldi, M., Leon, A., Costa, E.: Benzodiazepines: a tool to explore the biochemical and neurophysiological basis of anxiety. Fed. Proc. *39*, 3039–3042 (1980)

Karobath, M., Rogers, J., Bloom, F.E.: Benzodiazepine receptors remain unchanged after chronic ethanol administration. Neuropharmacology *19*, 125–128 (1980)

Leeb-Lundberg, F., Snowman, A., Olsen, R.W.: Barbiturate receptor sites are coupled to benzodiazepine receptors. Proc. Natl. Acad. Sci. U.S.A. (in press)

Mallorga, P., Tallman, J.F., Henneberry, R.C., Gallager, D.W.: Pharmacological characterisation of benzodiazepine binding sites in various cell cultures. Neurosci. Letters Suppl. *5*, 242 (1980)

Martin, I.L.: Endogenous ligands for benzodiazepine receptors. Trends Neurosci. *3*, 299–301 (1980)

Mimaki, T., Deshmukh, P.P., Yamamura, H.I.: An interaction of phenytoine (DPH) with benzodiazepine receptor in rat brain. J. Neurochem. *35*, 1473–1475 (1980)

Möhler, H., Battersby, M.K., Richards, J.G.: Benzodiazepine receptors in rat brain: localization in regions of synaptic contacts. Brain Res. Bull. *5*, 155–159 (1980)

Müller, W.E., Antoniadis, A., Wollert, U.: Penicillins and GABAergic transmission. GABA and benzodiazepine receptor interactions may be involved in the neurotoxicity of penicilline derivatives. Neurosci. Letters Suppl. *5*, 272 (1980)

Nielsen, M., Braestrup, C.: Ethyl β-carboline-3-carboxylate shows differential benzodiazepine receptor interaction. Nature *286*, 606–607 (1980)

Paul, S.M., Skolnick, P., Zatz, M.: Avermectin B_{1a}: an irreversible activator of the γ-aminobutyric acid benzodiazepine-chloride-ionophore receptor complex. Biochem. Biophys. Res. Commun. *96*, 632–638 (1980)

Paul, S.M., Marangos, P.J., Goodwin, F.K., Skolnik, P.: Brainspecific benzodiazepine receptors and putative endogenous benzodiazepine-like compounds. Biol. Psychiatry *15*, 407–428 (1980)

Reisine, T.D., Overstreet, D., Gale, K., Rossor, M., Iversen, L., Yamamura, H.I.: Benzodiazepine receptors: the effect of GABA on their characteristics in human brain and their alteration in Huntington's disease. Brain Res. *199*, 79–88 (1980)

Rommelspacher, H., Nanz, C.: Pharmacodynamic effects of harmane, a β-carboline formed in vivo. Arch. Pharmacol. *313*, R 34 (1980)

Rommelspacher, H., Nanz, C., Borbe, H.O.: Fehske, K.J.: 1-Methyl-β-carboline (harmane), a potent endogenous inhibitor of benzodiazepine receptor binding. Arch. Pharmacol. *314*, 97–100 (1980)

Saano, V.E., Urtti, A., Airaksinen, M.M.: The increase in the binding of ³H-flunitrazepam to rat brain benzodiazepine receptors in vitro and in vivo by tofizopam, a 3,4-benzodiazepine. Arch. Pharmacol. *313*, R 34 (1980)

Sherman-Gold, R., Dudai, Y.: Solubilization and properties of a benzodiazepine receptor from calf cortex. Brain Res. *198*, 485–490 (1980)

Sieghart, W., Karobath, M.: Molekulare Heterogenität von Benzodiazepinrezeptoren. Z. Physiol. Chem. *361*, 1345–1346 (1980)

Skolnick, P., Paul, S.T., Marangos, P.J.: Purines as endogenous ligands of the benzodiazepine receptor. Fed. Proc. *39*, 3050–3055 (1980)

Skolnick, P., Paul, S., Zatz, M., Eskay, R.: "Brain-specific" benzodiazepine receptors are localized in the inner layer of rat retina. Eur. J. Pharmacol. *66*, 133–136 (1980)

Sonawane, B.R., Yaffe, S.J., Shapiro, B.H.: Changes in mouse brain diazepam receptor binding after phenobarbital administration. Life Sci. *27*, 1355–1330 (1980)

Speth, R.C., Johnson, R.W., Regan, J., Reisine, T., The benzodiazepine receptor of mammalian brain. Fed. Proc. *39*, 3032–3038 (1980)

Supavilai, P., Karobath, M.: The effect of temperature and chloride ions on the stimulation of ³H-flunitrazepam binding by the muscimol analogues THIP and piperidine-4-sulfonic acid. Neurosci. Letters *19*, 337–341 (1980)

Taniguchi, T., Wang, J.K.T., Spector, S.: Properties of ³H-diazepam binding to rat peritoneal mast cells. Life Sci. *27*, 171–178 (1980)

Tenen, S.S., Hirsch, J.D.: β-Carboline-3-carboxylic acid ethyl ester antagonizes diazepam activity. Nature *288*, 609–610 (1980)

Thomas, S.R., Iversen, S.D.: Effects of lesions and infusions to the amygdaloid complex on anxiety tests in rats: relationship to ³H-diazepam binding distribution. Neurosci. Letters Suppl. *5*, 167 (1980)

Vogel, R.A., Frye, G.D., Wilson, J.H., Kuhn, C.M., Koepke, K.M., Mailman, R.B., Mueller, R.A., Breese, G.R.: Attenuation of the effects of punishment by ethanol: comparisons with chlordiazepoxide. Psychopharmacology *71*, 123–129 (1980)

Wang, J.K., Taniguchi, R., Spector, S.: Properties of ³H-diazepam binding sites on rat blood platelets. Life Sci. *27*, 1881–1888 (1980)

Williams, E.F., Rice, K.C., Paul, S.M., Skolnick, P.: Heterogeneity of benzodiazepine receptors in the CNS demonstrated with kenazepine, an alkylating benzodiazepine. J. Neurochem. *35*, 591–597 (1980)

Willow, M., Morgan, I.G.: Retinal benzodiazepine receptors are destroyed by kainic acid lesions. Neurosci. Letters *20*, 147–152 (1980)

Wu, P.H., Phillis, S.W., Bender, A.S.: Inhibition of [³H] diazepam binding to rat brain cortical synaptosomal membranes by adenosine uptake blockers. Eur. J. Pharmacol. *65*, 459–460 (1980)

Section AA

Tenen, S.S., Hirsch, J.D.: β-Carboline-3-carboxylic acid ethyl ester antagonizes diazepam activity. Nature *288*, 609–610 (1980)

General Pharmacology and Neuropharmacology of Propanediol Carbamates

W. Haefely, R. Schaffner, P. Polc, and L. Pieri

A. Introduction

Meprobamate is the most important representative of the chemical class of propanediol carbamates (Fig. 1). It was introduced into therapy in 1955 as the first agent specifically intended for the treatment of anxiety and related emotional disturbances and found immediate broad acceptance. After the development of benzodiazepines, the use of meprobamate steadily declined. Synthesis and development of meprobamate were the result of directed efforts to find a compound with higher potency and longer duration of action than mephenesin, which had interesting central muscle relaxant and tranquilizing properties (Ludwig and Potterfield, 1971). Struc-

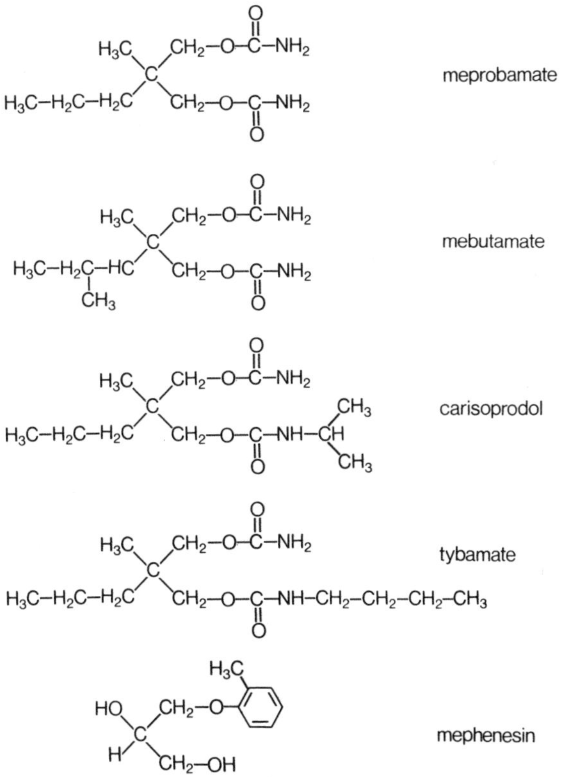

Fig. 1. Chemical structures of the main representatives of propanediol carbamates

Table 1. Acute lethal doses of meprobamate
$(mg \cdot kg^{-1})$

LD$_{50}$ i.v.	LD$_{50}$ i.p.	LD$_{50}$ p.o.
	Mouse	
482 ± 33 [a]	800 ± 15 [a]	$1,100 \pm 44$ [a]
450 ± 27 [b]	736 ± 53 [b]	$1,100 \pm 176$ [b]
	Rat	
–	545 ± 40 [a]	$1,600 \pm 163$ [a]

[a] Berger (1954)
[b] Randall et al. (1960)

ture-activity relationships for substituted propanediols were reported by Ludwig and Potterfield (1971).

We restrict our presentation of the general pharmacology and neuropharmacology of propanediols to meprobamate and mention other derivatives on only a few occasions, because they have very restricted use in therapy. Carisoprodol, a propanediol carbamate with a predominant effect on skeletal muscle tone, is not discussed in this review.

B. Acute Toxicity

As can be seen from Table 1, the absolute toxicity of meprobamate is rather low. The LD$_{50}$ values in rats and mice are in the order of magnitude reported for diazepam (Haefely et al., 1981). Acute lethal doses for other dicarbamate compounds were compiled by Ludwig and Potterfield (1971).

C. Cardiovascular System

I. Meprobamate

Arterial blood pressure was transiently lowered to a weak or moderate degree by meprobamate in anesthetized cats $(40 \text{ mg} \cdot kg^{-1}$ i.v., $50 \text{ mg} \cdot kg^{-1}$ i.m.) and dogs $(20 \text{ mg} \cdot kg^{-1}$ i.v.) as well as in conscious and anesthetized rabbits $(55 \text{ mg} \cdot kg^{-1}$ i.p., $25 \text{ mg} \cdot kg^{-1}$ i.v.) and conscious rats $(55 \text{ mg} \cdot kg^{-1}$ i.p.) (Berger, 1954; Berger et al., 1961; Takeda, 1960; Inoki et al., 1964). Whilst Berger (1954) and Takeda (1960) found heart rate to be minimally affected, tachycardia was observed by Chassaing and Duchene-Marullaz (1976) in conscious dogs after $50 \text{ mg} \cdot kg^{-1}$ meprobamate i.v.

Meprobamate $(20 \text{ mg} \cdot kg^{-1}$ i.v.) reduced ventricular arrhythmia induced in dogs by acute myocardial infarction (Arora, 1958; Arora et al., 1962), but had no effect on atrial flutter induced by electric stimulation or atrial fibrillation induced by aconitine (Arora, 1958).

Pressor responses of curarized dogs and cats to stimulation of hypothalamus, midbrain reticular formation, sciatic nerve or pneumogastric nerve were reduced or even reversed after 30–50 mg·kg^{-1} meprobamate i.v. (MERCIER and DESSAIGNE, 1959). The hypertensive response to pentetrazole or strychnine was diminished by 30–50 mg·kg^{-1} meprobamate i.v. (MERCIER and DESSAIGNE, 1959), but the pressor effect of adrenaline or noradrenaline or the depressor effect of acetylcholine were unaffected (BERGER, 1954; MERCIER and DESSAIGNE, 1959).

II. Mebutamate

In contrast to the weak effects of meprobamate, mebutamate was reported to have prominent cardiovascular effects. BERGER et al. (1961) described dose-dependent long-lasting hypotensive effects in conscious normotensive and hypertensive rabbits (18–37 mg · kg^{-1} i.v.), in DOCA and Goldblatt hypertensive rats (120 mg · kg^{-1} p.o.), and in hypertensive patients (300 mg p.o.). In anesthetized dogs 20 mg · kg^{-1} mebutamate i.v. produced a transient hypotension which was not altered by either atropine, removal of the carotid bodies, or by cutting the vagal nerves. No alterations of the ECG were observed. Peripheral and coronary vascular resistances were decreased; cardiac output remained unaffected. Blood pressure and blood flow in the renal arteries were slightly reduced. Mebutamate did not affect adrenaline-induced increase of arterial and venous blood flow or reduction of renal arterial blood flow, but consistently reduced the pressor effect of carotid artery occlusion. Blood pressure responses to adrenaline, histamine, and acetylcholine in anesthetized dogs were unchanged. VARAGIĆ and VOJVODIĆ (1962) reduced the pressor response to eserine (thought to be centrally mediated) by 10–20 mg·kg^{-1} mebutamate i.v. in rats. A slight reduction of the depressor response to peripheral vagal stimulation was found by BERGER et al. (1961). These authors, as well as SCHALLEK et al. (1964), reported reductions by 30 mg·kg^{-1} mebutamate i.v. of pressor responses to stimulation of the medulla, midbrain, hypothalamus, or central stump of the vagus nerve in curarized cats. No direct vasodilating effect of mebutamate was found in the perfused rabbit ear and the perfused hind limb of dogs; however, a centrally evoked vasodilation occurred in the dog hind limb in cross-circulation experiments (BERGER et al., 1961).

D. Effects on Respiration

Respiration seems to be minimally affected by meprobamate in pharmacologic doses. Respiratory rate and amplitude were unaltered or slightly increased in anesthetized cats after 140 mg·kg^{-1} meprobamate i.v. and i.m., respectively (BERGER, 1954). In anesthetized rabbits, TAKEDA (1960) observed a biphasic effect with 25 mg·kg^{-1} i.v., i.e., a brief depression followed by an increase.

E. Effects on Other Autonomic Functions

I. Gastrointestinal System

The formation of stomach ulcers in rats by intermittent electric shocks to the cage floor was reduced by 5 mg·kg^{-1} meprobamate (DESMAREZ and DOMB, 1960). No protection or only a small reduction of the severity of stomach ulcerations was reported in Shay rats with 20–200 mg·kg^{-1} meprobamate s.c. and of histamine-induced ulcerations in guinea pigs with 15 and 20 mg·kg^{-1} s.c. (Bornmann, 1961; Di Maggio, 1964). Repeated administration of 120–200 mg·kg^{-1} meprobamate s.c. induced dose-dependently an inflammatory process in the stomach of rats which led to severe hemorrhagic ulcerations and eventually death. Meprobamate (10^{-4}–10^{-3} mol·l^{-1}) reduced the contractions induced by vagus stimulation in the isolated vagus nerve–stomach preparation of the rat and the contractions induced by 5-hydroxytryptamine (serotonin, 5-HT) in rat stomach strips (Della Bella and Rognoni, 1960). Contractions of the isolated rat colon evoked by acetylcholine and 5-HT were depressed by the drug at 10^{-3} mol·l^{-1} (Berger et al., 1957, 1975). The isolated guinea-pig ileum was not relaxed (Berger, 1954); the contractile effects of acetylcholine, nicotine, barium chloride, and 5-HT were hardly affected at 10^{-3} mol·l^{-1} (Berger, 1954, 1957; Frommel et al., 1960; Theobald et al., 1965; Leeuwin et al., 1975), but an antihistamine effect was found at 10^{-5} mol·l^{-1} by Frommel et al. (1960). Berger and Neuweiler (1961) observed a relaxation of isolated human myometrium strips by meprobamate.

In rats with cannulated bile ducts Bornmann (1961) observed a dose-dependent, transient increase in bile flow with 80–160 mg·kg^{-1} meprobamate i.p.

No change in urinary excretion was observed with meprobamate in dogs and rats (Corson et al., 1960; Greene, 1963; Boris and Stevenson, 1967); glomerular filtration rate and renal plasma flow were unaltered (Greene, 1963).

Contractions of the nictitating membrane elicited in cats by stimulation of the preganglionic cervical sympathetic were unaffected by 40 mg·kg^{-1} meprobamate i.v. (Berger, 1954). The drug at a dose of 20 mg·kg^{-1} i.v. also did not change the spontaneous activity in the preganglionic cervical sympathetic nerve in anesthetized rabbits (Clubley and Elliott, 1977). High concentrations of meprobamate ($> 10^{-3}$ mol·l^{-1}) reduced the amplitude of evoked compound action potentials in the isolated cervical sympathetic nerve–superior cervical ganglion preparation of the rabbit (Clubley, 1978).

The increase of palmar skin conductance induced in mice by photostimulation was decreased by meprobamate (ED$_{50}$: 3 mg·kg^{-1} s.c., Marcy and Quermonne, 1975), whereas peripheral and central responses to tremorine remained unaffected by 100 mg·kg^{-1} p.o. (Frommel et al., 1960, 1961; Theobald et al., 1965). Meprobamate failed to affect pupil size in cats and mice (Berger, 1954; Bastian and Clements, 1961).

No effect on body temperature was found in mice and rabbits with doses of meprobamate that did not produce muscle relaxation (Berger, 1954; Bastian and Clements, 1961; Menon et al., 1977), but higher doses produced hypothermia (Berger, 1954; Frommel et al., 1960). These authors also found an antipyretic effect in rabbits (25 mg·kg^{-1} i.p.) and guinea pigs (200 mg·kg^{-1} p.o.).

The short-circuiting sodium current and the membrane potential of the isolated frog skin were increased or reduced depending on whether 1.5×10^{-2} mol·l^{-1} meprobamate was added to the epidermal or corial side (Rüberg-Schweer and Karger, 1970, 1974).

Meprobamate produced no antiemetic effect in dogs in doses up to 240 mg·kg^{-1} p.o. (Randall et al., 1960; Theobald et al., 1965).

A dipsogenic effect of 10–128 mg·kg^{-1} meprobamate i.p. was reported in fluid-deprived rats (Maickel and Maloney, 1973; Soubrié et al., 1976).

Increases (BAINBRIDGE, 1968) and no changes (STERNBACH et al., 1964) of food consumption in starved rats were found with doses of $100 \, \text{mg} \cdot \text{kg}^{-1}$ p.o. and $50 \, \text{mg} \cdot \text{kg}^{-1}$ s.c., respectively. In starved mice $25\text{--}200 \, \text{mg} \cdot \text{kg}^{-1}$ meprobamate s.c. dose-dependently increased food intake (STEPHENS, 1973). An increased food intake in fed mice and rats was also reported after $64 \, \text{mg} \cdot \text{kg}^{-1}$ i.p. or higher doses of meprobamate (SOUBRIÉ et al., 1975).

A questionable antinociceptive effect was found with $100 \, \text{mg} \cdot \text{kg}^{-1}$ meprobamate p.o. in guinea pigs in which tooth pulps were electrically stimulated (FROMMEL et al., 1960). Meprobamate was found inactive by WELLER et al. (1968) in four different analgesic tests in mice in doses up to $400 \, \text{mg} \cdot \text{kg}^{-1}$ (route of administration not indicated).

F. Effects on Neuromuscular Transmission

Neuromuscular transmission was unaffected by meprobamate in cats ($30\text{--}40 \, \text{mg} \cdot \text{kg}^{-1}$ i.v.) and rats ($20\text{--}100 \, \text{mg} \cdot \text{kg}^{-1}$ i.v.) (BERGER, 1954; INOKI et al., 1964). No direct effect on cat skeletal muscle was observed by BERGER (1954). In the isolated frog sartorius muscle, the drug at $10^{-4} \, \text{mol} \cdot \text{l}^{-1}$ had no effect on twitch responses, but it antagonized twitch augmentation by veratridine (ARORA, 1958). In single isolated frog skeletal muscle fibers, LOPEZ et al. (1979) observed an increase of twitch force and a delay in the twitch response with $5 \times 10^{-3} \, \text{mol} \cdot \text{l}^{-1}$ meprobamate. In muscle fibers injected intracellularly with the calcium-sensitive fluorescent aequorin the authors found an enhanced increase of light emission during the twitch and a delayed decay of light emission in the falling phase of the twitch, indicating an increased accumulation of Ca^{2+} in the myoplasm under the influence of meprobamate.

Meprobamate ($30\text{--}50 \, \text{mg} \cdot \text{kg}^{-1}$ i.v.) had a relatively weak protecting effect against local tetanus induced in rabbits by injection of tetanus toxin into the gastrocnemius muscle and by activating afferent inputs (WEBSTER, 1961).

G. Effects on the Endocrine System

ARON et al. (1967, 1968) observed an antiovulatory effect of $300 \, \text{mg} \cdot \text{kg}^{-1}$ meprobamate i.m. in rats. The effect was dependent on dose and time of injection as well as on the rat strain. The ovulatory action of exogenous gonadotrophin was not prevented by meprobamate.

In rats, $450 \, \text{mg} \cdot \text{kg}^{-1}$ meprobamate p.o. inhibited ascorbic acid depletion of the adrenal glands caused in acute conditions by psychic stress; during chronic treatment, tolerance to this effect occurred after 11–14 days (MÄKELÄ et al., 1959). The stress-induced increase of plasma corticosteroids in rats was blocked by $150 \, \text{mg} \cdot \text{kg}^{-1}$ meprobamate i.p.; diazepam was 30–40 times more potent in this respect (LAHTI and BARSUHN, 1974). In rats forced to swim in an unescapable situation, plasma corticosteroids were increased by approximately 120%; meprobamate in doses of 25, 50, and $100 \, \text{mg} \cdot \text{kg}^{-1}$ i.p. reduced this increased by about 50% without any dose relation (LE FUR et al., 1979). Benzodiazepines dose-dependently reduced the stress-induced elevation of plasma corticosteroids; the elevation was completely prevented by $0.5 \, \text{mg} \cdot \text{kg}^{-1}$ diazepam and $5 \, \text{mg} \cdot \text{kg}^{-1}$ chlordiazepoxide.

A nontoxic analogue of amphenone, 1-2-*bis*[3-pyridyl-]-2-methyl-1-propanone, elicits in man a release of pituitary corticotrophin which leads to a twofold rise in urinary 17-ketosteroids; meprobamate in clinical doses was able to reduce this rise (GOLD et al., 1960).

Dispersal of melanophore pigment in skin, which is under the control of the pituitary gland, occurred in frogs with muscle relaxant doses of meprobamate (100–150 mg $\cdot$ kg^{-1} i.p.); this effect was reversed by adrenaline. In hypophysectomized frogs and in the isolated frog skin, meprobamate did not induce melanophore dispersal (ROBINSON and SCOTT, 1960).

H. Anticonvulsant Activity

Meprobamate was the most potent compound of a series of propanediol derivatives in preventing convulsions caused by pentetrazole in mice (ED$_{50}$ determined after 30 min, 102 mg $\cdot$ kg^{-1} i.p.). In maximal electroshock seizures in mice the ED$_{50}$ was 165 mg $\cdot$ kg^{-1} i.p. Only at very high doses was meprobamate able to antagonize convulsions elicited by strychnine in mice (ED$_{50}$ at 30 min, 550 mg $\cdot$ kg^{-1} i.p.) (BERGER, 1954; BERGER et al., 1956; BERGER et al., 1964). The oral ED$_{50}$ values for meprobamate, tybamate, and carisoprodol were 67, 120, and 145 mg $\cdot$ kg^{-1} against pentetrazole (120 mg $\cdot$ kg^{-1} i.p.) and 470, 388, and >980 against strychnine (2.5 mg $\cdot$ kg^{-1} i.p.).

BERGER (1956) tried to correlate pharmacological actions with physical properties, i.e., melting points: He found a good correlation between paralyzing potency (i.e., induction of loss of righting reflex) and antipentetrazole effect on the one side and melting points of the different derivatives on the other side; no such correlation was found in the case of maximal electroshock. RANDALL et al. (1960) compared chlordiazepoxide with meprobamate in mice; ED$_{50}$ in the maximal electroshock test was 95 and 200 mg $\cdot$ kg^{-1} p.o., the ED$_{50}$ for antipentetrazole activity 18 and 133 mg, respectively, whereas the acute oral toxicity was lower for meprobamate than for chlordiazepoxide. FINK and SWINYARD (1959) and CHEN and BOHNER (1960) confirmed the effects against pentetrazole and maximal electroshock, and obtained values in good agreement with those reported above. FINK and SWINYARD (1959) reported the effectiveness of meprobamate against maximal audiogenic seizures in mice (ED$_{50}$: 29 mg $\cdot$ kg^{-1} p.o.). The withdrawal syndrome of rats made physically dependent on barbiturates is characterized by a loss of body weight and a susceptibility to sound-induced convulsions; spontaneous convulsions are also seen. Meprobamate was able to prevent these withdrawal symptoms (NORTON, 1970).

The anticonvulsant properties of meprobamate have also been investigated in patients undergoing electroconvulsive therapy (COOK and REID, 1962). In this study patients were given 800 mg meprobamate twice daily. The results indicated a highly significant difference in the incidence of fits between treated and untreated groups of patients, suggesting a strong anticonvulsant effect of meprobamate in this experimental situation.

I. Effects on Spontaneous and Imposed Motor Activity

Meprobamate at high doses decreased spontaneous locomotor activity (BORSY et al., 1960; DELLA BELLA and ROGNONI, 1960; WEAVER and MIYA, 1961). At 100 mg $\cdot$ kg^{-1} i.p. it was found inactive in mice (MENON et al., 1977).

However, in a study where the different phases of behavior of the "naive" mouse in the actograph were investigated, meprobamate increased the initial activity, which may be considered as orientational hypermotility or exploration (RAYNAUD et al., 1965). In the test of KNEIP (1960), which studies the climbing impulse of mice placed in an unfamiliar chamber with a wire netting on one wall, meprobamate was effective with an ED_{50} of about 150 mg·kg^{-1} and about 250 mg·kg^{-1} at 1 and 4 h, respectively. Meprobamate, at an intraperitoneal dose which per se elicits a decrease of spontaneous locomotor activity of mice, enhanced the amphetamine-induced increase of motor activity (SETHY et al., 1970). Meprobamate at 100 and 200 mg·kg^{-1} p.o. reduced performance of mice forced to swim (NIESCHULZ, 1963).

J. Effects on Muscle Tone and Coordination

BERGER (1954; BERGER et al., 1956) investigated propanediols for their effects on the righting reflex. The average effective dose producing loss of righting reflex in mice was 300 mg·kg^{-1} p.o. and 235 mg·kg^{-1} i.p. for meprobamate, whereas the mean lethal dose of meprobamate was 1,100 mg·kg^{-1} p.o. and 800 mg·kg^{-1} i.p. For tybamate an ED_{50} of 198 mg·kg^{-1} p.o. was determined (BERGER et al., 1964). BERGER and LYNES (1954) described a convulsant propranol derivative (W-181: 1-n-butylamino-3-p-toluidino-2-propranol) as a possible antagonist of anesthesia or paralysis induced by depressant drugs such as mephenesin. In mice, loss of righting reflex induced by phenobarbitone, mephenesin, and benzimidazole could be antagonized by nonconvulsant doses of this compound.

Meprobamate (150–300 mg·kg^{-1} i.p.) and diazepam (10–40 mg·kg^{-1} i.p.) produced a loss of righting reflex in mice when given alone. In subanesthetic doses the two compounds caused a parallel shift to the left of the phenobarbitone dose-response curve and the ED_{50} of phenobarbitone was reduced significantly (FRANK and JHAMANDAS, 1970 a).

In the inclined screen test in mice, meprobamate (ED_{50}: 282 mg·kg^{-1} p.o.) proved equally effective as chlordiazepoxide (RANDALL et al., 1960), with values in the range of those reported by ROBICHAUD et al. (1970). This value approximately corresponds to the ED_{50} for loss of righting reflex as indicated by BERGER (1954) and ROBICHAUD et al. (1970). Meprobamate in the same dose range reduced the ability of mice to hang from a horizontal grid (KONDZIELLA, 1964).

In contrast to chlordiazepoxide and other benzodiazepines, which had an ED_{50} p.o. in a mice rotarod test of 6–8 mg·kg^{-1}, meprobamate was reported either to be almost ineffective at 100 mg·kg^{-1} p.o. (WEAVER and MIYA, 1961) or to have an ED_{50} of about 100 mg·kg^{-1} i.p. (DELLA BELLA and ROGNONI, 1960).

Decerebrate rigidity in cats characterized by high-voltage, high-frequency potentials in the electromyogram of extensor muscles of the hind limb was completely abolished and a normal electromyogram reinstated after administration of 10 mg·kg^{-1} tybamate i.v. To obtain similar results with meprobamate and carisoprodol, 24 mg·kg^{-1} i.v. and 3 mg·kg^{-1} i.v., respectively, were required. In the case of spinal reflexes, 20 mg·kg^{-1} tybamate i.v. was strongly effective in depressing the flexor reflex in the hind limb, while not affecting the patellar reflex; in these experiments its effect was similar to that of meprobamate (BERGER et al., 1964).

Barbiturate synergism was studied in groups of 10 mice receiving jointly a dose of a propanediol and 100 mg·kg^{-1} hexobarbitone sodium, measuring the time during which the righting reflex was lost. Tybamate significantly prolonged sleeping time at $100 \text{ mg} \cdot \text{kg}^{-1}$ i.p., but half this dose had no marked effect. Meprobamate in similar doses produced comparable effects (BERGER et al., 1964).

K. Interactions with Various Centrally Active Agents

Meprobamate injected i.p. at $100 \text{ mg} \cdot \text{kg}^{-1}$ together with hexobarbitone significantly prolonged the duration of hexobarbitone anesthesia in mice, as measured by the duration of loss of righting reflex (BERGER et al., 1964) but was inactive on pentobarbitone (MENON et al., 1977). After repeated administration of large doses of meprobamate, a moderate decrease in the duration of hexobarbitone anesthesia became apparent (BERGER et al., 1964).

A potentiation of ethanol effects in mice was also observed; the minimal potentiating dose for meprobamate was $14 \text{ mg} \cdot \text{kg}^{-1}$ p.o. (FORNEY et al., 1962).

Meprobamate, at an intraperitoneal dose which per se elicited a decrease of spontaneous locomotor activity in mice, produced a greater increase of motor activity in combination with amphetamine than the same dose of amphetamine alone (SETHY et al., 1970).

L. Effects on Aggression

Rather high doses of meprobamate had to be given in order to detect antiaggressive effects in various animal species. Spontaneous aggressive cynomolgus and rhesus monkeys became quiet with doses of meprobamate ($100–200 \text{ mg} \cdot \text{kg}^{-1}$ p.o.) which induced a loss of motor coordination and spontaneous locomotor activity (BERGER, 1954; RANDALL et al., 1960). However, doses up to $200 \text{ mg} \cdot \text{kg}^{-1}$ p.o. affected neither the vicious behavior nor the aggression-associated vocalization in squirrel monkeys (SCHECKEL and BOFF, 1967). Meprobamate ($55 \text{ mg} \cdot \text{kg}^{-1}$ i.m.) was also ineffective in social dominance tests with pairs of a dominant and a submissive monkey (LEARY and STYNES, 1959). In line with the observations on monkeys, taming effects of meprobamate ($200 \text{ mg} \cdot \text{kg}^{-1}$ p.o.) in extremely vicious minks were found to be accompanied by sedation, muscle relaxation, and ataxia (BAUEN and POSSANZA, 1970). Doses of meprobamate which abolished the righting reflexes ($200 \text{ mg} \cdot \text{kg}^{-1}$ i.p.) were only slightly active in suppressing the muricide behavior of "killer" rats (HOROVITZ et al., 1966), a finding which is in agreement with an earlier observation made by KARLI (1959). On the other hand, meprobamate was more active ($20–64 \text{ mg} \cdot \text{kg}^{-1}$ p.o.) in reducing fighting among rabbits (WOLF and HAXTHAUSEN, 1960) and in a spontaneously aggressive strain of mice (BOISSIER et al., 1968) as well as in fighting Siamese fish ($10 \text{ μg} \cdot \text{ml}^{-1}$, WALASZEK and ABOOD, 1956).

Aggressive behavior which developed in mice previously kept in isolation was not very sensitive to the action of meprobamate, since isolation-induced aggressivity in mice was reduced only with doses of meprobamate ($200 \text{ mg} \cdot \text{kg}^{-1}$ p.o., $40–100 \text{ mg} \cdot \text{kg}^{-1}$ i.p.) which led to motor impairment (YEN et al., 1959; JANSSEN et al., 1960; DA VANZO et al., 1966; VALZELLI et al., 1967).

The original observation that meprobamate diminished foot-shock-induced aggression at dose levels below those depressing spontaneous motor activity in mice

(ED$_{50}$: 84 mg·kg^{-1} p.o., TEDESCHI et al., 1959) was not confirmed by other investigators. GRAY et al. (1961) and CHEN et al. (1963) found meprobamate to be effective in this test with doses (120 mg·kg^{-1} p.o.) producing sedation and ataxia in mice, while in another study the aggression-reducing effect of meprobamate in mice and rats was obvious only with doses (350 mg·kg^{-1} p.o.) which were almost as high as those inhibiting locomotor activity (CHRISTMAS and MAXWELL, 1970).

Rats with bilateral septal lesions become extremely aggressive (BRADY and NAUTA, 1953). Early studies with this preparation showed that meprobamate, given either orally (240 mg·kg^{-1}; HUNT, 1957) or intraperitoneally (95 mg·kg^{-1}, SCHALLEK et al., 1962), diminished hyperirritability of septal rats. However, in later investigations meprobamate was found to be ineffective in hyperreactive septal rats (STARK and HENDERSON, 1966; SOFIA, 1969) as well as in rats made aggressive by lesions in the ventromedial hypothalamus, olfactory bulbs (MALICK et al., 1969) or midbrain (CHRISTMAS and MAXWELL, 1970).

Conflicting reports also appeared on the effect of meprobamate on aggressive behavior elicited by electrical stimulation of the hypothalamus or the periaqueductal gray matter. BAXTER (1968), on the one hand, was unable to find a clear-cut effect of meprobamate on the hissing response in the hypothalamically stimulated cat at doses below those inducing ataxia (50 mg·kg^{-1} i.p.). On the other hand, the threshold for vocalization evoked by central gray stimulation in monkeys was elevated after 100 mg·kg^{-1} meprobamate i.p. (DELGADO et al., 1971), and the same dose of meprobamate markedly reduced the aggressiveness in gibbons induced by central gray stimulation (APFELBACH, 1971). In the latter two studies, however, no overall behavioral effects were mentioned, rendering questionable any interpretation about the possible specific action of this high dose of meprobamate on aggression elicited by electrical brain stimulation.

Pharmacologically induced aggression can be most consistently produced by pretreatment of mice with high intravenous doses of DOPA (250–500 mg·kg^{-1}), which elicits powerful attacks and repeated biting (VAN DER WENDE and SPOERLEIN, 1962). Increased biting after these high nonlethal doses of DL-DOPA was reduced by meprobamate (89–200 mg·kg^{-1} i.p., KLETZKIN, 1969; YEN et al., 1970). Increased irritability in rats, which follows the degeneration of central catecholaminergic neurons induced by intraventricular injection of 6-hydroxydopamine, was reduced by meprobamate (ED$_{50}$: 195 mg·kg^{-1} i.p.) and a series of other centrally active agents (NAKAMURA and THOENEN, 1972).

Summarizing the effects of meprobamate on different forms of aggression in animals, the statement can be made that meprobamate has antiaggressive actions in doses leading to sedation and muscle relaxation and, therefore, can hardly be ascribed to a specific influence on aggression-modulating mechanisms in the brain.

M. Effects on Spinal Cord Activities

Effects of meprobamate on spinal cord functions were first described by BERGER (1954). In chloralose-urethane anesthetized cats with intact neuraxis, 40 mg·kg^{-1} meprobamate i.v. abolished polysynaptic flexor and crossed extensor reflexes in the hind limb elicited by electrical stimulation of the sciatic nerve and recorded as contractions of the tibialis anterior and the quadriceps muscle, respectively. Since the monosynaptic reflex (knee jerk) evoked by mechanical stimulation of the patellar tendon was only slightly depressed or unaffected after this dose of meprobamate, Berger (1954) concluded that meprobamate selectively depressed spinal interneurons responsible for polysynaptic reflexes and proposed reduction of interneuronal activity as the mechanism of muscle relaxant properties of the drug.

Since this original study by Berger (1954), the specificity of action attributed to meprobamate in depressing interneuronal circuits at the spinal level has been questioned for several reasons. It was soon recognized that other centrally active compounds, such as pentobarbitone, phenobarbitone, morphine, and chlorpromazine in appropriate doses also diminished polysynaptic reflexes more readily than monosynaptic reflexes (Pfeiffer et al., 1957; Busch et al., 1960; De Salva and Oester, 1960). Furthermore, in additional studies using unanesthetized spinal as well as intact anesthetized cats, meprobamate depressed monosynaptic reflexes at doses (50–100 mg $\cdot$ kg^{-1} i.v.) which were only slightly higher than those inhibiting polysynaptic reflexes (Wilson, 1958; De Salva and Oester, 1960; Inoki et al., 1961). Ngai et al. (1966) reported that 20–40 mg $\cdot$ kg^{-1} meprobamate i.v. reduced ipsilateral and contralateral extensor reflexes to 20–50% of control in decerebrate cats without affecting the knee jerk, whereas in spinal animals 80–120 mg $\cdot$ kg^{-1} meprobamate were required to diminish the polysynaptic reflexes to a similar extent. In the latter preparations the knee jerk was also depressed, although less markedly than polysynaptic reflexes. An explanation for the relative selectivity of meprobamate for polysynaptic reflexes was offered by Wilson (1958), who recorded monosynaptic reflex potentials from the lumbosacral ventral roots upon stimulation of flexor and extensor muscle nerve afferents in spinal cats. Wilson (1958) suggested that a more pronounced reduction of polysynaptic responses as compared to monosynaptic reflexes was due not to the selective action of meprobamate on interneurons, but rather to a summation effect, i.e., that meprobamate depressed excitability of neurons indiscriminately and that polysynaptic pathways containing a greater number of neurons in series were consequently more affected than monosynaptic pathways. Inhibitory disynaptic pathways in the spinal cord, such as those involved in reciprocal and recurrent inhibition of motoneurons, were found to be more resistant to meprobamate than are excitatory polysynaptic pathways (recurrent facilitation, Wilson and Talbot, 1960). In line with this observation is the finding that meprobamate depressed facilitation of the knee jerk evoked by pontine reticular stimulation more easily than inhibition of the knee jerk elicited by stimulation of the bulbar reticular formation in intact anesthetized cats (Del Castillo and Nelson, 1960), again indicating that excitatory pathways were generally more sensitive to meprobamate than inhibitory pathways. However, this assumption was not confirmed by other studies which have demonstrated a similar marked depression by meprobamate and by its newer analogue, tybamate, of both excitatory and inhibitory pathways to motoneurons in decerebrate and spinal cats (Abdulian et al., 1960; Tseng et al., 1970).

In addition to its depressant effects on spinal cord reflexes, 20–40 mg $\cdot$ kg^{-1} meprobamate i.v. was found in decerebrate and slightly anesthetized intact cats to reduce the activity of γ-motoneurons and tonic α-motoneurons considered to be responsible for the maintenance of muscle tone (Busch et al., 1960); this effect would be an alternative mechanism for the muscle relaxant action of meprobamate.

The spinal cord effects discussed above were obtained predominantly in intact anesthetized or decerebrate animals. A direct spinal action of meprobamate has not been unequivocally demonstrated unless high doses (50–100 mg·kg^{-1} i.v.) were administered. In the case of tybamate, relatively low doses (5 mg·kg^{-1} i.v.) depressed the firing of unidentified interneurons in the dorsal horn evoked by dorsal root stimulation (KIRSTEN and TSENG, 1972). The effect of meprobamate on two electrophysiological correlates of presynaptic inhibition, dorsal root potentials (DRPs) and dorsal root reflexes (DRRs), was studied in unanesthetized spinal cats. Up to a dose of 100 mg·kg^{-1} i.v., meprobamate did not affect DRPs and DRRs (HAEFELY et al., 1978), and in another study even a depression of DRRs was observed (MURAYAMA et al., 1972).

Taken together, the effects of meprobamate on spinal cord activities appear to be primarily mediated through changes in supraspinal control mechanisms, in particular by a reduction of descending facilitatory influences. Very high doses are required for effects within the spinal cord, and these effects differ essentially from those of benzodiazepines and barbiturates by the complete absence of an enhancement of presynaptic inhibition. Whether the effect of meprobamate can be accounted for by a moderate generalized depression of neuronal excitability, as suggested by WILSON (1958), cannot be decided at present.

N. Effects on Evoked Potentials in the CNS

The finding that meprobamate up to 80 mg·kg^{-1} i.v. in unanesthetized immobilized cats did not affect evoked potentials in response to auditory stimuli, recorded in the specific ascending sensory system (medial geniculate body, temporal cortex) and in the nonspecific "arousal" system (reticular formation, centromedian thalamus) of the brain, led KLETZKIN and SWAN (1959) to exclude any effect of meprobamate on the arousal system of the reticular formation. However, meprobamate (50 mg·kg^{-1} i.v.) was found to depress the inhibition of click-evoked responses in the dorsal cochlear nucleus by conditioning reticular stimulation in unrestrained freely moving as well as unanesthetized immobilized cats (CHIN et al., 1965). Furthermore, in unrestrained rats meprobamate (40 mg·kg^{-1} i.p.) reduced visual evoked potentials in the tectotegmental midbrain area, which includes both the dorsal part of the reticular formation and ventral optic tectum (OLDS and BALDRIGHI, 1968).

FRANK and JHAMANDAS (1970 b) observed a depression by 20–40 mg·kg^{-1} meprobamate i.v. of the surface negative and the surface positive waves of the cortical potential evoked by nearby surface stimulation in neuronally isolated cortex slabs in decerebrate cats. Meprobamate (200 mg·kg^{-1} i.p.) clearly depressed cortical evoked potentials induced by single shocks applied to the tooth pulp, whereas the same dose had no effect on posttetanic potentiation of these potentials (BANSI et al., 1976).

Diencephalolimbic neuronal circuits were postulated to be the site of anxiolytic action of meprobamate (BERGER, 1968, 1977; LUDWIG and POTTERFIELD, 1971). In agreement with this finding, meprobamate significantly reduced the amplitude of the amygdalohippocampal evoked potentials with the high dose of 51 mg·kg^{-1} i.v. in unanesthetized immobilized cats (JALFRE et al., 1971). However, meprobamate (20–40 mg·kg^{-1} i.p.) did not affect potentials elicited in the hippocampus by single shocks applied to the fornix, potentials evoked in the hippocampus by stimulation of the amygdala, or hypothalamic activity in response to the hippocampal stimuli in *encéphale isolé* rats (TAKAGI and BAN, 1960). Meprobamate (30 mg·kg^{-1} i.v.) was also only slightly active in antagonizing the depression by bicuculline (0.3 mg·kg^{-1} i.v.) of the strio-nigral evoked potential in unanesthetized curarized cats (SCHAFFNER, unpublished work).

From studies of the action of meprobamate on brain evoked potentials no conclusive statements are possible. It seems, however, that the same doses of meprobamate which have depressant effect on some limbic structures also reduce the activity of the ascending reticular activating system, including the cortex.

O. Effects on the EEG

An early investigation of meprobamate in unanesthetized immobilized cats revealed a synchronization of the EEG (appearance of high-amplitude slow waves), which was more pronounced in the thalamus than in the neocortex after relatively low intravenous doses (20 mg·kg^{-1}). This observation led HENDLEY et al. (1954) to assume a thalamic site of action of meprobamate. In addition to the thalamus, later studies emphasized the sensitivity of other subcortical regions to the depressant action of meprobamate. BERGER et al. (1957) pointed out that the dose is a critical factor in determining sites of action of meprobamate, since doubling of the dose which elicited a spindle-like (10–15 Hz) activity in the thalamus (20 mg·kg^{-1} i.v. to 40 mg·kg^{-1} i.v.), produced a similar synchronization also in the cortex. In unanesthetized and anesthetized cats, 20–40 mg·kg^{-1} meprobamate i.v. induced EEG synchronization in the thalamus, amygdala, and basal ganglia (caudate nucleus and putamen), but not in the hypothalamus (BAIRD et al., 1957). Meprobamate (20–40 mg·kg^{-1} i.v.) was rather ineffective in elevating the threshold for the EEG arousal reaction in the neocortex upon high-frequency stimulation of the reticular formation in *encéphale isolé* cats (BRADLEY and KEY, 1959) and unanesthetized immobilized cats (GANGLOFF, 1959; KLETZKIN and BERGER, 1959). The same doses of meprobamate, however, markedly reduced the excitability of the thalamus, as shown by a depression of recruiting cortical response to the low-frequency stimulation of unspecific thalamic nuclei (GANGLOFF, 1959; HUKUHARA, 1962; KLETZKIN, 1962). In addition, the threshold for inducing EEG afterdischarges (high-amplitude epileptoid waves overlasting the stimulation period) in the limbic system upon stimulation of the septum, amygdala, and hippocampus was elevated after meprobamate (KLETZKIN and BERGER, 1959; SCHALLEK and KUEHN, 1960; KLETZKIN, 1962). Results virtually identical to those observed with meprobamate were obtained with intravenous injections of a newer analogue, tybamate (10–40 mg·kg^{-1} i.v.), in unanesthetized immobilized cats and rabbits (BERGER et al., 1964).

Other investigations, including those performed with unrestrained freely moving animals, questioned the selective sensitivity of the limbic system and thalamus to the depressant effect of meprobamate. In fact, rather low doses of meprobamate (20 mg·kg^{-1} i.v.) attenuated the cortical and thalamic arousal response to acoustic and hypothalamic stimuli in unrestrained rabbits (BOVET et al., 1957). In unanesthetized immobilized cats, meprobamate (25–50 mg·kg^{-1} i.v., 80 mg·kg^{-1} i.p.) was found to elevate the EEG arousal threshold in cortex, amygdala, and hippocampus to stimulation of the reticular formation, but not to stimulation of the hypothalamus and caudate nucleus (HUKUHARA, 1962; TAKAGI et al., 1967). High-amplitude waves (8–20 Hz) were observed in all cortical and subcortical leads after 25 mg·kg^{-1} meprobamate i.v. in these same cats (HUKUHARA, 1962). In freely moving cats, KIDO and YAMAMOTO (1962) found a synchronization (14–20 Hz) in the neocortical and thalamic EEG after meprobamate (30 mg·kg^{-1} i.v.). Intraperitoneal and oral administration of meprobamate (160 mg·kg^{-1}) induced slow waves in the hippocampus and cortex (SCHALLEK and KUEHN, 1965), but the threshold for cortical arousal by reticular stimulation was only slightly raised in unrestrained cats (SCHALLEK and KUEHN, 1965). In freely moving monkeys, DELGADO et al. (1971) observed after meprobamate (100 mg·kg^{-1} i.m.) an EEG synchronization in the caudate nucleus and amygdala, accompanied by a reduced excitability of central gray matter, thalamus, and amygdala.

In a recent study the effect of meprobamate was assessed by quantitative evaluation of the frequency distribution spectra of the EEG. GEHRMANN and KILLAM (1978) found that 100 mg·kg^{-1} meprobamate p.o. increased the power of higher frequencies (16–64 Hz) in the neocortex of monkeys, an effect which remained stable for several hours.

P. Effects on Sleep

Very few studies are concerned with the effects of meprobamate on sleep. KIDO and YAMAMOTO (1962) found a sleep-like behavior in cats after high doses of meprobamate (60–120 mg·kg^{-1} i.v.), but they did not further analyze the sleep patterns. GOLDSTEIN et al. (1967) in rabbits and GOGERTY (1973) in monkeys observed a small increase of the rapid eye movement sleep (REM sleep) after meprobamate (1 mg·kg^{-1} i.v. in rabbits, 60 mg·kg^{-1} p.o. in monkeys). In monkeys, the slow wave sleep was not consistently altered by meprobamate (GOGERTY, 1973). In contrast to these few reports of a possible REM sleep enhancing effect of meprobamate, the highest dose of meprobamate studied (30 mg·kg^{-1} i.v.) was without effects on a phasic phenomenon of REM sleep, the so-called ponto-geniculo-occipital (PGO) waves, induced by Ro 14–1284, a reserpine-like benzoquinolizine, in unanesthetized immobilized cats (RUCH-MONACHON et al., 1976 b).

Summarizing the effects of meprobamate on EEG and sleep, one may conclude that in unanesthetized immobilized cats, in which most studies with meprobamate were performed, the thalamus and limbic structures seem to be more affected by the drug than are the hypothalamus, reticular formation, and cortex. However, the few studies with meprobamate in unrestrained animals and in other species, which are in part contradictory to those performed in immobilized cats, do not yet allow one to make a definite statement on the assumed specific depressant action of meprobamate on the limbic system and thalamus.

Q. Effects on Specific Neurotransmitter Systems

Acetylcholine. MALHOTRA and METHA (1966) injected dogs with 50 mg·kg^{-1} meprobamate i.v. The acetylcholine content determined by bioassay was increased by 45% in the hypothalamus and by 71% in the hippocampus, but not significantly altered in the frontal cortex, cerebellar cortex, and midbrain.

Serotonin (5-HT). The urinary excretion of 5-hydroxyindoleacetic acid (5-HIAA) in rats was unaffected by 200 mg·kg⁻¹ meprobamate i.p. (BERGER et al., 1956). The 5-HIAA content in the brainstem of rats was slightly increased (by 30%) after 50 mg·kg⁻¹ meprobamate i.p. (DA PRADA and PLETSCHER, 1966). Meprobamate up to 10^{-4} mol·l⁻¹ did not affect the 5-HT content of isolated blood platelets of rabbits (PLETSCHER et al., 1966).

Dopamine (DA). The brain content of homovanillic acid (HVA), a major metabolite of dopamine, was unaffected in rats after 50 mg·kg⁻¹ meprobamate i.p. (DA PRADA and PLETSCHER, 1966). Measuring by histochemical and biochemical methods the decline of DA after an inhibitor of tyrosine hydroxylase, LIDBRINK et al. (1972, 1973) found that 200 mg·kg⁻¹ meprobamate i.p. reduced the turnover of DA in the striatum of unstressed rats and accentuated the decrease of turnover produced by immobilization stress. The stress-induced decrease of DA turnover in the median eminence was counteracted by meprobamate. The effects of meprobamate on DA turnover were similar to those of 100 mg·kg⁻¹ phenobarbitone i.p. The increased motor activity induced in mice by the combination of the monoamine oxidase inhibitor, iproniazid, and L-DOPA was potentiated by 75 and 150 mg·kg⁻¹ meprobamate i.p. (BERENDSON et al., 1976).

Noradrenaline (NA). In contrast to barbiturates and benzodiazepines (CORRODI et al., 1971), 200 mg·kg⁻¹ meprobamate i.p. failed to decrease the turnover of NA in the cerebral cortex of rats, measured histochemically and biochemically by the decrease of NA after tyrosine hydroxylase inhibition (LIDBRINK et al., 1972, 1973). However, the increase of NA turnover in all main parts provoked by immobilization stress was attenuated by meprobamate.

GABA. Meprobamate did not affect presynaptic inhibition in the cat spinal cord, suggesting that the compound does not affect GABAergic mechanism (POLC, unpublished work).

R. Effects on Brain Energy Metabolism

Meprobamate (200 mg·kg⁻¹ i.p.) did not affect the inorganic phosphate, phosphocreatinine, AMP, ADP, and ATP contents of rat brain, in contrast to 60 mg·kg⁻¹ chlordiazepoxide i.p., which produced a similar degree of muscle relaxation (KAUL and LEWIS, 1963) but increased phosphocreatinine and ADP and consequently reduced the ATP/ADP-ratio.

S. Concluding Remarks

The pharmacologic profile places meprobamate between barbiturates and benzodiazepines. Common to the three classes of drugs are sedative, anxiolytic, anticonvulsant, and muscle relaxant properties. In contrast to both barbiturates and benzodiazepines, meprobamate has not been used clinically as anticonvulsant. The compound resembles barbiturates more than benzodiazepines in its low potency and relatively narrow therapeutic range. It differs from barbiturates and resembles more benzodiazepines because of virtual absence of direct effects on autonomic functions and the inability to produce complete surgical anesthesia; however, if meprobamate acts on a specific receptor, this has to be quite different from the benzodiazepine receptor because it does not inhibit ^{3}H-diazepam binding in relevant concentrations (MÖHLER and OKADA, 1977; WILLIAMS and RISLEY, 1979) and the effects of meprobamate are not antagonized by specific benzodiazepine antagonists (HUNKELER et al., 1981).

Thirty years after the discovery of meprobamate, virtually nothing is known about the mechanism of its action. While barbiturates produce their effects by a combination of enhanced synaptic inhibition and depressed synaptic excitation, and benzodiazepines selectively enhance GABA-mediated synaptic inhibition through highly specific receptors (HAEFELY, 1977), neither molecular nor synaptic effects of meprobamate have been elucidated. The most likely basis of the action of meprobamate appears to be a moderate generalized depression of neuronal excitability. No enhancement of synaptic inhibition has yet been observed. The decreasing interest in meprobamate as a therapeutic agent is reflected by the declining number of recent experimental studies with this drug. In view of the urgent need of basic knowledge on the mechanisms of psychotropic drug actions for the rational development of new ones, it would be extremely important to understand why grossly similar effects of meprobamate, barbiturates, and benzodiazepines are produced in spite of apparently quite dissimilar synaptic and molecular actions.

References

Abdulian, D.H., Martin, W.R., Unna, K.R.: Effects of central nervous system depressants on inhibition and facilitation of the patellar reflex. Arch. Int. Pharmacodyn. Ther. *228*, 169–186 (1960)

Apfelbach, R.: Chemische Unterdrückung elektrisch ausgelöster Aggression. Naturwissenschaften *58*, 368 (1971)

Aron, C., Roos, J., Asch, G.: Données nouvelles sur l'action antiovulatoire du méprobamate chez la ratte. C.R. Soc. Biol. (Paris) *161*, 1325–1328 (1967)

Aron, C., Roos, J., Asch, G., Roos, M.: Données nouvelles sur les modalités chronologiques et quantitatives de l'action antiovulatoire du méprobamate chez la ratte. Acta Endocrinol. (Kbh.) *58*, 396–406 (1968)

Arora, R.B.: Antiarrhythmics. Quinidine-like activity of some ataraxic agents. J. Pharmacol. Exp. Ther. *124*, 53–58 (1958)

Arora, R.B., Somani, P., Lal, A.: Antiarrhythmics Part XIII. Effect of chloroquine and chloroquine-tranquillizing drug combination on ectopic ventricular tachycardia following acute myocardial infarction in dogs. Indian J. Med. Res. *50*, 720–731 (1962)

Bainbridge, J.G.: The effect of psychotropic drugs on food reinforced behaviour and on food consumption. Psychopharmacologia (Berl.) *12*, 204–213 (1968)

Baird, H.W., Szekely, E.G., Wycis, H.T., Spiegel, E.A.: The effect of meprobamate on the basal ganglia. Ann. N.Y. Acad. Sci. *67*, 873–894 (1957)

Bansi, D., Krug, M., Schmidt, J.: Der Einfluß von Psychopharmaka auf durch Zahnpulpareizung ausgelöste kortikale Potentiale und langhaltende posttetanische Erregbarkeitsänderungen. Acta Biol. Med. Germ. *35*, 613–625 (1976)

Bastian, J.W., Clements, G.R.: Pharmacology and toxicology of hydroxyphenamate (listica). Dis. Nerv. Syst. *22*, 9–16 (1961)

Bauen, A., Possanza, G.J.: The mink as a psychopharmacological model. Arch. Int. Pharmacodyn. Ther. *186*, 133–136 (1970)

Baxter, B.L.: The effect of selected drugs on the "emotional" behavior elicited via hypothalamic stimulation. Int. J. Neuropharmacol. *7*, 47–54 (1968)

Berendson, H., Leonard, B.E., Rigter, H.: The action of psychotropic drugs on DOPA induced behavioral responses in mice. Drug Res. *26*, 1686–1689 (1976)

Berger, F.M.: The pharmacological properties of 2-methyl-2-n-propyl-1,3-propanediol dicarbamate (Miltown), a new interneuronal blocking agent. J. Pharmacol. Exp. Ther. *112*, 413–423 (1954)

Berger, F.M.: The chemistry and mode of action of tranquilizing drugs. Ann. N.Y. Acad. Sci. *67*, 685–700 (1957)

Berger, F.M.: The relation between the pharmacological properties of meprobamate and the clinical usefulness of the drug. In: Psychopharmacology; a review of Progress 1957–1967. Efron, D.H. (ed.), U.S. Dept. Health Educ. Welfare, Washington D.C., 1968, pp. 139–152

Berger, F.M.: Meprobamate and other glycol derivatives. In: Usdin, E., Forrest, I.S. (Eds.): Psychotherapeutic Drugs, Part II, pp. 1089–1100. New York: Dekker 1977

Berger, F.M., Lynes, T.E.: The analeptic action of 1-n-butylamino-3-p-toluidino-2-propanol (W 181) in sleep or paralysis produced by certain central nervous system depressants. J. Pharmacol. Exp. Ther. *112*, 399–403 (1954)

Berger, F.M., Hendley, C.D., Ludwig, B.J., Lynes, T.E.: Central depressant and anticonvulsant activity of compounds with 2-methyl-2-n-propyl-1,3-propanediol dicarbamate (Miltown). J. Pharmacol. Exp. Ther. *116*, 337–342 (1956)

Berger, F.M., Campbell, G.L., Hendley, C.D., Ludwig, B.J., Lynes, T.E.: The action of tranquilizers on brain potentials and serotonin. Ann. N.Y. Acad. Sci. *66*, 686–694 (1957)

Berger, F.M., Douglas, J.F., Kletzkin, M., Ludwig, B.J., Margolin, S.: The pharmacological properties of 2-methyl-2-sec-butyl-1,3-propanediol dicarbamate (mebutamate, W-583), a new centrally acting blood pressure lowering agent. J. Pharmacol. Exp. Ther. *134*, 356–365 (1961)

Berger, F.M., Kletzkin, M., Margolin, S.: Pharmacologic properties of a new tranquilizing agent, 2-methyl-2-propyltrimethyline butylcarbamate carbamate (Tybamate). Med. Exp. *10*, 327–344 (1964)

Berger, M., Neuweiler, W.: Die medikamentöse Relaxation des menschlichen Uterus. Wissenschaftl. Ausstellung, 3. Weltkongreß der Intern. Fed. f. Gynäkol., Wien, Sept. 1961

Boissier, J.-R., Grasset, S., Simon, P.: Effects of some psychotropic drugs on mice from a spontaneously aggressive strain. J. Pharm. Pharmacol. *20*, 972–973 (1968)

Boris, A., Stevenson, R.H.: The effects of some psychotropic drugs on dehydration induced antidiuretic hormone activity in the rat. Arch. Int. Pharmacodyn. Ther. *166*, 486–498 (1967)

Bornmann, G.: Zum Einfluß einiger psychotroper Substanzen auf Magen und Gallefluß. Arzneim. Forsch. *11*, 89–90 (1961)

Borsy, J., Csanyi, E., Lazar, I.: A method of assaying tranquilizing drugs based on the inhibition of orientational hypermotility. Arch. Int. Pharmacodyn. Ther. *124*, 180–190 (1960)

Bovet, D., Longo, V.G., Silvestrini, B.: Les méthodes d'investigations électrophysiologiques dans l'étude des médicaments tranquillisants. Contribution à la pharmacologie de la formation réticulaire. In: Garattini, S., Ghetti, V. (Eds.): Psychotropic Drugs, pp. 193–206. Amsterdam: Elsevier 1957

Bradley, P.B., Key, B.J.: A comparative study of the effects of drugs on the arousal system of the brain. Brit. J. Pharmacol. *14*, 340–349 (1959)

Brady, J.V., Nauta, W.J.H.: Subcortical mechanisms in emotional behavior: affective changes following septal forebrain lesions in the albino rat. J. Comp. Physiol. Psychol. *46*, 339–346 (1953)

Busch, G., Henatsch, H.-D., Schulte, F.J.: Elektrophysiologische Analyse der Wirkungen neuroleptischer und tranquilisierender Substanzen (Phenothiazine, Meprobamat) auf die spinalmotorischen Systeme. Arzneim. Forsch. *10*, 217–223 (1960)

Chassaing, C., Duchene-Marullaz, P.: The influence of meprobamate on heart rate in the conscious dog. Arch. Int. Pharmacodyn. Ther. *220*, 45–50 (1976)

Chen, G., Bohner, B.: A study of certain CNS depressants. Arch. Int. Pharmacodyn. Ther. *125*, 1–20 (1960)

Chen, G., Bohner, B., Bratton, A.C., Jr.: The influence of certain central depressants on fighting behavior in mice. Arch. Int. Pharmacodyn. Ther. *142*, 30–34 (1963)

Chin, J.H., Killam, E.K., Killam, K.F.: Evoked interaction patterns in chronically implanted cats following chlorpromazine. Int. J. Neuropharmacol. *4*, 47–64 (1965)

Christmas, A.J., Maxwell, D.R.: A comparison of the effects of some benzodiazepines and other drugs on aggressive and exploratory behaviour in mice and rats. Neuropharmacology *9*, 17–29 (1970)

Clubley, M.: The action of CNS drugs on an isolated sympathetic nerve preparation of rabbit. Eur. J. Pharmacol. *50*, 175–181 (1978)

Clubley, M., Elliot, R.C.: Centrally active drugs and the sympathetic nervous system of rabbits and cats. Neuropharmacology *16*, 609–616 (1977)

Cook, G.E., Reid, A.A.: The anticonvulsant properties of meprobamate. Med.J. Aust. *49*, 877–878 (1962)

Corrodi, H., Fuxe, K., Lidbrink, P., Olson, L.: Minor tranquillizers, stress, and central catecholamine neurons. Brain Res. *29*, 1–16 (1971)

Corson, S.A., O'Leary Corson, E., Dykman, R.A., Peters, J.E., Reese, W.G., Seager, L.D.: Effect of meprobamate on conditioned antidiuretic and electrolyte retention responses. Fed. Proc. *19*, 21 (1960)

Da Prada, M., Pletscher, A.: On the mechanism of chlorpromazine-induced changes of cerebral homovanillic acid levels. J. Pharm. Pharmacol. *18*, 628–630 (1966)

Da Vanzo, J.P., Daugherty, M., Ruckart, R., Rang, L.: Pharmacological and biochemical studies in isolation-induced fighting mice. Psychopharmacologia (Berl.) *9*, 210–219 (1966)

Del Castillo, J., Nelson, T.E., Jr.: The mode of action of carisoprodol. Ann. N.Y. Acad. Sci. *86*, 108–142 (1960)

Delgado, J.M.R., Lico, M.C., Bracchitta, H., Snyder, D.R.: Brain excitability and behavioral reactivity in monkeys under meprobamate. Arch. Int. Pharmacodyn. Ther. *194*, 5–17 (1971)

Della Bella, D., Rognoni, F.: Proprietà farmacologiche di un nuovo derivato di sintesi ad attività depressiva centrale: Il 2,2-bis-chlorometil-1,3-propandiolo (dispranol). Boll. Chim. Farm. *99*, 67–78 (1960)

De Salva, S.J., Oester, Y.T.: The effect of central depressants on certain spinal reflexes in the acute high cervical cat. Arch. Int. Pharmacodyn. Ther. *124*, 255–262 (1960)

Desmarez, J.J., Domb, A.: A propos de l'action du méprobamate sur les ulcères gastriques expérimentaux obtenus par la méthode d'électrisation intermittente chez le rat blanc. C.R. Soc. Biol. *154*, 450–451 (1960)

Di Maggio, G.: Meprobamate ed ulcera gastrica sperimentale. Boll. Soc. Ital. Biol. Sper. *40*, 2007–2010 (1964)

Fink, G.B., Swinyard, E.A.: Modification of maximal audiogenic and electroshock seizures in mice by psychopharmacologic drugs. J. Pharmacol. Exp. Ther. *127*, 318–324 (1959)

Forney, R.B., Hulpieu, H.R., Hughes, F.W.: The comparative enhancement of the depressant action of alcohol by eight representative ataractic and analgesic drugs. Experientia *18*, 468–470 (1962)

Frank, G.B., Jhamandas, K.: Effects of drugs acting alone and in combination on the motor activity of intact mice. Brit. J. Pharmacol. *39*, 696–706 (1970a)

Frank, G.B., Jhamandas, K.: Effects of general depressant drugs on the electrical responses of isolated slabs of cat's cerebral cortex. Brit. J. Pharmacol. *39*, 707–715 (1970b)

Frommel, E., Fleury, C., Schmidt-Ginzkey, J., Béguin, M.: De la pharmacodynamie différentielle des thymoanaleptiques et des substances „neuroleptiques" en expérimentation animale. Thérapie *15*, 1175–1198 (1960)

Frommel, E., Gold-Aubert, P., Fleury, C., Schmidt-Ginzkey, J., Béguin, M.: De la pharmacodynamie d'un nouveau tranquillisant, d'effet relax et antitrémulant, de longue durée d'action, le Go 560 ou 3-[γ-butoxy,β-carbamyl,β-propranolol]-5-phényl, 5-éthylmalonylurée. Helv. Physiol. Acta *19*, 241–253 (1961)

Gangloff, H.: Effect of phenaglycodol and meprobamate on spontaneous brain activity, evoked EEG arousal and recruitment in the cat. J. Pharmacol. Exp. Ther. *126*, 30–40 (1959)

Gehrmann, J.E., Killam, K.F., Jr.: Studies of central functional equivalence. I. Time-varying distribution of power in discrete frequency bands of the EEG as a function of drug exposure. Neuropharmacology *17*, 747–759 (1978)

Gogerty, J.H.: Pharmacological methods and prediction of the clinical value of hypnotic agents. In: Koella, W.P., Levin, P. (Eds.): Sleep. Physiology, Biochemistry, Psychology, Pharmacology, Clinical Implication. 1st Europ. Congress Sleep Res. Basel, 1972, pp. 69–83. Basel: Karger 1973

Gold, E.M., Di Raimondo, V.C., Kent, J.R., Forsham, P.H.: Comparative effects of certain nonnarcotic central nervous system analgesics and muscle relaxants on the pituitary adrenocortical system. Ann. N.Y. Acad. Sci. *86*, 178–190 (1960)

Goldstein, L., Gardocki, J.F., Mundschenk, D.L., O'Brien, G.: The effect of psychotropic drugs on the occurrence of paradoxical sleep in rabbits and cats. Fed. Proc. *26*, 506 (1967)

Gray, W.D., Osterberg, A.C., Rank, C.E.: Neuropharmacological actions of mephenoxalone. Arch. Int. Pharmacodyn. Ther. *134*, 198–215 (1961)

Greene, F.E.: Absence of a renal effect from two substituted propanediols: meprobamate and mebutamate. Proc. Soc. Exp. Biol. Med. *114*, 165–168 (1963)

Haefely, W.E.: Synaptic pharmacology of barbiturates and benzodiazepines. Agents Actions *7*, 353–359 (1977)

Haefely, W., Keller, H.H., Pieri, L., Polc, P., Schaffner, R., Zihlmann, R.: Interaction of minor tranquillizers with synaptic processes mediated by GABA. In: Deniker, R., Radouco-Thomas, C., Villeneuve, A. (Eds.): Neuro-Psychopharmacology. Proc. of the X. Congr. of the Collegium Int. Neuro-Psychopharmacol. 1976, pp. 907–916. Oxford: Pergamon Press 1978

Haefely, W., Pieri, L., Polc, P., Schaffner, R.: General pharmacology and neuropharmacology of benzodiazepine compounds. Handbook of Experimental Pharmacology, Vol. 55, Part II. Stille, G., Hoffmeister, F. (Eds.). Berlin-Heidelberg-New York: Springer 1981, pp. 13–262

Hendley, C.D., Lynes, T.E., Berger, F.M.: Effect of 2-methyl, 2-n-propyl-1,3-propanediol di-carbamate (Miltown) on central nervous system. Proc. Soc. Exp. Biol. Med. *87*, 608–610 (1954)

Horovitz, Z.P., Piala, J.J., High, J.P., Burke, J.C., Leaf, R.C.: Effects of drugs on the mouse-killing (muricide) test and its relationship to amygdaloid function. Int. J. Neuropharmacol. *5*, 405–411 (1966)

Hukuhara, T.: Der Einfluß von Tranquilizern auf die elektrische Aktivität cortikaler und sub-cortikaler Substrate der Katze. Arzneim. Forsch. *12*, 1133–1143 (1962)

Hunkeler, W., Möhler, H., Pieri, L., Polc, P., Bonetti, E.P., Cumin, R., Schaffner, R., Haefely, W.: Selective antagonists of benzodiazepines. Nature *290*, 514–516 (1981)

Hunt, H.F.: Some effects of meprobamate on conditioned fear and emotional behavior. Ann. N.Y. Acad. Sci. *67*, 712–723 (1957)

Inoki, R., Otori, K., Kimura, I.: Comparison of the action of related compounds of soma. Folia Pharmacol. Jap. *57*, 280–288 (1961)

Inoki, R. et al.: Quoted in: "Animal Research in Psychopharmacology". Psychopharmacology Handbook, Vol. III. Washington, D.C.: U.S. Dept. of Health, Education and Welfare – Public Health Service Publication, 1964, pp. 383

Jalfre, M., Monachon, M.A., Haefely, W.: Effects on the amygdalohippocampal evoked potential in the cat of four benzodiazepines and some other psychotropic drugs. Naunyn Schmiedebergs Arch. Pharmacol. *270*, 180–191 (1971)

Janssen, P.A.J., Jageneau, A.H., Niemegeers, C.J.E.: Effects of various drugs on isolation-induced fighting behaviour of male mice. J. Pharmacol. Exp. Ther. *129*, 471–475 (1960)

Karli, P.: Action de substances dites „tranquillisantes" sur l'agressivité interspécifique rat–souris, C.R. Soc. Biol. *153*, 467–469 (1959)

Kaul, C.L., Lewis, J.J.: Effects of minor tranquillizers on brain phosphate levels in vivo. Biochem. Pharmacol. *12*, 1279–1282 (1963)

Kido, R., Yamamoto, K.: An analysis of tranquilizers in chronically electrode implanted cat. Int. J. Neuropharmacol. *1*, 49–53 (1962)

Kirsten, E.B., Tseng, T.C.: Effects of tybamate and pentylenetetrazol on spinal interneurons. Experientia *28*, 1459–1460 (1972)

Kletzkin, M.: Possible modes of action of psychotherapeutic agents in the treatment of mental disturbances. Ann. N.Y. Acad. Sci. *96*, 263–278 (1962)

Kletzkin, M.: An experimental analysis of aggressive-defensive behaviour in mice. In: Garattini, S., Sigg, E.B. (Eds.): Aggressive Behavior, pp. 253–262. Amsterdam: Excerpta Med. Foundation 1969

Kletzkin, M., Berger, F.M.: Effect of meprobamate on limbic system of the brain. Proc. Soc. Exp. Biol. Med. *100*, 681–683 (1959)

Kletzkin, M., Swan, K.: The effects of meprobamate and pentobarbital upon cortical and sub-cortical responses to auditory stimulation. J. Pharmacol. Exp. Ther. *125*, 35–39 (1959)

Kneip, P.: Kletter-Trieb und Kletter-Test. Arch. Int. Pharmacodyn. Ther. *126*, 238–245 (1960)

Kondziella, W.: Eine neue Methode zur Messung der muskulären Relaxation bei weißen Mäusen. Arch. Int. Pharmacodyn. Ther. *152*, 277–284 (1964)

Lahti, R.A., Barsuhn, C.: The effect of minor tranquilizers on stress-induced increases in rat plasma corticosteroids. Psychopharmacologia (Berl.) *35*, 215–220 (1974)

Leary, R.W., Stynes, A.J.: Tranquilizer effects in the social status, motivation and learning of monkeys. Arch. Gen. Psychiatry *1*, 499–505 (1959)

Leeuwin, R.S., Djojodibroto, R.D., Groenewoud, E.T.: The effects of three benzodiazepines and of meprobamate on the action of smooth muscle stimulants on the guinea-pig ileum. Arch. Int. Pharmacodyn. Ther. *217*, 18–21 (1975)

Le Fur, G., Guilloux, F., Mitrani, N., Mizoule, J., Uzan, A.: Relationships between plasma corticosteroids and benzodiazepines in stress. J. Pharmacol. Exp. Ther. *211*, 305–308 (1979)

Lidbrink, P., Corrodi, H., Fuxe, K., Olson, L.: Barbiturates and meprobamate: decreases in catecholamine turnover of central dopamine and noradrenaline neuronal systems and the influence of immobilization stress. Brain Res. *45*, 507–524 (1972)

Lidbrink, P., Corrodi, H., Fuxe, K., Olson, L.: The effects of benzodiazepines, meprobamate, and barbiturates on central monoamine neurons. In: Garattini, S., Mussini, E., Randall, L.O. (Eds.): The Benzodiazepines, pp. 203–223. New York: Raven Press 1973

Lopez, J.R., Helland, L.A., Wanek, L.A., Rudel, R., Taylor, S.R.: Calcium transients in skeletal muscle are not necessarily antagonized by muscle "relaxants". Biophys. J. *25*, 119a (1979)

Ludwig, B.J., Potterfield, J.R.: The pharmacology of propanediol carbamates. In: Garattini, S., Goldin, A., Hawking, F., Kopin, I.J. (Eds.): Advances in Pharmacology and Chemotherapy, Vol. 9, pp. 173–240. New York-London: Academic Press 1971

Mäkelä, S., Näätänen, E., Rinne, U.K.: The response of adrenal cortex to psychic stress after meprobamate treatment. Acta Endocr. *32*, 1–7 (1959)

Maickel, R.P., Maloney, G.J.: Effects of various depressant drugs on deprivation-induced water consumption. Neuropharmacology *12*, 777–782 (1973)

Malhotra, C.L., Metha, V.L.: The effect of meprobamate on the acetylcholine content of certain areas of dog brain. Br. J. Pharmacol. *27*, 440–442 (1966)

Malick, J.B., Sofia, R.D., Goldberg, M.E.: A comparative study of the effects of selected psychoactive agents upon three lesion-induced models of aggression in the rat. Arch. Int. Pharmacodyn. Ther. *181*, 459–465 (1969)

Marcy, R., Quermonne, M.A.: Benzodiazepines: a comparison of their effects in mice on the magnitude of the palmar skin conductivity response and on pentylenetetrazole-induced seizures. Experientia *31*, 954–955 (1975)

Menon, M.K., Dandiya, P.C., Bapna, J.S.: Modification of the effects of tranquilizers in animals treated with α-methyl-1-tyrosine. J. Pharmacol. Exp. Ther. *156*, 63–69 (1977)

Mercier, J., Dessigne, S.: Sur le mécanisme de l'action neurodépressive centrale du dicarbamate de méthyl-N-propyl propanediol (méprobamate). Arch. Int. Pharmacodyn. Ther. *121*, 38–58 (1959)

Möhler, H., Okada, T.: Benzodiazepine receptor: demonstration in the central nervous system. Science *198*, 849–851 (1977)

Murayama, S., Uemura, H., Suzuki, T.: Effects of benzodiazepines on spinal reflexes in cats. Jap. J. Pharmacol. *22*, 117 (1972)

Nakamura, K., Thoenen, H.: Increased irritability: a permanent behavior change induced in the rat by intraventricular administration of 6-hydroxydopamine. Psychopharmacologia (Berl.) *24*, 359–372 (1972)

Ngai, S.H., Tseng, D.T.C., Wang, S.C.: Effect of diazepam and other central nervous system depressants on spinal reflexes in cats: a study of site of action. J. Pharmacol. Exp. Ther. *153*, 344–351 (1966)

Nieschulz, O.: Über Schwimmversuche mit Mäusen. Med. Exp. *8*, 135–140 (1963)

Norton, P.: The effects of drugs on barbiturate withdrawal convulsions in the rat. J. Pharm. Pharmacol. *22*, 763–766 (1970)

Olds, M.E., Baldrighi, G.: Effects of meprobamate, chlordiazepoxide, diazepam, and sodium pentobarbital on visually evoked responses in the tectotegmental area of the rat. Int. J. Neuropharmacol. *7*, 231–239 (1968)

Pfeiffer, C.C., Riopelle, A.J., Smith, R.P., Jenney, E.H., Williams, H.L.: Comparative study of the effect of meprobamate on the conditioned response, on strychnine and pentylenetetrazol thresholds, on the normal electroencephalogram and on polysynaptic reflexes. Ann. N.Y. Acad. Sci. *67*, 734–745 (1957)

Pletscher, A., Da Prada, M., Foglar, G.: Differences between neuroleptics and tranquilizers regarding metabolism and biochemical effects. Proc. V. Int. Congr. Collegium Internationale Neuropsychopharmacologicum. Excerpta Medica Internat. Congress Series No. 129, 1966, pp. 101–107

Randall, L.O., Schallek, W., Heise, G.A., Keith, E.F., Bagdon, R.E.: The psychosedative properties of methaminodiazepoxide. J. Pharmacol. Exp. Ther. *129*, 163–171 (1960)

Raynaud, G., Ducrocq, J., Raoul, Y.: Etude de l'activité motrice de la souris, et en particulier du comportement explorateur. J. Physiol. (Paris) *58*, 749–761 (1965)

Robichaud, R.C., Gylys, J.A., Sledge, K.L., Hillyard, I.W.: The pharmacology of prazepam. A new benzodiazepine derivative. Arch. Int. Pharmacodyn. Ther. *185*, 213–227 (1970)

Robinson, M.A., Scott, G.T.: Frog melanophore dispersing action of meprobamate. Biochem. Biophys. Res. Commun. *2*, 19–21 (1960)

Ruch-Monachon, M.A., Jalfre, M., Haefely, W.: Drugs and PGO waves in the lateral geniculate body of the curarized cat. V. Miscellaneous compounds. Synopsis of the role of central neurotransmitters on PGO wave activity. Arch. Int. Pharmacodyn. Ther. *219*, 326–346 (1976)

Rüberg-Schweer, M., Karger, W.: Beeinflussung des Ionentransports an Membranen durch Tranquilizer. Eur. J. Physiol. *316*, R 74 (1970)

Rüberg-Schweer, M., Karger, W.: Beeinflussung des Na$^+$-Transportes an der isolierten Froschhaut durch Meprobamat, Carisoprodol, Oxazepam und Phenobarbital. Arzneim. Forsch. *24*, 1568–1574 (1974)

Schallek, W., Kuehn, A.: Effects of psychotropic drugs on limbic system of cat. Proc. Soc. Exp. Biol. Med. *105*, 115–117 (1960)

Schallek, W., Kuehn, A.: Effects of benzodiazepines on spontaneous EEG and arousal responses of cats. Prog. Brain Res. *18*, 231–238 (1965)

Schallek, W., Kuehn, A., Jew, N.: Effects of chlordiazepoxide (Librium) and other psychotropic agents on the limbic system of the brain. Ann. N.Y. Acad. Sci. *96*, 303–314 (1962)

Schallek, W., Zabransky, F., Kuehn, A.: Effects of benzodiazepines on central nervous system of cat. Arch. Int. Pharmacodyn. Ther. *149*, 467–483 (1964)

Scheckel, C.L., Boff, E.: Effects of drugs on aggressive behavior in monkeys. In: Brill, H. et al. (Eds.): Neuropsychopharmacology, pp. 789–795. Amsterdam: Excerpta Medica 1967

Sethy, V.H., Naik, P.Y., Sheth, U.K.: Effect of d-amphetamine sulphate in combination with CNS depressants on spontaneous motor activity of mice. Psychopharmacologia (Berl.) *18*, 19–25 (1970)

Sofia, R.D.: Effects of centrally active drugs on four models of experimentally-induced aggression in rodents. Life Sci. *8*, 705–716 (1969)

Soubrié, P., Kulkarni, S., Simon, P., Boissier, J.R.: Effets des anxiolytiques sur la prise de nourriture de rats et de souris placés en situation nouvelle ou familière. Psychopharmacologia (Berl.) *45*, 203–210 (1975)

Soubrié, P., De Angelis, L., Simon, P., Boissier, J.R.: Effets des anxiolytiques sur la prise de boisson en situation nouvelle et familière. Psychopharmacology *50*, 41–45 (1976)

Stark, P., Henderson, J.K.: Differentiation of classes of neurosedatives using rats with septal lesions. Int. J. Neuropharmacol. *5*, 385–389 (1966)

Stephens, R.J.: The influence of mild stress on food consumption in untrained mice and the effect of drugs. Br. J. Pharmacol. *49*, 146 P (1973)

Sternbach, L.H., Randall, L.O., Gustafson, S.R.: 1,4-Benzodiazepines (chlordiazepoxide and related compounds). Psychopharmacol. Agents *1*, 137–224 (1964)

Takagi, H., Ban, T.: The effect of psychotropic drugs on the limbic system of the cat. Jap. J. Pharmacol. *10*, 7–14 (1960)

Takagi, K., Kasuya, Y., Tachikawa, S.: The effect of certain psychotropic drugs on arousal responses in rats' EEG. Nippon Yakugaku Zasshi *87*, 781–787 (1967)

Takeda, Y.: Quoted in: "Animal Research in Psychopharmacology". Psychopharmacology Handbook, Vol. II, U.S. Dept. of Health, Education and Welfare – Public Health Service Publication, Washington, D.C., 1962, pp. 258

Tedeschi, R.E., Tedeschi, D.H., Mucha, A., Cook, L., Mattis, P.A., Fellows, E.J.: Effects of various centrally acting drugs on fighting behavior of mice. J. Pharmacol. Exp. Ther. *125*, 28–34 (1959)

Theobald, W., Büch, O., Kunz, H.A.: Vergleichende Untersuchungen über die Beeinflussung vegetativer Funktionen durch Psychopharmaka im akuten Tierversuch. Arzneim. Forsch. 15, 117–125 (1965)

Tseng, T.-C., Przybyla, A.C., Chen, S.T., Wang, S.C.: Locus of central depressant action of tybamate. Neuropharmacology 9, 211–218 (1970)

Valzelli, L., Giacalone, E., Garattini, S.: Pharmacological control of aggressive behavior in mice. Eur. J. Pharmacol. 2, 144–146 (1967)

Van der Wende, C., Spoerlein, M.T.: Psychotic symptoms induced in mice by the intravenous administration of solution of 3,4-dihydroxyphenylalanine (DOPA). Arch. Int. Pharmacodyn. Ther. 137, 145–154 (1962)

Varagić, V., Vojvodić, N.: Effect of guanethidine, hemicholinium, and mebutamate on the hypertensive response to eserine and catecholamines. Br. J. Pharmacol. 19, 451–457 (1962)

Walaszek, E.J., Abood, L.G.: Effect of tranquilizing drugs on fighting response of Siamese fighting fish. Science 124, 440–441 (1956)

Weaver, J.E., Miya, T.S.: Effects of certain ataraxic agents on mice activity. J. Pharm. Sci. 50, 910–912 (1961)

Webster, R.A.: Centrally acting muscle relaxants in tetanus. Br. J. Pharmacol. 17, 507–518 (1961)

Weller, C.P., Ibrahim, I., Sulman, F.G.: Analgesic profile of tranquillizers in multiple screening tests in mice. Arch. Int. Pharmacodyn. Ther. 176, 178–192 (1968)

Williams, M., Risley, E.A.: Enhancement of the binding of ^{3}H-diazepam to rat brain membranes in vitro by SQ 20009, a novel anxiolytic, γ-aminobutyric acid (GABA) and muscimol. Life Sci. 24, 833–842 (1979)

Wilson, V.J.: Action of meprobamate on spinal monosynaptic reflexes and on inhibitory pathways. J. Gen. Physiol. 42, 29–37 (1958)

Wilson, V.J., Talbot, W.H.: Recurrent conditioning in the cat spinal cord. Differential effect of meprobamate on recurrent facilitation and inhibition. J. Gen. Physiol. 43, 495–502 (1960)

Wolf, A., von Haxthausen, E.: Zur Analyse der Wirkung einiger zentral-sedativer Substanzen. Arzneim. Forsch. 10, 50–52 (1960)

Yen, C.Y., Stanger, L., Millman, N.: Ataractic suppression of isolation-induced aggressive behavior. Arch. Int. Pharmacodyn. Ther. 123, 179–185 (1959)

Yen, H.C.Y., Katz, M.H., Krop, S.: Effects of various drugs on 3,4-dihydroxyphenylalanine (DL-dopa)-induced excitation (aggressive behavior) in mice. Toxicol. Appl. Pharmacol. 17, 597–604 (1970)

CHAPTER 4

Behavioral Pharmacology of Anxiolytics

P. B. Dews

A. Introduction

Anxiety is a term applied by clinicians to certain manifestations in patients. Clinical anxiety has three components. First there is a verbal component: The patient says that he or she is anxious or fearful or gives a semantically similar description. Second, there is a somatic-autonomic component. The patient is restless and agitated, has a higher heart rate, and sweats. Third, there is an interference with normal productive activities. Clinical anxiety should probably not be diagnosed if any of these three components is entirely lacking. In the clinical assessment of anxiety by history and physical examination, all three components are taken into account.

There is a consensus among physicians that certain drugs alleviate anxiety without abolishing all behavioral activities, as occurs with general anesthesia. We will take this as our definition of anxiolytic agents. These drugs are certain barbiturates, notably phenobarbital and butethal (Butabarbital); meprobamate; and a variety of benzodiazepines, notably chlordiazepoxide and diazepam. Behavioral pharmacology is concerned with those behavioral effects of drugs that can be measured objectively, unequivocally, and reliably. This chapter, therefore, is concerned with the behavioral effects of the anxiolytic agents listed above.

Some attempts to measure anxiety and changes in anxiety due to drugs, particularly in human subjects, have sought a unitary "measure" of anxiety, as though anxiety were a particular one-dimensional inner state with external manifestations providing a more or less good indication of the magnitude of the anxiety. The assumption of a unitary state is gratuitous, and an analogy may help to make this point clear. We can talk about respiration and effects of drugs on respiration in terms of rate and depth of breathing, gas exchange, and blood flow through the lungs. None of these, in itself, is the measure of respiration, and in the absence of other information, none allows us to determine normality or abnormality. What is normal under one set of conditions, e.g., rest, may be quite abnormal under another set of conditions, such as vigorous exercise. The various aspects of respiration one can measure are related, however; for example, rate and depth of respiration do affect gas exchange. So it is with anxiety. Agitation and restlessness affect cardiovascular variables such as heart rate and sweating. Disruption of normal productive behavior will lead to changes in verbal behavior as manifested by complaints of a subject. That the manifestations are related does not justify the postulation of a single inner determining state any more than the interrelations of respiratory functions make one postulate a single inner determining respiratory state.

There is a large literature on the effects of anxiolytics, as befits the most frequently prescribed class of drug, comprised of studies on both humans and animals. Results of comparable experiments have been generally quite concordant, so there are few disputes regarding facts. How the results are to be put together and what new experiments are needed to understand the behavioral pharmacology of the anxiolytics is another matter, however.

Studies on drug effects on anxiety in human subjects have involved assessment of verbal and somatic-autonomic components, but have rarely attempted to measure interference with normal productive activities. Studies on anxiety in animals have involved the so-called avoidance behaviors, the somatic-autonomic component, and also the suppression of behavior.

B. History

Shortly after the introduction of curare for muscular relaxation in clinical anesthesia, BERGER and BRADLEY (1946) rediscovered that certain substituted ethers of glycerol produced profound muscular relaxation, superficially similar to that caused by curare. They studied particularly the 2-methylphenoxy compound, mephenesin (Myanesin), and suggested that the compound exerted its effects on the spinal cord rather than the myoneural junction as for curare. Spinal cord effects of mephenesin were demonstrated directly by HENNEMAN et al. (1949), who introduced the term "inter-neurone blocking agent." They also commented that mephenesin has "a more general effect which may be described as tranquilizing or sedative." This is probably the earliest use of the word "tranquilize" to describe the type of effect that characterizes the minor tranquilizers and antedates the introduction of chlorpromazine (Morphine and relatives had been described as tranquilizing by BARLOW as early as 1932). As a drug for clinical use, mephenesin had disadvantages, one being that it was not effective when given by mouth. The search for an orally active drug with similar pharmacologic effects culminated in the development of meprobamate, inaugurating the era of anxiolytics. A few years later, studies on the medicinal chemistry of benzodiazepines led to the synthesis and testing of chlordiazepoxide. In a series of animal assays, chlordiazepoxide was found to be more like meprobamate than other drugs. The drug was rapidly introduced clinically and was found, indeed, to be similar to but more effective than meprobamate. Chlordiazepoxide has been followed into the clinic by a continuing succession of benzodiazepines, and this class of compound has virtually displaced meprobamate in clinical use.

C. Behavioral Pharmacology in Humans

I. Effects on Verbal Behavior

Small daytime doses of barbiturates, notably the barbiturates (e.g., phenobarbital and butethal) with long or fairly long durations of action, 6–24 h, have been used for decades as "sedatives" in the treatment of clinical anxiety. It was assumed that the sedation was the first manifestation of a unidimensional central nervous system depression which, with increasing doses, led through progressively increasing depression to general anesthesia and death through suppression of respiratory and cardiovascular controls. When meprobamate was given to patients for relief of skeletal muscle spasms and stiffness, it was recognized by global clinical assessment that the drug relieved clinical anxiety. While it proved difficult in the early years to establish the effects by objective criteria (WEISS and LATIES, 1958), subsequent studies, mostly on the benzodiazepines, have established that the drugs can reduce clinical assessments of anxiety. That higher doses do not produce general anesthesia suggests that the sedative effects of barbituates may represent a pharmacologic effect qualitatively different from the general anesthetic effect.

Verbal descriptions can be made objective and quantitative by means of scales. An early example is the Taylor Manifest Anxiety Scale. For this, items were selected from the large number of items in the Minnesota Multiphasic Personality Inventory (MMPI) which were judged to be indicative of anxiety (TAYLOR, 1953). The MMPI consists of many statements that the patients respond to as "true" or "false" as applied to themselves. Examples of items relating to anxiety are: "I feel anxious about something or someone almost all the time" and "I do not often notice my heart pounding and I am seldom short of breath." A "true" to the former statement and a "false" to the latter represent two items scored positive for manifest anxiety. Another scale completed by the subject is the Hopkins Symptom Checklist (HSCL) (DEROGATIS et al., 1974), which asks patients to assess the personal applicability of concepts such as "feeling fearful" and "heart pounding or racing", using a rating of 1, not at all; 2, a little bit; 3, quite a bit; or 4, extremely. There are also scales to be completed by the observer such as the Hamilton Questionnaire which asks the physician to rate the patient on some dozens of items, including "worries" and "palpitations" on a five-point scale: 0, none; 1, mild; 2, moderate; 3, severe; and 4, grossly disabling (HAMILTON, 1959).

As examples of results obtained by use of these scales, RICKELS et al. (1978) have reported that 4 weeks' treatment of anxious family practice patients with chlordiazepoxide reduced the average HSCL Anxiety Score from 2.18 to 1.58 (with a placebo the average score went from 2.18 to 1.81). With the Hamilton scale, outpatients with at least a moderate degree of anxiety showed a fall in average score from 1.63 to 0.57 with 6 weeks of 5–10 mg/day diazepam; with placebo the average score went from 1.66 to 0.88 (RICKELS et al., 1977). In Australia, BURROWS et al. (1976) found that 15 mg/day diazepam reduced the average score on the Hamilton scale from 1.5 on day 1 to 0.95 on day 22, while placebo takers declined to 1.2.

Two points deserve emphasis. First, while the changes due to the drugs are undoubtedly significant, both statistically and biologically, they are modest in magnitude and placebo "effects" are appreciable. Second, the scales include many questions not related to specific descriptions of anxiety. The HSCL has clusters of questions that relate to somatization, to interpersonal sensitivity, and to depression; the changes in scores in these clusters are similar to those in the anxiety cluster. Other studies have yielded generally similar results. Thus, while effects of the drugs on anxiety scores are consistent and statistically significant, studies on the verbal behavior of patients suggest that the effects of the drugs on anxiety are neither dramatic nor specific.

II. Effects on Somatic-Autonomic Functions

The effects of anxiolytics on the restlessness and agitation component of anxiety have been little studied, despite the desirable possibility of objective measurement by physical methods. One study has used a simple kymograph technique to measure movements during sleep following meprobamate; no effect was found (BROCKLEHURST et al., 1978). Studies on heart rate and on the galvanic skin response (measuring sweating) do not show selective effects of the drugs. For example, 10 mg diazepam had no effect on the heart rate increase or the weight loss (due to sweating) of students undergoing a stressful oral examination (ALLEN et al., 1976). Substantial changes in heart rate and sweating take place as a result of relatively minor changes in activity; consequently, small changes in heart rate and sweating are uninterpretable when activity is unknown. No study has found large effects, and no study appears to have controlled for changes in autonomic function secondary to changes in bodily activity.

III. Effects on Productive Activities

There have been many studies on the effects of anxiolytics on psychomotor functions of normal subjects. Many studies have used a battery of tests and have been ingenious and well controlled. They have shown that therapeutic doses of the drug have only equivocal effects on psychomotor functions. Indeed, 5 or 10 mg diazepam improved performance on tasks similar to those involved in automobile driving (LINNOILA and MANTILLA, 1973).

Productivity and satisfaction for the vast majority of people in most of their activities are not appreciably affected by marginal changes in psychomotor capabilities. Consider the factors that generate work and play and creative activities. Conventional psychomotor batteries of tests provide no insight into such factors, and effects measured in such tests are more related to minor toxic side effects of the drugs than to the sought-after therapeutic effects. Unfortunately, there is very little information on the effects of the drugs on normal human productivity.

It is fair to summarize the studies in normal humans by saying that they give no grounds for identifying benzodiazepines as selective anxiolytics. It has been pointed out that it may be inappropriate to study the clinical pharmacology of the drugs in normal subjects. Yet, the studies in psychiatric patients gave no greater indication of selectively anxiolytic effects; moreover, the most extensive clinical use of the drugs is not in very sick psychiatric patients.

IV. Miscellaneous Effects

Both meprobamate and the benzodiazepines produce drowsiness and facilitate sleep. Certain compounds, e.g., nitrazepam, are marketed primarily as agents for the induction of sleep, although the evidence that they have significantly different behavioral pharmacologic effects from those of chlordiazepoxide and diazepam is lacking. Indeed, evidence for clinically significant qualitative differences between any of the clinically used benzodiazepines is not conclusive. When benzodiazepines are taken regularly, their tendency to cause sleepiness abates while the sought-after therapeutic effects may persist. This phenomenon is not a special characteristic of the drugs as an abatement of sleepiness with persistence of therapeutic effects is well known for phenothiazines in psychosis and for phenobarbital in epilepsy. Benzodiazepines are also effective anticonvulsant agents, and their efficacy in antagonizing pentylenetetrazole (Metrazole) seizures correlates with their clinical effectiveness as anxiolytics. But the relation between the two types of effect is unknown.

D. Behavioral Pharmacology in Animals

Prompted no doubt by the clinical reports of meprobamate as a "tranquilizer", there were early reports that the drug "tamed" wild animals such as fierce cats and rhesus monkeys. Unfortunately, taming is produced by any disabling action and lacks specificity. A number of tests were worked out, however, in industrial laboratories to recognize meprobamate-like activity, and these tests were sufficiently discriminating by 1957 for an astute pharmacologist, Randall, to recognize immediately when chlordiazepoxide came unexpectedly into his hands that it was an interesting agent of the meprobamate type (STERNBACH, 1979).

In 1960, GELLER and SEIFTER (1960) reported that meprobamate and a barbiturate, but not amphetamine or promazine, could increase a rate of responding that had been suppressed. They studied rats that had developed consistent rates of pressing a lever, responding under two different conditions in daily sessions. The rats were maintained on a limited food supply that kept their weight at about 80% of free-feeding weight. Under one condition, a food pellet was delivered to the rat occasionally when a response (a lever press) occurred, on the average once every 2 min, but with the individual intervals varying over a range. Such a program of food delivery in relation to responding generated a steady rate of responding of about one response every 2–4 s. At intervals during the session, an additional auditory stimulus was presented for 3 min, and during these periods, every response was followed by delivery of a food pellet. But each response was also immediately accompanied by an electric shock to the feet of the rat. The intensity of the shock affected the amount of suppression of responding during the signaled periods. Even at levels of shock that suppressed responding to very low rates, e.g. only one two responses in the 3-min auditory stimulus period, meprobamate or a barbiturate was able to increase the rate substantially. The rates outside the signaled periods were little affected. Neither amphetamine nor phenothiazines led to an increase in rate of responding during the signaled period, although amphetamine increased and promazine decreased the rate outside the signaled periods. It has been shown subsequently that all the clinically useful benzodiazepines increase the rate of a suppressed response and that the relative potency of the drugs in increasing the rate is well correlated with their clinical potency (SEPINWALL and COOK, 1978).

The phenomenon of selective increase of the rate of suppressed responding by anxiolytics has been shown to be of great generality. The procedure itself permits wide latitude. For example, not every response during the signaled period need be followed by a shock. Even when only occasional responses lead to shock, as determined by a variety of schedules, if suppression results, it is selectively attenuated by anxiolytic agents. Anxiolytic agents have this effect in every species in which they have been studied: rats, pigeons, dogs, cats, pigs, squirrel monkeys, rhesus monkeys, goldfish and humans. Finally, the suppression need not be produced by a noxious stimulus; suppression engendered by the characteristics of the reinforcement schedule itself (KELLEHER et al., 1961) or superstitiously (DEWS, 1976) is attenuated by anxiolytic agents.

There are technical limits to the selectivity of anxiolytic agents in attenuating suppression and amphetamine and of other classes of drugs in not attenuating suppression. But the limits are rather well defined and do not detract seriously from the impressive generality of the phenomenon (for a comprehensive technical discussion of the field, see SEPINWALL and COOK, 1978). The generality is so well established that each behavioral effect of an anxiolytic agent should be examined to see whether it can be accounted for as an attenuation of a suppression; other explanations should be considered only when such attenuation has been shown to be inadequate to account for the findings.

As noted, anxiolytic agents have been described as having a taming action, but specificity in this regard has not been established convincingly. Even the elaborate and very expensive and time-consuming methods of trying to record all the spontaneous behavioral activities of subjects such as rats, cats, or monkeys over some period of time, while certainly enabling investigators to detect changes due to anxiolytic agents in adequate doses, have provided little insight into the specific behavioral pharmacology of the anxiolytics. Characteristic changes in the interactions between subjects have been noted, however. Ethologists are able to distinguish convincingly between the elements (defense and offense) of what they call agonistic behavior, i.e., the interactions between two or more animals in conflict. Chlordiazepoxide is very effective in reducing defensive elements but appears not to interfere with offensive elements until doses causing ataxia are reached (MICZEK and KRSIAK, 1979). In rats, 5 mg/kg chlordiazepoxide actually increased various elements of attack while not affecting grooming (MICZEK, 1974). In cats, the topography of the offensive and defensive elements is quite different from that of rats, but the differential effects of chlordiazepoxide in preferentially attenuating the latter is the same in both species and also in mice (HOFFMEISTER and WUTTKE, 1969).

An unsolved problem in the integration of the findings in ethologic studies with the main body of behavioral pharmacology is the paucity of information on the absolute frequency of, for example, agonistic behavior and its consequences (MICZEK and KRSIAK, 1979). It is well established in behavioral pharmacology that the rate of responding on which a drug effect is superimposed, and the program of consequences of the response, usually have important influences on what the drug effect will be (DEWS and DEWEESE, 1977). It is consequently unsafe to make strong statements about differences in drug effects on different agonistic behaviors in the absence of information on the predrug frequencies of the respective behaviors, as such differences themselves may occasion a differential effect of the drug. Also, in dealing with more than one subject, the effect that changes in behavior in one subject has on the behavior of the second that will further modify the behavior of the first must be considered. For this reason, the usual practice of administering a drug to all of the interacting subjects has been questioned (MICZEK and KRSIAK, 1979). It is impossible at present to decide to what extent the effects of anxiolytic agents on innate behavior patterns reflect attenuation of suppression. The lack of effect on offensive behavior and the attenuation of defensive behavior (and its replacement by otherwise suppressed behavior) is not incompatible with such an interpretation. It is more difficult to reconcile the results of the more analytic ethologic studies with the apocryphal taming effects of anxiolytic agents.

E. Conclusion

The studies of effects of anxiolytic agents in human subjects, both normal and clinical patients, have not provided firm evidence of a specific anxiolytic action of the agents. Studies in animals also provide no plausible support for a specific anxiolytic action.

Studies in animals have established, however, a highly consistent selective effect in attenuating certain types of suppression in all species studied, an effect that may be the fundamental behavioral effect of the agents. Such a conclusion would in no way deny that the so-called anxiolytic agents are valuable therapeutic agents and that they may make patients less anxious. The conclusions do suggest that their therapeutic impact be reevaluated to determine the contribution of attenuation of suppressed behavior to their therapeutic efficacy. Patients who are enabled to be more effective and productive may understandably report their anxiety to be somewhat lowered. As there is inadequate evidence of a selective anxiolytic action and abundant evidence of a selective antisuppressant action, the name of the class of agents should be changed to antisuppressant agents to parallel antidepressant agents. An antisuppressant agent that may help a subject to be efficient and productive evokes a different public image from that of an anxiolytic agent that makes people expect him to be calm and indifferent. A change in name may allay some of the irrational public alarm about the widespread use of benzodiazepines. There is no good evidence that these agents, properly used, are other than beneficial to society.

References

Allen, J.A., Mewha, I.S., Roddie, I.C.: The effect of diazepam on performance and emotional response during viva examination. J. Physiol. (Lond.) *263*, 191P–192P (1976)

Barlow O.W.: The tranquilizing potency of morphine, pantopan, codeine, papaverine and narcotine. J. Am. Med. Ass. *99*, 986–988 (1932)

Berger, F.M., Bradley, W.: The pharmacological properties of α:β-dihydroxy-α-(2-methylphenoxy) propane (Myanesin). Br. J. Pharmacol. *1*, 265–272 (1946)

Brocklehurst, J.C., Carty, M.H., Skorecki, J.: The use of a kymograph in a comparative trial of flunitrazepam and meprobamate in elderly patients. Curr. Med. Res. Opin. *5*, 663–668 (1978)

Burrows, G.D., Davies, B., Fail, L., Poynton, C., Stevenson, H.: A placebo controlled trial of diazepam and oxprenolol for anxiety. Psychopharmacology *50*, 177–179 (1976)

Derougatis, L.R., Lipman, R.S., Rickels, J., Uhlenhuth, E.H., Covi, L.: The Hopkins Symptom Checklist (HSCL): a self-report symptom inventory. Behav. Sci. *19*, 1–15 (1974)

Dews, P.B.: Effects of drugs on suppressed responding. Br. J. Pharmacol. *58*, 451 P (1976)

Dews, P.B., DeWeese, J.: Schedules of reinforcement. In Handbook of Psychopharmacology. Iversen, L.L., Iversen, S.D., Snyder, S.H. (eds.), Vol. 7, pp. 107–150. New York: Plenum Press 1977

Geller, I.H., Seifter, J.: The effects of meprobamate, barbituates, D-amphetamine and promazine on experimentally induced conflict in the rat. Psychopharmacologia *1*, 482–502 (1960)

Hamilton, M.: The assessment of anxiety states by rating. Br. J. Med. Psychol. *32*, 50–55 (1959)

Henneman, E., Kaplan, A., Unna, K.: A neuropharmacological study on the effect of myanesin (Tolserol) on motor systems. J. Pharmacol. *97*, 331–341 (1949)

Hoffmeister, F., Wuttke, W.: On the actions of psychotropic drugs on the attack – and aggressive – defensive behavior of mice and cats. In Aggressive behavior. Garattini, S., Sigg, E.B. (eds.), pp. 273–280. New York: Wiley 1969

Kelleher, R.T., Fry, W., Deegan, J., Cook, L.: Effects of meprobamate on operant behavior in rats. J. Pharmacol. *133*, 271–280 (1961)

Linnoila, M., Mantilla, M.J.: Drug interaction or psychomotor skills related to driving: diazepam and alcohol. Eur. J. Clin. Pharmacol. *5*, 186–194 (1973)

Miczek, K.A.: Intraspecies aggression in rats: effects of D-amphetamine and chlordiazepoxide. Psychopharmacologia *39*, 275–301 (1974)

Miczek, K.A., Krsiak, M.: Drug effects on agonistic behavior. In Advances in behavioral pharmacology. Thompson, T., Dews, P.B. (eds.), Vol. 2, pp. 88–153. New York: Academic Press 1979

Rickels, K., Pereira-Ogan, J., Csanalosi, I., Morris, R.J., Rosenfeld, H., Sablosky, L., Schless, A., Werbowsky, J.H.: Halazepam and diazepam in neurotic anxiety: A double blind study. Psychopharmacology 52, 129–136 (1977)

Rickels, K., Downing, R.W., Winokur, A.: Antianxiety drugs: Clinical use in psychiatry. In Handbook of Psychopharmacology. Iversen, L.L., Iversen, S.D., Snyder, S.H. (eds.), Vol. 13, pp. 395–430. New York: Plenum 1978

Sepinwall, J., Cook, L.: Behavioral pharmacology of antianxiety drugs. In Handbook of Psychopharmacology. Iversen, L.L., Iversen, S.D., Snyder, S.H. (eds.), Vol. 13, pp. 345–385. New York: Plenum 1978

Sternbach, L.H.: The benzodiazepine story. J. Med. Chem. 22, 1–7 (1979)

Taylor, J.A.: A personality scale of manifest anxiety. J. Abnorm. Soc. Psychol. 48, 285–290 (1953)

Weiss, B., Laties, V.: A critical review of the efficacy of meprobamate (Miltown, Equanil) in the treatment of anxiety. J. Chronic. Dis. 7, 500–519 (1958)

CHAPTER 5

Biochemical Effects of Anxiolytics

C. BRAESTRUP

A. Introduction

Anxiolytic drugs, also called "minor tranquillizers" or anti-anxiety drugs, are substances which reduce pathological anxiety, tension and agitation without therapeutic effects on cognitive or perceptual processes. Most of these drugs are also potent anticonvulsants, sedatives and hypnotics. Several classes (groups) of drugs possess anxiolytic properties. The most important group is the benzodiazepines, which are remarkably non-toxic, much less toxic than the barbiturates. Meprobamate is an anxiolytic drug much used in the 1950s and 1960s but without a known mechanism of action at the biochemical or synaptic level (BERGER, 1975). Miscellaneous drugs, such as β-blockers, and some neuroleptic and antidepressant drugs possess anxiolytic properties in some clinical situations, but are not considered true anxiolytic drugs. The present chapter will focus on the benzodiazepines and emphasis will be given to biochemical effects pertinent to their mechanism of action.

B. Benzodiazepine Receptors

There is good evidence that the clinical and pharmacological effects of the benzodiazepines are mediated at the molecular level by interacting with brain specific receptors. These receptors are localized on neurons and all pharmacologically and clinically active benzodiazepines interact with them. The interaction between the receptors and benzodiazepines is very specific, and at present it is shared by only a very few non-benzodiazepine drugs.

I. General Properties

1. Binding Characteristics

Brain receptors for drugs and neurotransmitters have in recent years been successfully characterized by high affinity binding technique using tritium-labelled agonists or antagonists as binding ligands (YAMAMURA et al., 1978 b).

Quite unexpectedly, it was discovered in 1977 that ^{3}H-diazepam binds with high affinity to membranes prepared from rat brain and that this binding was displaced with low concentrations of several clinically active benzodiazepines (SQUIRES and BRAESTRUP, 1977; MÖHLER and OKADA, 1977 b; BOSMANN et al., 1977; MACKERER et al., 1978). One of these experiments (Fig. 1) shows that binding is saturable, indicating a limited number of binding sites; that the binding affinity is high, half maximal binding occurring at only ca. 3 nM ^{3}H-diazepam (K_D value) and that there appears to be

294

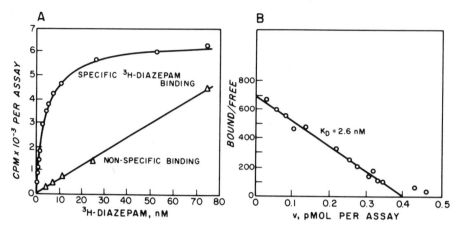

Fig. 1. A Saturation experiment with ^{3}H-diazepam. **B** Scatchard analysis of the same data. A whole rat forebrain was excised and homogenized in 20 vol. iced 0.32 M sucrose in a Potter-Elvehjem homogenizer fitted to 0.25 mm clearance. The homogenate was centrifuged for 5 min at 2,000 × g at 5 °C and the supernatant was recentrifuged for 10 min at 30,000 × g. The pellet from the second centrifugation (P$_2$ pellet) was resuspended in 20 times the original tissue weight of 50 mM Tris, HCl, pH 7.4, and used directly in the binding assays. Five hundred microlitres of this P$_2$ suspension (corresponding to 25 mg original tissue) was pre-incubated for 5 min; 25 μl ^{3}H-diazepam working solution (to give a final concentration of ca. 2 nM or approximately 14,000 cpm) was then added and the incubation was continued at 37 °C for an additional 15 min. The samples were then cooled in an ice bath for 30 min. Ten millilitres of iced 50 mM Tris, HCl, pH 7.4, was added to each sample immediately before it was filtered through Whatman GF/C glass fibre filters. The filters were washed immediately with an additional 10 ml iced buffer and counted for tritium by conventional scintillation counting. Other membrane preparations than the P$_2$ membranes described above exhibit similar but not identical binding properties. Crude homogenates or briefly centrifuged (1,000 × g for 10 min) homogenates, prepared directly in 50 vol. or more of either TrisHCl, sodium phosphate, Trismaleate, or Krebs-phosphate buffer, pH 7–7.5, can be used. Membranes can be washed repeatedly and assays with or without pre-incubation at 37 °C can be used. (Data from BRAESTRUP and SQUIRES, 1977)

only a single class of binding sites, since Scatchard analysis yields a single straight line. However, the occurrence of biphasic dissociation of ^{3}H-diazepam from the receptors and of biphasic heat inactivation of binding sites as well as Hill-coefficients of ca. 0.6 for some new drugs (i.e. CL 218,872, Fig. 2) have been interpreted as indicating the presence of a second type of binding site (SQUIRES et al., 1979b).

^{3}H-Flunitrazepam binds to the same receptors as ^{3}H-diazepam (BRAESTRUP and SQUIRES, 1978b) with even higher affinity than ^{3}H-diazepam; K_D for ^{3}H-flunitrazepam is 1–2 nM at 0 °C in rat or man (SPETH et al., 1978; BRAESTRUP and SQUIRES, 1978b).

The dissociation rate constant for the ^{3}H-diazepam receptor complex in rat is high, $k_{-1} = 0.06$–0.16 min^{-1} at 0 °C (BRAESTRUP and SQUIRES, 1978b; MACKERER et al., 1978). The rate for association k_{+1}, is ca. $7 \times 10^7 M^{-1}$ min^{-1} (MACKERER et al., 1978). The affinity constant calculated from the rate constants,

$K_D = \dfrac{k_{-1}}{k_{+1}} = 2.3$ nM, is in good agreement with that determined by equilibrium analyses.

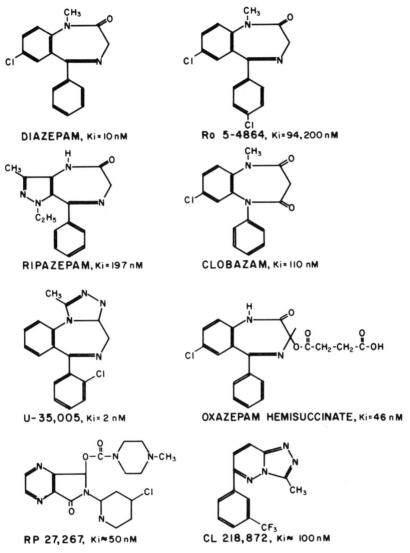

Fig. 2. Structure–activity relationships of some compounds with affinity for benzodiazepine receptors. The concentration causing 50% inhibition of specific binding (IC_{50}) was determined using ^{3}H-diazepam as ligand and rat brain membranes at 0 °C. $K_i = IC_{50} \times \left(1 + \dfrac{C}{K_D}\right)^{-1}$, where C = concentration of ^{3}H-diazepam = ca. 2 nM, K_D = affinity constant for ^{3}H-diazepam = 2.4–3.4 nM. (Data from BRÆSTRUP and SQUIRES, 1978a; LIPPA et al., 1979; BLANCHARD et al., 1979)

The binding site is a protein which can be destroyed by proteolytic enzymes (trypsin and chymotrypsin) (BRAESTRUP and SQUIRES, 1977; MÖHLER and OKADA, 1977a). Binding sites are rather thermostable, brain membranes can be stored for months at −18 °C, and the half life at 50 °C is about 2–3 h in Tris-HCl buffer, pH 7.4.

2. Distribution

The subcellular distribution of benzodiazepine receptors is characterized hy high levels in the "P_2" fraction, containing synaptosomes (pinched off nerve endings) (BRAESTRUP et al., 1978 a; MACKERER et al., 1978; BOSMANN et al., 1977). The "microsomal" fraction, however, also contains appreciable amounts of specific binding sites, together with several other kinds of binding sites (DEBLAS et al., 1978; BRAESTRUP et al., 1978 a). The membrane fraction on which benzodiazepine receptors are located sediments at a density between 0.8 M and 1.2 M sucrose together with the marker enzyme Na^+-K^+-ATPase, indicating that the binding sites are located in the cell plasma membranes as opposed to, for example, membranes from mitochondria, vesicles and endoplasmatic reticulum (BRAESTRUP et al., 1978 a; BOSMANN et al., 1978).

The brain concentration of benzodiazepine receptors show marked regional variations. Maximal levels are found in cortical areas of rat (BRAESTRUP and SQUIRES, 1977; MÖHLER and OKADA, 1977 b; MACKERER et al., 1978), baboon (SQUIRES et al., 1979 a) and man (BRAESTRUP et al., 1977; MÖHLER and OKADA, 1978; MÖHLER et al., 1978 a; SPETH et al., 1978). Mid-brain structures such as thalamus and caudate nucleus exhibit intermediate levels, while white matter areas and spinal cord contain low levels. It is of interest that there is no preferential localization in limbic structures (BRAESTRUP et al., 1977; MÖHLER and OKADA, 1978; MÖHLER et al., 1978 a).

3. Brain Specifity

Benzodiazepine receptors are brain specific (BRAESTRUP and SQUIRES, 1977).

Some diazepam binding is found in rat and baboon kidney, liver and lung, but not in intestine or skeletal muscle. Although the diazepam binding in kidney, liver and lung can be displaced by excess unlabelled diazepam, these peripheral binding sites display quite different properties from those in brain, e.g. the binding site in kidney has an affinity constant for diazepam of about 40 nM, at least ten times higher than in brain. Displacement of diazepam binding by clonazepam, one of the most potent diazepam displacers in brain, and by RO 5-4,864, one of the least potent displacers in brain, are just reversed with respect to their potencies in displacing diazepam binding to kidney membranes (BRAESTRUP and SQUIRES, 1977). It is striking that RO 5-4,864 differs structurally from diazepam by only one para chloro atom (see Fig. 2).

Serum albumin binds benzodiazepines with much lower affinity than the brain specific binding sites (MÜLLER and WOLLERT, 1973; MÜLLER and WOLLERT, 1976; BRODERSEN et al., 1977). Both brain specific ^{3}H-diazepam binding and binding to serum albumin exhibit stereoselectivity, the D-form of oxazepam being more potent in both binding and pharmacological tests than the L-form (WADDINGTON and OWEN, 1978; MÜLLER and WOLLERT, 1975 a).

4. Ontogenetic and Phylogenetic Development of Benzodiazepine Receptors

Benzodiazepine receptors are detectable in rat brain 8 days before birth. Their concentration rises rapidly just after birth to reach almost adult levels 1–2 weeks after birth (BRAESTRUP and NIELSEN, 1978).

Benzodiazepine receptors appear at a late stage in evolution. Specific diazepam binding is present among 15 tetrapods, including 2 species of amphibians, 2 reptiles,

3 birds, and 8 mammals. Receptor concentration in brain and affinity constants for ^{3}H-diazepam (K_D 2–4 nM) are similar in all tetrapods investigated. Benzodiazepine receptors are present in the brain of higher bony fishes (plaice, codfish, salmon and sturgeon), although in forms somewhat different from those found in higher vertebrates, while specific ^{3}H-diazepam binding sites are not detectable in lower fishes (hagfish, lamprey and shark) nor in invertebrates (NIELSEN et al., 1978; FERNHOLM et al., 1979).

II. Pharmacological Specificity

With the exception of a very few recently discovered substances (see below) the only identified compounds which potently displace ^{3}H-diazepam and ^{3}H-flunitrazepam from rat and human brain binding sites are other benzodiazepines (SQUIRES and BRAESTRUP, 1977; BRAESTRUP et al., 1977; MÖHLER and OKADA, 1977b; BRAESTRUP and SQUIRES, 1978a; SPETH et al., 1978; MACKERER et al., 1978). The affinities of different benzodiazepines for the binding sites (IC$_{50}$ values or K_i values) are highly correlated to the clinical and pharmacological potencies of these compounds. Figure 3 shows two such correlations. Cat muscle relaxant effect, inhibition of pentazol convulsions in mice, inhibition of mouse rotarod performance, inhibition of el-shock induced fighting in mice, inhibition of experimental human anxiety and restoration of behavior suppressed by punishment, effects which are indicative of anxiolytic effects in man, are all correlated with the affinity for the receptors (SQUIRES and BRAESTRUP, 1977; BRAESTRUP et al., 1977; MÖHLER and OKADA, 1977b; BRAESTRUP and SQUIRES,

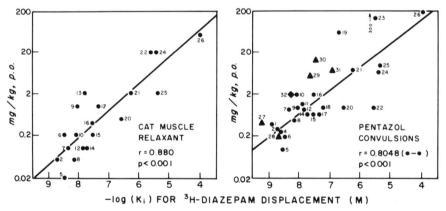

Fig. 3. Correlation between ^{3}H-diazepam displacement potency (K_i values) and *a* cat muscle relaxant effect (Minimum effective dose, mg/kg p.o.), *b* inhibition of mouse pentazol convulsions (ED$_{50}$, mg/kg p.o.). Drugs are: 1, KC-4-2,846; 2, clonazepam; 3, U 39,219; 4, U 35,005; 5, flunitrazepam; 6, lorazepam; 7, RO 5-3,027; 8, RO 5-3,590; 9, demethyl-diazepam; 10, diazepam; 11, estazolam; 12, RO 5-2,904; 13, flurazepam; 14, nitrazepam; 15, bromazepam; 16, chlorazepate; 17, oxazepam; 18, U 31,957; 19, ripazepam; 20, RO 5-4,528; 21, chlordiazepoxide; 22, RO 5-5,807; 23, RO 5-3,785; 24, medazepam, 25, RO 5-3,636; 26, RO 5-4,864; 27, RO 5-3,448; 28, alprazolam; 29, RO 5-6,227; 30, Sc 31,312; 31, RO 5-2,181; 32, midazolam; Data from BRAESTRUP and SQUIRES, 1978a (●–●) except triangles (▲) which are calculated from MACKERER and KOCHMANN (1978). Most chemical structures are presented in RANDALL et al. (1974)

298   C. Braestrup

1978a; Speth et al., 1978; Mackerer et al., 1978; Möhler et al., 1978a; Chang and Snyder, 1978). Several enantiomers of benzodiazepines exhibit stereoselectivity for the receptors paralleling their pharmacological potencies (Möhler and Okada, 1977b; Waddington and Owen, 1978).

The good in vivo/in vitro correlations suggest that the benzodiazepine receptors characterized in vitro mediate the clinical and pharmacological effects of benzodiazepines in vivo. Specific benzodiazepine receptor binding in vivo can be demonstrated with ^{3}H-flunitrazepam (Chang and Snyder, 1978).

A few benzodiazepines exhibit considerably lower affinity for the benzodiazepine receptors in vitro than expected from the pharmacological effects (oxazolam, cloxazolam, pinazepam and others), probably because they are metabolized in vivo to active compounds (Braestrup and Squires, 1978a).

Because of several hypotheses suggesting that benzodiazepines exert their pharmacological and clinical effects by interacting with certain presumed neurotransmitters, particularly GABA, glycine and serotonin (see below), it is of interest to determine whether the brain specific diazepam binding sites correspond to the receptor for any known or putative neurotransmitter substance. ^{3}H-Diazepam is not displaced by GABA, glycine, serotonin, noradrenaline, dopamine, histamine, metenkephalin, substance P, somatostatin, VIP (vasoactive intestinal polypeptide), cholecystokinin, glutamate, aspartate or their antagonists (when available). Among more than 200 chemical compounds tested, representing over 22 pharmacological classes, no ^{3}H-diazepam displacing compound was found with reasonably low K_i values, suggesting that none of these exert their pharmacological effects by interaction with the benzodiazepine receptors. These results indicate that the benzodiazepine receptor is not identical with the recognition site of any known or putative neurotransmitter receptor (Squires and Braestrup, 1977; Braestrup and Squires, 1978a).

The pharmacological selectivity of the benzodiazepine receptors can be used to select new compounds, chemically different from benzodiazepines but having some of their pharmacological properties (i.e. RP 27,267, Blanchard et al., 1979; CL 218,872, Lippa et al., 1979).

III. Neuronal Localization

Brain specific benzodiazepine receptors are not located on mouse primary astrocytes or on C_6-glioma cell lines, indicating the lack of benzodiazepine receptors on brain glia cells (Braestrup et al., 1978b; Syapin and Skolnick, 1979). The level of benzodiazepine receptors is reduced in rat substantia nigra and cerebellum following local injection of the neurotoxic agent kainic acid (Braestrup and Squires, 1978b; Braestrup et al., 1979b); it is also reduced in the cerebellum of Purkinje cell deficient "nervous" mouse mutants (Lippa et al., 1978; Braestrup et al., 1979b) and in the basal ganglia of patients dying with Huntington's chorea, a disease with profound neuronal degeneration (Möhler and Okada, 1978; Reisine et al., 1978). Taken together these results strongly indicate that benzodiazepine receptors are located on neurons in the CNS. The marginal effects of selective lesions, however, indicate that benzodiazepine receptors are probably located both on cell bodies and terminals of many different kinds of neurons (Braestrup et al., 1979b).

Techniques are available to isolate with some purity glia cells from brain tissue. Experiments with such isolated glia cells indicate that some benzodiazepine receptors might be located on glia cells (HENN and HENKE, 1978).

IV. In Vivo Receptor Modifications

Several neurotransmitter receptors respond to prolonged exposure to agonist or antagonist by changes in receptor number or affinities for their ligand (TATA, 1975; RAFF, 1976; NIELSEN et al., to be published, a; COOPER et al., 1978).

Prolonged administration of diazepam, lorazepam and chlordiazepoxide to rats (up to 90 mg/kg diazepam per day, p.o. for 8 weeks) do not greatly change benzodiazepine receptor number or affinities for ^{3}H-diazepam (BRAESTRUP et al., 1979a; MÖHLER et al., 1978b). A small decrease in receptor number may occur (CHIEU and ROSENBERG, 1978). Tolerance to benzodiazepines and occurrence of abstinence symptoms upon withdrawal are thus not clearly dependent on changes in affinity or number of benzodiazepine receptors.

It is difficult to change benzodiazepine receptor number or affinities for their ligand by application of experimental stresses to laboratory animals. Small and inconsistent effects have been presented (BRAESTRUP et al., 1979c; YAMAMURA et al., 1978a) after immobilization stress, isolation stress and electric foot shock stress. Experimental stresses are generally antagonized by benzodiazepines.

A small and short-lasting increase in the number of benzodiazepine receptors has been reported following seizures induced by electric shock or pentazol (PAUL and SKOLNICK, 1978).

V. In Vitro Receptor Modulation (see Table 1)

1. GABA (γ-Amino Butyric Acid)

Extensive evidence indicates that benzodiazepines enhance GABA-ergic transmission (see Sect. C) and several studies have investigated interaction between GABA and benzodiazepine receptors. GABA agonists, such as GABA itself (10^{-5}–10^{-4} M), muscimol (10^{-6}–10^{-5} M), trans-4-aminocrotonic acid (10^{-5}–10^{-4} M), and others increase the affinity (the affinity constant K_D is decreased) of ^{3}H-diazepam or ^{3}H-flunitrazepam for benzodiazepine receptors in vitro (TALLMAN et al., 1978; BRILEY and LANGER, 1978; WASTEK et al., 1978; MARTIN and CANDY, 1978; WILLIAMS and RISLEY, 1979; KAROBATH and SPERK, 1979; BRAESTRUP et al., 1979d; MAURER, 1979; CHIEU and ROSENBERG, 1979) and in vivo (GALLAGER et al., 1978). An increase in the association rate constant and a decrease in the dissociation rate constant is responsible for the increased affinity. The effects of GABA agonists are counteracted by bicuculline in a stereoselective manner (TALLMAN et al., 1978). These results indicate that the GABA receptor is functionally coupled to the benzodiazepine receptor.

There has been some controversy as to whether the GABA receptors involved in benzodiazepine receptor regulation were similar to or different from "classical" GABA-receptors. Several well described GABA agonists [imidazoleacetic acid (IAA), THIP, isoguvacine, 3-aminopropanesulphonic acid (APS), β-guanidinopropionic acid and piperidine-4-sulphonic acid (PSA)] increased ^{3}H-diazepam binding in vitro

Table 1. "Modulatory" effects and inhibiting effects of non-benzodiazepines on benzodiazepine receptors in vitro

Treatment	Effect on specific ^{3}H-diazepam or ^{3}H-flunitrazepam binding		Affected binding parameter	Ref.
Ni^{2+} (1–5 mM)	40%–80%	increase	K_D	[1, 14]
Hg^{2+} (0.1 mM)	30%	increase		[1]
Cu^{2+} (0.1 mM)	20%	increase		[1]
Zn^{2+} (0.1 mM)	20%	increase		[1]
Cd^{2+} (1 mM)	40%	increase		[14]
Mn^{2+} (100 mM)	30%	increase		[1]
Co^{2+} (1 mM)	25%	increase		[1]
I^- (10 mM)	20%–60%	increase	$K_D{}^a$	[2, 14]
Br^- (50 mM)	20%–80%	increase		[2, 14]
Cl^- (100 mM)	40%	increase		[2, 15]
No_2^- (100 mM)	50%	increase		[2]
SCN^- (10 mM)	25%	increase		[2]
Muscimol (10^{-5}–10^{-6} M)	30%–80%	increase	$K_D{}^b$	[3, 4, 5, 14]
GABA (10^{-4}–10^{-5} M)	30%–80%	increase	K_D	[3, 4, 5, 6, 14, 15]
SQ 20,009 (10^{-5}–10^{-6} M)	25%–40%	increase	K_D	[5]
SQ 65,396 (10^{-5}–10^{-6} M)	20%–30%	increase		[5]
Heating (10 min, 50 °C) (180 min, 37 °C)	40%–60%	increase	K_D	[7, 8, 14]
Repeated washing		Decrease	K_D	[9]
"Heat stabile protein" inhibitor, Mw 15,000 (10 µg)		Decrease	K_D?	[10]
Bicuculline (10^{-5}–10^{-4} M)		Decrease		[3, 4, 5, 14]
Strychnine (10^{-4} M)		Decrease	Competition?	[11]
Chlorpromazine (10^{-4} M)		Decrease	–	[12]
Chlorzoxazone (10^{-4} M)		Decrease	–	[12]
Hypoxantine (10^{-4} M)		Decrease	–	[13, 14]

Several compounds do not exhibit effects in the above experimental situations: DABA aspartate, glutamate, taurine, imidazol acetic acid, (3), F^- (2), IBMX, theophylline, kainic acid, nipecotic cid (5) and others.

References:

[1] Mackerer and Kochman (1978)
[2] Costa et al. (1979)
[3] Tallmann et al. (1978)
[4] Briley and Langer (1978)
[5] Williams and Risley (1979)
[6] Wastek et al. (1978)
[7] Braestrup and Squires (1977)
[8] H. Yamamura, personal communication
[9] M. Karobath, personal communication
[10] Guidotti et al. (1978a)
[11] Müller et al. (1978)
[12] Braestrup and Squires (1978a)
[13] Skolnick et al. (1978)
[14] Braestrup, unpublished; Klepner and Squires, unpublished
[15] Martin and Candy (1978)

---

^{a} Effect on dissociation rate (Ref. [2])
^{b} Effect on association rate (Ref. [3])

much less than would be expected from their GABA receptor agonist activity (TALL-MAN et al., 1978; KAROBATH et al., 1979; BRAESTRUP et al., 1979 d; MAURER, 1979) a finding claimed to indicate the presence of a novel type of GABA receptors with selective recognition properties. More recent data, however, are not in favour of a novel type of GABA-receptor. Rather, the GABA receptor recognition site is "classical" but the coupling between the GABA receptor and the benzodiazepine receptor is of a new kind, different from the coupling between the GABA-receptor and most of the chloride channels. This conclusion arises from studies showing that the apparently inactive GABA agonists in fact do interfere with the GABA receptor recognition site: They can inhibit the effect of muscimol and GABA on ^{3}H-diazepam binding (BRAESTRUP et al., 1979 d; KAROBATH and LIPPITSCH, 1979). IAA, THIP, isoguvacine, APS, β-guanidinopropionic acid, and PSA are thus partial agonist or even pure antogonist (depending on the agent and the conditions) to the GABA/benzodiazepine receptor complex (BRAESTRUP et al., 1979 d).

Another interaction between GABA receptors and benzodiazepine receptors may be exerted by GABA-modulin, a heat stable, 15,000 dalton protein found in brain and liver (TOFFANO et al., 1978). GABA-modulin is an inhibitor of both GABA and benzodiazepine receptors. Since benzodiazepines may increase the affinity of ^{3}H-GABA for rat brain GABA-receptors in vitro (GUIDOTTI et al., 1978 b), it was proposed that benzodiazepines increase the affinity of GABA for GABA receptors by releasing GABA-modulin, thereby disinhibiting GABA receptors (COSTA et al., 1978; GUIDOTTI et al., 1978 a). These findings indicate that the benzodiazepine receptor might be an allosteric modulatory site at or near the GABA receptor. However, the different regional brain distribution (BRAESTRUP and SQUIRES, 1977) and the dissimilar ontogenetic and phylogenetic developments (NIELSEN et al., 1978; BRAESTRUP and NIELSEN, 1978) of benzodiazepine receptors and GABA receptors is difficult to reconcile with the contention that there is always a functional link between benzodiazepine receptors and GABA receptors. Furthermore GABA-ergic drugs exhibit only very weak activity in conflict tests and they do not easily potentiate the effects of benzodiazepines (see below).

2. Miscellanous Modulators

Increase in affinity of ^{3}H-diazepam or ^{3}H-flunitrazepam for benzodiazepine receptors can be achieved in several other ways than those described in Sect. B.V.1. Simple heating of rat brain membranes (50 °C for 10 min) increases binding affinity (Fig. 4). Similarly, several divalent cations (MACKERER and KOCHMAN, 1978) and halides (COSTA et al., 1979) can increase binding affinity under certain conditions in in vitro assays.

It is striking that these different modulatory changes in benzodiazepine receptor affinity all obtain a maximal affinity of about $K_D = 2.5$–3 nM for ^{3}H-diazepam in the high-affinity form and very often $K_D \simeq 4$–6 nM in the low-affinity form, indicating that the receptor may exist in two or more conformations, depending on several factors.

VI. Endogenous Ligands

The discovery of opiate receptors in 1973 intensified the search for endogenous substances in brain tissue with opiate-like activity. Such compounds were later identified

C. BRAESTRUP

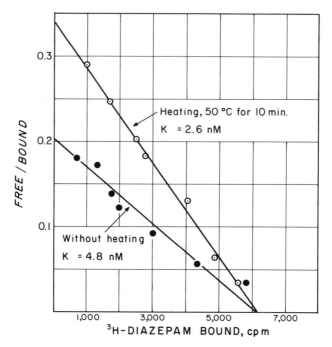

Fig. 4. Increased benzodiazepine receptor affinity after heating. Frozen rat whole brains were homogenized at 4 °C in 10 vol. 50 mM sodium phosphate, pH 7.4. The $P_1 + P_2$ pellet was prepared by centrifugation at 30,000 × g for 10 min and resuspended in 50 vol. buffer. Heated and non-heated aliquots were incubated with ^{3}H-diazepam (0.6–20 nM) for 60 min at 0 °C. Other details as described previously (BRAESTRUP and SQUIRES, 1977)

as peptides (the enkephalins and endorphines). The suspected endogenous ligand (endogenous diazepam-like compound) for benzodiazepine receptors (SQUIRES and BRAESTRUP, 1977) has not yet been identified. The "endogenous protein inhibitor" described above has been proposed as a "modulating ligand" (COSTA et al., 1978). Hypoxanthine, which is present in high concentrations in brain (MORI et al., 1973), and inosine and nicotineamide have been proposed as endogenous ligands for the benzodiazepine receptor (SKOLNICK et al., 1978; MÖHLER et al., 1979) even though the affinity of these compounds is extremely low. The K_i value for hypoxanthine is about 10^{-3} M (SKOLNICK et al., 1978; NIELSEN et al., 1979b) compared to about 10^{-8} M for active benzodiazepines. A neutral, lipophilic, low-molecular-weight, aromatic compound with high affinity for the benzodiazepine receptor has been obtained from human urine. The K_i value of this compound, ethyl β-carboline-3-carboxylate, for ^{3}H-diazepam displacement is about 4 nM (NIELSEN et al., 1979b; BRAESTRUP et al., 1980).

C. Benzodiazepines and GABA

I. Electrophysiological and Biochemical Interaction

HAEFELY et al. (1975) and COSTA et al. (1975a) suggested that GABA is involved in the mechanism of action of benzodiazepines. Extensive electrophysiological evidence now supports this contention. Benzodiazepines enhance GABA-mediated presynaptic inhibition in the spinal cord (SCHMIDT et al., 1967; POLC et al., 1974; STRATTEN and BARNES, 1971; SCHLOSSER, 1971; POLZIN and BARNES, 1976). In the central nervous system, benzodiazepines enhance GABA-mediated presynaptic inhibition, postsynaptic inhibition and recurrent inhibition (TSUCHIYA and FUKUSHIMA, 1978; POLC and HAEFELY, 1976; PIERI and HAEFELY, 1976; WOLF and HAAS, 1977, GALLAGER, 1978; SCHAFFNER and HAEFELY, 1975, CURTIS et al., 1976a). Postsynaptic inhibition in the spinal cord is mediated by glycine and this inhibition is not potentiated by benzodiazepines (SCHMIDT et al., 1967).

Iontophoretic application of chlordiazepoxide potentiates the inhibitory effect of GABA on single rabbit sensorimotor neurons (KOZHECHKIN and OSTROVSKAYA, 1977). Chlordiazepoxide (10^{-5}–10^{-4} M) and flurazepam ($< 10^{-5}$ M) (CHOI et al., 1977; FISCHBACH, personal communication) and iontophoretically applied chlordiazepoxide and diazepam (MACDONALD and BARKER, 1978) augment GABA actions in spinal cord neuron cultures.

Bicuculline is the most selective GABA-antagonist available. Benzodiazepines are antagonists to the effect of bicuculline on the firing rate of some neurons (BOWERY and DRAY, 1978; DRAY and STRAUGHAN, 1976; OSTROVSKAYA and MOLODAVKIN, 1976), but there is only weak antagonism on cerebellar Purkinje cells (LIPPA et al., 1979).

Some electrophysiological studies, however, find effects of benzodiazepines which are not "GABA-like" (STEINER and FELIX, 1976; GÄHWILER, 1976; DAVIES and POLC, 1978; BOAKES et al., 1977; LIPPA et al., 1979; CURTIS et al., 1976a).

Several non-benzodiazepine drugs, such as barbiturates (NICOLL, 1972, 1975a, 1975b, 1978; WOLF and HAAS, 1977; BOWERY and DRAY, 1976; BROWN and CONSTANTI, 1978; TSUCHIYA and FUKUSHIMA, 1978; CURTIS and LODGE, 1977a, 1977b; POLC and HAEFELY, 1976; EVANS, 1977; ECCLES et al., 1963), ethanol (MIYAHARA et al., 1966; HAEFELY et al., 1978), phenytoin (DEISZ and LUX, 1977; DAVIDOFF, 1972; RAABE and AYALA, 1976), possibly droperidol (MARUYAMA and KAWASAKI, 1976), and methaqualone (HAEFELY et al., 1978), but not meprobamate, enhance GABA-like effects or reverse the effects of GABA-antagonists in electrophysiological models (see also review by HAEFELY et al., 1978).

Several behavioral studies are consistent with a GABA-ergic mechanism of action of benzodiazepines (MAO et al., 1975b; COSTA et al., 1975a; HAEFELY et al., 1975; WADDINGTON, 1978), while other studies are not (JUHAZC and DAIRMAN, 1977; SOUBRIE et al., 1976; BOLME and FUXE, 1977; LIPPA and REGAN, 1977; STONE and JAVID, THIEBOT et al. 1979).

Results with "anticonflict tests" are controversial. Benzodiazepines selectively restore behaviors suppressed by punishment in these tests and their effects can sometimes be reduced by GABA antagonists (OSTROVSKAYA and VORONINA, 1977; ZAKUSOV et al., 1977; STEIN et al., 1977; BILLINGSLEY and KUBENA, 1978), but also by strychnine (STEIN et al., 1977) and by naloxone (BILLINGSLEY and KUBENA, 1978). Further, an inhibitor of GABA catabolism, cycloserine (WOOD et al., 1978), exhibits anticonflict properties (W. HAEFELY, personal communication). In contrast, other studies indicate that potentiation of GABA-ergic neurotransmission by the GABA transaminase inhibitors amino-oxyacetic acid or ethanolamine O-sulphate (FILE and HYDE, 1977; COOK and SEPINWALL, 1975) or by stimulation of the GABA receptors by muscimol (Sullivan et al., 1978; Thiebot et al., 1979) or THIP [4,5,6,7-tetrahy-droisoxazolo(5,4-c)pyridin-3-ol] does not elicit anticonflict activity in several conflict situations.

II. GABA Turnover

High doses of benzodiazepines reduce GABA turnover.

Diazepam (3–30 mg/kg) increases the levels of endogenous GABA in mouse cerebral cortex and whole forebrain, in rat substantia nigra and cat spinal cord, but not in rat caudate, cingulate cortex and pyriform cortex (Haefely et al., 1975; Saad, 1972; Pericic et al., 1977). The increased levels of GABA may indicate a reduced turnover.

Reduced GABA-turnover is more directly shown by isotope methods. Diazepam (1–30 mg/kg i.p.) reduces the incorporation of ^{14}C-glucose and ^{13}C-glucose into GABA in rat caudate nucleus and nucleus accumbens and mouse whole brain (Mao et al., 1977; Haefely et al., 1975).

The accumulation of GABA after inhibition of GABA metabolism by amino-oxyacetic acid or gabaculine is counteracted by diazepam (10 mg/kg, i.p.) (Fuxe et al., 1975; Bernasconi and Martin, 1978; Pericic et al., 1977; Tarver et al., 1975). Reduced turnover is also indicated by the benzodiazepine-induced reversal of GABA-disappearence after synthesis inhibition with isoniazid (Saad, 1972; Löscher and Frey, 1977; Guidotti, 1978). The effects of benzodiazepines on GABA level and turnover are partly shared by barbiturates and phenytoin (Saad et al., 1972; Pericic et al., 1977; Löscher and Frey, 1977) and by the direct GABA receptor agonist, muscimol (Mao et al., 1977).

The decreased GABA-turnover may be explained by assuming that benzodiazepines act either directly or indirectly as GABA-agonists thus leading to a compensatory, "feed-back inhibition" of GABA turnover (Pericic et al., 1977).

III. Enzymes

Clonazepam, diazepam and chlordiazepoxide do not inhibit the enzymes catabolizing GABA, GABA-transaminase [4-aminobutyrate: 2 oxoglutarate amino transferase (EC 2.6.1.19)] or succinic semialdehyde dehydrogenase (EC 1.2.1.16), to any great extent at concentrations about 10^{-4} M (Sawaya et al., 1975).

IV. GABA Uptake

Uptake of GABA in cerebral cortex slices of rats or brain synaptosomes is inhibited by diazepam and chlordiazepoxide only at high, unphysiological concentrations (0.05–0.5 mM) (Harris et al., 1973; Nelson-Krause and Howard, 1976; Iversen and Johnston, 1971; Olsen et al., 1977). Uptake of GABA into rat or cat cerebellar slices is not inhibited by diazepam, flurazepam or chlordiazepoxide at 10^{-5} M (Curtis et al., 1976a). Diazepam (10^{-4} and 10^{-6} M) increased the Ca^{2+}-independent and the low K^+ (15 mM) induced GABA-release from preloaded mouse or rat brain synaptosomes (Olsen et al., 1978b; Mitchell and Martin, 1978). Other studies using rat brain synaptosomes failed to show a spontaneous or K^+ (30 mM) induced GABA release by diazepam (10^{-5}–5×10^{-4} M) (Nelson-Krause and Howard, 1976; Maisov et al., 1976).

V. Interaction with GABA-Receptors

Benzodiazepines may increase the affinity of ^{3}H-GABA for fresh rat brain membranes (see Sect. B.V.1). Benzodiazepines do not, however, increase the affinity of ^{3}H-muscimol for its brain binding site (GUIDOTTI, unpublished), nor are ^{3}H-GABA and ^{3}H-muscimol binding sites inhibited by benzodiazepines (BEAUMONT et al., 1978; OLSEN et al., 1978a; ZUKIN et al., 1974). ^{3}H-Bicuculline binding sites (GABA receptors) are not inhibited by chlordiazepoxide and diazepam ($10^{-5} M$) (MÖHLER and OKADA, 1977c).

VI. Cyclic GMP

The level of cyclic GMP is decreased in cerebellum by several sedative drugs, such as benzodiazepines in small doses (0.1–5 mg/kg) (diazepam, chlordiazepoxide, desmethyl diazepam, clonazepam, flunitrazepam, chlordesmethyl diazepam), muscimol, barbiturates, ethanol, haloperidol and morphine (BIGGIO et al., 1977b; MAO et al., 1975b; OPMEER et al., 1976; MAILMAN et al., 1978; GOVONI et al., 1976; GUDIOTTI, 1978; LUNDY and MAGOR, 1978).

Cyclic GMP is increased in cerebellum by stimulant or convulsant compounds such as isoniazid, harmaline, pentazol, glutamate, picrotoxin, oxotremorin, soman and bicyclic phosphorous ester (EPTBO), and these increases are counteracted by benzodiazepines and also in most cases by barbiturates (BIGGIO et al., 1977b; MAO et al., 1975a, b; OPMEER et al., 1976; COSTA et al., 1975b; LUNDY and MAGOR, 1978; MATTSSON et al., 1977). Other treatments increase cyclic GMP levels in cerebellum without reported interactions with benzodiazepines (cold exposure, apomorphine, intracerebral glycine) (MAO et al., 1974a, b; VOLICER et al., 1977).

The second messenger cyclic GMP in cerebellum is confined mainly to Purkinje cells (COSTA et al., 1975c) and the level is apparently regulated by several factors, including the GABA input from basket cells, glutamate input from climbing fibres and remote factors such as stimulation and blockade of dopamine receptors in corpus striatum (BIGGIO et al., 1978; BIGGIO and GUIDOTTI, 1977). The effects of benzodiazepines on cyclic GMP in cerebellum is consistent with a GABA-potentiating effect (see review by GUIDOTTI, 1978).

Benzodiazepines have other biochemical effects proposed to be secondary to GABA-ergic stimulation (see Sect. F.II).

VII. Conclusion

Benzodiazepines and barbiturates enhance GABA-ergic transmission, but the mechanism of action is not yet clear. It cannot be excluded that benzodiazepines improve the stimulus-induced GABA-release (HAEFELY et al., 1978). Alternatively, benzodiazepines might enhance the sensitivity of GABA receptors.

D. Benzodiazepines and Serotonin

Pharmacological studies suggest that serotonin (5-hydroxytryptamine) is involved in the anxiolytic action of benzodiazepines. Serotonin antagonists (methysergide, cinanserin and d-2-bromlysergic acid diethyl amide) or serotonin synthesis inhibitors (*p*-chlorophenyl alanine) can restore behaviors suppressed by punishment in conflict tests (Stein et al., 1975; Stein et al., 1973; Cook and Sepinwall, 1975; File and Hyde, 1977; for a review, Stein et al., 1977).

I. Serotonin Receptors

Diazepam does not interact directly with serotonin receptors as measured by ^{3}H-LSD binding to brain membranes (Bennett and Snyder, 1975), nor does serotonin act on benzodiazepine receptors (see Sect. B.II).

II. Serotonin Level and Metabolism

Uptake of serotonin is not affected in brain tissue by diazepam or fludiazepam (Nakamura and Fukushima, 1977; Chase et al., 1970) or in blood platelets by chlordiazepoxide and diazepam (Pletscher, 1969; Lingjaerde, 1973).

Effects of benzodiazepines on endogenous brain serotonin level are variable. The brain serotonin has been reported to be unchanged (Pletscher, 1969; File and Velucci, 1978; Fennesy and Lee, 1972; Lidbrink et al., 1974; Dominic et al., 1975) or slightly increased (Jenner et al., 1975; Fennesy and Lee, 1972; Fernstrom et al., 1974; Rastogi et al., 1977) following chlordiazepoxide, clonazepam, nitrazepam, clobazam and diazepam.

The level of the major serotonin metabolite, 5-HIAA, is increased in rat and mouse brain after acute administration of clonazepam (2.5 mg/kg, i.p.) and diazepam (10 mg/kg, i.p.) (Fernstrom et al., 1974; Jenner et al., 1975; Rastogi et al., 1977).

The turnover of serotonin is reduced by benzodiazepines. The disappearance of intracerebrally injected ^{14}C-5-HT is decreased in rat brain by oxazepam (20 mg/kg, i.p.) and diazepam (20 mg/kg, i.p.) (Chase et al., 1970; Wise et al., 1972). Flurazepam (5 mg/kg, i.p.), diazepam (5 mg/kg, i.p.) and chlordiazepoxide (20 mg/kg, i.p.) reduce the formation of ^{3}H-5-HT from ^{3}H-tryptophan in mice (Dominic et al., 1975). Chlordiazepoxide (25 mg/kg) reduces the disappearance of endogenous serotonin after synthesis inhibition by α-propyldopacetamide (H 22/54) (Lidbrink et al., 1973). The formation of the serotonin precursor, 5-hydroxytryptophan, is decreased by diazepam (3 mg/kg) (Biswas and Carlsson, 1978).

Benzodiazepines may increase 5-HIAA and ^{14}C-5-HIAA in brain by a probenecid-like inhibition of the elimination from brain (Rastogi et al., 1977); the mechanism of action of other serotonin effects is not known.

Diazepam, oxazepam and chlordiazepoxide may increase free plasma tryptophan by competing for its serum albumin binding site (Bourgoin et al., 1975; Müller and Wollert, 1975b). Increased plasma level of free tryptophan may increase brain serotonin and 5-HIAA levels.

E. Benzodiazepines and Acetylcholine

Pharmacological evidence suggests that acetylcholine is involved in the anticonvulsant effects of benzodiazepines (see review by Ladinsky et al., to be published).

I. Acetylcholine Level

The levels of endogenous acetylcholine are increased by chlordiazepoxide, diazepam, flurazepam, triazolam, N-methyloxazepam, lorazepam, nitrazepam, N-desmethyl diazepam and oxazepam (5–100 mg/kg) in several but not all rat and mouse brain areas (CONSOLO et al., 1972, 1974, 1975, 1977; DOMINO and WILSON, 1972; SETHY, 1978; TONKOPY et al., 1978). Brain choline levels were not affected (CONSOLO et al., 1975; LADINSKY et al., 1973).

The level of acetylcholine may be related to impulse flow in cholinergic neurons and the increased level of acetylcholine after benzodiazepines suggests a decreased impulse-flow and reduced acetylcholine release. This conclusion is in keeping with a reduced turnover of acetylcholine after diazepam (3 mg/kg, i.p.) in various rat brain areas (ZSILLA et al., 1976).

The mechanism of benzodiazepine effects on brain acetylcholine is unclear, but pharmacological and biochemical evidence indicates that GABA is not involved (LADINSKY et al., to be published).

Barbiturates and several other drugs increase brain acetylcholine levels (GIARMAN and PEPEU, 1962; CONSOLO et al., 1972; DOMINO and WILSON, 1972; CONSOLO et al., 1975).

II. Acetylcholine Receptors

Diazepam and chlordiazepoxide $(10^{-5} M)$ do not act directly on muscarinic acetylcholine receptors as measured by binding of ^{3}H-quinuclidinyl-benzilate (^{3}H-QNB) to rat brain membranes (YAMAMURA and SNYDER, 1974). Conversely, muscarinic and antimuscarinic substances do not interfere with benzodiazepine receptors (see Sect. B.II).

F. Benzodiazepines and Catecholamines

There is no good evidence that catecholamines are involved in the mechanism of action of benzodiazepines. Other psychotropic drugs may have their major actions on catecholamines. For example, neuroleptics block dopamine and noradrenaline receptors, resulting in increased turnover of catecholamines. Antidepressant drugs may inhibit catecholamine uptake into nerve endings, inhibit oxidation by MAO or release catecholamines from nerve terminals.

I. Catecholamine Turnover

High doses (10–25 mg/kg) of diazepam, chlordiazepoxide, triazolam and nitrazepam decrease dopamine turnover in rat striatum or whole brain (CORRODI et al., 1971; TAYLOR and LAVERTY, 1969, 1973; PUGSLEY and LIPPMAN, 1976; SHIBUYA, 1976; FUXE et al., 1975; LIDBRINK et al., 1973; BISWAS and CARLSSON, 1978). Noradrenaline turnover was decreased in rat cortex or rat or mouse whole brain (FUXE et al., 1975; TAYLOR and LAVERTY, 1969, 1973; SHIBUYA, 1976; CORRODI et al., 1971; DOMINIC et al., 1975; LIDBRINK et al., 1973). The effects on catecholamine turnover were determined as the influence either on catecholamine disappearance rate following synthesis inhibition by α-methyl tyrosine, on disappearance rate of intracerebrally injected ^{3}H-dopamine, on accumulation of L-Dopa after inhibition of L-Dopa-decarboxylase by NSD 1015 or on semiquantitative fluorescence histochemistry.

The reported decrease in dopamine turnover is not substantially supported by measurements of the major dopamine metabolites, HVA and DOPAC. Brain levels of HVA and DOPAC are either decreased, probably because of hypothermia (BARTHOLINI et al., 1973; KARASAWA et al., 1978; RASTOGI et al., 1977; NAKAMURA and NAKAMURA, 1976; KELLER et al., 1976; DAPRADA and PLETCHER, 1966), or unchanged (KARASAWA et al., 1978; WESTERINK et al., 1977; RASTOGI et al., 1977; SHARMAN, 1966; SETOGUCHI et al., 1978) by diazepam (3–30 mg/kg), clonazepam (1–10 mg/kg), chlordiazepoxide (10–50 mg/kg), flunitrazepam (1 mg/kg) and clobazam (10 mg/kg).

The level of the major brain noradrenaline metabolite, MOPEG-SO$_4$ (3-methoxy-4-hydroxy-phenylglycol sulphate), is not decreased by diazepam (3–30 mg/kg, i.p.) or Y-7,131 (5 mg/kg, i.p.) (KARASAWA et al., 1978; CONSOLO et al., 1975; SETOGUCHI et al., 1978), indicating no major effects on noradrenaline turnover.

Experimental stresses increase catecholamine turnover. Benzodiazepines (diazepam, 2.5–20 mg/kg; N-desmethyldiazepam, 5 mg/kg; chlordiazepoxide, 10–25 mg/kg; nitrazepam, 20 mg/kg; RO 5,807, 5 mg/kg; Y-7,131, 0.3–2.5 mg/kg) counteract the increased brain catecholamine turnover in response to stress (TAYLOR and LAVERTY, 1969; CORRODI et al., 1971; SETOGUCHI et al., 1978; DOTEUCHI and COSTA, 1973; LIDBRINK et al., 1973).

II. Indirect Effect on Catecholamines

The effects of benzodiazepines on the catecholamines may be secondary to an inhibitory GABA-ergic action on dopamine cell bodies in substantia nigra and noradrenaline cell bodies in locus coeruleus (FUXE et al., 1975). Thus benzodiazepines (1–10 mg/kg) counteract the increase in HVA (KELLER et al., 1976) and the increase in tyrosine hydroxylase activity (GALE et al., 1978) induced by neuroleptic drugs. A low dose of diazepam (0.5 mg/kg) strongly potentiates the increase in mouse brain DOPAC induced by the GABA mimetic muscimol (BIGGIO et al., 1977a). Both diazepam (10 mg/kg) and muscimol inhibit the increased release of ^{3}H-dopamine from striatum of cats induced by the GABA antagonist, picrotoxin (CHERAMY et al., 1977). These studies indicate that benzodiazepines may potentiate the presumed GABA-ergic input into dopamine cell bodies in substantia nigra even though the great complexity of nigral neuronal connections (CHERAMY et al., 1978; SCHEEL-KRÜGER et al., 1978; ARNT and SCHEEL-KRÜGER, 1979) calls for caution.

III. Dopamine Receptors

Diazepam does not interact directly with dopamine receptors (^{3}H-haloperiodol and ^{3}H-dopamine binding to brain membranes) (BURT et al., 1976; SEEMAN et al., 1975) or noradrenaline β-receptors (^{3}H-dihydroalprenolol binding to brain membranes (BYLUND and SNYDER, 1976).

IV. Other Minor Tranquillizers

Barbiturates and meprobamate, like benzodiazepines, counteract stress-induced increased noradrenaline turnover (LIDBRINK et. al., 1972) and barbiturates alone decrease noradrenaline turnover (LIDBRINK et al., 1972; PERSSON and WALDECK, 1971).

G. Miscellaneous

I. Glycine Receptors

An interaction of benzodiazepines with glycine receptors was proposed because diazepam in a high concentration (26 μM) and other benzodiazepines displaced ^{3}H-strychnine from specific binding sites on rat brain membranes (YOUNG et al., 1974). Electrophysiological and biochemical studies have not confirmed the proposed interaction of benzodiazepines with glycine receptors (CURTIS et al., 1976 b; HUNT and RAYNAUD, 1977). Further, glycine and the antagonist, strychnine, exhibit low affinity for benzodiazepine receptors (BRAESTRUP and SQUIRES, 1978 a).

II. Phosphodiesterases

An interaction of benzodiazepines with the "second messenger" cyclic AMP was proposed because diazepam and other benzodiazepines inhibited phosphodiesterase, the enzyme responsible for cyclic AMP metabolism (BEER et al., 1972; HOROVITZ et al., 1972). Many other psychoactive substances, however, inhibit phosphodiesterases (SHEKOLDINA et al., 1978) in similar concentrations, while several potent benzodiazepines are weak phospodiesterase inhibitors.

III. Glucose Metabolism

Intracellular glucose levels in rat brain are reported to be increased by diazepam (4 mg/kg, i.p.) and chlordiazepoxide (10–30 mg/kg, i.p.) (RUTISHAUSER, 1963; NAHORSKI, 1972; GEY, 1973). The brain levels of glycogen, glucose-6-phosphate, fructose 1,6-diphosphate, dihydroxyacetone, pyruvate, lactate and malate are unchanged (GEY, 1973). These results indicated lack of effect of benzodiazepines on glycolysis. Increased glucose levels might reflect increased glucose uptake into the brain. In contrast the hypnotics and neuroleptics inhibited glycolysis.

IV. Chloride Channels

Barbiturates in rather high concentrations (1–100 μM) inhibit the binding of ^{3}H-dihydropicrotoxinin to rat brain membranes (OLSEN et al., 1978 c). This finding suggests that the GABA potentiating effect of barbiturates may involve a chloride channel which is coupled to the GABA receptor.

Acknowledgement. This study was aided by a grant from the Danish Medical Research Council Jr. Nr. 512-8405. I thank Dr. RICHARD F. SQUIRES for critical reading of this manuscript and for valuable cooperation in experimental studies.

References

Arnt, J., Scheel-Krüger, J.: GABA-ergic and glycinergic mechanisms within the Substantia Nigra. Pharmacological specificity of dopamine dependent counterlateral turning behavior and interaction with other neurotransmitters. Psychopharmacology *62*, 267–277 (1979)
Bartholini, G., Keller, H., Pieri, L., Pletscher, A.: Diazepam and cerebral dopamine. In: The benzodiazepines. Garattini, S., Mussini, E., Randall, L.O. (eds.), pp. 235–240. New York: Raven 1973

Beaumont, K., Chilton, W., Yamamura, H.I., Enna, S.J.: Muscimol binding in rat brain: Association with synaptic GABA receptors. Brain Res. 148, 153–162 (1978)

Beer, B., Chasin, M., Clody, D.E., Vogel, J.R., Horovitz, Z.P.: Cyclic adenosine monophosphate phosphodiesterase in brain: Effect on anxiety. Science 176, 428–430 (1972)

Bennett, J.P., Snyder, S.H.: Stereospecific binding of D-lysergic acid diethylamide (LSD) to brain membranes: Relationship to serotonin receptors. Brain Res. 94, 523–544 (1975)

Berger, F.M.: The pharmacology of antianxiety (anxiolytic) agents. In: Psychopharmacological treatment. Denber, H.C.B. (ed.), pp. 135–156. New York: Dekker 1975

Bernasconi, R., Martin, P.: Effects of diazepam and baclofen on the GABA turnover rate in various mouse brain regions. Arch. Pharmacol. [Suppl.] 302, R58 (1978)

Biggio, G., Casu, M., Corda, M.G., Vernaleone, F., Gessa, G.L.: Effect of muscimol, a GABA-mimetic agent, on dopamine metabolism in the mouse brain. Life Sci. 21, 525–532 (1977a)

Biggio, G., Guidotti, A.: Regulation of cyclic GMP in cerebellum by a striatal dopaminergic mechanism. Nature 265, 240–242 (1977)

Biggio, G., Brodie, B.B., Costa, E., Guidotti, A.: Mechanisms by which diazepam muscimol, and other drugs change the content of cGMP in cerebellar cortex. Proc. Natl. Acad. Sci. USA 74, 3592–3596 (1977b)

Biggio, G., Corda, M.G., Casu, M., Gessa, G.L.: Kainic acid-induced lesion of dopaminergic target cells in the striatum: Consequences on the dynamics of cerebellar cGMP. Naunyn-Schmiedebergs Arch. Pharmacol. 304, 5–7 (1978)

Billingsley, M.L., Kubena, R.K.: The effects of naloxone and picrotoxin on the sedative and anticonflict effects of benzodiazepines. Life Sci. 22, 897–906 (1978)

Biswas, B., Carlsson, A.: On the mode of action of diazepam on brain catecholamine metabolism. Naunyn Schmiedebergs Arch. Pharmacol. 303, 73–78 (1978)

Blanchard, J.C., Boireau, A., Jolon, L.: In Vitro and in Vivo Inhibition by zopiclone of benzodiazepine binding to rodent brain receptors. Life Sci. 24, 2417–2420 (1979)

Boakes, R.J., Martin, I.L., Mitchell, P.R.: Burst firing of cerebellar Purkinje neurones induced by benzodiazepines. Neuropharmacology 16, 711–713 (1977)

Bolme, P., Fuxe, K.: Possible involvement of GABA mechanisms in central cardiovascular and respiratory control. Studies on the interaction between diazepam, picrotoxin and clonidine. Med. Biol. 55, 301–309 (1977)

Bosmann, H.B., Case, K.R., DiStefano, P.: Diazepam receptor characterization: specific binding of a benzodiazepine to macromolecules in various areas of rat brain. FEBS Lett. 82, 368–372 (1977)

Bosmann, H.B., Penney, D.P., Case, K.R., DiStefano, P., Averill, K.: Diazepam receptor: specific binding of [³H]diazepam and [³H]flunitrazepam to rat brain subfractions. FEBS Lett. 87, 199–202 (1978)

Bourgoin, S., Héry, F., Ternaux, J.P., Hamon, M.: Effects of benzodiazepines on the binding of tryptophan in serum. Consequences on 5-hydroxyindoles concentrations in the rat brain. Psychopharmacol. Commun. 1, 209–216 (1975)

Bowery, N.G., Dray, A.: Barbiturate reversal of amino acid antagonism produced by consulsant agents. Nature 264, 276–278 (1976)

Bowery, N.G., Dray, A.: Reversal of the action of amino acid antagonists by barbiturates and other hypnotic drugs. Br. J. Pharmacol. 63, 197–215 (1978)

Braestrup, C., Squires, R.F.: Specific benzodiazepine receptor in rat brain characterized by high-affinity ³H-diazepam binding. Proc. Natl. Acad. Sci. USA 74, 3805–3809 (1977)

Braestrup, C., Albrechtsen, R., Squires, R.F.: High densities of benzodiazepine receptors in human cortical areas. Nature 269, 702–704 (1977)

Braestrup, C., Squires, R.F.: Pharmacological characterization of benzodiazepine receptors in the brain. Eur. J. Pharmacol. 78, 263–270 (1978a)

Braestrup, C., Squires, R.F.: Brain specific benzodiazepine receptors. Br. J. Psychiatry 133, 249–260 (1978b)

Braestrup, C., Squires, R.F., Bock, E., Torp Pedersen, C., Nielsen, M.: Benzodiazepine receptors: Cellular and subcellular localization in brain. Adv. Pharm. Ther. 7, 173–185 (1978a)

Braestrup, C., Nissen, C., Squires, R.F., Schousboe, A.: Lack of brain-specific benzodiazepine receptors on mouse primary astroglial cultures, which specifically bind haloperidol. Neurosci. Lett. 9, 45–49 (1978b)

Braestrup, C., Nielsen, M.: Ontogenetic development of benzodiazepine receptors in the rat brain. Brain Res. *147*, 170–173 (1978)

Braestrup, C., Nielsen, M., Squires, R.F.: No changes in rat benzodiazepine receptors after withdrawal from continuous treatment with lorazepam and diazepam. Life Sci. *24*, 347–350 (1979a)

Braestrup, C., Nielsen, M., Squires, R.F.: Neuronal localization of benzodiazepine receptors in cerebellum. Neurosci. Lett. *13*, 219–224, (1979b)

Braestrup, C., Nielsen, M., Nielsen, E.B., Lyon, M.: Benzodiazepine receptors in brain are affected by several different experimental stresses, the changes are small and not unidirectional. Psychopharmacologia, *65*, 273–277 (1979c)

Braestrup, C., Nielsen, M., Krogsgaard-Larsen, P., Falch, E.: Partial agonists for brain GABA/benzodiazepine receptor complex. Nature *280*, 331–333 (1979d)

Braestrup, C., Nielsen, M., Olsen, C-E.: Urinary and brain β-carboline-3-carboxylates as potent inhibitors of brain benzodiazepine receptors. Proc. Natl. Acad. Sci. USA 77, 2288–2292 (1980)

Briley, M.S., Langer, S.Z.: Influence of GABA receptor agonists and antagonist on the binding of ^{3}H-diazepam to the benzodiazepine receptor. Eur. J. Pharmacol. *52*, 129–132 (1978)

Brodersen, R., Sjödin, T., Sjöholm, I.: Independent binding of ligands to human serum albumin. J. Biol. Chem. *252*, 5067–5072 (1977)

Brown, D.A., Constanti, A.: Interaction of pentobarbitone and γ-aminobutyric acid on mammalian sympathetic ganglion cells. Br. J. Pharmacol. *63*, 217–224 (1978)

Burt, D.R., Creese, I., Snyder, S.H.: Properties of [^{3}H] haloperidol and [^{3}H]dopamine binding associated with dopamine receptors in calf brain membranes. Mol. Pharmacol. *12*, 800–812 (1976)

Bylund, D., Snyder, S.H.: Beta adrenergic receptor binding in membrane preparations from mammalian brain. Mol. Pharmacol. *12*, 568–580 (1976)

Chang, R.S.L., Snyder, S.H.: Benzodiazepine receptors: Labeling in intact animals with [^{3}H]flunitrazepam. Eur. J. Pharmacol. *48*, 213–218 (1978)

Chase, T.N., Katz, R.I., Kopin, I.J.: Effect of diazepam on fate of intracisternally injected serotonin-C^{14}. Neuropharmacology *9*, 103–108 (1970)

Chéramy, A., Nieoullon, A., Glowinski, J.: Blockade of the picrotoxin-induced in vivo release of dopamine in the cat caudate nucleus by diazepam. Life Sci. *20*, 811–816 (1977)

Chéramy, A., Nieoullon, A., Glowinski, J.: Gabaergic processes involved in the control of dopamine release from nigrostriatal dopaminergic neurons in the cat. Eur. J. Pharmacol. *48*, 281–295 (1978)

Chieu, T.H., Rosenberg, H.C.: Reduced diazepam binding following chronic benzodiazepine treatment. Life Sci. *23*, 1153–1158 (1978)

Chieu, T.H., Rosenberg, H.C.: GABA receptor-mediated modulation of ^{3}H-diazepam binding in rat cortex. Eur. J. Pharmacol. *56*, 337–345 (1979)

Choi, D.W., Farb, D.H., Fischbach, G.D.: Chlordiazepoxide selectively augments GABA action in spinal cord cell cultures. Nature *269*, 342–344 (1977)

Consolo, S., Ladinsky, H., Peri, G., Garattini, S.: Effect of central stimulants and depressant on mouse brain acetylcholine and choline levels. Eur. J. Pharmacol. *18*, 251–255 (1972)

Consolo, S., Ladinsky, H., Peri, G., Garattini, S.: Effect of diazepam on mouse whole brain and brain area acetylcholine and choline levels. Eur. J. Pharmacol. *27*, 266–268 (1974)

Consolo, S., Garattini, S., Ladinsky, H.: Action of the benzodiazepines on the cholinergic system. In: Mechanism of action of benzodiazepines. Costa, E., Greengard, P. (eds.), pp. 63–80. New York: Raven 1975

Consolo, S., Ladinsky, H., Bianchi, S., Ghezzi, D.: Apparent lack of a dopaminergic-cholinergic link in the rat nucleus accumbens septi-tuberculum olfactorium. Brain Res. *135*, 255–263 (1977)

Cook, L., Sepinwall, J.: Behavioral analysis of the effects and mechanisms of action of benzodiazepines. In: Mechanism of action of benzodiazepines. Costa, E., Greengard, P. (eds.), pp. 1–28. New York: Raven 1975

Cook, L., Sepinwall, J.: Relationship of anticonflict activity of benzodiazepines to brain receptor binding, serotonin, and GABA. ACNP December 1978

Cooper, B., Handin, R.I., Young, L.H., Alexander, R.W.: Agonist regulation of the human platelet α-adrenergic receptor. Nature *274*, 703–706 (1978)

Corrodi, H., Fuxe, K., Lidbrink, P., Olson, L.: Minor tranquillizers, stress and central catechol-amine neurons. Brain Res. *29*, 1–16 (1971)

Costa, E., Guidotti, A., Mao, C.C., Suria, A.: New concepts on the mechanism of action of benzodiazepines. Life Sci. *17*, 167–186 (1975a)

Costa, E., Guidotti, A., Mao, C.C.: Diazepam, cyclic nucleotides and amino acid neurotrans-mitters in rat cerebellum. In: Neuropsychopharmacology. Boissier, J.R., Hippius, H., Pichot, P. (eds.), pp. 849–856. Amsterdam: Excerpta Medica 1975b

Costa, E., Guidotti, A., Mao, C.C.: Evidence for involvement of GABA in the action of ben-zodiazepines. In: Mechanism of action of benzodiazepines. Costa, E., Greengard, P. (eds.), pp. 113–130. New York: Raven 1975c

Costa, E., Guidotti, A., Toffano, G.: Molecular mechanisms mediating the action of diazepam on GABA receptors. Br. J. Psychiatry. *133*, 239–248 (1978)

Costa, T., Rodbard, D., Pert, C.B.: The benzodiazepine receptor coupled to a chloride anionic channel. Nature *277*, 315–317 (1979)

Curtis, D.R., Lodge, D., Johnston, G.A.R., Brand, S.J.: Central actions of benzodiazepines. Brain Res. *118*, 344–347 (1976a)

Curtis, D.R., Game, C.J.A., Lodge, D.: Benzodiazepines and central glycine receptors. Br. J. Pharmacol. *56*, 307–311 (1976b)

Curtis, D.R., Lodge, D.: Pentobarbitone enhancement of the inhibitory action of GABA. Na-ture *270*, 543–544 (1977a)

Curtis, D.R., Lodge, D.: Effect of pentobarbitone on the inhibition of spinal interneurones, in the cat by glycine and GABA. J. Physiol. (Lond.) *272*, 48P–49P (1977b)

DaPrada, M., Pletscher, A.: On the mechanism of chlorpromazine-induced changes of cerebral homovanillic acid levels. J. Pharm. Pharmacol. *18*, 628–630 (1966)

Davidoff, R.A.: Diphenylhydantoin increases spinal presynaptic inhibition. Trans. Am. Neurol. Assoc. *97*, 193–196 (1972)

Davies, J., Polc, P.: Effect of a water soluble benzodiazepine on the responses of spinal neurones to acetylcholine and excitatory amino acid analogues. Neuropharmacology *17*, 217–220 (1978)

DeBlas, A., Mahler, H.R.: Studies on nicotinic acetylcholine receptors in mammalian brain. Characterization of a microsomal subfraction enriched in receptor function for different neurotransmitters. J. Neurochem. *30*, 563–577 (1978)

Deisz, R.A., Lux, H.D.: Diphenylhydantoin prolongs postsynaptic inhibition and ionto-phoretic GABA action in the crayfish stretch receptor. Neurosci. Lett. *5*, 199–203 (1977)

Dominic, J.A., Sinha, A.K., Barchas, J.D.: Effect of benzodiazepine compounds on brain amine metabolism. Eur. J. Pharmacol. *32*, 124–127 (1975)

Domino, E.F., Wilson, A.E.: Psychotropic drug influences on brain acetylcholine utilization. Psychopharmacology *25*, 291–298 (1972)

Doteuchi, M., Costa, E.: Pentylenetetrazol convulsions and brain catecholamine turnover rate in rats and mice receiving diphenylhydantoin or benzodiazepines. Neuropharmacology *12*, 1059–1072 (1973)

Dray, A., Straughan, D.W.: Benzodiazepines: GABA and glycine receptors on single neurons in the rat medulla. J. Pharm. Pharmacol. *28*, 314–315 (1976)

Eccles, J.C., Schmidt, R., Willis, W.D.: Pharmacological studies on presynaptic inhibition. J. Physiol. (Lond.) *168*, 500–530 (1963)

Evans, R.H.: GABA-potentiating action of pentobarbitone on the isolated superior cervical ganglion of the rat. J. Physiol. (Lond.) *272*, 49P–50P (1977)

Fennessy, M.R., Lee, J.R.: The effect of benzodiazepines on brain amines of the mouse. Arch. Int. Pharmacodyn. Ther. *197*, 37–44 (1972)

Fernholm, B., Nielsen, M., Braestrup, C.: Absence of brain specific benzodiazepine receptors in cyclostomes and elasmobranchs. Comp. Biochem. Pysiol. *62C*, 209–211 (1979)

Fernstrom, J.D., Shabshelowitz, H., Faller, D.V.: Diazepam increases 5-hydroxyindole concen-trations in rat brain and spinal cord. Life Sci. *15*, 1577–1584 (1974)

File, S.E., Hyde, J.R.G.: The effects of *p*-chlorophenylalanine and ethanolamine *O*-sulphate in an animal test of anxiety. J. Pharm. Pharmacol. *29*, 735–738 (1977)

File, S.E., Velucci, S.V.: Studies on the role of ACTH and of 5-HT in anxiety using an animal model. J. Pharm. Pharmacol. *30*, 105–110 (1978)

Fuxe, K., Agnati, L.F., Bolme, P., Hökfelt, T., Lidbrink, P., Ljungdahl, Å, Mora, P. de la, Ögren, S.V.: The possible involvement of GABA mechanisms in the action of benzodiazepines on central catecholamine neurons. In: Mechanism of action of benzodiazepines. Costa, E., Greengard, P. (eds.), pp. 45–61. New York: Raven 1975

Gähwiler, B.H.: Diazepam and chlordiazepoxide: powerful GABA antagonists in explants of rat cerebellum. Brain Res. *107*, 176–179 (1976)

Gale, K., Costa, E., Toffano, G., Hong, J.-S., Guidotti, A.: Evidence for a role of nigral γ-aminobutyric acid and substance P in the haloperidol-induced activation of striatal tyrosine hydroxylase. J. Pharmacol. Exp. Ther. *206*, 29–37 (1978)

Gallager, D.W.: Benzodiazepines: Potentiation of a GABA inhibitory response in the dorsal raphe nucleus. Eur. J. Pharmacol. *49*, 133–143 (1978)

Gallager, D.W., Thomas, J.W., Tallman, F.: Effect of GABAergic drugs on benzodiazepine binding site sensitivity in rat cerebral cortex. Biochem. Pharmac. *27*, 2745–2749 (1978)

Gey, K.F.: Effect of benzodiazepines on carbohydrate metabolism in rat brain. In: The Benzodiazepines. Garattini, S., Mussini, E., Randall, L.O. (eds.), pp. 243–255. New York: Raven 1973

Giarman, N.J., Pepeu, G.: Drug-induced changes in brain acetylcholine. Br. J. Pharmacol. *19*, 226–234 (1962)

Govoni, S., Fresia, P., Spano, P.F., Trabucchi, M.: Effect of desmethyldiazepam and chlordesmethyldiazepam on 3′,5′-cyclic guanosine monophosphate levels in rat cerebellum. Psychopharmacology *50*, 241–244 (1976)

Guidotti, A.: Synaptic mechanisms in the action of benzodiazepines. In: Psychopharmacology: A Generation of Progress. Lipton, M.A., DiMascio, A., Killam, K.F. (eds.), pp. 1349–1357. New York: Raven 1978

Guidotti, A., Toffano, G., Costa, E.: An endogenous protein modulates the affinity of GABA and benzodiazepine receptors in rat brain. Nature *275*, 553–555 (1978a)

Guidotti, A., Toffano, G., Costa, E.: A molecular mechanism for the action of benzodiazepines on GABA receptors. In: GABA-Neurotransmitters. Krogsgaard-Larsen, P., Scheel-Krüger, J., Kofod, H. (eds.), pp. 406–419, Copenhagen: Munksgaard 1978b

Haefely, W., Kulcsár, Möhler, Pieri, L., Polc, P., Schaffner, R.: Possible involvement of GABA in the central actions of benzodiazepines. In: Mechanism of action of benzodiazepines. Costa, E., Greengard, P. (eds.), pp. 131–151. New York: Raven 1975

Haefely, W., Polc, P., Schaffner, R., Keller, H.H., Pieri, I., Möhler, H.: Facilitation of GABA-ergic transmission by drugs. In: GABA-Neurotransmitters. The Alfred Benzon Symposium. Krogsgaard-Larsen, P., Scheel-Krüger, J., Kofod, H. (eds.), pp. 357–375. Copenhagen: Munksgaard 1978

Harris, M., Hopkin, J. M., Neal, M.J.: Effect of centrally acting drugs on the uptake of γ-aminobutyric acid (GABA) by slices of rat cerebral cortex. Br. J. Pharmacol. *47*, 229–239 (1973)

Henn, F.A., Henke, D.J., Cellular localization of [³H]-diazepam receptors. Neuropharmacology *17*, 985–988 (1978)

Horovitz, Z.P., Beer, B., Clody, D.E., Vogel, J.R., Chasin, M.: Cyclic AMP and anxiety. Psychosomatics *13*, 85–92 (1972)

Hunt, P., Raynaud, J.-P.: Benzodiazepine activity: is interaction with the glycine receptor, as evidenced by displacement of strychnine binding, a useful criterion? J. Pharm. Pharmacol. *29*, 442–444 (1979)

Iversen, L.L., Johnston, G.A.R.: GABA uptake in rat central nervous system: comparison of uptake in slices and homogenates and the effects of some inhibitors. J. Neurochem. *18*, 1939–1950 (1971)

Jenner, P., Chadwick, D., Reynolds, E.H., Marsden, C.D.: Altered 5-HT metabolism with clonazepam, diazepam and dipenylhydantoin. J. Pharm. Pharmacol. *27*, 707–710 (1975)

Juhasz, L., Dairman, W.: Effect of sub-acute diazepam administration in mice on the subsequence ability of diazepam to protect against metrazol and bicuculline induced convulsions. Fed. Proc. *36*, 377 (1977)

Karasawa, T., Furukawa, K., Ochi, Y., Shimizu, M.: Monoamine metabolites as indicators of the effect of centrally acting drugs on monoamine release in rat brain. Arch. int. Pharmacodyn. *231*, 261–273 (1978)

Karobath, M., Lippitsch, M.: THIP and isoguvacine are partial agonists of GABA-stimulated benzodiazepine receptor binding. Eur. J. Pharmacol. *58*, 485–488 (1979)

Karobath, M., Sperk, G.: Stimulation of benzodiazepine receptor binding by γ-aminobutyric acid. Proc. Natl. Acad. Sci. USA *76*, 1004–1006 (1979)

Karobath, M., Placheta, P., Lippitsch, M., Krogsgaard-Larsen, P.: Is stimulation of benzodiazepine receptor binding mediated by a novel GABA receptor? Nature *278*, 748–749 (1979)

Keller, H.H., Schaffner, R., Haefely, W.: Interaction of benzodiazepines with neuroleptics at central dopamine neurons. Naunyn-Schmiedebergs Arch. Pharmacol. *294*, 1–7 (1976)

Kozhechkin, S.N., Ostrovskaya, R.U.: Are benzodiazepines GABA antagonists? Nature *269*, 72–73 (1977)

Ladinsky, H., Consolo, S., Peri, G., Garattini, S.: Increase in mouse and rat brain acetylcholine levels by diazepam. In: The Benzodiazepines. S. Garattini, E. Mussini, Randall, L.O. (eds.), pp. 241–242. New York: Raven Press 1973

Ladinsky, H., Consolo, S., Bellantuono, C., Garattini, S.: Interaction of benzodiazepines and chemical mediators in the brain. To be published in Handbook of Biological Psychiatry, Rafaelsen and Lader (eds.) New York: Marcel Dekker, Inc. 1979 (in press).

Lidbrink, P., Corrodi, H., Fuxe, K., Olson, L.: Barbiturates and meprobamate: decreases in catecholamine turnover of central dopamine and noradrenaline neuronal systems and the influcence of immobilization stress. Brain Res. *45*, 507–524 (1972)

Lidbrink, P., Corrodi, H., Fuxe, K., Olson, L.: The effects of benzodiazepines meprobamate, and barbiturates on central monoamine neurons: In: The Benzodiazepines, pp. 203–220. Garattini, S., Mussini, E., Randall, L.O. (eds.). New York: Raven Press 1973

Lidbrink, P., Corrodi, H., Fuxe, K.: Benzodiazepines and barbiturates: Turnover changes in central 5-hydroxytryptamine pathways. Eur. J. Pharmacol. *26*, 35–40 (1974)

Lingjaerde, O.: Effect of benzodiazepines on uptake and efflux of serotonin in human blood patelets in vitro. In: The benzodiazepines. Garattini, S., Mussini, E., Randall, L.O. (eds.), pp. 225–233. New York: Raven 1973

Lippa, A.S., Regan, B.: Additional studies on the importance of glycine and GABA in mediating the actions of benzodiazepines. Life Sci. *21*, 1779–1784 (1977)

Lippa, A.S., Critchett, D., Sano, M.C., Klepner, C.A., Greenblatt, E.N., Coupet, J., Beer, B.: Benzodiazepine Receptors: Cellular and Behavioral Characteristics. Pharmacol. Biochem. Behav. *10*, 831–843 (1979)

Lippa, A.S., Sano, M.C., Coupet, J., Beer, B.: Evidence that benzodiazepine receptors reside on cerebellar purkinje cells: Studies with "nervous" mutant mice. Life Sci. *23*, 2213–2218 (1978)

Löscher, W., Frey, H.-H.: Effect of convulsant and anticonvulsant agents on level and metabolism of γ-aminobutyric acid in mouse brain. Naunyn-Schmiedebergs Arch. Pharmacol. *296*, 263–269 (1977)

Lundy, P.M., Magor, G.F.: Cyclic GMP concentrations in cerebellum following organophosphate administration. J. Pharm. Pharmacol. *30*, 251–252 (1978)

MacDonald, R., Barker, J.L.: Benzodiazepines specifically modulate GABA-mediated postsynaptic inhibition in cultured mammalian neurones. Nature *271*, 563–564 (1978)

Mackerer, C.R., Kochman, R.L.: Effects of cations and anions on the binding of ^{3}H-diazepam to rat brain. Proc. Soc. Exp. Biol. Med. *158*, 393–397 (1978)

Mackerer, C.R., Kochman, R.L., Bierschenk, A., Bremner, S.S.: The binding of [^{3}H] diazepam to rat brain. J. Pharmacol. Exp. Ther. *206*, 405–413 (1978)

Mailman, R.B., Frye, G.D., Mueller, R.A., Breese, G.R.: Thyrotropin-releasing hormone reversal of ethanol-induced decrease in cerebellar cGMP. Nature *272*, 832–833 (1978)

Maisov, N.I., Tolmacheva, N.S., Raevsky, K.S.: Liberation of ^{3}H-gamma-aminobutyric acid (^{3}H-GABA) from isolated nerve endings of the rat's brain under the effect of psychotropic substances (in Russian). Farmakol. Toksikol. *39*, 517–520 (1976)

Mao, C.C., Guidotti, A., Costa, E.: The regulation of cyclic guanosine monophosphate in rat cerebellum: possible involvement of putative amino acid neurotransmitters. Brain Res. *79*, 510–514 (1974a)

Mao, C.C., Guidotti, A., Costa, E.: Interactions between γ-aminobutyric acid and guanosine cyclic 3′,5′-monophosphate in rat cerebellum. Mol. Pharmacol. *10*, 736–745 (1974b)

Mao, C.C., Guidotti, A., Costa,: Inhibition by diazepam of the tremor and the increase of cerebellar cGMP content elicited by harmaline. Brain Res. *83*, 516–519 (1975 a)

Mao, C.C., Guidotti, A., Costa, E.: Evidence for an involvement of GABA in the mediation of the cerebellar cGMP decrease and the anticonvulsant action of diazepam. Naunyn-Schmiedebergs Arch. Pharmacol. *289*, 369–378 (1975 b)

Mao, C.C., Marco, E., Revuelta, A., Bertilsson, L., Costa, E.: The turnover rate of γ-aminobutyric acid in the nuclei of telencephalon: Implications in the pharmacology of antipsychotics and of a minor tranquilizer. Biol. Psychiatry *12*, 359–371 (1977)

Martin, I.L., Candy, J.M.: Facilitation of benzodiazepine binding by sodium chloride and GABA. Neuropharmacology *17*, 993–998 (1978)

Maruyama, S., Kawasaki, T.: Further electrophysiological evidence of the GABA-like effect of droperidol in the purkinje cells of the cat cerebellum. Jpn. J. Pharmacol. *26*, 765–767 (1976)

Mattsson, H., Brandt, K., Heilbronn, E.. Bicyclic phosphorus esters increase the cyclic GMP level in rat cerebellum. Nature *268*, 52–53 (1977)

Maurer, R.: The GABA agonist THIP, a muscimol analogue, does not interfere with the benzodiazepine binding site on rats cortical membranes. Neurosci. Lett. *12*, 65–68 (1979)

Mitchell, P.R., Martin, I.L.: The effects of benzodiazepines of K$^+$-stimulated release of GABA. Neuropharmacology *17*, 317–320 (1978)

Miyahara, J.T., Esplin, D.W., Zablocka, B.: Differential effects of depressant drugs on presynaptic inhibition. J. Pharmacol. Exp. Ther. *154*, 119–127 (1966)

Mori, A., Ohkusu, H., Kohsaka, M., Kurono, M.: Isolation of hypoxanthine from calf brain. J. Neurochem. *20*, 1291–1292 (1973)

Möhler, H., Okada, T.: Properties of ^{3}H-diazepam binding to benzodiazepine receptors in the rat cerebral cortex. Life Sci. *20*, 2101 (1977 a)

Möhler, A., Okada, T.: Benzodiazepine receptor: Demonstration in the central nervous system. Science *198*, 848–851 (1977 b)

Möhler, A., Okada, T.: GABA receptor binding with ^{3}H(+) bicuculline-methiodide in rat CNS. Nature *267*, 65–67 (1977 c)

Möhler, H., Okada, T.: The benzodiazepine receptor in normal and pathological human brain. Br. J. Psychiatry *133*, 261–268 (1978)

Möhler, H., Okada, T., Heitz, Ph., Ulrich, J.: Biochemical identification of the site of action of benzodiazepines in human brain by ^{3}H-diazepam binding. Life Sci. *22*, 985–996 (1978 a)

Möhler, H., Okada, T., Enna, S.J.: Benzodiazepine and neurotransmitter receptor binding in rat brain after chronic administration of diazepam or phenobarbital. Brain Res. *156*, 391–395 (1978 b)

Möhler, H., Polc, P., Cumin, R., Pieri, L., Kettler, R.: Nicotinamide is a brain constituent with benzodiazepine-like actions. Nature *278*, 563–565 (1979)

Müller, W., Wollert, U.: Characterization of the binding of benzodiazepines to human serum albumin. Naunyn-Schmiedebergs Arch. Pharmacol. *280*, 229–237 (1973)

Müller, W., Wollert, U.: High stereospecificity of the benzodiazepine binding site on human serum albumin. Mol. Pharmacol. *11*, 52–60 (1975 a)

Müller, W., Wollert, U.: Benzodiazepines: Specific competitors for the binding of 1-tryptophan to human serum albumin. Naunyn-Schmiedebergs Arch. Pharmacol. *288*, 17–27 (1975 b)

Müller, W., Wollert, U.: Interaction of benzodiazepine derivates with bovine serum albumin. J. Biochem. Pharmacol. *25*, 141–145 (1976)

Müller, W., Schläfer, U., Wollert, U.: Benzodiazepine receptor binding in rat spinal cord membranes. Neurosci. Lett. *9*, 239–243 (1978)

Nahorski, S.R.: Biochemical effects of the anticonvulsants trimethadione, ethosuximide and chlordiazepoxide in rat brain. J. Neurochem. *19*, 1937–1946 (1972)

Nakamura, K., Nakamura, K.: Interaction of benzodiazepine drugs with striatal dopaminergic neurons in the brain. Jpn. J. Pharmacol. [Suppl.] *26*, 101P (1976)

Nakamura, M., Fukushima, H.: Effect of benzodiazepines on central serotonergic neuron systems. Psychopharmacology *53*, 121–126 (1977)

Nelson-Krause, D.C., Howard, B.D.: Release of glycine and gamma aminobutyric acid from synaptosomes prepared from rat central nervous tissue. Fed. Proc. *35*, 543 (1976)

Nicoll, R.A.: The effects of anesthetics on synaptic excitation and inhibition in the olfactory bulb. J. Physiol. (Lond.) *223*, 803–814 (1972)

Nicoll, R.A.: Presynaptic action of barbiturates in the frog spinal cord. Proc. Natl. Acad. Sci. USA *72*, 1460–1463 (1975a)

Nicoll, R.A.: Pentobarbital: action on frog motoneurons. Brain Res. *96*, 119–123 (1975b)

Nicoll, R.A.: Pentobarbital: Differential postsynaptic actions on sympathetic ganglion cells. Science *199*, 451–452 (1978)

Nielsen, M., Braestrup, C., Squires, R.F.: Evidence for a late evolutionary appearance of brain-specific benzodiazepine receptors: an investigation of 18 vertebrate and 5 invertebrate species. Brain Res. *141*, 342–346 (1978)

Nielsen, M., Nielsen, E.B., Ellison, G., Braestrup, C.: Modification of dopamine receptors in brain by continuous amphetamine administrations to rats. IInd World Congress of Biol. Psychiatry. Barcelona 1979 to be published, a

Nielsen, M., Gredal, O., Braestrup, C.: Some properties of ^{3}H-diazepam displacing activity from human urine. Life Sci. *25*, 679–686 (1979b)

Olsen, R.W., Lamar, E.E., Bayless, J.D.: Calcium-induced release of γ-aminobutyric acid from synaptosomes: Effects of tranquilizer drugs. J. Neurochem. *28*, 299–305 (1977)

Olsen, R.W., Greenlee, D., Ness, P. van, Ticku, M.K.: Studies on the gammaaminobutyric acid receptor/ionophore proteins in mammalian brain. In: Amino acids as neurotransmitter. Fonnum, F. (ed.), pp. 467–486. New York: Plenum 1978a

Olsen, R.W., Ticku, M.K., Ness, P. van, Greenlee, D.: Effects of drugs on γ-aminobutyric acid receptors, uptake, release and synthesis in vitro. Brain Res. *139*, 277–294 (1978b)

Olsen, R.W., Ticku, M.K., Greenlee, D., Ness, P. van: GABA receptor and ionophore binding sites: Interaction with various drugs. In: GABA-Neurotransmitters. Alfred Benzon Symposium. Krogsgaard-Larsen, P., Scheel-Krüger, J., Kofod, H. (eds.), p. 28. Copenhagen: Munkgsgaard 1978c

Opmeer, F.A., Gumulka, S.W., Dinnendahl, V., Schönhöfer, P.S.: Effects of stimulatory and depressant drugs on cyclic guanosine 3′,5′-monophosphate and adenosine 3′,5′-monophosphate levels in mouse brain. Naunyn Schmiedebergs Arch. Pharmacol. *292*, 259–265 (1976)

Ostrovskaya, R.U., Molodavkin, G.M.: A study of the GABA-ergic action mechanism of diazepam on the cortical neurons (in Russian). Byul. Eksp. Bil. Med. *82*, 1073–1076 (1976)

Ostrovskaya, R.U., Voronina, T.A.: Antagonistic effects of bicuculline and thiosemicarbazide on diazepam tranquilizing action (in Russian). Byul. Eksp. Biol. Med. *83*, 293–295 (1977)

Paul, S.M., Skolnick, P.: Rapid changes in brain benzodiazepine receptors after experimental seizures. Science *202*, 892–894 (1978)

Pericic, D., Walters, J.R., Chase, T.N.: Effects of diazepam and pentobarbital on amino-oxyacetic acid-induced accumulation of GABA. J. Neurochem. *29*, 839–846 (1977)

Persson, T., Waldeck, B.: A reduced rate of turnover of brain noradrenaline during pentobarbitone anaesthesia. J. Pharm. Pharmacol. *23*, 377–378 (1971)

Pieri, L., Haefely, W.: The effect of diphenylhydantoin, diazepam and clonazepam on the activity of purkinje cells in the rat cerebellum. Naunyn Schmiedebergs Arch. Pharmacol. *296*, 1–4 (1976)

Pletscher, A.: Biochemistry and psychosomatic medicine: The effects of psychotropic drugs on neurohumoral transmitters. In: Psychotropic drugs in internal medicine. Pletscher, A., Marino, A., Pinkerton, P. (eds.), pp. 1–15. Amsterdam: Excerpta Medica 1969

Polc, P., Möhler, H., Haefely, W.: The effect of diazepam on spinal cord activities, possile sites and mechanisms of action. Naunyn Schmiedebergs Arch. Pharmacol. *284*, 319–337 (1974)

Polc, P., Haefely, W.: Effects of two benzodiazepines, phenobarbitone, and baclofen on synaptic transmission in the cat cuneate nucleus. Naunyn Schmiedebergs Arch. Pharmacol. *294*, 121–131 (1976)

Polzin, R., Barnes, C.D.: The effect of diazepam and picrotoxin on brainstem evoked dorsal root potentials. Neuropharmacology *15*, 133–137 (1976)

Pugsley, T.A., Lippmann, W.: Effects of pyrroxan and chlordiazepoxide on biogenic amine metabolism in the rat brain. Psychopharmacology *50*, 113–118 (1976)

Raabe, W., Ayala, G.F.: Diphenylhydantoin increases cortical postsynaptic inhibition. Brain Res. *105*, 597–601 (1976)

Raff, M.: Self regulation of membrane receptors. Nature *259*, 265–266 (1976)

Randall, L.O., Schallek, W., Sternbach, L.H., Ning, R.Y.: Chemistry and pharmacology of the 1,4-benzodiazepines. In: Psychoharmacological agents. Gordon, M. (ed.), Vol. 3, pp. 175–281. New York: Academic Press 1974

Rastogi, R.B., Agarwal, R.A., Lapierre, Y.D., Singhal, R.L.: Effects of acute diazepam and clobazam on spontaneous locomotor activity and central amino metabolism in rats. Eur. J. Pharmacol. 43, 91–98 (1977)

Reisine, T.D., Wastek, G.J., Yamamura, H.I.: Alterations in benzodiazepine binding sites in Huntington's disease. Pharmacologist 20, 240 (1978)

Rutishauser, M.: Beeinflussung des Kohlenhydratstoffwechsels des Rattenhirns durch Psychopharmaka mit sedativer Wirkung. Naunyn Schmiedebergs Arch. Pharmacol. 245, 396–413 (1963)

Saad, S.F.: Effect of diazepam on γ-aminobutyric acid (GABA) content of mouse brain. J. Pharm. Pharmacol. 24, 839–840 (1972)

Saad, S.F., El Masry, A.M., Scott, P.M.: Influence of certain anticonvulsants on the concentration of γ-aminobutyric acid in the cerebral hemispheres of mice. Eur. J. Pharmacol. 17, 386–392 (1972)

Sawaya, M.C., Horton, R.W., Meldrum, B.S.: Effects of anticonvulsant drugs on the cerebral enzymes metabolizing GABA. Epilepsia 16, 649–655 (1975)

Schaffner, R., Haefely, W.: The effects of diazepam and bicuculline on the striato-nigral evoked potential. Experientia 31, 732 (1975)

Scheel-Krüger, J., Arnt, J., Braestrup, C., Christensen, V., Magelund, G.: Development of new animal models for GABA-ergic actions using muscimol as a tool. In: GABA-Neurotransmitters. The Alfred Benzon Symposium. Kofod, H., Krogsgaard-Larsen, P., Scheel-Krüger, J. (eds.), pp. 447–464. Copenhagen: Munksgaard 1978

Schlosser, W.: Action of diazepam on the spinal cord. Arch. Int. Pharmacodyn. Ther. 194, 93–102 (1971)

Schmidt, R.F., Vogel, M.E., Zimmermann, M.: Die Wirkung von Diazepam auf die präsynaptische Hemmung und andere Rückenmarksreflexe. Naunyn Schmiedebergs Arch. Pharmacol. 258, 69–82 (1967)

Seeman, P., Chau-Wong, M., Tedesco, J., Wong, K.: Brain receptors for antipsychotic drugs and dopamine: Direct binding assays. Proc. Natl. Acad. Sci. USA 72, 4376–4380 (1975)

Sethy, V.H.: Effect of hypnotic and anxiolytic agents on regional concentration of acetylcholine in rat brain. Naunyn Schmidebergs Arch. Pharmacol. 301, 157–161 (1978)

Setoguchi, M., Takehara, S., Nakajima, A., Tsumagari, T., Takigawa, Y.: Effects of 6-(o-Chlorophenyl)-8-ethyl-1-methyl-4H-s-triazolo [3,4-c]thieno [2,3-e] [1,4]diazepine (Y-7,131) on the metabolism of biogenic amines in brain. Arzneim. Forsch. 28, 1165–1173 (1978)

Sharman, D.F.: Changes in the metabolism of 3,4-dihydroxyphenylethylamine (dopamine) in the striatum of the mouse induced by drugs. Br. J. Pharmacol. 28, 153–163 (1966)

Shekoldina, T.G., Vatolkina, O.E., Libinzon, R.E.: Effect of psychotropic preparations on the activity of cAMP phosphodiesterase in brain cortex (in Russian). Vopr. Med. Khim. 24, 166–169 (1978)

Shibuya, T.: Effects of benzodiazepines on brain monoamines. Jpn. J. Pharmacol. [Suppl.] 26, 102P (1976)

Skolnick, P., Marangos, P.J., Goodwin, P.K., Edwards, M., Paul, S.: Identification of inosine and hypoxanthine as endogenous inhibitors of ^{3}H diazepam in the central nervous system. Life Sci. 23, 1473–1480 (1978)

Soubrié, P., Simon, P., Boissier, J.R.: Antagonism of diazepam against central anticholinergic drug-induced hyperactivity in mice: involvement of a GABA mechanism. Neuropharmacology 15, 773–776 (1976)

Speth, R.C., Wastek, G.J., Johnson, P.C., Yamamura, H.I.: Benzodiazepine binding in human brain: Characterization using ^{3}H flunitrazepam. Life Sci. 22, 859–866 (1978)

Squires, R.F., Braestrup, C.: Benzodiazepine receptors in rat brain. Nature 266, 732–734 (1977)

Squires, R., Naquet, R., Riche, D., Braestrup, C.: Increased thermolability of benzodiazepine receptors in cerebral cortex of a baboon with spontaneous seizures. Epilepsia 20, 215–221, (1979a)

Squires, R.F., Beer, B., Benson, D.I., Coupet, J., Klepner, C.A., Lippa, A.S., Myers, V.: Some evidence for two or more brain-specific benzodiazepine receptors. Pharmacol. Biochem. Behav. 10, 825–830 (1979b)

Stein, L. Wise, C.D., Berger, B.D.: Antianxiety action of benzodiazepines. Drecrease in activity of serotonin neurons in the punishment system. In: The Benzodiazepines. Garattini, S., Mussini, E., Randall, L.O. (eds.), 299–326. New York: Raven 1973

Stein, L., Wise, C.D., Belluzzi, J.D.: Effects of benzodiazepines on central serotonergic mechanisms. In: Mechanism of action of benzodiazepines. Costa, E., Greengard, P. (eds.), pp. 29–44. New York: Raven 1975

Stein, L., Beluzzi, J.D., Wise, C.D.: Benzodiazepines: Behavioral and neurochemical mechanism. Am J. Psychiatry 134, 665–669 (1977)

Steiner, F.A., Felix, D.: Antagonistic effects of GABA and benzodiazepines on vestibular and cerebellar neurones. Nature 260, 346–347 (1976)

Stone, W.E., Javid, M.J.: Benzodiazepines and phenobarbital as antagonists of dissimilar chemical convulsants. Epilepsia 19, 361–368 (1978)

Stratten, W.P., Barnes, C.D.: Diazepam and presynaptic inhibition. Neuropharmacology 10, 685–696 (1971)

Sullivan, J.W., Sepinwall, J., Cook, L.: Anticonflict evaluation of muscimol, a GABA receptor agonist, alone and in combination with diazepam. Faseb 1978

Syapin, P.J., Skolnick, P.: Characterization of benzodiazepine binding sites in cultured cells of neural origin. J. Neurochem. 32, 1047–1051 (1979)

Tallman, J.F., Thomas, J.W., Gallager, D.W.: GABAergic modulation of benzodiazepine binding site sensitivity. Nature 274, 383–384 (1978)

Tarver, J., Bautz, G., Horst, W.D.: A new method for the determination of γ-aminobutyric acid (GABA) in brain. Fed. Proc. 34 (1975)

Tata, J.R.: Hormonal regulation of hormone receptors. Nature 257, 740–741 (1975)

Taylor, K.M., Laverty, R.: The effect of chlordiazepoxide, diazepam and nitrazepam on catecholamine metabolism in regions of the rat brain. Eur. J. Pharmacol. 8, 296–301 (1969)

Taylor, K.M., Laverty, R.: The interaction of chlordiazepoxide, diazepam, and nitrazepam with catecholamine and histamine in regions of the rat brain. In: The Benzodiazepines. Garattini, S., Mussini, E., Randall, L.O. (eds.), pp. 191–202. New York: Raven 1973

Thiebot, M.H., Jobert, A., Soubrie, P.: Effects compares du muscimol et du diazepam sur les inhibitions du comportements induite chez le rat par la nouveaute la punition et le nonreinforcement. Psychopharmacology 61, 85–89 (1979)

Toffano, G., Guidotti, A., Costa, E.: Purification of an endogenous protein inhibitor of the high affinity binding of γ-aminobutyric acid to synaptic membranes of rat brain. Proc. Natl. Acad. Sci. USA 75, 4024–4028 (1978)

Tonkopy, V.D., Sofronov, G.A., Alexandriiskaya, I.E., Brestkina, L.M.: Study of the mechanism of diazepam influence on acetylcholine level in the mouse brain (in Russian). Byul. Eksp. Biol. Med. 86, 38–40 (1978)

Tsuchiya, T., Fukushima, H.: Effects of benzodiazepines and pentobarbitone on the GABAergic recurrent inhibition of hippocampal neurons. Eur. J. Pharmacol. 48, 421–424 (1978)

Volicer, L., Puri, S.K., Choima, P.: Cyclic GMP and GABA levels in rat striatum and cerebellum during morphine withdrawal: Effect of apomorphine. Neuropharmacology 16, 791–794 (1977)

Waddington, J.L.: Behavioral evidence for GABAergic activity of the benzodiazepine flurazepam. Europ. J. Pharmacol. 51, 417–422 (1978)

Waddington, J.L., Owen, F.: Stereospecific benzodiazepine receptor binding by the enantiomers of oxazepam sodium hemisuccinate. Neuropharmacology 17, 215–216 (1978)

Wastek, G.J., Speth, R.C., Reisine, T.D., Yamamura, H.I.: The effect of γ-aminobutyric acid on ^{3}H-flunitrazepam binding in rat brain. Eur. J. Pharmacol. 50, 445–447 (1978)

Westerink, B.H.C., Lejeune, B., Korf, J., Praag, H.M. van: On the significance of regional dopamine metabolism in the rat brain for the classification of centrally acting drugs. Eur. J. Pharmacol. 42, 179–190 (1977)

Williams, M., Risley, E.A.: Enhancement of the binding of ^{3}H-diazepam to rat brain membranes in vitro by SQ 20,009 a novel anxiolytic, γ-aminobutyric acid (GABA) and muscimol. Life Sci. 24, 833–842 (1979)

Wise, D.C., Berger, B.D., Stein, L.: Benzodiazepines: Anxiety-reducing activity by reduction of serotonin turnover in the brain. Science 177, 180–183 (1972)

Wolf, P., Haas, H.L.: Effects of diazepines and barbiturates on hippocampal recurrent inhibition. Naunyn-Schmidebergs Arch. Pharmacol. 299, 211–218 (1977)

Wood, J.D., Peesker, S.J., Gorecki, D.K.J., Tsui, D.: Effect of L-cycloserine on brain GABA metabolism. Can. J. Physiol. Pharmacol. *56*, 62–68 (1978)

Yamamura, H.I., Snyder, S.H.: Muscarinic cholinergic binding in rat brain. Proc. Natl. Acad. Sci. USA *71*, 1725–1729 (1974)

Yamamura, H.I., Speth, R.C., Reisine, T.D., Wastek, G.J., Chen, F.M., Kobayashi, R.M.: Biochemical characterization of ^{3}H-flunitrazepam binding to benzodiazepine receptors in the rat brain. 7th Intern. Congr. Pharmacol., Paris 1978 a

Yamamura, H.I., Enna, S.J., Kuhar, M.J.: Neurotransmitter receptor binding. New York: Raven 1978 b

Young, A.B., Zukin, S.R., Snyder, S.H.: Interaction of benzodiazepines with central nervous glycine receptors: Possible mechanism of action. Proc. Natl. Acad. Sci. USA *6*, 2246–2250 (1974)

Zakusov, V.V., Ostrovskaya, R.U., Kozhechkin, S.N., Markovich, V.V., Molodavkin, G.M., Voronina, T.A.: Further evidence for GABA-ergic mechanisms in the action of benzodiazepines. Arch. Int. Pharmacodyn. Ther. *229*, 313–326 (1977)

Zsilla, G., Cheney, D.L., Costa, E.: Regional changes in the rate of turnover of acetylcholine in rat brain following diazepam or muscimol. Naunyn-Schmiedebergs Arch. Pharmacol. *294*, 251–255 (1976)

Zukin, S.R., Young, A.B., Snyder, S.H.: Gamma-aminobutyric acid binding to receptor sites in the rat central nevous system. Proc. Natl. Acad. Sci. USA *71*, 4802–4807 (1974)

CHAPTER 6

Pharmacokinetics and Metabolism of Anxiolytics

S. A. KAPLAN and M. L. JACK

A. Introduction

Anxiety may be defined as a prevailing feeling of apprehension and/or dread, sometimes associated with an immediately stressful or fearful stimulus. Frequently, anxiety overlaps with fear (TINKELBERG, 1977). Anxiety rarely occurs in isolation but is often accompanied by other emotions such as drepression and anger. Subjective and objective symptoms such as muscular tension, palpitations, headaches, dizziness, abdominal distress, chest pains, tremulousness, and nausea are often associated with anxiety. Many are drugs available for the treatment of anxiety. Anxiolytic agents encompass drugs from several drug classes, including benzodiazepines, propanediols, and some barbiturates and antidepressants. Ideally, these agents are used to reduce anxiety in the awake individual without inducing sedation.

HOLLISTER (1973) divides antianxiety agents into two major classes, namely sedative hypnotics and autonomic sedatives. The sedative hypnotics include all antianxiety agents that are relatively pure antianxiety or sedative agents lacking major autonomic side effects. The benzodiazepines, propanediols, and barbiturates would be classified as sedative hypnotics since they are sedative and antianxiety agents at low doses and induce sleep at higher dosages. The autonomic sedatives, such as the antidepressants and antihistamines, also induce sedation and reduce anxiety. However, these drugs are generally prescribed for other purposes and have anticholinergic and often adrenergic porperties. They are known to cause dry mouth, blurred vision, dysuria, hypotension, and tachycardia at some doses. Some of the differential pharmacologic properties of the drug classes most commonly prescribed as anxiolytic agents (sedative hypnotics and autonomic sedatives) are presented in Table 1.

Once a diagnosis is made, the clinician is then faced with a vast number of agents available for the treatment of anxiety. The benzodiazepines have emerged as the drug class of choice for the treatment of anxiety. The pharmacokinetic profiles for the benzodiazepine compounds presented herein are designed to highlight the similarities and differences between the anxiolytic benzodiazepines.

Pharmacokinetics is the study of the time course of drug absorption, distribution, biotransformation, and excretion and the relationship of these processes to the intensity and time course of therapeutic and toxicologic effects (GIBALDI, 1977). Knowledge of a pharmacokinetic profile of a drug in man is most useful to the clinician for several reasons. Such profiles permit estimation of the rates and extent of absorption, distribution, biotransformation, and excretion of a drug; allow for the prediction of drug level profiles on chronic administration; aid in optimizing dosage regimes in relatively healthy patients and in patients with various pathologic conditions; and assist in predicting potential drug interactions.

Table 1. Differential pharmacologic properties of antianxiety drugs (Cole, 1978)[a]

	Pheno-barbital	Mepro-bamate	Benzo-diazepines	Anti-histamines	Pheno-thiazines	Tricyclics
Antianxiety/sedative ratio	+	+ +	+ +	±	±	±
Muscle relaxation	±	+ +	+ + +	0	−	0
Anticonvulsant action	+ + +	+ +	+ + +	−	−	−
Duration of action	+ + +	+ + +	+ + +	+	+ +	+ +
Tolerance	+ +	+	+	0	0	0
Habituation	±	+ + +	±	0	0	0
Physical dependence	+	+ + +	+	0	0	0
Disturbed sleep pattern	+ +	+ +	±	+ +	+ +	+ +
Potential suicidal use	+ +	+ + +	0	+ +	0	+ + +

[a] Symbols indicate degree or probability, ranging from (−) opposite effect, (0) none, (±) minimal, (+) slight, (+ +) moderate, and (+ + +) great

B. Benzodiazepines

I. Biotransformation Pathways

The 1,4-benzodiazepines as a drug are extensively metabolized. Although some differences occur, the overall biotransformation pathways of the benzodiazepines are similar in that:

Substituents are removed from the B ring of the 1,4-benzodiazepine nucleus.

Position R_3 is hydroxylated.

The hydroxylated metabolite undergoes conjugation and subsequent elimination in the urine.

The biotransformation pathways for all the anxiolytic benzodiazepines discussed are presented in Fig. 1. The similarities in pathways are immediately apparent.

Chlordiazepoxide, diazepam, clorazepate, and prazepam all form nordiazepam by different pathways. Chlordiazepoxide is dealkylated in the liver in two steps with subsequent loss of the oxide to form nordiazepam. Diazepam is directly N-demethylated in the liver of form nordiazepam, its major metabolite. A minor pathway for diazepam bypasses nordiazepam with the formation of temazepam. Prazepam undergoes virtually complete presystemic dealkylation of the cyclopropylmethyl side chain in the liver to form nordiazepam. The very slow but complete presystemic formation of nordiazepam suggests possible binding of prazepam in the gastrointestinal tract or liver and slow release to metabolic sites most probably in the liver (Di Carlo et al., 1970). Clorazepate, on the other hand, undergoes acid hydrolysis to form nordiazepam in the gastric fluid prior to absorption.

Nordiazepam is hydroxylated in the 3-position by hepatic enzymes to form oxazepam which is subsequently conjugated and excreted in the urine. Temazepam can be conjugated directly or demethylated in the liver to form oxazepam. Lorazepam, the 2′-chloro derivative of oxazepam, is also metabolized by conjugation.

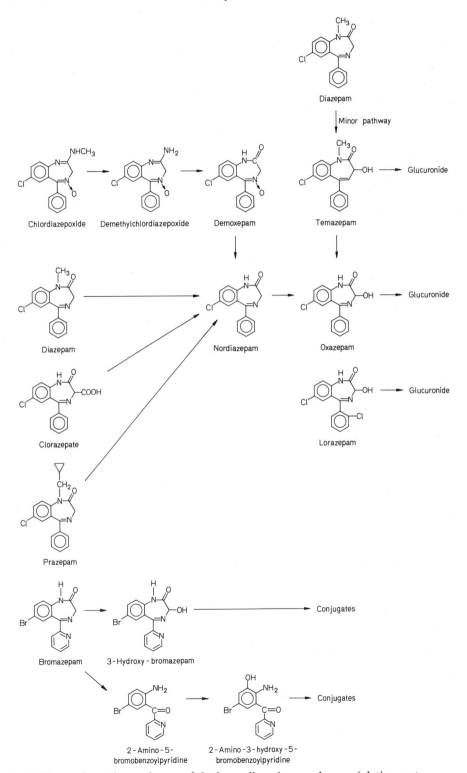

Fig. 1. Biotransformation pathways of the benzodiazepines used as anxiolytic agents

Bromazepam exhibits two major metabolic pathways: hydroxylation in the liver at the 3-position with subsequent conjugation of the 3-OH metabolite, and a ring opening to form the benzoypyridine derivative which is hydroxylated in the 3-position and conjugated.

II. Pharmacokinetic Profiles

All the benzodiazepine compounds discussed herein exhibit linear "apparent" first-order pharmacokinetic profiles over the therapeutic dose range. Such an observation is substantiated by the multiple dose data reported which confirm the predictability of steady-state levels from single dose pharmacokinetic parameters. Since the majority of drugs are administered orally, the rate and extent of absorption, i.e., the biovailability following oral administration are of primary concern. Biovailability is influenced by physicochemical and physiologic factors such as solubility, dissolution rate, permeability, and presystemic gastrointestinal and liver metabolism. The plasma peak times and heights may be used as an index of the rate of absorption, whereas the extent of absorption can be estimated by comparing the areas under the plasma level-time curves or cumulative urinary excretion data following oral and intravenous administration.

1. Single Dose Pharmacokinetics

The pharmacokinetic parameters for the benzodiazepine compounds are summarized in Tables 2 and 3 for intravenous and oral administrations, respectively.

Table 2. Mean pharmacokinetic parameters of the benzodiazepine anxiolytic agents following intravenous administration [a]

Parameter	Chlordiazepoxide hydrochloride	Brom-azepam [b]	Loraz-epam	Diaz-epam	Nordiazepam following diazepam
Dose (mg)	30	6	4	10	10
Peak time (h)	–	–	–	–	48
Peak height (µg/ml)	–	–	–	–	0.02–0.04
Volume of distribution as % of body wt.	31	90	84	186	110
Protein binding (%)	94	70.1	90.9	98.6	98.4
Half-life of elimination (h)	9.4	20.6	13.2	31.3	55–99 [c]
Total body clearance (ml/min)	45	–	55.3	26–35	–
% of dose exreted in urine as intact drug	< 1	2.3	1	< 0.05	< 0.05
Total excretion as known substances	34–61	70	69	5–10	5–10

[a] Information obtained from the following sources: Chlordiazepoxide, KOECHLIN et al., 1965; GREENBLATT and KOCH-WESER, 1975; BOXENBAUM et al., 1977a; GREENBLATT et al., 1977a; MACLEOD et al., 1977; ROBERTS et al., 1977, 1978. Bromazepam, RAAFLAUB and SPEISER-COURVOISIER, 1974. Lorazepam, GREENBLATT et al., 1977b, 1979b; JOHNSON et al., 1979. Diazepam, KAPLAN et al., 1973; KLOTZ et al., 1975; ANDREASEN et al., 1976; HENDEL et al., 1976; KLOTZ et al., 1976a, b; Drug Action, 1978. Nordiazepam, KAPLAN et al., 1973
[b] Radioactive drug used
[c] Determined following chronic administration

Table 3. Mean pharmacokinetic parameters of the benzodiazepine anxiolytic agents following oral administration[a]

Parameter	Chlordiazepoxide hydrochloride	Bromazepam	Lorazepam	Oxazepam	Temazepam	Diazepam	Nordiazepam following oral administration of:		
							Diazepam	Clorazepate	Prazepam
Dose (mg)	30	12	2	15	30	10	10	10	20
Peak time (h)	1 – 2	0.5–8	2.6	1–4	1–2	0.5–1.5	30–48	0.5–2	2.5–72
Peak height (µg/ml)	0.94– 1.94	0.13	0.023	0.1–0.4	0.5	0.14–0.19	0.03–0.04	0.14–0.25	0.14
Half-life of elimination (h)	6.5 –11.4	11.9	13.2	10.5	15–20	32	50–99	40–70	29–193
Bioavailability (% of dose)	100	84–98	100	41–89	–	100	–	–	–

[a] Information obtained from the following: Chlordiazepoxide, SCHWARTZ et al., 1971; GREENBLATT et al., 1974a, 1978; BOXENBAUM et al., 1977a; SHADER et al., 1977. Bromazepam, SCHWARTZ et al., 1973; KAPLAN et al., 1976. Lorazepam, GREENBLATT et al., 1976, 1977d, 1979a, b; KYRIAKOPOULOS, 1976; KYRIAKOPOULOS et al., 1978. Oxazepam, GREENBLATT et al., 1975; ALVÁN et al., 1977. Temazepam, FUCCELLA et al., 1972. Diazepam, KAPLAN et al., 1973; KLOTZ et al., 1975; EATMAN et al., 1977; Drug Action, 1978. Nordiazepam (Diazepam), KAPLAN et al., 1973; TOGNONI et al., 1975; SHADER and GREENBLATT, 1977. Nordiazepam (Clorazepate), ABRUZZO et al., 1977; CARRIGAN et al., 1977; CHUN et al., 1977; POST et al., 1977. Nordiazepam (Prazepam), GREENBLATT and SHADER, 1978a, ALLEN et al., 1979.

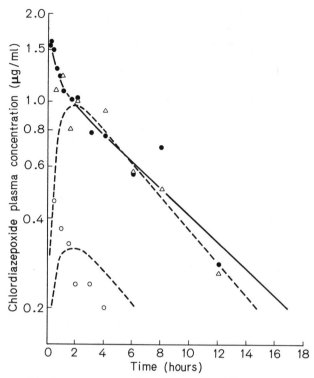

Fig. 2. Chlordiazepoxide plasma concentration–time profiles following intravenous administration of 30 mg ● and oral administration of 10 ○ and 30 mg △ (Boxenbaum et al., 1977a)

a) Chlordiazepoxide

A typical single dose intravenous and oral plasma level curve indicates rapid and complete absorption of an orally administered dose (Fig. 2). It should be noted that in contrast with diazepam, the metabolites of chlordiazepoxide are generally not detectable following a single dose administration.

b) Diazepam

The blood level curves of diazepam and nordiazepam following a 10-mg single intravenous and oral dose are presented in Fig. 3. The comparable areas under the diazepam intravenous and oral blood level curves indicate complete absorption, whereas the early and sharp blood level peak following oral administration is indicative of rapid absorption. The areas under the blood level curves of the metabolite, nordiazepam, following intravenous and oral administrations of diazepam are virtually the same, further reflecting the completeness of absorption of diazepam. The formation rate constants for nordiazepam after intravenous diazepam administration are reported in Table 4. It should be noted that the initial formation rate constant of nordiazepam is 10–20 times more rapid than the formation rate constant calculated after the 12 h postadministration. This slower formation rate constant of nordiazepam is equal to the overall elimination rate constant of diazepam. Such equivalency of rate constants

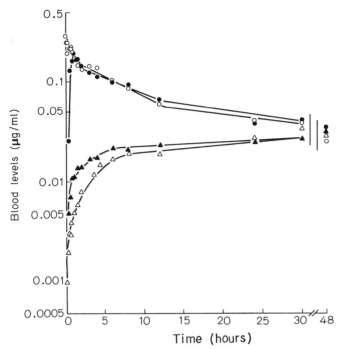

Fig. 3. Diazepam ○ and ● and nordiazepam (desmethyldiazepam) △ and ■ blood level-time curves following 10-mg intravenous and oral administrations to a healthy volunteer (Kaplan et al., 1973)

Table 4. Formation rate constants for nordiazepam. (KAPLAN et al., 1973)

	Subject			
	1	2	3	4
Overall elimination rate constant of diazepam (h^{-1})	0.019	0.026	0.024	0.021
Formation rate constant of nordiazepam after 12 h, (h^{-1})	0.020	0.028	0.030	0.016
Initial formation rate constant of nordiazepam (h^{-1}) mg	0.546	0.427	0.329	0.351

suggests that diazepam is virtually completely metabolized to nordiazepam in man; temazepam is a minor metabolite of diazepam.

Based on the data obtained following intravenous administration, an open three-compartment pharmacokinetic model system for diazepam was developed and is presented in Fig. 4 with the mean calculated rate constants (KAPLAN et al., 1973). Compartment 1 is the so-called central compartment into which a drug is administered and from which elimination occurs. Compartments 2 and 3 are peripheral compartments for which no anatomic designations are given as they merely reflect two distinguishable partition phenomena between the blood and distribution and/or binding sites. Overall, the characteristics of this deep peripheral compartment, compartment 3, may be of importance in understanding the physiologic disposition characteristics of diaze-

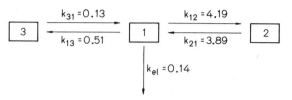

Fig. 4. The open three-compartment pharmacokinetic model and the mean calculated rate constants proposed for diazepam (Kaplan et al., 1973)

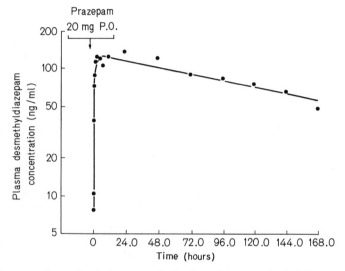

Fig. 5. Nordiazepam plasma level-time curve following a 20-mg oral administration of prazepam (Greenblatt and Shader, 1978 b)

pam in man. This results since the rate of return of drug from this compartment to the central compartment may be the rate-limiting step in terms of the elimination of diazepam and the formation of nordiazepam.

c) Prazepam

Prazepam undergoes virtually complete presystemic dealkylation most probably in the liver in which the cyclopropylmethyl side chain is removed to form nordiazepam (GREENBLATT and SHADER, 1978 a, b). GREENBLATT and SHADER (1978 b) found no intact prazepam level following 20-mg single doses of prazepam to fasting volunteers. Following the oral administration of 20 mg prazepam, drug levels of nordiazepam peaked between 2.5–72 h postadministration, indicating either slow gastrointestinal absorption, slow metabolism, or possible binding of prazepam at some site prior to the formation and passage of nordiazepam into systemic circulation (DI CARLO et al., 1970). A typical nordiazepam plasma curve following a 20-mg prazepam oral dose is presented in Fig. 5.

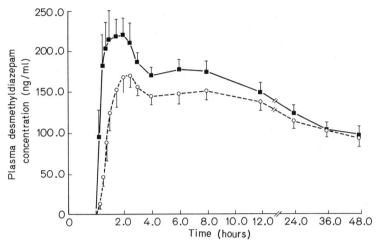

Fig. 6. Plasma level-time curves of nordiazepam (desmethyldiazepam) following the administration of 15 mg clorazepate with water ■ and with magnesium aluminum hydroxide (Maalox) ○ (Shader et al., 1978)

d) Clorazepate

Clorazepate undergoes hydrolysis in the acidic environment of the stomach to form nordiazepam which is subsequently rapidly absorbed (ABRUZZO et al., 1977; CHUN et al., 1977). Nordiazepam peak levels of 140–188 ng/ml occur at approximately 0.5–2 h following oral administration of a 15-mg dose chlorazepate (Table 3). Intact clorzepate is not readily absorbed (SHADER and GREENBLATT, 1977).

The early peak times of nordiazepam following the administeration of clorazepate suggest that nordiazepam is formed and absorbed rapidly. ABRUZZO et al. (1977) observed prolongation of blood level peak times and a decrease in blood level peak heights and areas under the blood level curves of nordiazepam in subjects whose gastric pH had been elevated with sodium bicarbonate. SHADER et al. (1978) observed similar effects in patients dosed concomitantly with magnesium aluminium hydroxide (Maalox) (Fig. 6).

Pharmacologically active nordiazepam is the major metabolite of diazepam and of the prodrugs prazepam and chlorazepate. The pharmacokinetic profile of nordiazepam following single dose oral administrations of diazepam, clorazepate, and prazepam are presented in Table 3 and comparative blood level curves are presented in Fig. 7.

The late peak times and low peak heights of nordiazepam following the administration of diazepam and prazepam reflect the slow dealkylation of these compounds to form nordiazepam. The differences in nordiazepam plasma concentrations and peak times observed following the administration of diazepam, prazepam, and clorazepate, therefore, reflect differences in the rate and extent of nordiazepam formation.

e) Lorazepam, Oxazepam, and Temazepam

The plasma level peaks of lorazepam, oxazepam, and temazepam each occur at approximately 2 h postadministration, suggesting rapid absorption with similar rates of

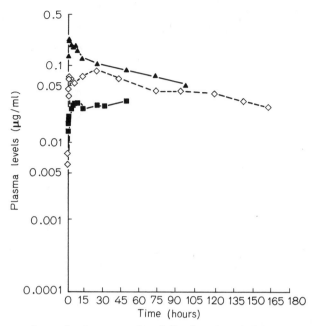

Fig. 7. Nordiazepam plasma levels versus time following the administration of clorazepate (–▲–), diazepam* (–■–), and prazepam (–◇–). Nordiazepam plasma levels are normalized with respect to dose of the parent compound, i.e., 14.4 mg clorazepate, 10 mg diazepam, and 11.4 mg prazepam, (*blood levels)

absorption for these compounds (Fig. 8–10). The plasma level peak heights reported in Table 3 for these three structurally related benzodiazepines are of the same order of magnitude when corrected for differences in dose. Although the reported urinary recovery following oral administration range from 40%–100%, there is nothing which suggests incomplete absorption of these compounds.

f) Bromazepam

Bromazepam is virtually completely absorbed following oral administration. The urinary excretion data following oral administration (KAPLAN et al., 1976) indicate a mean recovery of 70% of the dose in the urine. Oral and intravenous urine profiles following ^{14}C doses show that 70% of the dose is excreted in the urine following both administrations, indicating complete absorption of the oral dose (RAAFLAUB and SPEISER-COURVOISIER, 1974). The mean blood level maxima of bromazepam occur at 2.5 h, although the drug tends to exhibit flat rather than sharp peaks (KAPLAN et al., 1976). Typical blood level curves are presented in Fig. 11.

2. Distribution Characteristics

Protein binding and volume of distribution values of the benzodiazepines are reported in Table 2. The benzodiazepine anxiolytic agents are all extensively protein bound, all greater than 90% bound except for bromazepam which is 70% bound. The benzodiazepines are extensively distributed except for chlordiazepoxide which has a volume

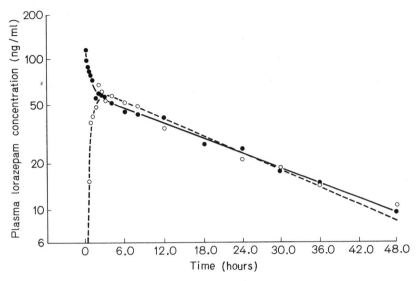

Fig. 8. Lorazepam plasma concentration-time profiles following 4-mg intravenous infusion ● and oral ○ administrations to a subject (Greenblatt and Shader, 1978 b)

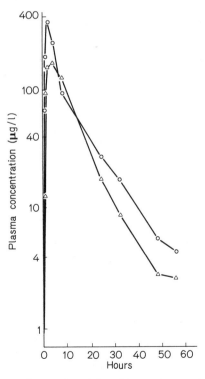

Fig. 9. Plasma concentrations of oxazepam (○) and its conjugates (△) following oral administration of 15 mg oxazepam to a subject (Alván et al., 1977)

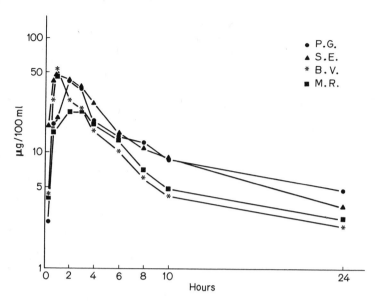

Fig. 10. Plasma levels versus time profiles of temazepam following the single oral administration of 30-mg capsules to four healthy volunteers (Fuccella et al., 1972)

of distribution approximately three times smaller than the other benzodiazepines. Generally the more lipophilic the compound, the greater the volume of distribution. Structurally, the $-NHCH_3$ and $N \to O$ substituents of chlordiazepoxide and the $-OH$ substituents of oxazepam on the benzodiazepine nucleus diminish lipophilicity; diazepam and nordiazepam lack such substituents.

Radioautograms obtained with benzodiazepines in several animal species indicated that labeled compound accumulates very rapidly in the brain. It localizes first in the gray matter, whereas shortly thereafter the radioactivity is primarily concentrated in the white matter (Morselli et al., 1973b). This is exemplified in the radioautograms obtained from the brain of the cat killed 1 min after intravenous injection of ^{14}C-diazepam. Initially, when the radioactivity was confined to the gray matter, the highest uptake was found in such sites as the thalamus, colliculi, geniculate bodies, midbrain nuclei, and cerebral and cerebellar cortex. At this time, the radioactivity in the white matter was low. As time progressed, the concentration of the labeled material tended to become more uniform throughout the whole brain, and the radioautograms obtained 30 min after drug administration did not show marked differences between gray and white matter. One and 4 h after the intravenous injection of ^{14}C-diazepam, radioactivity was much higher in the white than in the gray matter.

It is of interest to contrast these distribution and redistribution findings in the cat with the pharmacokinetics of diazepam in man. Immediately upon intravenous administration of diazepam to man, one observes sedation and amnesia during the 1st hour which is not observed following comparable oral doses (Driscoll et al., 1972). Such observations reflect the rapid distribution of intravenously administered diazepam into the central nervous system and subsequent redistribution. During this interval following intravenous administration, blood concentrations decline to approxi-

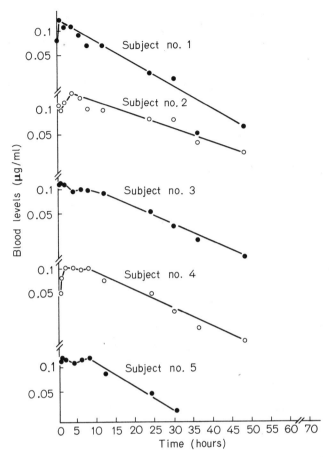

Fig. 11. Bromazepam blood level curves in man following the administration of single oral 12-mg doses (Kaplan et al., 1976)

mately one-half maximum values, whereas following oral administration blood concentrations increase due to absorption. In addition, since metabolite concentrations are very low or nonexistent during this interval, the clinical observations must be attributed to the high concentrations of diazepam per se.

3. Elimination Rate Characteristics

The benzodiazepines under consideration are all eliminated from the body by biotransformation via one or several steps. The "apparent" half-life elimination of the several benzodiazepines can vary from less than 10 h to over 100 h (Tables 2, and 3). The variability reflects differences in physicochemical properties, rates of presystemic metabolism, and the intricacies of the metabolic pathways.

Compounds such as oxazepam, lorazepam, temazepam, chlordiazepoxide, and bromazepam are eliminated fairly rapidly with apparent half-lives for each ranging from the teens to under 10 h. It is interesting to note that all these benzodiazepines

Table 5. Mean plasma diazepam levels (ng/ml) following a single 10 mg dose (ASSAF et al., 1974)

Number of patients	Route of Administration	Mean plasma levels of diazepam (ng/ml) at time (min) after administration			
		15	30	60	90[a]
40	Orally	75	100	208	177 ± 11.4
10	i.m. buttock	96	105	110	100 ± 5.1
33	i.m. thigh	80	110	152	149 ± 13.7
10	i.m. thigh (exercise)	214	284	272	243 ± 26.9

[a] Plasma levels at 90 min indicate mean results $\pm$ S.E.

have polar functional groups such as a 3-OH, a N_4-oxide, or a pyridine (bromazepam) in place of the 5-phenyl ring.

Diazepam and nordiazepam, however, exhibited much longer half-lives probably because they do not possess corresponding polar functional groups. The differences in apparent elimination rates of nordiazepam when observed after clorazepate, prazepam, or diazepam administration reflect the influence of the formation rate constant on the apparent elimination rate constant of the drug.

The elimination profiles of all the benzodiazepines can be characterized as "apparent" first-order processes, implying that the elimination rate is not dose dependent.

4. Intramuscular Absorption

Chlordiazepoxide, diazepam, and lorazepam are administered intramuscularly (GREENBLATT et al., 1974b, 1977c, 1978, 1979b; ASSAF et al., 1974; Drug Action, 1978; HILLESTAD et al., 1974). All three are completely absorbed from the intramuscular site; however, the rate of absorption and the corresponding peak plasma level will vary as a function of the site and depth of intramuscular administration, the amount of adipose tissue, and possible precipitation of drug at the injection site. Such variability may result in alterations in some "apparent" pharmacokinetic parameters.

An interesting study indicates that variability in the intramuscular diazepam administration can result in diazepam plasma levels that vary from one-half to two times the plasma levels observed following oral administration of diazepam at the same dose level (ASSAF et al., 1974). Differences were also observed in intramuscular absorption of diazepam in rested an exercised muscle (Table 5).

5. Multiple Dose Pharmacokinetics

Confirmation of the apparent first-order elimination kinetics of the benzodiazepines is based on the ability of each of the compounds to achieve predictable multiple dose steady-state drug level profiles. Overall, the experimental steady-state concentrations of the 1,4-benzodiazepines can be predicted from the single dose pharmacokinetic parameters. The ability of achieve such profiles confirms the constancy and reproducibility of absorption, distribution, metabolism, and elimination from administration to administration.

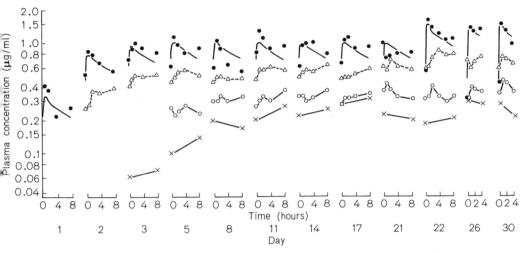

Fig. 12. Plasma concentration-time profiles of chlordiazepoxide, desmethylchlordiazepoxide, demoxepam, and desoxydemoxepam (nordiazepam) following oral administration of chlordiazepoxide HCl to a subject. On days 1–21, the dose was 10 mg every 8 h; on days 22–30, the dose was 30 mg once daily. *Abcissa*, time after the morning dose (Boxenbaum et al., 1977b). –●– Chlordiazepozide, –△– Desmethylchlordiazepoxide, –○– Demoxepam, ×–× Desoxydemoxepam

Interpretation of the pharmacokinetic profiles of the benzodiazepines following multiple dose administration in man must consider their extensive metabolism and accumulation of the parent compounds and metabolites following chronic dosing. The administered benzodiazepines are absorbed, accumulate to steady-state levels, and are metabolized at different rates; their respective metabolites are subsequently formed, metabolized, and excreted at rates differing from those of the parent compound. For some benzodiazepines, the metabolites are pharmacologically and pharmacokinetically unimportant following single dose administration, but become significant following chronic dose schedules.

a) Chlordiazepoxide

BOXENBAUM et al. (1977b) investigated the plasma level profiles of chlordiazepoxide following 10 mg t.i.d. and 30 mg once daily oral dosage regimens in man (Fig. 12). The pharmacokinetic parameters determined following single dose studies were used to predict the drug level profiles of chlordiazepoxide following chronic administration. Steady-state plasma levels of chlordiazepoxide are achieved within 72 h following the commencement of the t.i.d. chronic dosage regimen as evidenced in Fig. 12. The desmethylchlordiazepoxide metabolite also achieves steady state by day 3, while the demoxepam and desoxydemoxepam metabolites attain steady state by day 8. These metabolites are undetectable following single dose administration.

As anticipated, the average steady state levels following a 10 mg t.i.d. and 30 mg once-daily dosage regimen remain unchanged for chlordiazepoxide (BOXENBAUM et al., 1977b). It is interesting to note that metabolite plasma levels during both the t.i.d.

Table 6. Pharmacokinetic parameters k_{el}, clearance, and $t_{1/2}$ (β) following the administration of chlordiazepoxide as a 30 mg single dose, 10 mg t.i.d. for 21 days and 30 mg once daily chronic dose for 15 days (BOXENBAUM et al., 1977a, b)

Dose	Mean	Range
$k_{el} (h^{-1})$		
30 mg single dose	0.126	0.083– 0.157
10 mg t.i.d.	0.110	0.076– 0.159
30 mg once daily	0.112	0.060– 0.170
Clearance (1/h)		
30 mg single dose	2.74	1.60 – 3.54
10 mg t.i.d.	2.33	1.61 – 3.10
30 mg once daily	2.39	1.17 – 3.77
$t_{1/2}(\beta)$, (h)		
30 mg single dose	9.39	6.63 –13.6
10 mg t.i.d.	10.9	7.79 –16.1
30 mg once daily	11.5	6.24 –15.6

and once-daily dosage regimes remain constant and do not reflect the change in chlordiazepoxide dosage. Such data suggest that a once-daily administration is pharmacokinetically equivalent to the t.i.d. dosage regimen for chlordiazepoxide.

The pharmacokinetic parameters k_{el}, clearance, and $t_{1/2}$ (β) for chlordiazepoxide following a 30-mg single dose, 10 mg t.i.d., and 30 mg once-daily chronic dosage regimens remain unchanged (Table 6). Such findings confirm the constancy of absorption, distribution, metabolism and excretion of chlordiazepoxide following single and multiple dose therapy as well as confirm the lack of unpredicted drug accumulation with chronic doses of chlordiazepoxide.

b) Diazepam and Nordiazepam (Clorazepate and Prazepam)

Several investigators have studied the disposition profiles of diazepam and nordiazepam following chronic oral administration of diazepam to man. KAPLAN et al. (1973) studied the steady-state profile of diazepam following 10-mg once daily administration of diazepam for 15 days. Pharmacokinetic constants obtained after single dose intravenous studies allowed for the prediction of the typical oral steady-state blood level profile of diazepam presented in Fig. 13. Steady-state diazepam blood levels were achieved within 7 days, and the steady-state maximum and minimum blood levels are approximately twice the corresponding blood levels observed following single dose studies. The calculated elimination rate constant, β, observed following the last dose in the chronic administration approximated the corresponding rate constant observed following the single dose administration. The calculated and experimental minimum and maximum diazepam steady-state levels for four subjects are presented in Table 7. This finding of relatively constant steady-state diazepam blood levels substantiates the constancy of the absorption, distribution, metabolism, and excretion of diazepam

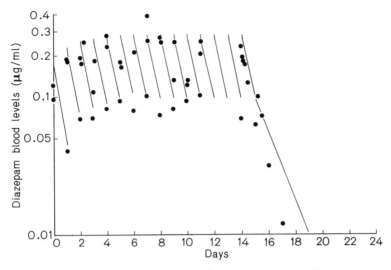

Fig. 13. Oral blood level data of diazepam in a subject receiving 10 mg diazepam every 24 h for 15 days. *Solid lines* represent calculated blood level curve; ●, the experimental data points (Adapted from Kaplan et al., 1973)

Table 7. Calculated and experimental diazepam steady-state blood levels (μg/ml) (KAPLAN et al., 1973)

	Subject			
	1	2	3	4
Calculated minimum steady-state level	0.088	0.066	0.099	0.094
Experimental minimum steady-state level	0.104	0.068	0.085	0.078
Calculated maximum steady-state level	0.212	0.204	0.289	0.277
Experimental maximum steady-state level	0.235	0.210	0.224	0.238

following chronic administration and indicates that unpredicted drug accumulation does not occur when diazepam is administered chronically.

Nordiazepam is the major metabolite formed following the administration of diazepam and of the prodrugs, clorazepate and prazepam, to human subjects. Certain aspects of the pharmacokinetic profile of nordiazepam following chronic administration of the parent drug are dependent on the origin of the nordiazepam.

KAPLAN et al. (1973) reported steady-state concentrations of nordiazepam following the administration of diazepam which were essentially equivalent to the mean steady-state blood levels of diazepam. The small range of maximum to minimum blood levels of nordiazepam reflects its slow formation and elimination following the administration and metabolism of diazepam (Fig. 14).

Following the chronic administration of clorazepate, the differences between the maximum and minimum nordiazepam blood levels at steady state are greater than those observed following chronic administration of diazepam (Fig. 15). Such findings

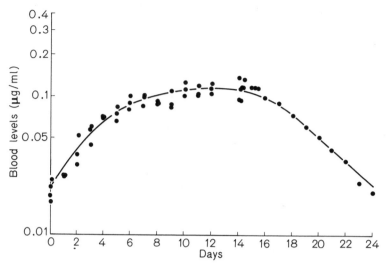

Fig. 14. Nordiazepam blood level data following the administration of 10 mg diazepam every 24 h for 15 days to a subject (Adapted from Kaplan et al., 1973)

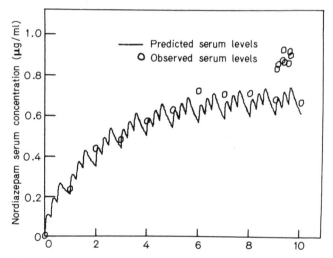

Fig. 15. Observed and predicted minimum steady-state serum levels of nordiazepam following the administration of 7.5 mg clorazepate dipotassium capsules every 6 h for three doses per day for 10 days (Carrigan et al., 1977)

reflect the more rapid rate of formation of nordiazepam from clorazepate than from diazepam.

It has been previously noted that the formation of nordiazepam following single dose administrations of prazepam is slow due to either slow gastrointestinal absorption, slow metabolism, and/or binding of prazepam prior to the formation of nordiazepam. Such characteristics should also be reflected in the pharmacokinetic profile of nordiazepam following the chronic administration of prazepam; however, there are very limited data available on the steady-state profile following prazepam administration. GLAZKO et al. (1979) report minimum steady-state nordiazepam plasma levels of 900 ng/ml and 463 ng/ml following the administration of 10 mg prazepam t.i.d. and b.i.d., respectively. In the same study, 10 mg diazepam administered b.i.d. produced comparable minimum steady-state levels of nordiazepam averaging 456 ng/ml.

It is interesting to note that following equivalent doses and dosage regimens, the minimum steady-state levels of diazepam were as anticipated, whereas the corresponding prazepam levels were below the 5-ng/ml sensitivity of the assay, confirming the lack of systematic availability of intact prazepam following single or multiple dose administrations (GREENBLATT and SHADER, 1978 a, b; GLAZKO et al., 1979).

c) Lorazepam, Oxazepam, Temazepam

Steady-state plasma level profiles of lorazepam and oxazepam and their conjugates following chronic administration are presented in Figs. 16 and 17. Based on their respective half-lives, both drugs will achieve steady-state within 48–72 h after drug therapy has been initiated.

Following single dose administrations, the plasma levels of oxazepam and its conjugate are essentially equivalent (ÁLVAN et al., 1977), while the plasma concentration of lorazepam glucuronide are somewhat greater than the plasma concentrations of the parent compound. With chronic doses, the steady-state plasma concentrations of oxazepam and its conjugate are again equivalent while the steady-state plasma levels of the conjugate of lorazepam are approximately twice those of the parent drug. The pharmacokinetic profile of lorazepam and lorazepam glucuronide presented by

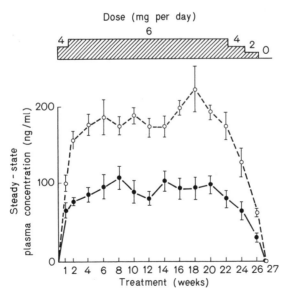

Fig. 16. Steady-state plasma concentrations of lorazepam ● and lorazepam glucuronide ○ determined 4 h following the morning oral administration of lorazepam. The subjects received lorazepam twice daily, 2 mg in the morning and 2 or 4 mg at bedtime (Greenblatt et al., 1977d)

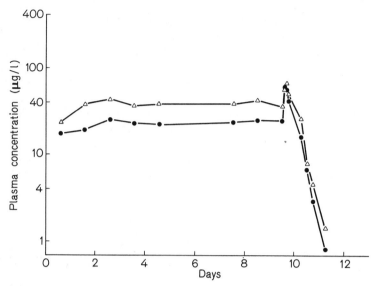

Fig. 17. Minimum steady-state plasma concentrations of oxazepam (●) and its conjugates (△) following multiple oral doses of oxazepam, 5 mg t.i.d. for 10 days (Alván et al., 1977)

Table 8. Elimination half-lives of oxazepan observed following single dose and chronic administrations and comparison of predicted and observed steady-state concentrations (C_{ss}) observed after 5 mg oxazepam orally t.i.d. (Adapted from ALVÁN et al., 1977)

Subject	Single dose $t_{1/2}$ (h)	Chronic dose $t_{1/2}$ (h)	Predicted C_{ss} (μg/ml)	Observed C_{ss} (μg/ml)
1	6.7	8.2	55	51.7
2	10.5	9.0	95	89.5
3	11.2	10.2	97	42.2
4	8.9	15.7	210	277.5
5	8.8	11.9	200	133.0
6	11.1	21.0	64	57.3
7	6.9	11.6	92	36.8
8	9.2	13.3	131	72.0
9	–	–	69	76.5

[a] Based on single dose kinetics

KYRIAKOPOULOUS (1976) indicates that the half-lives of lorazepam and lorazepam glucuronide are essentially the same; however, the volume of distribution of the glucuronide is smaller than that of the parent compound, resulting in higher plasma concentrations of the glucuronide.

The steady-state drug level profile may be predicted from single dose studies, provided the kinetics are first order and the plasma clearance, bioavailability, distribution profiles, and metabolism remain constant. The steady-state plasma concentrations of oxazepam were significantly lower ($P < 0.05$) in a majority of the subjects than the predicted levels based on single dose studies as shown in Table 8. This probably results from the somewhat slower half-life of oxazepam elimination following chronic administration. Such finding indicates some change in the pharmacokinetic profile of oxazepam on chronic dosing; however, the clinical significance, if any, of such a change is not known.

The pharmacokinetic profile of temazepam following multiple dose administrations has not been reported in the literature. Single dose studies indicate that temazepam is rapidly absorbed with a plasma peak time of 1–2 h and a peak height of 0.5 µg/ml following 30-mg single doses temazepam. Temazepam has a slower half-life of elimination (15–20 h) than either lorazepam or oxazepam (Fuccella et al., 1972). The single dose data indicate that temazepam exhibits apparent first-order kinetics, and therefore, following chronic administration, temazepam should achieve steady state in 3–5 days.

d) Bromazepam

A typical experimental blood level profile of bromazepam following a chronic oral administration is presented in Fig. 18. The solid line represents the simulated blood level profile based on the pharmacokinetic parameters obtained following a single dose

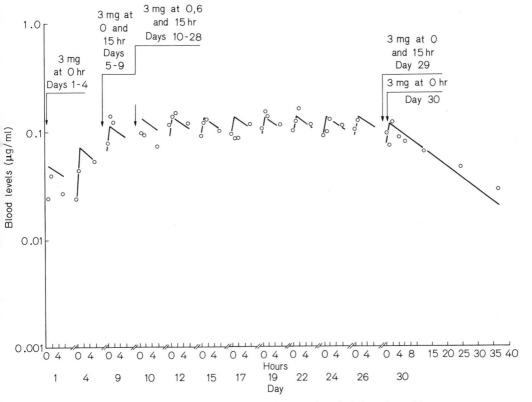

Fig. 18. Oral bromazepam blood level profile following the administration of bromazepam to a subject on the chronic dosage regimen indicated. The *solid lines* represent the simulated blood level curve (Kaplan et al., 1976)

Table 9. Steady-state blood concentrations (C) of bromazepam in man following chronic oral administration to six subjects (Adapted from Kaplan et al., 1976)

	Mean	SE
C maximum experimental (µg/ml)	0.120	0.011
C maximum theoretical (µg/ml)	0.130	0.012
C minimum experimental (µg/ml)	0.085	0.010
C minimum theoretical (µg/ml)	0.085	0.011

study. The experimental and theoretical steady-state maximum and minimum blood levels for six subjects are reported in Table 9.

The excellent agreement between the experimental and theoretical mean steady-state bromazepam blood levels indicates that all processes follow apparent first-order kinetics and substantiates the constancy of absorption, distribution, metabolism, and excretion with each administration of the drug. The steady-state profile confirms that the extent of absorption of bromazepam is constant in the 3–12-mg dose range and indicates that unpredicted drug accumulation will not occur.

III. Influence of Physiologic and Pathologic Variables on Pharmacokinetics

1. Age

The pharmacokinetic profiles discussed have been obtained in healthy volunteers. However, in a clinical setting, patients of various age groups may possess a variety of pathologic, genetic, and environmental characteristics. Age, disease state, and drug interactions may also affect the physiologic disposition profile of a drug. Such changes may be reflected in specific changes in the pharmacokinetic parameters which, in turn, may influence the clinical profile of the drug. For example, metabolic reactions such as oxidations, reductions, hydrolyses, and conjugations, which routinely occur within the livers of children and adults, occur at reduced rates in newborns (Vest and Rossier, 1963). Hydroxylation and glucuronidation capabilities, which are major metabolic pathways for the benzodiazepines, appear to be related to the degree of hepatic maturation. Such alterations in metabolism are reflected in the pharmacokinetic parameters of these drugs.

The urinary excretion profiles of diazepam metabolites in premature 8–81-day-old infants, full term infants who were 4–162 days old, and children 3.5–8 years old are presented in Fig. 19. The three groups all have the ability to demethylate diazepam to form nordiazepam. However, the ability to hydroxylate and conjugate is limited in the premature and full-term infant but not in older children.

It should be noted that diazepam, bromazepam, clorazepate, chlordiazepoxide, and prazepam all undergo demethylation, hydroxylation, and/or conjugation reactions in their metabolic pathways. Based on the results obtained following diazepam administration, one should anticipate that these drugs would also exhibit longer half-lives when administered to infants. Tomson et al. (1979) observed that the half-life of oxazepam and its metabolite was prolonged in the newborn as compared to the

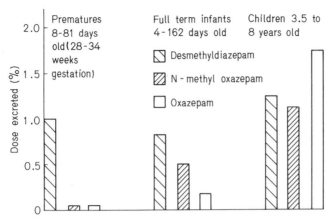

Fig. 19. The metabolites of diazepam excreted in the urine reported as percent of dose excreted following the administration of diazepam to premature 8–81-day-old infants, full term 4–162-day-old infants, and children 3.5–8 years old (Adapted from Morselli et al., 1973b)

Table 10. Half-lives of oxazepam and oxazepam conjugate in the newborn and the mother following the administration of 25 mg oxazepam to the mother prior to delivery (Tomson et al., 1979)

Subject	Oxazepam half-life (h)		Oxazepam conjugate half-life (h)	
	Newborn[a]	Mother[a]	Newborn	Mother
D.P.	–	5.3	–	5.6
L.E.	12.4	7.0	–	7.0
A.C.	27.0	–	549	–
S.B.	19.0	–	20.3	–
C.L.	20.7	–	40.9	–
P.E.	21.5	6.4	–	7.2
E.G.	27.2	6.4	23.4	4.6
N.M.	25.4	6.2	15.6	5.0
P.R.	–	7.8	–	6.7
N.I.	–	7.5	–	6.8
H.E.	–	5.8	–	4.7
Mean ± SD	21.9 ± 5.3	6.5 ± 0.8		

[a] Analyses performed on maternal plasma and neonatal blood

mother (Table 10). One should anticipate a comparable effect with other hydroxylated benzodiazepines.

The pharmacokinetic parameters of diazepam in prematures, children, and adults are presented in Table 11. The long half-life of diazepam in prematures reflects hepatic immaturity. The volume of distribution (Vd) is less for newborns than for adults. Differences in Vd may reflect the lesser amount of plasma proteins and protein binding capacity in newborns and/or differences in body composition, e.g., greater body water, low fat content.

Table 11. Pharmacokinetic parameters following the administration of diazepam to various age groups[a]

Subjects	$t_{1/2}$(h)	V_d(1/kg)
Prematures (8–81 days)	40–100	1.10
Children (3–7 years)	20– 45	1.99
Adult (25–43 years)	21– 46	1.86

[a] MORSELLI et al. (1973b) and KAPLAN et al. (1973)

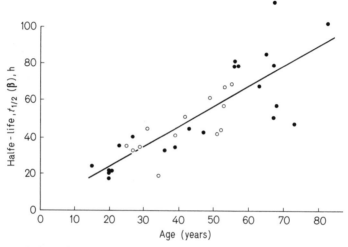

Fig. 20. The correlation of diazepam $t_{1/2}(\beta)$ and age in normal subjects. *Solid circles* refer to nonsmokers and *open circles* to smokers (more than 20 cigarettes per day) (Klotz et al., 1975)

The pharmacokinetic parameters of half-life and volume of distribution that differ in the infant also differ in geriatric patients when both groups are compared with young adults. The correlation between the half-life of diazepam and age shown in Fig. 20 indicates a marked increase in diazepam half-life with age. Figure 21 demonstrates that there is also an increase in volume of distribution of diazepam with age. Although these are the same pharmacokinetic parameters that were altered when diazepam was administered to newborns, these parameters are probably changing in the geriatric subject for different reasons. The prolonged half-lives of the benzodiazepines in aging normal subjects are probably due to changes in distribution characteristics (Vd) rather than hepatic dysfunction or alterations in protein binding. Such pharmacokinetic observations may reflect normal physiologic changes of aging, such as diminishing lean body mass. In addition, in the geriatric patients, absorption and metabolism are often slowed, and there is diminished renal function.

The pharmacokinetic profiles of several anxiolytics are known to change in the geriatric patient. In addition to diazepam, the half-lives of nordiazepam (desmethyldiazepam) (KLOTZ and MÜLLER-SEYDLITZ, 1979), chlordiazepoxide (SHADER et al., 1977; ROBERTS et al.; 1978), lorazepam (KYRIAKOPOULOS, 1976), amobarbital (IRVINE

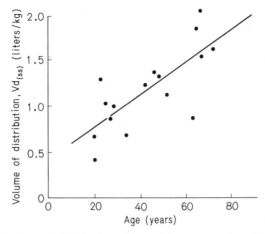

Fig. 21. Correlation of volume of distribution, Vd$_{(ss)}$, of diazepam and age in normal individuals (Klotz et al., 1975)

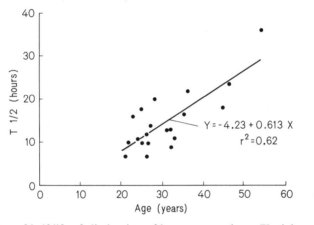

Fig. 22. Correlation of half-life of elimination of lorazepam and age (Kyriakopoulos 1976)

et al., 1974), and phenobarbital (TRAEGER et al., 1974) are known to increase with age in man. Figures 22 and 23 show the change in half-life with age for lorazepam (KYRIAKOPOULOS, 1976) and chlordiazepoxide (ROBERTS et al., 1978), respectively.

Pharmacokinetic parameters of particular interest are half-life and volume of distribution since they determine clearance. Although changes in half-life and volume of distribution may occur with age, if the clearance of a drug is age independent then unanticipated drug accumulation will not occur and chronic dosage regimen modifications based on pharmacokinetic considerations are unnecessary for the geriatric patient. Correlations of clearance and age for chlordiazepoxide and diazepam in adults are shown in Figs. 24 and 25, respectively. Whereas the clearance of lorazepam (KYRIAKOPOULOS, 1976) and chlordiazepoxide (ROBERTS et al., 1978) decreases with age, the clearance of diazepam is independent of age.

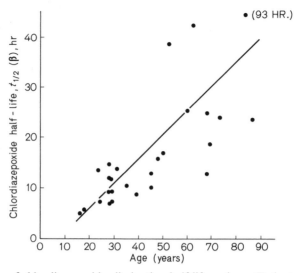

Fig. 23. Correlation of chlordiazepoxide elimination half-life and age (Roberts et al., 1978)

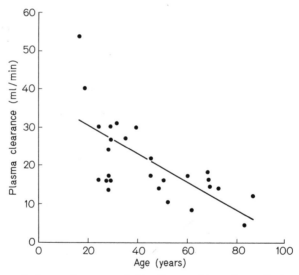

Fig. 24. Correlation of plasma clearance of chlordiazepoxide and age (Roberts et al., 1978)

2. Hepatic Disease

The pharmacokinetics of drugs may be altered in the presence of hepatic disease requiring adjustment in dose or dose frequency. The pharmacokinetic parameters affected by liver disease include binding, extraction ratio, hepatic clearance, and half-life of elimination of the administered drug. The pharmacokinetic profiles of some benzodiazepines in patients with acute and chronic parenchymal liver disease are presented in Table 12. Chlordiazepoxide and diazepam exhibit changes in half-lives,

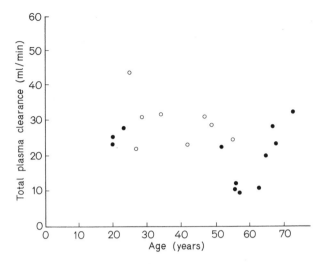

Fig. 25. Correlation of total plasma clearance of diazepam with age. *Solid circles* refer to non-smokers and *open circles* to smokers (more than 20 cigarettes per day) (Klotz et al., 1975)

Table 12. The half-lives, plasma clearances, and volumes of distribution of chlordiazepoxide, diazepam, lorazepam, and oxazepam in normal subjects and patients with hepatitis and cirrhosis[a]

	Chlordiazepoxide[b]	Diazepam[b]	Lorazepam	Oxazepam[b]
$t_{1/2}$ (h)				
Normals	11.1	32.7	24 (12)[c]	5.1
Hepatitis	91.0	60–75	25	5.3
Normals	23.8	46.6	24 (12)[c]	5.6
Cirrhosis	62.7	105.6	31.9	5.8
Plasma clearance (ml/min)				
Normals	18.1	26.6	0.75[d]	113
Hepatitis	6.1	13–18	0.81[d]	137
Normals	15.3	26.6	0.75[d]	136
Cirrhosis	7.7	13.8	0.74[d]	155
Volume of distribution (1/kg)				
Normals	0.27	–	1.28	0.64
Hepatitis	0.44	–	1.52	0.82
Normals	0.33	1.13	1.28	0.76
Cirrhosis	0.48	1.74	2.01	0.88

[a] Information obtained from the following sources: Chlordiazepoxide, ROBERTS et al., 1978; Diazepam, KLOTZ et al., 1975; Lorazepam, KYRIAKOPOLOUS, 1976 and KRAUS et al., 1978; Oxazepam, SHULL et al., 1976

[b] Age-matched controls

[c] Half-life values reported by KRAUS et al., 1978, of 24 h are at variance with all other studies. KYRIAKOPOLOUS, 1976 and GREENBLATT et al., 1977b, 1979b; where normals have reported half-lives of 12 h as indicated above

[d] Lorazepam, ml/min/kg; other drugs reported as ml/min

348   S. A. KAPLAN and M. L. JACK

Table 13. Dosage interval calculated to maintain steady-state plasma levels (µg/ml) equal to normal subjects in simulated cirrhotic patients exhibiting potential twofold or fivefold increase in half-life (KAPLAN and JACK, 1979)

Parameter	Normal	Cirrhotic		Cirrhotic (corrected)	
Half-life increase	–	2×	5×	2×	5×
Dosage interval	24 h	24 h	24 h	31 h	78 h
C_{min} (µg/ml)	0.144	0.225	0.607	0.166	0.163
C_{max} (µg/ml)	0.256	0.300	0.682	0.241	0.237

clearances, and volumes of distribution. There is a two–threefold decrease in clearance for both diazepam and chlordiazepoxide, suggesting that adjustments in dose schedules may be necessary in the presence of hepatic dysfunction.

The clearance values for lorazepam are essentially unchanged in the presence of liver disease; however, changes in half-life and volume of distribution are noted. Oxazepam exhibits slight changes in clearance and volume of distribution in patients with hepatitis and cirrhosis.

Changes in pharmacokinetic parameters of other anxiolytic agents have been observed. Meprobamate (HELD and VON OLDERSHAUSEN, 1969), amobarbital (MAWER et al., 1972), pentobarbital (HELD and VON OLDERSHAUSEN, 1969), and phenobarbital (ALVIN et al., 1975) have all been found to have longer half-lives in patients with liver disease.

Once the influence of disease on the pharmacokinetic parameters is established, a new dosage regimen may be calculated to yield desired plasma levels. The steady-state maximum and minimum plasma levels of a benzodiazepine following a once daily dosage regimen for normals and cirrhotics with a potential for two- and five-fold increases in half-life are reported in the first three columns of Table 13. As calculated, the steady-state maximum and minimum plasma levels for the cirrhotic patient would be high when compared to those of normals. To achieve comparable steady-state levels in the cirrhotic, the dosage regimen may be adjusted by taking into account changes in half-life. The resulting regimen for a two- and fivefold increase in half-life would be a change from a dosage once every 24 h to once every 31 and 78 h, respectively (columns five and six, Table 13). The steady-state maximum and minimum for the cirrhotic (corrected) would then be equivalent to the steady-state levels in normals, and unanticipated drug accumulation will not occur unless there are other changes in the pathologic state. Therefore, in spite of changes in the pharmacokinetic parameters of the benzodiazepines due to hepatic dysfunction or other pathologic states, new dosage regimens may be readily calculated to assure maintenance of plasma levels associated with clinical efficacy and safety of the drugs.

3. Renal Disease

In general, drugs which are extensively metabolized in vivo can be given in normal doses to uremic patients (REIDENBERG, 1971, 1975). However, in renal failure, water soluble drugs or metabolites will accumulate and, if pharmacologically active, may exhibit an enhanced or prolonged response. In addition, protein binding is reduced in

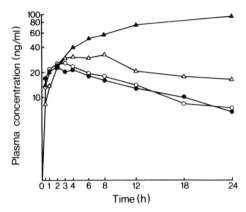

Fig. 26. Plasma concentration curves of the unchanged (●, ○) and conjugated (▲, △) lorazepam; data taken from six normal subjects (○, △) and seven patients with terminal renal insufficiency (●, ▲) after a 2.5-mg single oral dose of lorazepam (Verbeeck et al., 1976)

renal disease. Since the 1,4-substituted benzodiazepines are highly protein bound and extensively metabolized, the pharmacokinetics of these drugs may be affected by renal failure.

Lorazepam and oxazepam are metabolized to water soluble, pharmacologically inactive conjugates which are readily excreted in the urine of healthy subjects. However, when these drugs are administered to uremic patients, a somewhat different pharmacokinetic profile emerges. The plasma concentrations and half-life of lorazepam are essentially the same in uremic patients as in normals, suggesting that the metabolism of lorazepam to the glucuronide is uninhibited in uremia (VERBEECK et al., 1976). However, the urinary excretion of lorazepam glucuronide was decreased in these patients, resulting in a three- to sixfold increase in both plasma concentrations and half-lives of the metabolite (Fig. 26). Since the lorazepam glucuronide is pharmacologically inactive, the clinical significance of lorazepam glucuronide accumulation is not known.

Following single dose administrations of oxazepam to uremic patients (ODAR-CEDERLÖF et al., 1977), a two- to fivefold increase in half-life of oxazepam was observed, whereas the plasma clearance was not altered. However, accumulation of the conjugate, oxazepam glucuronide and a several-fold increase in half-life of this metabolite were both observed. The plasma level profiles and some pharmacokinetic parameters of oxazepam following single dose administration to normals and uremic patients are presented in Fig. 27 and Table 14.

The plasma levels of oxazepam following multiple doses to uremic patients were within the range found in normals as might be anticipated from the constancy of plasma clearance in the single dose study (ODAR-CEDERLÖF et al., 1977). However, the metabolite, oxazepam glucuronide, accumulated in the plasma following multiple doses of oxazepam (ODER-CEDERLÖF et al., 1977).

No data have yet been published on the pharmacokinetic profile of temazepam in uremic patients. However, the formation of the water-soluble glucuronide metabolite suggests that this metabolite will have a pharmacokinetic profile similar to that of lorazepam glucuronide and oxazepam glucuronide in uremic patients.

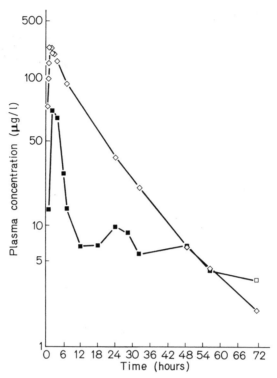

Fig. 27. Plasma levels of oxazepam following a 15-mg oral dose of oxazepam to a normal subject (◇) and a uremic patient (■) (Adapted from Odar-Cederlöf et al., 1977; Alván et al., 1977; and Wretlind et al., 1977)

Table 14. Pharmacokinetic parameters of oxazepam following oral administration to normal subjects and uremic patients[a]

Dose	Normals 15 mg	Uremics 0.2 mg/kg
Half-life of elimination (h)		
Mean	12.3	47.6
Range	7.5–24.9	23.7–91.2
Plasma clearance ($1 \ kg^{-1} \ h^{-1}$)		
Mean	0.108	0.141
Range	0.050–0.171	0.025–0.284
% protein binding	94.9–95.9	86.2–93.6
% of dose in the urine (0–72 h)		
Mean	67	21.5
Range	41–89	3.87–47.2
% of dose in feces (0–72 h)		
Mean	2.5	8.3
Range	0–3	0.1–19.1

[a] Adapted from ALVÁN et al. (1977) and ODARCEDERLÖF et al. (1977)

Diazepam and nordiazepam are highly protein bound benzodiazepines. KANGAS et al. (1976) report that the binding of both diazepam and nordiazepam is reduced in uremic patients from 98.4% and 98.3% to 92% and 94.5%, respectively. Such changes in protein binding have the potential to enhance the pharmacologic effect of diazepam and nordiazepam. Similar findings would be anticipated following the administration of clorazepate and prazepam to uremic patients.

C. Pharmacokinetic Profiles of Meprobamate and Propanediol Carbamates

Meprobamate was the first antianxiety agent of the propanediol carbamate drug class and for this reason may be considered the prototype drug. Meprobamate was originally synthesized as a potential muscle relaxant, a "longer acting" successor to mephenesin. Tybamate, another propanediol carbamate, is also marketed as an anxiolytic agent. The structures of meprobamate and tybamate are presented in Fig. 28. Meprobamate with a pKa of 14 is slightly soluble in water (0.34% w/w at 20 °C) and is stable in gastric and intestinal fluids (Merck Index, 1976). Tybamate is less water soluble and more lipophilic than meprobamate. The partition coefficient for tybamate is several orders of magnitude greater than for meprobamate.

I. Single Dose Pharmacokinetics

The pharmacokinetic profiles of meprobamate and tybamate in man are presented in Table 15. Meprobamate is not bound by plasma proteins and exhibits a half-life of 11.3 h. It is eliminated 3–4 times more slowly than tybamate. The substitution of a butyl group in place of a carbamyl hydrogen (tybamate) results in a compound with a 3-h half-life and which is 80% protein bound.

These differences in the physicochemical properties of meprobamate and tybamate influence the absorption, distribution, elimination, and protein binding profiles of these drugs. Following oral administration, the blood level peak times of meprobamate and tybamate occur at 2 h, suggesting rapid oral absorption of both drugs. The blood level peak height for meprobamate is greater than that of tybamate, reflecting differences in volume of distribution due to differences in physicochemical properties. Following whole-body radioautography in mice, tybamate distributes more rapidly than meprobamate into the brain and central nervous system (VAN DER KLEIJN, 1969). Such data reflect its greater lipophilicity. Meprobamate and tybamate

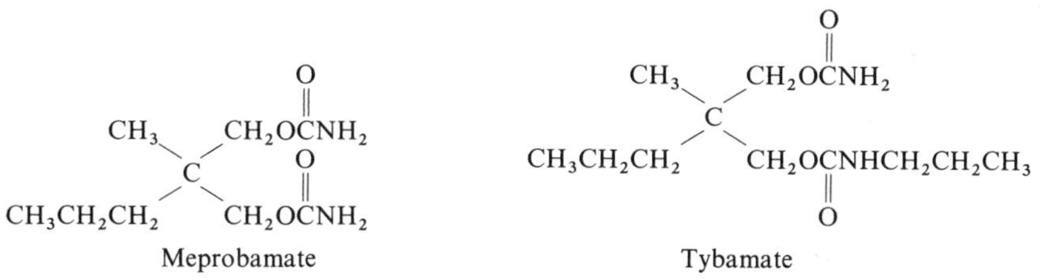

Fig. 28. Structures of meprobamate and tybamate

Table 15. Biopharmaceutical and pharmacokinetic profiles of meprobamate and tybamate[a]

	Meprobamate	Tybamate
Dose (mg)	800	1,050
Peak time (h)	1–2	2
Peak height (μg/ml)	16	12
Protein binding (%)	0	80
Half-life (h)	11.3	3
Clearance (ml/min)	100	–
Urinary excretion date		
Percent of dose in the 0–48-hour urine as:		
Intact drug	8–20	–
Metabolites and conjugates	10	–
Partition coefficient		
Chloroform/water	3.3	> 500
Cottonseed oil/water	0.3	> 20
pKa	14.0	–

[a] Information taken from the following sources: Meprobamate: LUDWIG et al., 1961; HOLLISTER, 1962; DOUGLAS et al., 1964; HOLLISTER and LEVY, 1964; VAN DER KLEIJN, 1969; LUDWIG and POTTERFIELD, 1971; RICE et al., 1972. Tybamate: DOUGLAS et al., 1964; HOLLISTER and CLYDE, 1968; VAN DER KLEIJN, 1969; LUDWIG and POTTERFIELD, 1971.

have also been shown to pass through the placenta into the fetuses of pregnant mice (VAN DER KLEIJN, 1969). Possible teratogenicity associated with meprobamate in humans has also been reported (MILKOVICH and VANDENBERG, 1974; ROSENBERG, 1975).

The urinary excretion profile of meprobamate is reported in Table 15. Of the dose 8%–20% is excreted as intact drug, suggesting extensive metabolism of meprobamate in vivo.

Meprobamate is metabolized in man to hydroxymeprobamate [2-methyl-2-(β-hydroxypropyl)-1,3-propanediol dicarbamate] and to the glucosyluronide of meprobamate (LUDWIG et al., 1961). Approximately 10% of the administered dose is excreted as metabolites and conjugates in the urine.

Little has been reported concerning the metabolism of tybamate in man; however, DOUGLAS et al. (1966) have shown that tybamate is metabolized to hydroxytybamate, hydroxymeprobamate, and meprobamate in the dog and the rat. These three metabolites, as well as unchanged tybamate, are excreted in the urine of these animals.

II. Multiple Dose Studies

It has been reported that the disposition profile of meprobamate changes on chronic administration. DOUGLAS et al. (1963) report that meprobamate induces its own metabolism on chronic administration as evidenced by the increased urinary excretion of metabolite following chronic administration of meprobamate. HOLLISTER (1964) and HOLLISTER and GLAZENER (1960), however, noted a two- to fivefold prolongation

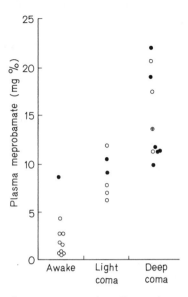

Fig. 29. Relationship between plasma concentration of meprobamate and state of consciousness (Maddock and Bloomer, 1967) ○ Meprobamate: alone, ● Meprobamate and complications, ⊗ Fatal case

in the half-life of meprobamate on chronic administration, suggesting inhibition of metabolism. Such differences remain to be resolved. There is no data available on tybamate following chronic administration.

III. Clinical Toxicology

MISRA et al. (1971) showed that chronic ethanol consumption results in acceleration of blood clearance of meprobamate. The average half-life of meprobamate decreased from 13.7 h to 8.2 h in the same subjects following 1 month of controlled alcohol ingestion.

Although HOLLISTER and CLYDE (1968) found no correlation between meprobamate blood or plasma level and antianxiety response, MADDOCK and BLOOMER (1967) demonstrated a correlation between meprobamate plasma levels and meprobamate intoxication (Fig. 29). At plasma concentrations below 5 mg-%, all patients were awake. Plasma concentrations greater than 10 mg-% are associated with deep coma, and plasma concentrations between 6 and 12 mg-% are associated with light coma.

Meprobamate has little or no affinity for plasma proteins, suggesting that hemodialysis and diuresis would be beneficial in meprobamate overdose (DOUGLAS et al., 1964; MADDOCK and BLOOMER, 1967).

IV. Structure Correlations

The extensive acceptance and success of meprobamate as an anxiolytic agent that did not decrease awareness or impair the physical and intellectual abilities of patients stimulated interest in the propanediol dicarbamate compounds. For this reason,

Table 16. Propanediol carbamate drug compounds (LUDWIG and POTTERFIELD, 1971).

$$
\begin{array}{c}
\text{CH}_3 \quad\quad \text{CH}_2\text{OCNH}_2 \\
\overset{\text{O}}{\underset{\parallel}{}} \\
\text{C} \\
\text{R}_1 \quad\quad \text{CH}_2\text{OCNHR}_2 \\
\overset{\parallel}{\text{O}}
\end{array}
$$

Drug	R_1	R_2
Meprobamate	$CH_3CH_2CH_2-$	H
Mebutamate	CH_3CH_2CH- $\quad\quad\quad\mid$ $\quad\quad\quad CH_3$	H
Carisoprodol	$CH_3CH_2CH_2-$	$-CH \overset{CH_3}{\underset{CH_3}{}}$
Tybamate	$CH_3CH_2CH_2-$	$-CH_2CH_2CH_2CH_3$

structurally related compounds in this drug class were investigated. Seemingly simple alkyl substitutions resulted in compounds with very different pharmacologic and pharmacokinetic properties. The propanediol carbamates structurally related to meprobamate are shown in Table 16.

Differences in half-life, protein binding, and distribution characteristics between meprobamate and tybamate have been previously noted. Substitution of a secondary butyl group in the R_1 position results in a compound (mebutamate) which, like meprobamate, is not protein bound but is pharmacologically active as an antihypertensive (LUDWIG and POTTERFIELD, 1971). Carisoprodol results from the substitution of an isopropyl group in the R_2 position. Tybamate and carisoprodol are protein bound (80% and 55%, respectively) and are more lipophilic than meprobamate or mebutamate. Carisoprodol has muscle relaxant and analgesic properties. The pharmacology of these compounds is discussed by LUDWIG and POTTERFIELD (1971). Such data indicate the difficulties encountered in any structure-activity correlations with propanediol carbamates.

D. Summary

The pharmacokinetic profiles of the benzodiazepine anxiolytic agents and the propanediol carbamates are presented.

Following single dose administrations, the pharmacokinetic profiles of the benzodiazepines suggest that these compounds exhibit "apparent" first-order pharmacokinetic profiles and the multiple dose profiles are predictable from the parameters obtained following single dose administration. The ability to achieve such predictable multiple dose profiles confirms the constancy and reproducibility of absorption, distribution, and elimination from administration to administration.

The effects of age and disease state on the pharmacokinetic profiles of the benzodiazepines are also discussed. With the exception of oxazepam, the overall elimination rate of the benzodiazepines and meprobamate is usually prolonged in the geriatric patient and in patients with hepatic dysfunction. The pharmacokinetic profiles of lorazepam, oxazepam, and their respective metabolites are altered in the presence of renal disease, while the pharmacokinetic profiles of the other benzodiazepines appear to be essentially unchanged. Understanding the influence of various pathologic conditions on the pharmacokinetic profiles of the benzodiazepines will aid the clinician in the proper selection of dose and dosage regimen to maintain efficacy.

References

Abruzzo, C.W., Macasieb, T., Weinfeld, R.W., Rider, J.A., Kaplan, S.A.: Changes in the oral absorption characteristics in man of dipotassium clorazepate at normal and elevated gastric pH. J. Pharmacokinet. Biopharm. 5, 377–390 (1977)

Allen, M.D., Greenblatt, D.J., Shader, R.I.: Single-dose kinetics of oral prazepam. Clin. Pharmacol. Ther. 25, 211–212 (1979)

Álvan, G., Sievers, B., Vessman, J.: Pharmacokinetics of oxazepam in healthy volunteers. Acta Pharmacol. Toxicol. 40 (Suppl. 1), 40–51 (1977)

Alvin, J., Mchorse, T., Hoyumpa, A., Bush, M.T., Schenker, S.: The effect of liver disease in man on the disposition of phenobarbital. J. Pharmacol. Exp. Ther. 192, 224–235 (1975)

Andreasen, P.B., Hendel, J., Greisen, G., Hvidberg, E.F.: Pharmacokinetics of diazepam in disordered liver function. Eur. J. Clin. Pharmacol. 10, 115–120 (1976)

Assaf, R.A.E., Dundee, J.W., Gamble, J.A.S.: Factors influencing plasma diazepam levels following a single administration. Br. J. Clin. Pharmacol. 1, P343–344 (1974)

Boxenbaum, H.G., Geitner, K.A., Jack, M.L., Dixon, W.R., Spiegel, H.E., Symington, J., Christian, R., Moore, J.D., Weissman, L., Kaplan, S.A.: Pharmacokinetic and biopharmaceutic profile of chlordiazepoxide HCl in healthy subjects: single dose studies by the intravenous, intramuscular, and oral routes. J. Pharmacokinet. Biopharm. 5, 3–23 (1977a)

Boxenbaum, H.G., Geitner, K.A., Jack, M.L., Dixon, W.R., Kaplan, S.A.: Pharmacokinetic and biopharmaceutic profile of chlordiazepoxide HCl in healthy subjects: multiple-dose oral administration. J. Pharmacokinet. Biopharm. 5, 25–39 (1977b)

Carrigan, P.J., Chao, G.C., Barker, W.M., Hoffman, D.J., Chun, A.H.C.: Steady-state biovailability of two clorazepate dipotassium dosage forms. J. Clin. Pharmacol. 17, 18–28 (1977)

Chun, A.H.C., Carrigan, P.J., Hoffman, D.J., Kershner, R.P., Stuart, J.D.: Effect of antacid on absorption of clorazepate. Clin. Pharmacol. Ther. 22, 329–335 (1977)

Cole, J.O.: Drug treatment of anxiety. South. Med. J. 71, 10–14 (1978)

Dicarlo, F.J., Viau, J.P., Epps, J.E., Haynes, L.J.: Prazepam metabolism by man. Clin. Pharmacol. Ther. 11, 890–897 (1970)

Douglas, J.F., Ludwig, B.J., Smith, N.: Studies on the metabolism of meprobamate. Proc. Soc. Exp. Biol. Med. 112, 436–438 (1963)

Douglas, J.F., Bradshaw, W.H., Ludwig, B.J., Powers, D.: Interaction of plasma protein with related 1,3 propanediol dicarbamates. Biochem. Pharmacol. 13, 537–538 (1964)

Douglas, J.F., Ludwig, B.J., Schlosser, A., Edelson, J.: The metabolic fate of tybamate in the rat and dog. Biochem. Pharmacol. 15, 2087–2095 (1966)

Driscoll, E., Smelack, Z., Lichtbody, P., Fiorucci, R.D.: Sedation with intravenous diazepam. J. Oral Surg. 30, 332–342 (1972)

Drug action. Pharmacokinetics of diazepam after I.V., I.M., and oral administration. Drug Intell. Clin. Pharm. 12, 626–627 (1978)

Eatman, F.B., Colburn, W.A., Boxenbaum, H.G., Posmanter, H.N., Weinfeld, R.E., Ronfeld, R., Weissman, L., Moore, J.D., Gibaldi, M., Kaplan, S.A.: Pharmacokinetics of diazepam following multiple dose oral administration to healthy human subjects. J. Pharmacokinet. Biopharm. 5, 481–494 (1977)

Fuccella, L.M., Tosolini, G., Moro, E., Tamassia, V.: Study of physiological availability of temazepam in man. Int. J. Clin. Pharmacol. Ther. Tox. 6, 303–309 (1972)

Gibaldi, M.: Biopharmaceutics and clinical pharmacokinetics, 2nd ed. Philadelphia: Lea and Febiger 1977

Glazko, A.J., Chang, T., Peterson, F.E., Johnson, E.L., Young, R.M., Hayes, A.G., Goulet, R.J., Smith, T.C.: Metabolic disposition of diazepam and prazepam in man: Multiple dose studies. Fed. Proc., Fed. Am. Soc. Exp. Biol. *38*, 742 (1979)

Greenblatt, D.J., Koch-Weser, J.: Clinical pharmacokinetics. N. Engl. J. Med. *293*, 702–705 (1975)

Greenblatt, D.J., Shader, R.I.: Prazepam, a precursor of desmethyldiazepam. Lancet *1*, 720 (1978a)

Greenblatt, D.J., Shader, R.I.: Pharmacokinetic understanding of antianxiety drug therapy. South Med. J. *71* (suppl. 2), 2–9 (1978b)

Greenblatt, D.J., Shader, R.I., Koch-Weser, J.: Pharmacokinetic determinants of the response to single doses of chlordiazepoxide. Am. J. Psychiat. *131*, 1395–1397 (1974a)

Greenblatt, D.J., Shader, R.I., Koch-Weser, J.: Slow absorption of intramuscular chlordiazepoxide. N. Engl. J. Med. *291*, 1116–1118 (1974b)

Greenblatt, D.J., Shader, R.I., Koch-Weser, J.: Pharmacokinetics in clinical medicine: Oxazepam versus other benzodiazepines. Dis. Nerv. Syst. **36**, 6–13 (1975)

Greenblatt, D.J., Schillings, R.T., Kyriakopoulos, A.A., Shader, R.I., Sisenwine, S.F., Knowles, J.A., Ruelius, H.W.: Clinical pharmacokinetics of lorazepam. I. Absorption and distribution of oral ^{14}C lorazepam. Clin. Pharmacol. Therap. *20*, 329–341 (1976)

Greenblatt, D.J., Shader, R.I., Franke, K., Maclaughlin, D.S., Ransil, B.J., Koch-Weser, J.: Kinetics of intravenous chlordiazepoxide: sex differences in drug distribution. J. Clin. Pharmacol. Ther. *22*, 893–903 (1977a)

Greenblatt, D.J., Comer, W.H., Elliott, H.W., Shader, R.I., Knowles, J.A., Ruelius, H.W.: Clinical pharmacokinetics of lorazepam. III. Intravenous injection. J. Clin. Pharmacol. *17*, 490–493 (1977b)

Greenblatt, D.J., Joyce, T.H., Comer, W.H., Knowles, J.A., Shader, R.I., Kyriakopoulos, A.A., Maclaughlin, D.S., Ruelius, H.W.: Clinical Pharmacokinetics of lorazepam. II. Intramuscular injection. Clin. Pharmacol. Ther. *21*, 222–230 (1977c)

Greenblatt, D.J., Knowles, J.A., Comer, W.H., Shader, R.I., Harmatz, J.S., Ruelius, H.W.: Clinical pharmacokinetics of lorazepam. IV. Long-term oral administration. J. Clin. Pharmacol. *17*, 495–500 (1977d)

Greenblatt, D.J., Shader, R.I., Macleod, S.M., Sellers, E.M., Franke, K., Giles, H.G.: Absorption of oral and intramuscular chlordiazepoxide. Eur. J. Clin. Pharmacol. *13*, 267–274 (1978)

Greenblatt, D.J., Allen, M.D., MacLaughlin, D.S., Huffman, D.H., Harmatz, J.S., Shader, R.I.: Single and multiple dose kinetics of oral lorazepam in humans: The predictability of accumulation. J. Pharmacokinet. Biopharm. *7*, 159–179 (1979a)

Greenblatt, D.J., Shader, R.I., Franke, K., MacLaughlin, D.S., Harmatz, J.S., Allen, M.D., Werner, A., Woo, E.: Pharmacokinetics and bioavailability of intravenous, intramuscular, and oral lorazepam in humans. J. Pharm. Sci. *66*, 57–63 (1979b)

Held, H., Oldershausen, H.F. von: Zur Pharmakokinetik von Meprobamat bei chronischen Hepatopathien und Arzneimittelsucht. Klin. Wochenschr. *47*, 78–80 (1969)

Hendel, J., Elsass, P., Andreasen, P.B., Gymoese, E., Hvidberg, E.F.: Neuropsychologic effects of diazepam related to single dose kinetics and liver function. Psychopharmacology *48*, 11–17 (1976)

Hillestad, L., Hansen, T., Melsom, H., Drivenes, A.: Diazepam metabolism in normal man. I. Serum concentrations and clinical effects after intravenous, intramuscular, and oral administration. Clin. Pharmacol. Ther. *16*, 479–484 (1974)

Hollister, L.E.: Studies of delayed-action medication. 1. Meprobamate administered as compressed tablets and as two delayed-action capsules. N. Engl. J. Med. *266*, 281–283 (1962)

Hollister, L.E.: Clinical use of psychotherapeutic drugs. Springfield, Illinois: Charles C. Thomas Publishers 1973

Hollister, L., Clyde, D.J.: Blood levels of pentobarbital sodium, meprobamate and tybamate in relation to clinical effect. Clin. Pharmacol. Ther. *9*, 204–208 (1968)

Hollister, L.E.: Glazener, F.S.: Withdrawal reactions from meprobamate alone and combined with promazine: a controlled study. Psychopharmacology *1*, 336–341 (1960)

Hollister, L.E., Levy, G.: Kinetics of meprobamate elimination in humans. Chemotherapia *9*, 20–24 (1964)

Irvine, R.E., Grove, J., Toseland, P.A., Trounce, J.R.: The effect of age on the hydroxylation of amylobarbitone sodium in man. Br. J. Clin. Pharmacol. *1*, 41–43 (1974)

Johnson, R.F., Schenker, S., Roberts, R.K., Desmond, P.V., Wilkinson, G.R.: Plasma binding of benzodiazepines in humans. J. Pharm. Sci. *68*, 1320–1322 (1979).

Kangas, L., Kanto, J., Forsstroem, J., Iisalo, E.: The protein binding of diazepam and *N*-desmethyldiazepam in patients with poor renal function. Clin. Nephrol. *5*, 114–118 (1976)

Kaplan, S.A., Jack, M.L.: Minor tranquilizer pharmacokinetics. In: The kinetics of psychiatric drugs. Schoolar, H., Claghorn, I. (eds.). New York: Brunner/Mazel, Inc. 1979

Kaplan, S.A., Jack, M.L., Alexander, K., Weinfeld, R.W.: Pharmacokinetic profile of diazepam in man following single intravenous and oral and chronic oral administration. J. Pharm. Sci. *62*, 1789–1796 (1973)

Kaplan, S.A., Jack, M.L., Weinfeld, R.W., Glover, W., Weissman, L., Cotler, S.: Biopharmaceutical and clinical pharmacokinetic profile of bromazepam. J. Pharmacokinet. Biopharm. *4*, 1–16 (1976)

Klotz, U., Müller-Seydlitz, P.: Altered elimination of desmethyldiazepam in the elderly. Br. J. Clin. Pharmacol. *7*, 119–120 (1979)

Klotz, U., Avant, G.R., Hoyumpa, A., Schenker, S., Wilkinson, G.R.: The effect of age and liver disease on the disposition and elimination of diazepam in adult man. J. Clin. Invest. *55*, 347–359 (1975)

Klotz, U., Antonin, K.H., Bieck, P.R.: Pharmacokinetics and plasma binding of diazepam in man, dog, rabbit, guinea pig, and rat. J. Pharmacol. Exp. Ther. *199*, 67–73 (1976a)

Klotz, U., Antonin, K.H., Bieck, P.R.: Comparison of the pharmacokinetics of diazepam after single and subchronic doses. Eur. J. Clin. Pharmacol. *10*, 121–126 (1976b)

Koechlin, B.A., Schwartz, M.A., Krol, G., Oberhansli, W.: The metabolic fate of C^{14}-labeled chlordiazepoxide in man, in the dog, and in the rat. J. Pharmacol. Exp. Ther. *148*, 399–411 (1965)

Kraus, J.W., Desmond, P.V., Marshall, J.P., Johnson, R.F., Schenker, S., Wilkinson, G.R.: Effects of aging and liver disease on disposition of lorazepam. Clin. Pharmacol. Ther. *24*, 411–419 (1978)

Kyriakopoulos, A.A.: Biovailability of lorazepam in humans. In: Pharmacokinetics of psychoactive drugs, Gottschalk, D., Merlis, S. (eds), New York: Spectrum Publications Inc. 1976

Kyriakopoulos, A.A., Greenblatt, D.J., Shader, R.I.: Clinical pharmacokinetics of lorazepam: a review. J. Clin. Psychiat. *39*, No. 10 Sec. 2, 16–23 (1978)

Ludwig, B.J., Potterfield, J.R.: The Pharmacology of propanediol carbamates. Adv. Pharmacol. Chemother. *9*, 173–240 (1971)

Ludwig, B.J., Douglas, J.F., Powell, L.S., Meyer, M., Berger, F.M.: Structures of the major metabolites of meprobamate. J. Med. Pharmacol. Chem. *3*, 53–64 (1961)

Macleod, S.M., Greenblatt, D.J., Sellers, E.M.: Determination of intravenous chlordiazepoxide (CDX) pharmacokinetics: plasma versus blood. Clin. Res. *25*, 273A (1977)

Maddock, R.K., Bloomer, H.A.: Meprobamate overdosage. J. Am. Med. Ass. *201*, 999–1003 (1967)

Mawer, G.E., Miller, N.E., Turnberg, L.A.: Metabolism of amylobarbitone in patients with chronic liver disease. Br. J. Pharmacol. *44*, 549–560 (1972)

The Merck Index.: (Ninth Edition), Rahway, N.J.: Merck & Co., Inc. 1976

Milkovich, L., Vandenberg, B.J.: Effects of prenatal meprobamate and chlordiazepoxide hydrochloride on human embryonic and fetal development. N. Engl. J. Med. *291*, 1268–1271 (1974)

Misra, P.S., Lefevre, A., Ishii, H., Rubin, E., Lieber, C.S.: Increase of ethanol, meprobamate and pentobarbital metabolism after chronic ethanol administration in man and rats. Am. J. Med. *51*, 346–351 (1971)

Morselli, P., Cassano, G., Placidi, G., Musscettola, G., Risso, M.: Kinetics of the distribution of ^{14}C-diazepam and its metabolites in various areas of cat brain. In: The benzodiazepines. Garattini, S., Mussini, E., Randall, L.O. (eds.), New York: Raven Press 1973a

Morselli, P.L., Principi, N., Tognoni, G., Reali, E., Belvedere, G., Standen, S.M., Sereni, F.: Diazepam elimination in premature and full term infants, and children. J. Perinatal. Med. *1*, 133–141 (1973b)

Odar-Cederlöf, I., Vessman, J., Alván, G., Sjoqvist, F.: Oxazepam disposition in uremic patients. Acta Pharmacol. Toxicol. *40 (Supppl. 1)*, 52–62 (1977)

Post, C., Lindgren, S., Bertler, A., Malmgren, H.: Pharmacokinetics of N-desmethyldiazepam in healthy volunteers after single daily does of dipotassium clorazepate. Psychopharmacology 53, 105–109 (1977)

Raaflaub, J., Speiser-Courvoisier, J.: Zur Pharmakokinetik von Bromazepam beim Menschen. Arzneim. Forsch. 24, 1841–1844 (1974)

Reidenberg, M.M.: Drug metabolism in uremia. Clin. Nephrol. 4, 83–85 (1975)

Reidenberg, M.M.: Renal function and drug action. Philadelphia: W.B. Saunders Company 1971

Rice, A.J., Gruhn, S.W., Gibson, T.P., Delle, M., Dibona, G.F.: Effect of saline infusion on renal excretion of secobarbital, glutethimide, meprobamate and chlordiazepoxide. J. Lab. Clin. Med. 80, 56–62 (1972)

Roberts, R.K., Wilkinson, G.R., Branch, R.A., Schenker, S.: Effect of age and cirrhosis on the disposition and elimination of chlordiazepoxide (Librium). Gastroenterology 73, A45/1243 (1977)

Roberts, R.K., Wilkinson, G.R., Branch, R.A., Schenker, S.: Effect of age and parenchymal liver disease on the disposition and elimination of chlordiazepoxide (Librium). Gastroenterology 75, 479–485 (1978)

Rosenberg, J.M.: Is it safe to utilize minor tranquilizers auch as Librium, Valium and meprobamate during pregnancy. N.Y. State J. Med. 75, 1334–1335 (1975)

Schwartz, M.A., Postma, E., Gaut, Z.: Biological half-life of chlordiazepoxide and its metabolite, demoxepam, in man. J. Pharm..Sci. 60, 1500–1503 (1971)

Schwartz, M.A., Postma, E., Kolis, S.J., Leon, A.S.: Metabolites of bromazepam, a benzodiazepine, in the human, dog, rat, and mouse. J. Pharm. Sci. 62, 1776–1779 (1973)

Shader, R.I., Greenblatt, D.J.: Clinical implications of benzodiazepine pharmacokinetics. Am. J. Psychiat. 134, 652–656 (1977)

Shader, R.I., Greenblatt, D.J., Harmatz, J.S., Franke, K., Koch-Weser, J.: Absorption and disposition of chlordiazepoxide in young and elderly male volunteers. J. Clin. Pharmacol. 17, 709–718 (1977)

Shader, R.I., Georgotas, A., Greenblatt, D.J., Harmatz, J.S., Allen, M.D.: Impaired absorption of desmethyldiazepam from clorazepate by magnesium aluminum hydroxide. Clin. Pharmacol. Ther. 24, 308–315 (1978)

Shull, H.J., Wilkinson, G.R., Johnson, R., Schenker, S.: Normal disposition of oxazepam in acute viral hepatitis and cirrhosis. Ann. Int. Med. 84, 420–425 (1976)

Tinklenberg, J.R.: Antianxiety medication and treatment of anxiety. In: Psychopharmacology from theory to practice (Barchas, J., Berger, P., Ciaranello, R, Elliot, G. (eds.), New York: Oxford University Press 1977

Tognoni, G., Gomeni, R., Demaio, D., Alberti, G.G., Franciosi, P., Scieghi, G.: Pharmacokinetics of N-desmethyldiazepam in patients suffering from insomnia and treated with nortriptyline. Br. J. Clin. Pharmacol. 2, 227–232 (1975)

Tomson, G., Lunell, N.O., Sundwall, A., Rane, A.: Placental passage of oxazepam and its metabolism in mothers and newborns. Clin. Pharmacol. Ther. 25, 74–81 (1979)

Traeger, A., Kiesewetter, R., Kunze, M.: Zur Pharmakokinetik von Phenobarbital bei Erwachsenen und Greisen. Dtsch. Ges. Wesen. 29, 1040–1042 (1974)

Van der Kleijn, E.: Kinetics of distribution and metabolism of ataractics of the meprobamate group in mice. Arch. Int. Pharmacodyn. 178, 457–480 (1969)

Verbeeck, R., Tjandramaga, T.B., Verberckmoes, R., Deschepper, P.J.: Biotransformation and excretion of lorazepam in patients with chronic renal failure. Br. J. Clin. Pharmacol. 3, 1033–1039 (1976)

Vest, M.F., Rossier, R.: Detoxification in the newborn: The ability of the newborn infant to form conjugates with glucuronic acid, glycine, acetate, and glutathione. Ann. N.Y. Acad. Sci. 111, 183–198 (1963)

Wretlind, M., Pilbrant, A., Sundwall, A., Vessman, J.: Disposition of three benzodiazepines after single oral administration in man. Acta Pharmacol. Toxicol. 40 (suppl. 1), 28–39 (1977)

CHAPTER 7

Toxicology and Side-Effects of Anxiolytics

L. R. HINES

A. Introduction

I. Ubiquity of Anxiety

Although we tend to regard anxiety as a product of twentieth century living, anxiety, stress, and tension in their various forms must have been with man throughout his entire history. Indeed, as early as about 380 B.C., a statement was made by Plato in *The Republic* associating anxiety with a disease state: "Man is always fancying that he is being made ill, and is in constant anxiety about the state of his body" (JOWETT, 1952). William Heberden also associated anxiety with disease in his celebrated lecture on angina pectoris to the Royal College of Physicians of London in 1768 (HEBERDEN, 1772). During the last 50 years, thousands of papers have appeared in medical and scientific journals and dozens, if not hundreds, of books and monographs have been published on the pervasive subject of anxiety. "Indeed, anxiety has become the cornerstone of both psychosomatic medicine and psychiatric theory and practice" (LIEF, 1967).

II. Use of Anxiolytic Drugs

It is, therefore, not surprising that when the practice of medicine and the related sciences became sufficiently sophisticated, efforts were directed toward the development of therapeutic agents for the management of these conditions. The subsequent extensive use by the medical profession of the anxiolytics or antianxiety drugs was therefore to be expected. During the past several years, the total number of prescriptions written in the United States for antianxiety drugs has been greater than that of any other class of medication; within the class of anxiolytics, the use made of the benzodiazepines has exceeded that of all other anxiolytics combined (BLACKWELL, 1973; LASAGNA, 1977; SHADER and GREENBLATT, 1977).

III. Scope of Present Discussion

In most countries, benzodiazepines are now the most widely prescribed anxiolytics. They are rapidly replacing the barbiturates, which have been deemed to be obsolete (KOCH-WESER and GREENBLATT, 1974; EDITORIAL, 1975; MATTHEW, 1975). Nonetheless, the latter class of drugs is still widely used and has great historical importance. The so-called nonbarbiturate anxiolytics, exemplified by meprobamate, hydroxyzine and others, are also currently in the process of being replaced by benzodiazepines.

Since the popularity of the nonbarbiturates was brief, and as they have little historical significance, only the benzodiazepines and barbiturates will be considered in the present discussion, and major emphasis will be placed on the benzodiazepines. Several reviews on the barbiturates have recently been published (ALMEYDA and LEVANTINE, 1972; BROWNING and MAYNERT, 1972; MATTHEW, 1975; GAULT, 1976; HOSKINS, 1976; LOUIS-FERDINAND, 1976; COOPER, 1977).

IV. Definition of Adverse Reactions

Side effects or adverse reactions have been defined in a number of ways (KARCH and LASAGNA, 1975; WESTON and WESTON, 1977); for present purpose, a side effect is taken to mean "an effect of a drug other than the one it was administered to evoke" (GOVE, 1963). Traditionally, we have assumed that when a side effect was observed, it was the fault of the drug, since if the drug had not been given, the side effect would not have occurred. However, there are two variables: the drug and the drug recipient.

Adverse effects of drugs are generally of three types. Pharmacodynamic adverse effects, the most common type by far, are simply an extension of known pharmacologic actions of the drugs. Many factors influence the prevalence of such reactions. Incorrect prescribing practices usually are not a major source of such reactions, but rather vagaries in the way drugs are handled by different patients. A small minority of patients show individual differences in the rates of absorption, excretion, and metabolism sufficient to provide a 20-fold or greater variation in the plasma level obtained from the identical dose of the same drug (HAMMER and SJÖQUIST, 1967; KUNTZMAN et al., 1968 b; LUND, 1973). Unwanted effects probably are more frequent and more severe in those patients with higher plasma levels. The greatest contribution from pharmacokinetic studies of anxiolytic drugs has been the realization that different patients require a wide range of doses. However, plasma concentrations of anxiolytics have not been very useful in gauging clinical efficacy. For example, KANTO et al. (1979) recently reported that they found no correlation between diazepam or oxazepam plasma levels and clinical effects in children.

Allergic and idiosyncratic adverse reactions, the other two types, are more attributable to the patient than to any property of the drug. Drugs do vary in their ability to act as haptens and combine with proteins in the body to form immunogens. Yet, factors in the patient seem to be of greater importance. A great variety of allergic reactions to drugs are possible. Idiosyncratic reactions imply that the major cause is something peculiar to the patient receiving the drug. It may be the genetic background of the person, the presence of concurrent drugs or diseases, the past history of exposure to other drugs, and very likely, other factors still unidentified.

Prevalence rates for adverse reactions to drugs are still extremely difficult to ascertain. We have poor numerators and uncertain denominators. Scarcely any reports of adverse reactions provide data that would allow one to deduce the rate of such reactions. The best one can do is to form some sort of estimate, based on the frequency of reports versus the known frequency of drug use. On such a basis, the incidence of serious side effects with the widely prescribed class of anxiolytic drugs, the benzosdiazepines, is remarkably low (BLACKWELL, 1973; HOLLISTER, 1973; AYD, 1975, SHADER et al., 1975; SHAPMAN, 1976; ZALL, 1978).

B. Benzodiazepines

Six benzodiazepines are currently marketed in the United States as anxiolytics and are listed in chronologic order of their introduction: chlordiazepoxide (Librium, 1960), diazepam (Valium, 1963), oxazepam (Serax, 1965), clorazepate dipotassium (Tranxene, 1972), prazepam (Verstran, 1977), and lorazepam (Ativan, 1977). Other benzodiazepines, for indications other than anxiety, are also referred to in the appropriate context. These are flurazepam (Dalmane) and nitrazepam (Mogadon), both hypnotics, and clonazepam (Clonopin), an anticonvulsant. Diazepam and chlordiazepoxide are by far the most widely used, and this will have a bearing on the frequency with which they are mentioned with regard to adverse reactions.

The various benzodiazepines share common pharamcologic actions, but differ in the relative spectrum of these effects. They also differ with regard to various kinetic parameters. Oxazepam and lorazepam are short-acting drugs (based on plasma half-life), while the remainder are long-acting drugs (with generally much longer plasma half-lives). The clinical significance of the differences in spectrum of pharmacologic actions and pharmacokinetic parameters is still uncertain; however, barbiturates with shorter half-lives have been more frequently abused than the longer-acting members of this class, such as phenobarbital (ISBELL and CHRUSCIEL, 1970; JAFFE, 1975; AMA DRUG EVALUATIONS, 1977).

I. Adverse Psychiatric Reactions

1. Tolerance/Dependence
a) Animal Studies

Several studies have indicated that under the proper experimental conditions, the benzodiazepines may produce tolerance in animals. MATSUKI and IWAMOTO (1966) demonstrated the development of tolerance to chlordiazepoxide in the rat, using the conditioned avoidance-escape response, and HOOGLAND et al. (1966) reported increased rates of tissue disappearance and excretion of ^{14}C-labeled chlordiazepoxide in rats made tolerant to chlordiazepoxide. GOLDBERG and his associates (1967) demonstrated the development of tolerance to chlordiazepoxide in rats and mice, using a variety of pharmacologic tests. BARNETT and FIORE (1971, 1973), using the linguomandibular reflex in the cat, described acute tolerance to diazepam. MARGULES and STEIN (1968) reported that rats developed tolerance toward the depressant action of oxazepam after three to four doses, while the disinhibitory action on punished behavior did not show tolerance. Similar observations were reported by STEIN and BERGER (1971), following lorazepam administration. CANNIZZARO et al. (1972) found that the short-term treatment of rats with flurazepam reduced spontaneous motor activity and unmasked the disinhibitory effect.

Evidence for physical dependence has been less clear. HARRIS et al. (1968) found that rats reduced their liquid intake when forced to drink water containing chlordiazepoxide, and later, when given a free choice, the animals returned to pure water with no evidence of either addiction or tolerance. However, when rats were conditioned to drink an aqueous solution of chlordiazepoxide to obtain food pellets, after 25 days of conditioning, the animals preferred the chlordiazepoxide solution to pure water. STOLERMAN and his associates (1971) later observed that when a 0.5 mg/ml aqueous solution of chlordiazepoxide was made freely available to rats, none developed dependence upon the drug.

A technique was employed by FINDLEY et al. (1972), using monkeys with an indwelling intravenous catheter providing a periodic forced choice between the self-infusion of chlordiazepoxide solution or saline. A preference for self-infusion of chlordiazepoxide over saline was demonstrated, using choice trials every 3 h and a dose of approximately 1 mg/kg per infusion. However, the animals addicted to chlordiazepoxide showed a decided preference for secobarbital over chlordiazepoxide, when offered a choice of the two drugs. In another series of experiments involving intravenous drug administration, YANAGITA and TAKAHASHI (1973) reported that the daily administration of chlordiazepoxide, diazepam, or oxazolam to monkeys produced physical dependence. However, during this experiment, the animals were not heavily depressed and did not exhibit marked withdrawal signs.

The evidence available indicates that both tolerance and physical dependence can be developed with the benzodiazepines in animals, under the proper experimental conditions, but it is more difficult with the benzodiazepines than with the barbiturates.

b) Human Studies

The extensive medical use made of the benzodiazepines since their introduction has provided innumerable opportunities for their misuse in almost every clinical situation and in every type of stable and unstable personality. Perhaps as many patients have taken at least one of the benzodiazepines as any other prescription drug in medical history. Such exposure certainly constitutes the ultimate test of their potential for abuse, and it is therefore to be expected that frequent reports of the abuse and misuse of benzodiazepines have appeared in the medical literature.

Experimental production of physical dependence on benzodiazepines has required more extensive efforts than the demonstration of the same phenomenon with barbiturates. Late in 1960, an unusual experiment was carried out. "For experimental purposes, a healthy male volunteer ingested 50 mg of chlordiazepoxide on the first day, 150 mg on the second day, 500 mg on the third day, and 1,000 mg daily for the remainder of the 12-day experiment. After the third day, the volunteer experienced mild euphoria, loss of appropriate and inappropriate anxiety, feeling of mild fatigue, feeling of loss of equilibrium and, temporarily, difficulty of concentration. During the last days of the experiment, the feeling of drug overdosage became progressive. The observing physician noted the following changes: Following the ingestion of 500–1,000 mg of chlordiazepoxide per day, the subject was euphoric most of the time; later he became irritable and hostile, but there was no obvious impairment of judgment, concentration or ability. Near the end of the experiment, ataxia and dysarthria were noted. The symptoms disappeared progressively over about 5 days after discontinuation of the medication; withdrawal symptoms were not observed" (ZBINDEN et al., 1961). The total amount of chlordiazepoxide ingested over the 12-day period was 9,700 mg.

HOLLISTER and associates (1961) were able to produce physical dependence on chlordiazepoxide. Ten of 11 patients treated for several weeks or months with daily oral doses of 300–600 mg, 8–20 times the usual therapeutic dose, experienced new symptoms and signs after being abruptly withdrawn by a single blind switch to placeobs. Depression, agitation, insomnia, loss of appetite, and nausea appeared between 2 and 8 days after withdrawal. Two patients had seizures, one 7 days after withdrawal, the other, 8 days. A third patient, not in the withdrawal study, had a seizure 12 days after discontinuation of a 300 mg daily dose. The important distinction to be made about the withdrawal syndrome from chlordiazepoxide, compared with that from short-acting barbiturates or drugs such as meprobamate, is that it is both milder and more attenuated than the acute explosive withdrawal reactions seen with short-acting drugs.

Diazepam was also employed in large doses in a similar study with schizophrenic patients. Clinical signs of a withdrawal reaction were seen in 6 of 13 patients abruptly switched to placebos after daily doses of 120 mg. One patient had a major seizure on the 8th day of withdrawal (HOLLISTER et al., 1963). The diazepam withdrawal reaction was also mild and attenuated. This subject has been reviewed by ISBELL and CHRUSCIEL (1970), COHEN (1976), PARE (1976), HOLLISTER (1977), GREENBLATT and SHADER (1978 b), MARKS (1978) and SELLERS (1978), who agree with HOLLISTER (1978) that the abuse potential of the benzodiazepines is low. Both the most comprehensive and the most recent review of this facet of the benzodiazepines is that of MARKS (1978). Marks, in his review of clinical dependence on benzodiazepines, counted 402 individual cases, many highly questionable. The majority were in the context of abuse of alcohol and other drugs. Only 56 cases showed signs of physical dependence. Considering the enormous clinical use of these drugs during the 17-year period surveyed, as well as the intensive interest in this problem, the number of cases reported seems to be rather small.

Based on the finding of this survey, Marks drew the following conclusions which are paraphrased here:

1) Physical dependence upon a benzodiazepine can be produced in man if given in excessive doses over a prolonged period, particularly to patients with unstable personalities.

2) The dependence risk factor is low and certainly less than that of the other commonly used sedatives and anxiolytics.

3) The risk factor and the dangers to society are of such a low order that no extension of controls is necessary.

4) In the interest of good medical care and to minimize the risks of dependence, patients should be carefully selected for benzodiazepine administration, and drug therapy should be discontinued as soon as it is therapeutically practical to do so.

Since the first medical use of chloral hydrate, well over 100 years ago, tens of thousands of chemical compounds have been synthesized in an attempt to produce better drugs with sedative-hypnotic properties. During the past 50 years, an enormous worldwide research commitment has been made toward the development of new sedative-hypnotic drugs free of any abuse potential. During this period, a variety of compounds, totally unrelated chemically, have been made available to the medical profession. In spite of this prodigious effort, the ideal drug has eluded the best twentieth century medical minds. Perhaps the reason for this is not a reflection on our science but, rather, on the fact that our idealistic goal is unattainable. "As far back as recorded history, every society has used drugs producing profound effects on mood, thought, and feeling. Moreover, there were always a few individuals who digressed from custom with respect to the time, the amount and the situation in which these drugs were to be used. Thus, both the non-medical use of drugs and the problem of drug abuse are as old as civilization itself" (JAFFE, 1975).

2. Overdose

Acute poisoning and overdose, both intentional and accidental, have been serious medical problems for many years. Early in the development of the benzodiazepines, animal studies suggested that the compounds in this series would have a wide margin of safety. RANDALL (1960) reported that chlordiazepoxide exhibited taming effects in monkeys at one-tenth the ataxic dose, whereas meprobamate and phenobarbital demonstrated a similar taming action only at doses that depressed their general activity or produced ataxia. In general, the pharmacologic profile indicated that an impressive difference in safety existed between the benzodiazepines and phenobarbital in all animal species studied (RANDALL et al., 1960, RANDALL and KAPPELL, 1973). The work of several investigators (LOEW and TAESCHLER, 1968; MALICK et al., 1969; BRUNAUD and ROCAND, 1972; SCHALLEK et al., 1972; COOK and DAVIDSON, 1973), using a variety of pharmacologic tests, reinforced the earlier conclusion of Randall.

In one of the first suicide attempts that occurred during the early clinical studies, a 30-year-old female took approximately 625 mg chlordiazepoxide in a single dose. This was followed by an uneventful recovery (KINROSS-WRIGHT et al., 1960), Shortly thereafter, a suicide attempt was made by a 47-year-old female who ingested 1,150 mg chlordiazepoxide within approximately 20 min. No treatment was given since the suicide attempt was not discovered until 45 h after the incident. Aside from ataxia and dysarthria, recovery was uneventful (SMITH, 1961). Another patient recovered after ingesting 2,250 mg chlordiazepoxide (ZBINDEN et al., 1961). GREENBLATT et al. (1978a) recently reported the recovery of a 28-year-old male following the ingestion of 2,000 mg diazepam.

A number of reports of overdose or suicide attempts with the various benzodiazepines have appeared, of which the following are representative: CLARKE et al., 1961; GILBERT, 1961; JENNER and PARKIN, 1961; PENNINGTON and SYNGE, 1961; THOMSON and GLEN, 1961; SCHAEFFER, 1962; Hillyer, 1965; Spark and GOLDMAN, 1965; AUSTIN, 1966; GJERRIS, 1966; SHIMKIN and SHAIVITZ, 1966; CRUZ et al., 1967; FELL and DENDY, 1968; TANNER and MOORHEAD, 1968; BARDHAN, 1969; CARROLL, 1970; GANGULI et al., 1970; ZILELI et al., 1972; CATE and JATLOW, 1973; CHAPALLAZ, 1973; O'NEIL and POGGE, 1973; BELL, 1975; RADA et al., 1975; GREENBLATT et al., 1977; VARMA et al., 1977. Many of these, as well as other related reports, have been discussed in the following reviews: ZBINDEN et al., 1961; DAVIS and TERMINI, 1969; GREENBLATT and SHADER, 1974; WHITLOCK, 1975; GREENBLATT et al., 1977.

Recently FINKLE et al. (1979) conducted an extensive survey to determine the role of diazepam in drug-related deaths. The survey included the offices of 27 medical examiners and coroners in the United States and Canada, with a jurisdictional population of 79,200,000. The presence of diazepam or its mjor metabolite, desmethyldiazepam, in each of the 1,239 cases included in the study was confirmed by toxicologic analysis. Drugs were believed to be the cause of death in 914 cases; the remainder were due to other causes in which the presence of the drug was incidental. Approximately two-thirds of the cases involved two or more agents. The combination of diazepam and ethanol was found in 51 fatalities. In slightly over half of the fatalities; diazepam concentrations were within the therapeutic range. Many cases had one or more other drugs present in concentrations that could have caused severe toxic or lethal consequences. Of the 914 deaths attributable to drugs, the authors conclude that diazepam alone was the responsible agent in two cases. Considering the fact that one is at risk of death in any comatose state, this small number must represent an irreducible minimum.

For some time the cholinesterase inhibitor, physostigmine, has been used in the management of delirium and central nervous system depression due to tricyclic antidepressant toxicity (SLOVIS et al., 1971; BURKS et al., 1974; HEISER and WILDBERT, 1974; SNYDER et al., 1974; NEWTON, 1975; HOLINGER and KLAWANS, 1976; CZECH et al., 1977). Physostigmine has also been used successfully in cases where either benzodiazepines, or benzodiazepines and tricyclics, have been taken in excessive amounts (BERNARDS, 1973; ROSENBERG, 1974; BLITT and PETTY, 1975; BRASHARES and CONLEY, 1975; DI LIBERTI et al., 1975; CHIN et al., 1976; MANOGUERRA and RUIZ, 1976; CZECH et al., 1977; LARSON et al., 1977; DAUNDERER, 1978). NAGY and DECSI (1978) reported that rats, rabbits, and cats respond promptly to intravenous or intraperitoneal injections of physostigmine salicylate following the administration of large intraperitoneal doses of diazepam. The mechanism(s) are obscure, since central cholinergic systems have not been considered to have a significant role in explaining the mechanism of action of the benzodiazepines. These observations may stimulate further research into the mechanism of action of the benzodiazepines. It has been suggested (VAN DER KOLK et al., 1978), however, that a central autonomic effect on the hypothalamus (SCHALLEK et al., 1972) may explain the reversal of benzodiazepine overdosage by physostigmine.

Accumulated clinical experience since the introduction of chlordiazepoxide in 1960 has demonstrated that the benzodiazepines are probably as safe as one can expect an active drug of this class to be, and their relative safety is now generally recognized (MATTHEW et al., 1969; BYCK, 1975; WHITLOCK, 1975; ABRAMOWICZ, 1976; LADER, 1976; SHAPIRO, 1976; COOPER, 1977; GREENBLATT et al., 1977; KOLB, 1977; RICKELS, 1977; ALLEN and GREENBLATT, 1978; GREENBLATT et al., 1978a; HOLLISTER, 1978). The successful suicide of a healthy adult, using a benzodiazepine as the only drug, is obviously difficult; however, suicide today is usually attempted with more than one drug and often, in addition, with that ubiquitous drug, alcohol. These facts should always be remembered in prescribing a benzodiazepine or any other medication. "The suicide rate has not fluctuated significantly over the past century. Man uses whatever means available for self-destruction; and the increased use of drugs reflects contemporary drug usage by the medical profession. It replaces other methods no longer available or in vogue" (BROPHY, 1967).

3. Disinhibiting Actions

Infrequent side effects, sometimes referred to as "behavioral toxicity," have been described (COLE, 1960; HOLLIDAY, 1967; SHADER and DiMASCIO, 1970). These include paradoxical excitement, hostility, or rage reactions rather than the expected sedation. In early clinical studies of chlordiazepoxide, three cases of rage reaction were described (TOBIN et al., 1960; TOBIN and LEWIS, 1960). Two additional patients in this study displayed increased irritability, as well as motor and psychomotor hyperactivity. Similar reports have subsequently appeared, including hostile and/or "acting-out" behavior (WALZER et al., 1960), hypermotor activity (SMITH, 1960), and increased irritability and assaultive behavior (INGRAM and TIMBURY, 1960). In its use as an anticonvulsant, oral clonazepam has been reported (BLADIN, 1973) to produce irritability, irrational social behavior, and outbursts of aggressive temper; however, such observations were not made in the short-term parenteral use of the drug. "Strange behavior" has been observed with oxazepan (ZUCKER, 1972). One patient reported unusual body sensations, another became unusually argumentative, and the third was arrested for disrobing in public. Two patients were reported (BLITT and PETTY, 1975) to have experienced postoperative delirium and hallucinatory-type CNS manifestations following parenteral lorazepam administration.

The incidence of these reactions cannot be estimated from the published literature, since authors frequently report interesting cases they have observed with no reference to the total number of patients treated. However, the recent experience of the Boston Collaborative Drug Surveillance Program 1966–1975 (GREENBLATT, 1976) indicated that of 2,086 patients treated with chlordiazepoxide, there were six cases (0.3%) of central nervous sytem excitation ("insomnia, agitation, hallucinations, etc."). In addition, 2,623 patients were treated with diazepam, and four cases (0.2%) of central nervous system excitation ("agitation, nightmares, etc.") were observed. Other benzodiazepines were not included in this study.

Whereas most investigators have thought of these reactions as being paradoxical, others have hypothesized that it may be only in patients with poor impulse control or with aggressive, destructive behavior tendencies that chlordiazepoxide may release sufficient hostility to result in a rage reaction (DiMASCIO and BARRETT, 1965; BARRETT and DiMASCIO, 1966; GUNDLACH et al., 1966; McDONALD, 1967; GARDOS et al., 1968; SALZMAN et al., 1969). Thus, in certain patients, rage reactions should not be considered as paradoxical but rather as predictable responses and part of the overall therapeutic effect (SHADER and DiMASCIO, 1970). Although these and other reports have appeared in the literature, the various paradoxical reactions described are not common in actual clinical practice (ZALL, 1978). Paradoxical reactions are not peculiar to the benzodiazepines. They have been observed with the phenothiazines (GOLDMAN, 1958; FREYHAN, 1959, KLERMAN et al., 1959, SARWER-FONER, 1960) and imipramine (DiMASCIO et al., 1968). Similar reactions to the barbiturates have been recognized for many years (LUNDY and OSTERBERG, 1929; GOODMAN and GILMAN, 1941).

4. Depression

Anecdotal accounts suggest that use of benzodiazepines in anxious patients may make them depressed. Nothing in the known pharmacologic actions of these drugs would suggest that they are "depressogenic," in the same sense as reserpine, for instance. As anxiety and depression are inextricably tied together, the more likely explanation is that the patients' conditions were misdiagnosed. If a depressed patient is mistakenly treated for the attendant anxiety, it is possible that as the latter symptom is alleviated, depression may be more evident.

II. Adverse Neurologic Reactions

As would be anticipated from their pharmacologic properties, the side effects most commonly observed are those associated with depression of the central nervous system, such as drowsiness, somnolence, fatigue, dysarthria, muscle weakness, and ataxia, which usually disappear within a few days or with an appropriate reduction of dosage (LADER, 1976; HOLLISTER, 1978). Although these side effects may occur in patients of any age group, they are more likely to be seen in the elderly and less likely to occur in individuals with a long history of cigarette smoking (BOSTON COLLABORATIVE DRUG SURVEILLANCE PROGRAM, 1973). In an earlier report in which 287 clinical studies of chlordiazepoxide involving 17,935 patients were reviewed, drowsiness was observed in 3.9%, ataxia in 1.7%, muscular weakness in 0.3%, and dysarthria in 0.2% of the patients (SVENSON and HAMILTON, 1966). Reports of similar side effects have appeared with diazepam (KERRY and JENNER, 1962; AIVAZIAN, 1964), oxazepam (TOBIN et al., 1964), clorazepate (MAGNUS, 1973; SKUPIN and FRANZKE, 1975), prazepam (GOLDBERG and FINNERTY, 1977; GREENBLATT and Shader, 1978a), and lorazepam (HAIDER, 1971; ELLISON and CANCELLARO, 1978).

III. Adverse Reactions Due to Drug Interactions

1. Ethanol

a) Animal Studies

Most laboratory studies have indicated that the depressant effects on the nervous system of the benzodiazepines and alcohol are at least additive. In an early study in mice, DANECHMAND et al. (1967) demonstrated that ethanol increased the muscle relaxant effects of chlordiazepoxide, chlorpromazine, and meprobamate. Similar observations were reported by GEBHARDT et al. (1969). ZBINDEN et al. (1961) reported that the hypnotic effects of ethanol were slightly or moderately potentiated by pretreatment with chlordiazepoxide. Similar observations were reported by NORIO et al. (1971) for diazepam. MILNER (1970) observed that in mice pretreated with ethanol, the length of time the righting reflex was lost, increased to about the same extent when the animals were treated with 5 mg/kg diazepam or trifluoperazine. In an earlier paper, MILNER (1968) reported that diazepam, phenobarbital, trifluoperazine, chlorpromazine, phenelzine, and thioridazine each potentiated the depressant effects of ethanol in mice. REGGIANI et al. (1968) reviewed many of these studies.

b) Human Studies

Conflicting reports have appeared in the literature concerning the interactive effect of ethanol and benzodiazepines in man. REGGIANI et al. (1968) reported that 10 mg dose chlordiazepoxide had no detrimental effect on the impairment produced by alcohol, either in a driving test or in the reaction time to stimuli. The subjects were volunteer policemen, between 25 and 40 years of age, who had consumed sufficient alcohol to produce a blood alcohol concentration of 0.08%. In a series of earlier reports (HOFFER, 1962; LAWTON and CAHN, 1963; MILLER et al., 1963; HUGHES et al., 1965; BERNSTEIN et al., 1967) in which ethanol and chlordiazepoxide were studied, significant impairment was produced by ethanol, but further significant impairment was not observed following the ingestion of chlordiazepoxide. BETTS et al. (1972) administered five 10 mg doses of chlordiazepoxide over 36 h, and ethanol 0.5 mg/kg body w., to normal volunteers participating in low-speed motor vehicle handling tests and observed significantly altered driving behavior. There was, however, little interaction between the drug and alcohol under the conditions of this study. LINNOILA and MATTILA (1973) studied the effects of combinations of diazepam (5 and 10 mg) and ethanol (0.5 and 0.8 mg/kg) on driving in 200 volunteer students. Individually, thes drugs either did not affect or slightly improved performance, but their combination impaired performance. These results are in general agreement with an earlier report of GOLDBERG (1966). In another study, LINNOILA and HAKKINEN (1974) showed that diazepam enhanced the effects of alcohol in nonanxious patients during a 40-min driving test.

Pharmacokinetic interactions between benzodiazepines and ethanol have been contradictory. CASIER and associates (1966) found that the administration of diazepam, 10 mg/day for 14 days, did not influence blood alcohol levels up to 4 h after ethanol ingestion. MACLEOD and his associates (1977) found that in subjects who had fasted for 8 h, higher plasma diazepam concentrations were obtained when diazepam (10 mg) was given immediately following the ingestion of ethanol (0.5 mg/kg) than when diazepam was taken alone. HAYES et al. (1977) also found that higher plasma concentrations were obtained when Valium powder (0.07 mg/kg body w.) was administered, suspended in 50% ethanol, than when the powder was given in distilled water. MORLAND et al. (1974) administered diazepam tablets with water and with a 15%–20% ethanol-water solution and found no difference in the plasma diazepam levels after 1 h. However, higher plasma diazepam levels were found after 3 h in five of eight subjects who had received the dilute ethanol solution. LINNOILA et al. (1974) examined the effect of 0.8 mg/kg ethanol on serum chlordiazepoxide (25 mg) and serum diazepam (10 mg) levels in volunteers who had fasted for 4 h. The chlordiazepoxide levels were slightly elevated over control values at 120 and 150 min but not before,whereas the diazepam levels were not significantly altered by alcohol at any time. GREENBLATT and his associates (1978 b) attempted to reproduce more nearly normal conditions under which diazepam and ethanol are consumed. They administered a 5-mg diazepam tablet with 120 ml of orange juice or with 120 ml of orange juice plus 45 ml of vodka (80 proof); no food or liquid was consumed for 3 h after each dose. Their results indicated the ethanol-orange juice cocktail tended to slow the rate, but not the completeness, of absorption.

Although the data available would indicate that experimental conditions can be designed where the ingestion of high concentrations of alcohol may increase the absorption of diazepam (and probably other benzodiazepines as well) on an empty stomach, it seems unlikely that with food in the stomach and with more dilute concentrations of alcohol being consumed, the absorption of diazepam would be altered sufficiently to be of any practical consequence. Obviously, alcohol should not be taken with any sedative-type drug, including the benzodiazepines.

2. Phenytoin

Many epileptic patients take more than one anticonvulsant drug, and interactions between these anticonvulsants, as well as with other medications, are common (KUTT, 1975). The biochemical basis for these interactions may involve one or more mechanisms, including absorption, plasma protein binding, biotransformation, and excretion. VAJDA et al. (1971) found that diazepam and chlordiazepam produced an increase in phenytoin levels, and ROGERS et al. (1977) reported phenytoin intoxication in two children during concurrent diazepam therapy. Conversely, HOUGHTON and RICHENS (1974) observed a small but significant reduction in phenytoin levels by diazepam. Later, RICHENS and HOUGHTON (1975) found a signifficant reduction in phenytoin levels by diazepam. These investigators also found that chlordiazepoxide lowered phenytoin levels, although too few patients were studied for the data to be statistically significant. Clonazepam has been found by EDWARDS and EADIE (1973) to lower phenytoin plasma levels. RICHENS (1977) suggests that a reduction in serum phenytoin concentration may be an effect shared by all of the benzodiazepines. Although the consensus of opinion appears to be that changes in phenytoin levels by the benzodiazepines are unlikely to be of great clinical importance in the majority of patients (RICHENS, 1977), the clinician should be aware that both increases and decreases in phenytoin levels have been reported.

3. Enzyme Induction

A substantial number of drugs and other chemicals have been found to stimulate their own metabolism or the metabolism of other compounds by increasing the availability of drug-metabolizing enzymes present in liver microsomes (CONNEY, 1967, 1969; GELEHRTER, 1976). This has been studied quite extensively with the benzodiazepines, in both animals and man, because of the frequency with which they are coadministered with other drugs.

a) Animal Studies

KATO and CHIESARA (1962) found that a single 50 mg/kg dose of chlordiazepoxide in rats had no effect upon barbiturate metabolism or sleeping time. In a similar study with the same dose, KATO and VASSANELLI (1962) found chlordiazepoxide to be without effect on meprobamate metabolism or sleeping time. A reduction in barbiturate sleeping time and an increase in liver weight was reported by HOOGLAND et al. (1966) when rats were pretreated with 100 mg/kg chlordiazepoxide for 5 days.

BERTE et al. (1969) found 20 mg/kg doses of oxazepam for 14–30 days to be without effect upon oxazepam or aminopyrine metabolism by homogenates of placental tissue. SZEBERENYI et al. (1969) reported that pretreatment of rats with 100 mg/kg diazepam for 5 days reduced the half-life of metyrapone. The pretreatment of rats with 40 mg/kg diazepam or nitrazepam did not significantly alter the pentobarbital sleeping time, the plasma half-life of ^{14}C-pentobarbital, the zoxazolamine paralysis time, nor the maximal velocity of N-demethylation of ethylmorphine by the liver microsomal enzymes. With chlordiazepoxide, however, the first three parameters were reduced and the fourth was significantly increased (ORME et al., 1972). However, the metabolism of warfarin was increased (RISTOLA et al., 1971) in rats after they received 10 mg/kg diazepam for 7 days. ALBANUS and co-workers (1971) pretreated beagles with phenobarbital (25 mg/kg), diazepam (35 mg/kg), and oxazepam (150 mg/kg) for 13 days and found that antipyrine half-life decreased following phenobarbital and diazepam but increased following oxazepam. After treating rats for 7 days with prazepam (100 mg/kg), VESSELL et al. (1972) observed an enhanced hepatic microsomal metabolism of ethylmorphine and aniline; also, the hepatic microsomal content of cytochrome P-450 was increased. However, after 4 days' treatment, only P-450 was elevated significantly and the plasma half-life of ^{14}C-prazepam was reduced.

b) Human Studies

The benzodiazepines and the coumarin anticoagulants are often used simultaneously in clinical medicine; this has stimulated a number of studies of their possible interaction. Chlordiazepoxide has been investigated by BIBAWI et al. (1963), VAN DAM and GRIBNAU-OVERKAMP (1967), LACKNER and HUNT (1968), ROBINSON and SYLVESTER (1970), SOLOMON et al. (1971), and ORME and his associates (1972). Diazepam has been studied by RISTOLA and co-workers (1971), SOLOMON et al. (1971), and ORME et al. (1972); nitrazepam was investigated by BRECKENRIDGE and ORME (1971), BIEGER et al. (1972), and ORME and his associates (1972). More recently, ROBINSON and AMIDON (1973) have reported on flurazepam. None of these investigations demonstrated that the benzodiazepines studied interfere with the clinical use of the anticoagulant, which is in agreement with the conclusions of KOCH-WESER and SELLERS (1971) and GREEN-BLATT and SHADER (1974).

Several additional studies have been carried out. O'MALLEY (1971) reported that the administration of nitrazepam, 5 or 10 mg/day for 14 days, did not significantly alter either plasma antipyrine half-life or the urinary 6β-hydroxycortisol: 17-hydroxycorticosteroid ratio when used as an index of drug metabolizing activity (KUNTZMAN et al., 1966, 1968a). Prazepam administrtion, 30 mg/day for 7 days, prolonged the plasma half-life of prazepam and antipyrine in man (VESSELL et al., 1972). Plasma antipyrine and phenylbutazone half-lives remained unaltered following the daily administration of 5 or 10 mg nitrazepam for 21 days (STEVENSON et al., 1972). Additional work by WHITFIELD and associates (1973) indicated that patients treated with barbiturates had increased plasma γ-glutamyl transpeptidase activity, indicating an increase in hepatic drug metabolizing activity. Patients receiving a benzodiazepine did not exhibit this change. Data indicate that at high doses the benzodiazepines induce enzymes in animals, but not in man, with therapeutic doses. The clinical significance of enzyme induction has been reviewed by BRECKENRIDGE and ROBERTS (1976).

IV. Adverse Reations Due to Allergy

1. Skin

The incidence of drug eruptions with the benzodiazepines is very low (BRUINSMA, 1973; GHOSH, 1977). However, because of their extensive use, such reactions have occasionally been reported.

After reviewing the cutaneous reactions to the benzodiazepines, ALMEYDA (1971) concluded that the majority were urticaria, angioneurotic edema, or maculopapular eruptions, but that such reactions were uncommon. MACKIE and MACKIE (1966) reviewed 179 allergic reactions believed to be due to a systemically administered drug and found that six nonurticarial reactions were due to a benzodiazepine. Five were with chlordiazepoxide alone, and one was due to chlordiazepoxide and diazepam. An early report (GAUL, 1961) described a fixed drug eruption in a 66-year-old female from chlordiazepoxide which reappeared upon rechallenge with the same drug. Two additional cases of fixed drug eruptions have also been reported (SAVIN, 1970). A photosensitivity reaction to chlordiazepoxide has been described (LUTON and FIN-CHUM, 1965) in a 53-year-old male who had taken chlordiazepoxide for about 7 days prior to the onset of a moderately severe eczematous reaction which reappeared when rechallenged with chlordiazepoxide and exposure to ultraviolet light. A report also appeared (RAPP, 1971) of a 65-year-old male who reacted with a swollen tongue to four doses of flurazepam. The patient had not previously responded in this way to either chlordiazepoxide or diazepam but had shown a similar reaction to both penicillin and tetracycline. A subsequent report (MILNER, 1977) of an allergic reaction to parenteral diazepam has been questioned (BLATCHLEY, 1977), since one of the ingredients, Cremophor El, contained in the Swedish diazepam preparation used by Milner, may be implicated in certain allergic reactions (PADFIELD and WATKINS, 1977). Hypersensitivity reactions to the benzodiazepines have been briefly reviewed by GHOSH (1977).

2. Hematology

The incidence of adverse hematologic effects with the benzodiazepines is low (SHADER and DiMASCIO, 1970; GREENBLATT and SHADER, 1974). Transient and benign leukopenias have been most often reported. Granulocytopenia (WBC 3,500; 28% granulocytes) was observed (BITNUM, 1969)in an infant whose mother had taken 100 mg chlordiazepoxide daily during pregnancy. After taking 100 mg chlordiazepoxide daily for at least 1 year, a female was reported (FAVAZZA, 1973) to have a WBC of 3,300. No additional details were provided regarding subsequent blood studies or prior exposure to other drugs. STRAUSE et al. (1974) reported the case of a 67-year-old female with hepatitis and leukopenia which disappeared after chlordiazepoxide was withdrawn and reappeared when it was reinstituted. HAERTEN und POETTGEN (1975) treated a 44-year-old male with penicillin and oxazepam (30 mg/day) precipitating leukopenia which disappeared shortly after the cessation of both drugs. Subsequent treatment with oxazepam again resulted in leukopenia which subsided when the latter was withdrawn. Treatment with penicillin plus diazepam (10 mg/day) also resulted in leukopenia. After cessation of diazepam, while continuing treatment with penicillin, the leukocyte count again returned to normal, indicating a cross sensitivity between these two benzodiazepines in this patient.

Shortly after the introduction of chlordiazepoxide, a case of agranulocytosis was reported (KAELBLING and CONRAD, 1960). This case is complicated by the fact that the patient, a 23-year-old female, exhibited a cutaneous sensitivity to chlorpromazine shortly before chlordiazepoxide therapy was begun. The patient recovered following the administration of antibiotics and corticosteroids. A second case was reported (WILCOX, 1962) in a 43-year-old female who, prior to the administration of chlordiazepoxide, had received aspirin, triflupromazine, and ethchlorvynol, and had had "some exposure to cleaning fluid." Four cases of agranulocytosis, possibly involving nitrazepam, were reported to the British Commitee on the Safety of Medicine, 1964–1973 (VERE, 1976). No details were provided. The author stated that "the publication of these reports does not imply that the Committee on Safety of Medicines accepts a cause/effect relationship exists in any individual case."

Nonthrombocytopenic purpura was reported (COPPERMAN, 1967) in a 65-year-old diabetic female who had received irregular courses of chlordiazepoxide for about 12 months. The purpuric rash subsided upon withdrawal of chlordiazepoxide. The purpura did not reappear when rechallenged with a 10 mg dose, but did reappear when 30 mg per day was given on a later admission.

Three cases of thrombocytopenia resulting from chlordiazepoxide and three from nitrazepam have been reported (New Zealand Committee on Adverse Drug Reactions, 1972). Three additional cases of thrombocytopenia involving chlordiazepoxide were also mentioned in a previous report (New Zealand Committee on Adverse Drug Reactions, 1969). No additional details were provided in either report. A case of thrombocytopenic purpura in an 18-year-old female was reported by BAUMES (1971). The etiology is not clear since the patient had been taking both aminopyrine and diazepam regularly. A 45-year-old female developed a diffuse petechial eruption and scattered ecchymoses 1 week after receiving oral penicillin, chlorpheniramine maleate, and diazepam (CIMO et al., 1977). The platelet count was $10,000/mm^3$. Red cell and white cell counts were normal, and bone marrow examination revealed normal cellularity and increased numbers of megakaryocytes. All medications were discontinued and prednisone therapy begun. During the next week the platelet count increased to $500,000/mm^3$, and studies of the patient's serum indicated the presence of diazepam-dependent platelet antibody, whereas tests with the other drugs being administered were negative. The platelet count remained normal, and prednisone was discontinued.

The porphyrias (SCHMID, 1966) are a group of syndromes characterized by the accumulation of the normal precursors of heme, or their by-products. The accumulation of these precursors may be associated with, but is not always causally related to, a variety of clinical manifestations (CHISOLM, 1972). The synthesis of these pigments in the porphyrias is greatly increased as a result of a failure of the control mechanisms that normally regulate heme synthesis (DeMATTEIS, 1967). A limited number of cases have been reported in the literature associating chlordiazepoxide with porphyria. EALES (1971) has reported on 145 porphyric attacks in 120 patients: 107 with variegate porphyria and 13 with acute intermittent porphyria. In his experience, chlordiazepoxide and diazepam given alone are not associated with any evidence of deterioration. An additional case has been described (SCOTT et al., 1973) in which progressive and fatal liver disease appeared to be a complication of erythropoietic protoporphyria. This 43-year-old female had a lifelong sensitivity to sunlight and had taken chlordiazepoxide for several years. The authors postulate that the massive overproduction of protoporphyrin which occurred during the patient's fatal illness may have been related to a reduced carbohydrate intake leading to a depression of delta-amino levulinic acid synthetase (KNUDSEN et al., 1967) or that dieting allowed chlordiazepoxide to induce the enzyme which previously may have been prevented by a "glucose effect" (TSCHUDY et al., 1964, WELLAND et al., 1964, REDEKER and STERLING, 1968). More recently, HORVATH et al. (1974) reported the case of a 27-year-old female who experienced an attack of acute porphyria following periodic use of glutethimide and the regular use of chlordiazepoxide for insomnia and restlessness. The patient had not previously experienced symtoms which could be described as a true attack of porphyria, and the family history was negative. The assigment of responsibility for the attack to either drug is difficult. Several reviews of the porphyrias have been published (DeMATTEIS, 1967, 1968; MAGNUS, 1968, TADDEINI and WATSON, 1968, TSCHUDY, 1968, ELDER et al., 1972, EISENBERG, 1973; BLOOMER, 1976; DOSS, 1976; EEROLA and BAER, 1976; MENNEAR, 1977). The assigment of a definitive role to chlordiazepoxide in porphyria cannot be made at this time. However, the drug should be used with caution in cases where a familial history of porphyrias exists, where the patient has a prior history of porphyria, or when chlordiazepoxide is to be used with a drug that may precipitate attacks of hepatic porphyria.

3. Hepatotoxicity

A relatively small number of reports have been published suggesting a relationship between the administration of one of the benzodiazepines and abnormal hepatic tests or liver disorders. Of 36 hospitalized psychiatric patients treated with 100–600 mg chlordiazepoxide daily for 1–7 months, four had an elevated serum glutamic oxaloacetic transaminase (SGO-T) titer; only one of the SGO-T titers remained elevated after rechecking, and none was associated with any other abnormal hepatic tests (HOLLISTER et al., 1961). Two groups (KURLAND et al., 1966; HOLDEN and ITIL, 1969) studied changes in liver function tests following the administration of chlordiazepoxide; neither found any significant changes attributable to the drug.

Cholestatic (hepatocanalicular) jaundice is a frequent form of allergic liver injury from drugs. After 11 tetanus patients were treated with diazepam for 2–3 weeks, all were reported (STACHER, 1973) to have liver function test results suggestive of cholestasis; four became jaundiced. There was a gradual return to normal liver function after medication was discontinued. Since all patients in this series exhibited liver damage, some etiology other than diazepam must be considered. Cholestatic jaundice was reported (FRANKS and JACOBS, 1975) in a 40-year-old female, but causation is difficult to determine since the patient received several drugs in addition to diazepam. More recently a case of cholestatic jaundice associated with flurazepam was reported in a 70-year-old male (FANG et al., 1978). Although the patient had taken several drugs, flurazepam was suspected since the liver enzyme tests returned to normal after flurazepam was withdrawn while other drugs were continued. In an additional report (LO et al., 1967), jaundice was observed in a 26-year-old female after 2 weeks of chlordiazepoxide therapy. The patient gave birth to a normal boy 3 days before beginning chlordiazepoxide, but she received no blood during labor or delivery. She was treated with penicillin for flu-like symptoms 2 days after beginning chlordiazepoxide treatment. A needle biopsy performed on the 19th day of jaundice showed moderate cholestasis but no parenchymal changes.

V. Teratogenic and Cytogenic Studies

The more ubiquitous the use of the drug, the greater the opportunity for possibly spurious correlations with birth defects. Interest in the teratogenic potential of the benzodiazepines is reflected in the increased number of studies, both experimental and epidemiologic, which have appeared. With only two exceptions, the experimental studies conducted to date in rodents and lagomorphs demonstrate that the different benzodiazepines do not produce malformations, even at high doses. Flurazepam and triazolam (TUCHMANN-DUPLESSIS, 1976) were not teratogenic in rabbits, rats, or mice at levels of 40 mg/kg and 30 mg/kg, respectively. Similarly, doses up to 40 mg/kg of tetrazepam, nitrazepam, chlorazepate, oxazepam, and lorazepam were without teratogenic effects in the species investigated (BRUNAUD 1970, 1976; OWEN et al., 1970; MILLER and BECKER, 1973). The slightly reduced fertility and decreased postnatal survival, as seen with compounds such as bromazepam (50 mg/kg/day), were due to modified maternal behavior (HUMMLER and THEISS, 1976) rather than a fetotoxic response. Although clonazepam was reported to produce enlarged cerebral ventricles in mice at doses of 0.2 and 1.8 mg/kg, levels which were approximately 3–18 times the human dose, resulting in a malformation rate (2.7%) twice that of controls (1.3%) (SULLIVAN and MCELHATTON, 1977), BLUM et al. (1973) reported no abnormalities in rats, mice, or rabbits. MILLER and BECKER (1975) were able to produce embryolethality and cleft palates in mice with daily diazepam levels of 400–500 mg/kg which killed 50% of the dams and incapacitated the remainder for as long as 36 h after dosing. On the other hand, BEALL (1972) could produce no malformations in rats with diazepam at daily levels of 200 mg/kg, whereas 100 mg/kg diazepam each day was sufficient to produce cleft palates only in the sensitive A/J mouse under conditions which kept the dam heavily sedated for 9–18 h (WALKER and PATTERSON, 1974). At much lower daily doses of diazepam (0.2 mg/kg) given to Balb/c mice on days 1–9 or 5–12 of gestation, STENCHEVER and PARKS (1975) were unable to produce a significant decrease in litter sizes or an increase in either resorption rate or gross abnormalities. Chlordiazepoxide given each day at 200 mg/kg produced cleft palates in the sensitive A/J mouse, but none in the C_3H or CD_1 strains of mice (WALKER and PATTERSON, 1974). Thus, it would appear that the experimental data do not support the possible teratogenicity of the benzodiazepines, unless the conditions were toxic to the dam or involved a strain already prone to the display of a malformation under control conditions.

Postnatal evaluation of the effects of prenatal administration of diazepam in rodents have produced conflicting results. LYUBIMOV et al. (1974) administered 10 mg/kg diazepam to rats each day throughout gestation and found both delayed development and impaired learning. FOX et al. (1977) demonstrated that although 20 and 100 mg/kg diazepam given daily to pregnant mice reduced the survival of their pups through weaning, those that did live exhibited enhanced learning. In the clearest demonstration of the postnatal effects of the prenatal administration of diazepam (BARLOW et al., 1979), rats exposed in utero to 1 mg/kg twice a day exhibited slightly enhanced learning when tested in a Y-maze, whereas those exposed to 10 mg/kg twice a day exhibited the negative effects upon learning that were seen in response to stress alone (BARLOW et al., 1978).

Studies designed to examine the effect of benzodiazepines upon chromosomes produced the claim that diazepam caused chromosomal aberations in human cells (STENCHEVER et al., 1969, 1970a). However studies by others failed to confirm these effects in either humn cells (COHEN et al., 1969; STAIGER 1969, 1970; WHITE et al., 1974; TUCHMANN-DUPLESSIS, 1975) or bone marrow from Chinese hamsters (SCHMID and STAIGER, 1969). No chromosomal aberrations were found following treatment with either chlordiazepoxide or medazepam in either human cells (COHEN et al., 1969; STAIGER, 1969, STENCHEVER et al., 1970b) or bone marrow from Chinese hamsters (SCHMID and STAIGER, 1969).

There are several reports in the literature of benzodiazepine-associated congential malformations (ISTVAN, 1970; RINGROSE, 1972; FEDRICK, 1973; BARRY and DANKS, 1974). But, in general, more than one drug was taken during the same interval, and no common pattern of malformation was seen, making the establishment of a positive relationship between benzodiazepines and the defects tenuous at best. However, reports such as the above have encouraged extensive epidemiologic review of the potential relationship. Retropective studies involving 19044 births (MILKOVICH and VAN DEN BERG, 1974), 590 births (SAXEN, 1975), 365 births (SPEIDEL and MEADOW, 1972), 278 births (SAFRA and OAKLEY, 1975), and 130 mothers with children exhibiting oral clefts only (AARSKOG, 1975) have suggested an association and have created interest in the potential teratogenicity of the benzodiazepines, although the findings are not conclusive. In contrast, studies by HARTZ et al. (1975) of 50,282 pregnancies, by LAKOS and CZEIZEL (1977) of 29,057 children on record in the Hungarian Congenital Malformation Register, a prospective study of combined English and French findings involving 21,911 children (CROMBIE et al., 1975), and one conducted by the Federal Republic of Germany (DEGENHART et al., 1972), together with the studies of FARKAS and FARKAS (1974) and GREENBERG et al. (1977), found no increased risk associated with the benzodiazepines studied and treatment during pregnancy.

Epidemiologic studies conducted in man are of two types: retrospective and prospective, neither totally satisfactory. Retrospective studies may be clouded by faulty recall of what occurred months before, by inadequately designed questionnaires, and by inadequate data analysis. Prospective studies are hampered by the need for a vast number of pregnancies to obtain significant data, as well as problems of design and data analysis. However, they are the only acceptable tools for examination and analysis of the effects of benzodiazepines in humans.

Evaluations of this substantial body of information have been conducted by MELLIN (1964), FORFAR and NELSON (1973), TUCHMAN-DUPLESSIS (1975, 1976), HEINONEN et al. (1977), PEARSON (1977), WILSON (1977), BODENDORFER (1978), and GOLDBERG and DiMASCIO (1978), who conclude that although the evidence conflicts, no causal relationship has been established between benzodiazepines and birth defects in humans. Nevertheless, it cannot be stated too emphatically that *no* drug should be given during the first trimester of pregnancy, unless the need is very great.

C. Barbiturates

Although barbituric acid was first synthesized by Baeyer in 1864, the first derivative with sedative-hypnotic properties, diethylbarbituric acid or barbital, was not introduced into medicine until 1903 by Fisher and Mering. The second important barbituric acid derivative, phenobarbital, was introduced in 1912, and it is still a useful central nervous system depressant, although its greatest use is probably as an anticonvulsant. At least 2,500 additional barbituric acid derivatives have been synthesized and approximately 50 have been used clinically, but not more than a dozen now have any extensive clinical use as orally administered sedative hypnotics. Their use as anxiolytics and hypnotics has declined substantially over the past several years and most authorities discourage their use for these indications (KOCH-WESER and GREENBLATT, 1974; EDITORIAL, 1975; MATTHEW, 1975; COOPER, 1977). Phenobarbital continues as an important anticonvulsant; thiopental sodium, the thioanalog of pentobarbital, is used extensively as an intravenous anesthetic. The adverse effects seen in these applications will not be considered here.

I. Adverse Psychiatric Reactions

1. Tolerance/Dependence

The ability of the barbiturates, when repeatedly taken in large doses, to produce tolerance and dependence in both animals and man is well documented (ISBELL, 1956; SHIDEMAN, 1961; JAFFE, 1975). However, therapeutic doses may be taken for extended periods by some undividuals with no problem (ISBELL, 1956; SHIDEMAN, 1961; JAFFE, 1975). The daily administration of 600–800 mg of one of the short- or intermediate-acting barbiturates for approximately 8 weeks will produce some degree of physical dependence in most subjects (SHIDEMAN, 1961; DEVENYI and WILSON, 1971). The administration of 600 mg secobarbital daily for 35–57 days to 18 patients produced convulsions in two patients, following abrupt withdrawal. However, 16 of 19 patients who were withdrawn from larger doses of secobarbital (1.0–2.2 g for a similar period) developed severe abstinence symptoms (FRASER et al., 1954). The amount of drug that barbiturate abusers take varies considerably, but an average daily intake of 1.5 g of a short-acting barbiturate is not unusual, and some individuals may take 2.5 g daily over several months (JAFFE, 1975). Although there may be considerable tolerance to the sedative and intoxicating effects, the lethal dose is not much greater in addicts than in nórmal individuals. Tolerance does not readily develop to the respiratory depressant action. An extensive discussion of acute barbiturate poisoning can be found in a volume edited by MATTHEW (1971).

2. Overdose

An overdose of one of the barbiturates results in marked depression of the central nervous system. Symptoms range from sleep to profound coma with marked depression of the respiratory center and ultimately, death. The lethal dose varies considerably depending upon the age and general health of the recipient, the presence of other drugs (especially alcohol), the specific barbiturate taken and, most of all, the availability of skilled medical management. A very severe reaction must be expected when 10–20 times the usual hypnotic dose has been taken (HARVEY, 1975; VICTOR and ADAMS, 1977). The short- and intermediate-acting barbiturates are more potent and more toxic than the long-acting compounds. Lethal blood levels determinded at autopsy may be as low as 1 mg/100 ml for short- and intermediate-acting, and 6 mg/100 ml for long-acting barbiturates The lethal concentration may be even lower if other depressant drugs or alcohol are also present (HARVEY, 1975).

Barbiturate blisters (bullae) are observed in approximately 6% of acute barbiturate intoxications. They most often appear where the skin surfaces have been in contact and, although not absolutely specific for the barbiturates, they greatly assist in attributing the unconsciousness to drug overdosage (MATTHEW, 1975).

Unfortunately, the barbiturates have become one of the drugs most frequently used in suicide attempts, but due to improved prescribing practices of physicians and the availability of the equally effective but less toxic benzodiazepine, this situation is changing. Suicides from poisoning by barbituric acid derivatives in the United States declined from 1,873 in 1970, to 905 in 1976 (GLASS, 1979). The number of barbiturate prescriptions (excluding phenobarbital) declined from 30,744,000 in 1970, to 11,407,000 in 1976. Coincidentally, during the same period, the prescriptions written for all benzodiazepines increased from 61,359,000 to 81,611,000, or approximately the same number which barbiturates prescriptions declined (NATIONAL PRESCRIPTION AUDIT, 1970–1976).

Although the number of hospital admissions for self-poisoning has risen in Britain from 964 in 1967, to 2,134 in 1976, the proportion of patients who had taken barbiturate hypnotics declined from 30% to 15% over the same period, while the proportion taking benzodiazepines rose from approximately 10%–40%. However, during this same period, the proportion of patients who were unconscious upon admission fell from 23% to 15% (PROUDFOOT and PARK, 1978). Hospital admissions due to acute barbiturate poisoning have decreased in England and Wales since 1965, at about the same rate as National Health Service prescriptions for barbiturates (JOHNS, 1977). "Admissions due to poisoning with other drugs have increased, but largely because the benzodiazepine hypnotics and tranquillizers are much less toxic than the barbiturates they are replacing, deaths from poisoning with all solids and liquids have decreased" (JOHNS, 1977).

3. Disinhibiting Actions

Relatively small hypnotic doses of the long-acting barbiturates may produce "hangover," especially in neurotic patients (LADER and WALTERS, 1971; WALTERS and LADER, 1971). Mood distortions, impaired motor skills, and impaired judgment may persist for several hours (HARVEY, 1975; WALTERS and LADER, 1971). Paradoxical excitement and restlessness have been reported (GREENBLATT and SHADER, 1972), especially in patients with severe pain. Hyperactivity and paradoxical excitements is frequently observed in children following phenobarbital. Care should be exercised in prescribing barbiturates for elderly patients who may react with excitement, confusion, or depression (AMA DRUG EVALUATION, 1977). Some patients report increased dreaming, nightmares, or increased insomnia when hypnotic doses of barbiturates are discontinued (GREENBLATT and SHADER, 1972).

4. Depression

As is the case with benzodiazepines, no direct evidence supports a primary "depressogenic" action of barbiturates. Depression may become clinically manifest during treatment, but due very likely to an incorrect diagnosis. Correct diagnosis is therefore very important, since barbiturates may be used more successfully for suicide than the benzodiazepines. They should only be used with great care, if at all, in patients with a history of depression, suicidal tendencies, or drug abuse (GREENBLATT and SHADER, 1972).

II. Adverse Neurologic Reactions

Side effects of the barbiturates include drowsiness, lethargy, somnolence, fatigue, and ataxia, as would be expected from their pharmacologic properties. These reactions are more commonly observed in the elderly, in patients with serious liver disease, or in patients taking excessive doses. Proper adjustment of dosage will usually minimize these conditions (HARVEY, 1975, AMA DRUG EVALUATIONS, 1977).

III. Adverse Reactions Due to Drug Interactions

1. Ethanol

The combined action of barbiturates and alcohol is, at the very least, additive and in certain cases, potentiative (POLACSEK et al., 1972; KISSIN, 1974; SEIXAS, 1975).

The sedative effects of alcohol are cross-tolerant with the barbiturates. Accordingly, a chronic alcoholic may require unusually large doses of barbiturates to supplant the sedative effects of alcohol. The situation is different when the alcoholic is drinking, since high prevailing levels of alcohol impair the metabolism of the barbiturate. Thus, one has more effect from any given dose of barbiturate (WIBERG et al., 1969; RUBIN et al., 1970; MISRA et al., 1971; COHEN and ARMSTRONG, 1974; PIROLA, 1978). Death may occur accidentally from respiratory depression caused by the barbiturate potentiated by alcohol. Such barbiturate-alcohol deaths have been associated toxicologically with sublethal blood levels of both drugs. To a lesser extent, such interaction may occur with benzodiazepines, but whether the mechanism is similiar is not established.

2. Other Drug Interactions

The barbiturates, and especially phenobarbital, are well-documented enzyme inducers (CONNEY, 1967; MARSHALL, 1978). The simultaneous administration of various drugs with the barbiturates may affect either the patient's response to the barbiturate or to the other drug. Phenobarbital treatment lowers the prothrombin time and increases the dose of anticoagulant required. Patients maintained on barbiturate and anticoagulant therapy should be carefully monitored to avoid hemorrhagic complications (SHEPHERD et al., 1972). Patients receiving both digitoxin and phenobarbital therapy may be underdigitalized, as phenobarbital may enhance the metabolism of digitoxin (SOLOMON and ABRAMS, 1972). The same situation applies with most corticosteroids (BROOKS et al., 1972). Phenobarbital has been reported to increase phenytoin levels in certain patients and to decrease it in others. However, marked changes in the phenytoin levels caused by phenobarbital are rare, and in the majority of patients these drugs may be safely given together (KUTT, 1975).

The long-term administration of phenobarbital and phenytoin can increase the metabolism of vitamin D and its biologically active metabolites, the hydroxycalciferols. ANAST (1975) has demonstrated a small but statistically significant reduction in serum 25-hydroxycalciferol and calcium in ambulatory, noninstitutionalized children receiving anticonvulsant medication. Whether barbiturates decrease the absorption of griseofulvin or increase its metabolism is uncertain, but the net result is decreased blood levels of griseofulvin (COHEN and ARMSTRONG, 1974). Other less intensively studied barbiturate effects are respiratory depression following ketamine anesthesia (KOPMAN, 1972) and the enhanced metabolism of chlorpromazine, phenylbutazone, testosterone, and bilirubin (GELEHERTER, 1976).

IV. Adverse Reactions Due to Allergy

1. Skin

Barbiturates have produced nearly every possible skin reaction, although the incidence of reactions is relatively low (BEERMAN and KIRSCHBAUM, 1975). The long-acting barbiturates are generally believed to cause more rashes than the short-acting barbiturates, but no unequivocal evidence for this exists (ALMEYDA and LEVANTINE, 1972). Allergic reactions to the barbiturates include angioneurotic edema, urticaria, morbilliform rash, and Stevens-Johnson syndrome (AMA DRUG EVALUATIONS, 1977). In addition, fever and serum sickness have been reported. Exfoliative dermatitis, which may be accompanied by hepatitis and jaundice, has rarely occurred (ALMEYDA and LEVANTINE, 1972). The barbiturate shold be discontinued whenever dermatologic reactions occur, since skin eruptions may precede potentially fatal reactions. Photosensitivity has rarely been reported.

2. Hematology

Therapeutic doses of the barbiturates are rarely responsible for blood dyscrasias, especially when the drugs are taken for relatively short periods. Megaloblastic anemia, which responds to folic acid, is not uncommon during the prolonged use of phenobarbital or mephobarbital in epileptic patients (HAWKINS and MEYNELL, 1958; SLATER, 1974). Aplastic anemia apparently has not been associated with the anticonvulsant barbiturates. Agranulocytosis has rarely been attributed to phenobarbital (DEVRIES, 1965), but has been reported following the use of other barbiturates (PLUMB, 1937). The barbiturates are contraindicated in patients with a history of porphyria (AMA DRUG EVALUATIONS, 1977), and may exacerbate acute intermittent porphyria (WITH, 1957, ALMEYDA and LEVANTINE, 1972) or porphyria variegata (ALMEYDA and Levantine, 1972).

3. Hepatotoxicity

In therapeutic doses, barbiturates do not impair normal liver function. Even in the large doses employed by addicts, barbiturates have little, if any, effect on the usual liver function tests (BROWNING and MAYNERT, 1972). Severe hepatic damage can occur from ordinary doses in hypersensitive patients. These reactions are usually associated with dermatitis and involvement of other organs (HARVEY, 1975).

V. Teratogenic Studies

WILSON (1977) reviewed the literature on the effects of barbiturates on laboratory animals and found little evidence of teratogenicity, which is in agreement with KALTER (1972) and SCHARDEIN (1976). However sodium pentobarbital and sodium barbital have been reported to be teratogenic in mice, but not in rats or rabbits (SETALA and NYYSSONEN, 1964; PERSAUD, 1965; PERSAUD and HENDERSON, 1969). McCOLL (1966) and McCOLL et al. (1967) found phenobarbital to be teratogenic in the rat and rabbit.

In a retrospective study of environmental influences thought to have been involved in 833 cases of human malformation, RICHARDS (1969) found no association with the barbiturates. TUCHMANN-DUPLESSIS and MERCIER-PAROT (1964) previously indicated that in view of the extensive use of these drugs and the lack of adverse reports, their teratogenic potential was low. However, NELSON and FORFAR (1971) found in a retrospective study of 458 infants with congenital abnormalities that a significantly larger number of these mothers took barbiturates than those in the control group with normal infants. A meaningful conclusion is difficult, since the mothers of the malformed children also took more analgesics, antacids, appetite suppressants, and other drugs than the control mothers of normal infants. This study clearly demonstrates the risk involved in taking any drug during the first trimester of pregnancy. SEIP (1976) recently reported facial dysmorphism, pre- and postnatal growth deficiency developmental delay, and minor malformations in two siblings following exposure to unusually high blood levels (5.0–8.6 mg/100 ml) of phenobarbital in utero. The usual therapeutic range is 1–3 mg/100 ml. SEIP indicated that the same clinical picture has been reported by others following the use of phenytoin in pregnancy and hypothesized that the two drugs may have a similar mechanism of action on the developing fetus.

A recent study raised the question of a possible etiologic role of barbiturates in the development of brain tumors in children. Mothers of children with brain tumors reported having used barbiturates more frequently during their pregnancy than did mothers of normal children or mothers of children with other cancers. In addition, more children with brain tumors were reported to have used barbiturates than normal children or children with other malignant diseases. "The results suggest that barbiturates may play an etiologic role, and it is estimated that as many as 8% of the brain tumors in children may be attributable to use of barbiturates either by the child or prenatally by the mother" (GOLD et al., 1978). This report urgently requires confirmation, since brain tumors account for approximately 20% of all cancers in children and are the second most frequent type of cancer in children (CUTLER and YOUNG, 1975).

D. Concluding Remarks

Barbiturates were for many years the most useful sedative-hypnotic drugs. These applications are now declining due to efforts in both the United States and the United Kingdom to discourage their prescription. This action is based not only on their propensity for abuse but also their history as effective suicidal agents. Numerous editorials and general articles have appeared decrying their use as other than induction agents in anesthesia, anticonvulsants, and in the management of hyperbilirubinemia in infancy. Phenobarbital, the first important anticonvulsant, remains an important drug.

Medical history indicates that the problems of suicide and drug abuse will always be with us; the benzodiazepines, if for no other reason than their remarkable safety, are a significant advance in the field of sedative-hypnotics. They have been in extensive use worldwide for nearly 2 decades, a time when drug abuse was more widespread than ever before. During this period, these drugs must have saved the lives of hundreds of people who would have died had they taken a barbiturate rather than a benzodiazepine in their suicide attempt. Their record of safety, when taken in overdose, is quite remarkable when one considers the relatively uneventful recoveries with no residual sequelae that are the rule. Most authorities conclude that the abuse potential of the benzodiazepines is low. For these reasons, as well as the fact that serious side effects are rare, one may conclude that these drugs will be used extensively for many years.

References

Aarskog, D.: Association between maternal intake of diazepm and oral clefts. Lancet *1975II/* 921

Abramowicz, M.: Benzodiazepine overdosage. Med. Lett. Drugs. Ther. *18*, 60 (1976)

Aivazian, G.H.: Clinical evaluation of diazepam. Dis. Nerv. Syst. *25*, 491–496 (1964)

Albanus, L., Jonsson, M., Sparf, B. Vessman, J.: A study of the induction effect of phenobarbital, diazepam und oxazepam in the dog. Acta Pharmacol. Toxicol. [Supp. 4] (Kbh), 55 (1971)

Allen, M.D., Greenblatt, D.J.: Hypnotics and sedatives. In: Side effects of drugs, Annual 2. Dukes, M.N.G. (ed.), pp. 36–44. Amsterdam: Excerpta Medica 1978

Almeyda, J.: Cutaneous reactions to imipramine and chlordiazepoxide. Br. J. Dermatol. *84*, 298–300 (1971)

Almeyda, J. Levantine, A.: Drug reactions XVII. Cutaneous reactions to barbiturates, chloral hydrate and its derivatives. Br. J. Dermatol. *86*, 313–316 (1972)

AMA Drug Evaluations: Sedatives and hypnotics, pp. 394–409. Antianxiety agents, 3rd ed., pp. 410–419. Littleton, Mass.: Publishing Sciences Group 1977

Anast, C.S.: Anticonvulsant drugs and calcium metabolism. N. Engl. J. Med. *292*, 587–588 (1975)

Austin, T.R.: Mixed drug overdosage with phenelzine, amytal, and chlordiazepoxide. A case report. Anaesthesia *21*, 249–252 (1966)

Ayd, F.J., Jr.: Oxazepam: An overview. Dis. Nerv. Syst. *36*, Suppl., 14–16 (1975)

Bardhan, K.D.: Cerebellar syndrome after nitrazepam overdosage. Lancet 2, 1319–1320 (1969)

Barlow, S.M., Knight, A.F., Sullivan, F.M.: Delay in postnatal growth and development of offspring produced by maternal restraint stress during pregnancy in the rat. Teratology *18*, 211–218 (1978)

Barlow, S.M., Knight, A.F., Sullivan, F.M.: Prevention by diazepam of adverse effects of maternal restraint stress on postnatal development and learning in the rat. Teratology *19*, 105–110 (1979)

Barnett, A., Fiore, J.W.: Acute Tolerance to diazepam in cats and its possible relationship to diazepam metabolism. Eur. J. Pharmacol. *13*, 239–243 (1971)

Barnett, A., Fiore, J.W.: Acute tolerance to diazepam in cats. In: The Benzodiazepines. Garattini, E.S., Mussini, E., Randall, L.O. (eds.), pp. 545–557. New York: Raven Press 1973

Barrett, J.E., DiMascio, A.: Comparative effects on anxiety of the "Minor Tranquilizers" in "High" and "Low" anxious student volunteers. Dis. Nerv. Syst. *27*, 483–486 (1966)

Barry, J.E., Danks, D.M.: Anticonvulsants and congenital abnormalities. Lancet *1974II*, 48–49

Baumes, R.M.: Cytopénies médicamenteuses: purpura, thrombopénique aigü et anticorps antiplaquettairs actifs en présence de Valium. Maroc. Med. *51*, 321–324 (1971)

Beall, J.R.: Study of the teratogenic potential of diazepam and SCH 12041. Can. Med. Assoc. J. *106*, 1061 (1972)

Beerman, H., Kirshbaum B.A.: Drug eruptions. In: Dermatology. Moschella, S.A., Phillsbury, D.M., Hurley, H.J. (eds.), pp. 350–384. Philadelphia: Saunders 1975

Bell, E.F.: The use of naloxone in the treatment of diazepam poisoning. J. Pediatr. *87*, 803–804 (1975)

Bernards, W.: Case history number 74: Reversal of phenothiazine-induced coma with physostigmine. Anesth. Anal. (Cleve) *52*, 938–941 (1973)

Bernstein, M.E., Hughes, F.W., Forney, R.B.: The influence of a new chlordiazepoxide analogue on human mental and motor performance. J. Clin. Pharmacol. *7*, 330–335 (1967)

Berte, F., Manzo, L., De Bernardi, M., Benzi, G.: Ability of the placenta to metabolize oxazepam and aminopyrine before and after drug stimulation. Arch. Int. Pharmacodyn. Ther. *182*, 182–185 (1969)

Betts, T.A., Clayton, A.B., MacKay, G.M.: Effects of four commonly used tranquilizers on low-speed driving performance tests. Br. Med. J. *4*, 580–584 (1972)

Bibawi, E., Girgis, B., Abu-Khatwa, H.: Effect of hypnotics and psychotropic drugs on prothrombin level. J. Egypt. Med. Assoc. *46*, 933–936 (1963)

Bieger, R., de Jonge, H., Loeliger, E.A.: Influence of nitrazepam on oral anticoagulation with phenprocoumon. Clin. Pharmacol. Ther. *13*, 361–365 (1972)

Bitnun, S., Possible effect of chlordiazepoxide on the fetus. Can. Med. Assoc. J. *100*, 351 (1969)

Blackwell, B.: Psychotropic drugs in use today. J. Am. Med. Ass. *225*, 1637–1641 (1973)

Bladin, P.F.: The use of clonazepam as an anticonvulsant – clinical evaluation. Med. J. Aust. *1*, 683–688 (1973)

Blatchley, D.: Allergy to diazepam. Br. Med. J. 2, 287 (1977)

Blitt, C.D., Petty, W.C.: Reversal of lorazepam delirium by physostigmine. Anesth. Analg. (Cleve) *54*, 607–608 (1975)

Bloomer, J.R., The hepatic prophyrias. Pathogenesis, manifestations, and management. Gastroenterology *71*, 689–701 (1976)

Blum, J.E., Haefely, W., Jalfre, M., Polc, P., Scharer, K.: Pharmakologie und Toxikologie des Antiepileptikums Clonazepam. Arzneim. Forsch. *23*, 377–389 (1973)

Bodendorfer, T.W.: Fetal effects of anticonvulsants drugs and seizure disorders. Drug. Intell. Clin. Pharm. *12*, 14–21 (1978)

Boston Collaborative Drug Surveillance Program: Clinial depression in the central nervous system due to diazepam and chlordiazepoxide in relation to cigarette smoking and age. N. Engl. J. Med. *288*, 277–280 (1973)

Brashares, Z.A., Conley, W.R.: Physostigmine in drug overdose. J. Am. Coll. Emerg. Physicians 4, 46–48 (1975)

Breckenridge, A.M., Orme, M.: Clinical implications of enzyme induction. Ann. N.Y. Acad. Sci. *179*, 421–431 (1971)

Breckenridge, A.M., Roberts, J.B., Clinical significance of microsomal enzyme induction. Pharmacol. Res. Commun. *8*, 229–242 (1976)

Brooks, S.M., Werk, E.E., Ackerman, S.J., Sullivan, I., Tracher, K.: Adverse effects of phenobarbital on corticosteroid metabolism in patients with bronchial asthma. N. Engl. J. Med. *286*, 1125–1128 (1972)

Brophy, J.J.: Suicide attempts with psychotherapeutic drugs. Arch. Gen. Psychiatry *17*, 652–657 (1967)

Browning, R.A., Maynert, E.W.: Phenobarbital, mephobarbital, and metharbital. In: Antiepileptic drugs. Woodbury, D.M., Penry, J.K., Schmidt, R.P. (eds.), pp. 345–351. New York: Raven Press 1972

Bruinsma, W.: A guide to drug eruptions. Amsterdam: Excerpta Medica 1973

Brunaud, M., cited by Tuchmann-Duplessis, H.: In: Influence des benzodiazepines sur la descendance. Rev. Med. *37*, 2013–2023 (1976)

Brunaud, M., Rocand, J.: Une nouvelle benzodiazepine, le lorazepam. Mise au point pharmacologique. Agressologie 213, 363–375 (1972)

Brunaud, M., Navarro, J., Salle, J., Siou, G.: Pharmalocogical, toxicological and teratological studies on dipotassium-7-chloro-3-carboxy-1,3-dihydro-2,2-dihydroxy-5-ühenyl-2H-1,4-benzodiazepine (dipotassium chloroazepate, 4306 Cb) a new tranquilizer. Arzneim. Forsch. *20*, 123–125 (1970)

Burks, J.S., Walker, J.E., Rumack, B.H., Ott, J.E.: Tricyclic antidepressant poisoning. J. Am. Med. Ass. *230*, 1405–1407 (1974)

Byck, R., Drugs and the treatment of psychiatric disorders. In: The pharmacological basis of therapeutics. Goodman, L.S., Gilman, A., (eds.), 5th ed., Chap. 12, pp. 152–200. New York. Macmillan 1975

Cannizzaro, G., Nigito, S., Provenzano, P.M., Vitikova, T.: Modification of depressant and disinhibitory action of flurazepam during short term treatment in the rat. Psychopharmacology *26*, 173–184 (1972)

Carroll, B.J., Attempted suicide: Hyponotics and sedatives. Med. J. Aust. *2*, 806 (1970)

Casier, H., Danechmand, L., De Schaepdryver, A., Hermans, W., Piette, Y.: Blood alcohol levels and psychotropic drugs. Arzneim. Forsch. *16*, 1505–1506 (1966)

Cate, J.C., Jatlow, P.I.: Chlordiazepoxide overdose: interpretation of serum drug concentrations. Clin. Toxicol. *6*, 553–561 (1973)

Chapallaz, S.: Intoxications aiguës par le nitrazépam (Mogadon). Schweiz. Apoth. Z. *111*, 95–99 (1973)

Chapman, A.H.: Textbook of Clinical Psychiatry, 2nd ed., pp. 432–435. Philadelphia: Lippincott 1976

Chin, L.S., Havill, J.H., Rothwell, R.P.G., Bishop, B.G.: Use of physostigmine in tricyclic antidepressant poisoning. Anaesth. Intensive care 4, 138–140 (1976)

Chisolm, J.J.: The porphyrias. In: The principles and practice of medicine. Harvey, A.M., Johns, R.J., Owens, A.H., Ross, R.S. (eds.), 18th ed., pp. 630–640. New York: Appleton-Century-Crofts 1972

Cimo, P.L., Pisciotta, A.V., Desai, R.G., Pino, J.L., Aster, R.H.: Detection of drug-dependent antibodies by the ^{51}Cr platelet lysis test: Documentation of immune thrombocytopenia induced by diphenylhydantoin, diazepam, and sulfisoxazole. Am. J. Hematol. 2, 65–72 (1977)

Clarke, T.P., Simpson, T.R., Wise, S.P., III: Two unsuccessful suicidal attempts with a new drug: methaminodiazepoxide (Librium). Tex. State. J. Med. 57, 24–26 (1961)

Cohen, M.M., Hirschorn, K., Frosch, W.A.: Cytogenetic effects of tranquilizing drugs in vivo and in vitro. J. Am. Med. Ass. 207, 2425–2426 (1969)

Cohen, S.N., Armstrong, M.A.: Drug interactions, p. 31. Baltimore: Williams & Wilkins 1974

Cohen, S.: Valium®: Its use and abuse. Drug. Abuse Alcohol News. 5, 1–4 (1976)

Cole, J.O.: Behavioral toxicology. In: Drugs and behavior. Uhr, L., Miller, J.G. (eds.), pp. 166–183. New York: Wiley & Sons 1960

Conney, A.H.: Drug metabolism and therapeutics. N. Engl. J. Med. 280, 653–660 (1969)

Conney, A.H.: Pharmacological implications of microsomal enzyme induction. Pharmacol. Rev. 19, 317–366 (1967)

Cook, L., Davidson, A.B.: Effects of behaviorally active drugs in a conflict-punishment procedure in rats. In: The benzodiazepines. Garattini, E.S., Mussini, E., Randall, L.O. (eds.), pp. 327–345. New York: Raven Press 1973

Cooper, J.R. (ed.): Sedative-hypnotic drugs. Risks and benefits. U.S. Department of Health, Education, and Welfar. National Institute on Drug Abuse, Rockville, Md., 1977

Copperman, I.B.: Purpura in a patient taking chlordiazepoxide. Br. Med. J. 4, 485–486 (1967)

Crombie, D.C., Pinsent, R.J., Fleming, D.M., Rumeau-Rouquette, C., Goujard, J., Huel, G.: Fetal effects of tranquilizers in pregnancy. N. Engl. J. Med. 293, 198–199 (1975)

Cruz, I.A., Cramer, N.C., Parrish, A.E., Hemodialysis in chlordiazepoxide toxicity. J. Am. Med. Ass. 202, 438–440 (1967)

Cutler, S.J., Young, J.L. (eds.): Third national cancer survey: Incidence data. Natl. Cancer Inst. Monogr. 41, 102–103 (1975)

Czech, K., Francesconi, M., Haimbock, E., Hruby, K.: Die akute Vergiftung durch trizyklische Antidepressiva und ihre Therapie mit physostigminsalzylat. Wien, Klin. Wochenschr. 89, 265–269 (1977)

Danechmand, L., Casier, H., Hebbelinck, M., DeShaepdryver, A.: Combined effects of ethanol and psychotropic drugs on muscular tone in mice. Q.J. Stud. Alcohol. 28, 424–429 (1967)

Daunderer, M.: Physostigmin als Antidot bei einer Limbatril-Valium-Intoxikation. Dtsch. Med. Wochensch. 103, 1245–1246 (1978)

Davis, J.M., Termini, B.A.: Attempted suicide with psychotropic drugs: Diagnosis and treatment (Part 1). Med. Counter Point 1, 43–49 (1969)

Degenhardt, K.H., Kerken, H., Knorr, K., Koller, S., Wiedemann, H.R.: Drug usage and fetal development: Preliminary evaluations of a prospective investigation. Adv. Exp. Med. Biol. 27, 467–479 (1972)

DeMatteis, F.: Disturbances of liver prophyrin metabolism caused by drugs. Pharmacol. Rev. 19, 523–557 (1967)

DeMatteis, F.: Toxic hepatic prophyrias. Semin. Hematol. 5, 409 (1968)

Devenyi, P., Wilson, M.: Barbiturate abuse and addiction and their relationship to alcohol and alcoholism. Can. Med. Assoc. J. 104, 215–218 (1971)

De Vries, S.I.: Haematological aspects during treatment with anticonvulsant drugs. Epilepsia 6, 1–15 (1965)

Di Liberti, J., O'Brien, M.L., Turner, T.: The use of physostigmine as an antidote in accidental diazepam intoxication J. Pediatr. 86, 106–107 (1975)

DiMascio, A., Barrett, J.E.: Comparative effects of oxazepam in "High" and "Low" anxious student volunteers. Psychosomatics 6, 298–302 (1965)

DiMascio, A., Meyer, R.E., Stifler, L.: Effects of imipramine on individuals varying in level of depression. Am. J. Psychiatry 125, 55–58 (1968)

Doss, M. (ed.): Prophyrins in human diseases. 1st Int. Porphyrin Meet., Freiburg IB, 1975. Basel: Karger 1976

Eales, L.: Acute porphyria: The precipitating and aggravating factors. S. Afr. J. Lab. Clin. Med. 17, 120–125 (1971)

Editorial: Barbiturates on the way out. Br. Med. J. *3*, 725–726 (1975)

Edwards, V.E., Eadie, J.M.: Clonazepam – a clinical study of its effectiveness as an anticonvulsant. Proc. Austr. Assoc. Neurol. *10*, 61–66 (1973)

Eerola, M., Baer, G.: Porphyrie und Anaesthesie. Fallbericht und Kurze Übersicht. Prakt. Anaesth. *11*, 160–165 (1976)

Eisenberg, J.: Die hepatischen Porphyrien. Med. Klin. *68*, 789–797 (1973)

Elder, G.H., Gray, C.H., Nicholson, D.C.: The prophyrias: A review. J. Clin. Pathol. *25*, 1013–1033 (1972)

Ellison, R.J., Cancellaro, L.A.: A study in the management of anxiety with lorazepam. J. Clin. Pharmacol. *18*, 210–219 (1978)

Fang, M.H., Ginsberg, A.L., Dobbins, W.O., III: Cholestatic jaundice associated with flurazepam hydrochloride. Ann. Intern. Med. *89*, 363–364 (1978)

Farkas, G., Farkas, G.: L'effet teratogene des medicaments psychotropes. J. Pharmacol. (Paris) *5*, Suppl. 2, 30 (1974)

Favazza, A.R.: Elevated erythrocyte sedimentation rates in chronic, mentally ill outpatients. Dis. Nerv. Syst. *34*, 110–112 (1973)

Fedrick, J.: Epilepsy and pregnancy. A report from the Oxford record linkage study. Br. Med. J. *2*, 442–448 (1973)

Fell, R.H., Dendy, P.R.: Severe Hypothermia and respiratory arrest in diazepam and glutethimide intoxication. Anaesthesia *23*, 636–640 (1968)

Findley, J.D., Robinson, W.W., Peregrino, L.: Addiction to secobarbital and chloridazepoxide in the rhesus monkey by means of self-infusion preference procedure. Psychopharmacology *26*, 93–114 (1972)

Finkle, B.S., McCloskey, K.L., Goodman, L.S.: Diazepam and drug associated deaths: A United States and Canadian Survey. J. Am. Med. Ass. *242*, 429–434 (1979)

Forfar, J.O., Nelson, M.M.: Epidemiology of drugs taken by pregnant women: Drugs that may affect the fetus adversely. Clin. Pharmacol. Ther. *14*, 632–642 (1973)

Foy, K.A., Abendschein, D.R., Lahcen, R.B.. Effects of benzodiazepines during gestation and infancy of Y-maze performance of mice. Pharmacol. Res. Commun. *9*, 325–338 (1977)

Franks, E., Jacobs, W.H.: Cholestatic jaundice possible due to benzodiazepine-type drugs. Mo. Med. *72*, 605–606 (1975)

Fraser, H.F., Isbel, H., Eisenman, A.J., Wikler, A., Pescor, F.T.. Chronic barbiturates intoxication; further studies. Arch. Intern. Med. *94*, 34–41 (1954)

Freyhan, F.A.: Therapeutic implications of differential effects of new phenothiazine compounds. Am. J. Psychiatry *115*, 577–585 (1959)

Ganguli, L.K., Sen, D., Chatterjee, P., Mandal, J.N.: Oxazepam overdosage. J. Indian Med. Assoc. *54*, 424–425 (1970)

Gardos, G., DiMascio, A., Salzman, C., Shader, R.I.: Differential actions of chlordiazepoxide and oxazepam on hostility. Arch. Gen. Psychiatry *18*, 757–760 (1968)

Gaul, L.E.: Fixed drug eruption from chlordiazepoxide. Arch. Dermatol. *83*, 1010–1011 (1961)

Gault, F.P.: A review of recent literature on barbiturate addiction and withdrawal. Bol. Estud. Med. Biol. *29*, 75–83 (1976)

Gebhart, G.F., Plaa, G.L., Mitchell, C.L.: The effects of ethanol alone and in combination with phenobarbital, chlorpromazine, or chlordiazepoxide. Toxicol. Appl. Pharmacol. *15*, 405–414 (1969)

Gelehrter, T.D.: Enzyme induction (first of three parts). N. Engl. J. Med. *294*, 522–526 (1976)

Gosh, J.S.: Allergy to diazepam and other benzodiazpines. Br. Med. J. *1*, 902–903 (1977)

Gibson, J.E., Becker, B.A.: Effect of phenobarbital and SKF 525A on the teratogenicity of cyclophosphamide in mice. Teratology *1*, 393–398 (1968)

Gilbert, J.E.: Ingestion of a massive dose of Librium. S.D. J. Med. *14*, 307–309 (1961)

Gjerris, F.: Poisoning with chlordiazepoxide (Librium). Dan. Med. Bull. *13*, 170–172 (1966)

Glass, E.: Personal communication 1979. Vital statistics of the United States, Mortality. US. Department of Health, Education, and Welfare

Gold, E. Gordis, L., Tonascia, J., Szklo, M.: Increased risk of brain tumors in children exposed to barbiturates. J. Natl. Cancer Inst. *61*, 1031–1034 (1978)

Goldberg, H.L., DiMascio, A.: Psychotropic drugs in pregnancy. In: Psychopharmacology: A generation of progress. Lipton, M.A., DiMascio, A., Killam, K.F. (eds.), pp. 1047–1055. New York. Raven Press 1978

Goldberg, H.L., Finnerty, R.J.: A double-blind study of prazepam versus placebo in single daily doses in the treatment of anxiety. Compr. Psychiatry *18*, 147–155 (1977)

Goldberg, L.: Psychopharmacological effects of ethanol and CNS-active drugs. In: 3rd Int. Pharmacol. Congr, Sao Paulo, Abstrs, pp. 61–62, 1966

Goldberg, M.E., Manian, A.A., Efron, D.H.: A comparative study of certain pharmacologic responses following acute and chronic administrations of chlordiazepoixde. Life Sci. *6*, 481–491 (1967)

Goldman, D.: The results of treatment of psychotic states with newer phenothiazine compounds effective in small doses. Am. J. Med. Sci. *235*, 67–78 (1958)

Goodman, L., Gilman, A.: The pharmacological basis of therapeutics. p. 145. New York: Macmillan 1941

Gove, P.B. (ed.): Websters' Third New International Dictionary of the English Language – Unabridged. Springfield Ill. Merriam 1963

Greenberg, G., Inman, W.H.W., Weatherall, J.A.C., Adelstein, A.M., Haskey, J.C.: Maternal drug histories and congenital abnormalities. Br. Med. J. *2*, 853–856 (1977)

Greenblatt, D.J.: Antianxiety agents. In: Drug effects in hospitalized patients. Miller, R.R., Greenblatt, D.J. (eds.), pp.193–205. New York: Wiley & Sons 1976

Greenblatt, D.J., Shader, R.I.: The clinical choice of sedative-hypnotics. Ann. Intern. Med. *77*, 91–100 (1972)

Greenblatt, D.J., Shader, R.I.: Benzodiazepines in clinical practice. New York: Raven Press 1974

Greenblatt, D.J., Shader, R.I.: Prazepam and lorazepam, two new benzodiazepines. N. Engl. J. Med. *299*, 1342–1344 (1978 a)

Greenblatt, D.J., Shader, R.I.: Dependence, tolerance, and addiction to benzodiazepines: Clinical and pharmacokinetic considerations. Drug. Metab. Rev. *8*, 13–28 (1978 b)

Greenblatt, D.J., Allen, M.D., Noel, B.J., Shader, R.I.: Acute overdose with benzodiazepine derivatives. Clin. Pharmacol. Ther. *21*, 497–514 (1977)

Greenblatt, D.J., Woo, E., Allen, M.D., Orsulak, P.J., Shader, R.I.: Rapid recovery from massive diazepam overdose. J. Am. Med. Ass. *240*, 1872–1874 (1978 a)

Greenblatt, D.J., Shader, R.I., Weinberger, D.R., Allen, M.D., MacLaughlin, D.S.: Effect of a cocktail on diazepam absorption. Psychopharmacology *57*, 199–203 (1978 b)

Gundlach, R., Engelhardt, D.M., Hankoff, L., Paley, H., Rudorfer, L., Bird, E.: A double-blind outpatient study of diazepam (Valium and placebo). Psychopharmacology *9*, 81–92 (1966)

Gupta, R.C., Kofold, J., Toxicological statistics for barbiturates, other sedatives, and tranquilizers in Ontario. A 10-year survey. Can. Med. Assoc. J. *94*, 863–865 (1966)

Haerten, K., Poettgen, W.: Leukopenie nach Benzodiazepin-Derivaten. Med. Welt *26*, 1712–1714 (1975)

Haider, I.: Evaluation of a new tranquilizer – Wy 4036 – in the treatment of anxiety. Br. J. Psychiatry *119*, 597–598 (1971)

Hammer, W. Sjöqvist, F.: Plasma levels of monomethylated tricyclic antidepressants during treatment with imipramine-like compounds. Life Sci. *6*, 1895–1903 (1967)

Harris, R.T., Claghorn, J.L., Schoolar, J.C.. Self administration of minor tranqzilizers as a function of conditioning. Psychopharmacology *13*, 81–88 (1968)

Hartz, S.C., Heinonen, O.P., Shapiro, S., Siskind, V., Slone, D.: Antenatal exposure to meprobamate and chlordiazepoxide in relation to malformations, mental development, and childhood mortality. N. Engl. J. Med. *292*, 726–728 (1975)

Harvey, S.C.: Hypnotics and sedatives. In: The pharmacological basis of therapeutics. 5th ed., Goodman, L.S., Gilman, A. (eds.), pp. 102–123. New York: Macmillan 1975

Hawkins, C.F., Meynell, J.J.: Macrocytosis and macrocytic anemia caused by anticonvulsant drugs. Q. J. Med. *27*, 45–63 (1968)

Hayes, S.L., Pablo, G., Radomski, T., Palmer, R.: Ethanol and oral diazepam absorption. N. Engl. J. Med. *296*, 186–189 (1977)

Heberden, W.: Some aspects of a disorder of the breast. Med. Trans. Royal Coll. Phys. Lond. *2*, 59–67 (1772) Cited by Lie, J.T.: Recognizing coronary heart disease – selected historical vignettes from the period of William Harvey (1578–1657) to Adam Hammer (1818–1878). Mayo Clin. Proc. *53*, 811–817 (1978)

Heinonen, O.P., Slone, D., Shapiro, S.: Birth defects and drugs in pregnancy, pp. 335–344. Littleton, Mass.: Publishing Sciences Group 1977

Heiser, J.F., Wilbert, D.E.: Reversal of delirium induced by tricyclic antidepressant drugs with physostigmine. Am. J. Psychiatry *131*, 1275–1277 (1974)

Hillyer, D.M.: An overdose of "Valium". Med. J. Aust. *1*, 565 (1965)

Hoffer, A.: Lack of potentiation by chlordiazepoxide (Librium®) of depression or excitation due to alcohol. Can. Med. Assoc. J. *87*, 920–921 (1962)

Holden, J.M.C., Itil, T.M.: Laboratory changes with chlordiazepoxide and thioridazine, alone and combined. Can. Psychiatr. Assoc. J. *14*, 299–301 (1969)

Holinger, P.C., Klawans, H.L., Reversal of tricyclic-overdosage-induced central anticholinergic syndrome by physostigmine. Am. J. Psychiatry *133*, 1018–1023 (1976)

Holliday, A.R.: The problem of a shifting definition of behavioral toxicity. In: Proc. Int. Congr. Coll. Int. Neuro-Psycho-Pharmacol. 1966. 5th ed., Brill, H., Cole, J.O., Diniker, P., Hippius, H., Bradley, P.B. (eds.), pp. 630–637. Amsterdam: Excerpta Medica Foundation 1967

Hollister, L.E.: Uses of psychotherapeutic drugs. Ann. Intern. Med. *79*, 88–98 (1973)

Hollister, L.E.: Valium: A discussion of current issues. Psychosomatics *18*, 44–58 (1977)

Hollister, L.E.: Clinical pharmacology of psychotherapeutic drugs. pp. 12–49. New York: Churchill Livingstone 1978

Hollister, L.E., Motzenbecker, F.P., Degan, R.O.: Withdrawal reactions from chlordiazepoxide (Librium). Psychopharmacology *2*, 63–68 (1961)

Hollister, L.E., Bennett, J.L., Kimbell, I., Savage, C., Overall, J.E.: Diazepam in newly admitted schizophrenics. Dis. Nerv. Syst. *24*, 746–750 (1963)

Hoogland, D.R., Miya, T.S., Bousouet, W.F.: Metabolism and tolerance studies with chlordiazepoxide-2-^{14}C in the rat. Toxicol. Appl. Pharmacol. *9*, 116–123 (1966)

Horváth, T., Gógl, A., Ruzsa, C., Ludány, A., Jávor, T.: Drug-induced manifestations of hereditary hepatopathy. Acta Med. Acad. Sci. Hung. *3*, 219–228 (1974)

Hoskins, N.M.: Current drug therapy-barbiturates. Am. J. Hosp. Pharm. *33*, 333–339 (1976)

Houghton, G.W., Richens, A.: The effect of benzodiazepines and pheneturide on phenytoin metabolism in man. Br. J. Clin. Pharmacol. *1*, 344–345 (1974)

Hughes, F.W., Forney, R.B., Richards, A.B.: Comparative effects in human subjects of chlordiazepoxide, diazepam, and placebo on mental und physical performance. Clin. Pharmacol. Ther. *6*, 139–145 (1965)

Hummler, H., Theiss, E.: Cited by Tuchmann-Duplessis, H.: In: Influence des benzodiazepines sur la descendance. Rev. Medecine *37*, 2013–2023 (1976)

Ingram, I.M., Timbury, G.C.: Side-effects of Librium. Lancet *2*, 766 (1960)

Isbel, H.: Abuse of barbiturates. J. Am. Med. Ass. *162*, 660–661 (1956)

Isbell, H., Chrusciel, T.L.: Dependence liability of "non-narcotic" drugs. Bull. WHO *43*, 49 (1970)

Istvan, E.J.: Drug-associated congenital abnormalities? Can. Med. Assoc. J. *103*, 1394 (1970)

Jaffe, J.H.: Drug addiction and drug abuse. In: The pharmacological basis o therapeutics. 5th ed., Goodman, L.S., Gilman, A. (eds.), pp. 284–324. New York: Macmillan 1975

Jenner, F.A., Parkin, D.: A large overdose of chlordiazepoxide. Lancet *2*, 322–323 (1961)

Johns, M.W.: Self-poisoning with barbiturates in England and Wales during 1959–1974. Br. Med. J. *1*, 1128–1130 (1977)

Jowett, B. (tr.), Plato: The Republic, Book III, Section 407. In: The dialogues of Plato, Encyclopedia Britannia. Great Books of the Western World. Hutchins, R.M. (ed.), p. 337. New York: Random House 1952

Kaebling, R., Conrad, F.G.: Agranulocytosis due to chlordiazepoxide hydrochloride, J. Am. Med. Ass. *174*, 1863–1865 (1960)

Kalter, H.. Teratogenicity, embryolethality, and mutagenicity of drugs of dependence. In: Chemical and biological aspects of drug dependence. Mule, S.J., Brill, H. (eds.), pp. 413–445. Cleveland: CRC Press 1972

Kanto, J., Iisalo, E.U.M., Hovi-Viander, M., Kangas, L.: A comparative study on the clinical effects of oxazepam and diazepam. Relationship between plasma level and effects. Int. J. Clin. Pharmacol. Biopharm. *17*, 26–31 (1979)

Karch, F.E., Lasagna, L.: Adverse drug reactions – a critical review. J. Am. Med. Ass. *234*, 1236–1241 (1975)

Kato, R., Chiesara, E.: Increase of pentobarbitone metabolism induced in rats pretreated with some centrally acting compounds. Br. J. Pharmacol. *18*, 2938 (1962)

Kato, R., Vassanelli, P.: Induction of increased meprobamate metabolism in rats pretreated with some neurotropic drugs. Biochem. Pharmacol. *11*, 779–794 (1962)

Kerry, R.J., Jenner, F.A.: A double blind crossover comparison of diazepam (Valium, RO 5-2,807) with chlordiazepoxide (Librium) in the treatment of neurotic anxiety. Psychopharmacology *3*, 302–306 (1962)

Kinross-Wright, J., Cohen, I.M., Knight, J.A.: The management of neurotic and psychotic states with Ro 5-0690 (Librium). Dis. Nerv. Syst. *21*, 23–26 (1960)

Kissin, B., Interactions of ethyl acohol and other drugs. In: The biology of alcoholism. Kissin, B., Bergleiter, H., (eds.), pp. 119–121, Vol. 3. New York: Plenum Press 1974

Klerman, G.L., DiMascio, A., Rinkel, M., Greenblatt, M.: The influence of specific personality patterns on the reactions of phrenotropic agents. In: Biological psychiatry. Masserman, J. (ed.), Vol. I, pp. 224–242. New York: Grune & Stratton 1959

Knudsen, K.B., Sparberg, M., Lecocq, F.: Porphyria precipitated by fasting. N. Engl. J. Med. *277*, 350–351 (1967)

Koch-Weser, J., Greenblatt, D.J.: The archaic barbiturate hyponotics. N. Engl. J. Med. *291*, 790–791 (1974)

Koch-Weser, J., Sellers, E.M.: Drug interactions with coumarin anticoagulants (second of two parts). N. Engl. J. Med. *285*, 547–558 (1971)

Kolb, L.C., Modern clinical psychiatry, p. 952. Philadelphia: Saunders 1977

Kopmann, A.F.: Letter to editor. Anesth. Analg. (Cleve.) *51*, 793–794 (1972)

Kuntzman, R., Jacobson, M., Conney, A.H.: Effect of phenylbutazone on cortisol metabolism in man. Pharmacologist *8*, 195 (1966)

Kuntzman, R., Jacobson, M., Levin, W., Conney, A.H.: Stimulatory effect of N-phenylbarbital (phetharbital) on cortisol hydroxylation in man. Biochem. Pharmacol. *17*, 565–571 (1968 a)

Kuntzman, R., Sernatinger, E., Tsai, I., Klutch, A.: New Methodology for studies of drug metabolism. In: Symposium "Importance of fundamental principles in drug evaluation". Tedeschi, D., Tedeschi, R. (eds.), pp. 87–103. New York. Raven Press 1968 b

Kurland, A.A., Bethon, G.D., Michaus, M.H., Agallianos, D.D.: Chlorpromazine-chlordiazepoxide and chlorpromazine-imipramine treatment: Side effects and clinical laboratory findings. J. New Drugs *6*, 80–95 (1966)

Kutt, H.: Interactions of antiepileptic drugs. Epilepsia *16*, 393–402 (1975)

Lackner, H., Hunt, V.E.: The effect of Librium on hemostasis. Am. J. Med. Sci. *256*, 368–372 (1968)

Lader, M.: Antianxiety drugs: Clinical pharmacology and therapeutic use. Drugs *12*, 362–373 (1976)

Lader, M., Walters, A.J.: Hangover effects of hypnotics in man. Br. J. Pharmacol. *41*, 412 (1971)

Lakos, P., Czeizel, E.: A teratological evaluation of anticonvulsant drugs. Acta Paediatr. Acad. Sci. Hung. *18*, 145–153 (1977)

Larson, G.F., Hurlbert, B.J., Wingard, D.W.: Physostigmine reversal of diazepam-induced depression. Anesth. Analg. (Cleve) *56*, 349–351 (1977)

Lasagna, L.: The role of benzodiazepines in nonpsychiatric medical practice. Am. J. Psychiatry *134*, 656–658 (1977)

Lawton, M.P., Cahn, B.: The effects of diazepam (Valium®) and alcohol on psychomotor performance. J. Nerv. Ment. Dis. *136*, 550–554 (1963)

Lief, H.I.: Anxiety Reactions. In: Comprehensive textbook of psychiatry. Freedman, A.M., Kaplan, H.I., (eds.), pp. 857–870. Baltimore: Williams and Wilkins Co. 1967

Linnoila, M., Hakkinen, S.: Effects of diazepam and codeine, alone and in combination with alcohol, on simulated driving. Clin. Pharmacol. Ther. *15*, 368–373 (1974)

Linnoila, M., Mattila, M.J.: Drug interaction on psychomotor skills related to driving: Diazepam and alcohol. Eur. J. Clin. Pharmacol. *5*, 186–194 (1973)

Linnoila, M., Otterström, S., Anttila, M.: Serum chlordiazepoxide, diazepam, and thioridazine concentrations after the simultaneous ingestion of alcohol or placebo drink. Ann. Clin. Res. *6*, 4–6 (1974)

Lo, K.-J., Eastwood, I.R., Eidelman, S.: Cholestatic jaundice associated with chlordiazepoxide hydrochloride (Librium) therapy: Report of a case and review of the literaure. Am. J. Dig. Dis. *12*, 845–949 (1967)

Loew, D.M., Taeschler, M.: Wirkungsspektren von Psychopharmaka: Ihre Ableitung und mögliche Bedeutung für die Therapie. Mod. Probl. Pharmacopsychiatry *1*, 118–137 (1968)

Louis-Fernand, R.T.: Barbiturates and psychotherapy. In: Psychotherapeutic drugs. Usdin, E., Forrest, I.S. (eds.), pp. 1318–1333. New York: Dekker 1975

Lund, L.: Effects of phenytoin in patients with epilepsy in relation to its concentration in plasma. In: Biological effects of drugs in relation to their plasma concentrations. Davies, D.S., Prichard, B.N.C. (eds.), pp. 227–238. Baltimore: University Park Press 1973

Lundy, J.S., Osterberg, A.E.: Review of the literature on derivates of barbituric acid; chemistry; pharmacology; clinical use. Proc. Staff Meet., Mayo Clin. *4*, Suppl., 386–416 (1929)

Luton, E.F., Finchum, R.N.: Photosensitivity reaction to chlordiazepoxide. Arch. Dermatol. *91*, 362–363 (1965)

Lyubimov, B.I., Smolnikova, N.M., Strekalova, S.N.: Effect of diazepam on the development of the progeny. Biull. Eksp. Biol. Med. *78*, 64–66 (1974)

Mackie, B.S., Mackie, L.E.: Antihistamines in the treatment of drug eruptions. Med. J. Aust. *2*, 1034–1037 (1966)

MacLeod, S.M., Giles, H.G., Patzalek, G., Thiessen, J.J., Sellers, E.M.: Diazepam actions and plasma concentrations following ethanol ingestion. Eur. J. Clin. Pharmacol. *11*, 345–349 (1977)

Magnus, I.A.: The cutaneous porphyrias. Semin. Hematol. *5*, 380–408 (1968)

Magnus, R.V.: Once-a-day potassium clorazepate in anxiety. Br. J. Clin. Pract. *27*, 449–452 (1973)

Malick, J.B., Sofia, R.D., Goldberg, M.E.: A comparative study of the effects of selected psychoactive agents upon three lesion-induced models of aggression in the rat. Arch. Int. Pharmacodyn. Ther. *181*, 459–465 (1969)

Manoguerra, A.S. Ruiz, E.: Physostigmine treatment of anticholinergic poisoning. J. Am. Coll. Emerg. Physicians. *5*, 125–127 (1976)

Margules, D.L., Stein, L.: Increase of "antianxiety" activity and tolerance of behavioral depression during chronic administration of oxazepam. Psychopharmacology *13*, 74–80 (1968)

Marks, J.: The benzodiazepines: Use, overuse, misuse, abuse. Baltimore: University Park Press 1978

Marshall, W.J.: Enzyme induction by drugs. Ann. Clin. Biochem. *15*, 55–64 (1978)

Matsuki, K., Iwamoto, T.: Development of tolerance to tranquillizers in the rat. Jpn. J. Pharmacol. *16*, 191–197 (1966)

Matthew, H.: Acute barbiturate poisoning. Amsterdam: Excerpta Medica 1971

Matthew, H.: Barbiturates. Clin. Toxicol. *8*, 495–513 (1975)

Matthew, H., Proudfoot, A.T., Aitken, R.L.B., Aitken, R.L.B., Raeburn, J.A., Wright, N.: Nitrazepam: A safe hypnotic. Br. Med. J. *3*, 23–25 (1969)

McColl, J.D.: Teratology studies. Appl. Ther. *8*, 48–52 (1966)

McColl, J.D., Robinson, S., Globus, M.: Effect of some therapeutic agents on the rabbit fetus. Toxicol. Appl. Pharmacol. *10*, 244–252 (1967)

McDonald, R.L.: The effects of personality type on drug response. Arch. Gen. Psychiatry *17*, 680–686 (1967)

Mellin, G.W.: Drugs in the first trimester of pregnancy and the fetal life of Homo sapiens. Am. J. Obstet. Gynecol. *90*, 1169–1180 (1964)

Mennear, J.H.: Familial pharmacology. Am. Fam. Physician *15*, 100–102 (1977)

Meyer, U.A., Schmid, R.: The Porphyrias. In: The metabolic basis of inherited disease, Stanbury, J.B., Wyngaarden, J.B., Fredrickson, D.S., (eds.), pp. 1166–1220. New York: McGraw-Hill Book Co. 1978

Milkovich, L., van den Berg, J.B.: Effects of prenatal meprobamate and chlordiazepoxide hydrochloride on human embryonic and fetal development. N. Engl. J. Med. *291*, 1268–1271 (1974)

Miller, A.I., D'Agostino, A., Minsky, R.: Effects of combined chlordiazepoxide and alcohol in man. Q. J. Stud. Alcohol. *24*, 9–13 (1963)

Miller, R.P., Becker, B.A.: The teratogenicity of diazepam metabolites in Swiss-Webster mice. Toxicol. Appl. Pharmacol. *25*, 453 (1973)

Miller, R.P., Becker, B.A.: Teratogenicity of oral diazepam and diphenylhydantoin in mice. Toxicol. Appl. Pharmacol. *32*, 53–61 (1975)

Milner, G.: The effect of antidepressants and "tranquilizers" on the response of mice to ethanol. Br. J. Pharmacol. *34*, 370–376 (1968)

Milner, G.: Interaction between barbiturates, alcohol, and some psychotropic drugs. Med. J. Aust. *1*, 1204–1207 (1970)

Milner, L.: Allergy to diazepam. Br. Med. J. *1*, 144 (1977)

Misra, P.S., Letevre, A., Ishii, H., Rubin, E., Lieber, C.S.: Increase of ethanol, meprobamate, and pentobarbital metabolism after chronic ethanol administration in man and rats. Am. J. Med. *51*, 346–351 (1971)

Morland, J., Setekleiv, J., Hattner, J.F.W., Stromsaether, C.E., Danielsen, A., Wethe, G.H.: Combined effects of diazepam and ethanol on mental and psychomotor functions. Acta Pharmacol. Toxicol. (Kbh.) *34*, 5–15 (1974)

Nagy, J., Decsi, L.: Physostigmine, a highly potent antidote for acute experimental diazepam intoxication. Neuropharmacology *17*, 469–475 (1978)

National Prescription Audit (U.S.A.), 1970–1976. I.M.S. International, Ambler, Pa

Nelson, M.M., Fortar, J.O.: Associations between drugs administered during pregnancy and congenital abnormalities of the fetus. Br. Med. J. *1*, 523–527 (1971)

Newton, R.W.: Physostigmine salicyclate in the treatment of tricyclic antidepressant overdose. J. Am. Med. Ass. *231*, 941–943 (1975)

New Zealand Committee on Adverse Drug Reactions: Reactions reported 1965–1968. NZ Med. J. *69*, 96–99 (1969)

New Zealand Committee on Adverse Drug Reactions: Three-year survey of reactions, 1969–1971. NZ Med. J. *75*, 100–104 (1972)

Norio, M., Isoaho, R., Idanpaan-Heikkila, J.: Interaction of benzodiazepines and ethanol on sleeping time in rats. Scand. J. Clin. Lab. Invest. *27*, Supp. 116, 76 (1971)

Olivecrona, H.: Embryo-destroying effect of injected phenobarbital in the mouse. Acta Anat. (Basel) *58*, 217–221 (1964)

O'Malley, K.: Safety of hypnotics. Br. Med. J. *1*, 729 (1971)

O'Neil, J.T., Pogge, R.C.: Relative safety of self-inflicted overdose with relatively newer medications. Ariz. Med. *30*, 484–485 (1973)

Orme, M., Breckenridge, A., Brooks, R.V.: Interactions of benzodiazepines with warfarin. Br. Med. J. *3*, 611–614 (1972)

Owen, G., Smith, T.H.F., Agersborg, H.P.K.: Toxicity of some benzodiazepine compounds with CNS activity. Toxicol. Appl. Pharmacol. *16*, 556–570 (1970)

Padfield, A., Watkins, J.: Allergy to diazepam. Br. Med. J. *1*, 575–576 (1977)

Pare, C.M.B.: Umwanted effects of long-term medication in schizophrenia and depression. Pharmakopsychiatr. Neuropsychopharmakol. *9*, 187–192 (1976)

Pearson, I.B.: Hypnotics and sedatives. In: Side effects of drugs. Dukes, M.N.G. (ed.), Annual I, pp. 21–29. Amsterdam: Excerpta Medica 1977

Pennington, G.W., Synge, V.M.: Chlordiazepoxide ("Librium") overdosage. J. Ir. Med. Assoc. *49*, 187–188 (1961)

Persaud, T.V.N.: Investigations on the teratogenic effect of barbiturates in experiments on animals. Acta Biol. Med. Ger. *14*, 89–90 (1965)

Persaud, T.V.N., Herderson, W.M.: The teratogenicity of barbital sodium in mice. Arzneim. Forsch. *19*, 1309–1310 (1969)

Pirola, R.D.: Drug metabolism and alcohol. P. 108. Baltimore: University Park Press 1978

Polacsek, E., Barnes, T., Turner, N., Hall, R., Weise, C.: Interactions of alcohol and other drugs. 2nd ed. Toronto: Addiction Research Foundation 1972

Plum, P.: Clinical and experimental investigations in agranulocytosis. London: Lervis & Co. 1937

Proudfoot, A.T., Park, J.: Changing patterns of drugs used for self-poisoning. Br. Med. J. *1*, 90–93 (1978)

Rada, R.T., Kellner, R., Buchanan, J.G.: Chlordiazepoxide and alcohol: A fatal overdose. J. Forensic Sci. *20*, 544–547 (1975)

Randall, L.O.: Pharmacology of methaminodiazepoxide. Dis. Nerv. Syst. *21*, Suppl., 7–10 (1960)

Randall, L.O., Kappell, B.: Pharmacological activity of some benzodiazepines and their metabolites. In: The benzodiazepines. Garattini, E.S., Mussini, E., Randall, L.O. (eds.), pp. 27–51. New York: Raven Press 1973

Randall, L.O., Schallek, W., Heise, G.A., Keith, E.F., Bagdon, R.E.: The psychosedative properties of methaminodiazepoxide. J. Pharmacol. Exp. Ther. *120*, 163–171 (1960)

Rapp, M.S.: Reaction to flurazepam. Can. Med. Assoc. J. *105*, 1020–1021 (1971)

Redeker, A.G., Sterling, R.E.: The "glucose effect" in erythropoietic protoporphyria. Arch. Intern. Med. *121*, 446–448 (1968)

Reggiani, G., Hürlimann, A., Theiss, E.: Some aspects of the experimental and clinical toxicology of chlordiazepoxide. Proc. Eur. Soc. Study Drug Toxic. *9*, 79–97 (1968)

Richards, L.D.G.: Congenital malformations and environmental influences in pregnancy. Br. J. Prev. Soc. Med. *23*, 218–225 (1969)

Richens, A.: Drug interactions in epilepsy. In: Drug interactions. Grahme-Smith, D.G. (ed.), pp. 239–249. Baltimore: University Park Press 1977

Richens, A., Houghton, G.W.: Effect of drug therapy on the metabolism of phenytoin. In: Clinical pharmacology of antiepileptic drugs. Schneider, H., Janz, D., Gardner-Thorpe, C., Meinardi, H., Scherwin, A.L. (eds.), pp. 87–96. Berlin-Heidelberg-New York: Springer 1975

Rickels, K.: Drug treatment of anxiety. In: Psychopharmacology in the practice of medicine. Jarvik, M.E. (ed.), pp. 309–324. New York: Appleton-Century-Crofts 1977

Ringrose, C.A.D.: The hazard of neurotropic drugs in the fertile years. Can. Med. Assoc. J. *106*, 1058 (1972)

Ristola, P., Pyoralo, K., Jalonen, K., Suhonen, O.: The effect of diazepam on the rate of warfarin metabolism in man, rabbit, and rat. Scand. J. Clin. Lab. Invest. *27*, Suppl. 116, 18 (1971)

Robinson, D.S., Amido, E.L.: Interaction of benzodiazepines with warfarin in man. In: The benzodiazepines. Garattini, E.D., Mussini, E., Randall, L.O. (eds.), pp. 641–646. New York: Raven Press 1973

Robinson, D.S., Sylvester, D.: Interaction of commonly prescribed drugs with warfarin. Ann. Intern. Med. *72*, 853–856 (1970)

Rogers, H.J., Haslam, R.A., Longstreth, J., Lietman, P.S.: Phenytoin intoxication during concurrent diazepam therapy. J. Neurol. Neurosurg. Psychiatry *40*, 890–895 (1977)

Rosenberg, H.: Physostigmine reversal of sedative drugs. J. Am. Med. Ass. *229*, 1168 (1974)

Rubin, E., Gang, H., Mirsa, P.S., Lieber, C.S.: Inhibition of drug metabolism by acute ethanol intoxication. Am. J. Med. *49*, 801–806 (1970)

Safra, M.J., Oakley, G.P., Jr.: Association between cleft lip with or without cleft palate and prenatal exposure to diazepam. Lancet *1975II*, 478–480

Salzman, C., DiMascio, A., Shader, I.R., Hazmatz, J.S.: Chlordiazepoxide, expectation and hostility. Psychopharmacology *14*, 38–45 (1969)

Sarwer-Foner, G.J.: Recognition and management of drug-induced extrapyramidal reactions and "paradoxical" behavioural reactions in psychiatry. Can. Med. Assoc. J. *83*, 312–318 (1960)

Savin, J.A.: Current causes of fixed drug eruptions. Br. J. Dermatol. *83*, 546–549 (1970)

Saxen, I.: Associations between oral clefts and drugs taken during pregnancy. Int. J. Epidemiol. *4*, 37–44 (1975)

Schaeffer, S.: Toxicity from drug overdosage in an eleven-year-old boy. Case report. Clin. Pediatr. (Phil.) *1*, 103–104 (1962)

Schallek, W., Schlosser, W., Randall, L.O.: Recent developments in the pharmacology of the benzodiazepines. Adv. Pharmacol. Chemother. *10*, 119–183 (1972)

Schardein, J.L.: Drugs as Teratogens. Pp. 149–150. Cleveland: CRC Press 1976

Schmid, R.: In: The metabolic basis of inherited disease. Stanbury, J.B., Wyngaarden, J.B., Fredrickson, D.S. (eds.), pp. 939–1012. New York: Blakiston Division, McGraw-Hill Book Co., 1966

Schmidt, W., Staiger, G.R.: Chromosome studies on bone marrow from Chinese hamsters treated with benzodiazepine tranquillizers and cyclophosphamide. Mutat. Res. *7*, 99–108 (1969)

Scott, A.J., Ansford, A.J., Webster, B.H., Stringer, H.C.W.: Erythropoietic protoporphyria with features of a sideroblastic anaemic terminating in liver failure. Am. J. Med. *54*, 251–259 (1973)

Seip, M.: Growth retardation, dysmorphic facies, and minor malformations following massive exposure to phenobarbitone in utero. Acta Paediatr. Scand. *65*, 617–621 (1976)

Seixas, F.A.: Alcohol and its drug interactions. Ann. Intern. Med. *83*, 86–92 (1975)

Sellers, E.M.: Addictive drugs: Disposition, tolerance and dependence. Drug Metab. Rev. *8*, 5–11 (1978)

Setala, K., Nyyssonen, O.: Hypnotic sodium pentobarbital as a teratogen for mice. Naturwissenschaften *51*, 413 (1964)

Shader, R.I., DiMascio, A.: Psychotropic drug side effects. Baltimore: Williams & Wilkins 1970

Shader, R.I., Greenblatt, D.J.: Clinical implications of benzodiazepine pharmacokinetics. Am. J. Psychiatry *134*, 652–656 (1977)

Shader, R.I., Greenblatt, D.J., Salzman, C., Kochansky, G.E., Harmatz, J.S.: Benzodiazepines: Safety and toxicity. Dis. Nerv. Syst. *36*, 23–26 (1975)

Shapiro, A.K.: Psychochemotherapy. In: Biological foundation of psychiatry. Grenell, R.G., Gabay, S. (eds.), Vol. 2, p. 819. New York: Raven Press 1976

Shepherd, M., Lader, M., Lader, S.: Hypnotics and sedatives. In: Side effects of drugs. Meyler, L., Herxheimer, A. (eds.), pp. 52–54. Amsterdam: Excerpta Medica 1972

Shideman, F.E.: Clinical pharmacology of hypnotics and sedatives. Clin. Pharmacol. Ther. *2*, 313–344 (1961)

Shimkin, P.M., Shaivitz, S.A.: Oxazepam poisoning in a child. J. Am. Med. Ass. *196*, 662–663 (1966)

Skupin, G., Franzke, H.G.: Tranxilium 20 (Dikalium-chlorazepat) als 24-Stunden-Tranquilizer. Med. Welt *26*, 956–959 (1975)

Slater, S.D.: Megaloblastic anemia and chronic bromide intoxication. Br. J. Clin. Pract. *28*, 97–100 (1974)

Slovis, T.L., Ott, J.E., Teitelbaum, D.T., Lipscomb, W.: Physostigmine therapy in acute tricyclic antidepressant poisoning. Clin. Toxicol. *4*, 451–459 (1971)

Smith, M.E.: A comparative controlled study with chlordiazepoxide. Am. J. Psychiatry *117*, 362–363 (1960)

Smith, M.E.: Suicidal attempt by oral ingestion of chlordiazepoxide (Librium). Clin. Med. *8*, 72–74 (1961)

Snyder, B.D., Blonde, L., McWhirter, W.R.: Reversal of amitiyptyline intoxication by physostigmine. J. Am. Med. Ass. *230*, 1433–1434 (1974)

Solomon, H.M., Abrams, W.B.: Interactions between digitoxin and other drugs in man. Am. Heart J. *82*, 277–280 (1972)

Solomon, H.M., Barakat, M.J., Ashley, C.J.: Mechanisms of drug interaction. J. Am. Med. Ass. *216*, 1997–1999 (1971)

Somers, G.F.: The evaluation of drugs for foetal toxicity and teratogenicity in the rat: A collaborative study by sixteen laboratories. Excerpta Medica Int. Congr. Ser. *115*, 216–220 (1966)

Somers, G.F.: The evaluation of drugs for foetal toxicity and teratogenicity in the rabbit: A collaborative study by four laboratories. Excerpta Medica Int. Congr. Ser. *181*, 227–234 (1968)

Spark, H., Goldman, A.S.: Diazepam intoxication in a child. Am. J. Dis. Child *109*, 128–129 (1965)

Speidel, B.D., Meadow, S.R.: Maternal epilepsy and abnormalities of the fetus and newborn. Lancet *1972II*, 839–843

Stacher, G.: Intrahepatische cholestase nach einer hochdosierten kombinations therapie mit Diazepam und Barbituraten bei Tetanus-Patienten. Wien. Klin. Wochenschr. *85*, 401–406 (1973)

Staiger, G.R.: Chlordiazepoxide and diazepam: Absence of effects on the chromosomes of diploid human fibroblast cells. Mutat. Res. *7*, 109–115 (1969)

Staiger, G.R.: Studies on the chromosomes of human lymphocytes treated with diazepam in vitro. Mutat. Res. *10*, 635–644 (1970)

Stein, L., Berger, B.D.: Psychopharmacology of 7-chloro-5-(0-chlorophenyl)-1, 3-dihydro-3-hydroxy-2H-1,4-benzodiazepin-2-one (lorazepam) in squirrel, monkey, and rat. Arzneim. Forsch. *21*, 1072–1078 (1971)

Stenchever, M.A., Parks, K.J.: Some effects of diazepam on pregnancy in the Balb/c mouse. Am. J. Obstet. Gynecol. *121*, 765–770 (1975)

Stenchever, M.A., Frankel, R.S., Jarvis, J.A., Veress, K.: Some effects of diazepam in human cells in vitro. Am. J. Obstet. Gynecol. *103*, 836–842 (1969)

Stenchever, M.A., Frankel, R.S., Jarvis, J.A.: Effect of diazepam on chromosomes of human leukocytes in vivo. Am. J. Obstet. Gynecol. *107*, 456–460 (1970a)

Stenchever, M.A., Frankel, R.S., Jarvis, J.A., Veress, K.: Effect of chlordiazepoxide hydrochloride on human chromosomes. Am. J. Obstet. Gynecol. *106*, 920–923 (1970b)

Stevenson, I.H., Browning, M., Cooks, J., O'Mally, K.: Changes in human drug metabolism after long-term exposure to hypnotics. Br. Med. J. *4*, 322–323 (1972)

Stolerman, I.P., Kumar, R., Steinberg, H.: Development of morphine dependence in rats: Lack of effect of previous ingestion of other drugs. Psychopharmacology *20*, 321–336 (1971)

Straus, D.J., Vance, Z.B., Kasdon, E.J., Robinson, S.H.: Atypical lymphoma with prolonged systemic remission after splenectomy. Description of three cases. Am. J. Med. *56*, 386–392 (1974)

Sullivan, F.M., McElhatton, P.R.: A comparison of the teratogenic activity of the antiepileptic drugs carbamazepine, clonazepam, ethosuximide, phenobarbital, phenytoin, and primidone in mice. Toxicol. Appl. Pharmacol. *40*, 365–378 (1977)

Svenson, S.E., Hamilton, R.G., A critique of overemphasis on side effects with the psychotropic drugs: An analysis of 18,000 chlordiazepoxide-treated cases. Curr. Ther. Res. Clin. Exp. *8*, 455–464 (1966)

Szeberenyi, S., Szalay, K.S., Garattini, S.: Removal of plasma metyrapone in rats submitted to previous pharmacological treatment. J. Pharm. Pharmacol. *21*, 201–202 (1969)

Taddeini, L., Watson, C.J.: The clinical porphyrias. sem. hematol. *5*, 335–369 (1968)

Tanner, T.B., Moorhead, S.H.: High dose poisoning with diazepam (Valium) and survival in a two-year-old child. J. Med. Assoc. Ga. *57*, 534–536 (1968)

Thomson, J., Glen, A.I.M.: A large overdosage of chlordiazepoxide. Lancet *1961 II*, 722–723

Tobin, J.M., Lewis, N.D.C.: New psychotherapeutic agent, chlordiazepoxide. J. Am. Med. Ass. *174*, 1242–1249 (1960)

Tobin, J.M., Bird, I.F., Boyle, D.E.: Preliminary evaluation of Librium (RO 5-0690) in the treatment of anxiety reactions. Dis. Nerv. Syst. *21*, 11–19 (1960)

Tobin, J.M., Lorenz, A.A., Brousseau, E.R., Conner, W.R.: Clinical evaluation of oxazepam for the management of anxiety. Dis. Nerv. Syst. *25*, 689–696 (1964)

Tschudy, D.P., Wellan, F.H., Collins, A., Hunter, G.: The effect of carbohydrate feeding on the induction of delta-aminolevulinic acid synthetase. Metabolism *13*, 396–406 (1964)

Tschudy, D.: Acute intermittent porphyria. Semin. Hematol. *5*, 370–379 (1968)

Tuchmann-Duplessis, H.: Influence des benzodiazepines sur la descendance. Rev. Medecine *37*, 2013–2023 (1976)

Tuchmann-Duplessis, H.: Drug effects on the fetus. Sydney: Adis Press 1975

Tuchmann-Duplessis, H., Mercier-Parot, L.: Repercussions des neruoleptics et des antitumoraux sur le development prenatal. Bull. Acad. Suisse Sci. Med. *20*, 490–526 (1964)

Vajda, F.J.E., Prineas, R.J., Lovell, R.R.H.: Interaction between phenytoin and the benzodiazepines. Br. Med. J. *1*, 346 (1971)

Van Dam, F.E., Gribnau-Overkamp, M.J.H.: The effect of some sedatives (phenobarbital, glutethimide, chlordiazepoxide, choral hydrate) on the rate of disappearance of ethyl biscoumacetate from plasma. Folia Med. Neerl. *10*, 141–145 (1967)

Van der Kleijn, E., Vree, T.B., Guelen, P.J.M.: 7-Chloro-1,4-benzodiazepines: diazepam, desmethyldiazepam, oxydiazepam, oxydesmethyldiazepam (oxazepam), and chlordiazepoxide. In: Psychotherapeutic drugs. Usdin, E., Forrest, I.S. (eds.), Part II: Applications. Chap. V-I, pp. 997–1037. New York: Dekker 1977

Van der Kolk, B.A., Shader, R.I., Greenblatt, D.J.: Autonomic effects of psychotropic drugs. In: Psychopharmacology: A generation of progress. Lipton, M.A., DiMascio, A., Killam, K.F. (eds.), pp. 1009–1020. New York: Raven Press 1978

Varma, A.J., Fisher, B.K., Sarin, M.K.: Diazepam-induced coma with bullae and eccrine sweat gland necrosis. Arch. Intern. Med. *137*, 1207–1210 (1977)

Vere, D.W.: Risks of everyday life-drugs. Proc. R. Soc. Med. *69*, 105–107 (1976)

Vesell, E.S., Passananti, G.T., Viau, J.P., Epps, J.E., Di Carlo, F.J.: Effects of chronic prazepam administration on drug metabolism in man and rat. Pharmacology *7*, 197–206 (1972)

Victor, M., Adams, R.D.: Barbiturates. In: Harrison's principles of internal medicine. Thorn, G.W., Adams, R.D., Braunwald, E., Isselbacher, K.J., Petersdorf, R.G. (eds.), pp. 721–725. New York: McGraw-Hill 1977

Walker, B.E., Patterson, A.: Induction of cleft palate in mice by tranquilizers and barbiturates. Teratology 10, 159–163 (1974)

Walters, A.J., Lader, M.H.: Hangover effects of hypnotics in man. Nature 229, 637–638 (1971)

Walzer, R.S., Kurland, M.L., Braun, M.: Clinical trial of methaminodiazepoxide (Librium). Am. J. Psychiatry 117, 456–457 (1960)

Welland, F.H., Hellman, E.S., Gaddis, E.M., Collins, A., Hunter, G.W., Jr., Tschudy, D.P.: Factors affecting the excretion of porphyrin precursors by patients with acute intermittent porphyria. 1. The effect of diet. Metabolism 13, 232–250 (1964)

Weston, J.K., Weston, K.: Adverse drug reactions. The scene revisited – An update. Clin. Toxicol. 10, 129–148 (1977)

White, B.J., Driscoll, E.J., Tjio, J., Smilack, Z.H.: Chromosomal aberration rates and intravenously given diazepam. J. Am. Med. Ass. 230, 414–417 (1974)

Whitfield, J.B., Moss, D.W., Neale, G., Orme, M., Breckenridge, A.: Changes in plasma glutamyl transpeptidase activity associated with alterations in drug metabolism in man. Br. Med. J. 1, 316–318 (1973)

Whitlock, F.A.: Suicide in Brisbane, 1956–1973: The drug-death epidemic. Med. J. Aust. 1, 737–743 (1975)

Wiberg, G.S., Colwell, B.B., Trenholm, H.L.: Toxicity of ethanol-barbiturate mixtures. J. Pharm. Pharmacol. 21, 232–236 (1969)

Wilcox, W.W.: A case of agranulocytosis. Alaska Med. 4, 31–32 (1962)

Wilson, J.G.: Embryotoxicity of drugs in man. In: Handbook of teratology. Wilson, J.G., Fraser, F.C. (eds.), Vol. I, pp. 309–355. New York: Plenum Press 1977

With, T.K.: Porphyrin metabolism and barbiturate poisoning: Observations on cases of acute and chronic poisoning. J. Clin. Pathol. 10, 165–167 (1957)

Yanagita, T., Takahashi, S.: Dependence liability of several sedativehypnotic agents evaluated in monkeys. J. Pharmacol. Exp. Ther. 185, 307–316 (1973)

Zall, H.: Chemotherapy of anxiety. In: Mind-influencing drugs. Goldberg, M., Eggelston, E. (eds.), pp. 153–223. Littleton: PSG 1978

Zbinden, G., Bagdon, R.E., Keith, E.F., Phillips, R.D., Randall, L.O.: Experimental and clinical toxicology of chlordiazepoxide (Librium®). Toxicol. Appl. Pharmacol. 3, 619–637 (1961)

Zileli, M.S., Telatar, F., Deniz, S., Ilter, E., Adalar, N.: Pseudohypersomolar nonketoacitotic coma due to oxazepam intoxication. Clin. Toxicol. 5, 337–341 (1972)

Zucker, H.S.: Strange behavior with oxazepam. N.Y. State J. Med. 72, 974 (1972)

CHAPTER 8

Dependence-Producing Effects of Anxiolytics

T. YANAGITA

A. Pharmacodynamic Profiles

Since the 1950s, a number of nonbarbiturate sedatives have been introduced, some categorized as tranquilizers or so-called minor tranquilizers. The first popular minor tranquilizer was meprobamate, which has sedative, hypnotic, and muscle-relaxant effects. At the time of its introduction into medical use, the drug was claimed to be specifically effective for anxiety and convulsive disorders, without having marked general depressant effects. But later it was found that meprobamate is nearly indistinguishable from the barbiturates in its pharmacologic effects. Such drugs as benactyzine, buclizine, and hydroxyzine are sometimes classified as anxiolytics, but their use as anxiolytics has become very limited in clinical practice. Therefore, these drugs will not be dealt with here.

True anxiolytics can be said to have been successfully developed when chlordiazepoxide was introduced into medical use in the mid-1950s, as the first of the group known as benzodiazepines. Chlordiazepoxide was found to have potent sedative, muscle-relaxant, taming, and anticonvulsant effects in animals (RANDALL et al., 1960) and potent antianxiety and anticonvulsant effects in man which, depending on the dose, could be demonstrated to have no significant general central nervous system (CNS) depressant effects (HARRIS, 1960; TOBIN and LEWIS, 1960). Although the benzodiazepines that have since been developed possess quantitatively different pharmacodynamic and/or pharmacokinetic characteristics from those of chlordiazepoxide, their pharmacodynamic profiles are qualitatively similar. In laboratory animals, benzodiazepines suppress aggressive behavior, disinhibit conditioned or conflictive behavior, reduce spontaneous motor activity, potentiate the anesthetic effect of barbiturates, suppress convulsions induced by electric shock or pentylenetetrazol, relax skeletal muscle rigidity induced by decerebration, incapacitate motor coordination, and produce tolerance and dependence. The biggest difference between benzodiazepines and barbiturates is that as the dose is increased, the depressant effects of benzodiazepines reach but do not surpass a certain plateau at which respiration is not significantly suppressed. Consequently, anesthesia, coma, or dealth are never produced by benzodiazepines alone. Clinically, benzodiazepines are used most widely as anxiolytics, but also as sleep inducers and anticonvulsants. Their use with sleep or convulsive disorders requires stronger effects than with anxiety. In many countries, each of the benzodiazepines is usually classified for clinical purposes either as anxiolytic or as sleep-inducing. But this classification is not necessarily reflective of the essential pharmacologic properties, and the choice of dose regimen for a particular drug sometimes seems to be more important in actual practice than the choice of the drug itself.

B. Dependence-Producing Properties

The dependence-producing properties of meprobamate and of most benzodiazepines are qualitatively similar to those of the barbiturates: They produce tolerance, physical dependence of the barbiturate type, and psychological dependence. Physical dependence on these anxiolytics is said to be of the barbiturate type because (1) cross physical dependence is demonstrable between barbiturates and benzodiazepines or meprobamate, (2) the withdrawal signs observed in subjects physically dependent on anxiolytics are very similar to those seen in subjects undergoing barbiturate withdrawal.

I. Tolerance

Both metabolic and functional tolerance are known to be developed to benzodiazepines and meprobamate in animals and man (KALANT et al., 1971; PEET and MOONIE, 1977). In those drugs that produce metabolic tolerance, the major mechanism is induction of drug-metabolizing enzymes in the liver occurring as a result of drug use. Barbiturates are among the best-known drugs exemplifying this mechanism. Even with barbiturates, however, it seems certain that functional tolerance plays the major role in the development of marked tolerance (OKAMOTO et al., 1975). With benzodiazepines and meprobamate, it has been reported that metabolic tolerance occurs to such a limited extent that it has no clinical significance.

Functional tolerance can be subdivided into tissue tolerance and behavioral tolerance. Tissue tolerance is the decrease in susceptibility of the nervous system to the depressant effects of drugs. Its mechanisms of development are not yet clear and have been the subject of postulation (KALANT et al., 1971; SMITH, 1977). Many theories support the view that tissue tolerance is developed by compensatory hyperactivity of the nervous system under drug influence. When the drug is eliminated from the nervous tissue, tissue tolerance gradually disappears (usually within a week) with no observable pathologic state. During the process of recovery from tissue tolerance, transient hyperactivity of the nervous system may often be observed in such rebound phenomena as a lowering of the seizure threshold beyond the normal level or an increase in spontaneous motor activity (RASTOGI et al., 1978). In this period, an increase in susceptibility of the nervous system to the drug's effects, termed "intolerance," can also be seen.

Behavioral tolerance, the second subdivision, refers to the increase in behavioral capability under a certain drug-induced depressed state. This increase is thought to occur as a behavioral adaptation to, or a relearning of, the particular behavior under that state (LEBLANC et al., 1973). In animals, functional tolerance to benzodiazepines and meprobamate is readily demonstrable in the depressant effects of the drugs on, for example, gross behavior, motor coordination, electrically or drug-induced convulsions, and EEG. Behavioral tolerance can be reflected in effects on gross behavior and motor coordination, but unlike tissue tolerance probably not in the anticonvulsant and EEG effects.

In man, definite tolerance to the antiepileptic or hypnotic effects of benzodiazepines has been observed (MATTSON, 1972), but tolerance to the is antianxiety effects has been reported not to be clearly observable. The extent of development of tolerance to CNS depressants is known to be a function of the dose regimen, i.e., the severity of the drug-induced depressed state, the amount of time spent daily in the depressed state, and the total period on the drugs (SMITH, 1977). Thus, the apparent non-development of tolerance to the antianxiety effects may be partially attributable to lower dose regimens when the drugs are used as anxiolytics.

II. Cross Tolerance

Cross tolerance theoretically should exist between benzodiazepines and barbiturates or alcohol, because cross physical dependence is readily demonstrable, and physical dependence on these drugs is believed to be developed by the same mechanisms as in tissue tolerance. However, data on cross tolerance between benzodiazepines and barbiturates or alcohol have been only scantily reported due to methodological difficulties.

III. Types of Dependence

1. Physical

Meprobamate and many benzodiazepines are known to produce physical dependence in animals and man. The physical dependence potential of meprobamate is very similar to that of the barbiturates (ESSIG, 1958, 1964; YANAGITA and TAKAHASHI, 1973). The development of physical dependence on benzodiazepines is usually slower and the withdrawal signs somewhat less severe than with barbiturates, but the development of severe withdrawal signs in animals is possible when they are withdrawn after treatment for several weeks under an intensive dose regimen. These withdrawal signs are very similar to those observed in barbital-dependent and withdrawn subjects and include apprehension, hyperirritability, tremor, muscle rigidity, motor impairment, and convulsions (YANAGITA et al., 1973, 1975a, b, c, 1977a). In man, a number of case reports clearly indicate that may benzodiazepines produce such barbiturate-alcohol type withdrawal signs as intensified anxiety, agitation, extreme insomnia, severe tremor, diaphoresis, pain, depression, nightmares, convulsions, hallucinations, disorientation, and delirium. Case reports are also available concerning withdrawal sign associated with diazepam and chlordiazepoxide (HOLLISTER et al., 1961; ESSIG, 1964, 1966; COVI et al., 1973; MALETZKY and KLOTTER, 1976; RIFIKIN et al., 1976; FLOYD and MURPHY, 1976; PEET and MOONIE, 1977; AGRAWAL, 1978). Several reports on newer benzodiazepines such as oxazepam, flurazepam, nitrazepam, and lorazepam are also available (GREENBLATT and SHADER, 1974a; MISRA, 1975; KORSGAARD, 1976). Based on these observations in animals and man, it can be said that almost all benzodiazepines possess physical dependence-producing properties of similar quality.

The mechanisms involved in the development of physical dependence on a drug are not yet clarified, but they probably resemble those of tissue tolerance. Details of these mechanisms have been discussed by MARTIN and SMITH in Vol. 45/I of this series (MARTIN and SLOAN, 1977; SMITH, 1977). The difference between physical dependence and tissue tolerance seems to be that compensatory hyperactivity of the nervous system is more strongly and persistently developed in the former, to the extent that the nervous system cannot adapt to the nondrug condition without manifestation of a certain disease state upon withdrawal. It is thought that the withdrawal syndrome is caused by the compensatory hyperactivity of the nervous system becoming so persistent that the system cannot immediately return to its normal excitation level. With barbiturates and to a certain extent with alcohol and benzodiazepines, it has been observed that the severity of the withdrawal syndrome is a function of:

1) The extent to which the nervous system is depressed by the drug during the administration period
2) The amount of time daily spent at a certain level of depression
3) The total duration of the administration period
4) The elimination speed of the drug upon withdrawal (Fraser and Isbell, 1954; Essig, 1966; Yanagita and Takahashi, 1970; Greenblatt and Shader, 1974a; Okamoto et al., 1976).

The first three factors seem to be relevant to the intensity of development of the compensatory hyperactivity in the nervous system, while the fourth seems to be relevant to the extent of imbalance in the nervous excitation level between the gradually decreasing hyperactivity of the nervous system and the reducing residual depressant effect of the drug. This view can be supported by the fact that gradual withdrawal from narcotics or barbiturates minimizes the development of withdrawal signs in subjects with severe physical dependence (Isbell and White, 1953). Thus, the differences in physical dependence potential of benzodiazepines, barbiturates, alcohol, and certain other nonbarbiturate sedative-hypnotics may be attributable to differences in their pharmacologic properties.

A further point important for understanding the development of withdrawal phenomena is that it is possible for withdrawal signs to be developed in physically dependent subjects before the drug has been completely withdrawn, or even during the period of ongoing drug use, if and when the blood level drops to a certain point or at a certain speed during the interval between doses. In fact, in animal studies on physical dependence or subacute/chronic toxicity in which repeated administration of some benzodiazepine once or twice daily is required, obvious withdrawal signs such as severe tremor (with or without convulsions) are frequently observable at the time of daily drug administration, particularly with those drugs having a relatively short duration of effect.

2. Cross Physical

Cross physical dependence between barbiturates and benzodiazepines, meprobamate, or alcohol is well known in animals and man (Isbell and White, 1953; Deneau and Weiss, 1968; Yanagita and Takahashi, 1973). In animals, all of the benzodiazepines that have been tested so far suppressed the barbital withdrawal signs in barbital-dependent and withdrawn monkeys (Yanagita and Takahashi, 1973; Yanagita et al., 1975 a, b, c, e, 1977 a, b). Table 1 shows that the doses of the benzodiazepines equipotent in suppressing barbital withdrawal signs in monkeys parallel fairly closely the clinical doses for each drug.

Benzodiazepines also possess potential cross physical dependence with alcohol (Kaim, 1973; Greenblatt and Shader, 1974b; Kissin, 1975; Miyasato, 1978). Today, benzodiazepines are widely used in the treatment of alcoholic patients, primarily to suppress the alcohol withdrawal syndrome. Fairly good suppression over a long period, without marked general depression, may be thereby obtained. But there is no well-documented evidence as to whether such a substitution is truly effective in the

Table 1. Classification of some anxiolytics, barbiturates, and alcohol by potency of suppressing barbital withdrawal signs in rhesus monkeys[a]

Group	I	II	III	IV	V
Equipotent dose (mg/kg, p.o.)	1–2	4–10	20–25	100–200	4,000
Generic name	Nitrazepam	Clorazepate	Chlordiazepoxide	Barbital	Alcohol
	Prazepam	Diazepam	Cloxazolam	Fletazepam	
	Triazolam	Lorazepam	Flurazepam	Meprobamate	
			Oxazolam		
			Pentobarbital (Na, i.v.)		

[a] Physical dependence maintained by oral doses of barbital at 75 mg/kg every 12 h

radical treatment of the disease, i.e., in treatment of the psychological dependence. Although it is not known whether the use of benzodiazepines in treating alcoholics is a significant factor in the spread of mixed abuse of benzodiazepines and alcohol, such abuse is increasing (ABELSON et al., 1977). Mixed use sometimes occurs unintentionally, for example when an anxiolytic is prescribed for daytime use and alcohol is additionally ingested in the evening, possibly with a hypnotic upon retirement at bedtime. In such a case, physical dependence may be rapidly developed due to cross physical dependency. Therefore, in examining the possibility of development of physical dependence on benzodiazepines, it is of practical importance to consider those drugs that are capable of interacting with them to produce physical dependence.

3. Psychological

Psychological dependence on a drug is the strong and compulsive desire for the drug's effects, as well as the state of experiencing the desired effects of the drug. This dependence may behaviorally result in abuse of the drug. In animals, psychological dependence is said to have been experimentally developed when strong behavior of seeking or taking a certain drug has been demonstrated, and the animals have overt signs of the drug's effects following self-administration of the drug (YANAGITA, 1976). Essential to the development of psychological dependence is that a drug having a meaningful reinforcing effect be ingested by a susceptible subject using an appropriate dose and method of intake. Pharmacologically, the properties of a drug that are relevant to psychological dependence may be divided into three categories, namely: the reinforcing effect, the subjective effects, and the other pharmacodynamic effects of the drug ingested in a self-administration dose regimen.

a) Reinforcing Effects

The term "reinforcement" refers to a behavioral consequence following subjective experience of the systemic pharmacologic effects of a drug. A drug is said to have a reinforcing effect when the response rate in a certain drug-seeking or drug-taking behavior increases as a result of subjective experience of the drug's effects. The intensity of the reinforcing effect is regarded as the best parameter for gauging the psychological dependence potential of a drug.

Table 2. Highest average daily doses self-administered by individual rhesus monkeys in 2-week period[a]

Group	Drug	Intravenous (mg/kg/inj × No./day)	Intragastric (mg/kg/inj × No./day)
I	Nitrazepam	–	$1 \times 32.4 = 32.4$
	Prazepam	–	$1 \times 8.4 = 8.4$
	Triazolam	–	$0.24 \times 15 = 3.6$
II	Clorazepate	$1 \times 14.5 = 14.5$	–
	Diazepam	$0.4 \times 35 = 14$	$2 \times 12.4 = 24.8$
	Lorazepam	–	$2.5 \times 17.6 = 44$
III	Chlordiazepoxide	$1 \times 20 = 20$	$10 \times 8.7 = 87$
	Cloxazolam	–	$5 \times 14.5 = 72.5$
	Flurazepam	$1 \times 30.4 = 30.4$	–
	Oxazolam		$10 \times 3 = 30$
	Pentobarbital (Na)	$5 \times 132 = 660$	–
	Pentobarbital (Ca)	–	$40 \times 11 = 440$
IV	Fletazepam	–	$5 \times 18.9 = 94.5$
V	Alcohol	$200 \times 44 = 8,800$	$1,000 \times 7.5 = 7,500$

[a] Since the unit doses and subjects were not equalized, the figures cannot serve for strict comparison

In the laboratory, the reinforcing effect can be assessed by self-administration experiments. Many benzodiazepines have been tested in rhesus monkeys, using intragastric or intravenous self-administration techniques. These studies have served to demonstrate the reinforcing effects of benzodiazepines (Table 2) (YANAGITA and TAKAHASHI, 1973; YANAGITA et al., 1975 a, b, c, d, e, 1977 a, b; HOFFMEISTER, 1977). The reinforcing effects of chlordiazepoxide, medazepam, and flurazepam have also been demonstrated by intravenous or intragastric self-administration experiments in rats, rhesus monkeys, and baboons (FINDLEY et al., 1972; GÖTESTAM, 1973; COLLINS et al., 1978). The most characteristic pattern of self-administration of benzodiazepines observed in rhesus monkeys was that the animals took the drug at relatively high daily dose levels at the beginning of the experiment, but the levels lowered considerably thereafter. The pattern observed with intravenous and intragastric self-administration of diazepam and nitrazepam, respectively, is illustrated in Fig. 1; this pattern is seldom observed with other drugs. The daily self-administration rates do not necessarily reflect the intensity of the reinforcing effect, because the rate is also a function of the unit dose, the potency of the general pharmacologic effects, and the elimination speed. Nonetheless, the gradual decrease seen in the daily doses with some benzodiazepines, and the relatively low rate overall, seem to indicate that the reinforcing intensities of the benzodiazepines are distinguishably weaker than those of pentobarbital. For more accurate assessment of the reinforcing intensity, it is necessary to employ special experimental techniques (WHO, 1978; JOHANSON and SCHUSTER, 1975; YANAGITA, 1976; GRIFFITHS et al., 1978) requiring intravenous self-administration of the drugs. However, since many of the benzodiazepines are unfortunately water insoluble, comparative data on the reinforcing intensities of the benzodiazepines are not yet available.

In man, the reinforcing effect has been indicated in many case reports and surveys on benzodiazepine abuse. Regardless of a number of negative views, there is ample

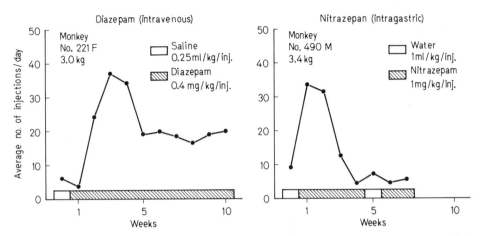

Fig. 1. Intravenous self-administration of diazepam and intragastric self-administration of nitrazepam. The daily numbers represent weekly averages. Self-administration of the vehicle preceded observation with the drugs

evidence that such benzodiazepines as diazepam, chlordiazepoxide, flurazepam, nitrazepam, and many others are subject to widespread abuse in man (HOLLISTER et al., 1961; ESSIG, 1964, 1966; COVI et al., 1973; GREENBLATT and SHADER, 1974a; MISRA, 1975; MALETZKY and KLOTTER, 1976; KORSGAARD, 1976; RIFIKIN et al., 1976; PEET and MOONIE, 1977). The most telling evidence for this is found in the survey of the Drug Abuse Warning Network (DAWN) of the United States. According to the survey for the period of April 1974–April 1975, diazepam was ranked first in instances of abuse and misuse, exceeding all of the prototypical drugs of abuse such as heroin, marihuana, synthetic analgesics, barbiturates, and stimulants (BRILL and JAFFE, 1978). The relative intensities of the reinforcing effects of various drugs in man cannot be rated solely on the basis of incidence of abuse, because the abuse of any particular drug is also greatly influenced by such nonpharmacologic factors as the availability of the drug and social attitude towards it. Nonetheless, it is quite evident that the reinforcing intensity of the benzodiazepines is strong enough for them to be widely abused in contemporary society.

Another aspect of the reinforcing effect of drugs in general is that it can be intensified by withdrawal discomfort, because the subject will attempt to avoid or escape from such discomfort. The intensification of the reinforcing effect by this process is known to be prominent in opioid dependence, but it is assumed to be much less prominent with the depressants (MARTIN and JASINSKI, 1977; FRASER and JASINSKI, 1977). In animals, this has been partially demonstrated by a progressive ratio test of intravenous self-administration of morphine and alcohol in physically dependent and nondependent rhesus monkeys (YANAGITA, 1976), but no confirming study on benzodiazepines has been carried out.

b) Subjective Effects

The reinforcing effect of a drug is thought to be developed as the result of perceiving the subjective effects of the drug as rewarding, regardless of whether the subject is intellectually aware of the role of such perception in shaping his drug-taking behavior. These subjective effects are usually described as euphoria or a sense of well-being. The subjective effects of benzodiazepines appear to be essentially similar to those of barbiturates and alcohol, but in a comparison of diazepam with alcohol, it was reported that diazepam produced stronger feelings of relaxation and more reduction of concentration than alcohol (HAFFNER et al., 1973).

In animals, the subjective effects are studied by a method called "drug discrimination." Here animals are trained to discriminate the subjective effects of a standard drug from those of saline or some other standard drug by operant behavioral procedures. The subjective effects serve as the stimulus for discrimination. Next, it is observed whether the subjects generalize the subjective effects of the standard drugs to those of test drugs. If generalization between a standard drug and a test drug is seen, the subjective effects of the test drug are regarded to be analogous to those of the standard drug. Intensive studies on drug discrimination in laboratory animals are presently being carried out (LAL, 1977; COLPERT and ROSENCRANS, 1978). In discrimination studies on benzodiazepines, similarities between the subjective effects of benzodiazepines and those of barbiturates and alcohol have been indicated. The equivalent doses of some benzodiazepines to chlordiazepoxide for discrimination of their subjective effects have been estimated in rats. The approximate ED_{50}s were lorazepam, 0.02; nitrazepam, 0.1; diazepam, oxazepam, and bromazepam, 1.0; chlordiazepoxide, 3.0; and flurazepam, 10 mg/kg p.o. (COLPERT et al., 1976). It is said that these values correlated well with ataxic doses in rats. Although the subjective effects themselves cannot be known directly in the animals, these methods will permit us to categorize, at the preclinical stage, the probable subjective effects of new compounds in relation to prototypical drugs. It is of great future interest whether animals will be able to discriminate each benzodiazepine from the others in such experiments.

c) Pharmacodynamic Effects in a Self-Administered Dose Regimen

Psychological dependence on a drug is dependence on its pharmacologic effects. When a drug is available, each subject empirically chooses his own doese regimen, according to preference for a certain intensity of drug effects. This intensity may vary from subject to subject, depending on the type of drug and the degree of development of psychological dependence. In man, for example, barbiturates and alcohol are used preferentially by some psychologically dependent subjects to levels effecting only mild depression or hypnosis, while other subjects consume them to the extent that drug effects such as slurred speech, ataxia, anesthesia, and coma are manifested. In contrast, nicotine is never self-administered up to acute toxic levels, even by heavy smokers. In assessing the degree of psychological dependence on any particular drug, it may be feasible to say that the severer the manifestation of self-administered drug effects, the stronger the psychological dependence.

In the abuse of meprobamate, the overt signs of the drug effects in the abusers were reported to be exactly the same as in barbiturate and alcohol abuse: drowsiness, sleep, slurred speech, staggering, failling down, coma, and death (ESSIG, 1964). Because the depressant effects of benzodiazepines are much weaker than those of barbiturates and meprobamate, severe depression to the point of anesthesia, coma, and death cannot occur through abuse of benzodiazepines alone, regardless of the dose. Drowsiness and ataxia, however, are frequently observed. These overt drug effects of barbiturates, alcohol, and benzodiazepines, as well as the lack of acute toxic manifestation with nicotine, all of which are found in man, are exactly reproducible by self-administration in rhesus monkeys (YANAGITA and TAKAHASHI, 1973; YANAGITA, 1977). Interestingly, the number of resistant´ or indifferent monkeys was greater with benzodiazepines and alcohol than with pentobarbital. In the susceptible subjects, the self-maintained dose levels of these drugs varied from animal to animal.

Because they are the major cause of social and individual harm resulting from drug abuse, an important aspect of the pharmacologic effects under self-administered dose regimens regards the problems of psychotoxic manifestation and influences on behavior. For example, evidence is rapidly accumulating that benzodiazepine use can cause traffic accidents, just as alcohol can. Although traffic accidents can also occur during prescribed medical use of the drugs, the risk appears to be much higher with non-medical use because of the larger doses and stronger effects involved. Another problem concerns psychotic manifestations with benzodiazepines. These seldom occur during the drug-maintained period, but are possible during the withdrawal period, as has been mentioned earlier.

C. Summary

As currently available prototypical anxiolytics, meprobamate and benzodiazepines have been dealt with the present chapter, including their pharmacodynamic profiles and their dependence-producing properties.

Metabolic tolerance can be developed to both meprobamate and benzodiazepines, but not to the extent of being of clinical importance. Functional tolerance has been reported to the hypnotic and antiepileptic effects.

The physical dependence-producing properties of meprobamate are very similar to those of barbiturates. Benzodiazepines also definitely produce barbituratelike withdrawal signs, the severity of which, however, is usually less prominent because of their weaker general CNS depressant effects and slower elimination speed. Ample evidence demonstrates that almost all benzodiazepines possess physical dependence-producing properties of similar quality.

Cross physical dependence among barbiturates, alcohol, meprobamate, and benzodiazepines is also well documented.

Three types of drug effects are regarded as the pharmacologic properties of drugs relevant to psychological dependence: The reinforcing effect, the subjective effects, and pharmacodynamic effects in the self-administered dose regimen. Benzodiazepines definitely possess reinforcing effect as demonstrated by a number of self-administration experiments in animals and the number of abuse case reports in man. Although in animals the reinforcing intensities of benzodiazepines seem to be generally weaker than that of pentobarbital, recent surveys on nonmedical use of benzodiazepines indicate a rapid increase in the number of abuse incidences.

The subjective effects of benzodiazepines are reported to be euphoria or a sense of well-being. In animals, the subjective effects cannot be known directly, but by experiments on drug discrimination, a categorization of the subjetive effects of drugs has become possible. The results to date indicate similarity in effect between benzodiazepines and barbiturates or alcohol.

Concerning the pharmacodynamic effects in a self-administered dose regimen, the benzodiazepines do not produce severe depression, but to produce drowsiness and ataxia in man. These drug effects are also observable in self-administration experiments in rhesus monkeys. The severity of the pharmacodynamic effects observable during the self-administration of drugs in animals may indicate the degree of psychological dependence in man. Also, it may serve to predict the extent of the mental and behavioral disturbances that man might develop.

References

Abelson, H.I., Fishburne, P.M., Cisin, I.: National survey on drug abuse. Vol. I. Rockville, Md.: National Institute on Drug Abuse 1977

Agrawal, P.: Diazepam addiction – A case report. Can. Psychiatr. Assoc. J. *23*, 35–37 (1978)

Brill, H., Jaffe, J.H.: Recent trends of abuse of therapeutics in U.S.A. Jpn. J. Clin. Pharmacol. *9*, 445–460 (1978) (Translated into Japanese)

Collins, R.J., Weeks, J.R., Good, P.I.: Evaluation of the reinforcing properties of psychoactive drugs using rats. In: Proc. 40th Annual Scientific Meeting of Committee on Problems of Drug Dependence. Hollister, L.E. (ed.), pp. 510–521. The Committee on Problems of Drug Dependence, Inc. 1978

Colpert, F.C., Desmedt, L.K.C., Janssen, P.A.J.: Discriminative stimulus properties of benzodiazepines, barbiturates and pharmacologically related drugs – relation to some intrinsic and anticonvulsant effects. Eur. J. Pharmacol. *37*, 113–123 (1976)

Colpert, F.C., Rosencrans, J.A. (eds.): Stimulus properties of drug – ten years of progress. Amsterdam, New York, Oxford: Elsevier/North-Holland 1978

Covi, L., Lipman, R.S., Pattion, J.H., Derogatis, L.R., Uhlenhuth, E.H.: Length of treatment with anxiolytic sedatives and response to their sudden withdrawal. Acta Psychiatr. Scand. *49*, 51–64 (1973)

Deneau, G.A., Weiss, S.: A substitution technique for determining barbiturate-like physiological dependence capacity in the dog. Pharmakopsychiatr. Neuropsychopharmacol. *1*, 270–275 (1968)

Essig, C.F.: Withdrawal convulsions in dogs following chronic meprobamate intoxication. Arch. Neurol. Psychol. *80*, 414–417 (1958)

Essig, C.F.: Addiction to nonbarbiturate sedative and tranquilizing drugs. Clin. Pharmacol. Ther. *5*, 334–343 (1964)

Essig, C.F.: Newer sedative drugs that can cause states of intoxication and dependence of barbiturate type. J. Am. Med. Assoc. *196*, 714–717 (1966)

Findley, J.D., Robinson, W.W., Peregrino, L.: Addiction to secobarbital and chlordiazepoxide in the rhesus monkey by means of a self-infusion preference procedure. Psychopharmacologia *26*, 93–114 (1972)

Floyd, J.B., Jr., Murphy, C.M.: Hallucinations following withdrawal of valium. J. Ky. Med. Assoc. *74*, 549–550 (1976)

Fraser, H.F., Isbell, H.: Abstinence syndrome in dogs after chronic barbiturate medication. J. Pharmacol. Exp. Ther. *112*, 261–267 (1954)

Fraser, H.F., Jasinski, D.R.: The assessment of the abuse potentiality of sedative/hypnotics. In: Drug addiction. Handbook of experimental pharmacology, Vol. 45/I, pp. 589–612. Berlin, Heidelberg, New York: Springer 1977

Götestam, K.G.: Intragastric self-administration of medazepam in rats. Psychopharmacologia *28*, 87–94 (1973)

Greenblatt, D.J., Shader, R.I.: The price we pay. In: Benzodiazepine in clinical Practice. Greenblatt, D.J., Shader, R.I. (eds.), pp. 263–268. New York: Raven Press 1974a

Greenblatt, D.J., Shader, R.I.: Benzodiazepines (Part I). N. Engl. J. Med. *271*, 1011–1015 (1974b)

Griffiths, R.R., Brady, J.V., Snell, J.D.: Progressive-ratio performance maintained by drug infusions: comparison of cocaine, diethylpropion, chlorphentermine, and fenfluramine. Psychopharmacology *56*, 5–13 (1978)

Haffner, J.F.W., Morland, J., Setekleiv, J., Stromsaether, C.E., Danielson, A., Frivik, P.T., Dybing, F.: Mental and psychomotor effects of diazepam and ethanol. Acta Pharmacol. Toxicol. (Kbh.) *32*, 161–178 (1973)

Harris, T.H.: Methaminodiazepoxide. J. Am. Med. Assoc. *172*, 1162–1163 (1960)

Hoffmeister, F.: Assessment of reinforcing properties of stimulant and depressant drugs in the rhesus monkey as a tool for the prediction of psychic dependence-producing capability in man. In: Predicting dependence liability of stimulant and depressant drugs. Thompson, T., Unna, K.V. (eds.), pp. 185–201. Baltimore, London, Tokyo: University Park Press 1977

Hollister, L.E., Motzenbecker, F.P., Degan, R.O.: Withdrawal reactions from chlordiazepoxide. Psychopharmacologia *2*, 63–68 (1961)

Isbell, H., White, W.M.: Clinical characteristics of addictions. Am. J. Med. *May*, 558–565 (1953)

Johanson, C.E., Schuster, C.R.: A choice procedure for drug reinforcers – cocaine and methylphenidate in the rhesus monkeys. J. Pharmacol. Exp. Ther. *193*, 676–688 (1975)

Kaim, S.C.: Benzodiazepines in the treatment of alcohol withdrawal state. In: The benzodiazepines. Garattini, S., Mussini, E., Randell, L.O. (eds.) pp. 571–575. New York: Raven Press 1973

Kalant, H., Leblane, A.E., Gibbins, R.J.: Tolerance to, and dependence on some non-opiate psychotropic drugs. Pharmacol. Rev. *23*, 135–191 (1971)

Kissin, B.: The use of psychoactive drugs in the long term treatment of chronic alcoholics. Ann. N.Y. Acad. Sci. *252*, 385–395 (1975)

Korsgaard,. S.: Abuse of lorazepam. Vgeskr. Leag. *138*, 164–165 (1976)

Lal, H. (ed.): Discriminative stimulus properties of drugs. New York, London: Plenum Press 1977

Leblanc, A.E., Gibbins, R.J., Kalant, H.: Behavioral augmentation of tolerance to ethanol in the rat. Psychopharmacologia *30*, 117–122 (1973)

Maletzky, B.M., Klotter, J.: Addiction to diazepam. Int. J. Addict. *11*, 95–115 (1976)

Martin, W.R., Jasinski, D.R.: Assessment of the abuse potential of narcotic analgesics in animals. In: Drug addiction. Handbook of experimental pharmacology, Vol. 45/I, pp. 43–158 Berlin, Heidelberg, New York: Springer 1977

Martin, W.R., Sloan, J.W.: Neuropharmacology and neurochemistry of subjective effects, analgesia, tolerance, and dependence produced by narcotic analgesics. In: Drug addiction. Handbook of experimental pharmacology, Vol. 45/I, pp. 43–158 Berlin, Heidelberg, New York: Springer 1977

Mattson, R.H.: The benzodiazepines: Antiepileptic drugs. New York: Raven Press 1972

Misra, P.C.: Nitrazepam dependence. Br. J. Psychiatry *126*, 81–82 (1975)

Miyasato, K.: Experimental study on development of physical dependence on alcohol and cross physical dependence liability of diazepam and harbital to alcohol in rhesus monkeys. Seishin Shinkeigaku Zasshi *80*, 657–667 (1978) (In Japanese with English summary and tables)

Okamoto, M., Rosenberg, H.C., Boisse, N.R.: Tolerance characteristics produced during the maximally tolerable chronic pentobarbital dosing in the cat. J. Pharmacol. Exp. Ther. *192*, 555–564 (1975)

Okamoto, M., Rosenberg, H.C., Boisse, N.R.: Withdrawal characteristics following chronic pentobarbital dosing in cat. Eur. J. Pharmacol. *40*, 107–119 (1976)

Peet, M., Moonie, L.: Abuse of benzodiazepines. Br. Med. J. *1/6062*, 714 (1977)

Randall, L.O., Schallek, W., Heise, G.A., Keith, E.F., Bagdon, R.E.: The psychoactive properties of methaminodiazepoxide. J. Pharmacol. Exp. Ther. *129*, 163–171 (1960)

Rastogi, R.B., Lapierre, Y.D., Singhal, R.L.: Some neurochemical correlates of "rebound" phenomenon observed during withdrawal after long term exposure to 1,4-benzodiazepines. Prog. Neuropsychopharmacol. *2*, 43–54 (1978)

Rifikin, A., Quitkin, F., Klein, D.F.: Withdrawal reaction to diazepam. J. Am. Med. Assoc. *236*, 2172–2173 (1976)

Smith, C.M.: The pharmacology of sedative/hypnotics, alcohol, and anesthetics – sites and mechanisms of action. In: Drug addiction. Handbook of experimental pharmacology, Vol. 45/I, pp. 413–587 Berlin, Heidelberg, New York: Springer 1977

Tobin, J.M., Lewis, N.D.C.: New psychotherapeutic agent, chlordiazepoxide. J. Am. Med. Assoc. *174*, 1242–1249 (1960)

World Health Organization: WHO expert committee on drug dependence. 21st Report. Technical Report Series, No. 618, 1978

Yanagita, T., Takahashi, S.: Development of tolerance to and physical dependence on barbiturates in rhesus monkeys. J. Pharmacol. Exp. Ther. *172*, 163–169 (1970)

Yanagita, T., Takahashia, S.: Dependence liability of several sedative-hypnotic agents evaluated in monkeys. J. Pharmacol. Exp. Ther. *185*, 307–316 (1973)

Yanagita, T., Takahashi, S., Oinuma, N.: Drug dependence potential of lorazepam (WY 4036) evaluated in the rhesus monkey. CIEA Preclin. Rpt. *1*, 1–4 (1975a)

Yanagita, T., Takahashi, S., Ito, Y., Miyasato, K.: Drug dependence potential of prazepam evaluated in the rhesus monkey. CIEA Preclin. Rpt. *1*, 257–262 (1975b) (In Japanese with English summary and tables)

Yanagita, T., Oinuma, N., Takahashi, S.: Drug dependence liability of pentazocine evaluated in the rhesus monkey. CIEA Preclin. Rpt. *1*, 51–57 (1975c) (In Japanese with English summary and tables)

Yanagita, T., Takahashi, S., Nakanishi, H., Oinuma, N.: Drug dependence potential of cloxazolazepam evaluated in the rhesus monkey. CIEA Preclin. Rpt. *1*, 223–230 (1975d) (In Japanese with English summary and tables)

Yanagita, T., Oinuma, N., Takahashi, S.: Drug dependence potential of Sch 12041 evaluated in the rhesus monkey. CIEA Preclin. Rpt. *1*, 231–235 (1975e)

Yanagita, T.: Some methodological problems in assessing dependence producing properties of drugs in animals. Pharmacol. Rev. *27*, 503–509 (1976)

Yanagita, T., Miyasato, K., Kiyohara, H.: Drug dependence potential of triazolam tested in rhesus monkeys. CIEA Preclin. Rpt. *3*, 1–7 (1977a) (In Japanese with English summary and tables)

Yanagita, T., Miyasato, K., Takahashi, S., Kiyohara, H.: Dependence potential of dipotassium clorazepate tested in rhesus monkeys. CIEA Preclin. Rpt. *3*, 67–73 (1977b) (In Japanese with English summary and tables)

Yanagita, T.: Brief review on the use of self-administration techniques for predicting drug dependence potential. In: Predicting dependence liability of stimulant and depressant drugs. Thompson, T., Unna, K.R. (eds.), pp. 231–242. Baltimore, London, Tokyo: University Park Press 1977

Gerontopsychopharmacological Agents

CHAPTER 9

Chemistry of Gerontopsychopharmacologic Agents

H. HAUTH

A. Introduction

The remarkable progress of medical science in this century has increased average human life expectancy, so that the shift in the age distribution of the population at large has been toward the older end of the spectrum. For this reason medical therapy has become more and more important in the last 20 years. Some reviews concerning pharmacologic and clinical aspects of this field have been published (SATHANANTHAN and GERSHON, 1975; WIECK and BLAHA, 1976; HAUTH and RICHARDSON, 1977; COLE and BRANCONNIER, 1978; BAN, 1978), but up to now no review of the chemical aspects of gerontopsychopharmacologic agents has appeared. The purpose of this chapter, therefore, is to provide the chemical background. As numerous compounds have been claimed to be gerontopsychiatric agents, it is inevitable that only those for which relevant clinical or pharmacologic investigations have been published could be taken into account. Patents have thus rarely been considered, whereas the results of metabolic studies have been included. It is not the purpose of this article to judge pharmacologic and clinical data; the references given are only intended to facilitate an approach to the literature for those with more specifically pharmacologic and clinical interests.

B. Alkaloids

I. Dihydroergopeptines

The ergot alkaloids occupy an outstanding position among natural products on account of their broad spectrum of biologic activity. The chemistry of this class of compounds has recently been exhaustively reviewed (RUTSCHMANN and STADLER, 1978). Within the bounds of the review, the dihydroergopeptines (1, Fig. 1) are of interest, above all co-dergocrine-mesylate [1] (Hydergine). The active principle contained in co-dergocrine-mesylate is dihydroergotoxine mesylate, which is an association of the mesylates of 9,10-dihydrogocornine (1 a, Fig. 1), 9,10-dihydroergocristine (1 b, Fig. 1), 9,10-dihydro-α-ergokryptine (1 c, Fig. 1), and 9,10-dihydro-β-ergokryptine (1 d, Fig. 1) in the ratio 3:3:2:1 (HARTMANN et al., 1978). Co-dergocrine was initially tested as a hypotensive because of its peripheral vasodilatory effects (KAPPERT, 1949) and later introduced with considerable success in the treatment of senile cerebral insufficiency (FANCHAMPS, 1979; MATEJCEK et al., 1979). In attempts to elucidate the mode of action of Co-dergocrine, the individual components have also been investigated in

---

1 generic name BAN; generic name USAN: ergoloid-mesylates

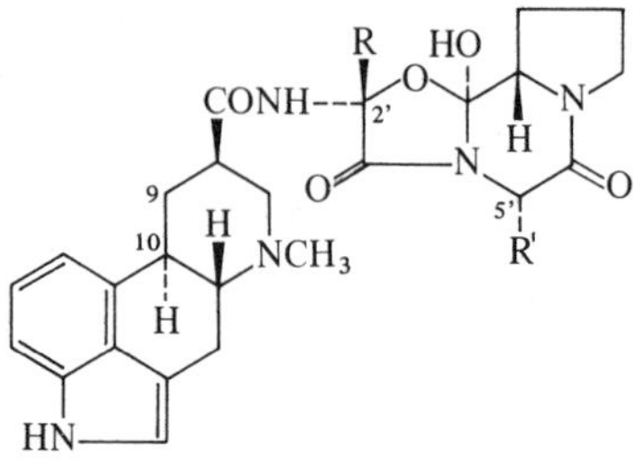

(1)

(1a) : 9,10–Dihydroergocornine	R=CH(CH$_3$)$_2$	R'=CH(CH$_3$)$_2$
(1b) : 9,10–Dihydroegocristine	R=CH(CH$_3$)$_2$	R'=CH$_2$C$_6$H$_5$
(1c) : 9,10–Dihydro–α–ergokryptine	R=CH(CH$_3$)$_2$	R'=CH$_2$CH(CH$_3$)$_2$
(1d) : 9,10–Dihydro–β–ergokryptine	R=CH(CH$_3$)$_2$	R'=CH(CH$_3$)CH$_2$CH$_3$
(1e) : 9,10–Dihydroergotamine, DHE	R=CH$_3$	R'=CH$_2$C$_6$H$_5$
(1f) : 9,10–Dihydro–β–ergosine, DQ 27–422	R=CH$_3$	R'=CH(CH$_3$)CH$_2$CH$_3$
(1g) : 9,10–Dihydroergostine, DE 145	R=CH$_2$CH$_3$	R'=CH$_2$C$_6$H$_5$
(1h) : 9,10–Dihydroergonine, DN 16–457	R=CH$_2$CH$_3$	R'=CH(CH$_3$)$_2$

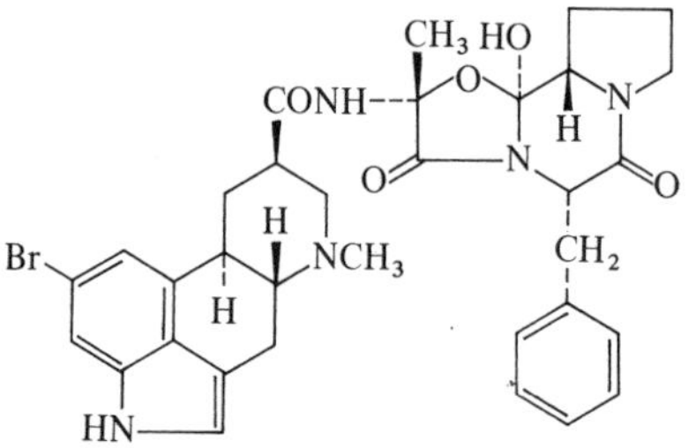

(2)

13–Bromo–9,10–dihydroergotamine, BZ 23–467

Fig. 1. Structure of 9,10-dihydroergopeptines

part (LOEW et al., 1978; KOHLMEYER and BLESSING, 1978). Parallel to these activities, an intensive study of dihydroergopeptines as a whole was made: 9,10-dihydroergotamine (DHE) (1 e, Fig. 1) (STOLL and HOFMANN, 1943) and 9,10-dihydro-β-ergosine (DQ 27-422) (1 f, Fig. 1) (STADLER and DEPOORTERE, 1976) influence the cortical EEG power spectrum and the sleep-wakefulness cycle in animals in an analogous way to co-dergocrine (LOEW et al., 1978). Similar effects were demonstraded in geriatric patients (LOEW et al., 1978) treated with either 9,10-dihydroergostine (DE 145) (1 g, Fig. 1) (HOFMANN et al., 1967) or 9,10-dihydroergonine (DN 16-457) (1 h, Fig. 1) (STADLER et al., 1971). As with the aforementioned dihydroergopeptines, 13-bromo-9,10-dihydroergotamine (BZ 23-467) (2, Fig. 1) (FEHR and HAUTH, 1973) produced inhibition of reserpine-induced ponto-geniculo-occipital (PGO) waves in the cat (ZUEGER et al., 1978).

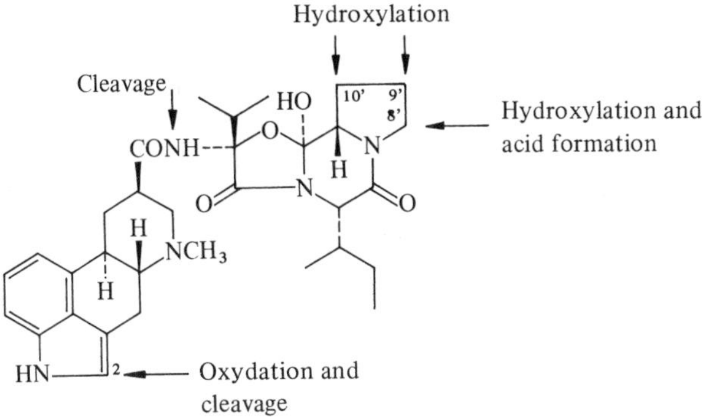

(3)

Fig. 2. Sites of biotransformation in 9,10-dihydro-β-ergokryptine

The biotransformation of 9,10-dihydro-β-ergokryptine (3, Fig. 2) has been exhaustively investigated (ECKERT et al., 1978). Apart from the oxidative opening of the indole ring and cleavage of the amide bridge, the major effect was oxidation of the proline ring. In addition, the proline ring was opened to yield a derivative of glutamic acid, which was in part further hydroxylated in positions 9′ and 10′. The pharmacodynamic effects of these metabolites have not yet been described.

The chemical, pharmacologic, and clinical investigation of this class of substances is at present being actively pursued. First attempts to characterize the binding site of 9,10-dihydroergotamine (1 e, Fig. 1) in calf and rat brain have been made (CLOSSE and HAUSER, 1978). As soon as information regarding the mode of action of dihydroergopeptines is available and suitable testing procedures have been developed, the description of some simple structure-activity relationships may become possible.

II. Ergolines

At the latest, the discovery of the central effects of lysergic acid diethylamide (LSD-25) showed clearly that even simple derivatives of lysergic acid can exhibit extensive actions on the central nervous system. But it was precisely this observation and the notoriety associated with it that for years hindered the exploitation of simple derivatives of lysergic acid. The first breakthrough came with nicergoline (MNE) (4 a, Fig. 3), the 5-bromo-nicotinic acid ester of 1-methyl-10-α-methoxy-dihydrolysergol, which was selected from a series of nicotinic acid esters because of its potent α-blockade (ARCARI et al., 1972; BERNARDI, 1979) and tested clinically as a peripheral and cerebrovascular vasodilator (BERNINI et al., 1977; HAUTH and RICHARDSON, 1977; SALETU et al., 1979). The α-blocking activity is associated with the stereochemistry at C-8 and C-10 and with the methyl group on N-1 and the methoxy group at C-10. Bromination at C-13 and replacement of the methyl group at N-6 by an ethyl group have minimal effects. Reduction of the double bond at position 2,3, substitution at C-2, and introduction of a double bond at position 8,9 lead to loss of activity (BERNARDI et al., 1975). Replacement of 5-bromo-nicotinic acid by 3,5-dimethyl-pyrrol-2-carboxylic acid yielded a derivative (4 b, Fig. 3), which was both more potent by the oral route and longer last-

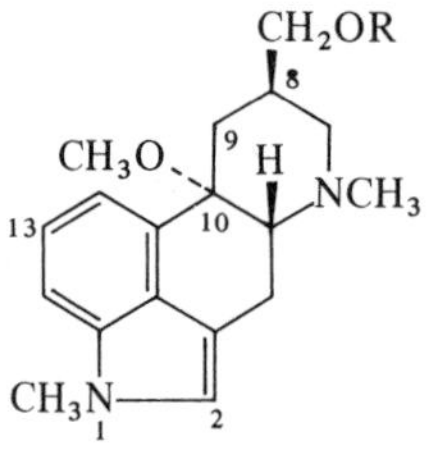

CH$_2$OR

CH$_3$O

H

NCH$_3$

13

10

9

8

CH$_3$N

1

2

(4)

(4a) : 1–Methyl–10α–methoxy–dihydrolysergol–
5–bromo–nicotinate, Nicergoline, MNE

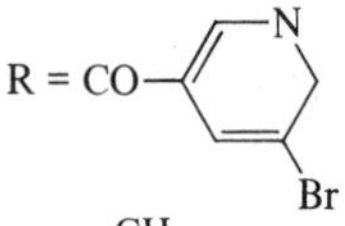

R = CO—

N

Br

(4b) : R = CO—

CH$_3$

N

CH$_3$

CH$_2$S—

N

H

NCH$_3$

HN—

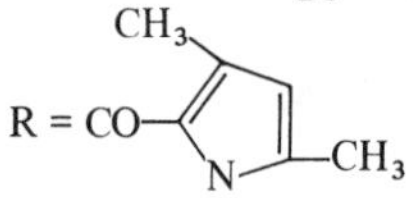

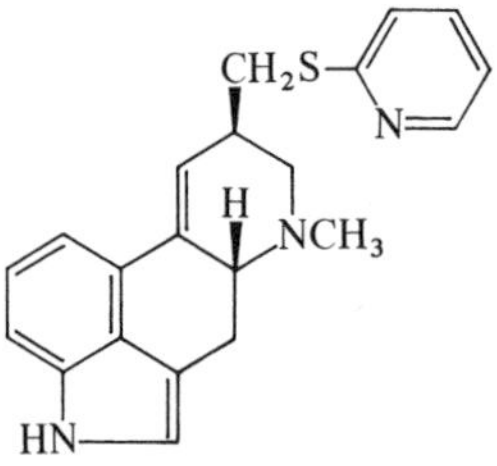

(5)

6–Methyl–8β–(2–pyridyl–
thiomethyl)–9–ergolene,
CF 25–397

CH$_2$OH

CONHCHCH$_2$CH$_3$

H

NCH$_3$

CH$_3$N—

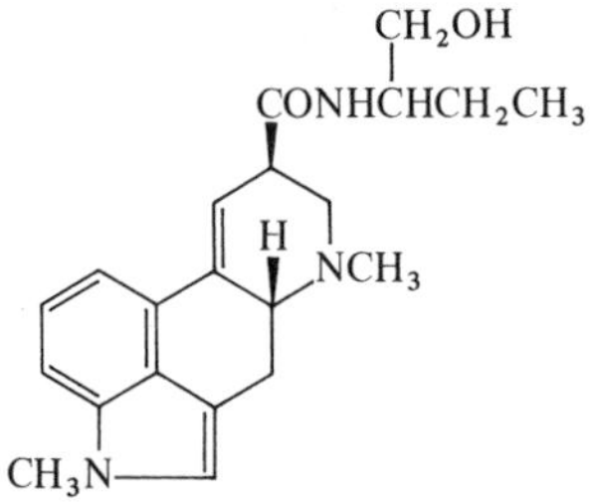

(6)

1–Methyl–d–lysergic acid–
L–2–butanolamide, Methysergide

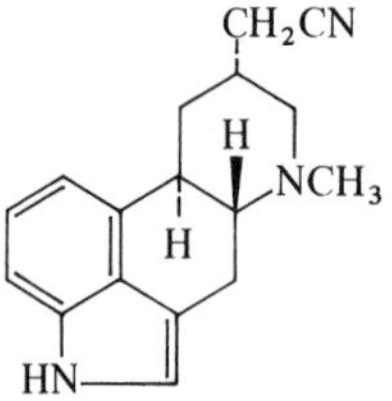

CH$_2$CN

H

NCH$_3$

H

HN—

(7)

6–Methyl–8β–cyanomethyl–
ergoline, CM 29–712

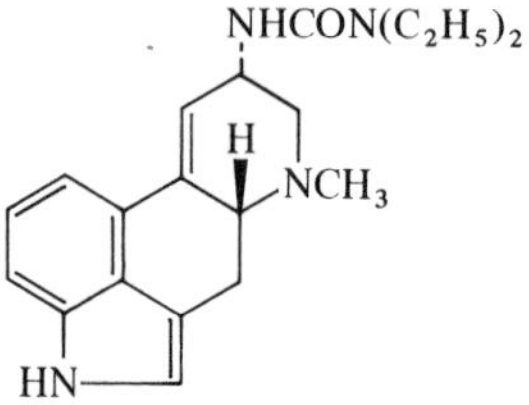

NHCON(C$_2$H$_5$)$_2$

H

NCH$_3$

HN—

(8)

N–[6–Methyl–8α–(9–ergolenyl)]–
N′,N′–diethylurea, Lisuride

Fig. 3. Structure of ergolines

ing in its effects (Bernardi et al., 1977). The metabolic degradation of nicergoline has been investigated, the major effects being hydrolysis of the ester linkage and N-de-methylation at position 1 (Arcamone et al., 1972).

The 6-methyl-8β-(2-pyridyl-thiomethyl)-9-ergolene (CF 25-397) (5, Fig. 3) (Stuetz et al., 1978) affects paradoxical sleep in the rat in a similar manner to dihy-droergotoxine (Loew et al., 1978). Likewise, methysergide (6, Fig. 3) (Hofmann and Troxler, 1965) and the central dopaminergic stimulant 6-methyl-8β-cyanomethlyer-goline (CM 29-712) (7, Fig. 3) (Stuetz et al., 1978) influence reserpine-induced PGO waves (Zueger et al., 1978). EEG is also influenced (Loew et al., 1978) by the 8α-amino-ergolenyl derivative lisuride (8, Fig. 3) (Zikan and Semonsky, 1960, 1968; Zi-kan et al., 1972).

Investigations of the effects of ergopeptines and ergolines on biogenic amines in the brain (LOEW et al., 1978; BUERKI et al., 1978), as well as the successful investigations of ergot derivatives with central dopaminergic activity (FLUECKIGER and DEL POZO, 1978; HAUTH, 1979) may justify the hope that further important discoveries as to the action of ergolines as gerontopharmacologic agents may be expected in future.

III. Vincamine Alkaloids

Vincamine (9 a, Fig. 4), the major alkaloid of periwinkle (*Vinca minor* L., Apocynaceae), after which the class of indole alkaloids eburnamine-vincamine was named (TAYLOR, 1965, 1968; TAYLOR and FARNSWORTH, 1973), was first isolated in 1953. Testing of vincamine (9 a, Fig. 4) in the therapy of cerebrovascular diseases (HAUTH and RICHARDSON, 1977; WITZMANN and BLECHACZ, 1977; THIERY et al., 1979) gave rise to increased interest in this compound, and many new syntheses were developed (TAYLOR, 1968; PFAEFFLI et al., 1975; SZANTAY et al., 1977; OPPOLZER et al., 1977, PARACCHINI and PESCE, 1978). Several of these are already being used for production-scale synthesis of vincamine.

The metabolism of vincamine has been studied in the rat. Vincamine was almost completely metabolized and two metabolites have been identified: 6-hydroxy- and 6-oxo-vincamine (9) (VIGANO et al., 1978).

Apart from vincamine, about 25 other alkaloids of the same structural class have been isolated from plants (TAYLOR and FARNSWORTH, 1973; BRUNETON et al., 1973, 1975; BOMBARDELLI et al., 1974; KUTNEY et al., 1974; KAN-FAN et al., 1976). These differ from each other mainly in substitution at C-14, C-17, and C-20, and in having a methoxy group in position 11 or 12. So far as is known, none of these alkaloids has been tested clinically. Little has been published on synthetic derivatives (KALAUS et al., 1978; PFAEFFLI and HAUTH, 1978; SZABO et al., 1979; CARON-SIGAUT et al., 1979). Patent registrations have, in contrast, been numerous, covering not only various salts of vincamine but also esters, amides, and aromatic substitutions. A report on clinical investigations (SOLTI et al., 1976) has appeared only for ethyl apovincaminate (vinpocetine, RGH-4405) (10 a, Fig. 4) (LOERINCZ et al., 1976). In a metabolic study, ethyl vincaminate (9 b, Fig. 4) was found among the minor metabolites; other metabolic products were apovincaminic acid (10 b, Fig. 4), hydroxylates, and conjugates (VERECZKEY and SZPORNY, 1976). Unchanged vinpocetine could not be detected in man (VERECZKEY et al., 1979).

In connection with ethyl apovincaminate (10 a, Fig. 4), various other derivatives, mainly stereoisomers of vincamine (9 a) and vincanol (11, Fig. 4), but also esters and amides of vincaminic acid (9 d, Fig. 4), apovincaminic acid (10 b, Fig. 4), dihydro-apovincaminic acid, and apovincaminol (10 c, Fig. 4) have been investigated, mainly for their peripheral effects (SZPORNY, 1977). *l*-Eburnamonine (vincamone) (12, Fig. 4) (NOVAK et al., 1977; BOELSING et al., 1979) stood out among the various vincamine derivatives tested for their effects on cerebral blood flow (AUROUSSEAU, 1971; LACROIX et al., 1979). It was more potent than *d*-eburnamonine (13, Fig. 4) (AUROUSSEAU et al., 1976 b). Vincanol (GESZTES and CLAUDER, 1968; BIRO and KARPATI, 1976) and (±)-16-desethyl-16-epi-eburnamonine (14 b, Fig. 4) (AUROUSSEAU et al., 1976 a) were also found to be active. Desoxy-vincaminamide (15 a, Fig. 4) and *N*-cyclopropyl-desoxyvincaminamide (15 b, Fig. 4) showed more potent alerting effects than vincamine

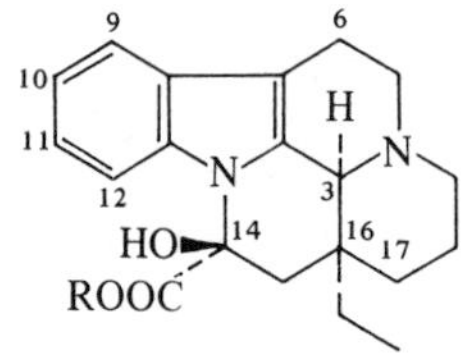

(9)

(9a) : Vincamine R = CH$_3$

(9b) : Ethyl vincaminate
       R = C$_2$H$_5$

(9c) : Isopropyl vincaminate
       R = CH(CH$_3$)$_2$

(9d) : Vincaminic acid
       R = H

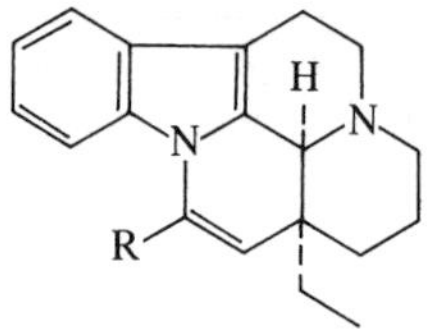

(10)

(10a) : Ethyl apovincaminate, Vinpocetine,
        RGH–4405, R = COOC$_2$H$_5$

(10b) : Apovincaminic acid R = COOH

(10c) : Apovincaminol R = CH$_2$OH

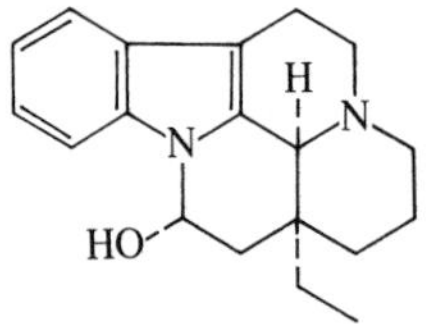

(11)

Vincanol

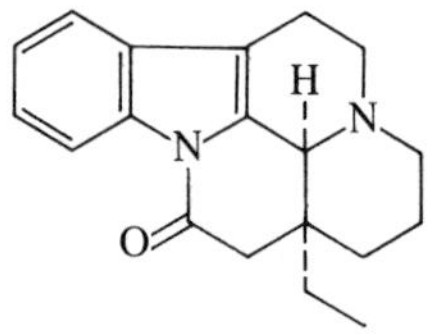

(12)

1–Eburnamonine, Vincamone

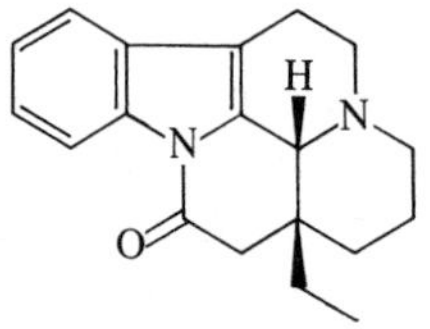

(13)

d–Eburnamonine

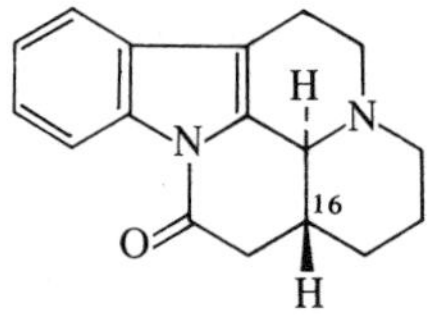

(14)

(+)–16–Desethyl–16–epi–
eburnamonine

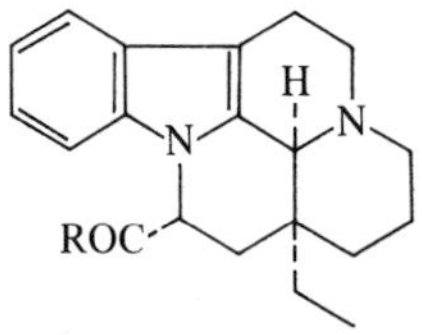

(15)

(15a) : Desoxy–vincaminamide R = NH$_2$

(15b) : N–Cyclopropyl–desoxy–
        vincamide

$$R = NH-CH\begin{matrix} \diagup CH_2 \\ | \\ \diagdown CH_2 \end{matrix}$$

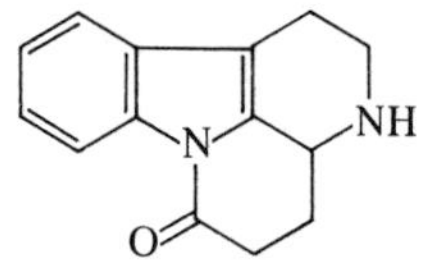

(16)

Hexahydrocanthinone

Fig. 4. Vincamine and derivatives

(DEPOORTERE et al., 1977). Isopropyl vincaminate (9c, Fig. 4) seems to have a similar cerebral vasodilator action in pharmacologic tests as vincamine (SZABO et al., 1979).

Vincamine and derivatives are at present being actively investigated from various directions. One may assume that simpler ring systems of the vincamine skeleton are being studied, since central nervous system effects may also be observed (KOVACH et al., 1969) with hexahydrocanthinone (16, Fig. 4) (TALYOR, 1968). Information from the literature suggests that various vincamine derivatives are presently undergoing clinical investigations. One can probably count on further discoveries in this class of substances in the near future.

IV. Isoquinoline Alkaloids

Papaverine (17, Fig. 5) which belongs to the class of benzylisoquinolines and was originally isolated from opium (SHAMMA, 1972; DYKE, 1978), has been given to geriatric patients because of its spasmolytic and vasodilating effects (HAUTH and RICHARDSON, 1977; SHAW and MEYER, 1978). Many derivatives have been studied only for peripheral effects; for example, various di- and tetra-hydro derivatives have been tested for β-sympathomimetic and spasmolytic effects (HOLTZ et al., 1968; PRUDHOMMEAUX et al., 1975; SIMON et al., 1977) or coronary arterial dilation (MERCIER et al., 1973). 3-Oxygenated derivatives of papaverine were tested as peripheral vasodilators (KREIGHBAUM et al., 1972) and structurally related compounds including two desmethyl papaverine metabolites have been tested for inhibition of phosphodiesterase (HANNA et al., 1972; BELPAIRE and BOGAERT, 1973). Although the first clinical results on papaverine were obtained some years ago, no further tests of compounds of this type in geriatric patients have been reported.

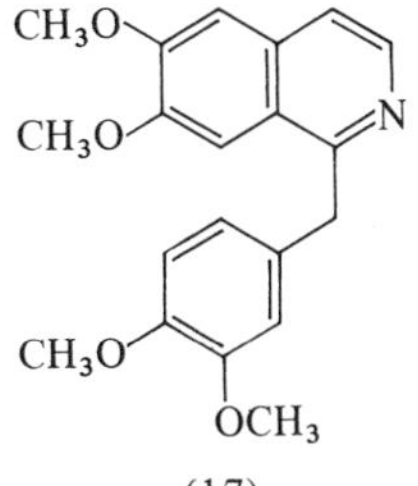

(17)

Papaverine

Fig. 5. Papaverine

C. Derivatives of Piperazine

The first representative of this class to be described as a gerontopsychiatric agent was the 1-cinnamyl-4-diphenylmethylpiperazine (cinnarizine, MD 516) (18a, Fig. 6), which was developed from a series of compounds with antihistaminic and sedative effects (JANSSEN, 1960). The later discovery of coronary arterial dilation (LOUBATIERES et al., 1965) led to its introduction for the treatment of disturbances in cerebral blood circulation (HAUTH and RICHARDSON, 1977). Investigations of the metabolism and excretion of cinnarizine in rats have not provided any new information (SOUDJIN and VAN WIJNGAARDEN, 1968). It is striking that of the numerous compounds similar to cinnarizine which have been patented, only a few have been published (ZIKOLOVA and NINOV, 1972 a, b, 1974), or pharmacologically tested (CIGNARELLA and TESTA, 1968; WRIGHT and MARTIN, 1968). Only flunarizine (18 b, Fig. 6), a difluoro derivative of cinnarizine, has come to clinical trial (STAESSEN, 1977; LEHR et al., 1978). It is also of interest that AS 2 (18 c, Fig. 6) a simple analogue of cinnarizine, also possesses coronodilatory activity and improves cerebral and peripheral blood flow in animals (NIKOLOV, 1976; KOVALYOV et al., KOVALYOV et al., 1976 a, b, c). It is impossible, however, to derive structure-activity relations for gerontopharmacologic activity on the basis of these few facts.

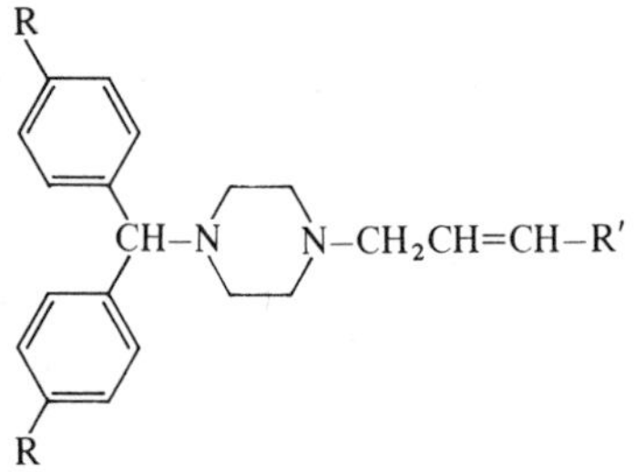

(18a) : 1–Cinnamyl–4–diphenylmethyl–
piperazine,Cinnarizine, MD 516
R = H, R'= C$_6$H$_5$

(18b) : 1–Cinnamyl–4–(4,4–difluoro–
diphenyl)–methylpiperazine,
Flunarizine
R = F, R'= C$_6$H$_5$

(18c) : 1–(2–Propenyl)–4–diphenylmethyl–
'piperazine, AS2
R = R'= H

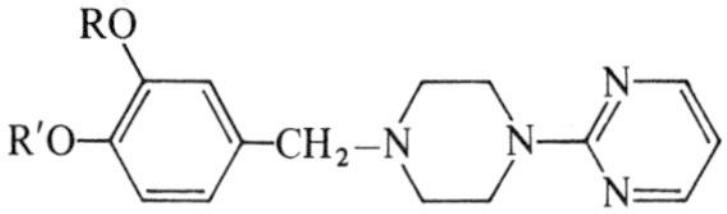

(19a) : 1–(3,4–Methylendioxybenzyl)–4–
(2–pyrimidyl) piperazine, Piri–
bedil, ET495
R + R'= CH$_2$

(19b) : 1–(3,4–Dihydroxybenzyl)–4–(2–
pyrimidyl) piperazine, S 584
R = R'= H

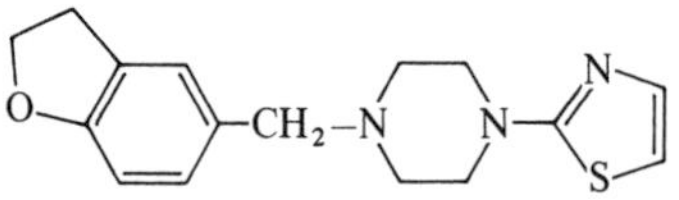

(20)   1–(Coumaran–5–yl–methyl)–4–
(2–thiazolyl) piperazine, S 3608

Fig. 6. Derivatives of piperazine

Further modifications of 4-substituted-1-arylalkyl-piperazines in the direction of vasodilating properties have led to the development of piribedil (ET 495) (19 a, Fig. 6) (REGNIER et al., 1968). After this compound was shown to be a centrally acting dopaminergic agonist (COSTALL and NAYLOR, 1973), interest in piribedil grew and led to clinical trials in the treatment of Parkinson's disease (SWEET et al., 1974) and cerebral insufficiency (SCHOLING and CLAUSEN, 1975, LASSERRE and COPPOLANI, 1980). It is interesting in this connection that significant improvements in senile dementia could also be achieved by application of L-Dopa (21, Fig. 7) (LEWIS et al., 1978). Metabolic investigations have demonstrated that the main metabolite of piribedil is the 3,4-dihy-droxyphenyl derivative S 584 (19 b, Fig. 6), which has also been shown to exhibit central dopaminergic stimulation (COSTALL and NAYLOR, 1974; MILLER and IVERSEN, 1974; POIGNANT et al., 1974; MAKMAN et al., 1975). Whether piribedil induces its activity directly or through its active metabolite S 584 could not yet be firmly established (CONSOLO et al., 1975). As a consequence of these observations, the coumaran derivative S 3608 (20, Fig. 6) was synthesized, which is also a central dopaminergic stimulant but which should not be metaboziled to a 3,4-dihydroxyphenyl derivative (POIGNANT et al., 1975).

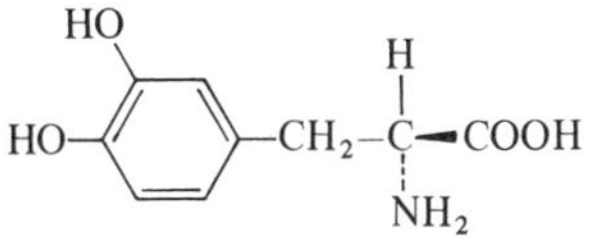

(21)

3–(3,4–Dihydroxyphenyl)
alanin, L–Dopa

Fig. 7. 3-(3,4-Dihydroxyphenyl)alanin, L-Dopa

A considerable number of aryl-substituted piperazines with adrenolytic, hypotensive, antihistaminic, and central sedative properties have been described. Derivatives around the piribedil structure are based on substitution on the piperazine ring (REGNIER et al., 1968; PINZA et al., 1976; CIGNARELLA et al., 1977) and variation of the N-aryl substituent (BOISSIER et al., 1963; REGNIER et al., 1968, 1972; CIGNARELLA et al., 1977) and of the benzyl group (REGNIER et al., 1968, 1972; RATOUIS et al., 1965; LINDNER, 1972; KOPPE et al., 1975; PINZA et al., 1976; CIGNARELLA et al., 1977). These substances have been investigated almost exclusively for their vasodilating properties. Since no information has been given on the more interesting and significant dopaminergic activity, a structure-activity relationship cannot at present be established.

D. Derivatives of Phenoxyacetic Acid

A number of basic esters and amides of phenoxyacetic acid have been synthesized as plant growth regulators, but stand out, among other things, as local anesthetics (THUILLIER and RUMPF, 1960). From these beginnings meclofenoxate (centrophenoxine, ANP 235, EN 1627) (22, Fig. 8) was developed as a central nervous system stimulant and tested in cerebrovascular insufficiency (MEIER, 1973; HOYER, 1979; NANDY, 1979). But the extent to which 2-(dimethylamino)ethanol (deanol) (25a, Fig. 9), one of its components easily split off in biologic systems and claimed to be active in senile dementia (FERRIS et al., 1977), can be held responsible for the activity of meclofenoxate (22, Fig. 8) is a question which remains open. This hypothesis receives support from investigations on cyprodenate (LB 125, Rd 406) (26, Fig. 10), (VALETTE, 1968), which has also been successfully tested in gerontopsychiatry (BERGENER and FREISTEIN, 1972) and has been demonstrated to rapidly release 2-(dimethylamino)ethanol via hydrolysis (DORMARD et al., 1975a, b).

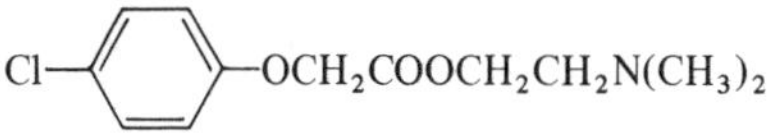

(22)

Cl—⬡—OCH₂COOCH₂CH₂N(CH₃)₂

(4–Chlorophenoxy) acetic acid
2–(dimethylamino) ethyl ester,
Meclofenoxate, Centrophenoxine,
ANP 235, EN 1627

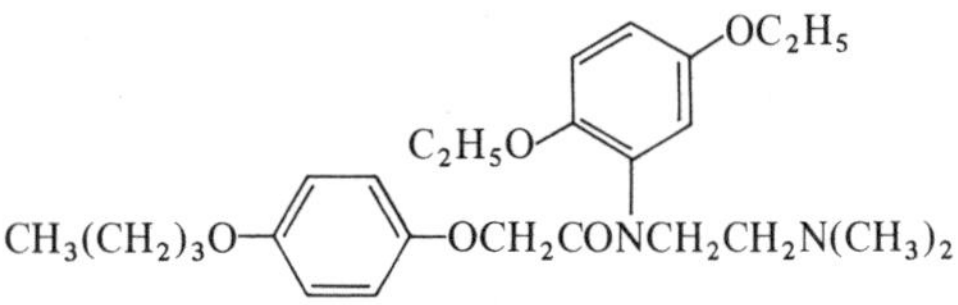

(23)

CH₃(CH₂)₃O—⬡—OCH₂CONCH₂CH₂N(CH₃)₂

2–(4–n–Butoxyphenoxy)–N–(2,5–
diethoxyphenyl)–N–[2–(diethyl–
amino) ethyl] acetamide, Fenoxe–
dil, ANP 3548

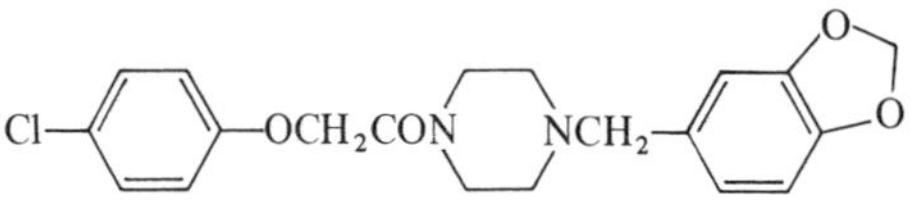

(24)

Cl—⬡—OCH₂CON⟨piperazine⟩NCH₂—⬡⟨O–CH₂–O⟩

1–(4–Chlorophenoxy) acetyl–1–
(3,4–methylendioxybenzyl) piperazine,
Fipexide

Fig. 8. Derivatives of phenoxyacetic acids

The transition from esters to more stable amides has led to the development of other compounds with vasodilatory activity (THUILLIER et al., 1975). Fenoxedil (ANP 3548) (23, Fig. 8), a member of this group, seems to induce cerebral vasodilation by vasculotropic and metabolic actions (BESSIN et al., 1975; LEVY et al., 1975). No metabolites have been identified in biopharmaceutical investigations (DORMARD et al., 1975c).

For the sake of completeness, fipexide (24, Fig. 8) should be mentioned, a piperazinamide structurally related to meclofenoxate and piribedil (BUZAS and PIERRE, 1970), which has apparently shown various clinical effects (SOULAIRAC, 1975).

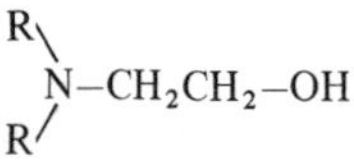

R\
  N–CH₂CH₂–OH
R/

(25)

(25a) : 2–(Dimethylamino) ethanol,
        Deanol
        R = R = CH₃
(25b) : 2–(Diethylamino) ethanol
        R = R = C₂H₅

Fig. 9. Derivatives of 2-aminoethanol

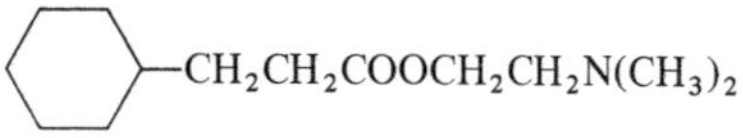

⬡—CH₂CH₂COOCH₂CH₂N(CH₃)₂

(26)

2–(Dimethylamino) ethyl–
3–cyclohexylpropionate,
Cyprodenate, LB 125, Rd 406

Fig. 10. 2-(Dimethylamino)ethyl
3-cyclohexylpropionate

Within the framework of a broad-ranging derivation of this class of substances, the aryl group, the aliphatic chain, and the N-substituent have been varied, and the ether oxygen atom has been replaced by sulphur and nitrogen, all of these in both the ester- and amide-series (THUILLIER and RUMPF, 1960; THUILLIER et al., 1963 a, b, 1975;

BRUNET et al., 1967). The published pharmacologic results (THUILLIER, 1966) do not, however, allow the establishment of a structure-activity relationship in respect of neurotropic activity.

E. Derivatives of Phenylethanolamine

Among the countless phenylethanolamines of the ephedrine type, compounds may also be found which have been clinically investigated for cerebrovascular effects by reason of their peripheral vasodilatory activity. The starting point for the investigation of this series was the N-stubstituted norephedrine derivative nylidrin (buphenine) (27, Fig. 11) (SCHOEPF and KUNZ, 1953), which was selected from a group of three derivatives and developed (KUELZ and SCHNEIDER, 1950) as far as clinical trial in patients with stroke and cerebral arteriosclerotic disturbances (PROBST and KEISER, 1969; GARETZ et al., 1979). Replacement of the 1-methyl-3-phenylpropyl substituent in nylidrin by the 1-methyl-3-phenoxyäthyl group (MOED and VAN DIJK, 1956) led to isoxsuprine (28, Fig. 11), which improves mental performance in cerebrovascular disease

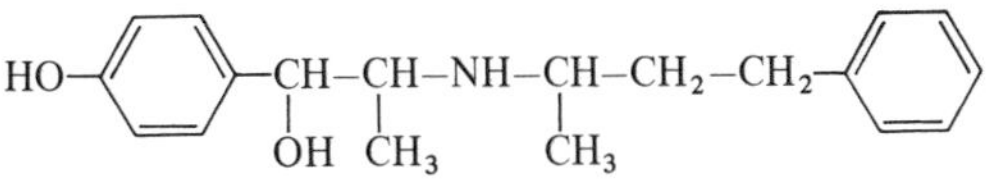

(27)

4−Hydroxy−a−[1−[(1−methyl−3−
phenylpropyl) amino]ethyl]
benzenemethanol, Nylidrin,
Buphenine

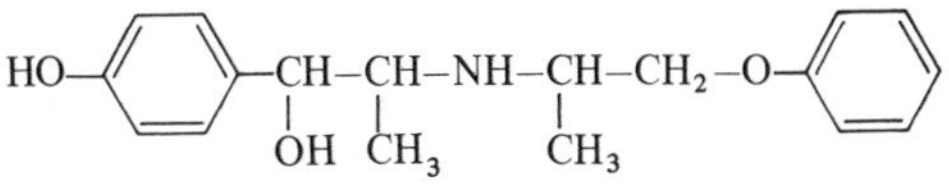

(28)

4−Hydroxy−a−[1−[(1−methyl−2−
phenoxyethyl) amino] ethyl]
benzenemethanol, Isoxsuprine

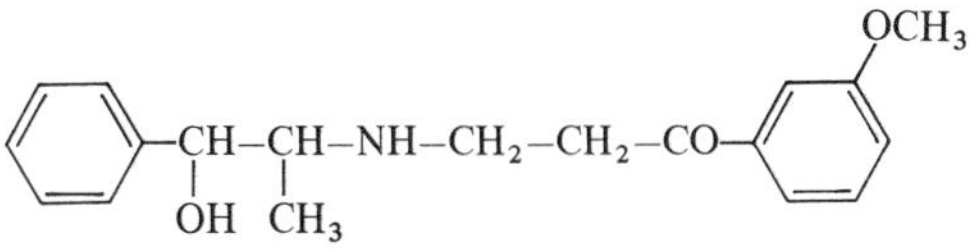

(29)

3−[(2−Hydroxy−1−methyl−2−
phenylethyl) amino]−1−(3−
methoxyphenyl)−1−propanone,
Oxyfedrine, D 563

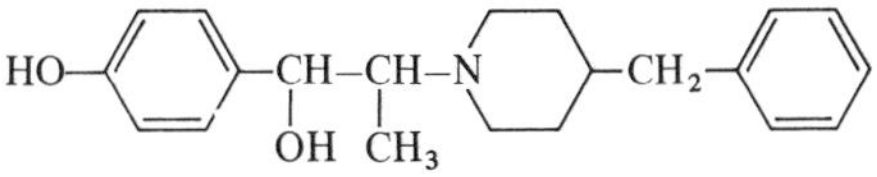

(30)

a−(4−Hydroxyphenyl)−β−methyl−
4−(phenylmethyl)−1−piperidine
ethanol, Ifenprodil, RC 61−91

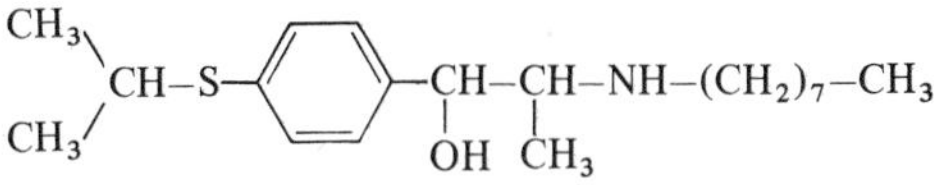

(31)

4−(1−Methylethyl) thiophenyl−a−[1−
(octylamino) ethyl] benzenemethanol,
Suloctidil, CP 556S

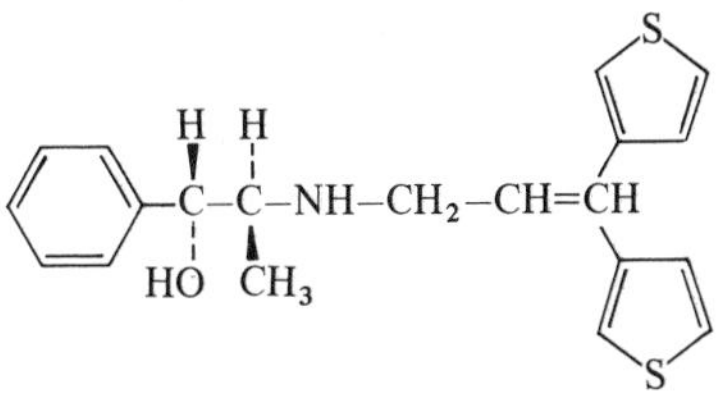

(32)

(+)−(R)−a−[(S)−1[(3,3−bis(3−
thienyl)−2−propenylamino] ethyl]
benzenemethanol, Tinofedrine,
D 8955

Fig. 11. Derivatives of phenylethanolamine

(TEUBNER, 1972; GUYER, 1978). For both nylidrin (VAN DIJK et al., 1963) and isoxsuprine (VAN DIJK et al., 1965), the enantiomers and diastereomers were prepared and the absolute configurations determined. Their vasodilatory activity seems to be associated with the erythro-configuration, the antipodes being distinguishable in respect of their β-stimulating and α-blocking activities (VAN DIJK and MOED, 1961; CLAASSEN, 1961). Some few derivatives, in which the substitution on the phenyl nucleus, at nitrogen, and in the aliphatic chain were varied, were tested for vascular activity (ARIENS et al., 1963; WAELEN et al., 1964; STANTON et al., 1965).

If the phenyl group in nylidrin is replaced by a benzoyl group, one obtains cardioactive β-aminoketones (THIELE et al., 1966) out of which oxyfedrine (D 563) (29, Fig. 11) has been developed (THIELE et al., 1968). The full activity of oxyfedrine resides in the L-form (HUELLER et al., 1972). Compounds derived from nylidrin by including the N-atom into a piperidine ring have been tested for vasodilation, α-blockade, and spasmolytic activity (CARRON et al., 1971). Of ten derivatives in which above all the ephedrine moiety was varied, ifenprodil (R 61-91) (30, Fig. 11) was selected for development of the basis of direct comparison with isoxsuprine and tested in cerebral insufficiency (MONTAUT et al., 1974). Replacement of the N-aryl substituent by an aliphatic chain (BUU-HOI et al., 1971) yielded the spasmolytic active suloctidil (CP 556 S) (31, Fig. 11) (ROBA et al., 1977), which has also been tested in cerebral insufficiency (VAN SCHEPDAEL, 1977; JACQUY and NOEL, 1977). If the aryl-alkyl chain in nylidrin is replaced by a diaryl-alkyl chain, compounds which increase coronary blood flow are obtained (THIELE et al., 1969). Some of these substances, especially thienyl-derivatives, also seem to have interesting activities in cerebral blood flow and brain-metabolism (THIELE et al., 1980a). The $1(+)$-form of the unsaturated dithienyl-derivative tinofedrine (D 8955) (32, Fig. 11), synthesized from l-norephedrine (THIELE et al., 1978, 1980b; SAUS and POSSELT, 1980), has influenced cerebral blood flow in pharmacologic testing (THIEMER et al., 1978) and cerebral energy metabolism (OBERMEIER et al., 1978a). Some effects of tinofedrine on the EEG of healthy volunteers (SPEHR, 1978) and its influence on blood parameters in patients with cerebral insufficiency (LECHNER and OTT, 1978) have been demonstrated. The metabolism of tinofedrine in rats and dogs occurs principally via conjugation, but traces of norephedrine could also be found (OBERMEIER et al., 1978b).

Up-till-now, the derivatives of phenylethanolamines have mainly been tested on their peripheral vasodilatory activity. Therefore no real structure-activity-relationship with respect to the activity in cerebral insufficiency can be established (THIELE et al., 1980a).

F. Derivatives of Vitamin B 6

Studies of vitamin B 6 (pyridoxine) (33a, Fig. 12) have led to the synthesis of pyritinol (pyrithioxin) (34, Fig. 12), which is a double molecule of pyridoxine linked via a disulphide bridge (ZIMA and SCHORRE, 1961; PETROVA and BELUSOVA, 1962; KURODA, 1964). Because of its effects on the central nervous system (HOTOVY et al., 1964), pyritinol has been tested for its effects on cerebral blood flow and glucose metabolism in patiens with senile dementia (COOPER and MAGNUS, 1980). In order to improve absorption and length of action, various mono-, di-, and tetraesters have been synthesized and tested with some success (KITAO et al., 1977), 29 mono- and dimeric pyridoxine derivatives, mainly substituted in position 4, have also been subjected to pharmacologic screening (KRAFT et al., 1961). But these investigations of central analgetic effects and the effects on the central nervous system afford very little insight into the relationship between pyridoxine derivatives and gerontopsychiatric agents.

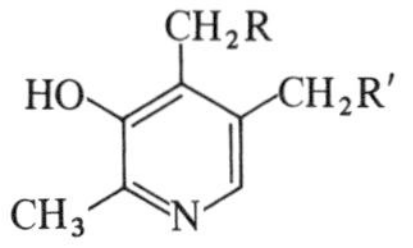

(33)

(33a) : 5–Hydroxy–6–methyl–3,4–pyridinedimethanol,
Pyridoxine, Vitamine B6
R = R = OH

(33b) : 3–Hydroxy–2–methyl–5–methylthiomethyl–4–pyridinemethanol,
EMD 17'246
R = OH, R'= SCH$_3$

(33c) : 3–Hydroxy–2–methyl–5–methylsulfinylmethyl–4–pyridine–
methanol
R = OH, R'= SOCH$_3$

(33d) : 4–Ethylaminomethyl–2–methyl–5–methylthiomethyl–3–
pyridinol, EMD 21'657
R = NHC$_2$H$_5$, R'= SCH$_3$

(33e) : (5–Hydroxy–4–hydroxymethyl–6–methyl–3–pyridinemethyl)–
2–(dimethylamino) ethyl succinate, Pyrisuccideanol
R = OH, R'= OCOCH$_2$CH$_2$COOCH$_2$CH$_2$N(CH$_3$)$_2$

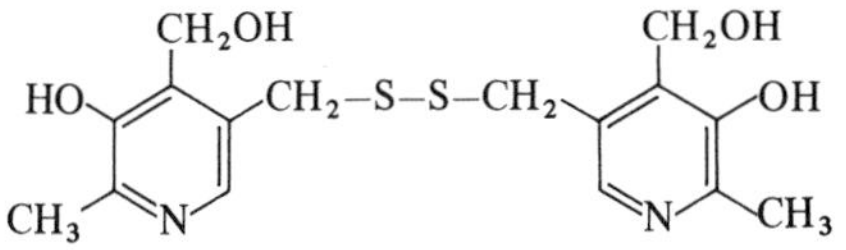

(34)

3,3–(Dithiodimethylene) bis
[5–hydroxy–6–methyl–4–
pyridinemethanol],
Pyritinol, Pyrithioxin

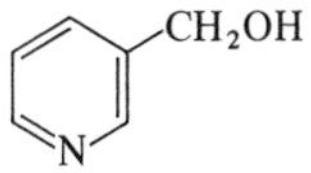

(35)

3–Pyridinemethanol,
β–Pyridylcarbinol,
Nicotinyl alcohol

Fig. 12. Derivatives of vitamin B 6

Pyritinol is completely metabolized in the rat, whereby the major excretory products are 3-hydroxy-2-methyl-5-methylthiomethyl- and 5-methylsulfinylmethyl-4-pyridine-methanol (33 b, 33 c, Fig. 12) (NOWAK and SCHORRE, 1969). 3-Hydroxy-2-methyl-5-methylthiomethyl-4-pyridinemethanol (EMD 17'246) (33 b, Fig. 12) has been investigated in respect of acute alcohol intoxication in rats (HILLBOM et al., 1973). On the basis of clinical studies, the 4-ethylaminomethyl derivative EMD 21'657 (33 d, Fig. 12) (SAIKO and KLUG, 1976) has been stated to have pronounced nootropic effects (SALETU et al., 1978 a, b). In judging derivatives of vitamin B 6 one should, however, note that nicotinyl alcohol (35, Fig. 12) (Jones and Kornfeld, 1951) has also been shown to have positive effects on patients with decreased cerebral blood flow (Cornu, 1969). It is by no means clear whether the actions (Hugelin et al., 1972; Devic, 1973) of pyrisuccideanol (33e, Fig. 12) (Esanu, 1973) should be ascribed to the compound itself or to the two individual components pyridoxine and 2-(dimethylamino)ethanol (25a, Fig. 9).

G. Derivatives of Xanthine

There has always been considerable interest in xanthines because of their actions as central nervous system stimulants, and on the cardiovascular system and the bronchi; a multitude of xanthine derivatives are on the market (Ritchie, 1975). Attempts have been made to influence their absorption, metabolism, and distribution, by substitution mainly in positions 1 and 7. These variations yielded 1-hexyl-3,7-dimethylxanthine (pentifylline, SK 7) (36a, Fig. 13) (Eidebenz and Schuh, 1952; Serchie, 1964),

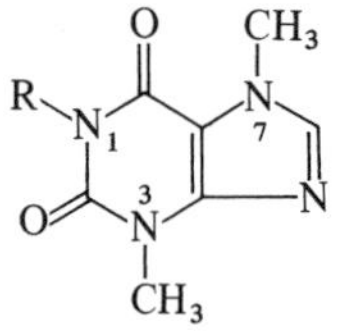

(36)

(36a) : 1–Hexyl–3,7–dimethyl–
           xanthine, Pentifylline, SK7
           R = (CH₂)₅CH₃

(36b) : 1–(5–Oxohexyl)–3,7–
           dimethylxanthine, Pentoxi–
           fylline, BL 191
           R = (CH₂)₄COCH₃

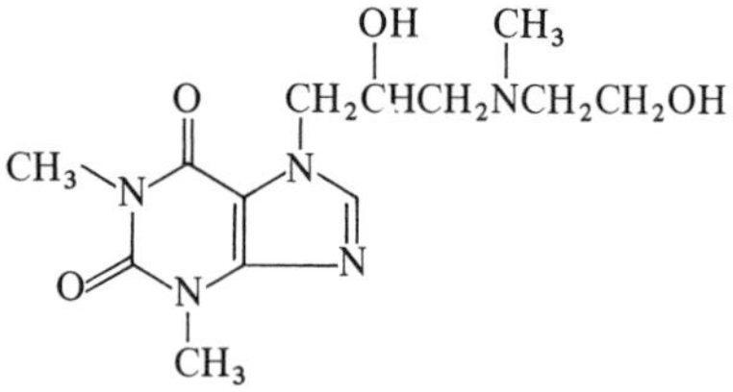

(37)

7–[2–Hydroxy–3–[N(2–hydroxy–
ethyl) methylamino] propyl]
theophylline, Xanthinol

Fig. 13. Derivatives of xanthine

which influences the brain metabolism of rats (Porsche and Stefanovich, 1979) and which has been developed as the nicotinate Cosaldon (Ramos et al., 1965). Investigations of the metabolic fate of pentifylline (Mohler et al., 1966a, b) have revealed 3,7-dimethyl-1-(5-oxohexyl)-xanthine (pentoxifylline, BL 191) (36b, Fig. 13) (Mohler and Soeder, 1971), which was initally developed as a peripheral vasodilator (Popendiker et al., 1971) and later tested for its effects on disturbances of cerebral blood flow (Theis et al., 1978; Harwart, 1979). Xanthinol (37, Fig. 13) (Bestian, 1961) also belongs to this class of compounds and was tested as the nicotinate (xanthinol niacinate) for treatment of cerebral insufficiency (Bartoli et al., 1977). Further derivatives were, however, compared with xanthinol niacinate for their hypotensive effects (Goi et al., 1973). In a further investigation, the effect of alkyl substitution of xanthines was tested, among other things, for its effect on spasmolytic and vasodilator activities (Serchi, 1964).

H. Miscellaneous Compounds

Bencyclane (38, Fig. 14) was developed from a series of basic cycloalkyl ethers (PALLOS, 1969; PALLOS et al., 1972, 1974) because of its spasmolytic and tranquilizing effects (KOMLOS and PETOECZ, 1970; PALLOS et al., 1974). Because of its effect on brain metabolism (HAPKE, 1973), bencyclane was subsequently tested, with conflicting results, for its effect in increasing cerebral blood flow in man (HAUTH and RICHARDSON, 1977). The attempt has been made to find a relationship between structure and spasmolytic, peripheral vasodilatory, tranquilizing, and local anesthetic effects (PALLOS et al., 1974), but no indications in respect of the possible development of a gerontopsy-

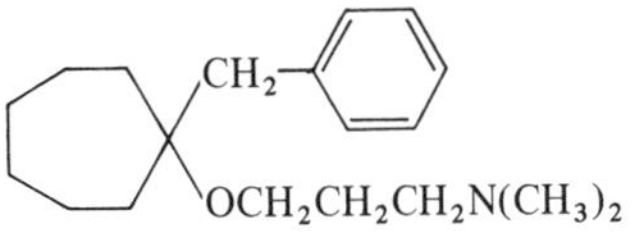

3–[(1–Benzylcycloheptyl) oxy]–
N,N–dimethylpropylamine, Bencyclane

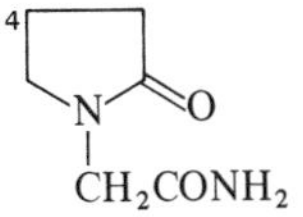

(38)

2–Oxo–1–pyrrolidineacetamide,
Piracetam, UCB 6215

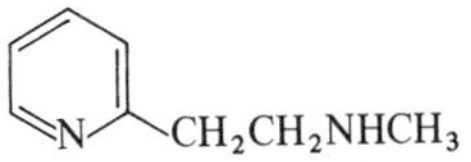

(39)

2–[2–(Methylamino) ethyl] pyridine,
Betahistine

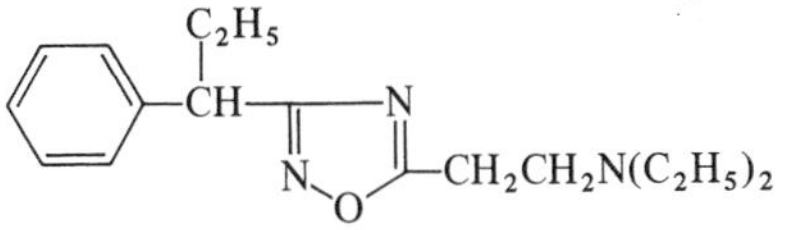

(40)

N,N–Diethyl–3–(1–phenylpropyl)–1,2,4–
oxadiazol–5–ethanamin, Proxazole,
Proxazoline, PZ 17'105

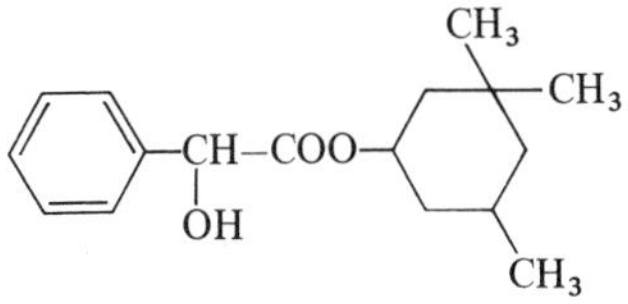

(41)

3,3,5–Trimethylcyclohexyl–α–hydroxy–
benzeneacetat, Cyclandelate, BS 572

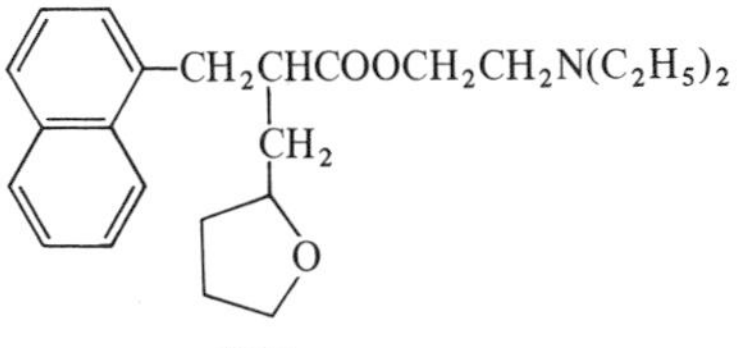

(42)

Tetrahydro–α–(1–naphthalenylmethyl)–
2–furanpropionic acid
2–(diethylamino) ethyl ester,
Nafronyl, Naftidrofuryl, LS 121

(43)

Fig. 14. Structure of miscellaneous compounds

chiatric agent can be gained from the fragmentary information given nor do metabolic studies provide clues (Kimura et al., 1979; Ono and Katsube, 1979).

Piracetam (UCB 6215) (39, Fig. 14), a pyrrolidine derivative structurally related to γ-aminobutyric acid (GABA), has been known as a chemical compound for a long time (Leuchs and Moebis, 1909), but has only recently been recognized to be both pharmacologically and clinically interesting (Giurgea, 1976; Giurgea and Salama, 1977), but with conflicting results (Lloyd-Evans et al., 1979). Metabolic studies indicate that the substance is excreted unchanged (Gobert, 1972). Derivatives have been registered in many patent applications. So far only of ISF-2522, the 4-hydroxy derivative of piracetam (39), some clinical investigations has been reported (Itil et al., 1979). Investigations which might give insight into a structur-activity relationship have not yet been published, which is not surprising in view of the special problems associated with nootropic substances.

Betahistine (40, Fig. 14), a histamine-like pyridine derivatives, has also been known for a long time (Walter et al., 1941). Its pharmacologic actions are similar to those of histamine. Because of ist activity in increasing cerebral blood flow, betahistine is clinically used in patients with cerebrovascular insufficiency (Hauth and Richardson, 1977).

Of a large series of 1,2,4-oxadiazoles (Palazzo et al., 1961), proxazole (proxazoline, AF 634, PZ 17'105) (41, Fig. 14) was developed (Silvestrini and Pozzati, 1963). Proxazole, papaverine-like in pharmacologic action, increases cerebral blood flow and improves the symptoms of cerebrovascular insufficiency (Esposito and De Gregorio, 1974). In pharmacologic tests both enantiomers, prepared by optical resolution, have shown properties very similar to those of the racemic proxazole (De Feo et al., 1971).

Salts and esters of mandelic acid are known to be of spasmolytic activity. Simple derivations (Brock et al., 1952) have led to cyclandelate (BS 572) (42, Fig. 14), the mandelic acid ester of 3,3,5-trimethylcyclohexanol (Funcke et al., 1953). On the basis of its effects on the peripheral circulation (Bijlsma et al., 1956), clinical studies for cerebrovascular action in geriatric patients have been made, but with variable results (Hauth and Richardson, 1977; Rao et al., 1977).

Because of their spasmolytic activity, derivatives of naphthalene alkylcarboxylic acids have been synthesized (Fontaine et al., 1965, 1968; Szarvasi et al., 1966, 1967). Of these compounds, naftidrofuryl (nafronyl, LS 121) (43, Fig. 14), an ester of 2-(diethylamino)ethanol (25b, Fig. 9), has been developed as a vasodilator (Fontaine et al., 1968). Naftidrofuryl, for which a cerebral metabolic stimulant activity has been demonstrated (Meynaud et al., 1975), has been tested in patients with cerebral arteriosclerosis (Bouvier et al., 1974; Gerin, 1974). Similar to the case of the aforementioned meclofenoxate (22, Fig. 8), cyprodenate (26, Fig. 9) and pyrisuccideanol (33e, Fig. 12), the 2-(diethylamino)ethanol (25b, Fig. 9) may be the active compound. The studies on the metabolism of naftidrofuryl are not incompatible with this hypothesis (Fontaine et al., 1969).

I. Conclusions

The substance which have been discussed are for the most part peripheral vasodilators which have been tested for cerebral vasodilation in geriatric patients. As no gerontopsychotherapeutic agent has been developed specifically for that purpose it has not yet been possible to establish a plausible structure-activity relationship for this indication. Compounds containing pyridine derivatives, e.g., nicotinic acid and nicotinyl alcohol, or 2-(dimethylamino)ethanol may be an exception. Against this background, it is understandable that lines of approach to the planned development of new compounds can only be extracted from the present body of knowledge with difficulty. Recently, however, serious attempts have been made to clarify the mode of action of such agents in the central nervous system, with the work on co-dergocrine leading the way. Ever-growing knowledge of the age-associated changes in brain and their therapy with gerontopsychotherapeutic agents has increased the chances of a relevant pharmacologic model being found; the efforts to isolate receptors belong in this area. Only when testing methods which are relevant to the effects on the central nervous system are rigorously applied will it become possible to describe and exploit sensible structure-activity relationships for gerontopsychotherapeutic agents.

References

Arcamone, F., Glässer, A.G., Grafnetterova, J., Minghetti, A., Nicolella, V.: Studies on the metabolism of ergoline derivatives. Metabolism of nicergoline in man and animals. Biochem. Pharmarcol. *21*, 2205–2213 (1972)

Arcari, G., Bernardi, L., Bosisio, G., Coda, S., Fregnan, G.B., Glässer, A.H.: 10-Methoxyergoline derivatives as α-adrenergic blocking agents. Experientia *28*, 819–820 (1972)

Ariens, E.J., Waelen, M.J.G.A., Sonneville, P.F., Simonis, A.M.: The pharmacology of catecholamines and their derivatives. Part I: Relationship between structure and activity as far as the vascular system is concerned. Arzneim. Forsch. *13*, 541–546 (1963)

Aurousseau, M.: Pharmacologie comparée des alcaloides indoliques et de leurs dérivés agissant sur la circulation cérébrale et le métabolisme du tissu nerveux. Chim. Ther. *6*, 221–234 (1971)

Aurousseau, M., Albert, O., Huet, Y.: First pharmacological data on an indolic compound active on cerebral blood flow: the (±)-epi-21 desethyl eburnamonine. In: Symposium on pharmacology of vinca alkaloids. 2nd Congress of the Hungarian Pharmacological Society. Knoll, J., Fekete, Gy. (eds.), vol. 5, pp. 5–8. Budapest: Akadémiai kiadó 1976a

Aurousseau, M., Linée, Ph., Albert, O., Lacroix, P.: Comparative pharmacology of vincamine and two optical antipodes with indolic structure: d- and l-eburnamonine. In: Symposium on pharmacology of vinca alkaloids. 2nd Congress of the Hungarian Pharmacological Society. Knoll, J., Fekete, Gy. (eds.), vol. 5, pp. 13–16. Budapest: Akadémiai kiadó 1976b

Ban, T.A.: Vasodilators, stimulants and anabolic agents in the treatment of geropsychiatric patients. In: Psychopharmacology – a generation of progress. Lipton, M.A., DiMascio, A., Killam, K.F. (eds.), pp. 1525–1533. New York: Raven Press 1978

Bartoli, G., Frandoli, G., Spreafico, P.L.: Langzeitbehandlung mit Xanthinol-nicotinat (Complamin regard) bei geriatrischen Patienten mit zerebraler Insuffizienz. Therapiewoche *27*, 575–585 (1977)

Belpaire, F.M., Bogaert, M.G.: Phospodiesterase inhibition and vascular activity of papaverine metabolites. Arch. Int. Pharmacodyn. Ther. *203*, 388–390 (1973)

Bergener, M., Freistein, H.: Die Anwendung der Wittenborn-Psychiatric-Rating Scales in der Gerontopsychiatrie. Arzneim. Forsch. *22*, 2058–2063 (1972)

Bernardi, L.: Von den Mutterkorn-Alkaloiden zum Nicergolin. Arzneim.-Forsch. *29* (II), 1204–1206 (1979)

Bernardi, L., Bosisio, G., Elli, C., Patelli, B., Temperilli, A., Arcari, G., Glaesser, H.A.: Ergoline derivatives. Note XIII: α-Adrenergic blocking drugs. Farmaco (Ed. Sci.) *30*, 789–801 (1975)

Bernardi, L., Bosisio, G., Croci, M., Elli, C., Temperilli, A., Arcari, G., Falconi, G., Glaesser, A.: Ergoline derivatives with oral, prolonged, α-adrenolytic activity. Farmaco (Ed. Sci.) *33*, 118–125 (1977)

426 H. HAUTH

Bernini, F.P., Muras, I., Maglione, F., Smaltino, F.: L'Azione della nicergolina sull' insufficenza del circolo cerebrale da arteriosclerosi. Vallutazione clinica e angioseriografica. Farmaco (Ed. Pr.) *32*, 32–46 (1977)
Bessin, P., Gillardin, J.-M., Thuiller, J.: Pharmacologie générale du Fénoxédil (ANP 3548). Nouveau vasodilateur cérébral. Eur. J. Med. Chem. *10*, 291–296 (1975)
Bestian, W.: Verfahren zur Herstellung eines Salzes von Theophyllinbasen. Ger. Auslegeschrift 1'102'750 (1961)
Bijlsma, U.G., Funcke, A.B.H., Tersteege, H.M., Rekker, R.F., Ernsting, M.J.E., Nauta, W.Th.: The pharmacology of cyclospasmol. Arch. Int. Pharmacodyn. Ther. *105*, 145–174 (1956)
Biró, K. Kárpáti, E.: Protective effect of synthetic vinca alkaloids on ischemic anoxia of the brain. In: Symposium on pharmacology of vinca alkaloids. 2nd congress of the Hungarian Pharmacological Society. Knoll, J., Fekete, Gy. (eds.), Vol. 5, pp. 51–54. Budapest: Akadémiai Kiadó 1976
Bölsing, E., Klatte, F., Rosentreter, U., Winterfeldt, E.: Stereoselektive Totalsynthese von Eburnamonin, Eburnamin und Eburnamenin. Chem. Ber. *112*, 1902–1912 (1979)
Boissier, J.R., Ratouis, R., Dumont, C.: Synthesis and pharmacological study of new piperazine derivatives. I. Benzylpiperazines. J. Med. Chem. *6*, 541–544 (1963)
Bombardelli, E., Bonati, A., Danieli, B., Gabetta, A., Martinelli, E.M., Mustich, G.: Decarbomethoxy apocuanzine, a new indole alkaloid from *Voacanga chalotiana*. Experientia *30*, 979–980 (1974)
Bouvier, J.B., Passeron, O., Chupin, M.P.: Psychometric study of praxilene. J. Int. Med. Res. *2*, 59–65 (1974)
Brock, N., Kühas, E,. Lorenz, D.: Untersuchungen über Spasmolytica. I. Zur Pharmakologie der Mandelsäureester. Arzneim. Forsch. *2*, 165–168 (1952)
Brunet, M.A., Boucherle, A., Badinand, A.: Amides et esters dérivés du naphtalène. Chim Thér. *2*, 246–249 (1967)
Bruneton, J. Bouquet, A. Cavé, A.: Alcaloides des écorces de racines de *Crioceras dipladeniiflorus*. Phytochem. *12*, 1475–1480 (1973)
Bruneton, J., Kan-Fen, Ch., Cavé, A.: La criocerine: Nouvel alcaloide isolé des tiges de *Crioceras dipladeniiflorus*. Phytochem. *14*, 569–571 (1975)
Bürki, H.R., Asper, H., Ruch, W., Züger, P.E.: Bromocryptine, dihydroergotoxine, methysergide, d-LSD, CF 25-397, and 29-712: Effects on the metabolism of the biogenic amines in the brain of the rat. Psychopharmacology *57*, 227–273 (1978)
Buu-Hoi, N.P., Lambelin, G., Roba, J., Jacques, G., Gillet, C.: Amino-alcools et leur préparation. Belg. Patent 755'688 (1971)
Buzas, A., Pierre, R.: Nouveaux dérivés amides de la pipéronyl-pipérazine pharmaceutiquement actifs. French Patent M 7'524 (1970)
Caron-Sigaut, C., Le Men-Olivier, L., Hugel, G., Lévy, J., Le Men, J.: Dérivés 14-hydroxyles de la vincadifformine et de la vincamine. Tetrahedron *35*, 957–960 (1979)
Carron, C., Jullien, A., Bucher, B.: Synthesis and pharmacological properties of a series of 2-piperidino alkanol derivatives. Arzneim. Forsch. *21*, 1992–1998 (1971)
Cignarella, G., Testa, E.: 2,6-Dialkylpiperazines. V. Synthesis of 2,6-Alkyl-piperazine derivatives structurally related to cinnarizine. J. Med. Chem. *11*, 612–615 (1968)
Cignarella, G., Pirisoni, G., Lorgia, M., Dorigotti, L.: 2,6-Dialkylpiperazines. VIII. N_1-Arylalkyl-N_4-(2'-pyridyl)-2,6-dimethylpiperazines as adrenolytic and vasodilator agents. Farmaco (Ed. Sci.) *32*, 296–302 (1977)
Claassen, V.: Stereospecific divergence in the actions on adrenergic α- and β-receptors. Biochem. Pharmacol. *8*, 116 (1961)
Closse, A., Hauser, D.: Evidence for an endogenous dihydroergotamine-like factor in calf and rat brain. Brain Res. *147*, 401–404 (1978)
Cole, J.O., Branconnier, R.: The therapeutic efficacy of psychopharmacological agents in senile organic brain syndrome. In: Senile dementia – a biomedical approach. Nandy, K. (ed.), pp. 271–286. Amsterdam, New York: Elsevier/North-Holland Biomedical Press 1978
Consolo, S., Fanelli, R., Garattini, S., Ghezzi, D., Jori, A., Ladinsky, H., Marc, V., Samanin, R.: Dopaminergic-cholinergic interaction in the striatum: studies with piribedil. Adv. Neurol. *9*, 257–272 (1975)

Cooper, A.J., Magnus, R.V.: A placebo-controlled study of pyritinol ("Encephabol") in dementia. Pharmatherapeutica 2, 317–322 (1980)

Cornu, F.: Zur Kreislaufphysiologie und Biochemie zerebraler Abbauprozesse und der Verhaltensbeeinflussung von Kranken durch Pharmakotherapie. Wien. Klin. Wochenschr. 81, 426–431 (1969)

Costall, B., Naylor, R.J.: Neuropharmacological studies on the site and mode of action of ET 495. Adv. Neurol. 3, 281–293 (1973)

Costall, B., Naylor, R.J.: Dopamine agonist and antagonist activities of piribedil (ET 495) and its metabolites. Naunyn Schmiedebergs Arch. Pharmacol. 285, 71–81 (1974)

De Feo, G., Giannangeli, M., Piccinelli, D., Sale, P.: Separazione e studio farmacologico dei due enantiomeri del proxazolo. Farmaco (Ed. Sci.) 26, 370–376 (1971)

Depoortere, H., Rousseau, A., Jalfre, M.: Action éveillante de la vincamine chez le rat. Rev. Electroencephalogr. Neurophysiol. Clin. 7, 153–157 (1977)

Devic, M.: Un médicament psychotonique, anxiolytique et activateur du métabolisme cérébral en neurologie. J. Méd. Lyon 54, 517–519 (1973)

Dormard, Y., Levron, J.C., Benakis, A.: Pharmacokinetic study of maleate acid of 2-(N,N-dimethylaminoethanol-$^{14}C_1$)-cyclohexylpropionate (cyprodenate) and of N,N-Dimethyl-aminoethanol-$^{14}C_1$ in animals. I. Localisation, distribution, and elimination of ^{14}C-cyprodenate and ^{14}C-dimethylaminoethanol in animals. Arzneim. Forsch. 25, 194–201 (1975a)

Dormard, Y., Levron, J.C., Le Fur, J.M.: Pharmakokinetic study of maleate acid of 2-(N,N-dimethylaminoethanol-$^{14}C_1$)-cyclohexylpropionate (cyprodenate) and of N,N-dimethyl-aminoethanol-$^{14}C_1$ in animals. II. Study and identification of the metabolites of ^{14}C-cyprodenate and ^{14}C-dimethylaminoethanol in animals. Arzneim. Forsch. 25, 201–207 (1975b)

Dormard, Y., Levron, J.C., Le Fur, J.M., Adnot, P.: Etude de la distribution, de l'élimination et de la biotransformation du Fénoxédil-^{14}C chez le rat et le porc. Eur. J. Med. Chem. 10, 302–308 (1975c)

Dyke. S.F.: The Isoquinoline Alkaloids. In: Rodd's chemistry of carbon compounds IV. Coffey, S. (ed.), Part H, pp. 1–258. Amsterdam, Oxford, New York: Elsevier 1978

Eckert, H., Kiechel, J.R., Rosenthaler, J., Schmidt, R., Schreier, E.: Biopharmaceutical aspects. Analytical methods, pharmakokinetics, metabolism and bioavailability. In: Ergot alkaloids and related compounds. Berde, B., Schild, H.O. (eds.), Handbook of Experimental Pharmacology, Vol. 49, pp. 719–803. Berlin, Heidelberg, New York: Springer 1978

Eidebenz, E. v. Schuh, H.G.: Verfahren zur Herstellung von 1-Hexyl-3,7-dimethylxanthin. Ger. Patent 860'217 (1952)

Esanu, A.: Salts of pyridoxine monoesters. US Patent 3'717'636 (1973)

Esposito, G., De Gregorio, M.: Proxazole in cerebrovascular insufficiency. Arzneim. Forsch. 24, 1692–1696 (1974)

Fanchamps, A.: Controlled studies with dihydroergotoxine in senile cerebral insufficiency. In: Geriatric Psychopharmacology, Developments in Neurology. Nandy, K. (ed.), Vol. 3, 195–212, New York: Elsevier North Holland, 1979

Fehr, T., Hauth, H.: A bromo ergot alkaloid. Br. Patent 1'451'904 (1973)

Ferris, S.H., Sathananthan, G., Gershon, S., Clark, C.: Senile dementia treatment with deanol. J. Am. Geriatr. Soc. 25, 241–244 (1977)

Flückiger, E., del Pozo, E.: Influence on the endocrine system. In: Ergot alkaloids and related compounds. Berde, B., Schild, H.O. (eds.), Handbook of Experimental pharmacology Vol. 49, pp. 615–690. Berlin, Heidelberg, New York: Springer 1978

Fontaine, L., Grand, M., Szarvasi, E.: Premiéres comparaisons, in vitro et in vivo, des activités antispasmodiques dans une série de dialcoylaminoesters et étheroxydes. C.R. Hebd. Séances Acad. Sci., Série D 262, 719–721 (1965)

Fontaine, L., Grand, M., Charbert, J., Szarvasi, E., Bayssat, M.: Pharmacologie générale d'une substance nouvelle vasodilatatrice le naftidrofuryl. Chim. Ther. 3, 463–469 (1968)

Fontaine, L., Belleville, M., Lechevin, J.C., Silie, M., Delahaye, J., Boucherat, M.: Etude du métabolisme du naftidrofuryl chez l'animal et chez l'homme. Chim. Ther. 4, 44–49 (1969)

Funcke, A.B.H., Ernsting, M.J.E., Rekker, R.F., Nauta, W.Th.: Untersuchungen über Spasmolytika. I. Mandelsäureester. Arzneim. Forsch. 3, 503–506 (1953)

Garetz, F.K., Baron, J.J., Barron, P.B., Bjork, A.E.: Efficacy of nylidrin hydrochloride in the treatment of cognitive impairment in the elderly. J. Am. Geriat. Soc. 27, 235–236 (1979)

Gerin, J.: Double-blind trial of naftidrofuryl in the treatment of cerebral arteriosclerosis. Br. J. Clin. Pract. *28*, 177–178 (1974)

Gesztes, L., Clauder, O.: *Vinca minor* L. Alkaloidjairól II. A vinkamin újabb lebontási termékei. Acta Pharm. Hung. *38*, 71–77 (1969)

Giurgea, C.: Piracetam: Nootropic pharmacology of neurointegrative activity. Curr. Dev. Psychopharmacol. *3*, 221–273 (1976)

Giurgea, C., Salama, M.: Nootropic drugs. Prog. Neuropsychopharmacol. *1*, 235–247 (1977)

Gobert, J.G.: Genèse d'un médicament: Le piracetam. Metabolisation et recherche biochimique. J. Pharm. Belg. *27*, 281–304 (1972)

Goi, A., Bruzzese, T., Ghielmetti, G., Riva, M.: Synthesis and pharmacological properties of pyridinecarbonyl derivatives of 7-substituted theophyllines. Chim. Ther. *8*, 634–637 (1973)

Guyer, B.M.: Cerebravscular disease in the elderly: Response to Isoxsuprine resinate (Defencin CP) therapy. Clin. Trial J. *15*, 49–53 (1978)

Hanna, P.E., O'Dea, R.F., Goldberg, N.D.: Phosphodiesterase inhibition by papaverine and structurally related compounds. Biochem. Pharmacol. *21*, 2266–2268 (1972)

Hapke, H.-J.: Tierexperimentelle Untersuchungen zur Charakterisierung zentralnervöser Wirkungen von Bencyclan. Arch. Int. Pharmacodyn. Ther. *202*, 231–243 (1973)

Hartmann, V., Rödiger, M., Ableidinger, W., Bethke, H.: Dihydroergotoxine: Separation and determination of four components by high performance liquid chromatography. J. Pharm. Sci. *67*, 98–103 (1978)

Harwart, D.: The treatment of chronic cerebrovascular insufficiency. A double-behind study with pentoxifylline ("Trental" 400"). Curr. Med. Res. Op. *6*, 73–84 (1979)

Hauth, H.: Chemical aspects of ergot derivatives with central dopaminergic activity. In: Dopaminergic ergot derivatives and motor functions. Wenner-Gren Center International Symposium Series. Fuxe, K., Calne, D.B. (eds.), Vol. 31, pp. 23–32. Oxford: Pergamon Press 1979

Hauth, H., Richardson, B.P.: Cerebral vasodilators. Annu. Rep. Med. Chem. *12*, 49–59 (1977)

Hillbom, M.E., Linkola, J., Nikander, P., Wallgren, H.: Effects of pyrithioxine, EMD 17246 and diethanolamine-rutin on acute alcoholic intoxication in rats. Acta Pharmacol. Toxicol. (Kbh) *33*, 65–73 (1973)

Hofmann, A., Troxler, F.: 1-Methyl ergotamines and ergocornines. U.S. Patent 3'218'324 (1965)

Hofmann, A., Frey, A., Ott, H.: Verfahren zur Herstellung von Lysergsäurederivaten. Ger. Patent 1'231'708 (1967)

Holtz, P., Langeneckert, W., Palm, D.: Sympathikomimetische Wirkungen von Papaverinderivaten. Naunyn Schmiedebergs Arch. Pharmakol. exp. Pathol. *259*, 290–306 (1968)

Hotovy, R., Enenkel, H.J., Gillissen, J., Jahn, M., Kraft, H.-G., Müller-Calgan, H., Mürmann, P., Sommer, S., Struller, R.: Zur Pharmakologie des Vitamins B6 und seiner Derivate. 2. Mitteilung: Pyrithioxin. Arzneim. Forsch. *14*, 26–29 (1964)

Hoyer, S.: Effects of centrophenoxine on cerebral circulation in geriatric patients. In: Geriatric Psychopharmacology, Developments in Neurology. Nandy, K. (ed.), Vol. 3, 261–274. New York: Elsevier North Holland, 1979

Hüller, H., Amon, I., Peters, R., Schmidt, D.: Zur Pharmakologie von L- und DL-Oxyfedrin. Pharmazie *27*, 242–245 (1972)

Hugelin, A. Legrain, Y., Willer, J.C., Clostre, F.: Action exitatrice du pyrisuccidéanol sur la formation réticulaire activatrice. Mécanisme noradrénergique. C.R. Hebd. Séances Acad. Sci. Soc. Biol. *166*, 1435–1442 (1972)

Itil, T.M., Soldatos, C., Bozak, M., Ramadanoglu, E., Dayican, G., Morgan, V., Menon, G.N.: CNS effects of ISF-2522, a new nootropic (A phase I safety and CNS efficacy study with quantitative pharmaco-EEG and pharmaco-psychology). Curr. Ther. Res. *26*, 525–538 (1979)

Jacquy, J., Noel, G.: Double blind trial with suloctidil, a new vasoactive agent, in elderly patients with psychoorganic brain syndrome. Acta Clin. Belg. *32*, 22–26 (1977)

Janssen, P.A.J.: Verfahren zur Herstellung von antihistaminaktiven, in 4-Stellung substituierten 1-Benzhydrylpiperazinen. Ger. Auslegeschrift 1'086'235 (1960)

Jones, R.G., Kornfeld, E.C.: Lithium aluminium hydride reduction of pyridine carboxylic esters: Synthesis of vitamin B6. J. Am. Chem. Soc. *73*, 107–109 (1951)

Kalaus, Gy., Györy, P., Szabó, L., Szántay, Cs.: Synthesis of vinca lakaloids and related compounds. IV. Synthesis of butyl group-containing ($\pm$)-vincamine analogue. Acta Chim. Acad. Sci. Hung. *96*, 385–391 (1978)

Kan-Fan, Ch., Husson, H.-P., Potier, P.: Plantes malgaches. XVI. La Craspidospermine, nouvel alcaloide de *Craspidosperum verticillatum* (Apocynacées). Bull. Soc. Chim. Fr. *1976*, 1227–1228

Kappert, A.: Untersuchungen über die Wirkung neuer dihydrierter Mutterkornalkaloide bei peripheren Durchblutungsstörungen und Hypertonie. Helv. Med. Acta *16*, Suppl. XXII, 5–163 (1949)

Kimura, K., Nagata, A., Miyawaki, H.: The metabolism of bencyclane in rat and man. Xenobiotica *9*, 119–127 (1979)

Kitao, K., Yata, N., Yamazaki, M., Iwane, J., Kamada, A.: Blood concentration and urinary excretion profiles following oral administration of esters of pyrithioxin to dogs. Chem. Pharm. Bull. (Tokyo) *25*, 1350–1356 (1977)

Kohlmeyer, K., Blessing, J.: Zur Wirkung von Dihydroergocristin-methansulfonat auf den Hirnkreislauf des Menschen im Akutversuch. Arzneim. Forsch. *28* (II), 1788–1797 (1978)

Komlos, E., Petöcz, L.E.: Pharmakologische Untersuchungen über die Wirkung von N-[3-(1-Benzyl-cycloheptyl-oxy)-propyl]-N,N-dimethylammonium-hydrogenfumarat. Arzneim. Forsch. *20*, 1338–1357 (1970)

Koppe, V., Poetsch, E., Schulte, K.: Phényl-4(pyrazolyl-3-akyl)-1-pipérazines substituées. Eur. J. Med. Chem. *10*, 154–161 (1975)

Kovách, A.G.B., Sándor, P., Biró, Z. Koltay, E., Mazán, K., Clauder, O.: Chemical structure and pharmacological properties of synthetic vincamine derivatives. Acta Physiol. Acad. Sci. Hung. *36*, 307–315 (1969)

Kovalyov, G.V., Nikolov, R., Tyurenkov, I.N., Tsakov, M.: Effect of the analog of cinnarizine AS 2 on the cardio-vascular-system. Acta Physiol. Pharmacol. Bulg. *2*, 27–31 (1976a); Chem. Abstr. *87*, 127′211 w (1977)

Kovalyov, G.V., Tyurenkov, I.N., Nikolov, R., Nikolova, M.: Effect of the analog cinnarizine AS2 on peripheral blood circulation. Acta Physiol. Pharmacol. Bulg. *2*, 33–39 (1976b); Chem. Abstr. *87*, 127′212x (1977)

Kovalyov, G.V., Tyurenkov, J.N., Nikolova, M., Nikolov, R.: Effect of the drug AS 2 on the central and peripheral mechanism of vascular tone regulation. Acta Physiol. Pharmacol. Bulg. *2*, 42–48 (1976c); Chem. Abstr. *86*, 100′959 p (1977)

Kraft, H.-G., Fiebig, L., Hotovy, R.: Zur Pharmakologie des Vitamin B 6 und seiner Derivate. Arzneim. Forsch. *11*, 922–929 (1961)

Kreighbaum, W.E., Kavanaugh, W.F., Comer, W.T., Deitchmann, D.: 3(2H)-Isoquinolones. 1.3-Oxygenated analogs of papaverine as peripheral vasodilators. J. Med. Chem. *15*, 1131–1135 (1972)

Külz, F., Schneider, M.: Über neue gefäßerweiternde Sympathomimetica. Klin. Wochenschr. *28*, 535–537 (1950)

Kuroda, T.: Synthetic studies of vitamin B 6 derivatives. VI. Synthesis of pyridoxine disulfide. Bitamin *30*, 431–435 (1964); Chem. Abstr. *62*, 10′402c (1965)

Kutney, J.P., Cook, G., Cook, J., Itoh, I., Clardy, J., Fayos, J., Brown, P., Svoboda, G.H.: Studies on vinca alkaloids. The structure of vincarodine. Heterocycles *2*, 73–78 (1974)

Lacroix, P., Quiniou, M.J., Linée, Ph., Le Polles, J.B.: Cerebral metabolic and hemodynamic activities of 1-eburnamonine in the anesthetized dog., Arzneim. Forsch. *29* (II), 1094–1101 (1979)

Lasserre, P., Coppolani, T.: Une étude nationale multiceutique mixte, Trivastal 50 retard. Vie méd. *61*, 39–50 (1980)

Lechner, H., Ott, E.: Die Wirkung von Tinofedrin auf Fibrinogen und spontane Thrombozytenaggregation bei Patienten mit zerebraler Insuffizienz. Klin. Wochenschr. *56*, 1137–1138 (1978)

Lehr, S., Sollberg, G., Schuhmacher, H.: Pharmakogene Erhöhung des Intelligenzniveaus. Überlegungen und eine Doppelblindstudie mit Flurnarizin (Sibelium). Pharmakopsychiatr. Neuropsychopharmakol. *11*, 134–146 (1978)

Leuchs, H., Möbis, E.: Verwendung von δ-Chlor-valerolactons zur Darstellung von Säuren und Lactonen. Ber. Dtsch. Chem. Ges. *42*, 1228–1238 (1909)

Levy, J.-C., Apffel, D., Desgroux, L., Pelas, J.: Etudes expérimentales des effets circulatoires et métaboliques cérébraux du Fénoxédil administré par voie digestive. Eur. J. Med. Chem. *10*, 297–301 (1975)

Lewis, C., Ballinger, B.R., Presly, A.S.: Trial of levadopa in senile dementia. Br. Med. J. *1978 I*, 550

Lindner, E.: Eine Reihe von Verbindungen mit α-sympathikolytischer, peripher gefäßerweiternder und sedierender Wirkung. Arzneim. Forsch. *22*, 1445–1448 (1972)

Lloyd-Evans, S., Brocklehurst, J.C., Palmer, M.K.: Piracetam in chronic brain failure. Curr. Med. Res. Op. *6*, 351–357 (1979)

Lörincz, Cs., Szabó, K., Kisfaludy, L.: The synthesis of ethyl apovincaminate. Arzneim. Forsch. *26*, 1907 (1976)

Loew, D.M., Van Deussen, E.B., Meier-Ruge, W.: Effects on the central nervous system. In: Ergot alkaloids and related compounds. Berde, B., Schild, H.O. (eds.), Handbook of Experimental Pharmacology, Vol. 49, pp. 421–531. Berlin, Heidelberg, New York: Springer 1978

Loubatiéres, A., Bouyard, P., Klein, M., Alric, R.: Action coronaro-dilatatrice de quelques dérivés de la pipérazine chez le chien anésthésié. C.R. Hebd. Séances Acad. Sci., Soc. Biol. *159*, 177–180 (1965)

Makman, M.H., Miskra, R.K., Brown, J.H.: The interactions with dopamine-stimulated adenylate cyclases of caudate nucleus and retina-direct agonist effect of a piribedil metabolite. Adv. Neurol. *9*, 213–222 (1975)

Matejcek, M., Knor, K., Piguet, P., Weil, C.: Electroencephalographic and clinical changes as correlated in geriatric patients treated three months with an ergot alkaloid preparation. J. Am. Geriat. Soc. *27*, 198–202 (1979)

Meier, C.: Centrophenoxin – ein Geriatrikum mit neurotroper Wirkung. Therapiewoche *23*, 3659–3662 (1973)

Mercier, J., Dessaigne, S., Lespagnol, A.: Sur le propriétés coronarodilatrices de dihydroisoquinoléines possédant un substituant xanthinique. C.R. Hebd. Séances Acad. Sci., Soc. Biol. *167*, 90–92 (1973)

Meynaud, A., Grand, M., Belleville, M., Fontaine, L.: Effet du naphtidrofuryl sur le métabolisme énergétique cérébral chez la souris. Thérapie *30*, 777–788 (1975)

Miller, R.J., Iversen, L.L.: Stimulation of a dopamine-sensitive adenylate cyclase in homogenates of rat striatum by a metabolite of pribedil (ET 495). Naunyn Schmiedebergs Arch. Pharmacol. *282*, 213–216 (1974)

Moed, H.D., Van Dijk, J.: Synthesis of β-phenylethylamine derivatives. IV. A new vasodilator. Rec. Trav. Chim. Pays-Bas *75*, 1215–1220 (1956)

Mohler, W., Bletz, I., Reiser, M.: Die Struktur von Ausscheidungsprodukten des 1-Hexyl-3,7-dimethylxanthins. Arch. Pharm. (Weinheim) *299*, 448–456 (1966 a)

Mohler, W., Popendiker, K., Reiser, M.: Resorption, Verteilung, Ausscheidung und Abbau von 1-Hexyl-3,7-dimethylxanthin. Arzneim. Forsch. *16*, 1524–1528 (1966 b)

Mohler, W., Söder, A.: Zur Chemie und Synthese von 3,7-Dimethyl-1-(5-oxo-hexyl)-xanthin. Arzneim. Forsch. *21*, 1159–1160 (1971)

Montaut, J., Martinelle, F., Hazeaux, C.: Action du vadilex injectable dans l'insuffisance circulatoire encéphalique. Ann. Med. Nancy *1974*, 1529–1533

Nandy, K.: Experimental studies on centrophenoxine in aging brain. In: Geriatric Psychopharmacology, Developments in Neurology, Nandy, K. (ed.), Vol. 3, pp. 247–260. New York: Elsevier North Holland 1979

Nikolov, R.: Pharmacological studies on derivatives of benzhydrylpiperazine. Farmatsiya (Sofia) *26*, 40–45 (1976); Chem. Abstr. *86*, 150′351 e (1977)

Novák, L., Rohály, J., Szántay, C.: Synthesis of vinca alkaloids and related compounds. VI. Synthesis of eburnamonine and isoeburnamonine. Heterocycles *6*, 1149–1156 (1977)

Novak, H., Schorre,, G.: Untersuchungen zum Metabolismus von Pyrithioxin. Arzneim. Forsch. *19*, 11–15 (1969)

Obermeier, K., Thiemer, K., von Schlichtegroll, A.: Einfluß von Tinofedrin auf den zerebralen Energiestoffwechsel von normotonen, hypotonen und hypoxämischen Ratten nach Carotis-Verschluß. Arzneim. Forsch. *28* (II), 1354–1360 (1978 a)

Obermeier, K., Niebch, G., Thiemer, K., Vergin, H.: Untersuchungen zu Pharmakokinetik and Metabolismus von Tinofedrin. Arzneim. Forsch. *28* (II), 1360–1367 (1978b)

Ono, K., Katsube, J.: Studies on vasodilators. I. Synthesis and stereochemistry of the metabolites of bencylane. Chem. Pharm. Bull. *27*, 1085–1093 (1979)

Oppolzer, W., Hauth, H., Pfäffli, P., Wenger, R.: A new enantioselective total synthesis of natural vincamine via an intramolecular Mannich reaction of a silyl enol ether. Helv. Chim. Acta *60*, 1801–1810 (1977)

Palazzo, G., Tavella, M., Strani, G., Silvestrini, B.: 1,2,4-Oxadiazoles, IV. Synthesis and pharmacological properties of a series of substituted aminoalkyl-1,2,4-oxadiazoles. J. Med. Pharm. Chem. *4*, 351–367 (1961)

Pallos, L.: Ergebnisse der Forschung über Herz- und Kreislaufmittel in den vereinigten Heil- und Nährmittelwerken, Budapest, in der Periode 1965–1968. Wiss. Beitr., Vol. 6, pp. 215–222, Martin-Luther-Univ. Halle-Wittenberg 1969

Pallos, L., Budai, Z. Zólyomi, G.: Basische Aether der 1-substituierten Cycloalkanole. Arzneim. Forsch. *22*, 1502–1509 (1972)

Pallos, L., Budai, Z. Zólyomi, G., Komlós, E., Petöcz, L.E.: Basische Aether der 1-substituierten Cycloalkan-1-ole. Therapiewoche *1974*, 2825–2826

Paracchini, S., Pesce, A.: Nuovo metodo di sintesi parziale della vincamina e di alcaloidi indolici correlati. Farmaco (Ed. Sci.) *33*, 573–582 (1978)

Petrova, L.A., Beltsova, N.N.: Synthesis of sulfar containing pyridoxin derivatives. Zh. Obshch. Khim. *32*, 274–277 (1962); Chem. Abstr. *57*, 16'543h (1962)

Pfäffli, P., Hauth, H.: Additionsreaktionen an der alicyclischen Doppelbindung von Eburnamenin und Apovincamin. Helv. Chim. Acta *61*, 1682–1695 (1978)

Pfäffli, P., Oppolzer, W., Wenger, R., Hauth, H.: Stereoselektive Synthese von optisch aktivem Vincamin. Helv. Chim. Acta *58*, 1131–1145 (1975)

Pinza, M., Dorigotti, L., Pifferi, G.: Synthesis, adrenolytic and vasodilator properties of new 2,2,6-trimetylpiperazines. Eur. J. Med. Chem. *11*, 395–398 (1976)

Poignant, J.-C., Lejeune, F., Malecot, E., Petitjean, M., Regnier, G., Canevari, R.: Effets comparés du piribédil et de trois de se métabolites sur le systéme extrapyramidal du rat. Experimentia *30*, 70–71 (1974)

Poignant, J.-C., Gressier, H., Petitjean, M., Regnier, G., Canevari, R.: A new central direct dopaminergic stimulant: 1-(Coumaran-5-yl-methyl)-4-(2-thiazolyl)piperazine hydrochloride (S 3608). Experimentia *31*, 1204–1205 (1975)

Popendiker, K., Boksay, J., Bollmann, V.: Zur Pharmakologie des neuen peripheren Gefäßdilatators 3,7-Dimethyl-1-(5-oxohexyl)-xanthin. Arzneim. Forsch. *21*, 1160–1171 (1971)

Porsche, E., Stefanovich, V.: Der Einfluß von Pentifyllin und Theophyllin auf die Reaktionskinetik von Katecholamin-stimulierbarer ATPase aus Rattenhirn. Arzneim. Forsch. *29* (II), 1089–1092 (1979)

Probst, G., Keiser, G.: Klinische Prüfung eines neuen Vasodilatans (Dihydrin) bei zerebralen Durchblutungsstörungen und apoplektischen Insulten. Praxis *58*, 1653–1658 (1969)

Prudhommeaux, E., Ernouf, G., Foussard-Blanpin, O., Viel, C.: Nouveaux analogues structuraux de la papavérine: benzyl-3 diméthoxy-6,7 isoquinoléines di- et tétra-hydrogénées. Eur. J. Med. Chem. *10*, 19–28 (1975)

Ramos, A.O., Ramos, L., Zanini, A.C., Slemer, O.: On the pharmacology of 1-hexyl-3,7-dimethylxanthine. Arch. Intern. Pharmacodyn. *153*, 430–435 (1965)

Rao, D.B., Georgiev, E.L., Paul, P.D., Guzmann, A.B.: Cyclandelate in the treatment of senile mental changes: A double-blind evaluation. J. Am. Ger. Soc. *25*, 548–551 (1977)

Ratouis, R., Boissier, J.R., Dumont, C.: Synthesis and pharmacological study of new piperazine derivatives. II. Phenethylpiperazines. J. Med. Chem. *8*, 104–107 (1965)

Regnier, G.L., Canevari, R.J., Laubie, M.J., De Douarec, J.C.: Synthesis and vasodilator activity of new piperazine derivatives. J. Med. Chem. *11*, 1151–1155 (1968)

Regnier, G., Canevari, R., Le Douarec, J.-C., Laubie, M.: Dépresseurs du systeme nerveux central. Etude de nouveaux dérivés de la purine. Chim. Thér. *7*, 192–205 (1972)

Ritchie, J.M.: Central nervous system stimulants. The xanthines. In: The pharmacological basis of therapeutics. Goodmann, L.S., Gilmann, A. (eds.), pp. 367–378. New York: Macmillan 1975

Roba, J., Roncucci, R., Lambelin, G.: Pharmacological properties of suloctidil. Acta Clin. Belg. *32*, 3–7 (1977)

Rutschmann, J., Stadler, P.A.: Chemical background. In: Ergot alkaloids and related compounds. Berde, B., Schild, H.O. (eds.), Handbook of Experimental Pharmacology, Vol. 49, pp. 29–85. Berlin, Heidelberg, New York: Springer 1978

Saiko, O., Klug, R.: Verfahren zur Herstellung eines schwefelhaltigen Pyridinderivates. Ger. Offenlegungsschrift 24′59′334 (1976)

Saletu, B., Grünberger, J., Linzmayer, L.: Bestimmung der enzephalotropen, psychotropen und pharmakodynamischen Eigenschaften von Nicergolin mittels quantitativer Pharmakoelektroenzephalographie und psychometrischer Analyse. Arzneim. Forsch. *29* (II), 1257–1261 (1979)

Saletu, B., Grünberger, J., Saletu, M., Mader, R., Volavka, J.: Treatment of the alcoholic organic brain syndrome with EMD 21,657. A derivative of a pyritinol metabolite: Double-blind clinical, quantitative EEG and psychometic studies. Int. Pharmacopsychol. *13*, 177–192 (1978a)

Saletu, M., Grünberger, J., Saletu, B., Mader, R.: Accelerated remission of the alcoholic organic brain syndrome with EMD 21,657. Double-blind clinical and psychometic trials. Arzneim. Forsch. *28* (II), 1525–1527 (1978b)

Sathananthan, G.L., Gershon, S.: Cerebral vasodilators – a review. In: Aging. Gershon, S., Raskin, A. (eds.), Vol. 2, pp. 155–168. New York: Ravens Press 1975

Saus, A., Posselt, K.: Synthese von radioaktiv markiertem Tinofedrin. Arzneim. Forsch. *30* (I), 917–918 (1980)

Schöpf, C., Kunz, K.J.: Pharmacologically valuable stereoisomers of certain aminoalcohols and their salts. US Patent 2′661′372 (1953)

Scholing, W.E., Clausen, H.D.: Langzeitbehandlung des neurovaskulären Psychosyndroms mit Trivastal. Med. Klin. *70*, 1522–1527 (1975)

Serchi, G.: Ricerche sulle dimetil-xantine. Nota V: Derivati alchilici e cycloalchilici della teofillina e della teobromina a cinque e sei atomi di carbonio. Chimica (Milan) *40*, 451–459 (1964); Chem. Abstr. *62*, 13′145c (1965)

Shamma, M.: The isoquinoline alkaloids. Chemistry and pharmacology. In: Organic chemistry, a series of monographs. Blomquist, A.T., Wassermann, H. (eds.), Vol. 25, 44–152, New York, London: Academic Press 1972

Shaw, T.G., Meyer, J.S.: Double-blind trial of oral papaverine in chronic cerebrovascular ischemia. Angiology *29*, 839–851 (1978)

Silvestrini, B., Pozzatti, C.: Pharmacological properties of 3-α-phenyl-5-β-diethylaminoethyl-1,2,4-oxazole citrate. Arzneim. Forsch. *13*, 798–802 (1963)

Simon, L., Pórszász, J., Gibiszerkatalin, P., Talpas, S.G.: Physikochemische Eigenschaften und Membranwirkung spasmolytisch wirksamer Isochinolin- bzw. 1,2,3,4-Tetrahydroisochinolinderivate. Pharmazie *32*, 235–239 (1977)

Solti, F., Iskum, M., Czakó, E.: Effect of ethyl apovincaminate on the cerebral circulation. Studies in patients with obliterative arterial disease. Arzneim. Forsch. *26*, 1945–1947 (1976)

Soudijn, W., van Wijngaarden, J.: The metabolism and excretion of cinnarizine by rats. Life Sci. *1968*, 231–238

Soulairac, A.: Etude des actions psychiques et psychomotrices du fipexide (Vigilor). Gaz. Méd. France *82*, 3547–3550 (1975)

Spehr, W.: Zur Zeitgestalt des Elektroenzephalogramms unter Tinofedrin. Arzneim. Forsch. *28* (II), 1312–1313 (1978)

Stadler, P., Depoortere, H.: Nouveaux amides peptidiques d'acides 6-alkyl-ergoline-8-carboxyliques, leur préparation et leur application comme médicaments. Belg. Patent 833′835 (1976)

Stadler, P., Hauth, H., Wersin, G., Guttmann, S., Hofmann, A., Stütz, P., Wilems, H.: Heterocyclische Verbindungen und Verfahren zu ihrer Herstellung. Ger. Offenlegungsschrift 1′795′022 (1971)

Staessen, A.J.: Treatment of circulatory disturbances with flunarizine and cinnarizine. A multicentre, double-blind and placebo-controlled evaluation. VASA *6*, 59–71 (1977)

Stanton, H.C., Dungan, K.W., Lish, P.M.: Some pharmacological comparisons of isoxsuprine with two structural analogues. Fed. Proc. *24*, 612 (1965)

Stoll, A., Hofmann, A.: Die Dihydroderivate der natürlichen linksdrehenden Mutterkornalkaloide. Helv. Chim. Acta 26, 2070–2081 (1943)

Stütz, P.L., Stadler, P.A., Vigouret, J.-M., Jaton, A.L.: Ergot alkaloids. New ergolines as selective dopaminergic stimulants. J. Med. Chem. 21, 754–757 (1978)

Sweet, R.D., Wasterlain, C.G., McDowell, F.H.: Piribedil, a dopamine agonist, in Parkinson's disease. Clin. Pharmacol. Ther. 16, 1077–1082 (1974)

Szabó, L., Kalaus, G., Nógradi, K., Szánty, C.: Synthesis of vinca alkaloids and related compounds. IX. Attempted assymetric synthesis of vincamine-5-carboxylic acid isopropylester. Acta Chim. Acad. Sci. Hung. 99, 73–80 (1979)

Szántay, C., Szabó, L., Kalaus, G.: Synthesis of vinca alkaloids and related compounds. II. Stereoselective and enantioselective synthesis of (+)-vincamine. Tetrahedron 33,, 1803–1808 (1977)

Szarvasi, E., Bayssat, M., Fontaine, L., Grand, M.: Quelques nouvelles structures naphtaléniques à activité antispasmodique. Bull. Soc. Chim. France 1966, 1838–1846

Szarvasi, E., Bayssat, M., Fontaine, L., Grand, M.: Diamines di-tertiaires naphtaléniques. Chim. Ther. 2, 407–409 (1967)

Szporny, L.: Pharmacologie de la vincamine et de ses dérivés. Actual. Pharmacol. (Paris) 29, 88–117 (1977)

Taylor, W.I.: The pentaceras and the eburnamine (hunteria)-vincamine alkaloids. In: The alkaloids. Manske, R.H.F. (ed.), Vol. 8, pp. 249–268. New York, London: Academic Press 1965

Taylor, W.I.: The eburnamine-vincamine alkaloids. In: The alkaloids. Manske, R.H.F. (ed), Vol. 11, pp. 125–143. New York, London: Academic Press 1968

Taylor,, W.I., Farnsworth, N.R. (eds.): The vinca alkaloids. New York: Dekker 1973

Teubner, W.: Isoxsuprin (Vasoplex). Literaturübersicht über experimentelle und klinische Ergebnisse. Fortschr. Med. 90, 517–521 (1972)

Theis, H., Lehrach, F., Müller, R.: A 5-year review of clinico-experimental and therapeutic experience with pentoxifylline. Pharmatherapeutica 2, Suppl. 1., 150–160 (1978)

Thiele, K., Schimassek, U., von Schlichtegroll, A.: Neue herzwirksame β-Aminoketone. Synthese und Betrachtungen über Zusammenhänge zwischen pharmakologischer Wirkung und Konstitution neuer Mannich-Basen I. Arzneim. Forsch. 16, 1064–1067 (1966)

Thiele, K., Koberstein, E., Nonnenmacher, G.: Neue herzwirksame β-Aminoketone. II. Ein physikalisch-chemischer Beitrag zur Charakterisierung von Oxyfedrin. Arzneim. Forsch. 18, 1255–1263 (1968)

Thiele, K., Posselt, K., Gross, A., Schuler, A.W.: Über neue basische Thienylalkanderivate mit coronargefäßerweiternder Wirkung. Chim. Ther. 4, 228–233 (1969)

Thiele, K., Posselt, K., Offermanns, H.: Zur Synthese der zerebroaktiven Substanz Tinofedrin. Arzneim. Forsch. 28 (II), 2047–2048 (1978)

Thiele, K., Posselt, K., Offermanns, H., Thiemer, K.: Neue zerebral wirksame basische Dithienyl-Verbindungen. Arzneim. Forsch. 30 (I), 747–757 (1980a)

Thiele, K., Posselt, K., Heese, J., Engel, J.: Spektroskopische Charakterisierung von Tinofedrin. Arzneim. Forsch. 28 (II), 1057–1059

Thiemer, K., Stroman, F., Szelenyi, I., von Schlichtegroll, A.: Pharmakologische Wirkung von Tinofedrin auf die zerebrale und periphere Hämodynamik des Hundes. Arzneim. Forsch. 28 (II), 1343–1354 (1978)

Thiery, E., Otte, G., Vander Eeken, H.: Comparative study of the clinical effect of vincamine versus papaverine given parenterally in the acute phase of stroke. Arzneim. Forsch. 29 (I), 571–574 (1979)

Thuillier, G.: Dérivés des acides aryloxyacétiques à activité neurotrope. Chim. Ther. 1, 82–86 (1966)

Thuillier, G., Rumpf, P.: Préparation de nouveaux esters et amides basiques des acides qui agissent comme régulateurs de croissance des végétaux. Relations entre la structure et l'activité biologique. Bull. Soc. Chim. Fr. 1960, 1786–1794

Thuillier, G., Marlier, S, Saville, B., Rumpf, P.: Préparation de nouveaux esters et amides basiques des acides qui agissent comme régulateurs de croissance des végétaux. II. Isostères soufrés et azotés. Bull. Soc. Chim. Fr. 1963a, 1084–1086

Thuillier, G., Dumont, J.-M., Vilar, A., Rumpf, P.: Préparation de nouveaux esters et amides basiques des acides qui agissent comme régulateurs de croissance des végétaux. III. Amides. Bull. Soc. Chim. Fr. *1963b*, 1087–1090

Thuillier, G., Geffroy, F., Bessin, P., Thuillier, J.: Synthèse d'aryloxyacétamides tertiaires. Vasodilateurs cérébraux et périphériques. Eur. J. Med. Chem. *10*, 286–290 (1975)

Valette, R.: β-Cyclohexylpropionsäure-2-dimethylamino-äthylester und seine Salze sowie Verfahren zu deren Herstellung. Ger. Auslegeschrift 1'283'233 (1968)

Van Dijk, J., Moed, H.D.: Synthesis of β-phenylethylamine derivatives VII. The enantiomers of erythro-1-(4'-hydroxyphenyl)-2-(1''-methyl-2''-phenoxyethylamino)-propanol-1. Rec. Trav. Chim. Pays-Bas *80*, 573–587 (1961)

Van Dijk, J., Keizer, V.G., Moed, H.D.: Synthesis of β-phenyläthylamine derivatives. VIII. Four diastereomers of 1-(4'-hydroxy-phenyl)-2-(1''-methyl-3''-phenylpropylamino)-propanol. Rec. Trav. Chim. Pays Bas *82*, 189–201 (1963)

Van Dijk, J., Keizer, V.G., Peelen, J.F., Moed, H.D.: Synthesis of β-phenylethylamine derivatives. IX. The enantiomers and diastereomers of N-phenoxyalkyl-β-(4-hydroxyphenyl) ethylamine derivatives. Rec. Trav. Chim. Pays Bas *84*, 521–539 (1965)

Van Schepdael, J.: Etude clinique de l'action du suloctidil sur la maladie cérébro-vasculaire chronique de la personne agée. Ars Med. *32*, 1505–1518 (1977)

Vereczkey, L., Szporny, L.: Metabolism of ethyl apovincaminate in the rat. Arzneim. Forsch. *26*, 1933–1938 (1976)

Vereczkey, L., Czira, G., Tamás, J., Szentirmay, Z., Botár, Z., Szporny, L.: Pharmacokinetics of vinpocetine in humans. Arzneim. Forsch. *29* (I), 957–960 (1979)

Vigano, V., Paracchini, S., Piacenza, G., Pesce, E.: Metabolismo della vincamina nel ratto. Farmaco (Ed. Sci.) *33*, 583–594 (1978)

Waelen, M.J.G.A., Sonneville, P.F., Ariens, E.J., Simonis, A.M.: The pharmacology of catecholamines and their derivatives. Part. II: An analysis of the actions on blood flow and oxygen exchange in skin and muscle. Arzneim. Forsch. *14*, 11–19 (1964)

Walter, L.A., Hunt, W.H., Fosbinder, R.J.: β-(2- and 4-Pyridylalkyl)-amines. J. Am. Chem. Soc. *63*, 2771–2773 (1941)

Wieck, H.H., Blaha, L.: Therapeutische Möglichkeiten bei zerebrovaskulärer Insuffizienz. Therapiewoche *26*, 5282–5290 (1976)

Witzmann, H.K., Blechacz, W.: Zur Stellung von Vincamin in der Therapie zerebrovaskulärer Krankheiten und zerebraler Leistungsminderungen. Arzneim. Forsch. *27* (I), 1238–1247 (1977)

Wright, H.B., Martin, D.L.: Hypocholesteremic agents. IV. Some substituted piperazines. J. Med. Chem. *11*, 390–391 (1968)

Zikan, V., Semonský, M.: Mutterkornalkaloide XVI. Einige N-(D-6-Methylisoergolenyl-8)-, N-(D-6-Methylergolenyl-8)- und N-(D-6-Methylergolin(I)-yl-8)-N'-substituierte Harnstoffe. Coll. Czech. Chem. Commun. *25*, 1922–1928 (1960)

Zikan, V., Semonský, M.: Mutterkornalkaloide 31. Mitteilung: Ein Beitrag zur Herstellung von N-(D-6-Methyl-8-isoergolenyl)-N',N'-diäthylharnstoff. Pharmazie *23*, 147–148 (1968)

Zikan, V., Semonský, M., Řezábek, K., Auskova, M., Seda, M.: Ergot alkaloids XL. Some N-(D-6-methyl-8-isoergolin-I-yl)- and N-(D-6-methyl-8-isoergolin-II-yl)-N'-substituted ureas. Coll. Czech. Chem. Commun. *37*, 2600–2605 (1972)

Zikolova, S., Ninov, K.: Analogs of N_1-benzhydryl-N_4-cinnamylpiperazine (cinnarizine). I. N_4-substituted-N_1-cinnamylpiperazines. Tr. Nauchnoizsled. Khim.-Farm. Inst. *8*, 49–58 (1972a); Chem. Abstr. *78*, 147'914v (1973)

Zikolova, S., Ninov, K.: Analogs of N_1-benzhydryl-N_4-cinnamylpiperazine (cinnarizine). II. N_1-substituted-N_4-benzhydryl-piperazines. Tr. Nauchnoizsled. Khim.-Farm. Inst. *8*, 59–67 (1972b); Chem. Abstr. *78*, 147'908w (1973)

Zikolova, S., Ninov, K.: Analogs of N_1-benzhydryl-N_4-cinnamylpiperazine (cinnarizine). III. N-Cinnamoyl- and N[(cinnamoyloxy)alkyl]piperazines. Tr. Nauchnoizsled. Khim.-Farm. Inst. *9*, 125–134 (1974); Chem. Abstr. *83*, 79'194m (1975)

Zima, O., Schorre, G.: Derivatives of vitamin B6. U.S. Patent 3'010'966 (1961)

Züger, P.E., Vigouret, J.-M., Loew, D.M.: Inhibition of reserpine-induced PGO waves in the cat by ergot derivatives. Experientia *34*, 637–639 (1978)

CHAPTER 10

Pharmacologic Approaches to Gerontopsychiatry

D. M. Loew and J. M. Vigouret

The increase in the number of aged individuals requiring medical treatment has resulted in a new speciality, geriatric medicine. In particular, today's physicians are increasingly confronted with patients presenting psychological and psychiatric problems. Some of these problems may appear independent of age but may present a particular symptomatology relating to the life situation, to the physical health condition, and to the socioeconomic status of the aged patient. Other conditions are considered to be not only frequent but typical in the older patient population.

A. Gerontopsychopharmacologic Agents

The pharmacologic treatment of psychological disorders in the elderly patient often involves the administration of psychotropic drugs such as anxiolytics, antidepressants, and neuroleptics which were originally developed for a younger population (Epstein, 1978). In addition, hypnotics and analgesics are frequently prescribed. Prien et al. (1975) surveyed prescriptions in 12 Veteran's Administration hospitals in the United States and reported that 55% of elderly veteran inpatients received at least one psychotropic medication. However, the prescription of psychotropic drugs in aged individuals requires particular attention as absorption, distribution, excretion, and tolerance in senescent patients may be different from those of younger individuals or modified by concomitant physical disease (Friedel, 1978).

In contrast to classic psychotropic drugs, gerontopsychopharmacologic agents are drugs with specific effects on the central nervous system that suggest they would be of particular value in the treatment of behavioral and mental disturbances often occurring in old people. The efficacy of existing agents is limited to symptomatic treatment. No preventive treatment that would delay the onset or the development of senescence is yet known (Kanowski, 1978).

Gerontopsychopharmacologic agents (Table 1) have been developed from plants (derivatives of ergot, vincamine, and xanthine) and from synthetic chemicals (e.g., piperazine, phenoxyacetic acid, and phenylethanolamine). Most of these agents have found their way into gerontopsychiatry based on some defined pharmacologic action (Table 2). Typically, vasodilation in animal experiments is given as their main pharmacologic action indicative of therapeutic efficacy. Increasingly, actions on brain metabolism are emphasized and other neuropharmacologic actions claimed to relate to a gerontopsychiatric use include effects on neurotransmission (e.g., co-dergocrine mesylate, deanol, piribedil) or a particular psychostimulant effect (fipexide, pemoline). Thus, there is no cohesive concept governing the pharmacologic basis of the therapeutic use of gerontopsychopharmacologic agents.

Table 1. Groups of gerontopsychopharmacologic agents
according to chemical structure.

1. *Alkaloids*
   Ergot-derivatives: Co-dergocrine mesylate Nicergoline
   Papaverine
   Vincamine derivatives

2. *Xanthines*
   Pentifylline
   Pentoxifylline
   Xanthinol

3. *Piperazines*
   Cinnarizine
   Flunarizine
   Piribedil

4. *Phenoxyacetic acid derivatives*
   Fenoxedil
   Fexicaine
   Meclofenoxate

5. *Phenylethanolamines*
   Isoxsuprine
   Nylidrin
   Oxyfedrine
   Tinofedrine

6. *Miscellaneous*
   Bencyclane
   Betahistine
   Cyclandelate
   Naftidrofuryl
   Piracetam
   Pyritinol

Most recent reviews on psychogerontopharmacology concentrate on clinical aspects of the subject. Kanowski (1978) in introducing a symposium at the 10th Congress of the Collegium Internationale Neuropsychopharmacologicum in Quebec, Canada, pointed out that the theoretical ideas are still on a high level of abstraction and offer few concrete possibilities for psychopharmacologic research and development. Eisdorfer (1973) recognized the value of existing drugs in the treatment of behavioral and affective disorders in the aged, but emphasized the need for a more efficacious pharmacotherapy of intellectual and cognitive alterations. Similar conclusions were reached by other authors reviewing clinical gerontopsychopharmacology (Ban, 1977; Cole and Branconnier, 1978; Fann and Wheless, 1976; Lemperiere, 1978; Petrie and Ban, 1978; Sathananthan et al., 1977; Yesavage et al., 1979). The only reviews that pay particular attention to chemical and pharmacologic aspects are those by Hauth and Richardson (1977) and by Horita (1978).

B. Gerontopsychiatric Patients

For didactic reasons, Prien and Cole (1978) divided the mental alterations of old age into two categories: the organic brain syndrome, which results from alterations of

Table 2. Presumed primary actions of gerontopsychopharmacologic agents

	Ref.
1. *Actions on brain vasculature*	
Bencyclane	KOMLOS and PETÖCZ (1970); KUKOVETZ (1975)
Betahistine	SEIPEL and FLOAM (1975)
Cinnarizine	VAN NUETEN (1969), GODFRAIND and KABA (1969)
Cyclandelate	BIJLSMA et al. (1956), RAO et al. (1977)
Fenoxedil	BESSIN et al. (1975)
Flunarizine	GODFRAIND (1977), VAN NUETEN and JANSSEN (1973)
Isoxsuprine	TEUBNER (1972)
Naftidrofuryl	FONTAINE et al. (1968), BRANCONNIER and COLE (1978)
Isonitol nicotinate	ROSNER (1973)
Nicotinyl alcohol	HEYCK (1962)
Nylidrine	EISENBERG (1960), LAWSON and MANLEY (1971)
Papaverine	DUVOISIN (1975), GYGAX et al. (1978), HÜNERMANN et al. (1975)
Pentoxifylline	KOMAREK and KARTHEUSER (1977), POPENDIKER (1971)
Proxazole	HEISS et al. (1973)
Suloctidil	GODFRAIND (1976)
Vincamine	KNOLL and FEKETE (1976), SZPORNY (1976)
Vinpocetin	KÁRPÁTI and SZPORNY (1976)
Viquidil	DE VALOIS (1973), HÜHNERMANN et al. (1973)
Xanthinol	BARTOLI et al. (1977)
2. *Actions on brain metabolism*	
Citicoline	YASUHARA and NAITO (1974), KASE et al. (1974)
Co-dergocrine mesylate	MEIER-RUGE et al. (1975), VENN (1978)
Cyprodenate	GENEVIEVE (1970)
Meclofenoxate	MEIER (1973), NANDY and LAL (1978)
Nicergoline	BENZI (1975)
Pyritinol	HOTOVY et al. (1964), HOYER et al. (1977)
3. *Other actions*	
Co-dergocrine mesylate	LOEW et al. (1979a), BÜRKI et al. (1978)
Deanol	RE (1974), FERRIS et al. (1977)
Fipexide	SOULAIRAC (1975)
Pemoline	PLOTNIKOFF (1970), GLASKY and SIMON (1966)
Piracetam	GIURGEA (1976), GOBERT (1972)
Piribedil	CORRODI et al. (1972), SCHOLING and CLAUSEN (1975)

brain cell function, and the so-called functional alterations, which have no known organic origin. The organic brain syndrome comprises impairment in orientation, memory, intellectual functions, comprehension, problem solving, learning, and judgment as well as lability and shallowness of affect. Functional alterations involve personality disorders, chronic neurotic reactions, depressions, and schizophrenia.

In contrast to a commonly held belief that progressive decline of emotional and cognitive function in the aged is related to vascular disease, WELLS (1978) found this to be the case in only 17 of 222 fully evaluated cases of organic brain syndrome (Table 3). TOMLINSON et al. (1970) performed autopsies on demented elderly patients and found that Alzheimer-type changes accounted for 50% of the cases, whereas changes due to arteriosclerosis accounted definitely for only 12%, and probably for an additional 6%. Thus it would appear that even if reductions in cerebral blood flow

Table 3. Diagnoses in organic brain syndrome (After Wells, 1978).

Diagnosis	%
Atrophy of unknown causes, possibly Alzheimer type	51
Vascular disease	8
Normal pressure hydrocephalus	6
Dementia in alcoholics	6
Intracranial masses	5
Huntington's chorea	5
Depression	4
Drug toxicity	3
Dementia (uncertain)	3
Other	9

do correlate with a failing mental performance in the elderly, the etiologic role of an overall vascular failure should not be overemphasized (Hachinski et al., 1976; De-Koninck et al., 1977).

The above-mentioned functional disorders are not exclusively found in old age. Depression, which occurs very frequently in elderly patients, presents a different symptomatology to that seen in younger patients. According to Epstein (1976) and Roth (1955) about 50% of older patients admitted to mental hospitals exhibit a type of depression that is characterized more by a preponderance of somatic complaints, apathy, and withdrawal than by overt changes in mood (Birkmayer et al., 1973; Salzman et al., 1975). The same appears to hold true for ambulatory geriatric patients (Smith et al., 1977). In addition, some individuals suffering from organic brain syndrome may respond to their mental deterioration with depression, agitation, or persecutory reactions. Severe forms of depression might even imitate the full picture of dementia ("pseudodementia," Post, 1975).

C. Current Theories of Aging

The numerous hypotheses on the aging process can be conveniently grouped according to the causative mechanisms. Exogenous and endogenous causes have been proposed. It should be borne in mind that studies of aging that entail singling out a particular level of organization cannot furnish an integral view of the problem, and the conclusions thereby reached must be regarded as possible contributions to the explanation of the aging process and not as possible explanations of the whole process.

I. Exogenous Causes

The stagnation in adult life expectancy in the industrialized countries in recent years has given prominence to the role of social factors in aging. The stress of daily life, sociocultural obligations, and taboos, and the failure to live according to the "biological clock" are claimed to increase sympathetic and endocrine tone which are capable of activating oxidative metabolism and simultaneously rendering certain areas hypoxemic. It Is conceivable that the increased formation of free radicals and the rupture of lysosomes are capable of accelerating the aging processes (LABORIT, 1975). The abuse of tobacco, alcohol, and other drugs; the consumption of adulterated food-stuffs; the exposure to environmental pollution, especially air and water pollution; and ionising radiation may also contribute to more rapid aging and hence to a reduction in life span (SACHER, 1956; KENT, 1976; NOEL, 1975).

II. Endogenous Causes

For a long time, aging was thought to be due to the complexity of the organisms as opposed to single cells. It was believed that if cells were isolated and correctly cultivated they could be immortal. This hypothesis was discarded after HAYFLICK (1961) demonstrated that cultures of human fibroblasts underwent a limited number of divisions, became senescent, and died. This phenomenon may be compared with the loss of weight of the aging brain, associated with anatomic changes (BOWEN and DAVISON, 1976). These findings were supported by results in the mouse which revealed a loss of neurons with age (JOHNSON and FERNER, 1972). By contrast, the number of glia cells was shown to increase with age in rats (VAUGHAN and PETERS, 1974). In man, the number of neurons and cerebral synapses appears to remain unchanged with increasing age (PRESTIGE, 1974; CRAGG, 1975). This observation questions the hypothesis advanced by BRODY (1955) that the loss of brain weight was due to a reduction in the number of nerve cells. In fact, MONAGLE and BRODY (1974) have shown that the number of nerve cells remains constant with increasing age, and thus the loss of brain weight could be due to a reduction in extracellular space (BONDAREFF, 1964; TREFF, 1974). Intraneuronal changes have also been observed, granulovascular degeneration (WISNIEWSKI and TERRY, 1973), lipofuscinosis (LAL et al., 1973), the appearance of Alzheimer fibrils, and cytoplasmic changes in the astroglia (BOWE and DAVISON, 1976) appearing to be fairly characteristic. Nevertheless, none of these morphological studies in man and in laboratory animals has resulted in the identification of a specific factor which could be responsible for the aging process.

The cross-linking theory (BUERGER, 1957; VERZAR, 1968) postulates the formation of intermolecular bridges under the influence of oxidizing agents, resulting in the formation of intermolecular bridges at free radicals, especially between lipid chains. These cross-links between molecules are a characteristic change in the aging of collagen (HARMAN, 1973), a process which leads to aging of all the connective tissues with deleterious consequences for the muscles, arteries, and serous membranes covering the viscera.

Other investigators believe that aging may result from mutations (SACHER and TRUCCO, 1962; BURNET, 1974) and assume that lesions of desoxyribonucleic acid are not detected by the control mechanism inherent in desoxyribonucleic acid, so that the cell becomes deficient in certain enzymes. The most discussed present theory of aging is the error catastrophe theory (ORGEL, 1963; PRICE and MAKINODAN, 1973; COMFORT, 1974; RYAN et al., 1974), which postulates that catastrophic errors occur in the mechanism of protein synthesis and that the accumulation of these errors in the amino-acid sequence of the proteins results in the deterioration and death of the cell. This hypothesis finds indirect support from the results of analyses that have shown a reduction

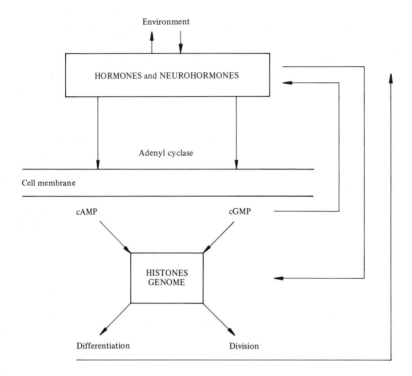

Fig. 1. An integrative view relating cellular aging to the reaction of the organism to its environment (Modified after LABORIT, 1975)

with age in various enzymes such as histone methylase (Lee and Duerre, 1974), acetylcholin esterase (Samorajski, 1972, 1973; Meier-Ruge, 1975), lactate dehydrogenase (Singh and Kanungo, 1968), Pyrophosphatase (Buruiana and Hadarag, 1973), and NA^+/K^+ ATPase (Velkow, 1973). Based on a review of their own and other investigators' results of age-dependent changes in enzyme activities in human brain autoptic material, Iwangoff et al. (1979) conclude that two systems are particularly affected. On the one hand, the decline in the activity of enzymes of the glycolytic pathways results in a reduction in glycolytic capacity which, under conditions of stress, is critical for an adequate energy supply. On the other hand, the reduction in the activity of neurotransmitter metabolizing enzymes lessens the brains capacity for information processing.

Recently, Laborit (1975) has put forward an attractive hypothesis to relate cellular aging with the reaction of an organism to its environment (Fig. 1). Bearing in mind that the cyclic nucleotide adenines cyclic adenosine monophosphate (cAMP) and cyclic guanosine monophosphate (cGMP) are involved in the transcription of the genome (cAMP facilitates cellular differentiation and cGMP promotes cell division) and that the synthesis of these two nucleotides is controlled by adenylate cyclase, the activity of which is governed by hormones and neurohormones, Laborit believes that cell division and differentiation could be a response to a neuroendocrine reaction of the organism to its environment. Through the mediation of cAMP, the sympatho-adrenergic reaction blocks cell division and facilitates cell differentiation and, therefore, aging. It is likewise conceivable that this cellular change could affect neurotransmission and thus also acclerate the preceding reaction.

D. Animal Models in Gerontopsychopharmacology

I. Models Derived from Current Theories

Most of the current theories on the causes of aging are not easily applicable to pharmacological and therapeutic intervention. As seen from the evidence reviewed by GRANICH (1972), a direct application to drug intervention in aging is highly speculative and lacks sufficient experimental foundation. However, a few examples may be mentioned which illustrate that exogenous factors can provide an approach to the study of drug effects on brain aging. NANDY and LAL (1978) have recently summarized their studies on cellular lipofuscin deposits and on learning deficits in aging mice subjected to a vitamin-E-deficient diet, and they have reported that some gerontopsychopharmacological agents may reduce lipofuscin pigments (NANDY and BOURNE, 1966; NANDY and SCHNEIDER, 1978a, b). As the prolonged administration of chlorpromazine also reduces lipofuscin content in mouse brain cells, direct membrane effects have been inferred (SAMORAJSKI and ROLSTEN, 1976). Another model consists of exposing animals to alcohol for a period of 2–3 months, which produces morphological alterations similar to those of aging (SAMORAJSKI et al., 1977, 1978; SUN et al., 1978). In these animals, concomitant administration of co-dergocrine mesylate prevented some of the physiologic and neurochemical changes caused by alcohol.

II. Models of Acute Brain Failure

In models of brain failure, an acute breakdown of central nervous system function is created by means of external manipulation such as ischemia, hypothermia, or hypoxia (HOYER, 1978). As has been pointed out by MEIER-RUGE (1975), these experimental models are a caricature of the aging process, as they may possibly represent only one selected aspect claimed to be specific for brain aging which is elicited under the time pressure of a short-term experiment. In addition, the procedures used and the parameters evaluated are often based on pathophysiologic mechanisms considered to be involved in acute breakdown of human brain function such as arterial hemorrhage or occlusion, and may therefore not reflect the insidious onset and slow progress found in senescence. It is true that an adequate oxygen supply and a sufficient macro- and micro-flow of brain circulation is critical for the maintenance of the high rate of brain metabolism and function. Cerebral oxygen consumption and blood flow have been shown to be reduced in old people with dementia (FREYAN et al., 1951; LASSEN et al., 1957), in particular in the frontotemporal region (INGVAR and GUSTAFSON, 1970; OBRIST et al., 1970). However, in normal aging, cerebral blood supply, oxygen consumption, and energy production are not necessarily impaired (SOKOLOFF, 1966; OLESEN, 1974; THOMPSON, 1976).

Numerous methods have been used to produce impairment of cerebral blood flow in animals (Kogure et al., 1975; Gygax et al., 1978), and typically cerebral vasodilators such as papaverine, cyclandelate, and isoxsuprine have been investigated. The question remains whether mental deterioration in old age is related to a reduction in blood supply due to atherosclerosis (Roth et al., 1967) and whether drugs that induce vasodilation really do dilate those vessels which supply the affected part of the brain. As pointed out by Lassen (1966, 1974), the local factors inducing vasodilation may already have induced maximal dilation, so that a vasodilator may either dilate healthy vessels outside the affected area or may cause an increased blood supply exceeding local demands.

Another model of acute brain failure relies on the assumption that brain aging is related to a reduced metabolic capacity (Meier-Ruge, 1975; Meier-Ruge et al., 1975). Studies in isolated brain preparations (Emmenegger and Meier-Ruge, 1968; Benzi et al., 1972) and whole animals subjected to different types of manipulation such as hypothermia, oligemia, or ischemia (Meier-Ruge et al. 1975; Gygax et al., 1978) indicate that ergot derivatives, in particular co-dergocrine mesylate and nicergoline, increase the metabolic capacity of the brain under conditions of an acute impairment of brain metabolism (Loew et al., 1978).

Acute hypoxia is another animal model frequently used in animals to induce failure of brain function. Various psychogerontologic drugs such as vincamine (Knoll and Fekete, 1976), piracetam (Giurgea, 1976), and ergot derivatives (Boismare et al., 1978) have been shown either to prolong survival time or to restore functional impairment due to hypoxia. As with the other models of acute brain failure, the question remains as to how well a protection against the noxious effects of acute hypoxia may predict the therapeutic efficacy of a gerontopsychopharmacologic agent.

III. Models Derived from Impairment of Synaptic Transmission

In contrast to the cited examples of acute brain failure, the interest in the effects of gerontopsychopharmacologic agents on synaptic neurotransmission stems from the fact that slowly progressing changes in neurotransmitter metabolism could correlate with the slow decline of mental function in the aged. An increasing body of evidence indicates that considerable changes in cerebral content of neurotransmitters and of the enzymes necessary for their metabolism are related to senescence (Samorajski, 1977; Domino et al., 1978; Vigouret, 1978). McGeer et al. (1971a) were the first to report a decrease in tyrosine hydroxylase in the striate nucleus of old rats and to suggest alterations in brain catecholamine metabolism in aging. Subsequently, a slowing of the metabolism of catecholamines, serotonin, and acetylcholine in animals was described by various authors (Finch, 1973; Simpkins et al., 1977; Meek et al., 1977; Vernadakis, 1975; Meier-Ruge et al., 1976). Similarly, a reduction of neurotransmitter metabolism was described in the human brain. Work of McGeer et al. (1971b, 1976) and of Lloyd and Hornykiewicz (1972) indicates that aging is accompanied by a reduction in the activity of tyrosine hydroxylase, Dopa decarboxylase, choline acetylase, and acetylcholinesterase. In addition, the reported increase in monoamine oxidase activity suggests an enhanced transmitter breakdown (Robinson, 1975). Indeed, the therapeutic effect of procaine hydrochloride has been attributed to its capacity to inhibit monoamine oxidase (MacFarlane, 1973, 1975).

Alterations of transmitter metabolism are particularly pronounced in brains of patients with senile dementia. Dopa decarboxylase activity is reduced by over 80% in paleostriatum, substantia nigra, and neostriatum. This amount of reduction in senile dementia is comparable to the changes reported in patients with Parkinson's disease. In addition, homovanillic acid and 5-hydroxyindoleacetic acid are lowered in certain parts of the brain, which suggests an additional impairment of dopaminergic and serotoninergic function (BOWEN and DAVISON, 1976; GOTTFRIES et al., 1973, 1974). Furthermore, the activities of choline acetylase, acetylcholinesterase and glutamic acid decarboxylase are considerably depressed in brains of patients with a previous diagnosis of senile dementia (BOWEN and DAVISON, 1976; DAVIES and MALONEY, 1976).

Impairment of neurotransmission in the aged brain can provide models of pharmacologic action of psychogeriatric agents. Precursors of neurotransmitters or agents imitating their effect have been investigated in old, mentally deteriorated patients. LEWIS et al. (1978) have reported an improvement in their ratings of demented patients treated with L-dopa. Similarly, ETIENNE et al. (1978) reported favorable results after administration of lecithin, the major dietary source of choline. Deanol, claimed to be a precursor of acetylcholine (ZAHNISER et al., 1977), was reported by FERRIS et al. (1977) to improve clinical ratings in patients with senile dementia. Isolated trials with bromocriptine, a dopamine agonist, have failed to give convincing evidence for a beneficial effect in demented patients (HONTELA et al., 1978; PHUAPRADIT et al., 1978).

Thus, the specific importance of one given neurotransmitter in aging of the human brain is not yet clear. It might be that in the normal aging brain and in senile dementia, different subgroups should be discerned according to deficiency of one particular transmitter. Alternately, as more than one transmitter is deficient, the ideal drug would have to act on several neurotransmitter systems.

The effects of psychogeriatric drugs acting on brain monoaminergic systems can be investigated in the animal using standard pharmacologic procedures. More recent studies of ergot derivatives may serve as examples (BÜRKI et al., 1978; CLEMENS and FULLER, 1978; LOEW et al., 1979a; VIGOURET et al., 1978). Co-dergocrine mesylate has been shown to imitate the effects of dopamine and serotonin at central synaptic receptor sites (LOEW et al., 1979a), and piribedil first found interest as a dopamine agonist (CORRODI et al., 1972). In addition, recent studies (CLEMENS and FULLER, 1978; CLEMENS, 1979) indicate that in the rat, lergotrile partly corrects age-dependent changes in monoamine-dependent neuroendocrine function which was proposed earlier to be a relevant indicator of central nervous system aging (FINCH, 1973; ASCHHEIM, 1976). A similar mechanism may also be involved in the increased life-span of mice reported under administration of L-dopa (COTZIAS et al., 1974, 1977).

E. Three Examples of Gerontopsychopharmacologic Agents

This section illustrates three typical approaches to the treatment of behavioral symptoms of gerontopsychiatric patients. The differences in the pharmacologic effects of the three agents chosen, vincamine, co-dergocrine mesylate, and piracetam, serve to underline the diversity of the present approaches to gerontopsychopharmacologic treatment. However, each of these agents has been found to offer some therapeutic benefit to patients suffering from organic brain syndrome, no matter how different their pharmacologic actions in animal experiments may be.

I. Vincamine

The preparation of the various alkaloids contained in periwinkle has led to the isolation of vincamine (1), first achieved in 1950 by Zabolotnaja (Le Men, 1971). Vincamine exerts its main pharmacodynamic actions on the circulatory system, in particular

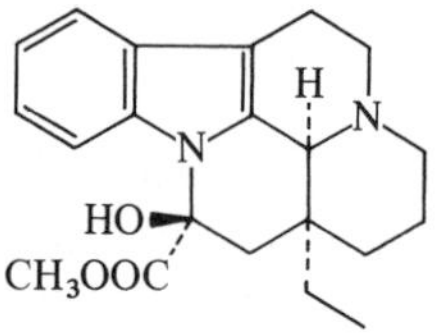

(1)

Vincamine

on cerebrovascular circulation (Szporny, 1976). Its therapeutic claims include the relief of symptoms of organic brain syndrome and the treatment of the symptoms consecutive to stroke (Witzmann and Blechacz, 1977). The typical daily therapeutic dose is 60 mg, orally.

In anesthetized rats, the effect of a dose of 2 mg/kg vincamine i.v. on arterial blood pressure develops in three phases. The first, a short-lasting drop in blood pressure due to a cholinergic effect, is followed by the second phase, an increase in blood pressure lasting 30 min, due to noradrenaline liberation. The third phase, starting after 40 min, consists of a long-lasting hypotension, probably related to noradrenaline depletion (Szporny and Görög, 1962). At doses of 50 mg/kg s.c., vincamine depletes adrenaline from the intestines and the suprarenal glands of the rat (Görög and Szporny, 1961).

The principal activity of vincamine justifying its use in geriatric patients is its effect on cerebral blood flow reported in animals and humans (Witzmann and Blechacz, 1977). In anesthetized dogs, Szporny (1976) demonstrated a decrease in total peripheral resistance and of resistance in the internal carotid artery, as well as an increase in brain oxygen consumption, after doses of 0.1–4 mg/kg i.v. Caravaggi et al. (1977) reported an increase in flow in the femoral and vertebral arteries of the dog. Furthermore, after ligation of the vertebral arteries of the dog, Rondeaux et al. (1972) showed an increase in cerebral blood flow using a rheoencephalographic method. Cahn and Herold (1972) found that vincamine increases cerebral blood flow and oxidative metabolism in dogs made hypocapnic by hyperventilation.

In monkeys *(Papio papio)*, Arfel et al. (1974) and Brailowski et al. (1975) found that vincamine increases blood flow in the brain and induces behavioral and electroencephalographic signs of increased arousal. In the rat, Quadbeck (1975) reported a reduction of electroencephalographic recovery after hypoxia. Similarly, Perrault et al. (1976) described a shortening of recovery time in the cat electroencephalogram after the production of transient ischemia by occlusion of carotid and basilar arteries. All these effects are observed after parenteral (mostly intravenous) administration of about 5 mg/kg vincamine.

At doses of 15 mg/kg i.p., vincamine enhanced survival time of mice subjected to hypobaric hypoxia (LINEE et al., 1977). In rats, 25 mg/kg i.p. appeared to partially reverse retrograde amnesia produced by hypobaric hypoxia (GOURET and RAYNAUD, 1976). This result, however, was not confirmed in studies of LINEE et al. (1977).

The arousing effects of vincamine, reported by ARFEL et al. (1974) in the monkey, might also be responsible for alterations of the sleep-wakefulness cycle. In cats and rats, DEPOORTERE et al. (1977) and DA COSTA et al. (1977) have reported that vincamine prolongs the duration of wakefulness at the expense of the sleep stages, in parenteral doses of 5–10 mg/kg. GLATT et al. (1978), however, found in the cat that an oral dose of 1 mg/kg tended to prolong rapid eye movement sleep.

Effects on brain monoamine metabolism have been reported only after high doses of vincamine. A short-lasting decrease followed by an increase in noradrenaline content, a weak decrease of serotonin content, and a prevention of the effects of iproniazid were reported after parenteral doses of 50–100 mg/kg (GÖRÖG and SZPORNY, 1961, 1962).

The primary action of vincamine, and a possible basis of its therapeutic effects in gerontopsychiatry, appears to be its well-documented ability to increase cerebral blood flow. Based on animal experiments, vincamine has also been suggested to influence brain metabolism which might be a consequence of its vascular effects.

II. Co-Dergocrine Mesylate

Co-dergocrine mesylate (Hydergine) is an ergot derivative and consists of a mixture of the methane sulfonates of dihydroergocornine, dihydroergocristine, dihydro-α-ergocryptine, and dihydro-β-ergocryptine in their natural ratio of 3:3:2:1 (Fig. 2). The

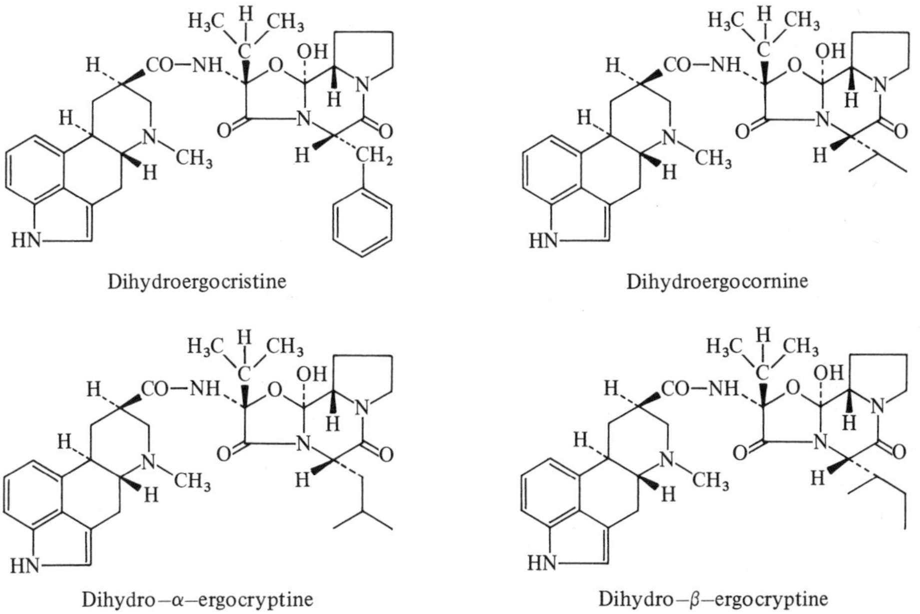

Dihydroergocristine

Dihydroergocornine

Dihydro−α−ergocryptine

Dihydro−β−ergocryptine

Fig. 2. Co-dergocrine mesylate (Hydergine)

various pharmacologic effects of ergot derivatives, in particular on the central nervous system, have been reviewed recently (Berde and Schild, 1978; Loew et al., 1978). Pharmacologic effects of co-dergocrine mesylate are seen on alpha-adrenoceptors, on serotonin and dopamine receptors, on the cardiovascular and central nervous systems, and on the uterus (Berde et al., 1980). In senile cerebral insufficiency, co-dergocrine mesylate at a daily dose of 3–4.5 mg p.o. reduces cognitive and emotional symptoms of organic brain syndrome (Venn, 1978; Fanchamps, 1979; MacDonald, 1980). Due to the multiple pharmacologic actions of co-dergocrine mesylate, the relationship between a pharmacologic effect and therapeutic efficacy is not fully established (Berde et al., 1980). In the context of the present review, effects on brain metabolism, synaptic transmission, and behavior are discussed.

1. Metabolic Effects

Studies with co-dergocrine mesylate on cerebral blood flow, recently reviewed by Loew et al. (1978), indicate that in animals with a normal cerebral blood flow, the evidence that co-dergocrine mesylate increases total cerebral blood flow is equivocal. In a series of experiments in cats subjected to oligemic hypotension, Gygax et al. (1975, 1976, 1978) measured cortical microflow and electrical energy of the electroencephalogram recorded from brain cortex. These authors found that, in contrast to vasodilators such as papaverine, co-dergocrine mesylate did not restore impaired microflow, but did increase EEG power that had been reduced by hypotension and also normalized cortical tissue pO_2 distribution (Wiernsperger et al., 1978). Thus, a metabolic effect was postulated which would result from an increased capacity of the neuron to maintain a functional steady state, even under conditions when its metabolic tolerance is limited (Meier-Ruge et al., 1975). Under various conditions of impaired brain function including oligemic hypotension (Gygax et al., 1978), temporary ischemia (Cerletti et al., 1973; Emmenegger et al., 1973; Perrault et al., 1976; Rossignol et al., 1972; Boulu, 1978), hypothermia (Emmenegger and Meier-Ruge, 1968; Emmenegger et al., 1973), respiratory arrest (Baldy-Moulinier and Passouant, 1967), and hypercapnia (Cahn and Borzeix, 1978), co-dergocrine mesylate increased the impaired electrical activity of the brain and, frequently, the supply of oxygen and energy-rich substrates to the brain cells.

In normal rats fed with 3.1–6.2 mg/kg co-dergocrine mesylate daily over 2 years, the concentration of cAMP in cortex and cerebellum was found to be lowered (Enz et al., 1975). In addition, an antagonism of noradrenaline-stimulated cAMP production was observed in rat cortex slices after treatment in vitro with 10^{-7} M co-dergocrine mesylate or after oral administration of 3 mg/kg per day for 3–6 weeks (Markstein and Wagner, 1978). This effect is possibly due to an α-adrenoceptor blocking effect in the rat brain cortex. Furthermore, an inhibition of cAMP phosphodiesterase, in particular of the membrane-bound fraction, was reported at concentrations of 10^{-6}–10^{-5} M. This effect appeared to be specific for the brain at lower concentrations (Iwangoff and Enz, 1973a, b; Iwangoff et al., 1975; Enz et al., 1978). In addition, maximal stimulation of cAMP-dependent protein kinase was abolished by co-dergocrine mesylate (Reichlmeier and Iwangoff, 1974).

Furthermore, activation of Na^+/K^+-adenosine triphosphatase, induced by noradrenaline, was inhibited by 10^{-5} M co-dergocrine mesylate in cat brain homogenates (MEIER-RUGE et al., 1975).

Direct effects on brain cell metabolism in vitro were reported by SAJI et al. (1978) and by NANDY and SCHNEIDER (1978a, b). In agreement with MEIER-RUGE and IWANGOFF (1976), HOSONO (1975) concludes that co-dergocrine mesylate acts directly on brain cells and allows the maintenence of brain metabolism under various pathologic conditions.

2. Synaptic Transmission

The interactions of co-dergocrine mesylate with brain neurotransmitters have been reviewed recently by LOEW et al. (1979a). At concentrations of 1–10 nM it displaces radioactive ligands from their specific binding sites in brain membranes in vitro and binds to receptors specific for noradrenaline and dopamine (GOLDSTEIN et al. (1978), LOEW et al., 1979a; VIGOURET et al., 1979). On the other hand, co-dergocrine mesylate inhibited cAMP elevations induced by noradrenaline in rat cortex slices (MARKSTEIN and WAGNER, 1978) and by dopamine in rat striatal homogenates (SPANO and TRABUCCHI, 1978). However, in the isolated rabbit retina, a stimulation of dopamine-sensitive cAMP was reported (SCHORDERET, 1978). After the intraperitoneal administration of 3 mg/kg to rats, an increase in cAMP of the striatum was observed (PORTALEONE, 1978).

In vivo, co-dergocrine mesylate reduced the content of 3,4-dihydroxyphenylacetic acid in the striate nucleus and that of 5-hydroxyindoleacetic acid in the cortex, and enhanced 4-hydroxy-3-methoxyphenylethylene sulfate (MOPEG-SO$_4$) in the brainstem of the rat (BÜRKI et al., 1978; HOFMANN et al., 1979; VIGOURET et al., 1978). These effects suggest a stimulation of postsynaptic dopamine and serotonin receptors. The elevation of MOPEG-SO$_4$ is related either to a postsynaptic blockade of adrenoceptors or to a facilitation of release of endogenous noradrenaline. Although no effects on brain dopamine or serotonin levels were seen, the neurochemical effects of morphine, haloperidol, and clozapine were antagonized (LOEW et al., 1976).

A number of functional studies support an effect on brain neurotransmission. Emesis observed in the dog (LOEW et al., 1978), the induction of contralateral turning in the Ungerstedt rat, the antagonism of the antinociceptive effect of morphine in the rabbit (VIGOURET et al., 1978), and a lowering of plasma prolactin levels in the rat (HOFMANN et al., 1979) are supportive evidence for dopamine agonist effects of co-dergocrine mesylate. In addition, like the dopamine agonists, L-Dopa, apomorphine, and bromocriptine, co-dergocrine mesylate partly reverses the behavioral changes induced in the rat by acute hypoxia (JÄGGI and LOEW, 1976). In contrast to dopaminergic stimulants, no motor excitation in animals is observed.

Co-dergocrine mesylate altered the sleep-wakefulness cycle of rats, as did 5-hydroxytryptophan (LOEW and SPIEGEL, 1976), and reduced the frequency of high voltage potentials induced by reserpine in the pons, lateral geniculate body, and occipital cortex of the cat (DEPOORTERE et al., 1975). As these so-called PGO-waves are under an inhibitory serotoninergic control (JOUVET, 1972), a reduction of their frequency is indicative of a serotonin agonist effect. As with 5-hydroxytryptophan, the effects of co-dergocrine mesylate on PGO-waves in the cat can be reduced by methiothepin administration, which is also consistent with an agonist effect at central serotonin receptors (Züger et al., 1978).

3. Behavior

Few behavioral effects have been reported in animals. Besides effects on rat behavior impaired by hypoxia (Jäggi and Loew, 1976; Boismare et al., 1978), an increased responsiveness to environmental stimuli was reported by Vigouret et al. (1978). In addition, experiments in rats acquiring reward-controlled behavior in a Lashley maze indicate that the effects of co-dergocrine mesylate on cognitive behavior may be dissociated from its action on motor function (Loew et al., 1979b; Jaton et al., 1979). At doses of 1–3 mg/kg s.c., administered once a day over 4 days of acquisition, co-dergocrine mesylate reduced the number of errors committed. This effect was independent of alterations in motor performance.

The results reviewed indicate that the pharmacologic basis of the therapeutic effect of co-dergocrine mesylate in gerontopsychiatry is probably its effects on brain cell metabolism and on brain synaptic transmission. An increase of cerebral blood flow has not been unequivocally demonstrated in acute animal experiments, but may occur as a secondary effect.

III. Piracetam

Piracetam is a derivative of γ-amino butyric acid and is considered to be the first representative of a new group of psychotropic drugs, a nootropic agent (Giurgea, 1972, 1976). A characteristic of nootropic drugs should be a selective action on integrative functions of the central nervous system, in particular on intellectual performance, learning capacity, and memory. Piracetam is given in an oral or parenteral daily dose of up to 10 g, which is the highest dosage of any gerontopsychiatric agent known. The therapeutic claims include organic brain syndrome and sequelae of acute head injury (Steginck, 1972; Dencker and Lindberg, 1977; Richardson and Bereen, 1977). Pharmacologic actions of piracetam are seen in neurophysiologic, metabolic, and behavioral investigations (2).

(2)

2–oxo–1–pyrrolidine acetamide
Piracetam, UCB 6215

1. Neurophysiologic Effects

The first recorded central effect of piracetam was a block of nystagmus provoked by electrical stimulation of the lateral geniculate body of the rabbit, observed after 2 mg/kg i.v. In doses of up to 3 g/kg, the agent had no other effects (Giurgea et al., 1967). At a dose of 45 mg/kg i.v., piracetam facilitated transcallosal evoked potentials in the cat provoked by homotopic cortical stimulation and recorded in the median suprasylvian gyrus (GIURGEA and MOYERSOONS, 1970). In addition, piracetam facilitated interhemispheric transfer of visual information (BURESOVA and BURES, 1972; GIURGEA, 1976) and facilitated "spinal fixation" in the rat (GIURGEA and MOURAVIEFF-LESUISSE, 1971).

2. Metabolic Effects

At doses of 100 and 300 mg/kg i.v., piracetam induced an elevation of ATP-turnover in the rat brain (GOBERT, 1972). This author assumes that piracetam increases "cell energy disponibility." During postanoxic recovery, 100 mg/kg i.p. accelerated restoration of ATP and DNA levels. In brains of aged rats, repeated administration of the agent rectified alterations in brain ribosome patterns, an effect not observed in young animals (GOBERT, 1972). A stimulation of ATP formation was also observed in liver mitochondria (PEDE et al., 1971). PLATT (1974) reported an increase of leucine incorporation into cerebral proteins and a decrease in activity of lysosomal enzymes. WOELK (1979) demonstrated that piracetam enhanced phospholipase-A_2 activity in neuronal and synaptosomal fractions of the rabbit brain and proposed a stimulation of synaptic transmission, mediated by a neurotransmitter. However, neurochemical investigations do not support this hypothesis. NYBÄCK et al. (1979) found that 5 g/kg piracetam i.p. elevated the content of metabolites of dopamine and noradrenaline in the rat brain. At the same dose, prolactin levels were enhanced. These authors postulate that piracetam blocks postsynaptic dopamine and noradrenaline receptors at high dose levels and resembles neuroleptic agents.

3. Behavioral Effects

Even at high doses of several grams per kilogram, piracetam is devoid of motor, autonomic, or toxic effects in normal animals (GIURGEA, 1976). However, a facilitation of learning in normal rats was observed at 30 mg/kg i.p. in a water maze (GIURGEA and MOURAVIEFF-LESUISSE, 1972) and at 100 mg/kg i.p. in a Y-maze and in a drinking test (WOLTHUIS, 1971). The same authors reported an improvement of learning impaired by age, alcohol, or repeated exposure to hypoxia (GIURGEA, 1976). Piracetam also protected newly acquired avoidance behavior against amnestic effects of anoxia and convulsive electroshock (GIURGEA et al., 1971; SARA and LEFEVRE, 1972).

Effects of piracetam on animal learning and protection from amnestic trauma occur at doses lower than that active in biochemical investigations. It has been proposed that the behavioral effects are related to the increase of intracerebral transfer of information, observed in neurophysiologic experiments, rather than to an effect on brain monoamine metabolism.

F. Concluding Remarks

In contrast to classic psychotropic drugs, gerontopsychopharmacologic agents have found their way into the treatment of cognitive and emotional symptoms of the elderly based on some defined pharmacologic action considered to be predictive of therapeutic efficacy in gerontopsychiatric patients. Typically, vasodilation is given as their main pharmacologic action, but an increasing number of agents are claimed to exert their main action on brain metabolism. As yet, the current theories on the causes of aging are of limited use for the creation of animal models for gerontopsychopharmacologic research. The models available derive mainly from external manipulations resulting in an acute breakdown of brain function. However, evidence is increasing that brain aging is related to a slow deterioration of synaptic neurotransmission, thus offering new possibilities for the development of new types of gerontopsychiatric drugs. It needs to be recognized that in patients suffering from organic brain syndrome or senile dementia, failure of cellular and synaptic function is more critical than alterations in the cerebrovascular system. New attempts at finding drugs with direct sites of action at cellular and synaptic effectors may lead to new gerontopsychopharmacologic agents with a more specific activity.

References

Ascheim, P.: Aging in the hypothalamic-hypophyseal axis in the rat. In: Hypothalamus, pituitary and aging. Everitt, B.J., Burgen, A.S. (eds.) pp. 376–418. Springfield: Thomas 1976

Arfel, G., De Pommery, J., De Pommery, H., De Larvarde, M.: Modifications de l'électrogénèse cérébrale suscitées par la vincamine. Rev. Electroencephalogr. Neurophysiol. *4*, 53–67 (1974)

Baldy-Moulinier, M., Passouant, P.: Modifications du débit sanguin du cortex cérébral par l'hydergine. C. R. Biol. (Paris) *161*, 2574–2578 (1967)

Ban, I.A.: Basodilators, stimulants and anabolic agents in the treatment of geropsychiatric patients. In: Psychopharmacology: A generation of progress. Lipton, M.A., DiMascio, A., Killiam, K.F. (eds.), pp. 1525–1533. New York: Raven 1977

Bartoli, G., Frandoli, G., Spreafico, P.L.: Langzeitbehandlung mit Yanthinol-nicotinat (Complamin retard) bei geriatrischen Patienten mit zerebraler Insuffizienz. Therapiewoche *27*, 575–585 (1977)

Benzi, G.: An analysis of the drugs acting on cerebral energy metabolism. Jpn. J. Pharmacol. *25*, 251–261 (1975)

Benzi, G., De Bernardi, M., Manzo, L., Ferrara, A., Panceri, P., Arrigoni, E., Berté, F.: Effect of lysergide and nicergoline on glucose metabolism investigated on the dog brain isolated in situ. J. Pharm. Sci. *61*, 348–352 (1972)

Berde, B., Schild, H.O.: Ergot alkaloids and related compounds. In: Handbook Exp. Pharmacol., Vol. 49, Berlin, Heidelberg, New York: Springer 1978

Berde, B., Schild, H.O., Weil, C.: Pharmacology and clinical pharmacology of hydergin. Berlin, Heidelberg, New York: 1980

Bessin, P., Gillardin, J.-M., Thuillier, G.: Pharmacologie générale du fénoxédil (ANP 3548). Nouveau vasodilateur cérébral. Eur. J. Med. Chem. Chim. Ther. *10*, 291–296 (1979)

Bijlsma, U.G., Funcke, A.B.H., Tersteege, H.M., Rekker, R.F., Ernsting, M.J.E., Nauta, W.Th.: The pharmacology of cyclospasmol. Arch. Int. Pharmacodyn. Ther. *105*, 145–174 (1956)

Birkmayer, W., Neumayer, E., Riederer, P.: Die larvierte Depression beim alten Menschen. In: Die larvierte Depression. Kielholz, P. (ed.) pp. 165–172. Bern: Huber 1973

Boismare, F., Le Poncin, M., Lefrançois, J.: Biochemical and behavioural effects of hypoxic hypoxia in rats: Studies of the protection afforded by ergot alkaloids. Gerontology *24*, Suppl. 1, 6–13 (1978)

Bondareff, W.: Histophysiology of the aging nervous system. Adv. Gerontol. Res. *1*, 1–22 (1964)

Boulu, R.G.: Effect of dihydroergotoxine on thalamic- and pyramidal-evoked responses in the cat under transient ischemia. Gerontology *24*, Suppl. 1, 139–148 (1978)

Bowen, D.M., Davison, A.N.: Biochemistry of brain degeneration. In: Biochemistry and neurological disease. Davison, A.N., (ed.), pp. 2–50. Oxford: Blackwell 1976

Brailowski, S., Walter, S., Vuillon-Cacciutolo, G., Serbanescu, T.: Alcaloides indoliques indui-sant on non un tremblement: Effects sur l'épilepsie photosensible du Papio papio. C.R. Soc. Biol. (Paris) *1969*, 1190–1193 (1975)

Branconnier, R.J., Cole, J.O.: The impairment index as a symptom independent parameter of drug efficacy in geriatric psychopharmacology. A double-blind study. J. Gerontol. *33*, 217–223 (1978)

Brody, H.: Organisation of the cerebral cortex; III: A study of aging in the human cerebral cor-tex. J. Comp. Neurol. *102*, 511–516 (1955)

Buerger, M.: Altern und Krankheit, Vol. 1. Leipzig: Thieme 1957

Bürki, H.R., Asper, H., Ruch, W., Züger, P.E.: Bromocriptine, dihydroergotoxine, methyser-gide, d-LSD, CF 25-397 and 29-712: Effects on the metabolism of the biogenic amines in the brain of the rat. Psychopharmacology *57*, 227–237 (1978)

Buresova, O., Bures, J.: Piracetam-induced facilitation of interhemispheric transfer of visual in-formation in rats. Psychopharmacologia *46*, 93–102 (1976)

Burnet, F.M.: Intrinsic mutagenesis: A genetic basis of aging. Pathology *6*, 1–11 (1974)

Buruina, L.M., Hadarag, H.E.: Modification of the brain's enzymogram of the pyrophos-phatase with age. Enzymologia *26*, 73–78 (1973)

Cahn, J., Borzeix, M.G.: Comparative effects of dihydroergotoxine (DHET) on CBF and me-tabolism changes produced by experimental edema, hypoxia and hypertension. Gerontol-ogy *24*, Suppl. 1, 34–42 (1978)

Cahn, J., Herold, M.: Pharmacologie des substances vasoactives cérébrales. Ann. Anesthesiol. Fr., Spécial 2, 185–191 (1972)

Garavaggi, A.M., Sardi, A., Baldoli, E., Di Francesco, G.F., Luca, C.: Hemodynamic profile of a new cerebral vasodilator, Vincamine and one of its derivatives, Apovincaminic acid ethylester (RGH-4405). Arch. Int. Pharmacodyn. Ther. *226*, 139–148 (1977)

Cerletti, A., Emmenegger, H., Enz, A., Iwangoff, P., Meier-Ruge, W., Musil, J.: Effects of ergot DH-alkaloids on the metabolism and function of the brain. An approach based on studies with DH-ergonine. In: Central nervous system – studies on metabolic regulation and func-tion. Genazzani, E., Herken, H. (eds.), pp. 201–212. Berlin, Heidelberg, New York: Springer 1973

Clemens, J.A.: CNS as a pacemaker of endocrine dysfunction in aging and its pharmacological intervention byv lergotrile mesylate. Interdisc. Topics Gerontol. *15*, 77–84 (1979)

Clemens, J.A., Fuller, R.W.: Chemical manipulation of some aspects of aging. In: Pharmaco-logical intervention in the aging process. Adv. Exp. Med. Biol. Roberts, J., Adelman, R.C., Cristofalo, V.J. (eds.), Vol. 97, pp. 187–206. New York: Plenum 1978

Cole, J.O., Branconnier, R.: The therapeutic efficacy of psychopharmacological agents in senile organic brain syndrome. In: Senile dementia: A biomedical approach. Nandy, K. (ed.), pp. 271–286. New York: Elsevier North-Holland, Biomedical Press 1978

Comfort, A.: The position of aging studies. Mech. Ageing Dev. *3*, 1–31 (1974)

Corrodi, H., Farnebo, L.O., Fuxe, K., Hamberger, B., Ungerstedt, U.: ET 495 and brain cat-echolamine mechanism: Evidence for stimulation of dopamine receptors. Eur. J. Pharma-col. *20*, 195–204 (1972)

Cotzias, G.C., Miller, S.T., Nicolson, A.R., Maston, W.H., Tang, L.C.: Prolongation of the life-span in mice adapted to large amounts of L-DOPA. Proc. Natl. Acad. Sci. USA *71*, 2466–2469 (1974)

Cotzias, G.C., Miller, S.T., Tang, L.C.: Levodopa, fertility and longevity. Science *196*, 549–550 (1977)

Cragg, B.G.: The density of synapses and neurons in normal, mentally defective ageing human brains. Brain *98*, 81–90 (1975)

Da Costa, L.M., Depoortere, H., Naquet, R.: Influence de la vincamine sur l'équilibre veille-sommeil du chat. Rev. Electroencephalogr. Neurophysiol. *7*, 158–164 (1977)

Davies, P.A., Maloney, A.J.F.: Selective loss of central cholinergic neurons in Alzheimer's dis-ease. Lancet *1976 II*, 1403 (1976)

Dekoninck, W.J., Collard, M., Noel, G.: Cerebral vasoreactivity in senile dementia. Gerontol-ogy *23*, 148–160 (1977)

Dencker, S.J., Lindberg, D.: A controlled double-blind study of piracetam in the treatment of senile dementia. Nord. Psykiatr. Tidsskr. *31*, 48–52 (1977)

Depoortere, H., Loew, D.M., Vigouret, J.M.: Neuropharmacological studies on Hydergine. Triangle 14, 73–79 (1975)
Depportere, H., Rousseau, A., Jalfre, M.: Action éveillante de la vincamine chez le rat. Rev. Electroencephalogr. Neurophysiol. 7, 153–157 (1977)
De Valois, J.C.: Increase in cerebral blood flow in the rabbit by Viquidil. Stroke 4, 218–220 (1973)
Domino, E.F., Dreu, A.T., Giardina, W.J.: Biochemical and neurotransmitter changes in the aging brain. In: Psychopharmacology: A generation of progress. Lipton, M.A., DiMascio, A., Killiam, K.F. (eds.), pp. 1507–1515. New York: Raven 1978
Duvoisin, R.C.: Antagonism of levodopa by papaverine. J. Am. Med. Assoc. 231, 845 (1975)
Eisdorfer, C.: Issues in the psychopharmacology of the aged. In: Psychopharmacology and aging Eisdorfer, C., Fann, W. (eds.), pp. 3–7. New York, London: Plenum 1973
Eisdorfer, S.: The effect of nylidrin hydrochloride (Arlidin) on the cerebral circulation. Am. J. Med. Sci. 240, 85–92 (1960)
Emmenegger, H., Meier-Ruge, W.: The actions of hydergine on the brain. A histochemical, circulatory and neurophysiological study. Pharmacology 1, 65–78 (1968)
Emmenegger, H., Gygax, P., Musil, J., Walliser, Ch.: Hydergine effects on the ischaemically disturbed EEG in the isolated cat head. Int. Res. Commun. System. Pharmacol. II, 7–10-4. (1973)
Enz, A., Iwangoff, P., Markstein, R., Wagner, H.: Die Wirkung von Hydergine auf die Enzyme des cAMP-Umsatzes im Gehirn. Triangle 14, 90–92 (1975)
Enz, A., Iwangoff, P., Chapuis, A.: The influence of dihydroergotoxine mesylate on the low-K_m phosphodiesterase of cat and rat brain in vitro. Gerontology 24, Suppl. 1, 115–125 (1978)
Epstein, L.J.: Anxiolytics, antidepressants, and neuroleptics in the treatment of geriatric patients. In: Psychopharmacol.: A generation of progress. Lipton, M.A., DiMascio, A., Killam, K.F. (eds.), pp. 1517–1523. New York: Raven Press 1978
Etienne, P., Gauthier, S., Dastoor, D., Collier, B., Ratner, J.: Lecithin in Alzheimer's Disease. Lancet 1978 II, 1206 (1978)
Fanchamps, A.: Controlled studies with dihydroergotoxine in senile cerebral insufficiency. In: Geriatric psychopharmacology. Nandy, K. (ed.). New York: Elsevier North-Holland 1979 (in press)
Fann, W.E., Wheless, J.C.: Effects of psychotherapeutic drugs on geriatric patients. In: Psychotherapeutic drugs. Usdin, E., Forrest, I.S. (eds.), Part I, pp. 545–565. New York: Decker 1976
Ferris, S.H., Sathananthan, G., Gershon, S., Clark, C.: Senile dementia: Treatment with deanol. Am. Geriatr. Soc. 25, 141–144 (1977)
Finch, C.E.: Catecholamine metabolism in the brains of aging male mice. Brain Res. 52, 261–276 (1973)
Gottfries, C.G., Roos, B.E., Winblad, B.: Monoamine and monoamine metabolites in the human brain post-mortem in senile dementia. Actuelle Gerontologie 5, 11–18 1874
Fontaine, L., Grand, M., Charbest, J., Szarvasi, E., Bayssat, M.: Pharmacologie générale d'une substance nouvelle vasodilatatrice, le naftidrofuryl. Chim. Ther. 3, 463–469 (1968)
Freyan, F.A., Woodford, R.R., Kety, S.S.: Cerebral blood flow and metabolism in psychosis of senility. J. Nerv. Ment. Dis. 115, 449–459 (1951)
Friedel, R.D.: Pharmacokinetics in the geropsychiatric patient. In: Psychopharmacology: A generation of progress. Lipton, M.A., DiMascio, A., Killam, K.F. (eds.), pp. 1499–1505. New York: Raven 1978
Geneviève, J.M.: Intérèt d'un nouvel activateur du métabolisme cérébral, le cyprodemanol, dans le domaine de la psychiatrie des vieillards. L'Encéphale 59, 90–95 (1970)
Giurgea, C.: Vers une pharmacologie de l'activité intégrative du cerveau. Tentative du concept noötrope en psychopharmacologie. Actual. Pharmacol. (Paris) 25, 115–156 (1972)
Giurgea, C.: Noötropic pharmacology of neurointegrative activity. Curr. Dev. Psychopharmacol. 3, 221–273 (1976)
Giurgea, C., Mouravieff-Lesuisse, F.: Pharmacologial studies on a elementary model of learning – the fixation of an experience at spinal level: Part I. Pharmacological reactivity of spinal cord fixation time. Arch. Int. Pharmacodyn. Ther. 191, 279–291 (1971)
Giurgea, C., Mouravieff-Lesuisse, F.: Effet facilitateur du piracetam sur un apprentissage répétitif chez le rat. J. Pharmacol. (Paris) 3, 17–30 (1972)

Giurgea, C., Moyersoons, F.: Differential pharmacological reactivity of three types of cortical evoked potentials. Arch. Int. Pharmacodyn. Ther. *188*, 401–404 (1970)

Giurgea, C., Moyersoons, F.E., Evraerd, A.C.: A GABA-related hypothesis on the mechanism of action of the antimotion-sickness drugs. Arch. Int. Pharmacodyn. Ther. *166*, 238–251 (1967)

Giurgea, C., Lefevre, D., Lescrenier, C., David-Remacle, M.: Pharmacological protection against hypoxia induced amnesia in rats. Psychopharmacologia *20*, 160–168 (1971)

Glasky, A.J., Simon, L.N.: Magnesium pemoline: Enhancement of brain RNA polymerases. Science *151*, 702–703 (1966)

Glatt, A., Krebs, K., Koella, W.P.: Influence of vincamine and piracetam on sleep-waking pattern of the cat. Biol. Psychiatry *13*, 417–427 (1978)

Gobert, J.C.: Genèse d'un médicament: Le piracétam. Métabolisation et recherche biochimique. J. Pharm. Belg. *27*, 281–304 (1972)

Godfraind, T.: Actions of sulocidil and of the Ca-antagonist cinarizine on the cat aorta. Arch. Int. Pharmacodyn. Ther. *221*, 342–343 (1976)

Godfraind, T.: Isoprenaline relaxation in vascular smooth muscle of aged rats. Effect of flunarizine. Arch. Int. Pharmacodyn. Ther. *230*, 331 (1977)

Godfraind, T., Kaba, A.: Blockade or reversal of the contraction induced by calcium and adrenaline in depolarized arterial smooth muscle. Br. J. Pharmacol. *36*, 549–560 (1969)

Goldstein, M., Lew, J.Y., Hata, F., Liebermann, A.: Binding interactions of ergot alkaloids with monoaminergic receptors in the brain. Gerontology 24, Suppl. 1, 76–85 (1978)

Görög, P., Szporny, L.: Effect of vincamin on the noradrenaline content of rat tissue. Biochem. Pharmacol. *8*, 259–262 (1961)

Görög, P., Szporny, L.: The depleting effect of vincamin on the cerebral serotonin level. Biochem. Pharmacol. 11, 165–166 (1962)

Gottfries, C.G., Roos, B.E.: Acid monoamines metabolites in cerebrospinal fluid from patients with presenile dementia. Acta Psychiat. Scand. *49*, 257–263 (1973)

Gouret, C., Raynaud, G.: Utilisation du test de la boîte à deux compartiments pour la recherche des substances protégeant le rat contre l'amnésie par hypoxie. J. Pharmacol. (Paris) 7, 161–175 (1976)

Granich, M.: Factors affecting aging: pharmacologic agents. In: Developmental physiology and aging. Timivas, P.S., Granich, M. (eds.), pp. 607–617. New York: Macmillan 1972

Gygax, P., Hunziker, O., Schulz, U., Schweizer, A.: Experimental studies on the action of metabolic and vasoactive substances in the brain. Triangle *14*, 80–89 (1975)

Gygax, P., Meier-Ruge, W., Schulz, U., Enz, A.: Experimental studies on the action of metabolic and vasoactive substances in the oligemically disturbed brain. Arzneim. Forsch. (Drug Res.) *26*, 1245–1246 (1976)

Gygax, P., Wiernsperger, N., Meier-Ruge, W., Baumann, T.: Effect of papaverine and dihydroergotoxine mesylate on cerebral microflow, EEG and pO_2 in oligemic hypotension. Gerontology 24, Suppl. 1, 14–23 (1978)

Hachinski, V.C., Illif, L., Zilkha, E., Duboulay, G., Marshall, J., Russel, R.: Cerebral blood flow in dementia. In: Cerebral vascular disease. Meyer, J.S., Lechner, H., Reivich, M. (eds.), pp. 75–78. Stuttgart: Thieme 1976

Harman, D.: Free radical theory of aging. Triangle *12*, 153–158 (1973)

Hauth, H., Richardson, B.P.: Cerebral vasodilators. Annu. Rep. Med. Chem. *12*, 49–59 (1977)

Hayflick, L.: The serial cultivation of human diploid cell strains. Exp. Cell Res. *25*, 585–621 (1961)

Heiss, W.D., Prosenz, P., Bruck, J.: Effect of proxazole on total and regional cerebral blood flow. Arzneim. Forsch. (Drug Res.) *23*, 772–775 (1973)

Heyck, H.: Der Einfluß der Nikotinsäure auf die Hirndurchblutung und den Hirnstoffwechsel bei Zerebralsklerosen und anderen diffusen Durchblutungsstörungen des Gehirns. Schweiz. Med. Wochenschr. *92*, 226–231 (1962)

Hofmann, M., Tonon, G.C., Spano, P.F., Trabucchi, M.: Mechanisms of dihydroergotoxine's effect on prolactin release. J. Pharm. Pharmacol. *31*, 42–44 (1979)

Hontela, S., Nair, N.R.U., Rosenberg, G., Schwartz, G., Guyda, H.: Bromocriptine: Effect on serum prolactin and growth hormone in psychogeriatric patients. J. Am. Geriatr. Soc. *26*, 49–52 (1978)

Horita, A.: Neuropharmacology and aging. Adv. Exp. Biol. *97*, 171–185 (1978)

Hosono, K.: Pharmacological studies on cerebral metabolism-activating drugs by tissue culture method. Acta Sch. Med. Univ. Gifu 23, No. 1, 1–44 (1975)

Hotovy, R., Enenkel, H.J., Gillissen, J., Jahn, U., Kraft, H.G., Müller-Calgan, H., Mürmann, P., Sommer, S., Struller, R.: Zur Pharmakologie des Vitamins B_6 und seiner Derivate. Arzneim. Forsch. (Drug Res.) 14, 26–29 (1964)

Hoyer, S.: Überlegungen zum Führen eines Wirkungsnachweises von Pharmaka beim organischen Psychosyndrom. Arzneim. Forsch. (Drug Res.) 28, (II), 2312–2315 (1978)

Hoyer, S., Oestereich, K., Stoll, K.D.: Effects of pyritinol on blood flow and oxidative metabolism of the brain in patients with dementia. Arzneim. Forsch. (Drug Res.) 27, 671–674 (1977)

Hühnermann, B., Felix, R., Wesener, K., Winkler, C.: Einfluß von Liquidil auf die Hirnzirkulation. Untersuchungen mit einem Szintillationskamera-Computer-System. Arzneim. Forsch. (Drug Res.) 23, 1074–1076 (1973)

Hühnermann, B., Felix, R., Wesener, K., Winkler, C.: Effect of papaverine hydrochloride on brain circulation. Studies using a szintillation-camera-computer system. Arzneim. Forsch. (Drug Res.) 25, 652–653 (1975)

Ingvar, D.H., Gustafson, L.: Regional cerebral blood flow in organ dementia with early onset. Acta Neurol. Scand. [Suppl. 43] 46, 42–73 (1970)

Iwangoff, P., Enz, A.: The brain specific inhibition of the cAMP-phosphodiesterase (PEase) of the cat by dihydroergotalkaloids in vitro. Int. Res. Commun. System. Med. Sci. 3, 1–9 (1973a)

Iwangoff, P., Enz, A.: Inhibition of phosphodiesterase by dihydroergotamine and hydergine in various organs of the cat in vitro. Experientia 29, 1067–1069 (1973b)

Iwangoff, P., Enz, E., Chappuis, A.: Inhibition of cAMP-phosphodiesterase of different cat organs by DH-ergotoxine in the micromolar substrate range. Int. Res. Commun. System. Med. Sci. 3, 403 (1975)

Iwangoff, P., Reichlmeier, K., Enz, A., Meier-Ruge, W.: Neurochemical findings in physiological aging of the brain. Interdiscipl. Topics Gerontol. 15, 13–33 (1979)

Jäggi, H.U., Loew, D.M.: Central dopaminergic stimulation and avoidance performance under hypoxia in rats. Experientia 32, 779 (1976)

Johnson, H.A., Ferner, S.: Neuron survival in the aging mouse. Exp. Gerontol. 7, 111–117 (1972)

Jaton, A.L., Vigouret, J.M., Loew, D.M.: Effects of hydergine and bromocriptine on maze acquisition in rats. Experientia 37, 38 (1979)

Jouvet, M.: The role of monoamines and acetylcholine-containing neurons in the regulation of the sleep-waking cycle. Ergeb. Physiol. 64, 166–307 (1972)

Kanowski, S.: The aging brain: Current theories and psychopharmacological possibilities. In: Neuropharmacology. Deniker, P., Radouco-Thomas, C., Villeneuve, A. (eds.), pp. 23–31. New York: Pergamon 1978

Karpati, E., Szporny, L.: General and cerebral haemodynamic activity of ethyl apovincaminate. Arzneim. Forsch. (Drug Res.) 26, 1908–1912 (1976)

Kase, M., Ono, J., Yoshimasu, N., Hiyamuta, E., Suginura, K., Ito, R., Hamasaki, K.: Effect of CDP-choline in experimental cerebral hemorrhage. Curr. Ther. Res. 16, 483–502 (1974)

Kent, S.: Neurotransmitters may be weak link in the aging brain's communication network. Geriatrics 31, 105–111 (1976)

Knoll, J., Fekete, G.: Symposium on pharmacology of vinca alkaloids. 2nd Congr. Hung. Pharm. Soc., Budapest 1974. Budapest: Akadémiai Kiado 1976

Kogure, K., Scheinberg, P., Matsumodo, A.: Catecholamines in experimental brain ischemia. Arch. Neurol. 32, 21–24 (1975)

Komarek, J., Cartheuser, C.: Der Effekt von Pentoxiphyllin, Xantinolnicotinat und Theophyllin auf das Kreislaufsystem, die myocardiale Dynamik und die linksventrikuläre Kontraktilität beim Hund im akuten Experiment. Arzneim. Forsch. (Drug Res.) 27, 1932–1942 (1977)

Komlos, E., Petöcz, L.E.: Pharmakologische Untersuchungen über die Wirkung von Benzyclan. Arzneim. Forsch. (Drug Res.) 20, 1338–1357 (1970)

Kukovetz, W.R.: Zum Wirkungsmechanismus von Benzyclan an der glatten Muskulatur. Arzneim. Forsch. (Drug Res.) 25, 722–726 (1975)

Laborit, H.: De la gériatrie à la gérontologie en passant par la biologie du comportement. Agressologie *16*, 203–217 (1975)

Lal, H., Pogacar, S., Daly, P., Puri, S.: Behavioral and neuropathological manifestations of nutritionally induced central nervous system aging in the rat. Prog. Brain Res. *40*, 129–141 (1973)

Lassen, N.A.: The luxury perfusion syndrome. Lancet *II*, 1113–1115 (1966)

Lassen, N.A.: Control of cerebral circulation in health and disease. Circ. Res. *34*, 749–760 (1974)

Lassen, N.A., Munck, O., Tottey, E.R.: Mental function and cerebral oxygen consumption in organic dementia. Arch. Neurol. Psychiatry *77*, 126–133 (1957)

Lawson, J.W., Manley, E.S.: Comparative cardiac effects of isoxuprine and nylidrin following administration of doses producing equivalent skeletal muscle vasodilation. Arch. Int. Pharmacodyn. Ther. *190*, 67–77 (1971)

Lee, T.C., Duerre, H.: Changes in histone methylase activity of rat brain and liver with aging. Nature *251*, 240–242 (1974)

Le Men, J.: Substances actives sur la circulation cérébrale et périphérique. Alcaloïdes indoliques et dérivés agissant sur la circulation cérébrale. Bull. Chim. Thér. 137–146 (1971)

Lempérière, T.: Cerebral protectors in psychogeriatrics. In: Neuropsychopharmacology. Deniker, P., Radouco-Thomas, C., Villeneuve, A. (eds.), pp. 59–65. New York: Pergamon 1978

Lewis, C., Ballinger, B.R., Presley, A.S.: Trial of levodopa in senile dementia. Br. Med. J. *1978I*, 550 (1978)

Linee, Ph., Perrault, G., Le Polles, J.B., Lacoix, P., Aurousseau, M., Boulu, R.: Activité protectrice cérébrale de la l-éburnamonine étudiée sur trois modèles d'aggression hypoxique aiguë. Comparaison avec la vincamine. Ann. Pharm. Fr. *35*, 97–106 (1977)

Lloyd, K.G., Hornykiewicz, O.: Occurence and distribution of aromatic ʟ-amino-acid (L-DOPA) decarboxylase in the human brain. J. Neurochem. *19*, 1549–1559 (1972)

Loew, D.M., Spiegel, R.: Polygraphic sleep studies in rats and in humans. Their use in psychopharmacological research. Arzneim. Forsch. (Drug Res.) *26*, 1032–1035 (1976)

Loew, D.M., Depoortere, H., Buerki, H.R.: Effects of dihydrogenated ergot alkaloids on the sleep-wakefulness cycle and on brain biogenic amines in the rat. Arzneim. Forsch. (Drug Res.) *26*, 1080–1083 (1976)

Loew, D.M., Van Deusen, E.B., Meier-Ruge, W.: Effects on the central nervous system. In: Ergot alkaloids and related compounds. Berde, B., Schild, H.O. (eds.), Handb. Exp. Pharmakol., Vol. 49, pp. 421–532. Berlin, Heidelberg, New York: Springer 1978

Loew, D.M., Vigouret, J.M., Jaton, A.L.: Effects of dihydroergotoxine mesylate (Hydergine) on cerebral synaptic transmission. Interdiscpl. Topics Gerontol. *15*, 85–103 (1979a)

Loew, D.M., Vigouret, J.M., Jaton, A.L.: Neuropharmacology of ergot derivatives. In: Dopaminergic ergot derivatives and motor function. Fuxe, K., Calne, D.B. (eds.), pp. 129–140. Oxford: Pergamon 1979b

MacDonald, R.J.: Hydergine. A review of 26 clinical studies. (to be published) (1980)

MacFarlane, M.D.: Possible rationale for procaine (Gerovital H-3) therapy in geriatrics: Inhibition of monoamine oxidase. J. Am. Geriatr. Soc. *21*, 414–418 (1973)

MacFarlane, M.D.: Procaine HCl (Gerovital H-3): A weak reversible fully competitive inhibitor of monoamine oxidase. Fed. Proc. *34*, 108–110 (1975)

McGeer, E.G., Fibiger, H.C., McGeer, P.L., Wickson, V.: Aging and brain enzymes. Exp. Gerontol. *6*, 391–396 (1971a)

McGeer, E.G., McGeer, P.L., Wada, J.A.: Distribution of tyrosine hydroxylase in human and animal brain. J. Neurochem. *18*, 1647–1659 (1971b)

McGeer, P.L., McGeer, E.G.: Enzymes associated with the metabolism of catecholamines, acetylcholine and JABA in human controls and patients with Parkinson's disease and Huntington's chorea. J. Neurochem. *26*, 65–76 (1976)

Markstein, R., Wagner, H.: Effect of dihydroergotoxine on cyclic AMP-generating systems in rat cerebral cortex slices. Gerontology *24*, Suppl. 1, 94–105 (1978)

Meek, J.L., Bertilsson, L., Cheney, D.L., Zsilla, G., Costa, E.: Aging-induced changes in acetylcholine and serotonin content of discrete brain nuclei. J. Gerontol. *32*, 129–131 (1977)

Meier, C.: Centrophenoxin – ein Geriatrikum mit neutroper Wirkung. Therapiewoche *23*, 3659–3660 (1973)

Meier-Ruge, W.: Experimental pathology and pharmacology in brain research and aging. Life Sci. *17*, 1627–1636 (1975)

Meier-Ruge, W., Iwangoff, P.: Biochemical effects of ergot alkaloids with special reference to the brain. Postgrad. Med. J. *52*, Suppl. 1, 47–54 (1976)

Meier-Ruge, W., Enz, A., Gygax, P., Hunziker, O., Iwangoff, P., Reichlmeier, K.: Experimental pathology in basic research of the aging brain. In: Aging. Gershon, S., Raskin, A. (eds.), Vol. 2, pp. 55–126. New York: Raven 1975

Meier-Ruge, W., Reichlmeier, K., Iwangoff, P.: Enzymatic and enzyme histochemical changes of the aging animal brain and consequences for experimental pharmacology on aging. In: Neurobiology of aging. Gershon, S., Terry, R.D. (eds.), pp. 379–387. New York: Raven 1976

Monagle, R.D., Brody, H.: The effects of age upon the main nuleus of the inferior olive in the human. J. Comp. Neurol. *155*, 61–66 (1974)

Nandy, K., Bourne, G.H.: Effect of centrophenoxine on the lipofuscin pigments in the neurons of senile guinea pigs. Nature *210*, 313–314 (1966)

Nandy, K., Lal, H.: Neuronal lipofuscin and learning deficits in aging mammals. In: Neuropharmacology. Deniker, P., Radouco-Thomas, C., Villeneuve, A. (eds.), pp. 1633–1645. New York: Pergamon 1978

Nandy, K., Schneider, F.H.: Effects of hydergine on aging neuroblastoma cells in culture. Pharmacology *16*, Suppl. 1, 88–92 (1978a)

Nandy, K., Schneider, F.H.: Effects of dihydroergotoxine mesylate on aging neurons in vitro. Gerontology *24*, Suppl. 1, 66–70 (1978b)

Noel, G.: Physiopathologie de la sénescence. J. Post. Univ. Gérontopsychiatrie, 29–38 (1975)

Nybäck, H., Wiesel, F.A., Skett, P.: Effects of piracetam on brain monoamine metabolism and serum prolactin levels in the rat. Psychopharmacology *61*, 235–238 (1979)

Obrist, W.D., Chivian, E., Cronquist, S., Ingvar, D.H.: Regional cerebral blood flow in senile and presenile dementia. Neurology (Minneap.) *20*, 315–322 (1970)

Olesen, J.: Methods for measurement of the cerebral blood flow. Acta Neurol. Scand. [Suppl. 1] *50*, 1–34 (1974)

Orgel, L.E.: The maintenance of the accuracy of protein synthesis and its relevance to aging. Proc. Natl. Acad. Sci. USA *49*, 517–521 (1963)

Pede, J.P., Schimpfessel, L., Crokaert, R.: The action of piracetam on the oxidative phosporylation. Arch. Int. Physiol. Biochim. Pharmacol. *79*, 1036–1037 (1971)

Perrault, G., Liutkus, M., Boulu, R., Rossignol, P.: Modification par l'hypoxie ischémique aiguë de la réponse cortico-pyramidale chez le chat. Application à l'étude des médicaments de l'insuffisance vasculaire cérébrale. J. Pharmacol. (Paris) *7*, 23–38 (1976)

Petrie, W.M., Ban, T.A.: Drugs in geropsychiatry. Psychopharmacol. Bull. *14*, No. 4, 7–19 (1978)

Phuapradit, P., Phillips, M., Lees, A.J., Stern, G.M.: Bromocriptine in presenile dementia. Br. Med. J. *1978 I*, 1052–1053

Platt, D., Hering, H., Hering, F.J.: Messungen lysosomaler Enzym-Aktivitäten sowie von Leuzin-Inkorparationsraten im Gehirn junger und alter Ratten nach Gabe von Pirazetam. Arzneim. Forsch. (Drug Res.) *24*, 1588–1590 (1974)

Plotnikoff, N.: Comparison of PMH (pemoline and magnesium hydroxide; Cylet) and pemoline activity after electroconvulsive shock. Arch. Int. Pharmacodyn. Ther. *184*, 175–185 (1970)

Popendiker, K., Boksay, J., Bollmann, V.: Zur Pharmakologie des neuen peripheren Gefäßdilatators 3,7-Dimethyl-1-(5-oxo-hexyl)-xanthin. Arzneim. Forsch. (Drug Res.) *21*, 1160–1171 (1971)

Portaleone, P.: Bromocriptine and hydergine: A comparison on striatal or hypothalamic adenylate cyclase activity. Pharmacology *16*, Suppl. 1, 207–209 (1978)

Post, F.: Dementia, depression and pseudo-dementia. In: Psychiatric aspects of neurologic disease. Benson, D.F., Blumer, D. (eds.), pp. 99–120. New York: Grune & Statton 1975

Prestige, M.C.: Axon and cells numbers in the developing nervous system. Br. Med. Bull. *30*, 107–111 (1974)

Price, G., Makinodan, T.: Aging: Alteration of DNA-protein information. Gerontology *19*, 58–70 (1973)

Prien, R.F., Cole, J.O.: The use of psychopharmacological drugs in the aged. In: Principles of psychopharmacology. Clark, N.G., Del Giudice, J. (eds.), pp. 593–606. New York: Academic Press 1978

Prien, R.F., Haber, P., Caffey, E.M., Jr.: The use of psychoactive drugs in elderly patients with psychiatric disorders: Survey conducted in twelve veterans administration hospitals. J. Am. Geriatr. Soc. 23, 104–112 (1975)

Quadbeck, G.: Rapport d'expertise sur l'influence de la pervincamine sur l'électroencéphalogramme du rat en anoxie. Méd. Pract. 571, 6–18 (1975)

Rao, D.B., Georgiev, E.L., Paul, P.D., Guzmann, A.B.: Cyclandelate in the treatment of senile mental changes: A double blind evaluation. J. Am. Geriatr. Soc. 25, 548–551 (1977)

Ré, O.: 2. Dimethylamino ethanol (Deaner). A brief review of its clinical efficacy and postulated mechanism of action. Curr. Ther. Res. 16, 1238–1242 (1974)

Reichlmeier, K., Iwangoff, P.: Influence of phosphodiesterase inhibitors on brain protein kinases in vitro. Experientia 30, 691 (1974)

Richardson, A.E., Bereen, F.J.: Effect of piracetam on level of consciousness after neurosurgery. Lancet 1977 II, 1110–1111

Robinson, D.S.: Changes in monoamine oxidase and monoamines with human development and aging. Fed. Proc. 34, 103–107 (1975)

Rondeaux, J.C., Dupont, M., Eyrand., Rondeaux, C., Aurousseau, M.: Etude comparative du rhéogramme cranien chez le chien normal ou soumis à un déficit circulatoire cérébral. J. Pharmacol. (Paris) 3, 289–308 (1972)

Rosner, J., Legros, J., Khalili-Varaste, H.: Meso-inosilol hexanicotinate induced protection against experimental anoxia and oedema. J. Int. Med. Res. 1, 13–14 (1973)

Rossignol, P., Boulu, R., Ribart, M., Paultre, C., Bache, S., Truelle, B.: Action de quelques médicaments de l'insuffissance vasculaire cérébrale sur les potentiels primaires somesthétiques evoqués au niveau du cortex et du thalamus chez le rat en état d'ischemie cérébrale aiguë. C.R. Acad. Sci. (Paris) Sér. D. 274, 3027–3029 (1972)

Roth, M.: The natural history of mental disorders in old age. J. Ment. Sci. 101, 281–301 (1955)

Roth, M., Tomlinson, B.E., Blessed, G.: The relationship between measures of dementia and of degenerative changes in cerebral gray matter of elderly subjects. Proc. R. Soc. Med. 60, 250–259 (1967)

Ryan, J.M., Ouada, G., Cristofalo, V.: Error accumulation and aging in human diploid cells. J. Gerontol. 29, 616–621 (1974)

Sacher, G.A.: On the statistical nature of mortality, with especial reference to chronic radiation mortality. Radiology 67, 250–258 (1956)

Sacher, G.A., Trucco, E.: The stochastic theory of mortality. Ann. N. Y. Acad. Sci. 96, 985–1007 (1962)

Saji, S., Misao, A., Kagawa, Y., Hosono, K., Sumi, Y., Omae, K., Yamada, H., Kunieda, T., Sakata, K.: Effect of dihydroergot alkaloids on experimental brain anoxia. Observations by tissue culture method and isolated perfusion method. Brain Nerv. 30, No. 1, 81–90 (1978)

Salzmann, C., Van der Kolk, B., Shader, R.T.: Psychopharmacology and the geriatric patient. In: Manual of psychiatric therapeutics. Shader, R.I. (ed.), pp. 171–184. Boston: Little, Brown 1975

Samorajsky, T.: Neurochemistry of aging. In: Aging and the brain. Gaitz, C.M. (ed.) New York: Plenum 1972

Samorajsky, T.: Central neurotransmitter substances and aging: A review. J. Geriat. Soc. 25, 337–348 (1977)

Samorajsky, T., Rolsten, C.: Age and regional difference in the chemical compositions of brains of mice, monkeys and humans. Prog. Brain Res. 40, 253–265 (1976)

Samorajsky, T., Strong, J.R., Sun, A.: Dihydroergotoxine (Hydergine) and alcohol-induced variations in young and old mice. J. Gerontol. 32, 145–152 (1977)

Samorajsky, T., Rolsten, C., Pratte, K.A.: Dihydroergotoxine (Hydergine) and ethanol-induced aging of C57BL/6J male mice. Pharmacology 16, Suppl. 1, 36–44 (1978)

Sara, S.J., Levèfre, D.: Hypoxia induced amnesia in one-trial learning and pharmacological protection by piracetam. Psychopharmacologia 25, 32–40 (1972)

Sathananthan, G.L., Ferris, S., Gershon, S.: Psychopharmacology of aging: Current trends. In: Current developments in psychopharmacology. Essmann, W., Valzelli, L. (eds.), Vol. 4, pp. 250–264. Spectrum 1977

Scholling, W.E., Clausen, H.D.: Langzeitbehandlung des neurovaskulären Psychosyndroms mit Trivastal. Med. Klin. 70, 1522–1527 (1975)

Schorderet, M.: Dopamine-mimetic activity of ergot derivatives, as measured by the production of cyclic AMP in isolated retinae of the rabbit. Gerontology 24, Suppl. 1, 86–93 (1978)

Seipel, J.H., Floam, J.E.: Rheoencephalographic and other studies of betahistine in humans: I. The cerebral and peripheral circulatory effects of single doses in normal subjects. J. Clin. Pharmacol. 15, 144–154 (1975)

Simpkins, J.W., Müller, G.P., Huang, H.H., Meites, J.: Evidence for depressed catecholamines and enhanced serotonin metabolism in aging male rats. Possible relation to gonotropin secretion. Endocrinology 100, 1672–1678 (1977)

Singh, S.N., Kanungo, A.: Alterations in lactate dehydrogenase of the brain, heart, skeletal muscle and liver of rats of various ages. J. Biol. Chem. 243, 4226–4529 (1968)

Smith, J.M., Bright, B., McCloskey, J.: Factor analytic composition of the geriatric rating scale (GRS). J. Gerontol. 32, 58–62 (1977)

Sokoloff, L.: Cerebral circulatory and metabolic changes associated with aging. Res. Publ. Assoc. Res. Nerv. Ment. Dis. 41, 237–253 (1966)

Soulairac, A.: Vigilor: Etude des actions psychiques et psychomotrice du fipexide. Gaz. Med. Fr. 30, 3547–3550 (1975)

Spano, P.F., Trabucchi, M.: Interaction of ergot alkaloids with dopaminergic receptors in the rat striatum and nucleus accumbens. Gerontology 24, Suppl. 1, 106–114 (1978)

Stegink, A.K.: The clinical use of piracetam, a new nootropic drug. Arzneim. Forsch. (Drug Res.) 22, 975–977 (1972)

Sun, G.Y., Creech, D.M., Sun, A.Y., Samorajsky, T.: Effects of ethanol and dihydroergotoxine on mouse brain myelin components. Res. Commun. Pathol. Pharmacol. 22, 617–620 (1978)

Szporny, L.: Pharmacologie de la vincamine et de ses derivés. Actual. Pharmacol. (Paris) 29, 87–117 (1976)

Szporny, L., Görög, P.: The effect of vincamine on the blood pressure of the rat. Arch. Int. Pharmacodyn. Ther. 138, 451–460 (1962)

Teubner, W.: Isoxsuprin (Vasoplex®). Literaturübersicht über experimentelle und klinische Ergebnisse. Fortschr. Med. 90, 517–521 (1972)

Thompson, L.M.: Cerebral blood flow, EEG and behavior in aging. In: Neurobiology of aging. Gershon, S., Terry, R.D. (eds.), pp. 103–119. New York: Raven 1976

Tomlinson, B.E., Blessed, G., Roth, M.: Observations on the brains of demented old people. J. Neurol. Sci. 11, 205–242 (1970)

Treff, W.M.: Das Involutionsmuster des Nucleus dentatus Cerebelli. In: Altern. Platt, D. (ed.), pp. 37–54. Stuttgart: Schattauer 1974

Van Nueten, J.M.: Comparative bioassy of vasoactive drugs using isolated perfused rabbit arteries. Eur. J. Pharmacol. 6, 286–293 (1969)

Van Nueten, J.M., Jansen, P.A.J.: Comparative study of the effects of flunarizine and cinnarizine on smooth muscles and cardiac tissues. Arch. Int. Pharmacodyn. Ther. 204, 37–55 (1973)

Vaughan, D.W., Peters, A.: Neurological cells in the cerebral cortex of rats from young adulthood to old age: an electron microscope study. J. Neurocytol. 3, 405–429 (1974)

Velkow, V.A.: Gerontological changes of ATP content and K^+Na^+ ATPase activity in rat brain. Folia Morphol. (Praha) 21, 345–347 (1973)

Venn, R.D.: Clinical pharmacology of ergot alkaloids in senile cerebral insufficiency. Handb. Exp. Pharmacol. 43, 533–566 (1978)

Vernadakis, A.: Neuronal-glial interactions during development and aging. Fed. Proc. 34, 1, 89–95 (1975)

Verzar, F.: Intrinsic and extrinsic factors of molecular aging. Exp. Gerontol. 3, 69–75 (1978)

Vigouret, J.M.: Altérations de la neurotransmission cérébrale avec la sénescence. In: Recherche Expérimentale et Investigations Cliniques dans la Sénescence Cérébrale. Lab. Sandoz-France (Ed.), pp. 9–36. Symposium à Bâle, 5.–6. juin, 1978

Vigouret, J.M., Bürki, H.R., Jaton, A.L., Züger, P.E., Loew, D.M.: Neurochemical and neuro-pharmacological investigations with four ergot derivatives: Bromocriptine, dihydroer-gotoxine, CF 25-397 and CM 29-712. Pharmacology *16*, Suppl. 1, 156–173 (1978)

Vigouret, J.M., Loew, D.M., Jaton, A.L., Markstein, R.: Actions des dérivés de l'ergot de seigle sur le système nerveux central. J. Pharmacol. (Paris) *10*, 4 bis, 503–515 (1979)

Wells, C.E.: Chronic brain disease: An overview. Am. J. Psychiatry *135*, 1–12 (1978)

Wiernsperger, N., Gygax, P., Danzeisen, M.: Corticol pO_2 distribution during oligemic hy-potension and its pharmacological modifications. Arzneim. Forsch. (Drug Res.) *28*, 768–770 (1978)

Wisniewski, H.M., Terry, R.D.: Morphology of the aging brain, human and animal. Progr. Brain Res. *40*, 167–186 (1973)

Witzmann, H.K., Blechacz, W.: Zur Stellung von Vincamin in der Therapie zerebrovaskulärer Krankheiten und zerebraler Leistungsverminderung. Arzneim. Forsch. (Drug Res.) *27*, 1238–1247 (1977)

Woelk, H.: Zum Einfluß von Piracetam auf die neuronale und synaptosomale Phospholipase-A_2-Aktivität. Arzneim. Forsch. (Drug Res.) *29*, 615–618 (1979)

Wolthuis, O.L.: Experiments with UCB 6215, a drug which enhances acquisition in rats: Its ef-fects as compared with those of metamphelamine. Eur. J. Pharmacol. *16*, 283–297 (1971)

Yasuhara, M., Naito, H.: Characteristic actions of CDP-choline on the central nervous system. Curr. Ther. Res. *16*, 346–347 (1974)

Yesavage, J.A., Tinklenberg, J.R., Hollister, L.E., Berger, P.A.: Vasodilators in senile de-mentias. A review of the literature. Arch. Gen. Psychiatry *36*, 220–223 (1979)

Zahniser, N.R., Chon, D., Hanin, I.: Is 2-dimethylaminoethanol (deanol) indeed a precursor of brain acetylcholine (Ach)? A gas chromatographic evaluation. J. Pharmacol. Exp. Ther. *200*, 545–559 (1977)

Züger, P.E., Vigouret, J.M., Loew, D.M.: Inhibition of reserpine induced PGO waves in the cat by ergot derivatives. Experientia *34*, 647–639 (1978)

CHAPTER 11

Experimental Behavioral Pharmacology of Gerontopsychopharmacological Agents

C. Giurgea, G. Greindl, and S. Preat

A. Introduction

"The trick is to die young but as late as possible."

ASHLEY MONTAGU

The above motto expresses the choice of the subject matter for this chapter. The authors are not going to discuss rejuvenating cures, nor elixirs or drugs claimed to be effective accordingly. Nor – other than incidentally – will the important scientific achievements in the knowledge of tissue, cellular, and metabolic age-related changes or possible drugs interactions at that level be dealt with. Those aspects of ageing are beyond the scope of this chapter and also beyond that of the authors' own competence.

Behavioral pharmacology is essentially, although not exclusively, CNS related; it will be viewed on the basis of a pragmatic experimental option: to manipulate and to facilitate efficacy of the CNS plasticity, which is reduced but still present in the elderly. The term "plasticity" – in the sense of KONORSKY (1967) – is one of the fundamental properties of the CNS: *Reactivity*, states KONORSKY, is the ability of the system to be activated, while *plasticity* is the capacity to change the reactivity as a function of previous stimulations. Homeostatic chronic adaptations and learning in the broadest sense of the word are typical examples of CNS plasticity.

In gerontopsychopharmacology, while taking advantage of any progress in fundamental research, the pragmatic option is to interfere essentially with concomitants of ageing. The basic and simple fact is that the elderly do retain mental capabilities, but that these are much too often partially masked by adverse economic, psychosocial, psychopathological, and physical factors.

A typical example of such factors is the psychosomatic vicious circle described by LEHMANN (1975). Severe or moderate psychiatric decompensations of the vulnerable aged CNS are usually induced by professional and social stresses as well as those caused by isolation from family and relatives. The resulting persistent negative affective responses of environment are in turn a source of stress. Stress impairs brain metabolism, usually by reducing demands on neurons, and decreases brain blood flow. These reactions aggravate the age-related enhanced loss of neurons; consequently, there is a further loss of noetic efficacy which reinforces, maintains, and somehow "justifies" the negative affective responses of and to environment.

Hence this cycle is self-perpetuating. Therefore intellectual and especially memory impairments may not be as inevitably associated with the ageing process per se as is generally believed (Jarvik et al., 1972; Kanowski, 1978). Intellectual performances are affected much more by illness than by strict chronological age on the basis of an equivalent genetic background. Moreover, humans, and in particular the elderly, show strong susceptibility to social factors.

Therefore, psychotropic drugs, together with other therapeutic tools, contribute to counteract at least partially the complex sociophysiopathological self-perpetuating destructive circle and consequently should help aged people to take advantage of undisturbed use of their mental capacities. If we cannot yet increase their years, we may, as Kass (1971) suggested, be able to help the elderly to enjoy their days.

Moreover it seems to be possible that a positive feedback or reinforcement such as success may even increase longevity in a given subject. In other words, and using the terminology of Kanowski (1978), the immediate pragmatic aim in this field is to look for "gerontotherapeutic" drugs, i.e., drug actions which help the elderly to compensate for some of their age-related deficits. Such drug effects may lead to "some sort of geroprophylaxis", i.e., causing the slowing down of intimate processes directly related to ageing. However realistic the possibility of gerotherapeutic intervention may be, even this is still a long-term aim.

It is easily understood that behavioral psychopharmacology faced with the task of dealing with extremely complex behavioral disturbances of the elderly certainly has difficulties in setting up appropriate analogue models in experimental animals for human ageing or the deficits occurring with human ageing. For example, one of the major problems for experimental behavioral pharmacology is whether or not old animals are the appropriate models. At first glance it seems obvious that the study of potential geropsychiatric drugs should be performed in old individuals. The problem is, however, much more complicated. Indeed, even laboratory standard animals are not, especially when old, a suitable, homogeneous population. A 2½- or 3-year-old rat is as old as Methuselah. Why is it alive when almost two-thirds of its congeners are dead? Moreover, most survivors have an individual differential pathological history which is ignored or unknown by the investigator. Some animals may be arthritic, others may have bronchitis or cardiac deficiencies. If an arthritic rat is given a performance task associated with lever pressing, the animal may fail simply because of his rigid and painful joints and not because of a brain deficit. Failure to perform a task may even be the result of a mixture of central and peripheral disturbances. Consequently it is impossible to ascribe the failure of one given individual to perform the task to deficits in some parts of the brain or to extracerebral forces. It is easily understood that such an attempt would be even more difficult using not a single individual, but a group.

For some tasks, an 8-month-old rat shows definite age-related deficits, while for others the animal has to be 14–20 months old. The same is true for higher mammalians such as rabbits, cats, and dogs. Moreover, the use of higher species in experimental gerontology and pharmacology is hardly suitable because of their long life-span (dogs, cats, and monkeys usually live more than 10 years). Thus, economic considerations have to be taken into account in order to make large-scale experimental gerontological studies feasible.

Accordingly, although of great value in particular experimental setups, old animals need not be exclusively used in psychogeriatric psychopharmacology. Relatively young adults in normal and/or deficient conditions are equally qualified for behavioral studies provided that two main requirements are fulfilled. First, in normal adults, parameters under investigation should be related to common psychogeriatric target symptoms such as mental fatigability (especially with accelerated rate of performance), memory retrieval failure, behavioral disinhibition, and homeostatic hypoplasticity, and to EEG and sleep pattern alterations. Secondly, if such deficits are induced in animals, they should mimic the usual concomitants of ageing in human beings such as cerebral hypoxia and ischemia, inhibition of protein synthesis, metabolic changes, and sociosensory deprivation.

Following these general considerations, this chapter will deal with experimental models relevant to behavioral psychogeriatry to be performed not only in old but also in young normal as well as in young animals made artificially behaviorally deficient.

Drugs will be referred to insofar as they are of potential clinical use, provided that sufficient data are available in the given experimental models. Since the nootropic drugs piracetam and etiracetam will often be mentioned, the concept of nootropics deserves definition: Nootropics form a class of CNS-active drugs whose functional direct impact is on the higher integrative mechanisms of the brain. They enhance the efficacy of these processes, there by producing direct improvement of mental, noetic functions.

The nootropic concept has been described in detail (GIURGEA, 1972, 1973). Consequently only the essential features of a nootropic drug will be mentioned (GIURGEA, 1978). A nootropic drug

1) Facilitates learning and enhances resistance to learning impairments from different causes [hypoxia, electroconvulsive shocks (ECS), chemicals such as 8-azaguanine].

2) Facilitates interhemispheric transfer of information (mainly across the corpus callosum, as assessed by electrophysiological and behavioral methods).

3) Enhances cerebral resistance, as demonstrated by other than noetic criteria (EEG, convulsions, pathology, survival), versus different noxious stimuli (hypoxia, high altitude, barbiturate and other chemical intoxications).

4) Induces even in very high dosages no significant behavioral (sedation or stimulation), electrophysiological (EEG: reticular or limbic excitability), or autonomic changes and is devoid of toxicity, even with long-term administration.

This unusual psychotropic profile is by no means an "animal" curiosity. Indeed, reliable, well-designed pharmacoclinical studies are now available that establish positive correlations with each of the four main features (GIURGEA and SALAMA, 1977).

The evident absence of interference of the nootropic drug with the functions of reticular formation of the brain, of the limbic system, or of other CNS functions detectable by the appropriate experimental methodology gives rise to the assumption that positive effects on learning or interhemispheric transfer or resistance to cerebral aggressions may be related to a certain degree to the functional telencephalic selectivity. The detailed mechanisms of such selectivity are still obscure, although it has been demonstrated that nootropic compounds such as piracetam readily pass physiological barriers such as the blood brain barrier and are able to enhance the energetic potential of the brain (GOBERT, 1972). Further, such compounds have a strong affinity to neuronal tissue,, especially to brain cortex and hippocampus (OSTROWSKI et al., 1975). More recently, NICKOLSON and WOLTHUIS (1976a, b) suggested that some of the nootropic compounds not only protect against hypoxia by activating brain adenylate kinase but also facilitate noetic functions by inhibiting the release of cortical proline.

Compounds such as hydergine, vincamine, and pyritinol which are generally accepted in geropsychiatry have also been included in the group of nootropic compounds (SALETU 1978; DOLCE et al., 1980; SALETU et al., 1980). Previously they have been referred to as cognitive activators (BARTUS, 1980) or antihypoxydotics (SALETU et al., 1980). Judged by their pharmacological profile, these compounds meet requirements 1 and 3 of the nootropic profile. Further, they have a high therapeutic index and low acute toxicity. They lack, however, the ability to facilitate interhemispheric connectivity.

The fact that a number of drugs most important for therapy of geriatric or gerontopsychiatric disorders meet, at least to some extent, the requirements of the nootropic concept seems to confirm that the notion underlying this may constitute an important strategy for the selection of compounds with possible gerontopsychiatric efficacy. Since at least a number of the important pharmacological properties of compounds belonging to this group can be demonstrated in young normal, young deficient, and in old animals, methods suitable for assessing their pharmacological profile in these three basic animals models will be described.

B. Studies in Old Animals

I. Life-Span Studies

Probably due to the economic and technical problems mentioned above, there are few studies that try to observe animals throughout their life-spans and to detect eventual drug effect of longevity. For the interested reader, three main sources of information are mentioned:

1) BERTHAUX and BECK (1975), in a general review, emphasize three lines of research: antioxidants and/or diets containing antioxidant ingredients; low-caloric diet; the attempt to enhance longevity in mice and rats by administration of psychoactive drugs such as meclofenoxate and its metabolite, the cholinergic substance DMAE (dimethylaminoethanol).

2) A possible correlation between alterations of the hormonal equilibrium and age has been reviewed by JARVIK and WILKINS (1978). The authors state that at present no conclusion about such correlation can be drawn from animal data. On the other hand, it seems clearly established that estrogens and extracts of the posterior pituitary are able to prolong life-span of rats, whereas treatment with androgens results in a shortening of life-span.

3) SEGALL and TIMIRAS (1976), in Long-Evans rats, demonstrate that survival is reduced in a group of animals on a tryptophan-deficient diet, while no significant effect is obtained with an excess of para-chlorphenylalanine (PCPA). Among other behavioral observations, it was seen that reproductive activity clearly decreased with age. This parameter should be taken into consideration when estimating a new potential psychogeriatric drug. The data, however, require replication since the number of rats per group was relatively small.

II. EEG and Evoked Potentials

Although electrophysiological changes are not necessarily correlated with behavior, these studies will be reviewed briefly because their results permit some correlation between EEG (electroencephalogram) and vigilance. Vigilance and its disturbances interfere with almost all behavioral parameters (SCHALLING et al., 1975; KANOWSKI and COPER, 1978).

In humans, age-dependent EEG changes occur. The most striking and constant finding is a slowing down of the rhythm, from a dominant frequency of about 10 cycles per second (cps) to 8 or 9 cps (OBRIST, 1972). The degree of reduced frequency is significantly correlated with general well-being and intellectual function, i.e., healthy and active old people show only minor deviations. This phenomenon seems to be significantly unrelated to concomitants of ageing, such as heart diseases (OBRIST, 1972). It also seems unrelated to intelligence and cultural level; a slowing down of the EEG dominant frequency is therefore likely to be an electrophysiological expression of brain ageing, presumably correlated with the concomitant reduction in vigilance and alertness.

Quantitative analysis of the EEG shows that decrease of the α-power spectrum is usually accompanied by an enhancement of slow waves and eventually of the occurrence of β frequencies (ROUBICEK et al., 1974; BENTE, 1977; ROUBICEK, 1977). DRECHSLER (1978) has described a progressive deterioration of the periodicity of occipital α-rhythm and a tendency to interhemispheric desynchronization with ageing.

Drugs like imipramine, pyritinol, hydergine, and piracetam were found to be effective as "stabilizers" of the ability to regulate vigilance in the elderly (SCHNELL and OSWALD, 1967; FÜNGFELD, 1970; KÜNKEL and WESTPHAL, 1970; FAIRCHILD et al., 1971; KANOWSKI, 1975; BENTE et al., 1978). The most recent general review concerning drugs and quantitative EEG, not necessarily in relation to age, has been published by FINK (1978).

Relatively few data are available on the influence of age on cortical evoked potentials. They seem, however, to be imparied in the elderly, thus indicating some alterations of the cortical signal processing (BECK et al., 1975). In this context it is interesting to note that drugs with a nootropic profile of pharmacology enhance interhemispheric functional connectivity both in man (DIMOND, 1975) and in animals (GIURGEA and MOYERSOONS, 1972; BURESOVA and BURES, 1973).

In animals, almost all studies using quantitative EEG measurements were done in young adults. For the sake of convenience they will be reviewed here rather than in Sect. D.

In the rat, ETEVENON et al. (1970) studied the EEG spectral analysis and ETEVENON and BOISSIER (1971, 1972) later applied quantitative EEG methods to neuropsychopharmacology. Since then, considerable progress has been made through the use of automated analysis of sleep patterns (KOHN et al., 1974; WINSON, 1976; JOHNS et al., 1977). On the basis of the advanced technique of EEG analysis DEVOS (1978) was able to develop a program for pharmacological studies and to describe the effects of several psychotropic drugs, including analeptics and antidepressants. Finally, LANDFIELD (1976) introduced a "three-dimensional approach" to the problem of studying the effects of analeptic drugs on different EEG patterns and memory in the rat.

In the rabbit, WILLINSKY (1974) studied the effects of cannabinoids on EEG by using power spectrum analysis. EFREMOVA and TRUSH (1973) investigated the chances of cortical power spectra in relation to the conditional reflex activity. Similar studies were done *in the cat* for amphetamine and barbiturates. GHERMANN and KILLAM (1975) described three qualitatively different drug-induced patterns in the EEG of *monkeys* using quantitative analysis. They differentiated barbiturates from nonbarbiturate hypnotics, meprobamate, and benzodiazepines and described further a specific pattern for chlorpromazine.

Presently, despite of obvious importance of this approach, pharmacological data on drug effects on the EEG of old animals are hardly available. It is, however, to be expected that research in this field will gain increasing importance, especially since old animals, like human beings, demonstrate a slowing of the EEG dominant frequencies.

III. Reactivity to Stress

Humans, like animals, respond to various stresses essentially in the same manner, i.e., by the so-called general adaptation syndrome (GAS) (SELYE, 1936). An important part of the GAS is the secretion of hormones, e.g., ACTH and cortisonelike substances.

Stress is related in many ways to ageing. One aspect is that it contributes significantly to the etiology and physiopathology of arterial hypertension, cardiac failure, and arthritis, diseases that are among the most usual concomitants of ageing (SELYE, 1970).

Another relation between stress and ageing is the reduction of homeostatic capacities in the old organism. It is generally assumed that the adaptability of homeostatic, regulatory processes decreases with ageing in man (LEHMANN, 1972) and in animals (VERZAR, 1957, 1963).

Thermoregulation has been studied by a number of authors. Thiss field of research seems important since it is known that there is a latent state of hypothermia in about 10% of human beings over 65. Moreover the lowered adaptive capacity of regulatory systems in the elderly may result in thermic decompensation caused by noxious stimuli such as drugs, disorders, affective stresses, etc. (EXTON-SMITH, 1964; FOX et al., 1973).

Whether or not old rats exposed to cold are able to maintain a stable central temperature when challenged with high or low environmental temperature is still controversial, probably because of the difference in the experimental approach. VERZAR (1957, 1963), for instance, described an age-related reduction of the thermoregulatory ability. On the other hand, COPER et al. (1978) using an experimental model based on an operant paradigm could not confirm an age-related instability of thermoregulation. However, general agreement exists that old rats subjected to cold are much more sensitive than young ones to decompensation by psychotropic drugs such as perazine, amphetamine, or phentolamine. This effect has been ascribed to a greater sensitivity of the receptors involved (ROMMELSPACHER et al., 1975; SCHULZE and BUERGEL, 1977).

Age-related changes in reactivity to drugs have been described by several authors. Chlorpromazine induced a greater hypothermia in old animals than in young, at the same brain drug levels (SAUNDERS et al., 1974). Older animals are more sensitive to morphine analgesia and to amphetamine-induced locomotor hyperactivity; they also need less hexobarbital than to young ones to suppress EEG activity (SAUNDERS et al., 1973). The authors conclude that an increase in CNS sensitivity appears to be an essential factor in this age-dependent effect. Age also interferes with an organism's ability to metabolize drugs. It is easily understood that changes in drug metabolism will interfere with an organism's reactivity to drugs to almost the same extent as changes in receptor sensitivity (BECK and VIGNALOU, 1975).

Resistance to more discrete metabolic stresses was studied in old animals. ADEL-MAN (1972) demonstrated that the maximal activity of a number of liver enzymes is not changed with increasing age. However, the organism's speed of responding to an enzymatic stimulus is significantly age-dependent delayed.

The above-reported and other existing data about the lowered adaptive responses to stress in old individuals point toward an eventual common neurochemical mechanism. Indeed there is strong evidence of an age-related decrease in the accumulation of dopamine in the CNS (particularly in the striatum) and in the norepinephrine turnover (FINCH, 1973).

This effect, together with other enzymatic age-related changes (MEIER-RUGE, 1975), results in desynchronized fluctuations in the activity of inhibitory and excitatory CNS mechanisms. These facts might contribute to a genetic and biochemical understanding of the decreased homeostatic capacities of the aged organism, which will become most obvious when exposed to stress. These neurochemical age concomitants, as well as reduced capacity for O_2 turnover and formation of ATP, might be the origin of decreased EEG activity; reduced locomotion, alertness, and short-term memory; also sleep impairment in the elderly (MEIER-RUGE, 1975).

IV. Learning and Memory

There are relatively few consistent studies available on age-dependent changes of cognitive functions of old animals. It appears that old animals generally do not exhibit learning deficits under all conditions of life and in all experimental situations. Like man, some old rats cope better with specific learning and memory tasks than do younger ones (JARVIK et al., 1972; LEHMANN, 1975; KRUSE and KOHLER, 1978), but as in man these findings are not consistent and reproducible in all individual organisms.

1. Thermic Decompensation

SCHULZE and BUERGEL (1977) and COPER et al. (1978) used a learning model to estimate the part of the higher nervous mechanisms that contributes to the thermic decompensation by a hypothermic drug to which old animals are particularly sensitive.

Animals were trained in a cold experimental chamber to press a lever in order to supply themselves with warm air. In such conditions, old rats will press more often and therefore will produce a higher room temperature than young ones. If treated with phentolamine, both young and old rats will increase lever pressing, thus maintaining a satisfactory ambient temperature.

Therefore it seems that old animals show a predominant peripheral neurovegetative disturbance which makes it difficult for them to thermoregulate in a cold environment and even more difficult when challenged with a hypothermic drug. Nevertheless, if appropriate conditions are available, they show good learning ability, which enables them to benefit from external heating facilities.

2. Passive Avoidance

KRUSE and KOHLER (1978) compared young and old rats in a passive avoidance task and in an active, shuttle-box avoidance task. They demonstrated that old Wistar rats (24 months) exhibit a "poor memory" under the conditions of the passive avoidance procedure but an "excellent memory" which is even better than that of younger animals when performing under the conditions of the shuttle-box task. Chronic treatment with a nootropic (piracetam, 350–400 mg/kg/day) did not affect the learning of young rats in either of the procedures. However, the poor performance of old rats in the passive avoidance task could be significantly improved by piracetam treatment. This finding again emphasizes the need for accurate models and control experiments in order to be able to assess a drug's effect in aged individuals.

Goodrick (1973) and others demonstrated the importance of the selection of the experimental procedure in gerontopsychopharmacology. They showed, for example, that old rats learn much better under massed trials than under the condition of distributed trials. Here again it becomes obvious that at least in the animal only certain abilities undergo changes with advancing age whereas other abilities are relatively age independent or may even improve with increasing age.

3. Appetitive Maze Learning

Nandy and Lal (1978) had mice perform a food-reinforced maze task followed by a reversal learning task. In terms of trials-to-criterion they found an age-related deficit of performance under their experimental conditions. This decrease in performance could be counteracted by chronic administration of centrophenoxine. The drug-treated mice also exhibited a reduction of lipofuscin pigments in the brain as compared to untreated animals. Further centrophenoxine treatment enhanced the life-span of these animals.

4. Conditioned Avoidance Response (CAR)

Nandy and Lal (1978) studied CAR in old rats and found reduced responses as compared to those in young rats. This model might be of use for pharmacological studies, but no data seem to be available as yet.

5. Short-Term Memory in Aged Monkeys

Bartus (1980) demonstrated that some cognitive functions of the rhesus monkey decrease with age. He used the measurement of response time as a model for short-term memory. He further showed that these age-related deficits could be improved by administration of physostigmine, piracetam, hydergine, vincamine, and centrophenoxine (Bartus, 1980).

6. "Threshold" Active Avoidance

Among the behavioral methods suitable for measuring age-related deficits, an active avoidance procedure based on the Randall-Selitto analgesic test has been proved to be most reliable (Greindl and Preat, 1971, 1976; Giurgea et al., 1978). In this test young adult Wistar rats (100–120 g, 1 ½–2 months old) are subjected to threshold determinations for pain produced by a standardized increasing, mechanical pressure on the hind paws of the animals. For this purpose Ugo Basile's analgesimeter is used. Retraction of the paw under pressure is considered as pain reaction and the pressure threshold expressed in grams is noted. A mean of two measurements (right and left hind paw) is noted for each rat as a "trial." Groups of a minimum of 10 rats are usually used, so that 20 determinations are averaged to give the basic threshold mean of the group (± 300 g). The individual dispersion at the first trial is very large, but if each animal is given two more trials with a 30-min interval, thresholds decrease highly significantly, dispersion is greatly reduced, and an analgesic drug can then be tested.

It has been assumed that rats retract the paws more quickly with each trial, i.e., with lower pressure, because they learn that a painful pressure will occur a few seconds after being placed in the analgesimeter. Consequently they anticipate the painful event and retract the paw more quickly. The validity of the hypothesis that this progressive decrease in threshold is due to a kind of active avoidance is based on several arguments:

1) There is an asymptote of learning, i.e., after three to four trials the threshold remains the same, independent of subsequent trials.

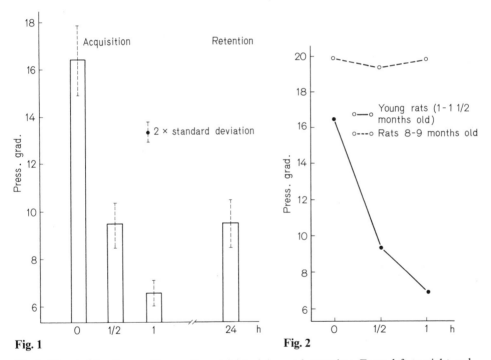

Fig. 1   **Fig. 2**

Fig. 1. Threshold active avoidance; three-trial training and retention. From left to right, columns show, before interruption, the mean thresholds (and standard deviations) determined three times (i.e., in three trials) at 30-min intervals ($n = 10$; many replications are available). Retention is seen as the mean threshold determined in the same group 24 h after training (after interruption). *Note: a* learning, seen as a progessive reduction in the thresholds, and *b* good retention 24 h later, when trained rats showed a clear-cut lower threshold than when they were naive

Fig. 2. Threshold active avoidance; age-induced impairment. (Ordinate and abscissa as in Fig. 1. Note that 8–9-month-old rats, trained in that way, do not show any tendency to learn ($n = 10$/group)

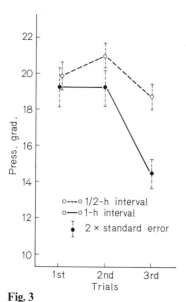

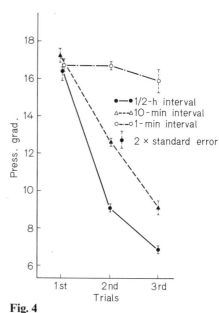

Fig. 3. **Fig. 4**

Fig. 3. Threshold active avoidance; ageing and "optimal" rhythm of learning. (*Ordinate* and *abscissa* as in Fig. 1, except that on the abscissa trials and not intertrial intervals are given; all rats were 8–9 months old ($n = 10$/group). Note that old rats show significant learning in the three-trial test if the intertrial interval is 60 min (●—●) instead of the regular 30 min (○---○)

Fig. 4. Threshold active avoidance; pessimal rhythm of training in young adults. (*Ordinate* and *abscissa* as in Fig. 1; all rats were 1–1½ months old ($n = 10$/group). Note the usual learning curve for the regular 30-min intertrial interval (●—●); significant learning, although impaired, is possible with an accelerated rhythm at 10-min intervals (△---△); no learning is seen with 1-min intertrial intervals, a much too accelerated pessimal training rhythm (○---○)

2) Twenty-four hours after a three-trial training there is excellent retention, as shown by the fact that the threshold is very close to the level reached at the end of the previous acquisition day (Fig. 1).

3) Learning of this particular active avoidance task is impaired by so-called amnesic interventions such as electroconvulsive shock (ECS) or protein inhibitors (see below).

This model is highly sensitive to ageing. Indeed, even 5–6-months-old rats show noticeable learning, retention, or retrieval impairment. However, a standard "old" population of 8–9-month-old rats is unable to "learn" under these conditions (Fig. 2). These so-called old rats are, however, not completely unable to learn under these experimental conditions. If the intertrial interval is extended as demonstrated in Fig. 3 they are able to "learn" at least to some extent. Since, however, young rats behave similarly when they are given shorter instead of longer intertrial intervals (Fig. 4), it is concluded that the "old" rats differ from "young" rats in that they need a slower rhythm of training.

This type of behavior seems to be related to behavior observed in humans of advanced age, i.e., a reduction of central nervous system plasticity. Insofar as intellectual

Table 1. Threshold active avoidance: drugs and old animals' pharmacological reactivity

Drug	Minimal dose[a]	Remarks
Deanol	17.8	
Dexamphetamine	> 1	Stereotypy and enhanced locomotion
Dihydroergotoxine	40	
Etiracetam	3.4	
Meclofenoxate	>200	
Methamphetamine	> 1.5	Stereotypy and enhanced locomotion
Pemoline-Mg	2.34	Enhanced locomotion
Piracetam	10	
Pyritinol	> 36.8	
Sulpiride	> 34.1	
Vincamine	35.4	

[a] The dose in mg/kg s.c. which enables old rats to show a significant acquisition pattern; note that > means the maximal dose used with a drug and that remained – as the lower ones – ineffective in this test. The given drug is then considered as inactive

functions are concerned, there is no doubt that the major concomitant of age is loss of speed depending on or generating a velocity decline in a series of fundamental biochemical reactions (JARVIK and COHEN, 1973; JARVIK and WILKINS, 1978). Consequently an experimental model permitting the measurement of speed of behavior or learning on the basis of a simple learning task seems to be a suitable tool for pharmacological studies.

Several psychotropic drugs which are said to be useful therapeutics in psychogeriatry are active in this methodological approach. Results are demonstrated in Table 1, and the activity of several drugs investigated is illustrated in Fig. 5. Table 1 and Fig. 5 demonstrate the high pharmacological sensitivity of the procedure. The active doses for some nootropic drugs are quite low as compared to those needed to demonstrate effects in other models (GIURGEA, 1976). Despite the sensitivity, this method is quite selective since in old rats only a few drugs are active.

C. Progeria Models

Several manipulations are claimed to accelerate normal ageing processes in animals. There are various rationales for such models:

1) To reveal critical changes (biochemical, subcellurlar, physicochemical) relevant to normal ageing.

2) To produce a relatively homogeneous population of accelerated geriatric subjects in which studies can be better programmed and followed than in spontaneous natural ageing.

3) To find drugs (or other tools) able to counteract the progeriatric manipulations, assuming that they will also be useful in natural ageing. Progeriatric manipulations may be physical, such as irradiations. or chemical in nature.

The approaches used by most of the available studies are either biochemical, morphological, or ontological. Among the studies using the biochemical approach is the dihydrotachysterol-increased glucose tolerance in rats which is accompanied by other

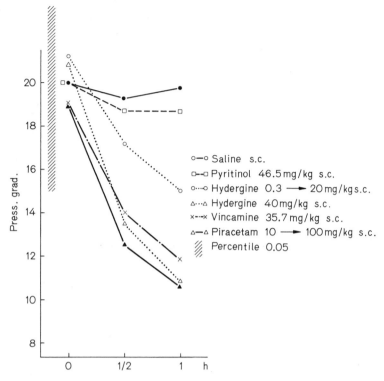

Fig. 5. Threshold active avoidance in "old" rats; 8 ½ to 9 months drug effects. Ordinate and abscissa as in Fig. 1; the percentile 0.5 is given for the first trial. Drugs or saline were injected subcutaneously ($n = 10$/group) 1 h before training. Note that pyritinol (46.5 mg/kg) is inactive, i.e., treated as control (saline) rats do not show any change in the thresholds with repeated, three trials. A weak effect is seen with the small doses of hydergine (0.3–20 mg/kg) while a clear-cut, highly significant learning is reached in rats treated with the high dose of hydergine (40 mg/kg) and of vincamine (35.7 mg/kg). Piracetam is active from 10 mg/kg. Old rats show, therefore, significant learning if they are treated, prior to learning, with an active compound

glucidic and calcium metabolism changes in the experimental animals (Schrieffer and Spratto, 1977). Morphological approaches are focussed for example, on accelerated lipofuscin accumulation in the brain of animals given a vitamin E-deficient diet (Puri et al., 1972). The rationale for this approach is that normal ageing in human beings is accompanied by increased lipofuscin deposits in the brain (Nandy, 1971). Another example is the use of the lathyrismlike lesions produced by chronic injections of β-amino-proprionitril (Bouissou et al., 1974). Ontological studies are usually focussed on measurement of life-span under certain conditions, for example, under a tryptophan-deficient diet (Segall and Timiras, 1976).

D. Studies in Young Adults

Studies in "Deficient" Animals. Here a persistent deficit – presumably related to concomitants of ageing or to ageing per se – is induced *prior* to the behavioral and/or electrophysiological investigation. Effects of treatment with CNS-active or other drugs is then evaluated either during the physiopathological manipulation and/or during the test procedure.

Studies in Standard Individuals. In these studies a deficit is induced which is contingent to the behavioral procedure. Drugs are administered to enhance in these young animals the efficacy of selected behavioral and/or electrophysiological functions that are known to be particularly age sensitive.

I. "Deficient" Animals

A great number of studies exist along this line. Here only those psychopharmacological models comprising behavioral and related parameters are commented on.

Three types of experiments are differentiated. Two of them *(brain ischemia and hypoxia)* are directly related to one of the most frequent concomitants of ageing, i.e., inadequate brain oxygen supply. This inadequacy is due to many causes which often coexist in the elderly: microinfarction, which might now replace the concept of atherosclerosis for the explanation of the causes of senile dementia (HACHINSKI et al., 1974); the consequences of sequelae of cerebrovascular accidents, pulmonary emphysema, and chronic bronchitis; cardiac insufficiency; atherosclerosis; enhanced platelet aggregability; impaired glucose utilization; and other deficient oxidative processes such as lack of physical exercise, etc. The third type of experiment involves deficits induced by a restricted *sociosensory environment.* Animal experiments along this line are relevant to psychogeriatrics since they mimic one of the concomitants of human ageing which occurs even in the relatively healthy elderly.

Indeed the aging subject is almost inexorably beset by increasing degrees of sociosensory deprivation (social and family disengagement, loss of relevant persons and responsibilities, reduced locomotion, etc.). One should also remember that simple sensory loss (e.g., visual and hearing troubles) may generate many of the behavioral changes in the elderly (BOTWINICK, 1975).

1. Brain Ischemia

Many studies are available in which a temporary brain ischemia is induced and recovery is measured by metabolic EEG or evoked potential parameters (MEIER-RUGE, 1975). Most of the pharmacological data are related to vasodilators or drugs such as hydergine, vincamine, and pyritinol. A typical paper illustrating this line of research is that of BOISMARE and STREICHENBERGER (1974) on the ergot alkaloids.

In curarized cats, brief carotid and vertebral occlusions block primary cortical evoked potentials for a few minutes after strangulation. Intracarotid, unilateral injection of the active compound significantly increases EPS recovery rate in the given hemisphere. Studies in hypercapnic, hypoventilated cats suggest that the protection seen with ergot alkaloid is due to a metabolic rather than a direct vasodilator effect.

Among the behavioral models for studying the consequences of brain ischemia is an experimental procedure in which both carotid arteries are ligated (GIURGEA and MOURAVIEFF-LESUISSE, 1978). The physiopathological changes induced by the bilateral carotid ligature are multiple and interrelated in temporospatial sequences that have not been sufficiently studied. Behavioral sedation and catatonia may suddenly change into myoclonic jerks and clonic seizures; various cardiac arrhythmic and respiratory

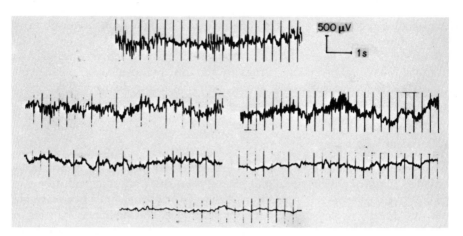

Fig. 6. Bilateral carotid ligation: cortical EEG recording. *Top:* EEG in a freely moving rat with electrodes implanted over the dura mater prior to carotid ligation. After this recording the rat was anesthetized, subjected to the procedure described in the text, and injected with saline. *Second row, left:* 8 min after ligation; EEG is still unchanged. *Second row, right:* 30 min after ligation; EEG shows frequent spindling while the rat makes no movement, apparently in inhibition of the righting reflex. *Third row, left:* 30 min later; righting reflex reappears; note important amplitude decrease in the EEG and some slow waves. *Third row, right:* 5 min later; the rat makes a first spontaneous movement and the EEG becomes much more flat. *Bottom:* 1 h later; almost isoelectric EEG. (Unpublished data of Mouravieff-Lesuisse)

irregularities are induced and most of the animals develop pulmonary edema and die within a few hours. Recently it has been shown that carotid ligated rats may at variable time intervals after the ligature develop an irreversible cortical flat EEG or an almost total electrical silence as demonstrated in Fig. 6. These electrophysiological experiments favor the assumption that bilateral carotid ligation in the freely moving rat may result in brain ischemia of various degrees. The principal available psychopharmacological data are shown in Table 2.

It is obvious that survival is increased by a great variety of drugs, presumably because they can interfere diversely and at various stages of the complex physiopathological syndrome induced by carotid ligatures. The model is therefore quite nonspecific, yet has potential previsional value for the initial phases in the search for new drugs.

2. Hypoxia

Three models of experimental hypoxia are reported (GIURGEA and MOURAVIEFF-LESUISSE, 1978): the "nitrogen" hypoxia and the "curarelike" hypoxia in mice (with DAUBY); the "catatoxic" model in rabbits (MOYERSOONS). Only the general schedule of the "catatoxic" model, i.e., the protection by a drug against a chemical intoxication, will be demonstrated in detail as a typical example for these types of studies. Figure 7 and Tables 3, 4, and 5 give effects of some drugs in the respective models. As in the ischemia studies, too many drugs are active to draw specific previsional implications from the hypoxia models.

Table 2. Psychotropic drugs and survival of rats, 24 h after bilateral carotid ligation

Drug	Dose (mg/kg i.p., $3 \times$)[a]	Survivors at 24 h	Activity[b]
Placebo	1 cm³–100 g	2/10	0
Atropine	34	3/18	0
Meclofenoxate	90	5/15	0
Chlordiazepoxide	3	4/15	0
Dexamphetamine	1.5	1/11	0
Dihydroergotoxine	3	13/18	+
Diphenylhydantoin	81	22/29	+
Deanol	28	3/16	0
Hydroxyzine	25	14/20	+
Metamphetamine	2.5	0/ 8	0
Piracetam	500	1/ 9	0
Etiracetam	54	11/17	+
Procainamide	200	26/36	+
Pyritinol	45	22/31	+
Sulpiride	110	3/22	0
Vincamine	3.5	0/ 9	0

[a] Maximal dose used
[b] Activity is established by the ratio between the number of survivors in drug-treated groups and in the placebo group; +, $p < 0.05$

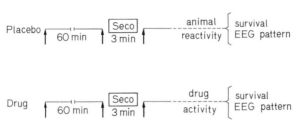

Fig. 7. Experimental schedule of the acute barbiturate intoxication; the "catatoxic" model: 33 mg/kg secobarbital in 3 min i.v. perfusion (rabbit). In rabbits preimplanted with cortical electrodes, drugs or placebo are given i.v. a suitable time (usually 1 h) before the secobarbital standard perfusion. Two rabbits are simultaneously run, one placebo treated and one drug treated. EKG is also usually recorded. Survival and EEG patterns are the criteria followed to assess drug activity. For details as well as for arguments relating this model to a hypoxic one, see Moyersoons and Giurgea, 1974

In two relatively recent studies the pharmacogenic changes of the brain's resistance to hypoxia are related to changes in brain biochemistry (BOISMARE et al., 1977) and to cognitive functions such as memory and learning (LINEE et al., 1977).

In spite of the obvious nonspecificity of both hypoxia and ischemia models one may tentatively admit that at least some gain may be derived for psychogeriatric pharmacology from these studies, provided that there is progress in terms of generality. This means that a compound should be active in all models and by different routes of administration and its effects should be well reproducible in each of the experiments. A further criterion is the intensity; that is, a compound has to have a low

Table 3. Psychotropic drugs and survival of mice in the nitrogen hypoxia model

Drug	Dose (mg/kg, p.o.)	Survival Placebo	Drug	Activity[a]
Atropine	34	5/40	2/40	0
Meclofenoxate	82	6/40	9/40	0
Chlordiazepoxide	11	5/40	4/40	0
Dexamphetamine	1	5/40	2/40	0
Dihydroergotoxine	15	2/40	6/40	0
Diphenylhydantoin	80	6/40	22/40	+
Deanol	28	5/40	6/40	0
Hydroxyzine	14	8/40	28/40	+
Metamphetamine	3	6/40	7/40	0
Piracetam	300	6/60	21/60	+
Procainamide	100	4/40	4/40	0
Pyritinol	46	7/40	23/40	+
Sulpiride	109	6/40	1/40	0
Vincamine	15	5/40	5/40	0

[a] Activity is established as in Table 2

N.B. Data referred here are taken out of many different experiments and selected to give a general image of the pharmacological reactivity of the model

Table 4. Psychotropic drugs and survival of mice in the curare hypoxia model

Drug	Dose (mg/kg, i.p.)	Survival Placebo	Drug	Activity[a]
Etiracetam	17	3/10	10/10	+
	0.17	3/10	7/10	0
Metamphetamine	0.6	1/10	7/10	+
Deanol	267	2/10	7/10	+
	89	2/10	3/10	0
Dihydroergotoxine	30	1/10	1/10	0
Vincamine	3	2/10	1/10	0
Hydroxyzine	1.4	1/10	7/10	+
Chlordiazepoxide	3.4	2/10	9/10	+
	0.34	3/10	2/10	0
Chlorpromazine	10	1/10	2/10	0
Imipramine	50	2/10	1/10	0
Procainamide	81	2/10	1/10	0
Meclofenoxate	29	2/10	8/10	+

[a] Activity is established as in Table 2

N.B. Data referred here are taken out of many different experiments and selected to give a general image of the pharmacological reactivity of the model

Table 5. Psychotropic drugs, survival, and EEG patterns in the acute barbiturate intoxication model

Drug	Dose (mg/kg)	Route	Activity		
			Survivors[a]	EEG patterns[b]	Conclusion
Placebo	1 cm³/kg	i.v.	2/10	0	Inactive
Meclofenoxate	50	i.v.	10/10	+	Active
Piracetam	19	i.v.	10/10	+	Active
	142	p.o.	9/10	+	Active
Pyritinol	100	p.o.	8/11	+	Active
Metamphetamine	2.5	i.v.	10/10	+	Active
Deanol	89	p.o.	10/10	+	Active
Dihydroergotoxine	0.03	i.v.	8/10	+	Active
Sulpiride	341	p.o.	4/10	0	Inactive

[a] Number of survivors, 30–60 min after secobarbital
[b] 0, long isolectric periods, very important EEG alterations; +, very important shortening of silences and more active EEG, similar to barbiturate sleep

minimal active dose and a large range of active doses and finally to compensate strongly the deficit under study. The third criterion is the therapeutic ratio; that is, a compound has to have a large gap between the minimal active dose and the doses producing side effects and/or death.

3. Sociosensory Deprivation

One of the usual psychophysiological deficits in the elderly is a progressive impairment of the central nervous system's inhibitory functions. Indeed, among common psychogeriatric symptoms one finds anterograde memory deficits, behavioral impulsivity, and distractibility. This might be partially related to the difficulty of forming new and stable memories, which is encountered with ageing. Even in relatively normal geriatric patients one might suspect a mild frontohippocampal-like syndrome. Moreover, on the basis of a large quantitative study, DRECHSLER (1978) concludes that with age, and especially in the dominant hemisphere, there is "a decrease of inhibitory cortical processes resulting in a spread of cortical excitability over the whole hemisphere" (op. cit. p. 212).

From this point of view, experiments with restricted sociosensory environment are of particular interest (MORGAN et al., 1975; GREENOUGH, 1976). This appears even more significant when one realizes that not only very young animals in a "critical period" but also adult individuals are sensitive to the minimization of their sensory, especially their social, universe (ROSENZWEIG, 1970). One might then compare behaviors of animals under such deprivations with the behaviors of elderly human beings under the influence of the inexorable sociosensory deprivation.

Particularly relevant from this point of view are the experiments of ROUSSEAU-LE-FEVRE (1977). Speculating upon her own and other authors' data on sensory-deprived rats, she tentatively attributes the behavioral induced symptomatology to a common factor, i.e., an impairment of the central inhibitory efficacy state that might be called "dys-inhibition." Only two aspects from ROUSSEAU-LEFEVRE's thesis which may also illustrate a possible nootropic "compensation" of this functional inhibitory "deficit" will be discussed here. For example, behavioral habituation to a sound was remarkably inconstant in young adults that were reared in a sensory-impoverished milieu. Piracetam (120 mg/kg i.p.) significantly increased retention over a few days of habituation. In a classic one-trial passive avoidance learning performance, the acquisition was excellent in both "impoverished" and "enriched" rats after 24 h, yet when tested again 96 h later, avoidance was almost completely absent in the impoverished group while still excellent in the enriched one. Nootropics such as piracetam (120 mg/kg i.p.) given to impoverished rats even once, before the second test, significantly enhanced maintenance of passive avoidance behavior.

If the passive avoidance behavior reflects a "memory trace" (or the memory trace availability), then nootropic drugs of the piracetam type are able to render this trace in the impoverished rats more stable or more available, at any rate less vulnerable to time decay. In other words, and within the limitations of the experiment, LEFEVRE showed that such drugs enhance the capability of deficient animals to form new, more stable memories. Other experiments showed that piracetam significantly compensated a learning deficit in sensory-deprived animals (MYSLIVICEK and HASSMANOVA, 1973)

These experiments demonstrated that it is possible to interfere by pharmacological means with the consequences of sensory deprivation. Thus they confirmed and enlarged previous studies which demonstrated that the brain weight gain and the enzymatic activity of the brain induced by an enriched environment in the rat are enhanced under the influence of amphetamine-type psychostimulants (BENNETT et al., 1973).

The fact that nootropic compounds of the piracetam type, that is, nonanaleptic drugs, are able to compensate for memory deficits in impoverished rats enhances the previsional psychogeriatric implications of both the drugs and the nootropic concept (GIURGEA, 1978). The influence of sensory deficits on behavior and cognitive functions was further demonstrated by experiments with environmentally impoverished rats subjected to changes in the external synchronizing signal (light-dark). These rats show typical impairments. For example, they follow the new "clock time" practically immediately but perform poorly in this respect. In other words, it seems that deprived rats lose a lot of their physiological autonomy, which results in a more pronounced dependence on environmental stimuli (WEYERS, personal communication). Biologically this can be considered as a kind of reversible regression not unlikely senile involution. WEYERS' experiments are, however, preliminary and deserve replication and further development.

II. Standard Young Adults

1. Preliminary Considerations

This section deals mainly with manipulations of memory in standard young animals by means of drugs. These manipulations are supposed, however, to be relevant for the aging organism too, inasmuch as drugs enhance CNS plasticity, which is impaired in the elderly. However, CNS low plasticity is not exclusive to the aged: is is caused as well by fatigue, illness, brain damage, etc. Amnesialike syndromes are common to cerebrovascular accidents (CVA), epilepsy, alcoholism, temporal lobe and hippocampal lesions, etc. Animal models in this field may consequently facilitate discovery of new drugs that will specifically enhance lability of memory processes, facilitating retrieval and counteracting the hypoplasticity syndrome common to so many brain dysfunctions, among which ageing is only one category.

In relation to memory, CNS hypoplasticity syndrome may be seen as difficulty in *retrieving*, i.e., disposing of memories that are readily available and adequate to environmental demands. Studies along this line, especially when aiming at previsional pharmacology, encounter at least two major difficulties. The first comes from the fact that for many, if not for most psychoactive drugs, we do not know the intimate mechanism of action, which is directly related to their eventual effect on memory.

The second difficulty arises because we infer from memory only by indirect estimations, i.e., through a behaving organism upon which the direct access of the experimenter is mainly on the level of motivation (hunger, thirst, pain, and, for human studies, verbal communication).

Behavior (latency and rate of responses, trials-to-criterion, and even electrophysiological events related to learning) is directly dependent upon engrams and the ability to retrieve them. However, a behavioral performance is also a function of motivational state, such as anxiety, perceptual capacity, locomotor abilities, and general level of cortical vigilance. It has been demonstrated that discrete electrical stimulation of the reticular formation (BLOCH, 1970) or of the hippocampus (McGAUGH and GOLD, 1976) under appropriate conditions facilitate learning and memory.

Most psychotropic drugs interfere in different ways with processes that modulate learning and memory, possibly directly or indirectly involving hippocampal pathways. Generally speaking, most drugs that impair learning are sedatives, while those that facilitate it are analeptics (McGAUGH, 1973; ALPERN and JACKSON, 1978). Apparently, nootropic drugs modulate memory without being sedative or stimulant, by possibly interfering directly with cortical vigilance (GIURGEA and SARA, 1978).

2. "Amnesic" Procedures

The reason for placing the word "amnesic" in quotation marks is that the literature is still controversial, especially when experimental paradigms assessing learning or retrieval disturbed by electroconvulsive shock such as the one-trial passive avoidance procedure are the variables of investigation. The most generally accepted position, however, is that electroconvulsive shock (ECS) interferes with adaptive integration of the learned material to previous knowledge and to environmental cues or, more simply, that ECS impairs memory by inducing a retrieval deficit and not a real amnesia (SARA and DAVID-REMACLE, 1974). If this is so, experimental models of this type should be related to experimental psychogeriatrics.

a) Physical Agents

The classic procedure is the passive avoidance, one-trial learning (step-through or step-down variants) in mice or rats. The general principle is that animals that received a painful shock in a specific part of a two-compartment cage will show retention (24 h later or more) by avoiding entry into the given compartment. If, however, contingent to learning, they are submitted to ECS or to other physical stimuli, such as hypoxia, a different situation will be encountered at the retention test. Most subjects will not

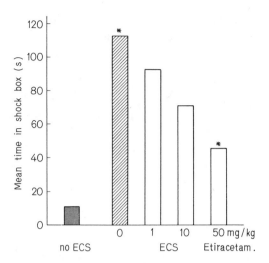

Fig. 8. One-trial, passive avoidance; etiracetam reversal of ECS-induced amnesia. *Ordinate*, mean time spent in the shock box at the retention test. Little time means good retention. Note that all non-ECS control rats *(black bar)* avoid the shock compartment 24 h after training. Rats subjected to ECS after training show amnesia *(striped bar)*. Rats treated with etiracetam (50 mg/kg, s.c.) 30 min prior to the retention test showed significant reversal of the amnesia (U = 40; n = 12.12; P<0.05); 1 mg/kg or 10 mg/kg had no significant effect. Similar results have been reported with piracetam (Sara and David-Remacle, 1974). (Courtesy of Giurgea and Sara, 1978)

avoid, thus showing that they either have really forgotten or that they have some difficulties in retrieving the experience from memory.

Many studies are available that have used drugs to counteract the *ECS-induced memory deficit*. As stated before, most experiments showed that analeptics, given in appropriate dosages at time-to-trial intervals, protect against ECS aggression. In the passive avoidance, nootropic drugs were found to be active against ECS-induced amnesia in rats submitted to the classic one-trial passive avoidance learning (GIURGEA, 1972). These findings were positively replicated by GOURET and RAYNAUD (1975) but not by WOLTHUIS (1971). However, SARA and DAVID-REMACLE (1974) found that the nootropic compound piracetam enhances recovery from ECS-induced amnesia when rats are exposed to training in the experimental environment. Another interesting finding was that the ECS-induced amnesia is prevented or reversed if the level of vigilance is increased during the retention test. This is obtained by injecting strychnine more than 23 h after learning acquisition, i.e., ½ h before the retention test (SARA and DAVID-REMACLE, 1977). Nootropic compounds (piracetam and etiracetam) are significantly efficient (Fig. 8).

The *active avoidance paradigm* is sensitive to ECS in the "three-trial" procedure. Contrary to old rats, in which no learning is seen, young adult rats show good learning and retention 24 h later. Learning is seen by a progressive threshold decrease, while retention is revealed by the fact that 24 h later most rats start performing almost at the level they reached at the end of the three-trial learning. If, however, ECS is applied 15 min after the last trial, retention on the next day is seriously impaired, i.e., the first

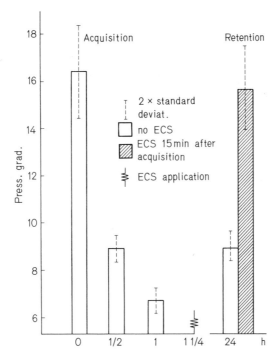

Fig. 9. Threshold active avoidance and ECS-Induced amnesia. See legend to Fig. 2. Note, as in Fig. 2, good learning in all rats ($n = 20$), as seen by the gradual decrease of the threshold. Half of the rats were then submitted to ECS (15 min after training); this is the group *(striped bar)* that showed amnesia (high threshold) when tested for retention 24 h after learning

threshold is high and relearning is required to reduce it (Fig. 9). Nootropic drugs (piracetam and etiracetam) protect against ECS-induced amnesia in a highly significant manner, as seen in Fig. 10. The *hypoxia-induced amnesia* as the ECS-induced amnesia strongly interferes with multitrial conditioned avoidance learning in the rat (GIURGEA et al., 1971). This has been demonstrated when animals were subjected to post-trial standard hypoxia sessions of 10-min-duration at 3.5% O_2 in a specially designed cage.

If the same procedure is followed, not immediately, but a few hours after a daily learning session of 30 min (delayed hypoxia), animals acquire normal CAR performances. Therefore, in those experiments immediate post-trial hypoxia acts as an amnesic agent and not as an unspecific, toxic one. Tolerance to hypoxia and conditioned performances under hypoxia were recently shown to depend on the central and peripheral "catecholamine status" of the animal (BOISMARE and LE PONCIN, 1978). Hypoxia-induced amnesia is equally observed in the one-trial passive avoidance learning in rats (SARA and LEFEVRE, 1972).

In both paradigms (multitrial active avoidance and one-trial passive avoidance), nootropic treatment is efficient in preventing hypoxia-induced amnesia (GIURGEA et al., 1971; SARA and LEFEVRE, 1972; MATTHIES and OTT, 1975; GOURET and RAYNAUD, 1976). Analeptic drugs protect against hypoxia-induced amnesia as they do in the ECS experiments (MATTHIES and OTT, 1975; GOURET and RAYNAUD, 1976).

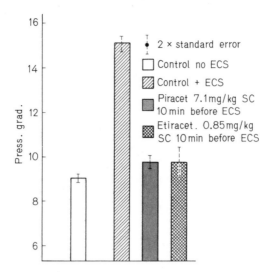

Fig. 10. Threshold active avoidance; ECS-induced amnesia is reversed by nootropics. See legend to Fig. 9, but only the retention test is shown here. ECS was supplied 15 min after training. *Note from left to right:* good retention in non-ECS group; nonretention in ECS-saline group; good retention in the ECS groups that received either piracetam or etiracetam 5 min after training

Hippocampal Seizures

It is generally agreed, that hippocampus and related limbic and frontal lobe structures play an important role in the ability to retrieve memories adequately to the environmental context (Lissak and Grastyan, 1957; Warrington and Weiskrantz, 1970; Isaacson, 1976). Little is done in previsional pharmacology in this field. However, Poschel (1977, personal communication) described a model related to the Korsakoff amnesic syndrome: Rats with electrodes implanted in the hippocampus are trained to run back and forth to obtain food pellets at either end of a special runway; in well-trained rats retrieval is blocked for about 10 min after noncontingent hippocampal seizures. Retrieval recovery was significantly speeded up by hydergine as well as by vincamine and piracetam.

b) Chemical Agents

Convulsants such as pentylentetrazol given even 7–8 h after learning (one-trial passive avoidance) were claimed to impair retention (Essman and Jarvik, 1961). However, the model seems insufficiently reproducible and is hardly ever used in previsional pharmacology.

Much more robust as experimental models, and also more closely related to psychogeriatric previsional pharmacology, are the studies in which memory impairment is provoked by interfering with *protein synthesis capacity* (synthesis inhibitors) and in which drugs are given to compensate the deficit. The fundamental rationales for studies along this line have been well discussed by Agranoff (1967), Barondes (1970), or Agranoff et al. (1978).

Generally, chemical interference with cognitive functions as an experimental model for psychogeriatry is of value provided that the basic mechanism of action of the given chemical compound is known. For example it has been shown that 8-azaguanine (8-AZA) interferes with the normal amino acid sequences in the newly formed RNA (DINGMAN and SPORN, 1961), while cycloheximide and other antibiotics are inhibitors of general protein synthesis (BARONDES, 1970). Further the administration of the intoxicating chemical substance should only interfere with the animals' cognitive functions without changing or deteriorating the animals' general behavior.

The psychogeriatric implications of these experiments are based on two groups of facts related to the biochemical memory concept of HYDEN (1967): In order to form new and stable memories the brain requires its optimal efficacy to synthesize correct RNA and proteins, Moreover, in man, as in other mammalians, there is an optimal age-dependent brain RNA functional efficiency, which decreases significantly in old individuals (GORDON, 1971). Thus age-related memory impairments might be at least partially due to the slowing down of RNA and protein synthesis turnover in the elderly. Consequently, drugs which compensate memory deficits due to protein synthesis inhibitors might be of use in psychogeriatric patients with memory deficits.

Behavioral previsional pharmacology in this field is insufficiently developed. The most conclusive results of our studies are that the threshold active avoidance procedure is sensitive to 8-azaguanine (5 and 10 mg/kg), cycloheximide (0.25 and 0.5 mg/kg) and streptomycin sulphate (25 and 50 mg/kg) and also the fact that piracetam among other compounds compensates the amnesic effect of all three inhibitors.

3. Memory-Related Psychophysiological Models

Two original approaches will be briefly presented in this section. Although the experimental subjects are young adult animals, these studies are theoretically relevant to behavioral psychogeriatric pharmacology because the functional cognitive deficit seems to be – at least from the behavioral point of view – strikingly similar to what is currently encountered in normal aged people. Indeed, normal aged people learn and perform relatively slowly. If they are "pushed," performance is poor, thus helping to maintain the psychogeriatric vicious circle. Studies on *"pessimal" rhythms of learning* are along this line. On the other hand, aged people are particularly sensitive to stress. One of the electrophysiological concomitants of stress is, as pointed out by GOLDSTEIN (1978), a relative degree of interhemispheric dysconnectivity. Consequently and whithin the framework of behavioral models relevant to geriatric psychopharmacology, the *"monolimb" input variant of the threshold active avoidance* might contribute an interesting model for pharmacological modulations of the brain's interhemispheric interactions.

a) Pessimal Rhythm of Learning

Within the framework of the Pavlovian classical learning it has long been known that dogs, even when well trained, do not support accelerated rhythms of conditional reflexes. The usual intertrial interval used by the Pavlovian school is of the order of magnitude of 5 min. Two-minute and especially one-minute intervals soon induce "supraliminal" inhibition or even neurosis (KUPALOV, 1952). This is true even for some nonmotivated conditional reflexes (CRS) involving direct cortical electrical stimulation for both unconditional and conditional stimulus (GIURGEA and RAICIULESCU,

1957; Doty and Giurgea, 1961). Therefore, impaired performances under pessimal rhythms seem to be intimately related to learning.

As shown in Figs. 3 and 4, a 30-min intertrial interval is already a pessimal rhythm in old rats, almost equivalent to a 1-min rhythm in young rats. We have considered that the psychogeriatric drugs listed in Table 1 might enhance the ability to cope with a higher rhythm of performance, i.e. to facilitate learning under "pessimal" speed and that, both in old and young individuals.

This was indeed the case when deanol, dexamphetamine, dihydroergotoxine, etiracetam, meclofenoxate, pemoline, piracetam, sulpiride and vincamine were given – in identical doses – to animals of both ages submitted to their respective "pessimal" speeds of learning.

b) Interhemispheric Transfer of Information
(the Threshold Active Avoidance Model with "Monolimb" Input)

Recently the possibility that the threshold active avoidance model may be of use to study the effects of drugs on the interhemispheric connectivity has been investigated. This new variant has been referred to as the "monolimb input," in analogy with monocular learning techniques (Buresova and Bures, 1976).

Wistar rats were tested using the "three-trial" variant of the threshold active avoidance paradigm. In this case, however, a "trial" consisted in the measurement of the threshold of only one paw, instead of both paws, as in the usual procedure. Therefore, only one paw was "trained." As illustrated in Fig. 11, after three successive trials at 30-min intervals, the threshold significantly decreased and the individual dispersion diminished, i.e., the paw "learned."

Subsequently the "naive" paw was tested either immediately ("immediate" transfer) or on the following day ("delayed" transfer). Figure 11 demonstrates that the "immediate" transfer is evident. Since it cannot be expected that it is the paw which learns, it can be inferred that during the monolimb input an interhemispheric transfer had occurred. The involvement of the corpus callosum in the immediate interhemispheric transfer was shown by the fact that callosotomy results in absence of this "immediate" transfer. As one might expect, the secondary engram is weaker and therefore more vulnerable to time decay, as demonstrated by the apparent absence of the "delayed" transfer (Fig. 12). As shown in Fig. 12 piracetam- and piritinol-treated rats preserve the "delayed" transfer in the same way as the control animals present the "immediate" transfer. These compounds therefore, when administered before retention test, enable retrieval of the weak, secondary, callosal-dependent engrams.

Another behavioral model is therefore available to study a callosal-dependent interhemispheric transfer of information, when initial learning takes place with unilateral, monosensorial ("monolimb") input. The last examples show that such models might be suitable for pharmacological research also. Moreover, relevant correlations can be observed between pharmacological results along this line. For example, piracetam was shown to enhance transcallosal EPs in the cat (Giurgea and Moyer-soons, 1972), callosal "writing-in" efficacy in the rat that learns through monocular input a visual discriminatory task (Buresova and Bures, 1976), and also to facilitate, in humans, verbal memory in a dichotic listening paradigm both in normal (Dimond, 1975) and in dyslexic subjects (Wilsher, 1979).

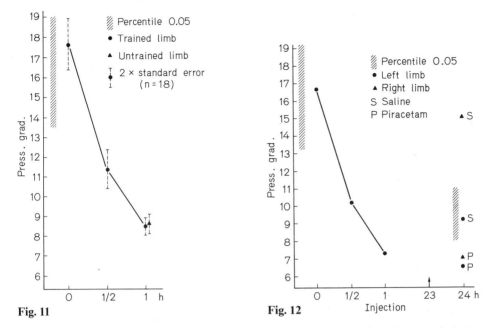

Fig. 11 　　　　　　　　　　　　　**Fig. 12** 　　　Injection

Fig. 11. Threshold active avoidance. Monolimb input immediate transfer. Ordinate and abscissa as in Fig. 1. Note that only one limb was trained (three trials) and that when the untrained limb was tested, it showed the same low threshold as the trained one. Immediate transfer is therefore present

Fig. 12. Piracetam retrieves "2delayed" interhemispheric transfer in monolimb learning of the threshold active avoidance Piracetam (28 mg/kg s.c.) or saline (S), given 1 h after the retention test which is performed 24 h after a three-trial learning with the left paw. *Retention test with the trained paw:* Saline group shows significant retention but piracetam group is significantly lower (improved retention). *Retention test with the untrained paw:* No retention in the S-group; "delayed" transfer is therefore absent. Note that a highly significant retention is seen in the piracetam-treated group, thus demonstrating that this drug is able to retrieve "delayed" transfer

E. Final Remarks

In the light of data and concepts presented in this chapter, behavioral, previsional, gerotherapeutic psychopharmacology appears to be a realistic, ongoing, therapeutic research purpose. Table 6 lists the main psychotropics drugs actually used.

However to date, no drug seems quite as beneficial as one would wish, either in clinical situations (LEHMANN, 1975) or in fundamental experiments. Indeed, most hormones respresented in Table 6 seem to enhance nonspecifically limbic vigilance by a moderate anxiogenic effect (FILE, 1978). Therefore, most studies agree that if a positive learning facilitation is seen (REISBERG et al., 1979), it is also usually accompanied by an extinction impairment of the learning material, thus somehow maintaining a behavior that is not longer adaptive (RIGTER and VAN RIEZEN, 1978). Various drugs, called "stimulants" in Table 6, do not form a homogeneous class: amphetamine derivatives, analeptics, cholinergic drugs like centrophenoxine, monoamine oxidase (MAO) inhibitors like procainamide, etc. Some of them have been shown to prevent lipofuscin accumulation in the brain (NANDY and LAL, 1978). Most of the stimulants

Table 6. Gerontopsychopharmacological agents

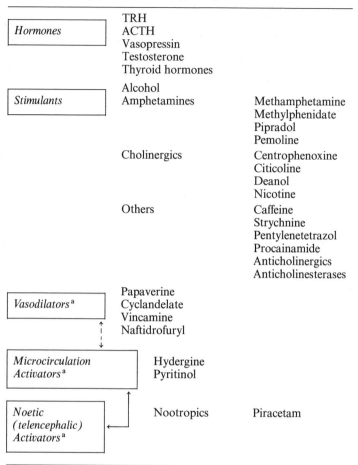

	TRH	
Hormones	ACTH	
	Vasopressin	
	Testosterone	
	Thyroid hormones	
	Alcohol	
Stimulants	Amphetamines	Methamphetamine
		Methylphenidate
		Pipradol
		Pemoline
	Cholinergics	Centrophenoxine
		Citicoline
		Deanol
		Nicotine
	Others	Caffeine
		Strychnine
		Pentylenetetrazol
		Procainamide
		Anticholinergics
		Anticholinesterases
Vasodilators[a]	Papaverine	
	Cyclandelate	
	Vincamine	
	Naftidrofuryl	
Microcirculation Activators[a]	Hydergine	
	Pyritinol	
Noetic (telencephalic) Activators[a]	Nootropics	Piracetam

[a] Synonyms: cognitive activators, antihypoxidotics metabolic drugs etc.

include the danger of tolerance and of state-dependent learning. They also provoke insomnia and REM alterations. Learning might be facilitated by weak doses but the safety margin to reach excitatory and dys-inhibitory side effects is usually rather narrow.

Cerebral vasodilators might produce a "steal"-effect, thus enhancing blood flow in normal rather than in ischemic brain areas. The brain glucose utilization impact of pyritinol or the glia-related microcirculatory mechanism of action of hydergine might be accompanied by a direct vasodilator effect (Ban, 1978, 1979). As for the nootropic approach more potent drugs than piracetam should be found. New openings are still expected in geriatric psychopharmacology. No specific geriatric antidepressant is yet available in spite of the clinical evidence of high incidence of depression in the elderly (Ban, 1978, 1979) which might be related to the experimental data showing a particularly elevated blood and brain MAO content (Robinson et al., 1972) in old animals.

In this context the suggestion of Lehmann (1977) for developing reliable, nontoxic euphoriants without disorganizing the vulnerable mental activity in the elderly is also to be considered. Further, drugs that increase the cortical vigilance in a specific way and are more potent than the existing nootropic drugs would be desirable. Anoxiosedatives that cause less impairment of mental faculties have yet to be found, as well as specifically designed neuroleptics for geriatric use.

From the experimental preclinical point of view, it seems evident that there is no single animal experimental model that will be able to assess the potential clinical value of neuropsychogeriatric drugs. This applies also to highly sophisticated techniques such as the quantiative electroencephalography. Only careful and competent evaluation by means of a relative large battery of models can be of previsional significance for this extremely complex field.

Acknowledgement. This work was partially supported by the Irsia Research Grant No. 2583.

References

Adelman, R.C.: Age-dependent control of enzyme adaptation. Adv. Gerontol. Res. *4*, 1–23 (1972)

Agranoff, B.W.: Agents that block memory. In: The neurosciences. A study program. Quarton, G.C., Melnechuk, T., Schmitt, F.O. (eds.), pp. 756–764. New York: Rockefeller University Press 1967

Agranoff, B.W., Burrell, H.R., Dokas, L.A., Springer, A.D.: Progress in biochemical approaches to learning and memory. In: Psychopharmacology: a generation of progress Lipton, M.A., Dimascio, A., Killam, K.F. (eds.), pp. 623–635. New York: Raven 1978

Alpern, H.P., Jackson, S.J.: Stimulant and depressant drugs effects on memory. In: Psychopharmacology: a generation of progress. Lipton, M.A., Dimascio, A., Killam, K.F. (eds.), pp. 663–675. New York: Raven 1978

Ban, A.Th.: Vasodilators, stimulants and anabolic agents in the treatment of geropsychiatric patients. In: Psychopharmacology: a generation of progress. Lipton, M.A., Dimascio, A., Killam, K.F. (eds.), pp. 1525–1533. New York: Raven 1978

Ban, A.Th.: Psychopharmacology in geropsychiatry: present and future. In: New frontiers in psychotropic drugs' research. Fielding and Effland (eds.), pp. 75–103. New York: Futura Publ. Comp. 1979

Barondes, S.H.: Cerebral protein synthesis inhibitors block long-term memory. Int. Rev. Neurobiol. *12*, pp. 177–205 (1970)

Bartus, R.T.: Animal models of age-related cognitive impairments. In: Abstracts of the 12th C.I.N.P. Congress (Götheburg), p. 72. Oxford, New York: Pergamon 1980

Beck, E.C., Dustman, R.E., Schenkenberg, T.: Life-span changes in the electrical activity of human brain as reflected in the cerebral evoked response. In: Neurobiology of ageing. (Advances in behavioural biology). Ordy, J.M., Brizzee, K.R. (eds.), Vol. 16, pp. 175–192. New York: Plenum 1975

Beck, H., Vignalou, J.: Pharmacocinétique des médicaments chez les personnes âgées. Thérapie *30*, 331–338 (1975)

Bennett, E.L., Rosenzweig, M.R., Wu, S.Y.C.: Excitant and depressant drugs modulate effects of environment on brain weight and cholinesterases. Psychopharmacology *33*, 309–328 (1973)

Bente, D.: Vigilanz: psychophysiologische Aspekte. Verh. Dtsch. Ges. inn. Med. 83. Kongress Wiesbaden, 17.–21.4. 1977. Schlegel, B. (ed.), pp. 945–952. München: Bergmann 1977

Bente, D., Glatthaar, G., Ulrich, G., Lewinsky, M.: Piracetam und Vigilanz. Arzneim. Forsch. *28/II*, 1529–1530 (1978)

Berthaux, P., Beck, H.: Etude critique des thérapeutiques du vieillissement. Thérapie *30*, 339–357 (1975)

Bloch, V.: Facts and hypothesis concerning memory consolidation. Brain Res. *24*, 561–575 (1970)

Boismare, F., Le Poncin, M.: Influence du blocage des enzymes de la chaîne des catécholamines centrales sur le réflexe conditionné du rat en hypoxie. J. Pharmacol. *9/1*, 45–62 (1978)

Boismare, F., Streichenberger, S.: The action of ergot alkaloids (ergotamine and dihydroergotoxin) on the functional effects of cerebral ischemia in the cat. Pharmacology *12*, 152–159 (1974)

Boismare, F., Le Poncin, M., Lefrançois, J., Marchand, J.C.: Biochemical and behavioral disturbances induced by hypoxic hypoxia in rats. Acta Neurol. Scand. (suppl.) *56*, 64 (1977)

Botwinick, J.: Behavioural processes. In: Ageing. Gershon, S., Raskin, A. (eds.), Vol. 2, pp. 1–18. New York: Raven 1975

Bouissou, H., Pieraggi, M.T., Julian, M.: Chronic lathyrism and experimental model of the ageing of human connective tissue. Experientia *30/2*, 210 (1974)

Buresova, O., Bures, J.: Mechanisms of interhemispheric transfer of visual information in rats. Acta Neurobiol. Exp. *33*, 673–688 (1973)

Buresova, O., Bures, J.: Piracetam-induced facilitation of interhemispheric transfer of visual information in rats. Psychopharmacologia (Berl.) *46/1*, 93–102 (1976)

Coper, H., Schulze, G., Bürgel, P.: Thermoregulation as a model in geriatric neuropsychopharmacology. In: Neuro-psychopharmacology. Deniker, P., Radouco-Thomas, C., Villeneuve, A. (eds.), Vol. 2, pp. 1661–1667. Oxford, New York: Pergamon 1978

Devos, J.E.: Evolution temporelle du signal électroencéphalographique. Applications en pharmacologie. Encéphale *4*, 267–279 (1978)

Dimond, S.J.: Use of a nootropic substance to increase the capacity for verbal learning and memory in normal man. In: Therapy in psychosomatic medicine, Vol. 3, Pharmacotherapeutic Tribune. Proceedings of the 3rd Congress of the international college of psychosomatic medicine, Rome, September 16–20 (1975), pp. 752–755. Roma: Edizioni Pozzi, L. 1977

Dingman, W., Sporn, M.B.: The incorporation of 8-azaguanine into rat brain RNA and its effect on maze-learning by the rat: an inquiry into the biochemical basis of memory. J. Psychiatr. Res. *1*, 1–11 (1961)

Dolce, G., Celloni, V., Cruccu, G., Zamponi, A.: Effect of a nootropic drug in patients affected by hemiplegia after stroke during rehabilitation treatment. In: Abstracts of the 12th C.I.N.P. congress (Götheburg), p. 308. Oxford, New York: Pergamon 1980

Doty, R.W., Giurgea, C.: Conditioned reflexes established by coupling electrical excitation of two cortical areas. In: Brain mechanisms and learning. Delafresnoy, J.F. (ed.), pp. 133–151. Oxford: Blackwell (1961

Drechsler, F.: Quantitative analysis of neurophysiological processes of the aging CNS. N. Neurol. *218*, 197–213 (1978)

Efremova, T.M., Trush, V.D.: Power spectra of cortical electric activity in the rabbit in relation to conditioned reflexes. Acta Neurobiol. Exp. *33*, 743–755 (1973)

Essman, W.B., Jarwik, M.E.: Impairment of retention for a conditioned response by ether anesthesia in mice. Psychopharmacology *2*, 172 (1961)

Etevenon, P., Boissier, J.R.: Statistical amplitude analysis of the integrated electrocorticogram of unrestrained rats before and after prochlorpromazine. Neuropharmacology *10*, 161–179 (1971)

Etevenon, P., Boissier, J.R.: Quantitative and computer EEG analysis in animal neuropharmacology. Psychopharmacology *26*, 10 (1972)

Etevenon, P., Kitten, G., de Barbeyrac, J., Goldberg, P.: Analyse de l'EEG du rat. Application en psychopharmacologie d'un programme de spectre moyen de puissance et du calcul de nouvelles données Spectrales caractéristiques. J. Pharmacol. *1/3*, 383–394 (1970)

Exton-Smith, A.N.: Accidental hypothermia in the elderly. Brit. Med. J. *II*, 1255–1258 (1964)

Fairchild, M.D., Jenden, D.J., Mickey, M.R.: Quantitative analysis of some drugs effects on the EEG by long-term frequency analysis. Proc. West. Pharmacol. Soc. *14*, 135–140 (1971)

File, S.E.: Anxiety, ACTH, and 5-HT. Trends in Neurosciences *1*, 9–11 (1978)

Finch, C.E.: Catecholamine metabolism in the brains of aging male mice. Brain Res. *52*, 261–276 (1973)

Fink, M.: Psychoactive drugs and the waking EEG, 1966–1976. In: Psychopharmacology: a generation of progress. Lipton, M.A., Dimascio, A., Killam, K.F. (eds.), pp. 691–698. New York: Raven 1978

Fox, R.H., Woodward, P.M., Exton-Smith, A.N., Green, M.F., Donnison, M.H.: Body temperatures in the elderly, A national study of physiological, social and environmental conditions. Brit. Med. J. *1*, 200–206 (1973)

Füngfeld, E.W.: Ergebnisse medikamentöser Therapie bei älteren Patienten mit cerebral organischen Störungen. Nervenarzt *41*, 352–354 (1970)

Ghermann, J.E., Killam, K.F.: Characterization of EEG effects produced by sedative-hypnotic agents using spectral analysis techniques. Fed. Proc. *34/3*, 779 (1975)

Giurgea, C.: Vers une pharmacologie de l'activité intégrative du cerveau. Tentative du concept nootrope en psychopharmacologie. Actual. Pharmacol. (Paris) *25*, 115–157 (1972)

Giurgea, C.: The "Nootropic" approach to the pharmacology of the integrative activity of the brain. Conditional Reflex *8/2*, 108–115 (1973)

Giurgea, C.: Piracetam; Nootropic pharmacology of neurointegrative activity. In: Current developments in psychopharmacology. Essman, W.B., Valzelli, L. (eds.), Vol. III, pp. 223–273. New York: Spectrum Publications 1976

Giurgea, C.: The pharmacology of nootropic drugs: Geropsychiatric implications. In: Neuropsychopharmacology. Deniker, P., Radouco-Thomas, C., Willeneuve, A. (eds.), Vol. I, pp. 67–72. Oxford, New York: Pergamon (1978)

Giurgea, C., Mouravieff-Lesuisse, F.: Central hypoxia models and correlations with aging brain. In: Neuropsychopharmacology. Deniker, P., Radouco-Thomas, C., Villeneuve, A. (eds.), Vol. 2, pp. 1623–1631. Oxford, New York: Pergamon 1978

Giurgea, C., Moyersoons, F.: On the pharmacology of cortical evoked potentials. Arch. Int. Pharmacodyn. Ther. *199/1*, 67–78 (1972)

Giurgea, C., Raiciulescu, N.: Etude électroencéphalographique du réflexe conditionné à l'excitation électrique corticale directe (EEG study of the conditioned reflex by direct cortical electrical stimulation). In: Van Bogaert, L., Radermecker, J., 1st international congress of neurological sciences, Brussels, July 21–28, 1957. Amsterdam: Excerpta Medica, p. 98 (1957)

Giurgea, C., Salama, M.: Nootropic Drugs. Prog. Neuropsychopharmacol. *1*, 235–247 (1977)

Giurgea, C., Sara, S.J.: Nootropic Drugs and Memory. In: Practical Aspects of Memory. Grüneberg, M.M., Morris, P.E., Sykes, R.N. (eds.), pp. 754–763. London: Academic Press (1978)

Giurgea, C., Lefevre, D., Lescrenier, C., David-Remacle, M.: Pharmacological protection against hypoxia-induced amnesia in rats. Psychopharmacology 20, 160–168 (1971)

Giurgea, C., Greindl, M.G., Preat, S.: Pharmacological reactivity of a new memory test in the rat in relation to major and minor tranquillizers. In: 11th C.I.N.P. Congress Vienna, July 9–14, 1978. Vienna: Interconvention, 1978, p. 248

Gobert, J.: Génèse d'un médicament: le piracetam. Métabolisation et recherche biochimique. J. Pharm. Belg. *27*, 281–304 (1972)

Goldstein, L.: Hemispheric EEG activity and psychopathology. In: Biological psychiatry today. Obiols, J. et al. (eds.), pp. 1242–1245. North Holland: Elsevier (1979)

Goodrick, C.L.: Maze learning of mature young and aged rats as a function of distribution of practice. J. Exp. Psychol. (Wash.) *98*, 344–349 (1973)

Gordon, P.: Molecular approaches to the drug enhancement of deteriorated functioning in the aged. In: Advances in gerontological research. Strechner, B.L. (ed.), Vol. 3, pp. 199. New York: Academic Press 1971

Gouret, C., Raynaud, G.: Psychopharmacological screening of different drugs effective on cerebral metabolism or vasomotricity. In: Tuomisto, J., Paasonen, M.K. (eds.), p. 238. Proceeding of the sixth international congress of New York: Pergamon 1975

Gouret, C., Raynaud, G.: Utilisation du test de la boîte à deux compartiments pour la recherche de substances protégeant le rat contre l'amnésie par l'hypoxie: intérêt et limites de la méthode. J. Pharmacol. (Paris) *7/2*, 161–175 (1976)

Greenough, W.T.: Enduring brain effects of differential experience and training. In: Neural mechanisms of learning and memory. Rozenzweig, M.R., Bennett, E.L. (eds.), pp. 255–278. Cambridge, Mass.: London: M.I.T. 1976

Greindl, M.G., Preat, S.: Contribution à l'étude des analgésiques par la méthode Randall et Se-
litto. Arch. Int. Pharmacodyn. Ther. *190/2*, 404–406 (1971)
Greindl, M.G., Preat, S.: A new model of active avoidance conditioning adequate for pharmacological studies. Arch. Int. Pharmacodyn. Ther. *223*, 168–170 (1976)
Hachinski, V.C., Lassen, N.A., Marshall, J.: Multi-infarct dementia; a cause of mental deterioration in the elderly. Lancet July 27, 1974, pp. 207–209
Hyden, H.: Biochemical changes accompanying learning. In: The neurosciences. A study program. Quarton, G.C., Melchenuk, T., Schmitt, F.O. (eds.), pp. 765–771. New York: Rocke-
feller University Press 1967
Isaacson, R.L.: Experimental brain lesions and memory. In: Neural mechanisms of learning
and memory. Rosenzweig, M.R., Bennett, E.L. (eds.), pp. 637. Cambridge, Mass., London:
M.I.T. 1976
Jarvick, L.F., Cohen, D.: A biobehavioral approach to intellectual changes with ageing. In: Psy-
chology of adult development on ageing. Eisdorfer, C., Lawton, M.P. (eds.), pp. 220–280.
Washington: Am Psychol. Association 1973
Jarvik, L.F., Wilkins, J.N.: Ageing, hormones and mental functioning. In: Neuropsychophar-
macology. Deniker, P., Radouco-Thomas, C., Villeneuve, A. (eds.), pp. 49–57. Oxford,
New York: Pergamon 1978
Jarvik, M.E., Gritz, E.R., Schneider, N.G.: Drugs and memory disorders in human ageing. Be-
hav. Biol. *7*, 643–668 (1972)
Johns, T.G., Piper, D.C., James, G.W.L., Birtley, R.D.M., Fischer, M.: Automated analysis
of sleep in the rat. Electroencephalogr. Clin. Neurophysiol. *43*, 103–105 (1977)
Kanowski, S.: Zum Wirkungsnachweis der enzephalotropen Substanzen (Pyrithioxin und Pira-
zetam). Z. Gerontol. *5*, 333–338 (1975)
Kanowski, S.: The aging brain: current theories and psychopharmacological possibilities. In:
Neuropsychopharmacology. Deniker, P., Radouco-Thomas, C., Villeneuve, A. (eds.),
Vol. I, pp. 23–31. Oxford, New York: Pergamon 1978
Kanowski, S., Coper, H.:Disturbed vigilance regulation as a model of geriatric neuropsycho-
pharmacology. In: Neuropsychopharmacology. Deniker, P., Radouco-Thomas, C., Vil-
leneuve, A. (eds.), Vol. 2, pp. 1669–1671. Oxford, New York: Pergamon 1978
Kass, L.R.: The new biology: what price relieving man's estate? Science *174*, 779–787 (1971)
Kohn, M., Litchfield, D., Branchey, M., Brebbia, D.R.: An autonomic hybrid analyser of sleep
stages in the rat. Electroencephalogr. Clin. Neurophysiol. *37*, 518–520 (1974)
Konorsky, J.: Integrative activity of the brain, p. 530. Chicago: University of Chicago Press
1967
Kruse, H., Kohler, H.: Memory enhancing effects of Piracetam in aged rats. Fed. Proc. *37/3*,
3548 (1978)
Künkel, H., Westphal, M.: Quantitative EEG analyses of Pyrithioxine action. Pharmakopsy-
chiatrie *3*, 41–49 (1970)
Kupalov, P.S.: On experimental neurosis in animals. (In Russian) Zh. Vyssh. Nerv. Deiat. *2*,
457–473 (1952)
Landfield, P.W.: Computer determined EEG patterns, associated with memory facilitating
drugs and with ECS. Brain Res. Bull. *1*, 9–17 (1976)
Lehmann, H.E.: Psychopharmacological Aspects of Geriatric Medicine. In: Ageing and the
brain. Gaitz, C.M. (ed.), pp. 193–208. New York: Plenum 1972
Lehmann, H.E.: Rational pharmacotherapy and geropsychiatry. Communication at the 10th
Intern. congress on Gerontology, Jerusalem, Israel, June 22–27, abstracts, pp. 22–23 (1975)
Lehmann, H.E.: Drugs of the Future. In: Psychotherapeutic drugs, Pat II. Usdin, E., Forrest,
I.S. (eds.), pp. 1470–1489. New York, Basel: Dekker 1977
Linee, Ph., Perrault, G., Le Polles, J.B., Lacroix, P., Aurousseau, M., Boulu, R.: Activité protectrice cérébrale de la L-éburnamonie, étudiée sur trois modèles d'agression hypoxique ai-
güe. Comparaison avec la vincamine. Ann. Pharm. Fr. *35/3–4*, 97–106 (1977)
Lissak, K., Grastyan, E.: The significance of activating systems and the hippocampus in the
conditioned reflex. In: The Ist. Intern. Congress of Neurological Sciences, Brussels, July 21–
28 (1957). Van Bogaert, L., Radermecker, J. (eds.), p. 93. Amsterdam: Excerpta Medica
1957

Matthies, H., Ott, T.: Differentiation of substances influencing acquisition and retention of learned behavior. In: Tuomisto, J., Paasonen, M.K. (eds.), p. 370. Proceedings of the sixth international congress of pharmacology, Helsinki, July 20–25, 1975. New York: Pergamon 1975

McGaugh, J.L.: Drug facilitation of learning and memory. Ann. Rev. Pharmacol. *13*, 229–241 (1973)

McGaugh, J.L., Gold, P.E.: Modulation of memory by electrical stimulation of the brain. In: Neural mechanisms of learning and memory. Rosenzweig, M.R., Bennett, E.L. (eds.), pp. 549–560. Cambridge, Mass., London: M.I.T. (1976)

Meier-Ruge, W.: Experimental pathology and pharmacology in brain research and ageing. Life Sci. *17*, 1627–1636 (1975)

Morgan, M.J., Einon, D.F., Nicholas: The effects of isolation rearing on behavioral inhibition in the rat. Q. J. Psychol. *27*, 611–634 (1975)

Moyersoons, F., Giurgea, C.: Protective effect of Piracetam in experimental barbiturate intoxication: EEG and behavioral studies. Arch. Intern. Pharmacodyn. Ther. *210/1*, 38–48 (1974)

Myslivicek, J., Hassmanova, J.: Early sensory deprivation treated with piracetam (ucb-Dipha 6215) in young rats. Acta Nerv. Super. *15/2*, 151–153 (1973)

Nandy, K.: Properties of lipofuscin pigment in mice. Acta Neuropathol. (Berl.) *19*, 25–32 (1971)

Nandy, K., Lal, H.: Neuronal lipofuscin and learning deficits in aging mammals. In: Neuropsychopharmacology. Deniker, P., Radouco-Thomas, C., Villeneuve, A. (eds.), Vol. 2, pp. 1633–1645. Oxford, New York: Pergamon 1978

Nickolson, V.J., Wolthuis, O.L.: Effect of the acquisition enhancing drug piracetam on rat cerebral energy metabolism. Comparison with naftidrofuryl and methamphetamine. Biochem. Pharmacol. *25*, 2241–2244 (1976a)

Nickolson, V.J., Wolthuis, O.L.: Differential effects of the acquisition enhancing drug pyrrolidone acetamide (piracetam) on the release of proline from visual and parietal cerebral cortex in vitro. Brain Res. *113*, 616–619 (1976b)

Obrist, W.D.: Cerebral physiology of the aged: Influence of circulatory disorders. In: Ageing and the brain. Gaitz, C.M. (ed.), pp. 117–133. New York, London: Plenum (1972)

Ostrowski, J., Keil, M., Schraven, E.: Autoradiographische Untersuchungen zur Verteilung von Piracetam ¹⁴C bei Ratte und Hund. Arzneim. Forsch. *25*, 589–596 (1975)

Puri, S.K., Pogacar, S., Lal, H.: Deficiency of memory and learning functions related to lipofuscin accumulation in brains of rats on chronic vitamine E deficient diet. Toxicol. Appl. Pharmacol. *22/2*, 334 (1972)

Reisberg, B., Ferris, S.H., Gershon, S.: Psychopharmacologic aspects of cognitive research in the elderly: Some current perspectives. Interdiscipl. Topics Geront., *15*, 132–152 (1979)

Rigter, H., Van Riezen, H.: Hormones and Memory. In: Psychopharmacology: a generation of progress. Lipton, M.A., Dimascio, A., Killam, K.F. (eds.), pp. 677–689. New York: Raven 1978

Robinson, D.S., Davis, J.M., Nies, A., Ravaris, C.L., Sylvester, D.: Relation of sex and ageing to menoamine oxidase activity of human brain, plasma and platelets. Arch. Gen. Psychiatry *24*, 536–539 (1972)

Rommelspacher, H., Schulze, G., Boldt, F.: Ability of young adult and aged rats to adapt to different ambient temperatures. In: Temperature and drug action. Lomax, J., Schönbaum, E., Jacob, J. (eds.), pp. 192–201. Basel: Karger 1975

Rosenzweig, M.: Evidence of anatomical and chemical changes in the brain during primary learning. In: Biology of memory. Pribam, K.M., Broadbent, D.E. (eds.), pp. 69–85. New York: Academic Press 1970

Roubicek, J.: The electroencephalogram in the middle-aged and the elderly. J. Am. Geriatr. Soc. *25*, 145–152 (1977)

Roubicek, J., Matejcek, M., Montague, S.: The electroencephalogram in old age. Electroencephalogr. Clin. Neurophysiol. *36*, 93 (1975)

Rousseau-Lefevre, D.: Modification de la plasticité comportementale par l'environnement: mise en évidence d'un syndrome de sysinhibition chez le rat. Thesis, University of Louvain, Belgium (1977)

Saletu, B.: Classification of psychotropic drugs by quantitative EEG, EP and sleep analyses, experiences with "Nootropic" substances. Abstracts of the 12th C.I.N.P. Congress (Vienna), p. 360 (1978)

Saletu, B., Grünberger, J., Berner, P.: CFF and assessment of pharmacodynamics; role and relation to psychometric, EEG and pharmacokinetic properties. Abstracts of the 12th C.I.N.P. Congress (Götheburg), p. 308 (1980)

Sara, S.J., David-Remacle, M.: Recovery from electroconvulsive shock-induced amnesia by exposure to the training environment: pharmacological enhancement by piracetam. Psychopharmacology 36, 59–66 (1974)

Sara, S.J., David-Remacle, M.: Strychnine-induced passive avoidance facilitation: a retrieval effect. Behav. Biol. 19, 465–475 (1977)

Sara, S., Lefevre, D.: Hypoxia-induced amnesia in one-trial learning and pharmacological protection by piracetam. Psychopharmacology 25, 32–40 (1972)

Saunders, D.R., Miya, T.S., Paolino, R.M.: Increased responsiveness of male rats to depressant and stimulant drugs as a function of age. Pharmacologist 15/2, 199 (1973)

Saunders, D.R., Paolino, R.M., Bousquet, W.F.: Age-related responsiveness of the rat to drugs effecting the central nervous system. proc. Soc. Exp. Biol. Med. 147/3, 593–595 (1974)

Schalling, D., Cronholm, B., Levander, S.: On models and measures of alertness and noetic functions. In: Antonelli, F., Therapy in psychosomatic medicine, Vol. 3, Pharmacotherapeutic tribune. Proceedings of the 3rd congress of the international college of psychosomatic medicine, Rome, September 16–20, 1975, pp. 709–715. Roma: Edizioni L. Pozzi 1977

Schnell, R., Oswald, W.D.: Geriatrische Pharmakotherapie des neurasthenischen Syndroms. Ärztl. Forsch. 21, 464–470 (1967)

Schrieffer, J.A., Spratto, G.R.: Dihydrotachysterol-induced progeria as on old age model for drug evaluation. Pharmacologist 19/2, 185 (1977)

Schulze, G., Buergel, P.: The influence of age and drugs on the thermoregulatory behavior of rats. Arch. Pharmacol. 293/2, 143–147 (1977)

Segall, P.E., Timiras, P.S.: Pathophysiologic findings after chronic tryptophan deficiency in rats: A model for delayed growth and ageing. Mech. Ageing Dev. 5, 109–124 (1976)

Selye, H.: A syndrome produced by diverse nocuous agents. Nature 138, 32 (1936)

Selye, H.: Stress and ageing. J. Am. Geriatr. Soc. 18, 669–680 (1970)

Verzar, F.: The ageing of connective tissue. Gerontology 1, 363 (1957)

Verzar, F.: The ageing of collagen. Sci. Am 208, 104–114 (1963)

Warrington, E.K., Weiskrantz, L.: Amnesic syndrome: consolidation or retrieval? Nature 228, 628–630 (1970)

Wilsher, C., Atkins, G., Manfield, P.: Piracetam as an aid to learning in dyslexia. Psychopharmacology 65, 107–109 (1979)

Willinsky, M.: Power spectral analysis in the evaluation of the central effects of the cannabinoids. J. Pharmacol. 5, 107 (1974)

Winson, J.A.: A simple sleep stage detector for the rat. Electroencephalogr. Clin. Neurophysiol. 41, 179–182 (1976)

Wolthuis, O.: Experiments with ucb 6215, a drug which enhances acquisition in rats: Its effects compared with those of methamphetamine. Eur. J. Pharmacol. 16, 283–297 (1971)

Erratum: Instead of "treshold active avoidance", please read throughout this Chapter: "treshold conditioned escape response".

CHAPTER 12

Cerebrovascular Agents
in Gerontopsychopharmacotherapy

F. HOFFMEISTER, S. KAZDA, and F. SEUTER

A. Introduction

Treatment of cerebral dysfunctions and disorders occurring mainly in the elderly by cerebral vasodilating agents seemed to gain its justification when KETY (1956) concluded that cerebral blood flow and oxygen consumption declines with age (Fig. 1). In an attempt to differentiate the extent to which decrease of cerebral blood flow is due to age or the effect of disease, DASTUR et al. (1963) excluded effects of disease by selecting old persons in good health. Cerebral blood flow in these selected elderly persons did not differ from that of young ones. Since cerebral blood flow was low even in diseased elderly subjects with mild disorders, it was concluded that pathology is the main cause for decreased cerebral circulation in old age.

Cerebral pathology of the elderly may, however, have its origin in primary cerebrovascular or primary parenchymatous changes or comprise vascular disease and

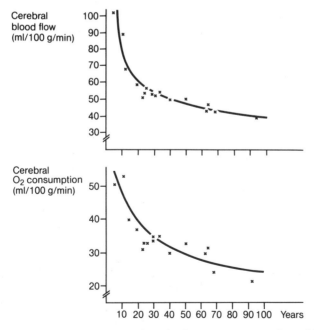

Fig. 1. Changes in cerebral blood flow and cerebral oxygen consumption with age in normal human males. (Modified from KETY, 1956)

cell damage – one disorder depending on the other. Thus, because vasodilatory therapy is primarily directed toward vessel functions, it should be indicated in those diseases of the elderly which have pathophysiologic mechanisms of cerebrovascular origin. Since, however, cerebrovascular interventions eventually are directed to improvement of brain dysfunction including psychological disturbances, a number of drugs with vascular sites of action may, simply as a consequence of their use, be included in the group of gerontopsychopharmacologic agents.

Due to the lack of exact diagnosis cerebral vasodilators very often have been used more or less *ex juvantibus* under the notion that pharmacologic intervention in cerebral vessel functions would be of benefit for the patient in any case. Very rarely was therapeutic use directed toward selected patients with diseases which could have been exactly attributed to a primary vascular damage. It is thus not surprising that the existing evidence on therapeutic results with vasodilators in cerebral disorders of the elderly is contradictory and confusing.

Drugs with effects on the cerebral vascular bed traditionally have been considered to be nonspecific vasodilators. The finding that vasodilation may cause hyperfusion of the unaffected areas and lower the perfusion of ischemic areas, in this way "stealing" blood from the injured region, has been generalized to cerebral circulation.

As a consequence the rationale underlying vasodilating therapy in cerebral dysfunctions has been severely doubted (see also HOYER, p. 533, this volume). In addition, the assumption that an arteriosclerotic vessel has to be considered unresponsive to pharmacologic actions contributed to a discrediting of therapy with vasodilators.

Pharmacologic analysis of the modes and sites of action of drugs referred to as vasodilators reveals, however, that the cerebrovascular pharmacotherapeutic approach comprises, at least theoretically, much more than simple undirected vasodilation. Generally speaking the term "vasodilator" has become obsolete. It originates from that time when only a few compounds such as papaverine, nitroglycerin, or nicotinic acid were known to relax vascular smooth muscle in vitro and to increase blood flow through some vascular areas. Recent progress in knowledge of physiology and pathophysiology of cerebro- and cardiovascular regulation has demonstrated that it is necessary to classify vasoactive compounds according to their modes and sites of action instead of referring to them simply as vasodilators. The vascular system does not represent an uniform homogeneous set of tubes differentiable only by lumen diameter or by thickness and construction of the vascular wall. It has been shown that the neurally and metabolically determined regulation of arteries is different in various vascular beds. Differences in regulation and responsiveness to stimuli between conductance and resistance vessels have been demonstrated. It became obvious that extramural arteries differ in sensitivity to stimuli from intramural vessels, although both have the same caliber and morphology. Finally, first, second, or third messengers may have various importance or cause alternating effects depending on the vascular beds they are acting on.

It thus became clear that vasodilators or, to use a better term, *vasoactive drugs* may influence cerebral or peripheral oxygen supply through very different mechanisms. They may influence regulation of cerebral vessels of various sizes in different ways through interference with autonomic nervous receptors in the vessel wall or by a variety of direct effects on the vascular smooth muscle. They may further prevent or ameliorate reoxygenation damages occurring after ischemic periods through effects on the vascular cell membrane. Prevention of ischemia or hypoxia is made further possible by inhibition of platelet aggregation, thus interfering with one of the mechanisms of thrombus formation. Vascular tone is also influenced by thromboxane (TXA_2), a strong vasoconstrictor and platelet aggregation inducer, and prostacyclin (PGI_2), a vasodilator and powerful platelet aggregation inhibitor. The same applies for drug-induced changes in rheologic properties of blood, and there is some evidence that vascular damages occurring with arteriosclerosis may be influenced or in part even prevented.

Although the possible therapeutic implications of these mechanisms for gerontopsychopharmacology are still obscure and far from being proven, an attempt will be made to review the pharmacologic and clinical-pharmacologic evidence on vasoactive drugs applied for therapy of cerebral disorders in the light of pharmacologic mechanisms which may play a role in gerontopsychopharmacology. Some examples which may represent the different approaches to vascular therapy are discussed.

B. Some Mechanisms of Vasoactive Pharmacologic Intervention in Cerebrovascular Disorders

I. Receptor Agonistic and Antagonistic Mechanisms

Neurotransmitters such as noradrenaline, adrenaline, dopamine, and histamine, as well as serotonin, play an important role in the regulation of cerebral blood flow both in normal and diseased states such as hypoxia or ischemia (ZERVAS et al., 1975; EDVINSSON and OWMAN, 1975). During brain ischemia monoamines are released in excess into the cerebral parenchyma. The effects of *serotonin* and noradrenaline are spasmogenic whereas the effects of *dopamine* may depend on concentration, being spasmogenic with high and spasmolytic with low levels (EKSTRÖM-JODAL et al., 1973). Thus α-adrenergic or serotonergic receptor stimulation seems to be the most common and powerful vasoconstricting factor in the cerebrovascular area. Consequently, blockades of the vascular effects of these neurotransmitters have been expected to decrease vascular tone to produce vasodilation and to prevent or release spasm, in this way reducing vascular resistance to flow and improving tissue perfusion. Pial vessels are accompanied by *cholinergic* fibers (LAVRENTIEVA et al., 1968). The effect of increased cholinergic tone is vasodilation and increased cerebral blood flow and cerebral metabolic rate of oxygen (PURVES, 1972; MATSUDA et al., 1974; MEYER et al., 1976). Stimulation of *β-adrenoreceptors* will result in the reduction of cerebral vascular tone and vasodilation. Simultaneously, β-adrenergic stimulation increases heart contractility and cardiac output, thus contributing to improved cerebral circulation. Stimulation of *vascular histamine receptor* (H_1) may result in cerebrovascular dilation, apart from peripheral vascular effects (WALTER et al., 1941; ANDERSON and KUBICEK, 1971).

II. Direct Effects on Cerebrovascular Smooth Muscle

In contrast to many other excitable tissues, the only second messenger directly involved in the activation of vascular smooth muscle appears to be calcium. The increase in calcium concentration required to induce contraction can be brought about in several ways. Some agents such as *angiotensin* or *noradrenaline* release intracellular cal-

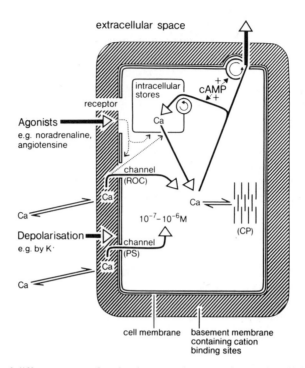

Fig. 2. Schema of different ways of activating vascular smooth muscle cell for contraction or relaxation. Receptor stimulating by agonists releases calcium from intracellular stores and opens receptor-operated channels *ROC*. Depolarization opens potential-sensitive *PS* channels. Both *ROC* and *PS* enhance the transmembrane calcium influx, thus increasing the intracellular concentration of free calcium necessary for activating contractile proteins *CP*. Activation of cAMP increases the calcium efflux and/or its reuptake in the intracellular stores, diminishing free calcium concentration and initiating relaxation of contraction. Relaxation (vasodilation) may be induced also by blocking receptors and/or by blocking channels. (Towart, 1981)

cium to initiate contraction and, in addition, open membrane calcium gates to sustain contraction. These gates have been called "receptor-operated channels" (Bolton, 1979). *Cell depolarization* results in the opening of voltage-sensitive or "potential-sensitive gates" (Bolton, 1979; Rosenberger and Triggle, 1978). As a consequence of these mechanisms there are different ways to pharmacologically relax the vascular smooth muscle cell (Fig. 2). Decreasing the concentration of adrenergic neurotransmitters or blocking their receptors will relax vascular smooth muscle tone.

Cyclic adenosine monophosphate (cAMP), an intracellular intermediate of adenonucleotide metabolism, seems to diminish intracellular concentration of activator calcium by stimulating either transmembrane calcium efflux (Fig. 2) or calcium reuptake in the intracellular calcium stores, or both. Thus, each event resulting in increase of intracellular cAMP, either enhancing its synthesis or blocking its degradation, will relax the muscular tone of the vessel, decrease vascular resistance, and increase blood flow. *β-adrenergic stimulation* of membrane receptors will activate adenylcyclase with consequently enhanced synthesis of cAMP. *Inhibition of phosphodiesterase (PDE)* will result in the same effect (Fig. 2). Availability of intracellular activator calcium as a basic denominator for contraction of the vascular smooth cell may also be achieved by pharmacologic *inhibition of transmembrane calcium influx* (Fig. 2). Excitation of the membrane of the smooth muscle cell enhances the calcium entry, thus increasing free calcium concentration for producing contraction. Some of the gates in the cellular membrane necessary for calcium entry are receptor operated (VAN BREEMEN and SIEGEL, 1980; HENRY et al., 1979), and others are essentially potential sensitive. The excitation-contraction uncoupling is the main effect of a number of compounds which are referred to as calcium entry blockers. Sensitivity to drugs may be entirely different in different vascular areas. It has been shown that Ca^{++} entry in vitro via receptor-operated channels of cerebral vessels (basilar artery) is much more susceptible to certain calcium entry blockers than entry via the corresponding channels in the peripheral vascular bed (TOWART, 1980a, b). In this way some compounds may have specific vasospasmolytic effects in the brain without affecting the peripheral vascular system (ALLEN and BANGHART, 1979). Other compounds may inhibit potential-dependent calcium channels only, in this way exerting vasospasmolytic activities based on a different mechanism (Fig. 2). Lack of oxygen in hypoxia or ischemia will result in damage to the cell membrane, thereby producing a loss of intracellular potassium. Increased extracellular potassium concentration depolarizes the cell membrane and further enhances transmembrane calcium influx (NAYLER et al., 1980; HENRY et al., 1979). For this reason "calcium antagonism" may contribute to the prevention of ischemia-induced damage to the brain, which may also occur when blood flow is restored to an area already damaged by ischemia.

III. Mechanisms Involving Blood and Blood Vessel Wall Interactions

Until 2 decades ago it was assumed that ischemic cerebral vascular disorders might be caused by hemodynamic factors only. It is still a matter of controversy whether cerebral multiinfarction or transient ischemic attacks are of hemodynamic or *thromboembolic origin* (FIELDS, 1977). On the other hand, there is no doubt that thromboembolic processes in the carotid arteries contribute to acute and chronic cerebrovascular disease (BARNETT, 1976; GENTON et al., 1977; HARRISON, 1978; GAUTIER, 1979; BANSAL et al., 1978; GÄNSHIRT, 1978). An arteriosclerotic plaque in the carotid artery very often is the primary cause of the induction of thrombogenesis (IMPARATO et al., 1979).

Platelet aggregation, blood coagulation, hemorheologic properties, and fibrinolysis are considered basic mechanisms for hemostasis as well as thrombogenesis, the pathological exaggeration of hemostasis (Fig. 3). Platelets are able to adhere to foreign surfaces such as exposed collagen of an injured vessel or an arteriosclerotically altered extracranial vessel. They release constituents which make further platelets sticky, forming platelet thrombi, and other compounds with procoagulant activity (Figs. 3 and 4). Such aggregates as well as mixed thrombi containing fibrin, platelets, and other blood cells or atheromatous debris, may embolize and downstream obstruct vessels of the intracranial circulation (RODVIEN and MIELKE, 1978).

Aggregate formation normally is a temporary process, the platelet plaque being dissolved within a very short time. Short-lasting syndromes such as amaurosis fugax may be considered the functional correlate of the existence of aggregates which are visible in the retinal vessels during seizure. Similar observations were made in animal

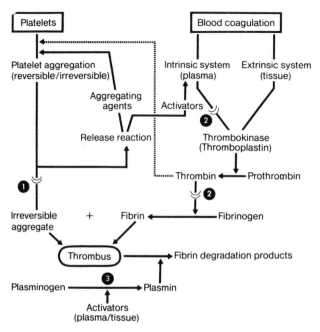

Fig. 3. Thrombogenesis and fibrinolysis. *1*, antiplatelet drugs; *2*, anticoagulants such as heparin; *3*, fibrinolytics

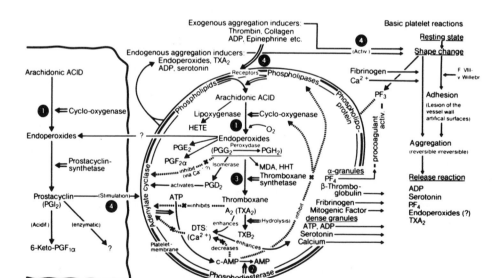

Fig. 4. Mechanisms regulating platelet function and platelet/vessel wall interaction. *DTS*, dense tubular system; *MDA*, malondialdehyde; *HHT*, 12-L-hydroxy-5,8,10-heptadecatrienoic acid; *HETE*, 12-L-hydroxy-5,8,10,14-eicosatetraenoic acid; for further explanations of the abbreviations (see text). Platelet-function-influencing drugs: *1*, Nonsteroidal anti-inflammatory agents; *2*, phosphodiesterase inhibitors; *3*, thromboxane synthetase inhibitors; *4*, prostaglandins

experiments using the pial window technique with aggregating agents such as ADP (adenosindiphosphate) or arachidonic acid (FIESCHI et al., 1977, 1978; ROSENBLUM and EL-SABBAN, 1977). Reinforcement of physiologic platelet reactions may be caused by hyperaggregable platelets or platelets with enhanced adhesive properties (PRENCIPE et al., 1974; JOBIN, 1978; TS'AO et al., 1978; TEN CATE et al., 1978). An increase in number of platelet aggregates was shown in the circulating blood of patients with cerebral infarction (ACHESON, 1974; MEYER and WELCH, 1974; WU and HOAK, 1975).

Thus cerebrovascular disorders may have their cause not only in primary vascular actions or reactions, but may also occur through interaction of blood and blood constituents with an altered vessel wall. This notion has been supported by the discovery of *thromboxane* A_2 (TXA_2) and prostacyclin (PGI_2) (MONCADA and VANE, 1977, 1979; VANE, 1978; SAMUELSSON et al., 1978). Arachidonic acid is liberated from phospholipids in cell membranes of platelets by phospholipase activated by aggregating agents such as thrombin, collagen, or ADP (Fig. 4). Arachidonic acid is metabolized by the *fatty acid cyclooxygenase* to the labile endoperoxides prostaglandin G_2/H_2 (PGG_2, PGH_2). *Thromboxane synthetase* rapidly transforms the endoperoxides to *thromboxane* A_2, which causes vasoconstriction and platelet aggregation. Arachidonic acid also serves as a substrate for the *lipoxygenase*. In this way 12-L-hydroxy-5,8,10,14-eicosatetraenoic acid (HETE) is generated (Fig. 4). Prostacyclin (PGI_2), an antagonist of thromboxane A_2, is the most active *inhibitor of platelet aggregation* known so far and a potent vasodilator (Fig. 4). This compound is synthesized in the vessel wall, predominantly in the microsomal fraction of the intima. PGI_2 is generated by prostacyclin synthetase from its own precursor arachidonic acid via endoperoxides. It is rapidly metabolized to the degradation product 6-keto-$PGF_{1\alpha}$. These findings (HAMBERG et al., 1975; MONCADA et al., 1976; GRYGLEWSKI et al., 1976) have generated the hypothesis that thromboxane A_2 and prostacyclin, in addition to adenine nucleotides and thrombin (COOPER et al., 1979; BORN, 1980), contribute to the control of local intravasal thrombus formation. Accordingly, disturbances of the equilibrium of these two substances might easily lead to fatal consequences. Cyclooxygenase inhibitors influence both thromboxane formation in platelets *and* prostacyclin generation in the vessel wall (Fig. 4). Thromboxane synthetase inhibition would not interfere with prostacyclin formation. Thromboxane synthetase inhibition, in contrast to interference with cyclooxygenase, would not impair prostacyclin synthesis, thus leaving intact an important endogenous vasodilating and antiaggregational mechanism. Thus, cyclooxygenase inhibitors, just as drugs inhibiting the thromboxane synthetase, would be promising pharmacotherapeutic approaches to cerebrovascular disease. As stated above, thromboxane A_2 has been shown to be a potent vasoconstrictor and prostacyclin a potent vasodilator.

It is thus easily understood that the *thromboxane-prostacyclin system* not only has an important function in thromboregulation, but may also contribute to *local regulation of vascular tone*. Thus, pharmacologic intervention in an imbalance of this system occurring in cerebrovascular disease seems to be promising, although relatively little is known about the significance of the TXA_2-PGI_2 balance for the local cerebral blood flow. As yet there is little information on the formation of prostaglandins and thromboxanes in brain tissue, but TXB_2 (degradation product of TXA_2) has been found in the brain tissue of animals and TXB_2 content in the blood increases after pentetrazol-induced seizures (mouse) (WOLFE, 1978; STEINHAUER et al., 1980). Pretreatment with TXA_2-synthetase inhibitors (imidazole or 1-carboxy-heptyl-imidazole) inhibited dose-dependently the increase in TXB_2 occurring with seizure. Shimamoto et al. (1977) demonstrated that injection of fluids containing TXA_2 in the carotid artery resulted in strokes. Thus it may be concluded that pharmacologic intervention with thromboxane synthesis, thromboxane antagonism, or stimulation of prostacyclin synthesis or release may be reasonable therapeutic approaches to cerebrovascular disorders.

The thrombogenic theory of atherosclerosis presumes that thrombosis precedes the development of the atherosclerotic plaque. Damage of the endothelial lining of the vessel results in formation of microthrombi, which are organized, infiltrated with cholesterol, and eventually become atherosclerotic plaques. This theory (Rokitanski, 1842; Duguid, 1949) has received renewed attention (Spaet et al., 1974), because a number of observations support it: Platelets and fibrin as the major constituents of thrombi are found in atherosclerotic plaques. As was expected, fibrous tissue or collagen, rather than lipids, is the major component of structured atherosclerotic plaques. In the experimental animal (Seuter et al., 1980) thrombogenic stimuli produce intimal thickening by proliferation of the medial smooth muscle. Consequently pharmacologic interventions aimed at this chain of events leading to development of atherosclerotic plaques will have much in common with antithrombotic therapy.

Disturbances and disorders of microcirculation may be caused by changed functional states of the blood vessel (constriction, dilatation, atherosclerotic plaques, etc.), as well as by changes in the function of the blood itself, especially of the red blood cells (RBC) (Schmid-Schönbein, 1977; Thomas, 1979). Changes of the flow properties of blood have been found to accompany disorders such as cerebrovascular disease, myocardial infarction, vascular diseases, or diabetes (Müller, 1980; Schmid-Schönbein, 1978). Whole-blood viscosity depends to a certain extent on plasma viscosity, but is decisively influenced by the ability of RBC to be easily deformed and by the formation of red blood cell aggregates. RBC aggregation is influenced by hematocrit and fibrinogen level in the plasma. It is easily understood that a change in the *deformability of the erythrocytes* may influence the oxygen or nutrition supply of tissues. The RBC which has a diameter of 7–8 μm when situated in larger blood vessels is able, by its physiologic fluidity or deformability, to pass through small capillaries with diameters of 2–3 μm. RBC deformability has been found to be decreased by changes in osmolarity, lactate concentration, and changes of the pH occuring in ischemic areas. *Red blood cell aggregation* is a reversible phenomenon. Under normal flow conditions there are no aggregates in larger vessels. However, under pathologic conditions RBC aggregation may be enhanced to such an extent that disturbances of blood flow may occur which sometimes result in stasis.

It thus appears quite probable that *pharmacologic improvement of rheologic properties* of blood may be of benefit in cerebrovascular disorders or in geriatric patients. This is especially the case when, as a consequence of major changes in the vascularization of an area, vasomotor compensation seems impossible. The rheologic effects caused by drugs are measurable but admittedly far from dramatic. The question remains open whether a number of reported pharmacotherapeutic successes in cerebrovascular disease may be ascribed to rheologic interventions. On the other hand there may exist undetected changes in rheologic properties of the blood due to the paucity of the experimental methodology.

C. The Drugs

I. Drugs with Vascular Receptor-Agonistic and Antagonistic Properties

Codergocrine mesylate, a mixture of hydrogenated ergot alkaloids (see also LOEW and VIGOURET, this volume, p. 435, possesses α- and β-adrenoreceptor blocking properties (TAESCHLER et al., 1952). As an α-blocker it inhibits noradrenaline-induced vasoconstriction but produces bradycardia instead of tachycardia. Similar to β-blocking agents codergocrine mesylate antagonizes the hypoglycemic effect of adrenaline and the adrenaline-induced inhibition of intestinal motility. It does, however, not modify the inotropic effect of adrenaline. Antiarrhythmic effects have been reported. Because of cerebral serotonergic and dopaminergic effects of codergocrine mesylate (see also LOEW and VIGOURET, this volume, p. 435), effects on cerebral as well as on peripheral circulation should be expected. Moreover, the preparation interferes with low k_m phosphodiesterase activity of the brain (ENZ et al., 1975), an effect which could lead to direct cerebral vascular smooth vessel actions (k_m is the substrate concentration at which the respective isoenzyme works with half maximal velocity).

It has been shown that codergocrine mesylate is able to increase cerebrovascular flow for a short time through a decreasing effect on the cerebrovascular resistance in a number of experimental animals such as rabbit, cat, dog, and baboon. Simultaneously, an increase in the cerebral metabolic rate of oxygen consumption (CMRO$_2$) has been reported (ROTHLIN and TAESCHLER, 1951; SCHNEIDER and WIEMERS, 1951; TAESCHLER et al., 1952; SZEWCZYKOWSKI et al., 1970, POURRIAS et al., 1972). Cerebrovascular resistance of normocapnic dogs is not influenced whereas the reduced cerebrovascular flow induced by hypocapnia is strongly increased. It has therefore been supposed that the preparation has a direct musculotropic vasodilating effect, especially in vessels with high muscular tone (SCHNEIDER and WIEMERS, 1951). In experimental cerebrovascular insufficiency of the cat produced by hypovolemic oligemia the preparation improves the cerebrocortical PO$_2$, thereby stabilizing EEG power without influencing cerebral blood flow (CBF). Since phenoxybenzamine, an α-antagonist, protected the brain in the same experimental procedure it has been concluded that the codergocrine mesylate induced protection is in part due to regulating effects on CNS catecholamines (GYGAX et al., 1978).

Clinical pharmacological evidence of codergocrine mesylate as affecting cerebral blood flow is controversial, possibly because different techniques have been used and different populations of healthy persons and patients investigated. After acute intravenous administration of a single dose almost no changes in human CBF have been observed (GOTTSTEIN, 1969; MCHENRY et al., 1971; OLESEN and SKINHOJ, 1972; HERRSCHAFT, 1977). HERZFELD and WITTGEN (1971) were unable to observe changes in brain circulatory time (99 MTC) of patients with cerebrovascular disease with intramuscular administration of single doses.

However, daily administration of codergocrine mesylate for 6 weeks shortened cerebral circulatory time in patients older than 65 years (HERZFELD et al., 1972). Cerebrovascular resistance to flow was clearly decreased after 6 weeks' therapy with codergocrine mesylate in patients with "cerebrovascular sclerosis." A similar effect of long-lasting therapy was observed in patients with cephalic hypertension (KLEIN and SIEDEK, 1966). There is a vast literature describing cerebral effects of codergocrine mesylate in geriatric and/or cerebrovascular patients that was recently reviewed by SPAG-

NOLI and TOGNONI (1979). Although there seems to be no doubt that codergocrine mesylate exerts a number of clinical-pharmacologic and therapeutic effects it is doubted that those actions described are due to vascular effects. It is now generally accepted that codergocrine mesylate exerts its actions mainly through metabolic and neurotransmitter effects on brain parenchyma rather than on brain vasculature (HYAMS, 1978).

Nicergoline is another ergot alkaloid derivative used in treating cerebrovascular dysfunctions (BERNARDI, 1979). It has been shown that its α-adrenolytic potency is more pronounced than that of other ergot alkaloids and that of phentolamine. The compound increases blood flow in various vascular beds including the cerebral. This has been demonstrated in the formal and cephalic (vertebral) arteries. In dogs phenylephrine-induced vasoconstriction of the vertebral vascular bed is inhibited as well as the epinephrine- and norepinephrine-induced blood pressure increase (LIEVRE et al., 1979). In the in situ isolated perfused normoxic brain of the dog nicergoline decreases cerebrovascular resistance to flow and increases $CMRO_2$. During the recovery perfusion period after a 15-min hypoxic perfusion, nicergoline increases glucose uptake and decreases pyruvate formation without changing lactate outflow in the same preparation (MORETTI, 1979). It is therefore concluded that nicergoline acts at least in part through parenchymatous metabolic effects. Single-dose administration of nicergoline in patients did not increase the regional or total cerebral blood flow (HERRSCHAFT, 1977). On the other hand, JLIFF et al. (1979) reported that nicergoline increased regional blood in some patients with multi-infarct dementia or transient ischemic attacks. A number of studies have demonstrated effects on behavior and cognitive functions in geriatric patients (for review see ALIPRANDI and TANTALO, 1979; BORGIOLI et al., 1979). As with codergocrine mesylate differentiation of vascular from nonvascular neurotransmitter effects is difficult. As an ergot alkaloid derivative nicergoline should not be very different from the former in this respect.

The chemical structure of *vincamine* (see also LOEW and VIGOURET, this volume, p. 435), one of the alkaloid constituents of vinca minor (Apocyanies), was first described by SCHLITTLER and FURLENMEIER (1953) as being related to the structure of reserpine. Although long known as a therapeutic remedy it was not used before 1960 in the treatment of cerebrovascular diseases. Vincamine and its analogues decrease peripheral resistance to flow via α-sympatholytic effects (SZPORNY and GÖRÖG, 1962), although a parasympathomimetic mode of action has also been postulated. Vasodilating effects of vincamine have been shown mainly in the cerebral and coronary vascular beds whereas flow in skeletal muscle is only slightly increased and splancnic vessels seem to remain unaffected (AUROUSSEAU, 1971; KARPATI and SZPORNY, 1976). Effects on CBF have been reported by WITZMANN and BLECHAZ (1977) as well as by SZPORNY (1976), ARFEL et al. (1974), and BRAILOWSKI et al. (1975). Besides its α-receptor antagonistic effects vincamine seems to exert a number of cerebral actions such as inhibition of spontaneous motility, prolongation of barbiturate anesthesia, and antagonism of amphetamine excitation (AUROUSSEAU, 1971; AUROUSSEAU et al., 1972; DUPONT and AUROUSSEAU, 1970). These effects might be due to direct cerebrometabolic actions and probably are independent of vascular smooth muscle effects.

The vincamine analogues ethyl-apovincaminate (KARPATI and SZPORNY, 1976) and L-eburnamomine (LINEE et al., 1979) increase the cerebral metabolic rate of oxygen ($CMRO_2$) in dogs. Other effects such as increased survival of mice in hypobaric hypoxia and inhibition of the amnesic effects of exposure to hypoxia in rats might be attributed to "oxygen-saving mechanisms." Vinca alkaloids have been shown to improve the metabolic status and the energy charge potential in the cerebral cortex of dogs during hypoxia and/or ischemia (VILLA et al., 1979), and metabolic effects in the brains of cats, rats, and dogs have been reported by BIRO et al. (1976), KANIG and HOFFMANN (1979), and GLATT et al. (1979).

In man, e.g., in healthy volunteers as well as in "arteriosclerotic patients," vincamine increases CBF as measured by ^{133}Xe clearance (ESPAGNO et al., 1969; ARBUS, 1972; GOSSETTI et al., 1979; LIM et al., 1980). In some patients the cerebral arteriovenous difference in oxygen content seemed to be increased after vincamine, an effect which has been interpreted as being caused by improved oxygen extraction of the brain (ESPAGNO et al., 1979). A number of clinical-pharmacologic and clinical studies on vincamine and vincamine analogues described improvement of carbohydrate metabolism in cerebrovascular patients, amelioration of the EEG of patients with advanced cerebral sclerosis, and improvement of cognitive deficits (TESSERIS et al., 1975; VAMOSI et al., 1977; MIKUS et al., 1973; MIKUS, 1980; MAROLDA et al., 1979). Further improvement of neurologic symptoms following stroke and attenuation of the Meniere syndrome as well as decrease of disturbances of psychomotor performance in encephalopathic children have been reported (PECH and GITENET, 1972; FOSSEY and PASQUIER, 1972). It appears that vinca alkaloids increase CBF through vasospasmolytic effects. Nevertheless there are no clearly defined metabolic actions which might contribute to the therapeutic effects reported.

Naphtidrophuryl is a spasmolytic and vasodilating compound with a potency 30–40 times greater than that of papaverine (SZARVASI et al., 1965; FONTAINE et al., 1966). Antiserotonergic activities were described by FONTAINE et al. (1968, 1969). Further naphtidrophuryl decreased the ^{45}Ca uptake of the membrane fraction of the rabbit aorta (BARON and KREYE, 1973). Besides vascular effects other pharmacologic properties such as local anesthesia, antifibrillatory actions, and ganglioplegic, analeptic, and antidepressant properties have been reported (ARNAUD et al., 1965; FONTAINE et al., 1968, 1969). FONTAINE demonstrated cerebral vasodilating effects in dogs. POURRIAS and RAYNAUD (1972) measured increased subcortical blood flow in the rabbit and the dog after naphtidrophuryl using a thermoelectric method. The same applies for cerebral blood flow of cats as measured by thermocouple probes. The reactive hyperemia occurring after short-lasting bilateral carotid occlusion seemed to be attenuated (LEVY and WALLACE, 1977). According to MEYNAUD et al. (1972, 1973) and KANIG et al. (1979) naphtidrophuryl exerts cerebral metabolic effects such as increased glucose concentration, decreased tissue lactate in the mouse brain, and changes in enzyme activity.

This is little information on the effects of naphtidrophuryl on the CBF in man. Cerebral transition time was found to be decreased in patients with internal carotid thrombosis, cerebral sclerosis, and stenotic carotid disease as measured by ^{51}Cr-radiocirculography (EICHHORN, 1969). Further release of spasms of the carotid artery occurring during angiography has been reported (FOURNIER and MOUROU, 1972). On the other hand, HERRSCHAFT (1977) found a slight decrease of regional cerebral blood flow after administration of naphtidrophuryl (^{133}Xe). A variety of reports on the clinical efficacy of the compound are available. Improvements in patients with acute cerebral ischemia (EICHHORN, 1969) and chronic arteriosclerosis have been claimed after treatment for several months (DANIELCZYK, 1971). Evidence of the clinical efficacy of naphtidrophuryl was reviewed recently by BEGHI (1979), who concluded that the reports available are not sufficient to prove therapeutic efficacy of the compound.

Isoxuprine is a catecholamine derivative with β-adrenomimetic properties. Accordingly, it dilates arterial vessels, lowers blood pressure, and increases heart rate and contractility. Isoxuprine dilates cerebral vessels in cats (WAREMBOURG et al., 1961) and increases CBF in monkeys (KARLSBERG et al., 1963) and in humans (GLONING and KLAUSBERGER, 1958; HORTON and JOHNSON, 1964; MIYAZAKI, 1971).

In cerebrovascular patients isoxuprine prevented abnormal slow waves in the EEG usually induced by hyperventilation. Vasodilating effects were postulated to occur (WHITTIER and DHRYMIOTIS, 1962) in cerebrovascular and/or geriatric patients. Improved performance (HUSSAIN et al., 1976) as well neurological symptoms (DHRYMIOTIS and WHITTIER, 1962; AFFLECK et al., 1961) were described. Beneficial effects on behavioral, psychiatric, and neurological criteria in a number of patients were reported (ELLIOT et al., 1973; GUYER, 1977, 1978).

Tinophedrine, an experimental compound being clinically investigated, exerts β-adrenomimetic actions (see also p. 495, this volume). This property becomes evident in positive ino- and chronotropic as well as vasodilating effects which can be antagonized by β-adrenergic blocking agents (ACHENBACH et al., 1979; STROMAN and THIEMER, 1981). Tinophedrine increases the vertebral artery blood flow and total CBF in the dog, as measured by ^{133}Xe clearance (THIEMER et al., 1978). Tinophedrine further antagonizes metabolic disturbances caused by controlled hypotension hypoxia and bilateral carotid occlusion through increasing cerebral glucose utilization and enhancing tissue concentration of ATP and CP in the rat. The "energy charge potential" was significantly increased (OBERMEIER et al., 1978). Besides slight sedative, anxiolytic, local anesthetic, and antiphlogistic effects, no other important pharmacologic effects have been reported (JAKOVLEV et al., 1978).

No significant effects on total hemispheric CBF occurred after intravenous injection of 0.2 mg/kg tinophedrine in humans (HEISS and ZEILER, 1978). However, in patients with reduced CBF in the course of multiinfarct dementia tinophedrine increased cerebral blood flow by an average of 28% (MERORY et al., 1978). A number of clinical-pharmacologic and therapeutic studies some of them reporting beneficial effects, have assessed EEG changes, changes in performance, cognitive functions, and vigilance (SPEHR, 1978; SALETU and ANDERER, 1980 a, b). Tinophedrine exhibits an interesting pharmacologic profile characterized by β-stimulant properties which contribute to its cerebrovascular dilating properties. Its cerebrometabolic effects are not yet clearly defined and proof of therapeutic value is not yet established.

Betahistine is a histamine analogue with a comparatively selective stimulating effect on H_1 (vascular) receptors (WALTER et al., 1941). The compound increases flow in the basilar artery of the dog as measured by electromagnetic flowmeter. At the same time the systemic blood pressure decreases (ANDERSON and KUBICEK, 1971). Further, an increasing effect on cochlear blood flow has been demonstrated (SUGA and SNOW, 1969). In patients with various forms of chronic cerebrovascular disease betahistine was reported to increase regional cerebral blood flow remarkably in most of the regions measured (MEYER et al., 1974). In addition to this study some improvement in vigilance and cognitive functions has been shown after betahistine therapy (PATHY et al., 1977; BOTEZ, 1975; SPRUILL et al., 1975). At present betahistine is used clinically to some extent. The appropriate indications and therapeutic value are not fully established.

II. Drugs with Direct Vascular Smooth Muscle Effects

Papaverine has been used in pharmacotherapy for decades due to its musculotropic, vasodilating, and spasmolytic effects. Its vasodilating effects are explained by the phosphodiesterase inhibitory activity (KUKOVETZ and POECH, 1970; TRINER et al., 1970) (for further explanation see p. 496, this volume). When administered parenterally papaverine dilates peripheral and cerebral vessels in normal animals and in humans (SOKOLOFF, 1959; BETZ, 1972; OLESEN, 1974). In rabbits with reduced cerebral blood flow papaverine increased CBF dose dependently (MUCCI and STERNIERI, 1968). In cats with unilateral occlusion of the middle cerebral artery papaverine increased CBF only in the nonischemic hemisphere. In other models mimicking cerebral ischemia, CBF seemed decreased – a result which was explained as being the consequence of a drop in mean arterial blood pressure due to general vasodilation (REGLI et al., 1971). Electrophysiologic phenomena, such as speed of recovery of evoked potentials during reperfusion periods after ischemic episodes, seemed to be improved by papaverine during hypocapnia. There was no effect in normocapnic animals (STREICHENBERGER et al., 1970). The immediate postischemic reactive cerebral hyperemia of the cat is prolonged by papaverine, but there is no influence on the subsequent postischemic impaired reperfusion hyperemia (KAZDA and HOFFMEISTER, 1979).

Although there is no doubt that papaverine exerts cerebral vasodilating effects in animals and normal subjects the clinical pharmacologic and therapeutic reports on the actions of the compound in chronic cerebrovascular disease are controversial. MEYER et al. (1965), GOTTSTEIN (1965), and WERNITZ (1969) reported favorable effects on cerebral blood flow and metabolism in patients suffering from stroke. Further, it has been shown that papaverine increased the regional blood flow in areas with low perfusion due to vasospasms. Despite this effect on cerebral perfusion the clinical symptoms accompanying vasospasm were not changed by papaverine infusion (McHENRY, 1972). Increase of cerebral blood flow was further reported by HÜNERMANN et al. (1975). Increased CBF in normally perfused areas, and decreased flow in ischemic areas, was demonstrated (OLESEN and PAULSON, 1971). For this reason it was recommended that vasodilator therapy should be avoided because of the "steal phenomenon." Although this finding has never been confirmed beyond doubt and McHENRY (1972) demonstrated an increase in regional cerebral blood flow in both healthy and ischemic areas in patients, the notion of the "steal phenomenon" as an inevitable consequence of pharmacogenic cerebral vasodilation greatly influenced clinical-pharmacologic and therapeutic attitudes toward cerebral vasodilation as means of pharmacologic intervention in cerebrovascular disease (HOYER, p. 533, this volume). The therapeutic effect of papaverine in geriatric patients with chronic cerebrovascular disease has been investigated repeatedly (DUNLOP, 1968; SMITH et al., 1968; RITTER et al., 1971). Favorable effects in those patients have been reported, but due to the poor design of these studies no conclusions as to the efficacy or nonefficacy of the compound can be drawn.

Cyclandelate is also a direct musculotropic vasodilator active in 3 times-lower concentrations than papaverine. As is to be expected, the compound as a phosphodiesterase inhibitor nonspecifically antagonizes acetylcholine-, histamine-, and barium-produced spasms of the guinea pig intestine.

When administered intravenously to humans cyclandelate increased CBF in the internal carotid artery. This increasing effect was more pronounced than the concomitant increase in the brachial artery. The effect lasted longer than that obtained with papaverine (MIYAZAKI, 1971). Increased CBF in the frontotemporal–parietal regions of elderly persons has been found as measured by ^{133}Xe clearance after administration of cyclandelate (O'BRIEN and VEALL, 1966). A 1-month treatment of elderly patients resulted in significant improvement in mental performance (BALL and TAYLOR, 1967). At the same time CBF was increased. A number of behavioral and cognitive improvements following cyclandelate therapy have been reported (HALL, 1976; CAPOTE and PARIKH, 1978; WESTREICH et al., 1975; FINE et al., 1970; DAVIES et al., 1977; JUDGE et al., 1973).

The *methylxanthines*, among them theophylline, caffeine, and a variety of other xanthine derivatives, are known as cerebral stimulants and vasodilators. In addition to papaverine they are the prototype of cyclic AMP phosphodiesterase inhibitors (see also p. 496, this volume), and most of their vascular and stimulatory effects seem to be related to this basic property. There is little evidence of a direct cerebrovascular dilatory activity of the xanthine derivatives. Moreover, WECHSLER et al. (1950), GOTTSTEIN (1962, 1965), FAZEKAS et al. (1953), and HERRSCHAFT (1977) found that xanthine derivatives such as aminophylline as well as theophylline exerted cerebral vasoconstriction.

The assumption that cerebral vasoconstriction after xanthines is due to hypocapnia occurring as a result of amino(theo)-phylline-induced hyperventilation could not be proven, because SKINHOJ and PAULSON (1970) demonstrated that the xanthines also exert a direct vasoconstrictor effect on brain vessels at physiologic $PaCO_2$ levels.

In patients the xanthines seem to have an inhomogeneous effect on cerebral circulation which possibly depends on the metabolic and circulatory state of a given region (PAULSON, 1970). Redistribution phenomena (see also p. 494, this volume) of cerebral blood flow in the sense of an "inverted steal phenomenon" have been demonstrated (HEISS, 1973). This effect, referred to as the "Robin Hood phenomenon," is considered to be responsible for some positive therapeutic effects reported in patients following stroke. Such effects (including improved EEG, performance, and cognitive functions) are described by JOVANOVIC (1972), KOPPENHAGEN et al. (1977), LEHRACH and MÜLLER (1971), FEINE-HAAKE (1977), KELLNER (1976), HARWART (1979), and SEN and CHAKRAVARTY (1977). Further therapeutic effects in ophtamologic (HEINSIUS and FLAMM, 1973; KÜCHLE, 1977) and otologic (WACKENHEIM, 1976) patients have been reported using pentoxithylline. The xanthines, also comparatively weak in action, are still, with some justification, used in the pharmacotherapeutic management of chronic cerebrovascular disorders. To which extent, however, whether the effects reported are due to cerebrovascular or other cerebral or peripheral actions remains unsolved.

Xanthinol-nicotinate exerts vascular effects and interferes with cerebral metabolism (BRENNER and BRENNER, 1972). Among the reported effects are increased oxygen uptake in brain homogenates in vitro as well as ex vivo. This does not apply to the xanthinol base and nicotinic acid. Metabolic actions are explained as being caused by stimulation of the biosynthesis of the oxygenated pyridine-nucleotides in tissues (BRENNER, 1974).

Xanthinol-nicotinate has been shown to inhibit spontaneous platelet aggregation in patients with parenteral but not enteral administration (STEGER, 1973). With long-term administration only collagen-induced platelet aggregation was inhibited; ADP-induced aggregation remained unaffected (SEIDEL and ENDELL, 1977). The compound was ineffective preventing aggregation of platelets in human platelet-rich plasma in vitro (SEUTER, 1976).

Increase of CBF after xanthinol-nicotinate was not shown convincingly. Investigations with (^{131}I-albumin) demonstrated an increase of radioactivity in the scintigram in cerebral sclerotic patients. This effect was interpreted in terms of improved CBF (BIRKMAYER et al., 1965). Ophtalmotemporal dynamographic analysis revealed decreased vascular resistance in the internal as well as external carotid vascular bed when xanthinol-nicotinate was administered intravenously (KLEIN and SIEDEK, 1965). Cephalic venous outflow increased after continuous intravenous infusion of xanthinol-nicotinate (thermocouple measurement) (BECKMANN and HERRMANN, 1970). As with other methylxanthines total CBF decreased in patients with chronic cerebrovascular disease after an intravenous bolus injection (^{133}Xe) (HERRSCHAFT, 1979). This finding could not be confirmed in patients treated orally with xanthinol-nicotinate for 4 weeks. In contrast, in demented patients with initially low CBF values (Kety-Schmidt method), a significant increase of CBF was found parallel to increased oxygen and glucose uptake. In patients with normal initial CBF values no changes have been found (QUADBECK and LEHMANN, 1978). In clinical pharmacologic and therapeutic investigations effects on attention, visuomotor coordination, self-care, general performance have been observed in some cases (HELD et al., 1973; HELD, 1973; REICHERTZ et al., 1967; BRAVERMANN and NAYLOR, 1975; BRÜCKNER and JANSEN, 1979; HAUPT and ISERMANN, 1976). Positive effects on xanthinol-nicotinate in the treatment of the Meniere syndrome, acute loss of hearing, and ophtalmologic vascular diseases have also been reported.

Bencyclane is an antiserotonergic compound with a potency similar to that of methylsergide (DAVID and KENEDI, 1967; CSABA et al., 1969). Mild sedative, tranquilizing, and analgesic effects were described (GRASSER et al., 1966; CSABA et al., 1969). Bencyclane has spasmolytic effects on isolated intestine preparations and on the uterus in situ. Coronary vessels of the dog are dilated and blood flow and O_2 delivery to extremities increase (SOLTI, 1970; SOLTI et al., 1970; MOLNAR and KELLER, 1970; SZEKERES, 1970; KISS et al., 1972). Later the cardiovascular effects of bencyclane were explained by calcium-antagonistic properties (KUKOVETZ et al., 1975; FLECKENSTEIN and FLECKENSTEIN-GRÜN, 1977) (for explanation see p. 496, this chapter). In situ bencyclane produced electromechanical uncoupling in the coronary artery strip and negative ino- and chronotropic effects in the isolated guinea pig heart. The negative inotropic action can be antagonized by increased calcium concentration. In the anesthetized cat bencyclane diminishes the force of heart contractions, lowers blood pressure, and increases the PQ and QT interval in the ECG (KÖHLER et al., 1975).

The diameter of pial vessels of cats is enlarged by bencyclane, and the cortical blood flow and pO_2 of cats and pigs is increased (SARATIKOV et al., 1971; GÄRTNER et al., 1975). Reduction of cerebral blood flow as a consequence of embolism in cats can be counteracted by appropriate doses of bencyclane (SARATIKOV et al., 1971). Its vasodilatory effects are different in various vascular beds. Main effects have been found to be in vessels of the heart and skeletal muscle. Less vasodilatory effects are seen in the brain and liver (NISHINO, 1974). Serotonin-induced spasms of rabbit basilar and saphenous artery can be counteracted by bencyclane. The compound's serotonin-spasmolytic effect is much more pronounced in the saphenous artery than in the basilar artery. Its vasospasmolytic potency is, however, identical in both vascular beds when K^+ ion is used as a spasmogen (KAZDA and TOWART, 1981). Bencyclane was claimed to have metabolic effects. In bovine lens homogenate O_2 consumption and formation of CO_2 are increased and ATP, ADP, and AMP levels are stabilized (HOCKWIN et al., 1977). These metabolic effects become evident in very high concentrations of the drug (10^{-2} M) only.

Bencyclane was shown to inhibit the ADP-, collagen-, and epinephrine-induced platelet aggregation in vitro (SEUTER, 1976; KOVACS et al., 1971; JÄGER et al., 1975; PONARI et al., 1976) as well as the spontaneously enhanced aggregation (BREDDIN et al., 1976) in 10^{-5} M concentration (JÄGER et al., 1975). However, no significant ex vivo activity was revealed (SEUTER, 1976; JÄGER et al., 1975; RIEGER et al., 1978).

Controversial findings on the influence of bencyclane on CBF in humans have been published. In patients with reduced CBF bencyclane increased the regional and total CBF (KOHLMEYER, 1972). Using ^{133}Xe clearance, HERRSCHAFT et al. (1975) could find no effects on CBF of healthy persons whereas there was some decrease in total and regional CBF in patients with cerebrovascular disorders. KLAUSBERGER and RAJNA (1970) demonstrated bencyclane-induced shortening of the passage time of contrast agents through cerebral vessels in patients with cerebrovascular disorders.

As with other compounds there is a vast literature on therapeutic results with bencyclane in a number of disorders and diseases occurring in the elderly. Improvement of symptoms such as vertigo, insomnia, depression, and tinnitus and further effects on performance and cognitive functions have been described (HOEFT, 1972; BÖHLAU, 1975; GARCIA GUERRA, 1978; DINKHOFF, 1975; BARTELS and SCHNEIDER, 1978; SCHNEIDER et al., 1977). Not all of these studies were controlled and controversial opinions as to their relevance as proof of therapeutic efficacy do exist.

Cinnarizine is also a musculotropic vasodilator which inhibits the contractile response of isolated arteries to calcium in depolarizing solution but not noradrenaline-induced contractions in calcium-free medium. It is therefore postulated that cinnarizine acts on the cell membrane, reducing the availability of free Ca^{++} to the contractile proteins (GODFRAIND and KABA, 1969). In this sense cinnarizine belongs by definition to the class of Ca-antagonistic compounds (see p. 496, this chapter). This basic effect is modulated by other actions which may contribute to its overall pharmacologic profile. Cinnarizine inhibits the contractions of isolated smooth muscle and heart preparations induced by a number of agonists including noradrenaline in a noncompetitive way. Histamine-induced contractions, however, are inhibited both competitively and noncompetitively (VAN NUETEN and JANSSEN, 1933). The occurrence of isoproterenol-induced multifocal necrotic lesions in rat myocardium is markedly reduced (GODFRAIND and STURBOIS, 1972), an effect which might be due to cinnarizine's calcium-antagonistic properties. Some effects on CBF in the dog and rabbit have been described (POURRIAS and RAYNAUD, 1972; COSNIER et al., 1977). These effects seem to be pCO_2 independent (COSNIER et al., 1977). Obviously cinnarizine does not specifically or predominantly act on cerebral vessels because it affects CBF less and for a shorter time than femoral artery flow (ITO et al., 1980). In patients with intracranial space-occupying lesions or cerebral edema cinnarizine (i.v.) increased the rCBF

(^{133}Xe clearance) to some extent (ITO et al., unpublished work). The CBF as measured by ophthalmodynamometry increased after drug administration in patients with cerebrovascular disease (WEIGELIN and SAYEGH, 1969). Prolonged brain circulation time was shortened in patients when treated 3–4 weeks. Improvement of neurologic symptoms was also reported (WILCKE, 1966). Similar results were observed in other open studies (BEHRENS, 1966; REIMANN-HUNZIKER and REIMANN-HUNZIKER, 1969). In patients with chronic cerebrovascular disease treated with cinnarizine for 4–6 weeks the signs of disturbed circulation in rheoencephalography were significantly improved (YARULLIN et al., 1972). Again, a number of reports are available demonstrating the clinical efficacy of cinnarizine in geriatric patients with or without chronic cerebrovascular disease. Cinnarizine was found to reduce blood viscosity in vascular patients, and the increased viscosity was even normalized after long-term administration (DI PERRI et al., 1977; DE CREE et al., 1979). It was suggested that this effect is due to changes in red cell deformability. Improvement of performance, cognitive functions, and neurological symptoms was reported (MEER-VAN MANEN, 1967; BERNARD and GOFFART, 1968; TOLEDO et al., 1972). There are also a number of studies in which no therapeutic effect could be demonstrated (IRVINE et al., 1970; BODEN et al., 1973). Clinical evidence on cinnarizine is controversial, probably because pivotal clinical therapeutic studies were not well designed.

Flunarizine is a difluoro derivative of cinnarizine. It possesses pharmacological qualities similar to those of cinnarizine, but flunarizine is more active than cinnarizine (VAN NUETEN and JANSSEN, 1973). In cats flunarizine increases the cerebrocortical oxygen tension as well as CBF (implanted thermocouple) and decreases cerebrocortical pCO_2 despite a fall in blood pressure, indicating that the increase in CBF is due to cerebral vasodilation. The effects are comparable to those of papaverine (TOYODA et al., 1975). Flunarizine was shown to improve RBC deformability in patients under normal as well as hyperosmolar conditions (DE CREE et al., 1979). More recently (VAN NUETEN and VANHOUTTE, 1980) these effects were explained by the ability of cinnarizine and flunarizine to inhibit Ca^{2+} influx, because increased levels of intracellular calcium diminish RBC deformability. Such a decrease in deformability occurs during hypoxia, causing insufficient ATP and oxygen supply to maintain the Ca^{2+} efflux.

Nicardipine (IWANAMI et al., 1979) and *nimodipine* (KAZDA and HOFFMEISTER, 1979) are experimental dihydropyridine derivatives chemically related to nifedipine (VATER et al., 1972), which is used for treatment of ischemic heart disease. The vasodilating effect of nicardipine is in part caused by the inhibition of cyclic AMP phosphodiesterase (SAKAMOTO et al., 1977). Comparable effects have been demonstrated with nimodipine (SCHINDLER, 1979). Nimodipine inhibits calcium-induced contraction of K^+ depolarized aortic strip with no effect on norepinephrine-induced contractions in vitro (TOWART and KAZDA, 1979). K^+- and serotonin-induced contractions of the basilar artery are inhibited at low concentrations whereas in the saphenous artery the serontonin-induced spasm is less inhibited than the depolarization contraction (TOWART and KAZDA, 1980) (further explanation, see p. 495, this volume). In anesthetized dogs both compounds have stronger vasodilatory effects in both cerebral and coronary vascular beds than in the femoral vessels. Pretreatment with nimodipine prevents impaired postischemic reperfusion after global cerebral ischemia in the cat (KAZDA et al., 1979), thereby improving postischemic survival rate and EEG changes (HOFFMEISTER et al., 1979). The vasodilating effect of nimodipine is more pronounced in baboons with breakdown of the blood-brain barrier (Craigen et al., 1981; Teasdale, 1980). In cats topical administration of nicardipine solution rapidly reverses spasms of the basilar artery induced with subarachnoid application of autogenous blood, serotonin, or prostaglandin F_2 (Handa, 1976; Handa et al., 1975). Nicardipine increased CBF in patients with chronic cerebrovascular disease (^{133}Xe clearance) (intracarotid and intravenous injection) (Takenaka and Handa, 1979). Spasms of the internal carotid or the middle cerebral artery in cranial surgery are reversed by topical application of nicardipine (Handa, 1976).

Improvement of subjective and objective symptoms in patients with chronic cerebrovascular disorders by nicardipine has been reported (Handa et al., 1979). Nimodipine increased CBF (^{133}Xe clearance) in ischemic brain regions of patients (Ott and Lechner, 1981).

Nicardipine and nimodipine are still experimental drugs and their therapeutic value has not been proven. Nevertheless this therapeutic approach seems to be – at least from the pharmacologic point of view – an interesting one.

Suloctidil, a compound with very complex pharmacologic properties, dilates vessels, affects lipid metabolism, and inhibits platelet aggregation, thrombus formation, and inflammation. As ionophore-mediated calcium translocation as well as glucose-stimulated ^{45}C uptake is inhibited in isolated pancreatic islets and in myocardial tissue (Malaisse, 1977), suloctidil shares effects of calcium antagonists. In the isolated rat aorta both the Ca^{2+} and norepinephrine-induced contractions are attenuated, but Ca^{2+} channels in the cell membrane are not blocked (Godfraind, 1976). Thus, suloctidil is another type of calcium-antagonist with direct smooth vascular muscle effects (Roba et al., 1976a). In rabbits suloctidil antagonizes spasms of pial vessels induced by the intracarotid injection of barium. In dogs subjected to transient respiratory hypoxia and cerebral ischemia suloctidil lowered brain lactate concentrations during recovery and increased the energy charge potential. No changes in the brain metabolism during hypoxia-ischemia occurred (Benzi, 1978). In curarized rats during iterative hypercapnic anoxia suloctidil increased the "brain resistance" (time to onset of cerebral electric silence) and accelerated electric recovery during the first anoxic exposure, but not during subsequent anoxic periods (Van den Driessche et al., 1979). Increased enzyme activities in rat brain homogenates and mitochondria (maleate, NADH cytochrome c reductase, cytochrome oxidase, citrate synthetase and LDH) have been reported after treatment from the 16th to the 20th week of age. Treatment in advanced age increased mitochondrial activity only (Benzi, 1979).

Suloctidil inhibited platelet aggregation in human PRP in vitro, when the aggregation was induced by thrombofax (partial thromboplastin) or collagen (De Gaetano et al., 1976). The drug was also active by repeated oral administration to volunteers (deGaetano et al., 1976). Ex vivo efficacy has not been observed in the rat (Seuter, unpublished results). The bleeding time and platelet retention to glass were not modified after ingestion of suloctidil (De Gaetano et al., 1976).

Antithrombotic properties of the compound in experimental thrombosis have been described (Roba et al., 1976b, c; Gurewich and Lipinski, 1976).

There are almost no reports available on a cerebral vasodilating effect of suloctidil in humans. Geriatric inpatients with mental deterioration of vascular origin showed improvement in concentration, attention, psychomotor capacities, and recognition. No neuropsychiatric changes were observed by Thiery et al. (1977). Symptoms such as dizziness, sleep disturbances, headache, fatigue, concentration disorders, and loss of interest seemed to be improved by suloctidil when administered to elderly patients (JANSEN, 1980). In multicenter studies of patients with chronic cerebrovascular disease several therapeutic effects were described (VAN SCHEPDAEL, 1977). Further, vertigo has been claimed to be susceptible to suloctidil treatment (NORRE, 1977). Therapeutic effects of suloctidil have been reviewed by CANDELISE (1979), who stressed the need for more and better controlled studies in order to provide better judgment of its clinical value, which presently is considered to be unclear.

III. Nonspecific Vasodilators

Hexobendine is an arterial vasodilating compound which increases coronary blood flow without changes in the systemic arterial blood pressure. In spite of the increased cardiac work, O_2 consumption of the heart remained unchanged. Increased glucose uptake parallel to decreased lactate consumption was explained through a possible activation of cardiac phosphofructokinase (KRAUPP et al., 1966 a, b). Hexobendine also increases the CBF, as evaluated by electromagnetic flow measurements in the internal maxillary vein. Its effects on substrate uptake were similar in the brain and heart, the most striking feature being the high increase in glucose consumption. The AV difference in pCO_2 decreases parallel to the increased cerebral release of hydrogen ion. It was postulated that this primary metabolic effect may contribute to the cerebral vasodilating effect of hexobendine, probably through an increased tissue CO_2 tension (KRAUPP, 1969). In cats with unilateral carotid occlusion hexobendine increased CBF only in the healthy hemisphere, but to a lesser degree than papaverine (REGLI, 1972). In patients with ischemic cerebrovascular disease, CBF in both the diseased and the healthy hemisphere was reported enhanced. Cerebral oxygen and glucose consumption and lactate and pyruvate production were unchanged (MEYER, 1971). An increase of CBF in patients with cerebrovascular disease was found also by MCHENRY (1970, 1972) and by HEISS (1970). HERRSCHAFT (1977) did not find changes in CBF in patients with CVD after hexobendine.

Instenon, a combination of hexobendin with vanillinic acid, diethylamide, and theophylline, improved the CBF to a greater extent than hexobendine alone. This was explained by the fact that the decrease of blood pressure observed with hexobendine was not observed with instenon. In some patients with focal vascular lesions the focal CBF was improved together with an increase of the total CBF. In other cases blood was shunted to other regions and the pathologic area was enlarged. The danger of intracerebral "steal phenomenon" was considered as a possible limitation of the therapeutic value of hexobendine (HEISS, 1970). Inteston is described as increasing the loading tolerance of the brain as measured by flicker frequency in 24 healthy volunteers (AMBROZI, 1971). In patients with "general brain symptoms" and with transient disorders in the vertebrobasilar system instenon normalized asymmetry of EEG waveforms and of desynchronization (LEBEDEVA, 1975). The combination significantly improved mood and memory and there was some improvement in headaches, dizziness, and insomnia.

Nicotinyl alcohol is considered to be a predrug. In its metabolism an active nicotinic acid is released which results in a prolonged pharmacologic effect (RAAFLAUB, 1966). The pharmacology of nicotinyl alcohol is complex. Besides arteriolar vasodilation, antilipidemic as well as fibrinolytic effects have been described. CBF-increasing effects in dogs were shown by means of rheography (KAINDL, 1954). By means of the Kety-Schmidt method increased CBF due to a decrease in cerebrovascular resistance was found after a single intravenous injection as well as after longterm therapy in patients with chronic cerebrovascular disease (HEYCK, 1962). However, GOTTSTEIN (1962) could not confirm increased CBF in patients with cerebral arteriosclerosis, either after an intravenous bolus or continuous infusion, although using the same method. HERRSCHAFT et al. (1975) reported a decrease in CBF in patients with chronic cerebrovascular disease applying ^{133}Xe clearance. There are no well-controlled therapeutic studies with nicotinyl alcohol in geriatric patients with chronic cerebrovascular disorders.

IV. Antiplatelet Drugs

Many investigators have described the inhibitory effect of *acetylsalicyclic acid (ASA)* on platelet aggregation (BUSSE and SEUTER, 1979; MONCADA and VANE, 1979; SEUTER, 1976; JOBIN, 1978; WEISS et al., 1968; ROSENBERG et al., 1971; MUSTARD and PACKHAM, 1975; WEISS, 1976; BAUMGARTNER, 1977; TSU, 1978). ASA acetylates plasma proteins and donates the acetate group for incorporation in platelet components (AL-MONDHIRY et al., 1970). Recent studies suggest that the arachidonate pathway is important for the platelet aggregation inhibitory action of ASA. Formation of prostaglandin endoperoxides increases the tendency of platelets to aggregate. ASA inhibits cyclooxygenase, the enzyme controlling the formation of endoperoxides from arachidonic acid. It was therefore suggested that the platelet aggregation inhibitory activity of ASA is due to irreversible inhibition of the platelet cyclooxygenase (MONCADA and VANE, 1979; HAMBERG et al., 1974; WILLIS, 1974). ASA, depending upon the experimental conditions (JOBIN, 1978; BAUMGARTNER and MUGGLI, 1974; CAZENAVE et al., 1978), is an inhibitor of platelet adhesion and retention to foreign surfaces or to altered elements of the vessel wall. The substance attenuates platelet release reaction, including the procoagulatory activity. It inhibits the second phase of ADP- and of epinephrine-induced aggregation as well as collagen-, thrombin-, and serotonin-induced platelet aggregation. Ex vivo ASA proved to be antiaggregatory in oral doses of 3 mg/ kg when administered to rats. These effects persisted for up to 2 days when the animals were given doses of 30 mg/kg orally (SEUTER, 1976). ASA also prevents venous as well as arterial thrombus formation in different animal species (MENG, 1975, 1976; SCHMIDT, 1975; MENG and SEUTER, 1977). Rabbits pretreated with ASA are protected against arachidonic-acid-induced thromboembolic death (SILVER et al., 1974; SEUTER and BUSSE, 1979).

ASA is considered to have good therapeutic effects in prophylactic treatment of transient ischemic attacks (TIA), as well as in chronic cerebrovascular disease (FIESCHI et al., 1977; MILLIKAN and MCDOWELL, 1978; MUSTARD and PACKHAM, 1975; WEISS, 1976; YATSU, 1977). In most TIA studies the positive results consisted of protection against an additional TIA and a trend to lower the incidence of stroke or death. Two of the most appreciated trials on TIAs within the last years are the AITIA studies (Aspirin in Transient Ischemic Attacks), performed by FIELDS (FIELDS, 1977; FIELDS and LEMAK, 1978; FIELDS et al., 1977, 1978) and the Canadian trial reported by BARNETT et al. (1978). FIELDS, in his studies with nonsurgical and surgical patients, found statistically significant differences in favor of ASA when death, infarction, and continuation of TIA activity were considered together. ASA therapy seemed particularly successful in patients with a history of multiple episodes of TIAs. In individuals having symptoms referable to stenotic lesions in the carotid artery territory, the "aspirin takers" had markedly fewer TIAs. But there was no distinct difference in the rate of stroke mortality and cerebral infarction when considered separately. In the Canadian collaborative double-blind trial (BARNETT, 1978; BARNETT et al., 1978; BARNETT and Canadian Cooperative Study Group, 1978) with ASA and sulfinpyrazone (see p. 513) in threatened stroke, ASA was effective ($p < 0.05$) when TIA and death/stroke were considered as endpoints together or separately, respectively. But only men benefited (48% reduction in the risk of stroke or death), whereas it was negative in female patients. Sulfinpyrazone alone was completely ineffective and did not further diminish the incidence of stroke and death when administered in combination with ASA (BARNETT et al., 1978; BARNETT, 1979). Consistent with previous findings was the reduction of stroke incidence by ASA in two recently finished prospective trials with ASA – the AMIS (Aspirin Myocardial Infarction Study) and PARIS (Persantin-Aspirin Reinfarction Study) (see p. 514) studies (ASPIRIN MYOCARDIAL INFARCTION STUDY RESEARCH GROUP, 1980; PERSANTIN-ASPIRIN-REINFARCTION STUDY RESEARCH GROUP, 1980).

Other nonsteroidal antiinflammatory agents (NSAIA) such as amidopyrine, flufenamic acid, indomethacin, ibufenac, ibuprofen, mefenamic acid, paracetamol, phenylbutazone, sodium salicylate, and suprofen exert antiinflammatory activity and inhibition of collagen-induced platelet aggregation (DE CLERCK et al., 1975; O'BRIEN, 1968). The typical NSAIAs are inhibitors of the release reaction only and differ from each other primarily in potency, with the exception of ASA which has a unique long-lasting effect. The safety margin of most of them is low and their widespread use as antithrombotic agents is therefore doubtful.

Sulfinpyrazone is a pyrazole compound structurally related to phenylbutazone. Like ASA, sulfinpyrazone is a cyclooxygenase inhibitor (BAILEY et al., 1977) which inhibits collagen-induced platelet aggregation and the release of platelet contents at high concentrations in vitro (BUSSE and SEUTER, 1979; SEUTER, 1976). However, ex vivo effects were not found at therapeutic dose levels in patients (WEISS, 1976). Sulfinpyrazone was shown to be a competitive inhibitor of prostaglandin synthesis in platelets (ALI and McDONALD, 1977). Its ability to protect rabbits from arachidonate-induced death (SEUTER and BUSSE, 1979) may be due to its interference with the arachidonic acid metabolism. Sulfinpyrazone prolongs decreased platelet survival time and restores platelet survival values to normal in patients (SACLE et al., 1975; MUSTARD et al., 1964; WEILY and GENTON, 1970; WEILY et al., 1974). Adherence of pig platelets to fibrinogen-coated surfaces (PACKHAM et al., 1971) is decreased as well as adherence of rabbit platelets to the vessel wall (DAVIES and MENYS, 1979). In contrast to the positive results found in the "Anturane Reinfarction Trial," a multicenter clinical trial, in cardiac death (Anturane Reinfarction Trial Research Group, 1978) sulfinpyrazone was ineffective in threatened stroke (BARNETT et al., 1978; compare this chapter, p. 513).

Dipyridamole, developed as a vasodilator of coronary vessels, and other pyrimido-pyrimidines (RA 233, RA 433) as well as the thienopyrimidines (VK 744, VK 774) inhibit the first- and second-wave aggregation-induced by ADP at high concentrations in vitro (BUSSE and SEUTER, 1979; SEUTER, 1976; EMMONS et al., 1965; GRIGUER et al., 1975; RIFKIN and ZUCKER, 1973; DIDISHEIM and FUSTER, 1978; HORCH et al., 1970; CUCUIANU et al., 1971). However, in ex vivo clinical doses dipyridamole does not inhibit platelet aggregation (SEUTER, 1976; WEISS, 1976; BAUMGARTNER, 1977). Its antiaggregatory effects are explained by inhibition of the platelet phosphodiesterase (ASANO et al., 1977; MILLS and SMITH, 1971; ROZENBERG and WALKER, 1973; McELROY and PHILP, 1975). This effect may be of importance in reinforcing the adenyl cyclase-stimulating activity of compounds such as prostaglandins (MONCADA and KORBUT, 1978). Dipyridamole also inhibits erythrocytic adenosine deaminase and blocks uptake of adenosine by platelets and red blood cells (PHILP et al., 1973; BUNAG et al., 1963; BORN and MILLS, 1969; SUBBARAO et al., 1977), thereby causing an increase in the platelet aggregation inhibitor adenosine. Reduced platelet adhesion and retention to glass beads was found by some authors (RIFKIN and ZUCKER, 1973; HORCH et al., 1970; MUSTARD and PACKHAM, 1975; WEISS, 1976; TSU, 1978), both in vitro and ex vivo in patients. Dipyridamole normalizes decreased platelet survival (HARKER and SLICHTER, 1974). Antithrombotic properties were found in some experimental models of thrombosis (DIDISHEIM, 1968; HORCH et al., 1970; DIDISHEIM and OWEN, 1970). Recently, potentiation of the antiaggregatory effect of PGI_2 production has been reported (see p. 499, this chapter) (MONCADA and KORBUT, 1978; MASOTTI et al., 1979; DI MINNO et al., 1979; PEDERSEN, 1978; HORROBIN et al., 1978; BEST et al., 1978). Further, inhibition of TXA_2 formation has been described (HORROBIN et al., 1978; BEST et al., 1978, 1979; ALLY et al., 1977; MONCADA et al., 1978; NERI SENERI et al., 1979), although these effects are not unequivocal as yet.

The first clinical trials with dipyridamole derivatives were less encouraging (SIXMA et al., 1972; TEN CATE et al., 1972), whereas dipyridamole itself is an agent very often administered in cerebrovascular disease alone or in combination with ASA. Dipyridamole, similar to sulfinpyrazone, causes a prolongation of platelet survival time in patients (HARKER and SLICHTER, 1970, 1974; WEILY et al., 1974). In most of the other successful studies dipyridamole has been used in combination with other drugs (anticoagulants and platelet aggregation inhibitors). There is at present no evidence that dipyridamole alone is effective in cerebral ischemic disease (amaurosis fugax, TIA, stroke) (MUSTARD and PACKHAM, 1975; WEISS, 1976; TSU, 1978; HARRISON et al., 1971; ACHESON et al., 1969). In the PARIS study (Persantine-Aspirin Reinfarction Study Research Group, 1980) the incidence of definite stroke was reduced from 2.0% in the placebo group to 1.1% in the ASA and 1.2% in the ASA/dipyridamole group.

Prostaglandins such as PGE_1 inhibit aggregation of platelets (KLOEZE, 1969). This effect is attributed to PGE_1-induced stimulation of adenyl cyclase and subsequent accumulation of cyclic AMP. PGE_1 is one of the most potent inhibitors of the primary phase of ADP-induced platelet aggregation known so far; it is active at $5 \times 10^{-8} M$ (see also p. 498/9, this chapter). Prostaglandins in general are rapidly eliminated from the circulation, and thus their application in antithrombotic therapy is limited.

V. Inhibitors of Thromboxane Synthesis and Thromboxane Antagonists

Imidazole and methylimidazole are inhibitors of platelet aggregation at relatively high concentrations, but are also selective inhibitors of thromboxane synthetase (PUIG-PARELLADA and PLANAS, 1977), which from a theoretical point of view may be a better approach in the treatment of thromboembolic diseases (BUSSE and SEUTER, 1979). Pyridinolcarbamate and phthalazinol are considered as TXA_2 antagonists (BUSSE and SEUTER, 1979; SHIMAMOTO et al., 1976). Their potency in influencing platelet function is very weak in vitro, particularly that of pyridinolcarbamate (BUSSE and SEUTER, 1979; SEUTER, 1976; NN 1972).

VI. Defibrinating Agents, Fibrinolytics, and Anticoagulants

Defibrinating agents such as arvine are considered to improve the hemorheologic properties of blood, but do not seem to be more advantageous than heparin (GALLUS and HIRSH, 1976). Also, dextrane as a rheologic drug was not found to be clinically effective (GALLUS and HIRSH, 1976). Theoretically *thrombolytic therapy* would appear to be a promising and rational therapeutic approach to the destruction of occlusive thrombi in extra- or intracranial vessels by thrombolytic agents. On the other hand it is known that *fibrinolytic drugs* involve a higher risk of bleeding than anticoagulants. As a consequence the possibility exists that hemorrhages are provoked and/or that emboli will result from the dissolution of an extracranial thrombus. Thus the administration of the fibrinolytic enzymes such as plasmin, streptokinase, and urokinase is limited to a few cases (HOSSMANN, 1977), because the benefit risk/ratio is considered sufficiently high and clinical emergency care must be at hand when this therapy is in use.

The results obtained with *anticoagulants* (coumarin derivatives, heparin) are controversial; the more recent randomized trials show negative results (PERKIN, 1979; SANDOK et al., 1978; MILLIKAN and McDOWELL, 1978; GENTON et al., 1977; GOTSHALL and HARKER, 1977). They do not reduce stroke mortality in TIA patients, nor do they prevent recurrent strokes (GOTSHALL and HARKER, 1977). However, in some studies it does reduce the frequency of TIAs (HASS, 1977). Anticoagulants like heparin may be valuable in an active thrombotic state (progressing stroke) as well as in cerebral infarction caused by thrombotic material of cardiac or peripheral origin, but not in a completed stroke. Prevention of recurrent thrombosis may be attempted by oral anticoagulants (e.g., coumarin derivatives). The use of anticoagulants is always potentially associated with a risk of hemorrhage, which should be born in mind. In some cases anticoagulants also may temporarily be a completion of the antiplatelet therapy.

D. Conclusions

The vasoactive drugs presently in use for treatment of gerontoneurologic and psychiatric disorders belong to very different chemical classes and have different sides and modes of action. Moreover, most of these drugs have a multifunctional pharmacologic profile which includes smooth vascular effects together with a variety of other pharmacologic properties such as influence on carbohydrate metabolism, oxygen consumption, and interference with neurotransmitter regulation, which result in changes in vigilance, attention, and emotions. Even cerebrovascular effects are caused by very different modes of action involving transmitter-dependent vascular smooth cell regulation as well as direct smooth vascular relaxation. Finally, a number of vasoactive drugs exert therapeutic results through actions on blood and blood constituents.

Because of the comparatively broad spectrum of pharmacologic properties, single mechanisms of action influence the experimental or clinical pharmacologic profile of these vasoactive substances only to a limited extent. As a consequence, due to their multiple pharmacodynamic effects, the majority of the drugs in therapeutic use do not allow one to establish the clinical-pharmacologic or therapeutic relevance of pharmacologic actions on individual regulatory functions. Thus, further research is necessary and new compounds with "tailor-made" pharmacologic properties might help to assess the benefit of the individual approaches to vasoactive treatment in gerontopsychiatry more clearly. In this respect it should be mentioned that the therapeutic efficacy of the "antithrombotic approach" obviously has been much more reliably assessable than that of vasodilators acting by qualitatively different smooth muscle effects. Progress toward solving these questions, however, does not depend on pharmacologic and clinical-pharmacologic research alone. A sort of vicious circle develops as the patients to be treated are generally multimorbid. As a result the pathophysiology and etiology of the vascular parenchymatous-morphological or metabolic changes in the brain of individual patients underlying the symptoms or syndromes indicating a decrease in their physical and mental capacity are almost impossible to describe in detail. It is therefore difficult to select those specific pharmacologic interventions which could be expected to be of benefit for the individual patient according to his pathophysiologic state.

As a consequence, clinical trials with vasoactive compounds are very often performed on ill-diagnosed multimorbid collectives of patients, collectives which are not preselected to include only certain diagnosed diseases and to exclude all others.

Moreover some of these clinical trials do not have a well-defined strategy to answer questions such as: Does a compound improve the blood supply in ischemic regions and if so, what does this mean from a functional point of view? Or is it effective in preventing new ischemic foci and if so, what is the functional importance of this effect? And, finally, what benefit does restoring the total cerebral blood flow to normal value have for the patient? We are still far from meeting those prerequisites and as long as the clinical methodology for assessing possible therapeutic effects in gerontoneurology and psychiatry is not sufficiently developed, therapeutic trials will yield little information on the important question as to which direction pharmacology should take to achieve therapeutic progress (HOFFMEISTER, 1981).

Thus, at present we have to state that results of pharmacologic treatment of gerontopsychiatric disorders with vasoactive drugs are far from satisfactory. This does, however, not mean that the theoretical basis of this therapeutic approach has to be considered invalid. Our understanding of the regulation of the cerebrocardiovascular system under normal and diseased conditions continues to increase. Hitherto-unknown regulatory mechanisms for cerebral vessels as well as for cerebral blood vessel interactions have been established, and these mechanisms open up new possibilities for pharmacotherapeutic interventions. It is certainly worthwhile to investigate their relevance with regard to the treatment of gerontopsychiatric disorders involving malnutrition of the cerebral tissue.

It is hoped that further research both in the clinical as well as in the experimental field will give more insight into the possibilities of pharmacotherapy and will essentially solve the question as to the "sense" or "nonsense" of vasoactive therapy in a number of gerontoneurologic and psychiatric diseases.

References

Achenbach, C., Klemme, E., Schueller, H., Ziskoven, R.: Tinofedrin and contraction. Eur. J. Physiol. *382*, Suppl., R 6 (1979)

Acheson, E.J.: Platelet adhesiveness and cerebral vascular disease revisited. In: Platelet aggregation in the pathogenesis of cerebrovascular disorders (Abstracts: Round Table Conference, Rome – 1974), Fazio, C. (ed.), pp. 21–23

Acheson, E.J., Danta, G., Hutchinson, E.C.: Controlled trial of dipyridamole in cerebral vascular disease. Br. Med. J. *1969 I*, 614–615

Affleck, D.C., Treptow, K.R., Herrick, H.D.: The effects of isoxsuprine hydrochloride (Vasodilan) on chronic cerebral arteriosclerosis. J. Nerv. Ment. Dis. *132*, 335–338 (1961)

Ali, M., McDonald, J.W.D.: Effects of sulfinpyrazone on platelet prostaglandin synthesis and platelet release of serotonin. J. Lab. Clin. Med. *89*, 868–875 (1977)

Aliprandi, G., Tantalo, V.: Physiopathologie des Innenohrs und Therapie der Perzeptionstaubheit. Arzneim. Forsch. *29*, 1287–1295 (1979)

Allen, G.S., Banghart, S.B.: Cerebral arterial spasm: Part 9. In vitro effects of nifedipine on serotonin-, phenylephrine-, and potassium-induced contractions of canine basilar and femoral arteries. Neurosurgery *4*, 37–42 (1979)

Ally, A.I., Manku, M.S., Horrobin, D.F.: Dipyridamole: A possible potent inhibitor of thromboxane A_2 synthetase in vascular smooth muscle. Prostaglandins *14*, 607–609 (1977)

Al-Mondhiry, H., Marcus, A.J., Spaet, T.H.: On the mechanism of platelet function inhibition by acetylsalicyclic acid. Proc. Soc. Exp. Biol. Med. *133*, 632–636 (1970)

Ambrozi, L., Neumayer, E.: Zerebrovaskuläre Insuffizienz und Hirnleistung. Wien. Klin. Wochenschr. *83*, 188–192 (1971)

Anderson, W.D., Kubicek, W.G.: Effects of betahistine HCl, nicotinic acid, and histamine on basilar blood flow in anaesthetized dogs. Stroke *2*, 409–415 (1971)

Anturane Reinfarction Trial Research Group: Sulfinpyrazone in the prevention of cardiac death after myocardial infarction. New Engl. J. Med. *298*, 289–295 (1978)

Arbus, L.: Circulation cérébrale et drogues. Médecine Practicienne *478*, 147–152 (1972)

Arfel, G., de Pommery, J., de Pommery, H., de Lavarde, M.: Modifications de l'électrogenèse cérébrale suscitées par la vincamine. Rev. Electroencephalogr. Neurophysiol. Clin. *4*, 53–67 (1974)

Arnaud, P., Kofman, J., Frederich, A., Faucon, G.: Sur les propriétés antifibrillantes des anesthésiques locaux. Compt. Rend. Soc. Biol. *159*, No. 12, 2427–2430 (1965)

Asano, T., Ochiai, Y., Hidaka, H.: Selective inhibition of separated forms of human platelet cyclic nucleotide phosphodiesterase by platelet aggregation inhibitors. Mol. Pharmacol. *13*, 400–406 (1977)

Aspirin Myocardial Infarction Study Research Group: A randomized, controlled trial of aspirin in persons recovered from myocardial infarction. J. Am. Med. Assoc. *243*, 661–669 (1980)

Aurousseau, M.: Pharmacologie comparée des alcaloides indolique et de leurs derivés agissant sur la circulation cérébral et le métabolisme du tissu nerveux. Chim. Thér. *6*, 221–234 (1971)

Aurousseau, M., Dupont, M., Rondeaux, C., Rondeaux, J.C.: Variation de l'irrigation sanguine cérébrale sous l'influence de quelques dérivés indoliques apparentes à la vincamine. Chim. Thér. *7*, 235–243 (1972)

Bailey, J.M., Bryant, R.W., Feinmark, S.J., Makheja, A.N.: Differential separation of thromboxanes from prostaglandins by one and two-dimensional thin layer chromatography. Prostaglandins *13*, 479–492 (1977)

Ball, J.A.C., Taylor, A.R.: Effect of cyclandelate on mental functions and cerebral blood flow in elderly patients. Brit. Med. J. *1967 III*, 525–528

Bansal, B.C., Prakash, C., Arya, R.K., Gulati, S.K., Mittal, S.C.: Serum lipids, platelets, and fibrinolytic activity in cerebrovascular disease. Stroke *9*, 137–139 (1978)

Barnett, H.J.M.: Pathogenesis of transient ischemic attacks. In: Cerebrovascular diseases. Scheinberg, P. (ed.), pp. 1–21. New York: Raven Press 1976

Barnett, H.J.M.: Aspirin and sulfinpyrazone in threatened stroke – the results of the cancidian collaborative double-blind trial. In: Acetylsalicylic acid in cerebral ischemia and coronary heart disease. Breddin, K., Dorndorf, W., Loew, D., Marx, R. (eds.), p. 93. Stuttgart, New York: Schattauer 1978

Barnett, H.J.M.: The pathophysiology of transient cerebral ischemic attacks. Therapy with platelet antiaggregants. Med. Clin. North Am. *63*, 649–679 (1979)

Barnett, H.J.M., and the Canadian Cooperative Study Group: A randomized trial of aspirin and sulfinpyrazone in threatened stroke. New Engl. J. Med. *299*, 53–59 (1978)

Barnett, H.J.M., McDonald, B.W.D., Sackett, D.L.: Aspirin-effective in males threatened with stroke. Stroke *9*, 295–298 (1978)

Baron, G.D., Kreye, V.A.W.: Effects of drugs on ^{45}Ca uptake by isolated vascular smooth muscle membranes. Eur. J. Physiol. *343*, Suppl. R 54 (1973)

Bartels, H., Schneider, B.: Kontrolle der pharmakodynamischen Wirkung von Fludilat bei der Behandlung der cerebrovasculären Insuffizienz. Med. Welt *29*, 1056–1060 (1978)

Baumgartner, H.R.: Wirkungsmechanismen von Plättcheninhibitoren. Ther. Umsch. *34*, 341–346 (1977)

Baumgartner, H.R., Muggli, R.: Effect of acetylsalicyclic acid on platelet adhesion to subendothelium and the formation of mural thrombi. Thromb. Diath. Haemorrh. Suppl. *60*, 345 (1974)

Beckmann, G., Herrmann, E.: Untersuchungen zur Beeinflußbarkeit der Innenohrdurchblutung. Arch. Klin. Exp. Ohren-Nasen-Kehlkopfheilkd. (Kongreßbericht II. Teil) *194*, 534–538 (1970)

Beghi, E.: Naftidrofuryl in drug treatment and devention in cerebrovascular disorders. In: Tognoni, G., Garattini, S. (eds.), pp. 211–222. Amsterdam: Elsevier North Holland Biomedical Press 1979

Behrens, E.: Medikamentöse Beeinflussung der Hirndurchblutung durch Stutgeron. Med. Welt *38*, 2029–2031 (1966)

Benzi, G.: Drugs action on cerebral energy state during and after various hypoxic conditions. Arch. Int. Pharmacodyn. *236*, 234–251 (1978)

Benzi, G.: Effects of chronic treatment with some drugs on the enzymatic activities of the rat brain. Biochem. Pharmacol. *28*, 2703–2708 (1979)

Bernard, A., Goffart, J.M.: A double-blind cross-over clinical evaluation of cinnarizine. Clin. Trials J. *5*, 945–947 (1968)

Bernardi, L.: Von den Mutterkorn-Alkaloiden zum Nicergolin/Chemische Gesichtspunkte. Arzneim. Forsch. *29*, 1204–1206 (1979)

Best, L.C., Martin, T.J., McGuire, M.B., Preston, F.E., Russell, R.G.G., Segal, D.S.: Dipyridamole and platelet function. Lancet *1978 II*, 846

Best, L.C., McGuire, M.B., Jones, P.B.B., Holland, T.K., Martin, T.J., Preston, F.E., Segal, D.S., Russell, R.G.B.: Mode of action of dipyridamole of human platelets. Thromb. Res. *16*, 367–379 (1979)

Betz, E.: Pharmakologie des Gehirnkreislaufs. In: Der Hirnkreislauf. Gänshirt, H. (ed.), pp. 412–440. Stuttgart: Thieme 1972

Birkmayer, W., Seemann, D., Zita, G.: Objektivierung des zerebralen Nutritionseffektes. Szintigraphische Untersuchungen. Münch. Med. Wochenschr. *107*, 2410–2413 (1965)

Biro, K., Karpati, E., Szporny, L.: Protective activity of ethyl apovincaminate on ischaemic anoxia of the brain. Arzneim. Forsch. *26*, 1918–1920 (1976)

Boden, U., Boden, C., Ruehland, W.: Zur klinischen Wirksamkeit von Zinnarizin bei geriatrischen Patienten. Doppelter Blindversuch. Zentralbl. Pharm. Pharmakother. Laboratoriumsdiagn. *111*, 1257–1266 (1973)

Böhlau, V.: Beitrag zur medikamentösen Therapie in der Rehabilitation vorzeitiger Altersbeschwerden. Med. Welt *26*, 233–235 (1975)

Bolton, T.B.: Mechanisms of action of transmitter and other substances on smooth muscle. Physiol. Rev. *59*, 606–718 (1979)

Borgioli, M., Merendino, E., Ricci, B.: Therapeutische Wirksamkeit von Nicergolin in der Ophthalmologie/Fluoreszenzretinolographischer Beitrag. Arzneim. Forsch. *29*, 1311–1316 (1979)

Born, G.V.R.: Haemodynamic and biochemical interactions in intravascular platelet aggregation. In: Blood cells and vessel walls functional interactions, pp. 61–77. Amsterdam, Oxford, New York: Excerpta Medica 1980

Born, G.V.R., Mills, D.C.: Potentiation of the inhibitory effect of adenosine on platelet aggregation by drugs that prevent its uptake. J. Physiol. (Lond.) *202*, 41 (1969)

Botez, M.: Betahistidine hydrochloride in the treatment of vertebro-basilar insufficiency. Encephale *1*, 279–286 (1975)

Brailowski, S., Walter, S., Vuillon-Cacciutolo, G., Serbanescu, T.: Alcaloïdes indoliques induisant on non un tremblement: Effets sur l'épilepsie photosensible du papio papio. C.R. Soc. Biol. *1969*, 1190–1193 (1975)

Bravermann, A.M., Naylor, R.: Vasoactive substances in the management of elderly patients suffering from dementia. Mod. Geriatrics *5*, 20–29 (1975)

Breddin, K.: Die Thrombozytenfunktion bei hämorrhagischen Diathesen, Thrombosen und Gefäßkrankheiten. Stuttgart: Schattauer 1968

Breddin, K., Grun, H., Krzywanek, H.J., Schremmer, W.P.: On the measurement of spontaneous platelet aggregation. The platelet aggregation test III. Methods and first clinical results. Thromb. Haemostas. *35*, 669–691 (1976)

Brenner, G.: Vergleichende Untersuchungen über die Beeinflussung der O_2-Aufnahme von Leber- und Hirnhomogenaten der Ratte durch Xantinol-nicotinat und Nikotinsäure. Arzneim. Forsch. *24*, 321–325 (1974)

Brenner, G., Brenner, H.: Die Einwirkung von Xantinol-nicotinat auf den Stoffwechsel des Gehirns. Tierexperimentelle Untersuchungen über die Beeinflussung der Glukose-^{14}C-Permeation und der Pyridin- und Adenin-nucleotide. Arzneim. Forsch. *22*, 754–759 (1972)

Brückner, G.W., Jansen, W.: Zur Therapie der zerebrovaskulären Insuffizienz. Eine psychometrische Doppelblindstudie mit Xantinol-Nicotinat. Münch. Med. Wochenschr. *121*, 861–864 (1979)

Bunag, R.D., Douglas, C.R., Imai, S., Berne, R.M.: In vitro inhibition of adenosine deaminase by persantin. Fed. Proc. *22*, 642 (1963)

Busse, W.-D., Seuter, F.: Influence on thromboxane and malondialdehyde synthesis in human thrombocytes by various inhibitors of platelet function. In: Arachidonic acid metabolism in inflammation and thrombosis. Brune, K., Baggiolini, F. (eds.), pp. 127–137. Stuttgart: Birkhäuser 1979

Candelise, L.: Suloctidil and bencyclane in drug treatment and prevention in cerebrovascular disorders. In: Tognoni, G., Garattini, S. (eds.), pp. 205–210. Amsterdam: Elsevier North Holland Biomedical Press 1979

Capote, B., Parikh, N.: Cyclandelate in the treatment of senility: A controlled study. J. Am. Geriatr. Soc. *26*, 360–362 (1978)

Cazenave, J.P., Kinlough-Rathbone, L., Packham, M.A., Mustard, J.F.: The effect of acetylsalicyclic acid and indomethacin on rabbit platelet adherence to collagen and the subendothelium in the presence of a low or high hematocrit. Thromb. Res. *13*, 971–981 (1978)

Clerck, F. de, Vermylen, J., Reneman, R.: Effects of suprofen, an inhibitor of prostaglandin biosynthesis, on platelet function, plasma coagulation and fibrinolysis. I. In vitro experiments. Arch. Int. Pharmacodyn. *216*, 263–279 (1975)

Cooper, D.R., Lewis, G.P., Lieberman, G.E., Webb, H., Westwick, J.: ADP metabolism in vascular tissue, a possible thrombo-regulatory mechanism. Thromb. Res. *14*, 901–914 (1979)

Cosnier, M., Cheucle, M., Rispat, G., Streichenberger, G.: Influence of hypercapnia on the cerebrovascular activities of some drugs used in the treatment of cerebral ischemia. Arzneim. Forsch. *27*, 1566–1569 (1977)

Craigen, L., Harper, A.M., Kazda, S.: Effect of a calcium antagonist (nimodipine) on CBF and metabolism. (in press) (1981)

Csaba, B., Toth, S., Molnar, G.: Benzcyclan, a new anti-serotonin drug. A pharmacological study on the effect of benzcyclan in relationship to its anti-serotonin properties. Arzneim. Forsch. *19*, 1726–1728 (1969)

Cucuianu, M.P., Nishizawa, E.E., Mustard, J.F.: Effect of pyrimidopyrimidine compounds on platelet function. J. Lab. Clin. Med. *77*, 958–974 (1971)

Danielczyk, W.: Neue therapeutische Aspekte bei der Rehabilitation zerebraler Gefäßkranker. Therapiewoche *21*, 307–312 (1971)

Dastur, D.K., Laen, M.H., Hansen, D.B., Kety, S.S., Butler, R.N., Perlin, S., Sokoloff, L.: Effects of ageing on cerebral circulation and metabolism in man. In: Human ageing: A biological and behavioral study. PHS Publication Nr. 986, pp. 57–76. Washington D.C.: US Government Printing Office 1963

David, G., Kenedi, I.: The antiserotonin effect of benzcyclan. Acta Physiol. Hung. *33*, Suppl. 2, 75 (1967)

Davies, G., Hamilton, S., Hendrickson, E., Levy, R., Post, F.: The effect of cyclandelate in depressed and demented patients: A controlled study in psychogeriatric patients. Age Ageing *6*, 156–162 (1977)

Davies, J.A., Menys, V.C.: Effect on sulphinpyrazone (SP) aspirin (ASA), and dipyridamole (DP) on platelet-vessel wall interaction after oral administration to rabbits. Thromb. Haemostas. *42*, 197 (1979)

De Cree, J., De Cock, W., Geukens, H., De Clerck, F., Beerens, M., Verhaegen, H.: The rheological effects of cinnarizine and flunarizine in normal and pathologic conditions. Angiology *30*, 505–515 (1979)

Dhrymiotis, A.D., Whittier, J.R.: Die Wirkung eines Vasodilatans, Isoxsuprin, auf Zustände von cerebraler Ischämie. Curr. Therap. Res. *4*, 1–7 (1962)

Didisheim, P.T.: Inhibition by dipyridamole of arterial thrombosis in rats. Thromb. Diath. Haemorrh. *20*, 257–266 (1968)

Didisheim, P.T., Fuster, V.: Actions and clinical status of platelet-suppressive agents. Semin. Hematol. *15*, 55–72 (1978)

Didisheim, P.T., Owen, C.A.: Effect of dipyridamole (Persantin^R) and its derivatives on thrombosis and platelet function. Thromb. Diath. Haemorrh. Suppl. *42*, 267–275 (1970)

Di Minno, G., De Gaetano, G., Silver, M.J.: Dipyridamole (D) reduces the effectiveness of prostaglandin (PG)I$_2$, PGD$_2$, and PGE$_1$ as inhibitors of platelet aggregation in human platelet-rich plasma (PRP). Thrombos. Haemostas. *42*, 198 (1979)

Di Minno, G., Silver, M.J., de Gaetano, G.: Ingestion of dipyridamole reduces inhibitory effect of prostacyclin on human platelets. Lancet *1979 II*, 701–702

Dinkhoff, U.: Fludilat-Therapie bei zerebraler Mangeldurchblutung. Med. Welt *26*, 522–524 (1975)

Di Perri, T., Forconi, S., Guerrini, M., Loghi Pasini, F., Del Cipolla, R., Rossi, C., Agnusdei, D.: Action of cinnarizine on the hyperviscosity of blood in patients with peripheral obliterative arterial disease. Proc. R. Soc. Med. *70*, Suppl. 8, 25–28 (1977)

Duguid, J.B.: Pathogenesis of atherosclerosis. Lancet *1949 II*, 925

Dunlop, E.: Chronic cerebrovascular insufficiency treated with papaverine. J. Am. Geriat. Soc. *16*, 343–349 (1968)

Dupont, M., Aurousseau, M.: Variations de la circulation cérébrale sous l'influence de quelques dérivés indoliques apparentes à la vincamine. Chim. ther. *5*, 366 (1970)

Dyken, M.L.: Clinical studies of cerebral ischaemia and antiplatelet drugs. In: Acetylsalicyclic acid in cerebral ischaemia and coronary heart disease. Breddin, K., Dorndorf, F.W., Loew, D., Marx, R. (eds.), pp. 79–84. Stuttgart, New York: F.K. Schattauer 1978

Edvinsson, L., Owman, C.H.: Pharmacological identification of adrenergic α- and β, cholingeric (muscarine and nicotinic), histaminergic H$_1$ and H$_2$, and serotonergic receptors in isolated histaminergic H$_1$ and H$_2$, and serotonergic receptors in isolated intra- and extracranial vessels. In: Blood flow and metabolism in the brain. Harper, A.M., Jennett, W.B., Miller, J.D., Rowan, J.O. (eds.), pp. 118–125. Edinbourgh, London: Churchill Livingstone 1975

Eichhorn, O.: Zur Behandlung der ischämischen Hirnschädigung. Med. Welt *42*, 2314–2318 (1969)

Ekström-Jodal, B., von Essen, C., Haggendal, E., Roos, B.E.: Effects of noradrenaline, 5-hydroxytryptamine, and dopamine on the cerebral blood flow in the dog. Stroke *4*, 367–368 (1973)

Elliott, C.G., Brown, A.L., Smith, T.C.G.: Multi-centre general practitioner trial of isoxsuprine in cerebrovascular disease: a pilot study. Curr. Med. Res. Opinion *1*, 554–562 (1973)

Emmons, P.R., Harrison, M.J.G., Honour, A.J., Mitchell, J.R.A.: Effect of dipyridamole on human platelet behavior. Lancet *1965 II*, 603–606

Enz, A., Iwangoff, P., Markstein, R., Wagner, H.: The effect of hydergine on the enzymes involved in cAMP turnover in the brain. Triangle *14*, 90–92 (1975)

Espagno, S., Lazorthes, Y., Arbus, L.: Techniques d'étude hémodynamique et métabolique d'un médicament à visée vasculaire cérébrale. Thérapeutique *45*, 888–890 (1969)

Fazekas, J., Bessman, A., Cotsonas, N., Jr., Alman, R.: Cerebral hemodynamics in cerebral arteriosclerosis. J. Gerontol. *8*, 137–145 (1953)

Feine-Haake, G.: Zur Objektivierung der therapeutischen Wirksamkeit von Trental 400. Fortschr. Med. *95*, 48–58 (1977)

Fields, W.S.: Transient cerebral ischemic attackes (TIA's). In: Brain and heart infarct. Zülch, K.J., Kaufmann, W., Hossmann, K.-A., Hossmann, V. (eds.), pp. 281–283. Berlin, Heidelberg, New York: Springer 1977

Fields, W.S., Lemak, N.A.: Controlled trial of aspirin in cerebral ischemia; study design, surveillance, and results. In: Acetylsalicyclic acid in cerebral ischemia and coronary heart disease. Breddin, K., Dorndorf, W., Loew, D., Marx, R. (eds.), pp. 85–91. Stuttgart, New York: Schattauer 1978

Fields, W.S., Lemak, N.A., Frankowski, R.F., Hardy, R.J.: Controlled trial of aspirin in cerebral ischemia, Part I. Stroke *8*, 301–316 (1977)

Fields, W.S., Lemak, N.A., Frankowski, R.F., Hardy, R.J.: Controlled trial of aspirin in cerebral ischemia, Part II: Surgical group. Stroke *9*, 309–319 (1978)

Fieschi, C., Volante, F., Battistini, N., Passero, S.: Experimental cerebral ischemia by arachidonic acid-induced platelet emboli. In: Brain and heart infarct. Zülch, K.J., Kaufmann, W., Hossmann, K.-A., Hossmann, V. (eds.), pp. 261–270. Berlin, Heidelberg, New York: Springer 1977

Fieschi, C., Battistini, N., Nardini, M., D'Ettore, M., Volante, F., Zanette, E.: Clinical management of cerebrovascular disease. In: Atherosclerosis reviews. Paoletti, R., Gotto, A.M., jr. (eds.), vol. 2, pp. 155–174. New York: Raven Press 1977

Fieschi, C., Battistini, N., Volante, F., Passero, S.: Protective effects of drugs against embolic TIA in an animal model. In: Acetylsalicyclic acid in cerebral ischemia and coronary heart disease. Breddin, K., Dorndorf, W., Loew, D., Marx, R. (eds.), pp. 119–125. Stuttgart, New York: Schattauer 1978

Fine, E.W., Lewis, D., Villa Landa, I., Blakemore, C.B.: The effect of cyclandelate on mental function in patients with arteriosclerotic brain disease. Brit. J. Psychiat. *117*, 157–161 (1970)

Fleckenstein, A., Fleckenstein-Grün, G.: Zur kombinierten Anwendung von Herzglykosiden und Ca-Antagonisten. Arzneim. Forsch. *27*, 736–742 (1977)

Fontaine, L., Grand, M., Szarvasi, E.: Premières comparaisons, in vitro et in vivo, des activités antispasmodiques dans une série de dialcoylaminoesters et éthéroxydes. Compt. Rend. *262*, 719–721 (1966)

Fontaine, L., Grand, M., Chabert, J., Szarvasi, E., Bayssat, M.: Pharmacologie générale d'une substance nouvelle vasodilatrice, le naftidrofuryl. Bull. Chim. Thér. *6*, 463–469 (1968)

Fontaine, L., Grand, M., Szarvasi, E., Bayssat, M.: Etude de l'activité vasodilatrice du naftidrofuryl. Bull. Chim. Thér. *1*, 39–43 (1969)

Fossey, F., Pasquier, Ch.: Utilisation, dans les encéphalopathies chroniques, d'un médicament oxygénateur cérébral. Rev. Neuropsychiatr. Infant. *20*, 887–891 (1972)

Fournier, A.M., Mourou, M.: Naftidrofuryl et spasmes carotidiens. J. Radiol. Electrol. Med. Nucl. *53*, 897–901 (1972)

Gänshirt, H.: Zerebrale Durchblutungsstörungen. Therapiewoche *28*, 835–839 (1978)

Gärtner, E., Enzengross, H.G., Vlahov, V., Schanzenbächer, P., Brandt, H., Betz, E.: Durchblutung, Sauerstoffdruck und pH des zerebralen Kortex unter Einwirkung von Fludilat. Arzneim. Forsch. *25*, 887–891 (1975)

Gaetano, G. de, Miragliotta, G., Roncucci, R., Lansen, J., Lambelin, G.: Suloctidil: A novel inhibitor of platelet aggregation in human beings. (1). Thromb. Res. *8*, 361–371 (1976)

Gallus, A.S., Hirsh, J.: Antithrombotic drugs. Drugs *12*, 21–68, 132–157 (1976)

Garcia Guerra, C.M.: Evaluacion clinica del fludilat en la insuficienca vascular cerebral. Prensa Med. Mex. *42*, 504–508 (1978)

Gautier, J.C.: Arterial pathology in cerebral ischaemia and infarction. In: Progress in stroke. Greenhalgh, R.M., Rose, F.C. (eds.), pp. 28–39. Kent: Pitman Medical 1979

Genton, E., Barnett, H.J.M., Fields, W.S., Gent, M., Hoak, J.C.: Cerebral ischemia: The role of thrombosis and of antithrombotic therapie. Stroke *8*, 150–175 (1977)

Glatt, A., Klebs, K., Koella, W.P.: Influence of vincamine and piracetam on sleep-waking pattern of the cat. Biol. Psychiatry *13*, 417–427 (1979)

Gloning, K., Klausenberger, E.M.: Untersuchungen über die Hirngefäßfunktion im Bewegungsfilm. Wien. Klin. Wochenschr. *70*, 145–149 (1958)

Godfraind, T.: Actions of suloctidil and of the Ca-antagonist cinnarizine on the rat aorta. Arch. Int. Pharmacodyn. *221*, 342–343 (1976)

Godfraind, T., Kaba, A.: Blockade or reversal of the contraction induced by calcium and adrenaline in depolarized arterial smooth muscle. Br. J. Pharmacol. *36*, 549–560 (1969)

Godfraind, T., Sturbois, X.: Les lésions du myocarde provoquées par L'Isoprénaline et leur pré-´vention par la cinnarizine. Arch. Int. Pharmacodyn. *199*, 203–205 (1972)

Gossetti, B., Ventura, M., Damiano, M., Bait, C., Zaccaria, A.: CBF changes after (−) ebur-namonine infusion in patients with cerebrovascular insufficiency. Eur. Neurol. *17*, 171–172 (1979)

Gotshall, R.K., Harker, L.A.: Using antithrombotic therapy in ischemic cerebrovascular disease. Geriatrics *32*, 101–104 (1977)

Gottstein, U.: Der Hirnkreislauf unter dem Einfluß vasoaktiver Substanzen. Einzeldarstellungen aus der theoretischen und klinischen Medizin, Bd. 15. Heidelberg: A. Hüthig 1962

Gottstein, U.: Pharmacological studies of total cerebral blood flow in man with comments on the possibility of improving regional cerebral blood flow of drugs. Acta Neurol. Scand. Suppl. *14*, 136–141 (1965)

Gottstein, U.: The effect of drugs on cerebral blood flow especially in patients of older age. Pharmakopsychiatr. Neuro-Psychopharmakol. *2*, 100–109 (1969)

Grasser, K., Petocz, L., Komlos, E.: Effect of basic ethers of cycloalkanol derivatives on gastric juice secretion and experimental ulcer in the rat. Acta Physiol. Hung. *30*, 369 (1966)

Griguer, P., Brochier, M., Raynaud, R.: Étude de l'effet inhibiteur du dipyridamole sur l'adhe-´sivite et l'agrégation plaquettaires „in vitro" et „in vivo". Ann. Cardiol. Angeiol. *24*, 2–36 (1975)

Gryglewski, R.J., Bunting, S., Moncada, S., Flower, R.J., Vane, J.P.: Arterial walls are protected against deposition of platelet thrombi by a substance (prostaglandin X) which they make from prostaglandin endoperoxides. Prostaglandins *12*, 685–713 (1976)

Gurewich, W., Lipinski, B.: Evaluation of antithrombotic properties of suloctidil in comparison with aspirin and dipyridamole. Thromb. Res. *9*, 101–108 (1976)

Guyer, B.M.: The management of cerebrovascular disease with isoxsuprine resinate (Defencin CP). Clin. Trials. J. *14*, 159–163 (1977)

Guyer, B.M.: Cerebrovascular disease in the elderly: Response to isoxsuprine resinate (Defencin CP) therapy. Clin. Trials J. *15*, 49–53 (1978)

Gygax, P., Wiernsperger, N., Meier-Ruge, W., Baumann, T.: Effect of papaverine and dihydroergotoxine mesylate on cerebral microflow EEG, and pO_2 in oligemic hypotension. Gerontology *24*, 14–22 (1978)

Hall, P.: Cyclandelate in the treatment of cerebral arteriosclerosis. J. Am. Geriatr. Soc. *24*, 41–45 (1976)

Hamberg, M., Svensson, J., Samuelsson, B.: Mechanism of antiaggregating effect of aspirin on human platelets. Lancet 1974, II, 223–224

Hamberg, M., Svensson, J., Samuelsson, B.: Thromboxanes: A new group of biologically active compounds derived from prostaglandin endoperoxides. Proc. Natl. Acad. Sci. U.S.A. *72*, 2994–2998 (1975)

Handa, J.: Cerebral vascular effects of a new derivative of 1,4-dihydropyridine (YC-93), with special reference to its effect on the experimental basilar artery spasm in cats. Arch. Jpn. Chir. *44*, 343–351 (1976)

Handa, J., Yoneda, S., Koyama, T., Matsuda, M., Handa, H.: Experimental cerebral vasospasm in cats: Modification by a new synthetic vasodilator YC-93. Surg. Neurol. *3*, 195–199 (1975)

Handa, J., Koyama, T., Tsuji, H., Ishijima, Y., Teraura, T.: Clinical effect of a new 1,4-dihydropyridine derivative, YC-93, in patients with cerebrovascular diseases. Arch. Jap. Chir. *48*, 400–403 (1979)

Harker, I.A., Slichter, S.J.: Studies of platelet and fibrinogen kinetics in patients with prosthetic heart valves. New Engl. J. Med. *283*, 1302–1305 (1970)

Harker, I.A., Slichter, S.J.: Arterial and venous thromboembolism: Kinetic characterization and evaluation of therapy. Thromb. Diath. Haemorrh. *31*, 188–203 (1974)

Harrison, M.J.G.: Evidence for thromboembolism as a cause of transient cerebral ischemia. In: Acetylsalicylic acid in cerebral ischemia and coronary heart disease. Breddin, K., Dorndorf, F.W., Loew, D., Marx, R. (eds.), pp. 75–77. Stuttgart, New York: F.K. Schattauer 1978

Harrison, M.J.G., Marshall, J., Meadows, J.C., Ross Russel, R.W.: Effect of aspirin in amaurosis fugax. Lancet 1971. II, 743

Harwart, D.: The treatment of chronic cerebrovascular insufficiency: A double-blind study with pentoxifylline ("Trental" 400). Curr. Med. Res. Opin. 6, 73–84 (1979)

Hass, W.K.: Aspirin for the lumping brain. Stroke 8, 299–301 (1977)

Haupt, R., Isermann, H.: Zur Lern- und Konzentrationsfähigkeit von Patienten in höherem Lebensalter mit depressivem Syndrom bei cerebralen Durchblutungsstörungen. Nervenarzt 47, 269–271 (1976)

Heinsius, E., Flamm, P.: Ophthalmologische Erfahrungen mit dem neuen Xanthin-Körper BL 191. Med. Klin. 68, 1540–1542 (1973)

Heiss, W.D.: Drug effect on regional cerebral blood flow in focal cerebrovascular disease. J. Neurol. Sci. 19, 461–482 (1973)

Heiss, W.D., Zeiler, K.: Medikamentöse Beeinflussung der Hirndurchblutung. Pharmakotherapie 1, 137–144 (1978)

Heiss, W.D., Prosenz, P., Gloning, K., Tschabitscher, H.: Regional and total cerebral blood flow under vasodilating drugs. In: Brain and blood flow. Ross Russell, R.W. (ed.), pp. 270–276. London: Pitman 1970

Held, K.: Experimentelle Untersuchungen über Wirkung und Wirkungsmechanismus von Xantinol-nicotinat beim Menschen im Sauerstoffmangel. Therapiewoche 23, 3270–3272 (1973)

Held, K., Wünsche, O., Reuter, N.: Die Wirkung von Xantinol-Nicotinat auf den Menschen im Sauerstoffmangel der Höhe. Ärztl. Prax. 25, 91–93 (1973)

Henry, P.D., Borda, L., Schuchlieb, R.: Chronotropic and inotropic effects of vasodilators. In: International Adalat® Pannell discussion. Lichtlen, P.R., Kimura, E., Taira, N. (eds.), pp. 14–23. Amsterdam: Excerpta Medica 1979

Herrschaft, H.: Kann die Hirndurchblutung medikamentös verbessert werden? Schweiz. med. Wochenschr. 107, 581–583 (1977)

Herrschaft, H.: Möglichkeiten der medikamentösen Behandlung der zerebralen Mangeldurchblutung. Therapiewoche 27, 4525–4534 (1979)

Herrschaft, H., Gleim, F., Schmidt, H., Duss, P.: Das Verhalten der regionalen Hirndurchblutung unter dem Einfluß von Bencyclan. Quantitative örtliche Hirndurchblutungsmessungen bei Gesunden und Kranken mit zerebrovaskulärer Insuffizienz im Wachzustand und leichter Allgemeinnarkose. Med. Klin. 70, 896–903 (1975)

Herzfeld, U., Wittgen, M.: Veränderung der zerebralen Zirkulationszeit unter dem Einfluß von Hydergin. Ärztl. Forsch. 25, 224–230 (1971)

Herzfeld, U., Christian, W., Oswald, W.D., Ronge, J., Wittgen, M.: Zur Wirkungsanalyse von Hydergin im Langzeitversuch. Med. Klin. 67, 1118–1125 (1972)

Heyck, H.: Der Einfluß der Nikotinsäure auf die Hirndurchblutung und den Hirnstoffwechsel bei Cerebralsklerosen und anderen diffusen Durchblutungsstörungen des Gehirns. Schweiz. Med. Wschr. 92, 226–231 (1962)

Hockwin, O., Korte, I., Loth, C., Ohrloff, Ch., Fuss, R., Schmidt, G.: Action of bencyclane-hydrogen-fumarate on the carbohydrate metabolism of bovine lens homogenates. Arzneim. Forsch. 27, 1417–1420 (1977)

Hoeft, H.J.: Fludilat im Doppelblindversuch zur Behandlung zerebraler und peripherer Durchblutungsstörungen. Therapiewoche 22, 905–911 (1972)

Hoffmeister, F.: Cerebrovascular diseases: Drugs and methods. Proceedings of the International Symposium "Experimental and clinical methodologies for study of acute and chronic cerebrovascular diseases, pp. 243–247. Oxford, New York: SIR Pergamon Press 1981

Hoffmeister, F., Kazda, S., Krause, H.P.: Influence of nimodipine (BAY e 9736) on the postischaemic changes of brain function. Acta Neurol. Scand. 60, 358–359 (1979)

Horch, U., Kadatz, R., Kopitar, Z., Ritsehard, J., Weisenberger, H.: Pharmacology of dipyridamole and its derivatives. Thromb. Diath. Haemorrh. Suppl. 42, 253–266 (1970)

Horrobin, D.F., Ally, A.I., Manku, M.S.: Dipyridamole and platelet aggregation. Lancet 1978 II, 270

Horton, G.E., Johnson, P.C.: The application of radioisotopes to the study of cerebral blood flow, comparison of three methods. Angiology 15, 70–74 (1964)

Hossmann, V.: Coagulation disturbanas in cerebroviscular disorders. In: Brain and heart infarct. Zülch, K.J., Kaufmann, W., Hossmann, K.-A., Hossmann, V. (ed.), pp. 81–92. Berlin, Heidelberg, New York: Springer 1977

Hünermann, B., Felix, R., Wesener, K., Winkler, C.: Zur Wirkung von Papaverinhydrochlorid auf die Hirnzirkulation. Arzneim. Forsch. 25, 652–653 (1975)

Hussain, S.M.A., Gedye, J.L., Naylor, R., Brown, A.L.: The objective measurement of mental performance in cerebrovascular disease. Practicioner *216*, 222–228 (1976)

Hyams, D.E.: Cerebral function and drug therapy: The use of cerebral vasodilators "vasorelaxans", "haemokinators", and "activators". In: Textbook of geriatric medicine and gerontology, IInd Edition, J.C. Brocklehurst (ed.), pp. 671–711. Edinbourgh: Churchill Livingstone 1978

Iliff, L.D., Du Boulay, G.H., Marshall, I., Ross Russel, R.W., Symon, L.: Wirkung von Nicergolin auf die Gehirndurchblutung. Arzneim. Forsch. *29*, 1277–1279 (1979)

Imparato, A.M., Riles, T.S., Gorstein, F.: The carotid bifurcation plaque: pathologic findings associated with cerebral ischemia. Stroke *10*, 238–245 (1979)

Irvine, R.E., Greenfield, P.R., Griffith, D.G.C., Paget, S.C., Strouthidis, T.M., Vaughan, V.St.G.: Cinnarizine in cerebrovascular disease. Geront. Clin. *12*, 297–301 (1970)

Iwanami, M., Shieanuma, T., Fujimoto, M., Kawai, R., Murakami, M.: Synthesis of new water-soluble dihydropyridine vasodilators. Chem. Pharm. Bull. *27*, 1426–1440 (1979)

Jäger, W., Scharrer, I., Satkowski, U., Breddin, K.: Thrombozyten-aggregationshemmende Wirkung von Bencyclan in vitro und in vivo. Arzneim. Forsch. *25*, 1938–1944 (1975)

Jakovlev, V., Thiemer, K., Habersang, S., Achterrath-Tuckermann, U., von Schlichtegroll, A., Sofia, R.D.: Über allgemeine pharmakologische Untersuchungen mit Tinofedrin. Arzneim. Forsch. *28*, 1335–1343 (1978)

Jansen, W.: Die zerebrale Leistungsschwäche im Blickpunkt therapeutischer Bemühungen doppelblinde Vergleichsprüfung mit encephabol forte und weiteren neurotropen Substanzen bei ambulanten geriatrischen Patienten. Therapiewoche *30*, 1126, 1129–1131 (1980)

Jobin, F.: Acetylsalicylic acid, hemostasis and human thromboembolism. Semin. Thromb. Hemostas. *4*, 199–240 (1978)

Jovanovic, U.J.: Polygraphische Registrierungen nach parenteraler Applikation von 3,7-dimethyl-1(5-oxo-hexyl)-xanthin (BL 191). Arzneim. Forsch. *22*, 994–999 (1972)

Judge, T.G., Urquart, A., Blakemore, C.B.: Cyclandelate and mental function, a double blind crossover trial in normal elderly subjects. Age Ageing *2*, 121–124 (1973)

Kaindl, F.: Rheographie peripherer Arterien – eine neue Methode zur Beurteilung arterieller Gefäße. Arch. Kreisl.-Forsch. *20*, 247–286 (1954)

Kanig, K., Hoffmann, Kh.: Der 32 P-Einbau in Adenosinphosphate des Rattengehirns nach zweiwöchiger oraler Verabreichung von Vincamin. Arzneim. Forsch. *29*, 33–34 (1979)

Kanig, K., Nitschki, J., Peiler-Ischikawa, K.: Der Einfluß von Naftidrofuryl auf den 32 P-Einbau in Nukleinsäuren und Adenosinphosphate des Rattengehirns. Arzneim. Forsch. *29*, 33–34 (1979)

Karlsberg, P., Elliott, H.W., Adams, J.E.: Effect of various pharmacologic agents on cerebral arteries. Neurology (Minneap.) *13*, 772–778 (1963)

Karpati, E., Szporny, L.: General and cerebral haemodynamic activity of ethyl apovincaminate. Arzneim. Forsch. *26*, 1908–1912 (1976)

Kazda, S., Hoffmeister, F.: Effect of some cerebral vasodilators on the postischaemic impaired cerebral reperfusion in cats. Arch. Pharmacol. Suppl. *307*, R 43 (1979)

Kazda, S., Towart, R.: Differences in the effects of the calcium antagonists nimodipine (BAY e 9736) and bencyclan on cerebral and peripheral vascular smooth muscle. Brit. J. Pharmacol. *72*, 582-3 P (1981)

Kazda, S., Hoffmeister, F., Garthoff, B., Towart, R.: Prevention of the postischemic impaired reperfusion of the brain by nimodipine (BAY e 9736). Acta Neurol. Scand. *60*, 302–303 (1979)

Kellner, H.: Zur Behandlung chronischer arterieller Durchblutungsstörungen. Doppelblindversuch mit Trendal 400. Münch. Med. Wochenschr. *118*, 1399–1402 (1976)

Kety, S.S.: Human cerebral blood flow and oxygen consumption as related to ageing. Res. Publ. Assoc. Nerv. Ment. Dis. *35*, 31–45 (1956)

Kiss, T., Szmolenszky, T., Lelkes, J., Tekeres, M.: Die Wirkung der Vasodilatatoren Bencyclan und Tolazolin auf die Muskeldurchblutung im pharmakologischen und klinischen Experiment. Therapiewoche *22*, 2791–2792 (1972)

Klausberger, E., Rajna, P.: Cerebrale Zirkulationsvorgänge unter der Einwirkung von Bencyclan. Arzneim. Forsch. *20*, 1457–1460 (1970)

Klein, K., Siedek, H.: Zur Erfassung intra- und extrazerebraler Kreislaufveränderungen mit neuen Methoden. Med. Welt *21*, 1167–1171 (1965)

Klein, K., Siedek, H.: Zum Verhalten des zerebralen Gefäßwiderstandes unter sympathikolytischem Einfluß. Wien. Med. Wochenschr. *116*, 20–22 (1966)

Kloeze, J.: Relationship between chemical structure and platelet-aggregation activity of prostaglandins. Biochim. Biophys. Acta *187*, 285–292 (1969)

Köhler, E., Motzer, S., Greeff, K.: Die kardiodepressive Wirkung des Bencyclans. Res. Exp. Med. *165*, 111–125 (1975)

Kohlmeyer, K.: Der Einfluß eines neuen Vasodilatators (Bencyclan) auf die allgemeine und regionale Hirndurchblutung. Herz Kreisl. *4*, 196–203 (1972)

Koppenhagen, K., Wenig, H.G., Müller, K.: The effect of pentoxifylline ("Trental") on cerebral blood flow: a double blind study. Curr. Med. Res. Opin. *4*, 681–684 (1977)

Kovacs, I.B., Csalay, L., Csakvary, G.: Antithrombotic and fibrinolytic effect of bencyclane. Arzneim. Forsch. *21*, 1553–1556 (1971)

Kraupp, O., Wolner, E., Adler-Kastner, L., Chirikdjian, J.J., Ploszczanski, B., Tuisl, E.: Die Wirkung von Hexobendin auf Sauerstoffverbrauch, Energetik und Substratstoffwechsel des Herzens. I Versuche mit intravenös verabreichten Einzeldosen. Arzneim. Forsch.*16*, 692–696 (1966a)

Kraupp, O., Wolner, E., Adler-Kastner, L., Chirikdjian, J.J., Ploszczanski, B., Tuisl, E.: Die Wirkung von Hexobendin auf Sauerstoffverbrauch, Energetik und Substratstoffwechsel des Herzens. II. Versuche mit intravenösen Infusionen: Arzneim. Forsch. *16*, 697–705 (1966b)

Kraupp, O., Nell, G., Raberger, G., Stühlinger, W.: The effect of hexobendine on cerebral blood flow and metabolism. Arzneim. Forsch. *19*, 1691–1698 (1969)

Küchle, H.J.: Zur Therapie der akuten arteriellen Durchblutungsstörungen von Netzhaut und Sehnerv. Klin. Monatsbl. Augenheilkd. *171*, 395–400 (1977)

Kukovetz, W.R., Poech, G.: Inhibition of cyclic-3′,5′-nucleotide-phosphodiesterase as a possible mode of action of papaverine and similarly acting drugs. Arch. Pharmakol. *267*, 189–194 (1970)

Kukovetz, W.R., Pölch, G., Holzmann, S., Paietta, E.: Zum Wirkungsmechanismus von Bencyclan an der glatten Muskulatur. Arzneim. Forsch. *25*, 722–726 (1975)

Lavrentieva, N.B., Mchedlishvili, G.I., Plechkova, E.K.: Distribution and activity of cholinesterase in nervous structures of the pial arteries (a histochemical study). Bull. Biol. Med. Exp. U.R.S.S. *64*, 110–113 (1968)

Lebedeva, N.V., Makarova, G.V.: Izmenenie parametra asimmetrii frontov voln EEG u bolnych s naruschenijami mozgovogo krovoobraschchenija pri lechenii istenonom: Z. Nevropatol. Psikhiatr. *75*, 1619–1624 (1975)

Lehrach, F., Müller, R.: Ergebnisse der klinischen Prüfung des Vaostherapeuticums 3,7-Dimethyl-1-(5-oxo-hexyl)-xanthin (BL 191). Arzneim. Forsch. *21*, 1171–1174 (1971)

Levy, L.L., Wallace, J.D.: Cerebral blood flow regulation. II. Vasodilator mechanisms. Stroke *8*, 189–193 (1977)

Lievre, M., Ollagnier, M., Faucon, G.: Einfluß auf die zerebrale Durchblutung und α-sympatholytische Eigenschaften von Nicergolin. Arzneim.Forsch. *29*, 1227–1231 (1979)

Lim, C.C., Cook, P.J., James, I.M.: The effect of an acute infusion of vincamine and ethyl apovincaminate on cerebral blood flow in healthy volunteers. Br. J. Clin. Pharmacol. *9*, 100–101 (1980)

Linee, P., Lacroix, P., Le Polles, J.B., Aurousseau, M., Boulu, R., van den Driessche, J., Albert, O.: Cerebral metabolic, hemodynamic and antihypoxic properties of l-eburnamonine. Eur. Neurol. *17*, 113–120 (1979)

Malaisse, W.J.: Calcium-antagonists and islet function. X. Effect of suloctidil. Arch. Int. Pharmacodyn. *228*, 339–344 (1977)

Marolda, M., Fragassi, N., Buscaino, G.A.: Clinical evaluation of (−) Eburnamonine in comparison with nicergoline in patients suffering from chronic brain ischemia. Eur. Neurol. *17*, 159–166 (1979)

Masotti, G., Poggesi, L., Galanti, G., Neri Serneri, G.G.: Stimulation of prostacyclin by dipyridamole. Lancet *1979 I*, 1412

Matsuda, M., Meyer, J.S., Ott, E.O., Aoyagi, M., Tagashira, Y.: Cholinergic influence on auto-regulation and CO_2 responsiveness of the brain. Circulation *50*, III-90 (Abstr.) (1974)

McElroy, F.A., Philp, R.B.: Relative potencies of dipyridamole and related agents as inhibitors of cyclic nucleotide phosphodiesterases: possible explanation of mechanism of inhibition of platelet function. Life Sci. *17*, 1479-1494 (1975)

McHenry, L.C.: Cerebral vasodilator therapy in stroke. Stroke *3*, 686-691 (1972)

McHenry, L.C., Jaffe, M.E., Kawamura, J., Goldberg, H.I.: Hydergine effect on cerebral circulation in cerebrovascular disease. J. Neurol. Sci. *13*, 475-480 (1971)

McHenry, L.C., Jaffe, M.E., West, J.W., Cooper, E.S., Kenton, E.J., Kawamura, J., Oshino, T., Goldberg, H.I.: Regional cerebral blood flow and cardiovascular effects of hexobendine in stroke patients. Neurology (Minneap.) *22*, 217-223 (1972)

Meer-Van Manen van der, A.H.E.: Klinische evaluatie van cinnarizine bij geriatrische patieen-ten. Ned.Tijdschr. Geneesk. *111*, 256-261 (1967)

Meng, K.: Tierexperimentelle Untersuchungen zur antithrombotischen Wirkung von Acetylsa-licylsäure. Ther. Ber. *47*, 69-79 (1975)

Meng, K.: Tierexperimentelle Thrombose und Behandlung mit Acetylsalicylsäure. Med. Welt *27*, 1359-1362 (1976)

Meng, K., Seuter, F.: Effect of acetylsalicylic acid on experimentally induced arterial thrombo-sis in rats. Naunyn-Schmiedebergs Arch. Pharmacol. *301*, 115-119 (1977)

Merory, J., Du Bonlay, G.H., Marshall, J., Morris, J., Ross Russell, R.W., Symon, L., Thomas, D.J.: Effect of tinofedrin (Homburg D 8955) on cerebral blood flow in multi-infarct de-mentia. J. Neurol. Neurosurg. Psychiatry *41*, 900-902 (1978)

Meyer, J.S., Deshmuch, V.D., Welch, K.M.A.: Experimental studies concerned with the patho-genesis of cerebral ischaemia and infarction. In: Cerebral Arterial Disease. Ross Russell, R.W. (ed.), pp. 57-84. Edinbourgh, London: Churchill Livingstone 1976

Meyer, J.S., Gotoh, F., Gilroy, J., Nara, N.: Improvement in brain oxygenation and clinical improvement in patients with stroke treated with papaverin hydrochlorid. J. Am. Med. As-soc. *194*, 957-961 (1965)

Meyer, J.S., Kanda, T., Shinohara, Y., Fukuuchi, Y., Shimazu, K., Ericsson, A.D., Gordon, W.H.: Effect of hexobendine on cerebral hemispheric blood flow and metabolism. Neurol-ogy (Minneap.) *21*, 691-702 (1971)

Meyer, J.S., Mathew, N.T., Hartmann, A.: Orally administered betahistine and regional cere-bral blood flow in cerebrovascular disease. J. Clin. Pharmacol. *14*, 280-289 (1974)

Meyer, J.S., Welch, K.M.A.: Contribution of platelet aggregation and serotonin release to pro-gressive cerebral infarction. In: Platelet aggregation in the pathogenesis of cerebrovascular disorders (Abstracts: Round Rable Conference, Rome, 1974). Fazio, C. (ed.), pp. 67-75 (1974)

Meynaud, A., Grand, M., Fontaine, L.: Beeinflussung der Hirndurchblutung und des Hirn-stoffwechsels durch Naftidrofuryl. Presented at International Symposium on CBF. Tou-louse 1972

Meynaud, A., Grand, M., Fontaine, L.: Effect of naftidrofuryl upon energy metabolism of the brain. Arzneim. Forsch. *23*, 1431-1436 (1973)

Mikus, P.: Klinische, physiologische und neurophysiologische Ergebnisse einer Doppelblind-studie mit Vincamin-Cromesilat bei Patienten mit cerebraler Durchblutungsinsuffizienz. Arzneim. Forsch. *28*, 2165-2168 (1980)

Mikus, P., Polak, O., Ochsenreither, A.M.: Klinische und elektroenzephalographische Ergeb-nisse eines Doppelblindversuches mit Vincamin (Pervincamin®) bei fortgeschrittener Zere-bralsklerose. Pharmakopsychiatry *6*, 39-49 (1973)

Millikan, C.H., McDowell, F.H.: Treatment of transient ischemic attacks. Stroke *9*, 299-308 (1978)

Mills, D.C.B., Smith, J.B.: The influence on platelet aggregation of drugs that affect the accu-mulation of adenosine 3',5'-cyclic monophosphate in platelets. Biochem. J. *121*, 185-196 (1971)

Miyazaki, M.: Effect of cerebral circulatory drugs on cerebral and peripheral circulation, with special reference to aminophylline, papaverine, cyclandelate, and isoxuprine. Jpn. Circulat. J. *35*, 1053-1057 (1971)

Molnar, G., Keller, L.: Die Wirkung von Bencyclan auf die Durchblutung der Extremitäten von Hunden nach intraarterieller Gabe. Arzneim. Forsch. 20, 1370–1371 (1970)

Moncada, S., Korbut, R.: Dipyridamole and other phosphodiesterase inhibitors act as antithrombotic agents by potentiating endogenous prostacyclin. Lancet 1978 I, 1286–1289

Moncada, S., Vane, J.R.: The discovery of prostacyclin – A fresh insight into arachidonic acid metabolism. In: Biochemical aspects of prostaglandins and thromboxanes. Kharash, N., Fried, J. (eds.), pp. 155–177. New York, San Francisco, London: Academic Press 1977

Moncada, S., Vane, J.R.: Mode of action of aspirin-like drugs. Adv. Intern. Med. 24, 1–22 (1979)

Moncada, S., Gryglewski, R.J., Bunting, S., Vane, J.R.: An enzyme isolated from arteries transforms prostaglandin endoperoxides to an unstable substance that inhibits platelet aggregation. Nature 263, 663–665 (1976)

Moncada, S., Flower, R.F., Russell-Smith, N.R.: Dipyridamole and platelet function. Lancet 1978 II, 1257–1258

Moretti, A.: Metabolische und neurochemische Wirkung von Nicergolin auf das Zentralnervensystem: Übersicht über die experimentellen Untersuchungen. Arzneim. Forsch. 29, 1213–1223 (1979)

Mucci, P., Sternieri, E.: Influenza della papaverina sulla irrorazione cerebrale del coniglio. Boll. Soc. Ital. Biol. Sper. 44, 965–969 (1968)

Müller, R.: Zum gegenwärtigen Stand der Hämorheologie aus klinisch-pharmakologischer Sicht. Therapiewoche 30, 2440–2451 (1980)

Mustard, J.F., Packham, M.A.: Platelets, thrombosis, and drugs. Drugs 9, 19–76 (1975)

Mustard, J.F., Murphy, E.A., Robinson, G.A., Roswell, H.C., Ozge, A., Crookston, J.H.: Blood platelet survival. Thromb. Diath. Haemorrh. 13, 245–275 (1964)

Nayler, W.G., Ferrari, R., Williams, A.: Protective effect of pretreatment with verapramil, nifedipine, and propranolol on mitochondrial function in the ischaemic and reperfused myocardium. Am. J. Cardiol. 46, 242–248 (1980)

Neri Seneri, G.G., Gensini, G.F., Abbate, R., Favilla, S., Laureano, R.: Modulation by dipyridamole of the arachidonic acid metabolic pathway in platelets. An in vivo and in vitro study. Thromb. Haemostas. 42, 197 (1979)

Nishino, H.: Effects of vasodilators on tissue blood flow. Folia Pharmacol. Jpn. 70, 621–628 (1974)

N.N.: Pyridimolcarbamat. Wien. Klin. Wochenschr. 84, 200–201 (1972)

Norre, M.: Suloctidil in vertigo: een dubbel-blind studie tegenover placebo. Ars. Medici 6, 1383–1391 (1977)

Obermeier, K., Thiemer, K., Schlichtegroll, V.A.: Einfluß von Tinofedrin auf den zerebralen Energiestoffwechsel von normotonen, hypotonen und hypoämischen Ratten nach Carotis-Verschluß. Arzneim. Forsch. 28, 1354–1360 (1978)

O'Brien, J.R.: Effect of antiinflammatory agents on platelets. Lancet 1968 I, 894–895

O'Brien, M.D., Veall, N.: Effects of cyclandelate on cerebral cortex perfusion-rates in cerebrovascular disease. Lancet 1966 II, 729–730

Olesen, J.: Cerebral blood flow. Methods for measurement. Regulation, effects of drugs and changes in disease. Acta Neurol. Scand. 50, 1–34 (1974)

Olesen, J., Paulson, O.B.: The effect of intra-arterial papaverine on the regional cerebral blood flow in patients with stroke or intracranial tumor. Stroke 2, 148–149 (1971)

Olesen, J., Skinhoj, E.: Effects of ergot alkaloids (hydergine) on cerebral haemodynamics. Acta Pharmacol. Toxicol. 31, 75–85 (1972)

Ott, E., Lechner, H.: The influence of nimodipine on cerebral blood flow in patients with subacute cerebral infarction. In: Pathophysiology and pharmacotherapy of cerebrovascular doisorders. Betz, E. (ed.). in press 1981

Packham, M.A., Jenkins, C.S.P., Kinlough-Rathbone, R.L., Mustard, J.F.: Agents influencing platelet adhesion to surfaces and the release reaction. Circulation 44, 67 Suppl. 2 (Abstr.) (1971)

Pathy, J., Menon, G., Reynolds, A., Van Strik, R.: Betahistine hydrochloride (serc) in cerebrovascular disease: A placebo-controlled study. Age Ageing 6, 179–184 (1977)

Paulson, O.: Mechanism of action of aminophylline and of hypocapnia on cerebrovascular disease. Acta Neurol. Scand. 46, 251 (1970)

Pech, A., Gitenet, P.: La pervincamine en O.-R.-L. Ann. Otol-Laryngol. *89*, 469–474 (1972)
Pedersen, A.K.: Dipyridamole and platelet aggregation. Lancet *1978 II*, 270
Perkin, G.D.: Anticoagulants in transient ischaemic attacks. In: Progress in Stroke. Greenhalgh, R.M., Rose, F.C. (eds.), pp. 181–203. Kent: Pitman Medical 1979
Persantine-Aspirin Reinfarction Study Research Group: Persantine and Aspirin in coronary heart disease. Circulation *62*, 449–461 (1980)
Philp, R.B., Francey, I., McElroy, F.: Effects of dipyridamole and five related agents on human platelet aggregation and adenosine uptake. Thrombos. Res. *3*, 35–50 (1973)
Ponari, O., Civardi, E., Dettori, A.G., Megha, A., Poti, R., Bulletti, G.: In vitro effects of bencyclan on coagulation, fibrinolysis, and platelet function. Arzneim. Forsch. *26*, 1532–1538 (1976)
Pourrias, B., Raynaud, G., Courbevoie, Fr.: Action de quelques agents vaso-actifs sur l'irrigation sous corticale du lapin et du chien. Thérapie *27*, 849–860 (1972)
Prencipe, M., Pisarri, F.M., Cecconi, V., Agnoli, A.: Platelet aggregation in cerebrovascular patients. In: Platelet aggregation in the pathogenesis of cerebrovascular disorders (Abstracts: Round Table Conference, Rome 1974). Fazio, C. (ed.), pp. 49–53
Puig-Parellada, J., Planas, J.M.: Action of selective inhibitor of thromboxane synthetase on experimental thrombosis induced by arachidonic acid in rabbit. Lancet *1977 I*, 40
Purves, M.J.: The physiology of the cerebral circulation. Cambridge: Cambridge University Press 1972
Quadbeck, H., Lehmann, E.: Die Veränderung des oxidativen Glukosestoffwechsels des Gehirns unter langfristiger Xantinol-nicotinat-Medikation. Arzneim. Forsch. *28*, 1531–1532 (1978)
Raaflaub, J.: Zur Umwandlung von β-Pyridylcarbinol in Nikotinsäure im tierischen Organismus. Experientia *22*, 258–259 (1966)
Regli, F., Yamaguchi, T., Waltz, A.G.: Cerebral circulation. Effects of vasodilating drugs on blood flow and the microvasculature of ischemic and nonischemic cerebral cortex. Arch. Neurol. *24*, 467–474 (1971)
Regli, F., Yamaguchi, T., Waltz, A.: Cerebral circulation, effects of vasodilating drugs on blood flow and the microvasculature of ischemic and non-ischemic cerebral cortex. Arch. Neurol. *24*, 476–484 (1972)
Reichertz, P.L., Kruskemper, G., Fröhlich, W.D., Stadeler, J., Konrad, D., Schaar, W., Overall, J.E., Dickhöfer, C.: Untersuchungen des physischen und psychischen Verhaltens und deren medikamentöse Beeinflußbarkeit bei Altersheiminsassen. Sonderdruck aus „Verhandlungen der Deutschen Gesellschaft für innere Medizin", 73. Kongreß. München: J.F. Bergmann 1967
Reimann-Hunziker, R., Reimann-Hunziker, G.J.: Wirkung von Cinnarizin bei Arteriosclerosis cerebri. Besserung der Symptome durch vermehrte Sauerstoffzufuhr und -ausnützung mittels Cinnarizin. Praxis *39*, 1239–1242 (1969)
Rieger, H., Klose, H.J., Schmid-Schönbein, H., Wurzinger, L.: The effects of orally administered bencyclane on spontaneous platelet aggregation (PA) as a function of bencyclane concentration in coded samples. Thrombos. Res. *12*, 353–356 (1978)
Rifkin, P.L., Zucker, M.B.: The effect of dipyridamol and RA 233 on human platelet function in vitro. Thrombos. Diathes. Haemorrh. *29*, 694–700 (1973)
Ritter, R.M., Nail, H.R., Tatum, P., Blazi, M.: The effect of papaverine on patients with cerebral arteriosclerosis. Clin. Med. *78*, 18–22 (1971)
Roba, J., Reuse Blom, S., Lambelin, G.: In vivo antispasmodic activity of suloctidil. Arch. Int. Pharmacodyn. *221*, 54–59 (1976a)
Roba, J., Claeys, M., Lambelin, G.: Antiplatelet and antithrombogenic effect of suloctidil. Eur. J. Pharmacol. *37*, 265–274 (1976b)
Roba, J., Bourgain, R., Andries, R., Claeys, M., Van Opstal, W., Lambelin, G.: Antagonism by suloctidil of arterial thrombus formation in rats. Thrombos. Res. *9*, 585–594 (1976c)
Rodvien, R., Mielke, C.H.: Platelet and antiplatelet agents in strokes. Stroke *9*, 403–405 (1978)
Rokitansky, C.: Von: Handbuch der pathologischen Anatomie, vol. 4. (1842)
Rosenberg, F.J., Gimber-Phillips, P.E., Groblewski, G.E., Davison, C., Phillips, D.K., Goralnick, S.J., Canhill, E.D.: Acetylsalicyclic acid: Inhibition of platelet aggregation in the rabbit. J. Pharmacol. Exp. Ther. *179*, 410–418 (1971)

Rosenberger, L., Triggle, D.J.: Calcium, calcium translocation, and specific calcium antagonists. In: Calcium in drug action. Weiss, G.B. (ed.), pp. 3–31. New York: Plenum Press 1978

Rosenblum, W.J., El-Sabban, F.: Platelet aggregation in the cerebral microcirculation. Circ. Res. *40*, 320–328 (1977)

Rothlin, E., Taeschler, M.: Zur Wirkung von Adrenalin und Hydergin auf die Hirndurchblutung. Helv. Physiol. Pharmacol. Acta *9*, 37–39 (1951)

Rozenberg, M.C., Walker, C.M.: The effect of pyrimidine compounds on the potentiation of adenosine inhibition of aggregation, on adenosine phosphorylation and phosphodiesterase activity of blood platelets. Br. J. Haematol. *24*, 409–418 (1973)

Sacle, P., Battock, D., Genton, E.: Effects of clofibrate and sulfinpyrazone on platelet survival in coronary artery disease. Circulation *52*, 473–476 (1975)

Sakamoto, N., Terai, M., Takenaka, T., Maeno, H.: Inhibition of cyclic AMP phosphodiesterase by 2,6-dimethyl-4-(3-nitrophenyl)-1,4-dihydropyridine-3,5-dicarboxylic acid 3-2-(N-benzyl-N-methylamino) ethyl ester 5-methyl ester hydrochloride (YC-93), a potent vasodilator. Biochem. Pharmacol. *27*, 1269–1274 (1977)

Saletu, B., Anderer, P.: Zur Vigilanzförderung bei geriatrischen Patienten durch Tinofedrin i.v./ Doppelblinde, Plazebo-kontrollierte quantitative Pharmako-EEG-Untersuchungen. Arzneim. Forsch. *30*, 1218 (1980 a)

Saletu, B., Anderer, P.: Double-blind placebo-controlled quantitative pharmaco-EEG investigations after tinofedrine i.v. in geriatric patients. Curr. Ther. Res. *28*, 1–15 (1980 b)

Samuelsson, B., Folco, G., Granström, E., Kindahl, H., Malmsten, C.: Prostaglandins and thromboses: Biochemical and physiological considerations. In: Advances in Prostaglandin and Thromboxane Research. Coceanin, F., Olley, P.M. (eds.), vol. 4, pp. 1–25. New York: Raven Press 1978

Sandok, B.A., Furlan, A.J., Whisnant, P., Sundt, I.M., jr.: Guidelines for the management of transient ischemic attacks. Maro Clin. Proc. *53*, 665–674 (1978)

Saratikov, A.S., Usov, L.A., Filimonova, L.T., Gorshkova, V.K., Dimitrienko, V.F.: Galidore action on the hemodynamics and oxidative metabolism of the brain. Farmakol. Toksikol. *34*, 668–671 (1971)

Schindler, M.: Über die Wirkung von Papaverin, Hydergin, BAY e 9736 und Nifedipin auf die Aktivität der zytoplasmatischen („High-K_M"-) und membrangebundenen („Low K_M"-) cAMP-Phosphodiesterasen des Rattenhirns und -herzens. Inaugural-Dissertation zur Erlangung des Doktorgrades der Medizin der Fakultät für theoretische Medizin am Universitätsklinikum der Gesamthochschule Essen, 1979

Schlittler, M., Furlenmeier, A.: Vincamine, ein Alkaloid aus Vinca minor L. (Apocyanaceae). Helv. Chim. Acta *36*, 2017–2020 (1953)

Schmid-Schönbein, H.: Rheological properties of the blood under normal and pathological conditions. In: Brain and heart infarct. Zülch, K.J., Kaufmann, W., Hossmann, K.-A., Hossmann, V. (eds.), pp. 96–106. Berlin, Heidelberg, New York: Springer 1977

Schmid-Schönbein, H.: Der gegenwärtige Stand der Hämorheologie – Methoden, Befunde und Bedeutung für die Physiologie und Pathologie des Blutkreislaufs. Wien. Klin. Wochenschr. *90*, 245–253 (1978)

Schmidt, R.: Eine neue Methode zur Erzeugung von Thromben durch Unterkühlung der Gefäßwand und ihre Anwendung zur Prüfung von Acetylsalicylsäure und Heparin. Inaugural-Dissertation, Gießen, 1975

Schneider, E., Fischer, P.A., Jacobi, P.: Bencyclan (Fludilat) in der Behandlung lokaler Hirndurchblutungsstörungen. Med. Klin. *71*, 1611–1616 (1977)

Schneider, M., Wiemers, K.: Über die Wirkung der hydrierten Mutterkornalkaloide auf die Gehirndurchblutung. Klin. Wochenschr. *29*, 580–581 (1951)

Seidel, G., Endell, W.: Effect of xanthinol nicotinate treatment on platelet aggregation. Int. J. Clin. Pharmacol. *15*, 139–143 (1977)

Sen, S., Chakravarty, A.: Clinical experience with pentoxifylline in occlusive cerebrovascular disorders. Angiology *28*, 340–344 (1977)

Seuter, F.: Inhibition of platelet aggregation by acetylsalicylic acid and other inhibitors. Haemostasis *5*, 85–95 (1976)

Seuter, F., Busse, W.D.: Arachidonic acid induced mortality in animals – An appropriate model for the evaluation of antithrombotic drugs? In: Arachidonic acid metabolism in inflammation and thrombosis. Agents and actions. Brune, K., Baggiolini, E. (eds.), Suppl. 4, pp. 175–183. Basel, Boston, Stuttgart: Birkhäuser 1979

Seuter, F., Sitt, R., Busse, W.-D.: Experimentally induced thromboatherosclerosis in rats and rabbits. Folia Angiologica 28, 85–87 (1980)

Shimamoto, T., Takashima, Y., Kobayashi, M., Moriya, K., Takabashi, T.: A thromboxane A_2-antagonistic effect of pyridinolcarbamate and phthalazinol. Proc. Jpn. Acad. 52, 591 (1976)

Shimamoto, T., Kobayashi, M., Takahashi, T., Takashima, Y., Motomiya, T., Morooka, S., Numano, F.: The production of heart attacks and cerebral stroke by thromboxane A_2 mixtures and their prevention with EG 626 (phthalazinol). Thromb. Haemostas. 38, 132 (1977)

Silver, M.J., Hoch, W., Kocsis, J.J., Ingerman, C.M., Smith, J.B.: Arachidonic acid causes sudden death in rabbits. Science 183, 1085–1087 (1974)

Sixma, J.J., Trieschnigg, A.M.C., De Graaf, S., Bouma, B.N.: In vivo inhibition of human platelet function by VK 744. Scand. J. Haemat. 9, 226–230 (1972)

Skinhoj, E., Paulson, O.B.: The mechanism of action of aminophylline upon cerebral vascular disorders. Acta Neurol. Scand. 46, 129–140 (1970)

Smith, W.L., Philippus, M.J., Lowrey, J.B.: A comparison of psychological and psychophysical test patterns before and after receiving papaverine HCl. Cur. Therap. Res. 10, 428–431 (1968)

Sokoloff, L.: The action of drugs on the cerebral circulation. Pharmacol. Rev. 11, 1–85 (1959)

Sokoloff, L.: Effects of normal ageing on cerebral circulation and energy metabolism. In: Brain function in old age. Hoffmeister, F., Müller, C. (eds.), pp. 368–384. Berlin, Heidelberg, New York: Springer 1979

Solti, F.: Die Wirkung von Bencyclan auf die Blutdurchströmung der Extremitäten. Arzneim. Forsch. 20, 1358–1360 (1970)

Solti, F., Krasznai, F., Iskum, M., Gyertyanfi, G.: Die Neuverteilung des Herzminutenvolumens auf einzelne Organe unter der Wirkung von Bencyclan. Arzneim. Forsch. 20, 1360–1361 (1970)

Spaet, T.H., Gaynor, E., Stermerman, M.B.: Thrombosis, atherosclerosis, and endothelium. Am Heart J. 87, 661–668 (1974)

Spagnoli, A., Tognoni, G.: Ergot-alcaloids in clinical pharmacology and drug epidemiology. In: Tognoni, G., Garattini, S. (eds.), pp. 223–243. North Holland: Elsevier 1979

Spehr, W.: Zur Zeitgestalt des Elektroencephalogramms unter Tinofedrin. Arzneim. Forsch. 28, 1312–1313 (1978)

Spruill, J.H., Toole, J.F., Kitto, W., Miller, H.E.: A comparison of betahistine hydrochloride with placebo for vertebral-basilar insufficiency: A double-blind study. Stroke 6, 116–120 (1975)

Steger, W.: Die Beeinflussung des Plättchenagglutinationstestes durch Xantinol-nicotinat. Med. Welt 24, 301–302 (1973)

Steinhauer, H.B., Anhut, H., Hertting, G.: Inhibition of thromboxane-synthesis in mouse brain in vivo. Arch. Pharmacol. Suppl. 311, R 30–117 (1980)

Streivhenberger, G., Boismare, F., Lauressergues, H., Lechat, P.: Modification par certains médicaments doués d'action vasculaire, des effets d'une anoxie ischémique encéphalique chez le chat. Thérapie 25, 1004–1016 (1970)

Stroman, F., Thiemer, K.: Untersuchungen zur allgemeinen Herz- und Kreislaufwirkung des Tinofedrin. In press 1981

Subbarao, K., Rucinsky, B., Rausch, M.A.: Binding of dipyridamole to human platelets and to alpha 1 acid glycoprotem and its significance for the inhibition of adenosine uptake. J. Clin. Invest. 60, 936–943 (1977)

Suga, F., Snow, J.B.: Cochlear blood flow in response to vasodilating drugs and some related agents. Laryngoscope 79, 1956–1979 (1969)

Szarvasi, E., Bayssat, M., Fontaine, L.: Dialcoylamino-esters et -éthéroxydes à activité antispasmodique. Compt. Rend. 260, 3095–3098 (1965)

Szekeres, L.: Die hämodynamische Wirkung von Bencyclan. Arzneim. Forsch. 20, 1362–1367 (1970)

Szewczykowski, J., Meyer, J.S., Kondo, A., Nomura, F., Teraura, T.: Effects of ergot alkaloids (hydergine) on cerebral hemodynamics and oxygen consumption in monkeys. J. Neurol. Sci. *10*, 25–31 (1970)

Szporny, L.: Pharmacologie de la vincamine et de ses dérivés. Actual. Pharmacol. *29*, 87–117 (1976)

Szporny, L., Görög, P.: The effect of vincamine on the blood pressure of the rat. Arch. Int. Pharmacodyn. *138*, 451–461 (1962)

Taeschler, M., Cerletti, A., Rothlin, E.: Zur Frage der Hyderginwirkung auf die Gehirnzirkulation. Helv. Physiol. Pharmacol. Acta *10*, 120–137 (1952)

Takenaka, T., Handa, J.: Cerebrovascular effects of YC-93, a new vasodilator, in dogs, monkeys and human patients. Int. J. Clin. Pharmacol. Biopharm. *17*, 1–11 (1979)

Teasdale, G.: Cerebrovascular effects of nimodipine. 2nd Beaune Conference. 1980

Ten Cate, J.W., Gerritsen, J., van Geet-Weijers, J.: In vitro and in vivo experiences with VK 774. A new platelet function inhibitor. Path. Biol. *20*, 76–81 (1972)

Ten Cate, J.W., Vos, J., Oosterhuis, H., Prenger, D., Jenkins, C.S.P.: Spontaneous platelet aggregation in cerebrovascular disease. Thromb. Haemostas. *39*, 223–229 (1978)

Tesseris, J., Roggen, G., Caracalos, A., Triandafillou, D.: Effects of vincamin on cerebral metabolism. Eur. Neurol. *13*, 195–202 (1975)

Thiemer, K., Stroman, F., Szelenyi, I., Schlichtegroll v., A.: Pharmakologische Wirkung von Tinofedrin auf die zerebrale und periphere Hämodynamik des Hundes. Arzneim. Forsch. *28*, 1343–1354 (1978)

Thiery, E., Verwerft, E., van der Eecken, H.: Étude comparative en double aveugle avec permutation croisée suloctidil/placébo d'une population agée, présentant une détérioration mentale étiologie cérébro-vasculaire. Ars. Medici *32*, 73–81 (1977)

Thomas, D.J.: The influence of blood viscosity on cerebral blood flow and symptoms. In: Progress in stroke. Greenhalgh, R.M., Rose, F.C. (eds.), pp. 47–55. Kent: Pitman Medical 1979

Toledo, J.B., Pisa, H., Marchese, M.: Clinical evaluation of cinnarizine in patients with cerebral circulatory deficiency. Arzneim. Forsch. *22*, 448–451 (1972)

Towart, R.: New pharmacological aspects of calcium antagonists. In: New aspects of unstable angina pectoris. Lichtlen, P.R., Balcon, R. (eds.). In press 1981

Towart, R., Kazda, S.: The cellular mechanism of action of nimodipine (BAY e 9736), a new calcium antagonist. Br. J. Pharmacol. *67*, 409 (1979)

Towart, R., Kazda, S.: Selective inhibition of serotonin-induced contractions of rabbit basilar artery by nimodipine (BAY e 9736) IRCS. Med. Sci. Nervous Syst. *8*, 206 (1980)

Toyoda, M., Takagi, S., Seki, T., Takeoka, T., Gotoh, F.: Effect of a new vasodilator (Flunarizine) on the cerebral circulation. J. Neurol. Sci. *25*, 371–375 (1975)

Triner, L., Vulliemoz, Y., Schwartz, I., Nahas, G.G.: Cyclic phosphodiesterase activity and the action of papaverine. Biochem. Biophys. Res. Commun. *40*, 64–69 (1970)

Ts'ao, Ch., Ali, N., Kolb, T.: "Spontaneous" platelet aggregation: Its characteristics and relation to aggregation by other agents. Thromb. Haemostas. *39*, 379–385 (1978)

Tsu, E.C.: Antiplatelet drugs in arterial thrombosis: A review. Am. J. Hosp. Pharm. *35*, 1507–1515 (1978)

Vamosi, B., Moln'ar, L., Demeter, J., T'ury, F.: Comparative study of the effect of ethyl apovincaminate and xantinol nicotinate in cerebrovascular diseases. Immediate drug effects on the concentrations of carbohydrate metabolites and electrolytes in blood and CSF. Arzneim. Forsch. *26*, 1980–1984 (1977)

Van Breemen, C., Siegel, B.: The mechanism of action of α-adrenergic activation of the dog coronary artery. Circulat. Res. *46*, 426–429 (1980)

Van den Driessche, J., Lacroix, P., Linee, Ph., Le Polles, J.B., Pape, D., Allain, H.: Activity of some drugs on the electroencephalogram of curarized rats during acute and iterative hypercapnic anoxia hypotheses on mechanisms of action. Arch. Int. Pharmacodyn. *239*, 62–77 (1979)

Vane, J.R.: Inhibitors of prostaglandin, prostacyclin, and thromboxane synthesis. In: Advances in Prostagoandin and Thromboxane research. Coceani, F., Olley, P.M. (eds.), vol. 4, pp. 27–43. New York: Raven Press 1978

Van Nueten, Janssen, P.A.J.: Comparative study of the effects of flunarizine and cinnarizine on smooth muscles and cardiac tissues. Arch. Int. Pharmacodyn. *204*, 37–55 (1973)

Van Nueten, J.M., Vanhoutte, P.M.: Improvement of tissue perfusion with inhibitors of calcium ion influx. Biochem. Pharmacol. *29*, 479–481 (1980)

Van Schepdael, J.: Étude clinique de l'action du suloctidil sur la maladie cérébro-vasculaire chronique de la personne agée. Ars. Médici *32*, 1506–1518 (1977)

Vater, W., Kroneberg, G., Hoffmeister, F., Kaller, H., Meng, K., Oberdorf, A., Puls, W., Schloßmann, K., Stoepel, K.: Zur Pharmakologie von 4-(2'-Nitrophenyl)-2,6-dimethyl-1,4-dihydropyridin-3,5-dicarbonsäuredimethylester (Nifedipine), BAY a 1040. Arzneim. Forsch. *22*, 1–170 (1972)

Villa, R.F., Strada, P., Marzatico, F., Dagani, F.: Effect of (−) eburnamonine, papaverine, and UDP-glucose on cerebral energy state during and after experimental hypoxia and ischaemia in beagle dogs. Eur. Neurol. *17*, 97–112 (1979)

Wackenheim, A.: Le traitement de l'insuffisance vertébrobasilaire par le torental. Med. Act. *3*, 6–8 (1976)

Walter, L.A., Hunt, W.H., Fosbinder, R.J.: Beta-(2- and 4-pyridyalkyl)-amines. J. Am. Chem. Soc. *63*, 2771–2773 (1941)

Warembourg, H., Pruvot, P., Sueur, A., Lekieffre, J.: An experimental study of a vasodilator drug, CAA 40. Its effect on the vascularization of the brain, on the arterial blood pressure and on the electro-encephalogram. Thérapie *16*, 125–129 (1961)

Wechsler, R.I., Kleiss, I.M., Kety, S.S.: The effects of intravenously administered aminophyllin on cerebral circulation and metabolism in man. J. Clin. Invest. *29*, 28–80 (1950)

Weigelin, E., Sayegh, F.: Zur Objektivierung des cerebralen durchblutungsfördernden Effektes vasoaktiver Substanzen unter besonderer Berücksichtigung von Cinnarizin. In: Aktuelle Probleme der psychiatrischen Pharmakotherapie in Klinik und Praxis. Heinrich, K. (ed.), pp. 20–26. Stuttgart, New York: Schattauer 1969

Weily, H.S., Genton, E.: Altered platelet function in patients with prosthetic mitral valves: Effects of sulfinpyrazone therapy. Circulation *42*, 967–972 (1970)

Weily, H.S., Steele, P.P., Davies, H., Pappas, G., Genton, E.: Platelet survival in patients in substitute heart valves. New Engl. J. Med. *290*, 534–539 (1974)

Weiss, H.J.: Antiplatelet drugs – A new pharmacologic approach to the prevention of thrombosis. Am. Heart J. *92*, 86–102 (1976)

Weiss, H.J., Aledort, L.M., Kochwa, S.: The effect of salicylates on the hemostatic properties of platelets in man. J. Clin. Invest. *47*, 2169–2180 (1968)

Wernitz, W.: Die Wirkung von Monotrean und seinen Komponenten auf die Hirndurchblutung. Vorläufige Mitteilung über die Untersuchungen mit Radiojod. Med. Welt *33*, 1799–1801 (1969)

Westreich, G., Alter, M., Lundgren, S.: Effect of cyclandelate on dementia. Stroke *6*, 535–538 (1975)

Whittier, J.R., Dhrymiotis, A.D.: Prevention of slow wave response to hyperventilation in the human electroencephalogram by a vasodilator. Angiology *13*, 324–327 (1962)

Wilcke, O.: Ergebnisse der Behandlung zerebraler Durchblutungsstörungen mit Cinnarizin. Med. Welt *27*, 1472–1477 (1966)

Willis, A.L.: An enzymatic mechanism for the antithrombotic and antihemostatic actions of aspirin. Science *183*, 325–327 (1974)

Witzmann, H.K., Blechacz, W.: Zustellung von Vincamin in der Therapie cerebrovasculärer Krankheiten und cerebraler Leistungsverminderung. Arzneim. Forsch. *27*, 1238–1247 (1977)

Wolfe, L.S.: Some facts and thoughts on the biosynthesis of prostaglandins and thromboxanes in brain. In: Advances in prostaglandin and thromboxane research. Coceani, F., Olley, P.M. (eds.), vol. 4, pp. 215–220. New York: Raven Press 1978

Wu, K.K., Hoak, J.C.: Increased platelet aggregates in patients with transient ischemic attacks. Stroke *6*, 521–524 (1975)

Yarullin, K.K., Khadzhiev, D., Penyazeva, G.A., Levchenko, N.I.: The influence of stutgeron on the cerebral hemodynamics in patients with disorders of the cerebral circulation. Klin. Med. *50*, 62–69 (1972)

Yatsu, F.M.: Stroke therapy: Status of anti-platelet aggregation drugs (editorial). Neurology *27*, 503–504 (1977)

Zervas, N.T., Lavyne, M.H., Negoro, M.: Neurotransmitters and the normal and ischaemic cerebral circulation. New Engl. J. Med. *293*, 812–816 (1975)

CHAPTER 13

Biochemical Effects
of Gerontopsychopharmacological Agents

S. Hoyer

A. Introduction

Discussion of the biochemical effectiveness of gerontopsychopharmacological agents in gerontopsychiatric (i.e. demented) patients should be based on criteria concerning cerebral blood flow, cerebral oxygen consumption and cerebral glucose uptake as biologically important brain parameters which might be predominantly altered in dementia. Physiologically, a close relationship exists between cerebral blood flow on the one hand and the cerebral metabolic rates of oxygen and glucose on the other (ALBERTI et al., 1975; ALEXANDER et al., 1965, 1968; COHEN et al., 1964, 1968; FOLBERGROVA et al., 1972; GOTTSTEIN et al., 1977, 1976; GRANHOLM et al., 1969; GRANHOLM and SIESJÖ, 1969, 1971; HAMER et al., 1976, 1978; HOYER et al., 1974; KAASIK et al., 1970; KOGURE et al., 1970; SIESJÖ and MESSETER, 1971; SIESJÖ et al., 1971; SIESJÖ and ZWETNOW, 1970; ZWETNOW, 1970). Therefore these parameters should not be considered separately in dementia. Cerebral blood flow variations should also be discussed in dementia although the disturbances of the metabolic brain parameters might be of greater importance in this disease (see below).

B. Pathobiochemical and Pathophysiological Variations
of Brain Functions in Gerontopsychiatry: General Considerations

The most common disease in gerontopsychiatry is dementia due to degenerative or cerebrovascular changes in brain tissue. Degenerative changes are the cause in 60% of dementia patients. Cerebrovascular disturbances alone are responsible for dementia in only 20%–25%, while both degenerative and cerebrovascular variations are present in 15%–20% (JELLINGER, 1976; TOMLINSON et al., 1970). Nosologically, "simple" senile dementia, Alzheimer's senile dementia and Alzheimer's presenile dementia might be regarded as variations of the same degenerative brain disease (ALBERT, 1964; ARAB, 1960; CONSTANTINIDIS, 1978; KATZMAN, 1976; LAUTER and MEYER, 1968; NEWTON, 1948; TERRY, 1976, 1978). It is evident that the cerebrovascular (multi-infarct) brain processes mentioned may be related to disturbances in cerebral microcirculation which might lead to circumscribed nerve cell loss with gliosis (CORSELLIS, 1969). Rheological factors such as arteriosclerosis or thrombosis of the larger arterial brain vessels, which would lead primarily to neurological disorders such as strokes, may be of marginal relevance in the development of the dementias. Therefore it might be expected that the pathological variations in brain tissue, i.e. more diffuse or more patchy nerve cell loss, might produce disturbances, firstly in brain metabolism and secondly in brain blood flow.

The variations of cerebral blood flow, cerebral oxygen consumption and cerebral glucose uptake were not found to be homogeneous. They are dissimilar in the different types of distinct morphological disturbances, i.e. degenerative or cerebrovascular variations (HACHINSKI et al., 1975; HOYER et al., 1975). In general, cerebral blood flow and cerebral oxygen consumption are rather more decreased in patients suffering from a cerebrovascular (multi-infarct) dementia than in patients in whom the dementia is due to a degenerative brain process.

The degree of changes in cerebral blood flow and metabolism is influenced by the duration of the dementia process. In both types of dementia the first and major pathological changes are found in cerebral glucose metabolism rather than in cerebral oxygen consumption or cerebral blood flow. In the further course of both types, all these biological brain parameters decrease more and more and approach a pathologically low level of about 50% of normal (HOYER, 1978 a, 1978 b).

The variations in cerebral blood flow and metabolism parallel the deranged functional state of the brain. In general, mild to moderate dementia symptoms accompany mild to moderate decreases in brain blood flow and metabolism, and severe dementia symptoms accompany severe variations [both decreases and (pathological) increases] of the biologic brain parameters (HOYER et al., 1978 b).

There is no doubt that these different factors may interfere and thus produce a larger number of factors determining the variations of brain blood flow and metabolism as well as clinical symptoms in dementia.

The preponderance of changes in brain tissue over changes in brain vessels along with the predominance of disturbances in oxidative brain metabolism over disorders of brain blood flow in dementia patients (HOYER, 1970; 1978 b) make it seem reasonable to treat dementia patients with gerontopsychopharmacological agents which would mainly act on the different disturbances in oxidative brain metabolism, i.e. the metabolism of glucose and oxygen and energy production in the brain, rather than on a disturbed cerebral circulation.

C. Studies of Drug Effects in Gerontopsychiatric Patients

Earlier investigations studying drug effects on disturbed brain blood flow and metabolism in dementia patients had two important failings:

1) The patients were not classified into the two major different types of dementia (degenerative or cerebrovascular), but were investigated as "organic brain syndromes" or "arteriosclerosis of the brain vessels." Since the pharmacological drug effects on the different pathophysiological disturbances in brain blood flow and metabolism and other factors in the dementia types were not studied, positive or negative drug effects could hardly be related to investigations in which the dementia types, the duration of dementia, the functional state of the brain etc. were examined.

2) Most drug studies in patients suffering from dementia were performed as acute experiments, i.e. drug effects were mostly investigated after only one single administration and within only a few minutes after the administration. It seems, however, to be questionable whether a drug can show any effect on generally investigated subchronically disturbed brain functions within such a short time. As a consequence, many drug effects on brain blood flow and metabolism, positive and negative, should

therefore be regarded with a certain circumspection. With these reservations the effectiveness of distinct gerontopsychopharmacological agents on brain blood flow and metabolism in patients suffering from primary or secondary dementia will be discussed here in more detail.

I. Sympathicomimetic Drugs

These drugs, such as adrenaline, noradrenaline, angiotensin and amphetamine, failed to influence brain blood flow and metabolism after intravenous injection. Intracarotid injections of adrenaline, noradrenaline or angiotensin in moderate dosages showed no effect on these biological brain parameters (AGNOLI et al., 1965, 1968; GOTTSTEIN, 1962, 1963, 1969; OLESEN, 1972, 1974; SOKOLOFF, 1959). Intravenous infusions of high dosages of adrenaline provoked an increase in both cerebral blood flow and cerebral oxygen consumption in humans not suffering from organic brain diseases. It was assumed that these effects were due to anxiety and sensations of apprehension which were observed under high dosages of adrenaline (KING et al., 1952).

II. Sympathicolytic Agents

This large group of drugs was extensively studied. *Rauwolfia alkaloids* showed no effect on cerebral blood flow and cerebral metabolic rate (CMR)-oxygen, despite various means of administration: intravenous infusion, intramuscular injection along with or immediately following control measurements and oral application over a period of 3 weeks (GOTTSTEIN, 1962, 1963, 1969; SOKOLOFF, 1959). Other sympathicolytic drugs with α-receptor blocking effects, such as tolazoline, phentolamine and phenoxybenzamine, did not show any effects on brain blood flow and metabolism (GOTTSTEIN, 1962, 1965, 1969; HEISS et al., 1971; HERRSCHAFT, 1973, 1975; SKINHØJ, 1971/72; SOKOLOFF, 1959). HACHINSKI et al. failed to find any effect of ergotamine on cerebral blood flow, but did not perform metabolic studies (HACHINSKI et al., 1978). The effect of another Secale alkaloid, *dihydroergotoxine*, was investigated by GOTTSTEIN (GOTTSTEIN, 1962, 1963, 1969), by McHENRY et al. (1971) and by OLESEN (1974) who performed intravenous as well as intracarotid infusions. These investigators could not find any influence of dihydroergotoxine on cerebral blood flow and CMR-oxygen. On the other hand HEYCK described an increase of the pathologically decreased cerebral blood flow depending on the degree of the disturbance, whereas CMR-oxygen remained unchanged (HEYCK, 1961).

The intravenous administration of *adenosine compounds* (ATP, AMP) revealed no changes of cerebral blood flow and CMR-oxygen. The intracarotid infusion of AMP did cause an increase in cerebral blood flow, but CMR-oxygen remained unchanged (GOTTSTEIN, 1962, 1965, 1969).

The spasmolytic drug *papaverine* administered as an intravenous or intracarotid infusion increased cerebral blood flow, but not CMR-oxygen, which was not influenced (GOTTSTEIN, 1962, 1969; McHENRY, 1972; OLESEN and PAULSON, 1971). However, the effect on cerebral blood flow seemed to be short lasting. On the other hand SHENKIN failed to show any effects of papaverine on cerebral circulation and metabolism (SHENKIN, 1951).

Neither *serotonin* nor *histamine* influenced cerebral blood flow and CMR-oxygen (ALMAN et al., 1952; OLESEN, 1974; SHENKIN, 1951).

As an interim result, one might conclude that sympathicomimetic drugs, sympath-icolytic drugs and biogenic amines have no effects on disturbed cerebral blood flow and metabolism in dementia patients. The beneficial effects of intracarotid infusions of adenosine bodies and of papaverine may be almost negligible because of the kind of application and because of the side effects of both drugs.

III. Miscellaneous Vasoactive and Metabolically Active Drugs

Several investigations of brain blood flow and metabolism were performed to study the effect of *xanthine derivatives* on the above-mentioned parameters. In most studies no improvement of the disturbed cerebral blood flow and metabolism could be found, but often a further decrease of cerebral blood flow due to vasoconstriction was de-scribed (Gottstein, 1962, 1965, 1969; Gottstein and Paulson, 1972; Heiss et al., 1971; Herrschaft, 1973, 1975). In only a very few cases could an inverse steal phenomenon of cerebral blood flow be observed in patients with acute stroke (Herr-schaft, 1975; Skinhøj et al., 1970).

The results of investigations concerning the effects of *xanthinole + nicotinic acid* derivatives on brain blood flow and metabolism are somewhat conflicting. While Gottstein, Gottstein et al., Lennartz, Herrschaft and Heiss et al. (Gottstein, 1962, 1969; Gottstein et al., 1962; Heiss et al., 1971; Herrschaft, 1975; Lennartz, 1962) were not able to demonstrate any effects of these substances on brain blood flow and metabolism, Hoyer and co-workers found a normalization of the disturbed CMR-oxygen after a 2-week treatment. An influence of this drug on CMR-glucose could be suspected but could not be proved statistically (Hoyer et al., 1978a) (Table 1). Recently Quadbeck and Lehmann described a positive effect of xanthinole nicotinate on disturbed cerebral glucose uptake after a 4-week treatment, but this ef-fect depended on the degree of the disturbance (Quadbeck and Lehmann, 1978). Nicotinic acid on its own could not be shown to have any influence on cerebral blood flow and metabolism (Gottstein, 1962, 1969; Gottstein et al., 1962).

While *naphtidrofuryle* did not show an effect on cerebral blood flow (Herrschaft, 1975), divergent influences of *bencyclane* and *proxazole* were reported. Herrschaft

Table 1. Mean values of cerebral blood flow (CBF) and oxidative brain metabolism in patients with organic brain disorders under treatment with xanthinole + nicotinic acid

	Age (years)		CBF	CMR-oxygen	CMR-glucose
			ml/100 g min		mg/100 g min
Patients with predomi-nant disturbances in CBF and CMR-oygen $(n=10)$	64	Resting rate	40.3	2.31	5.87
		After a 2-week treatment	41.5	3.66[a]	4.83
Patients with predomi-nant disturbances in cerebral glucose metabolism $(n=10)$	56	Resting rate	43.0	3.01	2.30
		After a 2-week treatment	45.1	3.03	6.10

[a] $=0.05$

Table 2. Mean values of cerebral blood flow (CBF) and oxidative brain metabolism in patients with organic brain disorders under treatment with pyritinol-HCl (900 mg/die)

	Age (years)		CBF	CMR-oxygen	CMR-glucose
			ml/100 g min		mg/100 g min
Patients with predominant disturbances in CBF and CMR-oxygen (n=18)	52	Resting state	42.1	2.18	5.99
		After a 4-week treatment	40.6	2.62	3.95
Patients with predominant disturbances in cerebral glucose metabolism (n=27)	49	Resting state	53.7	3.12	2.47
		After a 4-week treatment	52.7	3.10	4.76[a]

[a] $\alpha=0.01$

could not find any effects of these drugs on cerebral blood flow (HERRSCHAFT, 1975; HERRSCHAFT et al., 1974a), but HEISS described dose-dependent increases of cerebral blood flow under proxazole (HEISS, 1973) and KOHLMEYER reported improvements of decreased cerebral flow rates under bencyclane (KOHLMEYER, 1972).

The investigations of MEYER et al. (1971) showed an increase of cerebral blood flow under *hexobendine*, while cerebral metabolism remained unaffected (MEYER et al., 1971). HEISS et al. and McHENRY et al. confirmed these findings as far as cerebral blood flow was concerned (HEISS et al., 1971; McHENRY et al., 1972). On the other hand HERRSCHAFT was not able to demonstrate any effect of this drug on cerebral blood flow (HERRSCHAFT, 1976).

The effect of *vincamine*, the alkaloid from vinca minor, on global and regional cerebral blood flow was studied by HERRSCHAFT, by KOHLMEYER and by HEISS et al. (HEISS et al., 1977; HERRSCHAFT, 1977; KOHLMEYER, 1977). This drug obviously increased the disturbed blood flow rate dose dependently, especially in areas of the brain which are extremely underperfused.

The effects of drugs such as *pyritinol-HCl, centrophenoxine, extractum sanguinum deproteinatum siccum* and *piracetam* on cerebral blood flow alone and on cerebral blood flow along with the CMRs of oxygen and glucose were investigated by HERRSCHAFT et al., by BECKER and HOYER and by HOYER et al. (BECKER and HOYER, 1966; HERRSCHAFT, 1975, 1976; HERRSCHAFT et al., 1974b, 1977; HOYER et al., 1977, 1978a). HERRSCHAFT and co-workers observed an increase of the grey matter flow under the influence of pyritinol-HCl, centrophenoxine, and extractum sanguinum deproteinatum siccum, whereas the flow in the white matter of the brain was not affected. This flow increase in grey matter was regarded as secondary to an improvement of the oxidative brain metabolism. BECKER and HOYER (1976) and HOYER et al. (1977) found a normalization of the predominantly decreased CMR-glucose in patients suffering from organic brain disorders (Table 2).

Based on more detailed, clinicopsychometrically different findings (HACHINSKI et al., 1975), HOYER et al. (1978a) classified their patients into multi-infarct dementias or primary degenerative (Alzheimer) dementias. As mentioned above, this classification seems to be useful for nosological und also pharmacotherapeutic reasons.

Table 3. Mean values of cerebral blood flow (CBF), CMR-oxygen and CMR-glucose in patients with organic brain disorders (MI, multi-infarct dementia; PD, primary degenerative dementia; AD, dementia due to alcoholism) before and after a 3-week treatment with extr. sanguin. deprot. sicc., centrophenoxin or piracetam

	Age (years)	Resting rate			After treatment		
		CBF	CMR-oxygen	CMR-glucose	CMF	CMR-oxygen	CMR-glucose
		ml/100 g min		mg/100 g min	ml/100 g min		mg/100 g min
Extr. sanguin. deprot. sicc.							
MI (n=6)	71	29.9	2.50	2.69	36.1	2.73	3.50
PD (n=4)	63	52.0	3.90	4.83	47.0	3.14	4.93
AD (n=10)	47	28.0	1.99	3.03	45.1[a]	3.23[a]	4.14
Centro-phenoxin							
MI (n=9)	68	33.3	2.50	3.39	47.5[a]	2.92	4.43
PD (n=4)	65	32.1	2.36	3.14	37.8	2.25	3.60
AD (n=7)	43	50.1	3.62	3.70	37.7	2.40	3.64
Piracetam							
MI (n=7)	59	33.3	2.41	3.26	49.5[a]	3.83[a]	4.88[a]
PD (n=4)	62	32.3	2.23	3.57	38.3	3.15	3.83
AD (n=9)	44	42.1	3.56	4.77	46.2	3.44	4.83

[a] $\alpha = 0.05$

Centrophenoxine increased the disturbed cerebral blood flow in multi-infarct dementias. It also seems to have an effect on the decreased cerebral metabolic rate of glucose, but this increase was not statistically significant (Table 3).

Extractum sanguinum deproteinatum siccum improved cerebral blood flow and CMR-oxygen in dementia due to chronic alcoholism when these parameters were decreased to about 50%–60% of normal. CMR-glucose was also augmented, but this increase was just below the level of statistical significance (Table 3).

Piracetam produced an improvement of cerebral blood flow, CMR-oxygen and CMR-glucose to the normal range in patients suffering from multi-infarct dementia (Table 3). All improvements in the biological brain parameters found by Hoyer and co-workers were accompanied by improvements in the clinical findings.

D. Concluding Remarks

In all drug-induced improvements of biological and clinical brain parameters is should be noted that an improvement both of brain blood flow and metabolism and the dementia symptoms occur spontaneously in about one-third of the dementia patients, while in two-thirds the biological parameters as well as the clinical findings increasingly deteriorate (Hoyer, 1976; Hoyer et al., 1978a). Therefore the possibility of a spontaneous improvement should be taken into account when evaluating therapeutic effects of agents which are directed towards brain blood flow and metabolism. In performing such studies it seems to be more necessary to compare the findings between a treated and a non-treated group of patients in a randomized study. It would seem insufficient merely to compare the findings before and after treatment in one group of patients.

Gerontopsychopharmacological agents which are claimed to have almost 100% positive effects on brain blood flow and metabolism and/or dementia symptoms should be treated with much scepticism because of the pathophysiologically different underlying process and because of the possibility of spontaneous improvement. Results on improvements of the biological brain parameters and the clinical symptoms showing a success rate of 50%–60% after pharmacotherapeutic treatment are much more convincing and might also be explained in pathophysiological terms.

In future investigations on the effectiveness of agents on brain blood flow and metabolism one should differentiate more thoroughly between neurological brain diseases (strokes) and psychiatric brain diseases (dementias), which have different pathophysiological mechanisms. There is no doubt that strokes are primarily the result of rheological disturbances, whereas dementias are due more to diseases of the brain tissue itself.

By taking into account such (patho)biological and clinical suppositions and by using well-established biological and clinical methods, it should be possible to find ranges of indications for gerontopsychopharmacological agents which should be successful in the treatment of metabolic and circulatory disturbances in organic brain disorders.

References

Agnoli, A., Battistini, N., Bozzao, L., Fieschi, C.: Drug action on regional cerebral blood flow in cases of acute cerebro-vascular involvement. Acta Neurol. Scand. [Suppl. 14] *41*, 142–144 (1965)

Agnoli, A., Fieschi, C., Bozzao, L., Battistini, N., Prencipe, M.: Autoregulation of cerebral blood flow. Studies during-induced hypertension in normal subjects and in patients with cerebral vascular diseases. Circulation *38*, 800–812 (1968)

Albert, E.: Senile Demenz und Alzheimersche Krankheit als Ausdruck des gleichen Krankheitsgeschehens. Fortschr. Neurol. Psychiatr. *32*, 625–673 (1964)

Alberti, E., Hoyer, S., Hamer, J., Stoeckel, H., Packschiess, P., Weinhardt, F.: The effect of carbon dioxide on cerebral blood flow and cerebral metabolism in dogs. Br. J. Anaesth. *47*, 941–947 (1975)

Alexander, S.C., Cohen, P.J., Wollman, H., Smith, T.C., Reivich, M., van der Molen, R.A.: Cerebral carbohydrate metabolism during hypocarbia in man. Studies during nitrous oxide anesthesia. Anesthesiology *26*, 624–632 (1965)

Alexander, S.C., Smith, T.C., Strobel, G., Stephen, G.W., Wollman, H.: Cerebral carbohydrate metabolism of man during respiratory and metabolic alkalosis. J. Appl. Physiol. *24*, 66–72 (1968)

Alman, R.W., Rosenberg, M., Fazekas, J.F.: Effects of histamine on cerebral hemodynamics and metabolism. Arch. Neurol. Psychiatr. (Chic.) *67*, 354–356 (1952)

Arab, A.: Unité nosologique entre démence sénile et maladie d'Alzheimer d'après une étude statistique et anatomo-clinique. Sist. Nerv. *12*, 189–201 (1960)

Becker, K., Hoyer, S.: Hirnstoffwechseluntersuchungen unter der Behandlung mit Pyrithioxin. Dtsch. Z. Nervenheilkd. *188*, 200–209 (1966)

Cohen, P.J., Alexander, S.C., Wollman, H.: Effects of hypocarbia and of hypoxia with normocarbia on cerebral blood flow and metabolism in man. Scand. J. Clin. Lab. Invest. [Suppl. 102] *22*, IV:A (1968)

Cohen, P.J., Wollman, H., Alexander, S.C., Chase, P.E., Behar, M.G.: Cerebral carbohydrate metabolism in man during halothane anesthesia. Effects of pa CO_2 on some aspects of carbohydrate utilization. Anesthesiology *25*, 185–191 (1964)

Constantinidis, J.: Is Alzheimer's disease a major form if senile dementia? Clinical, anatomical and genetic data. In: Alzheimer's disease: Senile dementia and related disorders. Katzman, R., Terry, R.D., Bick, K.L. (eds.), pp. 15–25. New York: Raven 1978

Corsellis, J.A.N.: The pathology of dementia Br. J. Hosp. Med. *3*, 695–703 (1969)

Folbergrova, J., MacMillan, V., Siesjö, B.K.: The effect of moderate and marked hypercapnia upon the energy state and upon the cytoplasmatic NADH/NAD$^+$-ratio of the rat brain. J. Neurochem. *19*, 2497–2505 (1972)

Gottstein, U.: Der Hirnkreislauf unter dem Einfluß vasoaktiver Substanzen. Heidelberg: Hüthig 1962

Gottstein, U.: Der Hirnkreislauf unter dem Einfluß sympathikomimetischer, sympathikolytischer und ganglioplegischer Substanzen. In: Kreislaufmessungen. pp. 1–15. München: Werk 1963

Gottstein, U.: Physiologie und Pathophysiologie des Hirnkreislaufs. Med. Welt *15*, 715–726 (1965)

Gottstein, U.: The effect of drugs on cerebral blood flow especially in patients of older age. Pharmakopsychiatr. Neuropsychopharmakol. *2*, 100–109 (1969)

Gottstein, U., Paulson, O.B.: The effect of intracarotid aminophylline infusion on the cerebral circulation. Stroke *3*, 560–565 (1962)

Gottstein, U., Bernsmeier, A., Steiner, K.: Die Wirkung von Nikotinsäure auf Hirndurchblutung und cerebralen Stoffwechsel des Menschen. Klin. Wochenschr. *40*, 772–778 (1962)

Gottstein, U., Gabriel, F.H., Held, K., Textor, Th.: Continuous monitoring of arterial and cerebralvenous glucose concentrations in man. Advantage, procedure and results in: Blood glucose monitoring. Methodology and clinical application of continuous in vivo glucose analysis, pp. 127–135. Stuttgart: Thieme 1977

Gottstein, U., Zahn, U., Held, K., Gabriel, F.H., Textor, Th., Berghoff, W.: Einfluß der Hyperventilation auf Hirndurchblutung und cerebralen Stoffwechsel des Menschen. Untersuchungen bei fortlaufender Registrierung der arterio-hirnvenösen Glucosedifferenz. Klin. Wochenschr. *54*, 373–381 (1976)

Granholm, L., Siesjö, B.K.: The effects of hypercapnia and hypocapnia upon the cerebrospinal fluid lactate and pyruvate concentrations and upon lactate, pyruvate, ATP, ADP, phosphocreatine and creatine concentrations of cat brain tissue. Acta physiol. scand. *75*, 257–266 (1969)

Granholm, L., Siesjö, B.K.: The effect of combined respiratory and non-respiratory alkalosis on energy metabolites and acid-base parameters in the rat brain. Acta physiol. Scand. *81*, 307–314 (1971)

Granholm, L., Lukjanova, L., Siesjö, B.K.: The effect of marked hyperventilation upon tissue levels of NADH, lactate, pyruvate, phosphocreatine and adenosine phosphates of rat brain. Acta Physiol. Scand. *77*, 179–199 (1969)

Hachinski, V.S., Iliff, L.D., Zilkha, E., Du Boulay, G.H., McAllister, V.L., Marshall, J., Ross-Russell, R.W., Symon, L.: Cerebral blood flow in dementia. Arch. Neurol. *32*, 632–637 (1975)

Hachinski, V., Norris, J.W., Edmeads, J., Cooper, W.P.: Ergotamine and cerebral blood flow. Stroke *6*, 594–596 (1978)

Hamer, J., Hoyer, S., Alberti, E., Weinhardt, F.: Cerebral blood flow and oxidative brain metabolism during and after moderate and profound arterial hypoxaemia. Acta Neurochir. (Wien) *33*, 141–150 (1976)

Hamer, J., Wiedemann, K., Berlet, H., Weinhardt, F., Hoyer, S.: Cerebral glucose and energy metabolism, cerebral oxygen consumption and blood flow in arterial hypoxaemia. Acta Neurochir. (Wien) *44*, 151–160 (1978)

Heiss, W.-D.: Drug effects on regional cerebral blood flow in focal cerebrovascular disease. J. Neurol. Sci. *19*, 461–482 (1973)

Heiss, W.-D., Prosenz, P., Gloning, K., Tschabitscher, H.: Regional and total cerebral blood flow under vasodilating drugs. In: Brain and blood flow. Ross-Russell, R.W. (ed.), pp. 270–276. London: Pitman 1971

Heiss, W.-D., Podreka, I., Samec, P.: Die Wirkung von Vincamin auf die Hirndurchblutung in Abhängigkeit von der Applikationsgeschwindigkeit. Arzneim. Forsch. (Drug Res.) *27/1*, 1291–1293 (1977)

Herrschaft, H.: Regional cerebral blood flow changes effected by vasoactive substances. In: Cerebral vascular disease. Meyer, J.S., Reivich, M., Lechner, H., Eichhorn, O. (eds.), pp. 101–114. Stuttgart: Thieme 1973

Herrschaft, H.: The efficacy and course of action of vaso- and metabolic-active substances on regional cerebral blood flow in patients with cerebrovascular insufficiency. In: Blood flow and metabolism in the brain. Harper, A.M., Jennett, W.B., Miller, J.D., Rowan, J.O. (eds.), pp. 11.24–11.28. Edinburgh, London, New York: Livingstone 1975

Herrschaft, H.: Gehirndurchblutung und Gehirnstoffwechsel. Meßverfahren, Physiologie, Pathophysiologie, Veränderungen bei den hirnorganischen Erkrankungen, Pharmakologie. Stuttgart: Thieme 1976

Herrschaft, H.: Der Einfluß von Vincamin auf die globale und regionale Gehirndurchblutung bei der akuten und subchronischen zerebralen Ischämie des Menschen. Arzneim. Forsch. (Drug Res.) 27/I, 1278–1284 (1977)

Herrschaft, H., Gleim, F., Duus, P.: Der Einfluß von Bencyclan auf die regionale Hirndurchblutung bei Kranken mit zerebraler Mangeldurchblutung. Klin. Wochenschr. 52, 293–295 (1974a)

Herrschaft, H., Gleim, F., Duus, P.: Die Wirkung von Centrophenoxin auf die regionale Gehirndurchblutung bei Patienten mit zerebrovaskulärer Insuffizienz. Dtsch. Med. Wochenschr. 99, 1707–1714 (1974b)

Herrschaft, H., Kunze, U., Gleim, F.: Die Wirkung von Actovegin auf die Gehirndurchblutung und den Gehirnstoffwechsel des Menschen. Med. Welt (N.S.) 28, 339–345 (1977)

Heyck, H.: Der Einfluß der Ausgangslage auf sympathikolytische Effekte am Hirnkreislauf bei cerebro-vasculären Erkrankungen. Ärztl. Forsch. 15, 243–251 (1961)

Hoyer, S.: Der Hirnstoffwechsel und die Häufigkeit cerebraler Durchblutungsstörungen beim organischen Psychosyndrom. Dtsch. Z. Nervenheilkd. 197, 285–292 (1970)

Hoyer, S.: Hirndurchblutung und Hirnstoffwechsel im Verlauf eines organischen Psychosyndroms bei nichtbehandelten Patienten. In: Hirnstoffwechsel und Hirndurchblutung. Hoyer, S. (ed.), pp. 1–8. Amsterdam, Oxford: Excerpta Medica 1976

Hoyer, S.: Das organische Psychosyndrom. Überlegungen zur Hirndurchblutung, zum Hirnstoffwechsel und zur Therapie. Nervenarzt 49, 201–207 (1978a)

Hoyer, S.: Blood flow and oxidative metabolism of the brain in different phases of dementia. In: Alzheimer's disease: Senile dementia and related disorders. Katzman, R., Terry, R.D., Bick, K.L. (eds.), pp. 219–226. New York: Raven 1978b

Hoyer, S., Hamer, J., Alberti, E., Stoeckel, H., Weinhardt, F.: The effect of stepwise arterial hypotension on blood flow and oxidative metabolism of the brain. Pflügers Arch. 351, 161–172 (1974)

Hoyer, S., Oesterreich, K., Weinhardt, F., Krüger, G.: Veränderungen von Durchblutung und oxydativem Stoffwechsel des Gehirns bei Patienten mit einer Demenz. J. Neurol. 210, 227–237 (1975)

Hoyer, S., Krüger, G., Oesterreich, K., Weinhardt, F.: Effects of drugs on cerebral blood flow and oxidative metabolism in patients with dementia. In: Cerebral vascular disease. Meyer, J.S., Lechner, H., Reivich, M. (eds.), pp. 25–28. Amsterdam: Excerpta Medica 1978a

Hoyer, S., Krüger, G., Weinhardt, F.: Brain blood flow and metabolism in relation to psychiatric status in patients with organic brain syndromes. In: Cerebral vascular disease 2. Meyer, J.S., Lechner, H., Reivich, M. (eds.), pp. 151–154. Amsterdam: Excerpta Medica 1979

Hoyer, S., Oesterreich, K., Stoll, K.-D.: Effects of pyritinol-HCl on blood flow and oxidative metabolism of the brain in patients with dementia. Arzneim. Forsch. (Drug Res.) 27, 671–674 (1977)

Jellinger, K.: Neuropathological aspects of dementias resulting from abnormal blood and cerebrospinal fluid dynamics. Acta Neurol. Belg. 76, 83–102 (1976)

Kaasik, A.E., Nilsson, L., Siesjö, B.K.: The effect of arterial hypotension upon the lactate, pyruvate and bicarbonate concentration of the brain tissue and cisternal CSF and upon the tissue concentrations of phosphocreatine and adenine nucleotides in anesthetized rats. Acta Physiol. Scand. 78, 448–458 (1970)

Katzman, R.: The prevalance and malignancy of Alzheimer disease. Arch. Neurol. 33, 217–218 (1976)

King, B.D., Sokoloff, L., Wechsler, R.L.: The effects of 1-epinephrine and 1-nor-epinephrine upon cerebral circulation and metabolism in man. J. Clin. Invest. 31, 273–279 (1952)

Kogure, K., Scheinberg, P., Reinmuth, O.M., Fujishima, M., Busto, R.: Mechanisms of cerebral vasodilatation in hypoxia. J. Appl. Physiol. 29, 223–229 (1970)

Kohlmeyer, K.: Der Einfluß eines neuen Vasodilatators (Bencyclan) auf die allgemeine und regionale Hirndurchblutung. Untersuchungen mit der Xenon-133-Clearance-Methode. Herz Kreisl. 5, 196–203 (1972)

Kohlmeyer, K.: Zur Wirkung von Vincamin auf die Gehirndurchblutung des Menschen im Akutversuch. Untersuchungen mit der ^{133}Xenon-Clearance. Arzneim. Forsch. (Drug Res.) 27/1, 1285–1290 (1977)

Lauter, H., Meyer, J.E.: Clinical and nosological concepts of senile dementia. In: Senile dementia. Müller, C., Ciompi, L. (eds.), pp. 13–27. Bern: Huber 1968

Lennartz, H.: Das Verhalten des cerebralen Durchströmungsvolumens und des Stoffwechsels bei Hirngefäßerkrankungen und degenerativ-involutiven Hirnprozessen während der Behandlung mit 7-[2-Hydroxy-3-(N-2-hydroxy-äthyl-N-methylamino)-propyl]-1,3-dimethyl-xanthin-pyridin-3-carboxylat. Arzneim. Forsch. (Drug Res.) 12, 675–679 (1972)

McHenry, L.C., Jr.: Cerebral vasodilator therapy in stroke. Stroke 3, 686–691 (1972)

McHenry, L.C., Jr., Jaffe, M.E., Kawamura, J., Goldberg, H.J.: Hydergine effect on cerebral circulation in cerebrovascular disease. J. Neurol. Sci. 13, 475–481 (1971)

McHenry, L.C., Jr., Jaffe, M.E., West, J.W., Cooper, E.S., Kenton, E.J.III., Kawamura, J., Oshira, T., Goldberg, H.J.: Regional cerebral blood flow and cardiovascular effects of hexobendine in stroke patients. Neurology (Minneap.) 22, 217–223 (1972)

Meyer, J.S., Kanda, T., Shinohara, Y., Fukuuchi, Y., Shimazu, K., Ericsson, A.D., Gordon, W.H., Jr.: Effect of hexobendine on cerebral hemispheric blood flow and metabolism. Neurology (Minneap.) 21, 691–702 (1971)

Newton, R.D.: The identity of Alzheimer's disease and senile dementia and their relationship to senility. Br. J. Psychiatr. 94, 225–249 (1948)

Olesen, J.: Cerebral blood flow. Methods for measurement, regulation, effects of drugs and changes in disease. Acta Neurol. Scand. [Suppl. 57] 50, 49–58 (1974)

Olesen, J.: The effect of intracarotid epinephrine, norepinephrine and angiotension on the regional cerebral blood flow in man. Neurology (Minneap.) 22, 978–987 (1972)

Olesen, J., Paulson, O.B.: The effect of intraarterial papaverine on the regional cerebral blood flow in patients with stroke or intracranial tumor. Stroke 2, 148–159 (1971)

Quadbeck, H., Lehmann, E.: Die Veränderung des oxidativen Glukosestoffwechsels des Gehirns unter langfristiger Xantinol-nicotinat-Medikation. Arzneim. Forsch. (Drug Res.) 28/2, 1531–1532 (1978)

Siesjö, B.K., Messeter, K.: Factors determining intracellular pH. In: Ion homeostasis of the brain. Siesjö, B.K., Sørensen, S.C. (eds.), pp. 244–262. Copenhagen: Munksgaard 1971

Siesjö, B.K., Zwetnow, N.N.: The effect of hypovolemic hypotension on extra- and intracellular acid-base parameters and energy metabolism in the rat brain. Acta Physiol. Scand. 79, 114–124 (1970)

Siesjö, B.K., Nilsson, L., Rokeach, M., Zwetnow, N.N.: Energy metabolism of the brain at reduced cerebral perfusion pressures and in arterial hypoxaemia. In: Brain hypoxia. Brierley, J.B., Meldrum, B.S. (eds.), pp. 79–93. London: Heinemann 1971

Shenkin, H.A.: Effects of various drugs upon cerebral circulation and metabolism of man. J. Appl. Physiol. 3, 465–471 (1951)

Skinhøj, E.: The sympathetic nervous system and the regulation of cerebral blood flow. Eur. Neurol. 6, 190–192 (1971/72)

Skinhøj, E., Paulson, O.B.: The mechanism of action of aminophylline upon cerebral vascular disorders. Acta Neurol Scand. 76, 129–140 (1970)

Sokoloff, L.: The action of drugs on the cerebral circulation. Pharmacol. Rev. 11, 1–85 (1959)

Terry, R.D.: Dementia. A brief and selective review. Arch. Neurol. 33, 1–4 (1976)

Terry, R.D.: Aging, senile dementia and Alzheimer's disease. In: Alzheimer's disease: Senile dementia and related disorders. Katzman, R., Terry, R.D., Bick, K.L. (eds.), pp. 11–14. New York: Raven 1978

Tomlinson, B.E., Blessed, G., Roth, M.: Observations on the brains of demented old people. J. Neurol. Sci. 11, 205–242 (1970)

Zwetnow, N.N.: The influence of an increased intracranial pressure on the lactate, pyruvate, bicarbonate, phosphocreatine, ATP, ADP and AMP concentrations of the cerebral cortex of dogs. Acta Physiol. Scand. 79, 158–166 (1970)

Psychomotor Stimulants

CHAPTER 14

The Pharmacological Profile
of Some Psychomotor Stimulant Drugs
Including Chemical, Neurophysiological,
Biochemical, and Toxicological Aspects

S. GARATTINI and R. SAMANIN

A. Introduction

Psychostimulant agents are an ill-defined class of drugs in which the potential danger of abuse is greater than the therapeutic benefits. Yet it would be very important to have select drugs available for stimulation of psychomotor functions with the aim of achieving, among other effects, relief of fatigue and improvement of learning-memory capacities. Unfortunately, no such ideal drugs presently exist although there are some, such as amphetamine, which have played a historically important role in elucidating central biochemical and physiologic functions, particularly those connected with the neurochemical transmission linked to monoamines. In contrast, psychostimulants have only a limited role in therapy in the treatement of obesity, narcolepsy, and hyperkinesis in children (ANGRIST and SUDILOVSKY, 1978; MARTINDALE, 1977).

The space allotted to this review imposes several limitations. For instance, the effects of methylxanthines (theobromine and caffeine) and nicotine will not be taken into account because, although they are used as psychostimulants, their intake occurs in complex mixtures (beverages and smoking). Many psychostimulants are simply minor chemical variations in the structure of amphetamine; usually there is relatively little information to differentiate their actions from those of amphetamine, and therefore these drugs will not be discussed in detail. Whenever possible, quotations will be made from reviews dealing with specialized aspects of the actions of psychostimulants.

d-amphetamine, methylphenidate, nomifensine, mazindol, and amineptine are therefore the drugs considered to be of primary importance for this review, because they have clinical applications even if some (nomifensine and amineptine) are primarily used as antidepressants.

B. Chemistry

The chemical structures of some psychostimulants mentioned in this review are presented in Fig. 1. It will be noted that several compounds such as methylphenidate, pipradol, and nomifensine contain in their structures a phenylethylamine or a phenylisopropylamine skeleton, chracteristic of the prototypical sympathetic stimulant d-amphetamine; mazindol does not contain a phenylethylamine structure. Another notable exception to this common feature of psychostimulants is amineptine which has an easily recognizable tricyclic structure. Several thousand molecules have been

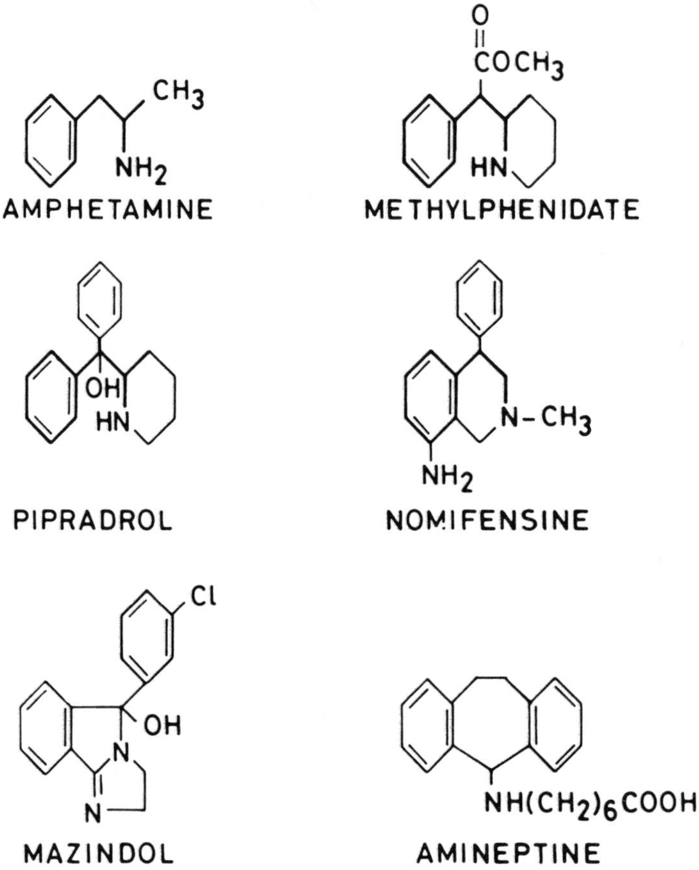

Fig. 1. Chemical structures of some psychostimulant drugs

synthesized since the discovery of amphetamine in the hope of finding a more potent and/or more specific agent.

Numerous reviews discuss the possible relationship between chemical structure and pharmacologic effects of amphetamines with special emphasis on locomotor stimulation and anorexia (Biel and Bopp, 1978; Biel, 1970; Shulgin, 1978; Van Rossum and Simons, 1969; Änggård, 1977). Briefly, the asymmetry of the α-carbon of the side chain of amphetamine makes possible two stereoisomers of which the d-form is several times more active than the l-isomer (Taylor and Snyder, 1971; Svensson, 1971; Lawlor et al., 1969). The length of the side chain is crucial because its shortening or lengthening diminishes the stimulant effect (Van Rossum and Simons, 1969). Substitution of the primary nitrogen with groups greater than methyl also results in a loss of activity (Änggård, 1977); substitution in the aromatic group has produced molecules such as fenfluramine (or its metabolite, norfenfluramine) where a trifluoromethyl group in meta position completely eliminates the stimulant activity without substantially affecting the anorectic effect (Beregi et al., 1970; Le Douarec and Neveu, 1970).

Incorporation of the aminoalkyl side chain into a ring structure led to synthesis of two well-known stimulants, methylphenidate and pipradrol. These piperdine derivatives have been reviewed by KRUEGER and MCGRATH (1964). Of the two diasterioisomers of methylphenidate, the threo form is the active one (KRUEGER and MCGRATH, 1974; SHAFI'EE and HITE, 1969; SHAFI'EE et al., 1967), while of the two enantiomers of pipradrol, the *l*-form exerts all the stimulant activity of the drug (PORTOGHESE et al., 1968). No structure-activity relationships have yet been reported for nomifensine, a stimulant drug utilized for treatment of depression (NICHOLSON and TURNER, 1977) or for mazindol, used as an anorectic agent (HADLER, 1972).

C. Kinetics and Metabolism

I. Amphetamine

The main factor influencing the kinetics of amphetamine is urinary pH. An acidic pH favors renal clearance of unchanged amphetamine, while a more basic pH favors the retention of amphetamine and therefore its metabolism (ASATOOR et al., 1965; BECKETT and ROWLAND, 1965a, b, c; BECKETT et al., 1965, 1969). For instance, when the urine is acidic, almost 70% of the administered amphetamine is eliminated in urine over a period of 4 days, the remaining 30% being metabolized; the plasma half-life is 5–6 h (DAVIS et al., 1971; ÄNGGÅRD et al., 1970a, b). In less acidic conditions, excretion of amphetamine as such amounts to only 30% with a plasma half-life of about 20–30 h (ÄNGGÅRD et al., 1970a). According to ÄNGGÅRD (1977), it is considered that each unit of increase in urinary pH prolongs the plasma half-life for *d*-amphetamine by about 7 h. This information has practical value in the treatment of amphetamine intoxication when it is important to keep a high flow of acidic urine to achieve maximum clearance of the drug (ÄNGGÅRD et al., 1970a).

In rats, *d*-amphetamine declines in plasma with a half-life $(t_{1/2})$ of 0.5 h (first phase) and 3 h (second phase) (MAICKEL et al., 1969; LEWANDER, 1971a; JONSSON and LEWANDER, 1973).

BAGGOT and DAVIS (1973) studied the pharmacokinetics of *d*-amphetamine in various animal species and concluded that the plasma $t_{1/2}$ of *d*-amphetamine was longer in carnivorous (dog and cat) than in herbivorous (pony, rabbit, and goat) species. Other information on the parmacokinetics of amphetamines can be found in the reviews by VREE (1973) and ÄNGGÅRD (1977).

Amphetamine and its congeners are readily absorbed in man (BECKETT and ROWLAND, 1965c; ASATOOR et al., 1965; QUINN et al., 1967; WILKINSON and BECKETT, 1968); in plasma the protein binding of *d*-amphetamine is about 20% (BAGGOT et al., 1972; FRANKSSON and ÄNGGÅRD, 1970). Amphetamine distributes extensively in the extravascular compartment with an apparent volume of distribution in man of 3.5–4.6 l/kg (ROWLAND, 1969). The drug rapidly penetrates the brain where it accumulates with a brain-to-plasma ratio of 7–12, depending on the animal species (JORI et al., 1978a; MAICKEL et al., 1970; ELLISON et al., 1968). Within the rat brain, *d*-amphetamine is uniformly distributed in the various areas (YOUNG and GORDON, 1962; JORI and CACCIA, 1974), as shown in Table 1. Similar results were obtained in cats (SIEGEL et al., 1968) where, however, at shorter times after amphetamine administration, the drug was localized more in the gray than in the white matter (LATINI et al., 1977).

548   S. GARATTINI and R. SAMANIN

Table 1. Distribution of d-amphetamine and its hydroxylated metabolites in various areas of the rat brain after intravenous administration of 15 mg/kg i.p. d-amphetamine (JORI and CACCIA, 1974)[a]

Area	Interval between treatment and death (h)	Levels (ng/g ± SE)		
		Amphetamine	p-Hydroxy-amphetamine	p-Hydroxy-norephedrine
Striatum	1	11,615 ± 874	92 ± 6	25
	5	1,099 ± 86	46 ± 5	57 ± 3
	12	100 ± 11	< 25	31 ± 1
Brainstem	1	14,763 ± 778	105 ± 18	32 ± 3
	5	852 ± 87	37 ± 6	168 ± 15
	12	75 ± 8	25	53 ± 1
Cerebellum	1	9,663 ± 777	83 ± 9	32 ± 5
	5	596 ± 56	< 25	84 ± 8
	12	82 ± 5	–	43 ± 3
Hemispheres	1	13,413 ± 488	105 ± 6	27 ± 2
	5	628 ± 44	< 25	120 ± 5
	12	91 ± 14	–	41 ± 5

[a] Determination by a gas chromatographic method developed by BELVEDERE et al. (1963)

Within any given brain area, such as the striatum or brainstem, indirect evidence indicates that d-amphetamine may be preferentially stored in the catecholaminergic nerve terminals (JORI et al., 1977), a finding which may explain some of this compound's neurochemical effects.

Studies of the subcellular localization of d-amphetamine have revealed higher concentrations of the drug in the cytoplasm than in the synaptosomal fraction (OBIANWU et al., 1968; WONG et al., 1972; PFEIFFER et al., 1969; MAGOUR et al., 1974). AZZARO et al. (1974) reported that d-amphetamine uptake may occur in vitro in the synaptosomal fraction when the drug is present at relatively low concentrations in the medium. The main metabolic pathway of amphetamine is depicted in Fig. 2; general surveys of the comparative metabolism of amphetamine in various animal species (WILLIAMS et al., 1973; SMITH and DRING, 1970; CASTAGNOLI, 1978) and in man (SMITH and DRING, 1970; GORROD, 1973) are available.

Aromatic hydroxylation of d-amphetamine in para position is well known in vivo (AXELROD, 1954b; DRING et al., 1966; ALLEVA, 1963) and in vitro (JONSSON, 1974; ROMMELSPACHER et al., 1974) with the formation of p-hydroxyamphetamine, a metabolite which has only weak central stimulant effects (TAYLOR and SULSER, 1973) because it does not easily cross the blood-brain barrier (JORI and CACCIA, 1974; JORI et al., 1978c). p-Hydroxyamphetamine is unevenly distributed in the brain (JORI and CACCIA, 1974; DANIELSON et al., 1976; LINDENBAUM et al., 1975) and disappears more slowly from the rat striatum ($t_{1/2}$, 8 h) than from the brainstem ($t_{1/2}$, 2 h), probably because it is stored in the dopaminergic system (JORI et al., 1978c; DANIELSON et al., 1976) which is present more in the striatum than the brainstem. This metabolite may have an affinity for dopamine structures as is borne out by reports of its uptake and storage by synaptic vesicles (L'HERMITE et al., 1973; EL GUEDRI et al., 1975), particu-

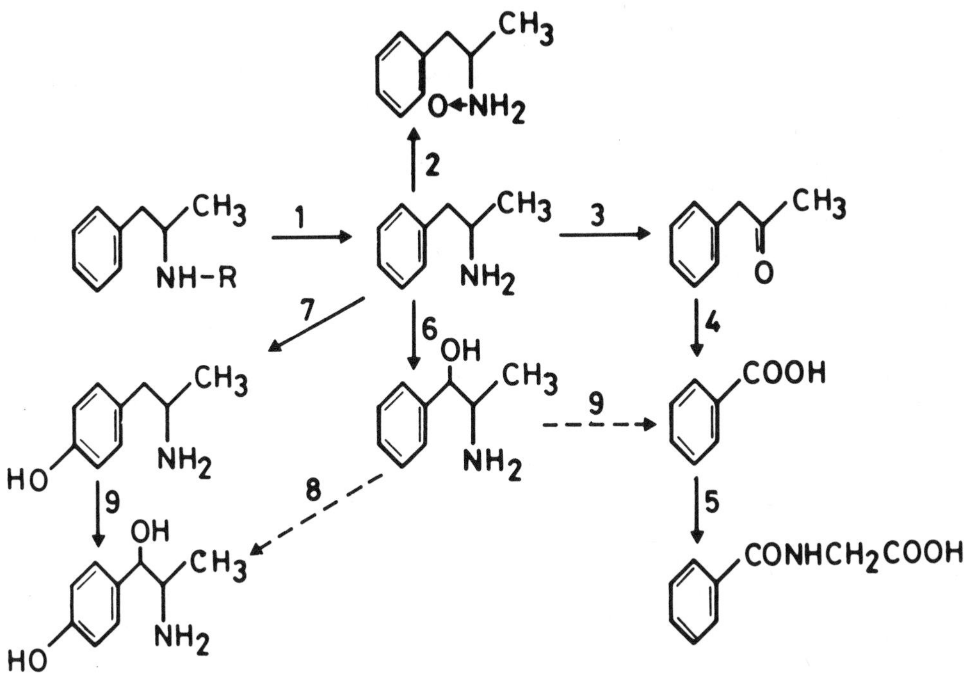

Fig. 2. Metabolism of *N*-alkylated amphetamines and amphetamine. *1*, *N*-dealkylation occurring, for instance, after administration of methamphetamine. *2*, formation of *N*-oxide derivatives. This metabolite has been shown only in vitro (BECKETT et al., 1973). *3*, oxidative deamination. Only the final product, phenylacetone, is shown in this scheme. *4*, oxidation of phenylacetone to benzoic acid. *5*, conjugation of benzoic acid with glycine to yield hippuric acid. *6–9*, aliphatic hydroxylation with formation of norephedrine or *p*-hydroxynorephedrine. This reaction is catalyzed by dopamine-*β*-hydroxylase. *7–8*, aromatic hydroxylation with formation of *p*-hydroxyamphetamine or *p*-hydroxynorephedrine. *9*, transformation of norephedrine to benzoic acid, probably with formation of the intermediate 1-hydroxy,1-phenylpropan-2-one (FELLER and MALSPEIS, 1971)

larly in striatal preparations (CHO et al., 1975). *p*-Hydroxyamphetamine, in fact, accumulates in the striatum (JORI et al., 1979) where its level is reduced by destruction of the dopaminergic nerve terminals as a consequence of intracerebral 6-hydroxydopamine treatment or catecholamine depletors such as tetrabenazine and reserpine or pimozide (JORI et al., 1979) a powerful specific and long-lasting dopamine receptor blocker (JANSSEN et al., 1968) which causes release of dopamine by a feedback response (NYBÄCK et al., 1967; WESTERINK and KORF, 1975).

Aliphatic hydroxylation of amphetamine is carried out by dopamine-*β*-hydroxylase (GOLDSTEIN and CONTRERA, 1962; CREVELING et al., 1962), an enzyme localized in the adrenergic neurons, with the formation of norephedrine (CALDWELL et al., 1972 b). *β*-Hydroxylation is stereo-specific for the *d*-form of amphetamine (GOLDSTEIN et al., 1964; TAYLOR, 1974) and *p*-hydroxyamphetamine is a better substrate than amphetamine. This suggests that amphetamine is first hydroxylated in the aromatic ring by the liver and then hydroxylated in the *β*-position in the adrenergic terminals with formation of *p*-hydroxynorephedrine (pOHNE) (GOLDSTEIN and ANAG-

Table 2. Metabolism of amphetamine in various animal species (Änggård, 1977)

Species	Percent of amphetamine excreted as			Ref.
	Unchanged	Aromatic hydroxylated	Deaminated	
Man				
acidic urine	65	5	15	DAVIS et al. (1971)
alkaline urine	22	9	27	DAVIS et al. (1971)
Monkey (squirrel)	29–42	1– 2	7–9	ELLISON et al. (1966)
Monkey rhesus	34	6	27	DRING et al. (1970)
Dog (beagle)	42–49	10–17	18–20	ELLISON et al. (1966)
Dog (grey hound)	30	6	30	DRING et al. (1966, 1970)
Rabbit	3	6	55	DRING et al. (1966, 1970)
Guinea pig	22	0	62	DRING et al. (1966, 1970)
Rat	14	48	3	DRING et al. (1966, 1970)
Mouse	33	14	31	DRING et al. (1966, 1970)

NOSTE, 1965; CAVANAUGH et al., 1970; CALDWELL et al., 1972 b); in fact, more pOHNE can be found in the brainstem than in striatum (CATTABENI et al., 1973; JORI and CACCIA, 1974) (see Table 1), paralleling the richness in noradrenergic terminals in these two discrete brain areas.

Oxidative deamination of amphetamine leads to the formation of phenylacetone and ammonia in the presence of rabbit liver microsomes fortified with nicotinamide adenine dinucleotide phosphate (NADPH) (AXELROD, 1954 b, 1955). The various mechanisms proposed to expalain the intermediate pathway of this oxidative process (DRING et al., 1966; BRODIE et al., 1958) have been recently summarized by ÄNGGÅRD (1977).

N-Dealkylation is a metabolic pathway common to several amphetamines which are substituted in the nitrogen (BOISSIER et al., 1970). Methamphetamine, for instance, is N-demethylated (AXELROD, 1954 a) by liver microsomal enzymes (for review see LA DU et al., 1971), the extent of this reaction varying from one animal species to another (CALDWELL et al., 1972 a, c).

N-Oxidation has been mostly described in vitro (BECKETT et al., 1973), with considerable differences between species. A review on oxidation of aliphatic amines is available (BRIDGES et al., 1972).

Any summary of knowledge of the metabolism of amphetamines must underline the considerable importance of the species in the predominance of any one pathway (WILLIAMS et al., 1973), as illustrated in Table 2. In rabbits and guinea pigs, deamination is the most important metabolic process, but aromatic hydroxylation predominates in rats.

Particular attention should be given to the metabolism of amphetamine in dependent subjects since it has been suggested that amphetamine psychosis depends on the formation of metabolites rather than on amphetamine itself. Änggård (1977) has recently summarized the arguments in favor of such a hypothesis showing that (1) amphetamine psychosis does not occur immediately; (2) it is not related to amphetamine plasma levels; (3) it is more intense under conditions which lead to increased metabolism; and (4) there is a positive correlation between excretion of hydroxylated amphetamine metabolites and the intensity of the psychosis.

II. Methylphenidate

Threo-methylphenidate is extensively metabolized in man, dogs, and rodents (FARAJ et al., 1974) and easily penetrates the brain, with a brain-to-plasma ratio ranging from 2 to 8 (FARAJ et al., 1974; BERNHARD et al., 1959; SHEPPARD et al., 1960; GAL et al., 1977). The half-life of plasma methylphenidate is around 2 h in dogs (FARAJ et al., 1974) and 25 min (GAL et al., 1977) or 105 min (SEGAL et al., 1976) in rats. A formal kinetic study in rats was made by GAL et al., (1977) using a specific gas-liquid chromatography mass spectrometry method. The principal metabolite of methylphenidate is ritalinic acid (BERNHARD et al., 1959; SHEPPARD et al., 1960; FARAJ et al., 1974; DAYTON et al., 1970), a product deriving from hydrolysis by plasma and tissue esterases. In addition, microsomal enzymes hydroxylate methylphenidate in the para position similarly to what has been found for d-amphetamine. The hydroxymethylphenidate may, after hydrolysis, yield p-hydroxyritalinic acid (FARAJ et al., 1974), a metabolite found in conjugated form in the urine.

Another important metabolic route is 6-oxomethylphenidate (BARTLETT and EGGER, 1972), which in turn is transformed into 6-oxoritalinic acid (FARAJ et al., 1974). The metabolism of methylphenidate differs according to the animal species (FARAJ et al., 1974). In man, the principal metabolite is ritalinic acid; in the dog it is oxoritalinic acid; and in rats it is p-hydroxyritalinic acid. All the metabolites described were found in the rat brain, p-hydroxymethylphenidate predominating. However, both p-hydroxymethylphenidate and 6-oxomethylphenidate can be regarded as inactive metabolites, at least judging by their locomotor stimulant activity in mice (FARAJ et al., 1974). A review on the kinetics and metabolism of methylphenidate appeared recently (PEREL and DAYTON, 1977).

III. Nomifensine

This compound is rapidly absorbed by the gastrointestinal tract after oral administration to rats, dogs, and monkeys (KELLNER et al., 1977). In these species, plasma protein binding is around 60%. In rats the drug does not seem to concentrate in brain, compared to plasma levels (KELLNER et al., 1977). In man, when nomifensine was determined with a specific GLC method (VERECZKEY et al., 1976), the opparent half-life was about 2–4 h (VERECZKEY et al., 1975; RINGOIR et al., 1977), but it is considerably longer in subjects with impaired renal function (RINGOIR et al., 1977).

The metabolism of nomifensine has been studied in several animal species (KELLNER et al., 1977; HEPTNER et al., 1978). In man, as in monkeys, nomifensine is hydroxylated in the unsubstituted aromatic ring in position 4 and then in position 3; 3-hydroxy, 4-methoxy, and 3-methoxy, 4-hydroxymetabolites have been isolated (KELLNER et al., 1977; HEPTNER et al., 1978). The dihydroxy metabolite of nomifensine may have a role in vivo, since it has been shown to stimulate striatal adenylate cyclase (POAT et al., 1978).

IV. Mazindol

Very little information is available on the kinetics and metabolism of this anorectic and stimulant agent. The drug is absorbed after oral administration, giving a peak level in blood at about 2–4 h and a half-life ranging from 33 to 55 h in man and in four animal species (HADLER, 1972).

V. Amineptine

This compound is rapidly absorbed in rats (intraperitoneally) and man (orally). The levels in rat brain are lower than in blood and they disappear very rapidly (SBARRA et al., 1979). In man, orally administered amineptine results in peak plasma levels around 30–45 min, with an apparent plasma $t_{1/2}$ of about 45 min (FANELLI, unpublished).

In rats and man, a metabolite forms with five carbon atoms in the side chain (β-oxidation), this has a plasma $t_{1/2}$ of about 90 min, a finding which explains why during repeated administration to man, the metabolite exceeds the level of the parent compound in plasma (FANELLI, unpublished).

D. Interaction with Central Chemical Transmitters

I. Catecholamines

The bulk of available data for psychostimulant agents concerns their effect on brain catecholamines (dopamine and noradrenaline), and therefore our comments will be mostly confined to this aspect of these drugs' complex effects in the brain. Many reviews are available and readers are referred to them for further details (COSTA and GARATTINI, 1970; LEWANDER, 1977a; MOORE, 1978; SULSER and SANDERS-BUSH, 1971; WEINER, 1972; KATZ and CHASE, 1970). The following preliminary comments are pertinent:

(1) The literature gives the impression of many contradictory findings concerning interactions between psychostimulants and central catecholaminergic mechanisms (ÄNGGÅRD, 1977). This is because of differences in animal species, doses, schedules of treatment, and/or intervals between drug administration and the determination of biochemical parameters reported. It is also evident that while d-amphetamine has been widely studied, for other psychostimulants the literature is scanty and much important information is lacking.

(2) To observe an effect, the doses of psychostimulants are frequently pushed up to toxic levels. As the dose increases, there is an increase of nonspecific effects. This point is clearly illustrated in Fig. 3, which reports the effect of d-amphetamine on the uptake of noradrenaline (NA), dopamine (DA), and serotonin (5HT) as a function of the drug concentration. The figure also shows the levels of d-amphetamine present in the rat brain after different doses of the drug are given in vivo. At lower doses (0.7 mg/kg), NA is affected more than DA uptake, but at higher doses there may also be an effect on 5HT uptake. At the dose of 15 mg/kg, the levels of amphetamine in the brain inhibit the uptake of all three amines (GARATTINI et al., 1978).

(3) Most of the biochemical data available refer to the whole brain or to large areas such as the striatum, but relatively small areas may also be affected by drugs in a specific manner and these effects are obviously missed when the determination of drug effect is diluted in a larger brain area or in the whole brain.

(4) Recent findings indicate a number of interactions among the various neurotransmitters in the brain (GARATTINI et al., 1977), so that no single monoaminergic system can be seen as isolated from the influence of the other chemical mediators. For instance, an increase of striatal homovanillic acid may depend on a direct effect on

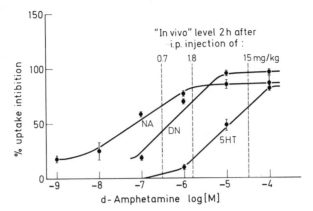

Fig. 3. Log-dose response curves for *d*--amphetamine inhibition of monoamine uptake. The dotted lines represent the concentration of *d*-amphetamine reached in the brain 2 h after i.p. injection of 0.7 mg/kg (CHO et al., 1973), 1.8 mg/kg (JORI et al., 1978a), and 15 mg/kg (BELVE-DERE et al., 1973) *d*-amphetamine sulfate in rats. The concentrations are calculated from the levels of the drug per gram of brain tissue, assuming a density of 1. Each point represents the mean ±SE of four replications

the dopaminergic system, but it may be the result of an interaction of the drug with the serotonergic system (CRUNELLI et al., 1980). An increase in striatal acetylcholine may be the result of direct action on the cholinergic system or of an effect on the dopaminergic (LADINSKY and CONSOLO, 1979) or serotonergic (SAMANIN et al., 1978 b) systems. The effect of a drug on a single chemical mediator can only be described for didactic purposes.

With these limitations, Table 3 gives a somewhat arbitrary selection of data to illustrate the effects of psychostimulants, namely *d*-amphetamine, methylphenidate, nomifensine, mazindol, and amineptine, on the noradrenergic system of the rat brain. The bulk of data is consistent with the hypothesis that *d*-amphetamine acts as an indirect noradrenergic agonist. There is, in fact, a release of NA and inhibition of NA uptake, both leading presumably to increased availability of NA at the postsynaptic receptor sites. The direct effects of *d*-amphetamine on dopamine-β-hydroxylase and on tyrosine hydroxylase are of doubtful significance because no consistent results have been found (ÄNGGÅRD, 1977). Several authors (GROPPETTI and COSTA, 1969; BRODIE et al., 1970; THOENEN et al., 1966; LEWANDER, 1977a; TAYLOR and SULSER, 1973) have suggested a role of *p*-hydroxynorephedrine, the amphetamine metabolite formed in the noradrenergic terminals, in explaining the release of NA, particularly during repeated treatments. For the other stimulants, the predominant effect seems to be a marked inhibition of brain NA uptake.

Table 4 sets out the effects of the various psychostimulants on the dopaminergic system in the rat striatum. The picture is now clearer for *d*-amphetamine. This drug is a releaser of DA, both in vitro and in vivo, and this results in an increase of 3-methoxytyramine and homovanillic acid (HVA), the extraneuronal metabolites of DA. Inhibition of monoamine oxidase (MAO) is probably responsible for inhibition of the intraneural metabolite of DA, dioxyphenylacetic acid (DOPAC). The inhibitory effect on DA uptake is not very marked and is certainly less than the inhibition

Table 3. Effects of single doses of psychostimulant agents on the rat noradrenergic system

Biochemical parameter (brain)	Effect of d-Amphetamine	Methylphenidate	Nomifensine	Mazindol	Amineptine
Noradrenaline	↘ [f] McLEAN and McCARTNEY (1961), MOORE and LARIVIERE (1963), JORI et al. (1978b)	– SCHEEL-KRÜGER (1971, 1972a)	– SAMANIN et al. (1975)	– SAMANIN et al. (1977), ENGSTROM et al. (1975), CARRUBA et al. (1976)	– SAMANIN et al. (1977c), DANKOVA et al. (1977)
Normetanephrine	↗ CARLSSON et al. (1966), CARLSSON (1970)[a]	↗ SCHEEL-KRÜGER (1971, 1972a)[a]		↗ ENGSTROM et al. (1975)	
MOPEG-SO$_4$	– CALDERINI et al. (1975), ↗ BAREGGI et al. (1978)	– BRAESTRUP and SCHEEL-KRÜGER (1976)	↗ BRAESTRUP and SCHEEL-KRÜGER (1976)		↗ BRAESTRUP and SCHEEL-KRÜGER (1976), SAMANIN et al. (1977c)
NA uptake (in vitro)	↘ FERRIS et al. (1972), HORN and SNYDER (1972), HENDLEY et al. (1972)	↘ FERRIS et al. (1972), HENDLEY et al. (1972)	↘ ALGERI et al. (1978), KRUSE et al. (1977), HUNT et al. (1974)	↘ HEIKKILA et al. (1977), GARATTINI et al. (1978)	
NA uptake (in vivo)	↘ TAYLOR and SNYDER (1971), CARLSSON (1969), SAMANIN et al. (1979)		↘ SAMANIN et al. (1975)	↘ GARATTINI et al. (1978), SUGRUE et al. (1978)	↘ SAMANIN (unpublished)[f]
NA release (in vitro)	↗ FERRIS et al. (1972), AZZARO and RUTLEDGE (1973), HEIKKILA et al. (1975b), BESSON et al. (1969a), GLOWINSKI (1970a)	↗ FERRIS et al. (1972)	– SCHACHT and HEPTNER (1974)	– HEIKKILA et al. (1977)	– SAMANIN (unpublished)
NA release (in vivo)	↗ STEIN and WISE (1970), TILSON and SPARBER (1972)	↗ CARR and MOORE (1970)[c]		– ENGSTROM et al. (1975)	

Table 3 (continued)

Biochemical parameter (brain)	Effect of				
	d-Amphetamine	Methylphenidate	Nomifensine	Mazindol	Amineptine
Tyrosine hydroxylase	↗ HARRIS et al. (1975), KUCZENSKI (1975)[d], BESSON et al. (1969b)	KUCZENSKI and SEGAL (1975)	− DI GIULIO et al. (1978)[e]		− ALGERI et al. (1978)[e]
COMT	− AXELROD and TOMCHICK (1960)			− ENGSTROM et al. (1975)	
Dopamine β-hydroxylase	↘ GOLDSTEIN and CONTRERA (1962), STOLK and RECH (1970)				
Monoamineoxidase	↘ BLASCHKO (1952), FULLER (1972)	↘ SZPORNY and GÖRÖG (1961)[f]		− ENGSTROM et al. (1975)	
Turnover of NA	− GERHARDS et al. (1974), CARENZI et al. (1975)[b], COSTA et al. (1972)		↗ GERHARDS et al. (1974)	↘ CARRUBA et al. (1976)	

[a] In MAO-blocked animals
[b] A variety of results including increase and decrease were obtained by other authors (GLOWINSKI, 1970b); FULGINITI and ORSINGHER, 1971)
[c] Experiments in cats
[d] Amphetamine inhibits this enzyme in vitro (BESSON et al., 1973; HARRIS and BALDESSARINI, 1973)
[e] Repeated treatments
[f] Large doses compared to behavioral effects
↗, ↘, and − indicate significant increase, decrease, or no effect, respectively.
COMT = catechol-o-methyl transferase

Table 4. Effects of single doses of psychostimulant agents on the rat dopaminergic system

Biochemical parameter (striatum)	Effect of				
	d-Amphetamine	Methylphenidate	Nomifensine	Mazindol	Amineptine
Dopamine	– SCHEEL-KRÜGER (1972a), SAMANIN et al. (1977c), GARATTINI (1973)	– SCHEEL-KRÜGER (1971, 1972a)	– ALGERI et al. (1978), SAMANIN et al. (1975)	– GARATTINI et al. (1978), CARRUBA et al. (1978), SAMANIN et al. (1977a)	– SAMANIN et al. (1977c), DANKOVA et al. (1977)
3-Methoxytamine	↗ DI GIULIO et al. (1978), SCHEEL-KRÜGER (1972a)[c]	↗ SCHEEL-KRÜGER 1971, 1972a)[c]	↗ ALGERI et al. (1978), DI GIULIO et al. (1978)		
DOPAC	↘ DI GIULIO et al. (1978), JORI et al. 1978b)	↗ BRAESTRUP (1977), BRAESTRUP and SCHEEL-KRÜGER (1976)	↘ ALGERI et al. (1978), DI GIULIO et al. (1978)		– DI GIULIO et al. (1978)
HVA	↗ DI GIULIO et al. (1978), JORI et al. (1978b), JORI et al. (1973)	↗ BRAESTRUP (1977), BRAESTRUP and SCHEEL-KRÜGER (1976), FANELLI (unpublished)	↗ ALGERI et al. (1978), DI GIULIO et al. (1978)	↗ JORI and DOLFINI (1974), JORI et al. (1978b), JORI and DOLFINI (1977)	↗ SAMANIN et al. (1977c), DANKOVA et al. (1977)
DA uptake (in vitro)	↘ FERRIS et al. (1972)	↘ FERRIS et al. (1972)	↘ ALGERI et al. (1978), KRUSE et al. (1977) HUNT et al. (1974)	↘ HEIKKILA et al. (1977), PEREL and DAYTON (1977)	↘ SAMANIN (unpublished), ALGERI et al. (1978)
DA uptake (in vivo)	– GARATTINI et al. (1978)		↘ SAMANIN et al. (1975)	↘ GARATTINI et al. (1978), CARRUBA et al. (1978)	↘ SAMANIN et al. (1977c)
DA release (in vitro)	↗ FERRIS et al. (1972), RAITERI et al. (1975), HEIKKILA et al. (1975a)	↗ FERRIS et al. (1972)	– SCHACHT and HEPTNER (1974)	– HEIKKILA et al. (1977), ↗ CARRUBA et al. (1978)	
DA release (in vivo)	↗ CHIUEH and MOORE (1975b)[d], BESSON et al. (1971)[d]	↗ CHIUEH and MOORE (1975b)[d]			

Table 4 (continued)

Biochemical parameter (striatum)	Effect of d-Amphetamine	Methylphenidate	Nomifensine	Mazindol	Amineptine
Tyrosine hydroxylase	↘ Kuczenski and Segal (1975)	– Di Giulio et al. (1978)[b], Kuczenski and Segal (1975)	– Di Giulio et al. (1978)[b]		– Algeri et al. (1978)[b]
COMT	– Axelrod and Tomchick (1960)			– Engstrom et al. (1975)	
MAO	↘ Blaschko (1952), Fuller (1972)	↘ Szporny and Görög (1961)[e]		– Engstrom et al. (1975)	
Turnover of DA	↗ Gerhards et al. (1974), Carenzi et al. (1975), Costa et al. (1972)	– Kuczenski and Segal (1975)	↗ Gerhards et al. (1974)	↗ Carruba et al. (1978)	↘ Algeri et al. (1978)
DA-adenylate cyclase	↗ Carenzi et al. (1975), Iversen et al. (1975)[a]	– Di Giulio et al. (1978)[b]	↘ Di Giulio et al. (1978)[b]		↘ Algeri (unpublished)
Haloperidol binding	– Di Giulio et al. (1978)[b]	– Di Giulio et al. (1978)[b]	– Di Giulio et al. (1978)[b]		– Algeri (unpublished)

[a] Increase of cyclic AMP in the striatum in vivo (Carenzi et al., 1975) although d-amphetamine is not active in vitro (Iversen et al., 1975) or after repeated treatments (Di Giulio et al., 1978)

[b] Repeated treatment

[c] In MAO-blocked animals

[d] In cats

[e] Only at very large doses

↗, ↘, and – indicate significant increase, decrease, or no effect, respectively

COMT = catechol-o-methyl transferase

of NA uptake (Garattini et al., 1978), but it may contribute to increasing the availability of DA at the postsynaptic receptor sites. Indeed, levels of the DA-mediated adenylate cyclase increase at shorter times after d-amphetamine administration (Carenzi et al., 1975). That this effect is due to the release of DA and not to a direct effect of d-amphetamine on DA receptors is shown by the inability of the latter to activate adenyl cyclase in vitro (Iversen et al., 1975). The other DA receptor, studied by means of haloperiodol binding, is not directly affected by d-amphetamine (Burt et al., 1976).

Methylphenidate is very similar to d-amphetamine in its effects on the dopaminergic system, with the difference that it increases DOPAC levels, a finding which may be related to its releasing DA intraneuronally from a storage pool.

The other psychostimulants induce much less DA release than d-amphetamine but except for amineptine, they are just as effective as amphetamine in inhibiting DA uptake. Other differences are less important or have still to be confirmed and evaluated.

The fact that a number of biochemical catecholaminergic parameters behave similarly under the effect of the various psychostimulants does not mean that the intimate mechanisms of action must be similar. Some recent findings concerning differences between d-amphetamine and methylphenidate are good examples of this point. When catecholamines are taken up by nerves of animals pretreated with reserpine and nialamide, they are mostly located extragranularly in the axoplasm (Malmfors, 1965; Stitzel and Lundborg, 1966; Jonsson and Sachs, 1969). In this experimental condition, d-amphetamine releases DA more powerfully than from tissues of untreated animals (Farnebo, 1971) Therefore, it may be concluded that d-amphetamine preferentially releases newly synthesized (reserpine-resistant) DA. In contrast, methylphenidate, and possibly nomifensine (Braestrup, 1977; Braestrup and Scheel-Krüger, 1976), do not release catecholamines from tissues pretretated with reserpine. These data have been recently confirmed in vivo by Chiueh and Moore (1975 a, b) and represent the biochemical equivalent of the fact that stereotypy induced by methylphenidate and nomifensine, but not by d-amphetamine, is inhibited by reserpine (Braestrup, 1977).

II. Serotonin

As previously indicated (see Fig. 3), d-amphetamine at high concentrations may inhibit 5 HT uptake (Garattini et al., 1978). However, the effects on levels of 5 HT, 5-hydroxyindoleacetic acid (5 HIAA), or on 5 HT turnover are inconsistent (for review see Lewander, 1977 a). Conversely, mazindol is a strong inhibitor of 5 HT uptake in vitro and partially in vivo (Garattini et al., 1978; Samanin et al., 1977 a) but does not affect brain 5 HT and 5 HIAA levels (Garattini et al., 1978). However, the effect of high doses of mazindol on the serotonergic system probably has no significance for the anorectic activity (Garattini et al., 1978). For nomifensine, methylphenidate, and amineptine, no effects have been described in relation to the serotonergic system.

III. Acetylcholine

d-Amphetamine has been reported to increase acetylcholine (ACh) release from the cortex of cats (Pepeu and Bartolini, 1967; Beani et al., 1968) and rats (Hemsworth and NEAL, 1968 a, b), probably indirectly through release of catecholamines because this effect is blocked by undercutting of the cerebral cortex (DEFFENU et al., 1970; PEPEU et al., 1970), septal lesions (NISTRI et al., 1972), or by administration of chlorpromazine (NISTRI et al., 1972; PEPEU and BARTOLINI, 1968), haloperidol (DEFFENU et al., 1970) or α-methyltyrosine (PEPEU et al., 1970; NISTRI et al., 1972). In the rat striatum, ACh is reduced by d-amphetamine at low doses (CARENZI et al., 1975; DOMINO and OLDS, 1972; DOMINO and WILSON, 1972) but raised at higher doses (CONSOLO et al., 1974; GLICK et al., 1974) with a consequent decrease of ACh turnover (TRABUCCHI et al., 1975). Amphetamine does not act on choline acetylase or acetylcholinesterase (HO and GERSHON, 1972; MANDELL and KNAPP, 1972), but it affects the cholinergic system through an activation of the striatal dopaminergic-cholinergic link (CONSOLO et al., 1975). In fact, the increase of striatal ACh induced by d-amphetamine is prevented by destruction of the presynaptic catecholaminergic terminals (CONSOLO et al., 1975; LADINSKY et al., 1975), and also by pimozide (LADINSKY et al., 1975), a specific dopaminergic antagonist. No studies of this kind are available for methylphenidate and mazindol, but amineptine had no effect on striatal ACh (SAMANIN et al., 1977 c) and nomifensine increased striatal ACh only at high doses (GARATTINI et al., 1976 a).

E. Pharmacology

In animals and man, psychostimulants in general increase alertness and locomotor activity, depress appetite, and at higher doses induce stereotyped behavior (for reviews see ÄNGGÅRD, 1977; LEWANDER, 1977 a; PEREL and DAYTON, 1977; BROOKES, 1977). It was long believed that appetite depression (anorexia) and central stimulation were closely associated, until the discovery of fenfluramine, an amphetamine analog with anorectic but no stimulant activity (LE DOUAREC et al., 1966; GARATTINI, 1973; GARATTINI et al., 1978). Table 5 shows this difference, indicating, in addition, that

Table 5. Pharmacologic effects of anorectic agents

Drug	Effects induced [a]		
	Locomotor stimulation	Stereotypy	Anorexia
d-Amphetamine [b]	+ + +	+ + +	+ + +
Methylphenidate	+ + +	+ + +	+
Nomifensine	+ +	+ +	+
Mazindol	+ + +	+ +	+ + +
Amineptine	+ + +	+	−
Fenfluramine	−	−	+ + +

[a] Ratings based on prevalent responses in various species; + + +, intense; + +, moderate; +, poor; −, absent
[b] Amphetamine analogs such as diethylpropion and phentermine are qualitatively similar to d-amphetamine (GARATTINI et al., 1978; SAMANIN et al., 1979; BORSINI et al., 1979)

there may be a stimulant effect without anorexia as in the case of amineptine (Samanin et al., 1977c).Recent findings show that even with *d*-amphetamine, by appropriate manipulation of the central monoaminergic systems, it is possible to dissociate the stimulant from the anorectic effect. Electrolytic lesion of the ventral noradrenergic bundle, but not of the locus ceruleus (Quattrone et al., 1977), antagonized the anorectic effect of low doses of *d*-amphetamine (Quattrone et al., 1977; Ahlskog and Hoebel, 1973), leaving intact the stimulant activity (Samanin et al., 1978a; Quattrone et al., 1977) and the stereotyped behavior induced by higher doses (Samanin et al., 1978a). In contrast, penfluridol, a long-acting specific dopaminergic antagonist (Nose and Takemoto, 1975), blocked locomotor stimulation and stereotyped behavior without antagonizing the anorectic activity of low doses of *d*-amphetamine (Samanin et al., 1978a; Quattrone et al., 1977). It was shown, in addition, that the anorectic effect of higher doses of *d*-amphetamine may have a dopaminergic component because it was partially blocked by penfluridol (Samanin et al., 1978a; Quattrone et al., 1977). These findings are summarized in Table 6.

I. Anorexia

Much work has been put into analyzing the mechanisms involved in depression of food intake. Table 7 summarizes a large amount of data on the effects of different procedures affecting central monoaminergic mechanisms on anorectic activity of amphetamine and mazindol (Kruk and Zarrindast, 1976; Garattini et al., 1978; Garattini and Samanin, 1976; Garattini et al., 1979; Blundell and Latham, 1978). Similar conclusions may also apply as regards the anorectic activity of *d*-aphetamine analogs such as diethylpropion (Hoekenga et al., 1978) and phentermine (Jenden et al., 1978; Garattini et al., 1978). In summary, it appears that the anorectic effect of amphetamine-like drugs requires an intact catecholaminergic system. Small differences may exist between the various compounds since for *d*-amphetamine and mazindol, NA and, to a lesser extent, DA may be involved, while for diethylpropion, DA apparently plays no role (Garattini et al., 1978). An important anatomic site for the action of *d*-amphetamine is probably the lateral hypothalamus, as shown by several authors (Booth, 1968; Leibowitz, 1970a, b; Blundell and Leshem, 1973) who indicated that *d*-amphetamine may interact with β-adrenergic receptors (Leibowitz, 1970a, b).

Table 7 sets out the different mechanisms of action of fenfluramine in depressing food intake. This drug should be considered the prototype of a new class of drugs which depress appetite through interaction with the serotonergic system (Blundell and Latham, 1978; Garattini et al., 1979; Clineschmidt et al., 1977; Samanin et al., 1978a; Garattini, 1979; Samanin et al., 1977b).

II. Locomotor Stimulation

It is impossible to summarize the large literature existing in this field, since *d*-amphetamine is widely used in studying locomotor acitivity. An attempt to cover the field was made recently by Lewander (1977a) and by Moore (1978). A basic concept is that the extent of the locomotor activity induced by *d*-amphetamine depends on many vari-

Table 6. Dissociation of various pharmacologic effect of *d*-amphetamine in rats

Dose (mg/kg i.p.)	Pharmacologic effect	Effect of			
		Striatum lesion [a]	NAS lesion [a]	Penfluridol (2.5 mg/kg p.o.) [b]	VNB lesion [c]
1.25	Anorexia	No effect (GARATTINI et al., 1978)	No effect (KOOB et al., 1979)	No effect (GARATTINI et al., 1978; SAMANIN et al., 1978a)	Antagonism (SAMANIN et al., 1978a, 1979)
2.50	Anorexia	–	–	Partial antagonism (SAMANIN et al., 1978a, 1979)	No effect (SAMANIN et al., 1978a, 1979)
1.50	Locomotor stimulation	No effect (KELLY et al., 1975)	Antagonism (KELLY et al., 1975)	Antagonism (SAMANIN et al., 1978a, 1979)	No effect (SAMANIN et al., 1978a, 1979)
5.00–10.00	Stereotypy	Antagonism (KELLY et al., 1975)	No effect (KELLY et al., 1975)	Antagonism (SAMANIN et al., 1978a, 1979)	No effect (SAMANIN et al., 1978a, 1979)

[a] Striatum and NAS (nucleus accumbens) lesions produced by 6-hydroxydopamine
[b] Penfluridol is a long-acting specific dopaminergic antagonist
[c] Electrolytic lesion of the ventral noradrenergic bundle (VNB)

Table 7. Effects of procedures affecting central monoaminergic mechanisms on anorectic activity of amphetamine, mazindol, and fenfluramine in the rat

Experimental condition [a]	Function of			Anorexia induced by		
	5-HT	NA	DA	Amphetamine	Mazindol	Fenfluramine
5-HT antagonists	D [b]			Unchanged	Unchanged	Reduced
MR lesion	D			Unchanged	Unchanged	Reduced
Pargyline + 6-OHDA		D	D	Reduced	Reduced	Unchanged
VNB lesion		D		Reduced	Reduced	Unchanged
Striatal 6-OHDA			D	Unchanged	Reduced	Unchanged
DA antagonists			D	Reduced or unchanged	Reduced	Unchanged

[a] See GARATTINI and SAMANIN (1976) für references regarding the various experimental conditions
[b] D, decreased
MR = MEDIAN RAPHE

ables. For instance, certain strains of mice (e.g., C3H, Balb/cJ) are insensitive to the effects of amphetamine (YEN and ACTON, 1973; JORI and GARATTINI, 1973; MOISSET and WELCH, 1973), young rats are less sensitive than adults (HEIMSTRA and McDON-ALD, 1962; SOFIA, 1969); grouped animals are more sensitive than isolated mice (GUNN and GURD, 1940; CHANCE, 1946); and individual animals respond differently to d-amphetamine, depending on their level of spontaneous activity (ISAAC, 1971; SEEGAL and ISAAC, 1971), their normal behavior (SALAMA and GOLDBERG, 1969), their degree of starvation (CAMPBELL and FIBIGER, 1971; FIBIGER et al., 1972; FIBIGER, 1973), and their thyroid function (MANTEGAZZA et al., 1968a; McDOWELL et al., 1967).

Much effort has gone into investigating the mechanisms involved in the locomotor stimulation induced by d-amphetamine. Many of these studies utilize interactions between drugs with known effects on given chemical mediators and d-amphetamine. The danger of this approach is that the interacting drugs may themselves modify the availability of d-amphetamine for the brain structures where it acts (GARATTINI et al., 1976b). The following example stresses this point. The locomotor hyperactivity or hyperthermia induced by d-amphetamine is potentiated by tricyclic antidepressant agents (e.g., desipramine); this has been suggested as a test to distinguish this class of psychotropic drugs from neuroleptics (MORPURGO and THEOBALD, 1965). The hypothesis to explain the interaction between desipramine and d-amphetamine was based on the fact that by blocking NA uptake at nerve terminals (CARLSSON et al., 1966; CARLSSON et al., 1969), tricyclic antidepressant agents would increase the amounts of NA released by d-amphetamine at the receptor sites. This attractive hypothesis is untenable, however, because tricyclic antidepressant drugs interact with d-amphetamine by increasing the concentration of d-amphetamine in the brain (VAL-ZELLI et al., 1967)., They do this by blocking hydroxylation of d-amphetamine (DIN-GELL and BASS, 1969; CONSOLO et al., 1967) by liver microsomal enzymes, thus limiting the major metabolic pathway of d-amphetamine in rats. That the potentiating effect of desipramine is almost entirely related to inhibition of amphetamine hydroxylation is indirectly confirmed by the fact that in mice (DOLFINI et al., 1969), a species in which amphetamine is poorly hydroxylated, desipramine does not potentiate d-amphetamine and it does not increase brain amphetamine concentrations. Furthermore, iprindole, a tricyclic antidepressant drug that does not inhibit NA uptake in brain (GLUCKMAN and BAUM, 1969), nevertheless increases brain amphetamine concentration and potentiates locomotor stimulation induced by d-amphetamine (MILLER et al., 1970).

The bulk of available data indicates that the locomotor stimulation induced by d-amphetamine is linked to an effect on central catecholamines. As expected, MAO inhibitors, by blocking the inactivation of catecholamines, tend to increase the stimulant effect of d-amphetamine (RECH and STOLK, 1970; SPENGLER, 1962), while α-methyltyrosine, by inhibiting catecholamine synthesis, completely blocks the stimulant effect (BUUS LASSEN, 1973; ERNST, 1969; HOLLISTER et al., 1974; MAJ et al., 1973; SIMON et al., 1970; SULSER et al., 1968). Reserpine, a depletor of granular stores of monoamines, does not inhibit d-amphetamine stimulation (BUUS LASSEN, 1973; ERNST, 1969; CORRODI et al., 1970; BANARJEE and LIN, 1973), a finding which agrees with the fact that d-amphetamine releases catecholamines from the nongranular pool (MOORE, 1978). Neuroleptic agents, blockers of postsynaptic catecholamine receptors, inhibit the stimulant activity of d-amphetamine (BORELLA et al., 1969 a, b; IRWIN et al., 1958; MAJ et al., 1974; ROLINSKI and SCHEEL-KRÜGER, 1973). It is important to underline that d-amphetamine stimulation is inhibited by neuroleptics such as haloperidol (ROLINSKI and SCHEEL-KRÜGER, 1973; TSENG and LOH, 1974), pimozide (ROLINSKI and SCHEEL-KRÜGER, 1973; MAJ et al., 1972), and penfluridol (SAMANIN et al., 1978 a; QUATTRONE et al., 1977), all of which are specific inhibitors of dopaminerigic receptors, with little effect on noradrenergic receptors.

The importance of dopamine for d-amphetamine-induced locomotor stimulation is further supported by the fact that extensive destruction of the catecholaminergic terminals by 6-hydroxydopamine reduced the effect of d-amphetamine (ERNST, 1969; FIBIGER, 1973; ESTLER et al., 1970; FIBIGER et al., 1973; CREESE and IVERSEN, 1973; GARATTINI et al., 1976b) even when only dopaminergic terminals were destroyed (HOLLISTER et al., 1974). Further studies support this view. For instance, injection of 6-hydroxydopamine into the ventral portion of the midbrain selectively destroys dopamineric neurons and blocks the stimulant activity of d-amphetamine (CREESE and IVERSEN, 1975), Whereas selective destruction of the noradrenergic neurons has no such effect (CREESE and IVERSEN, 1975; SAMANIN et al., 1978a; QUATTRONE et al., 1977). An important dopaminergic site for the locomotor stimulation induced by small doses of d-amphetamine is the nucleus accumbens [KELLY et al., 1975) (for a review see COOLS, 1977)]. Lesions of the n. accumbens with 6-hydroxydopamine make rats unresponsive to the stimulant effect of d-amphetamine although they are still sensitive to its anorectic effect (KOOB et al., 1979).

The data collected for d-amphetamine constitute an important basis for examining possible differences between the stimulant activity of this drug and that of other psychostimulants. For instance, reserpine is inactive on d-amphetamine stimulation but it markedly reduces the locomotor hyperactivity induced by methylphenidate (SCHEEL-KRÜGER, 1971), diethylpropion (OFFERMEIER and DU PREZ, 1978), and mazindol (OFFERMEIER and DU PREZ, 1978). In contrast, α-methyltyrosine, which blocks amphetamine, has little or no effect on the stimulation induced by methylphenidate (DOMINIC and MOORE, 1969; MOORE et al., 1970), diethylpropion (OFFERMEIER and DU PREZ, 1978), or mazindol (OFFERMEIER and DU PREZ, 1978).

III. Stereotypy

All the psychostimulants cause stereotyped behavior at doses usually higher than those required to induce locomotor stimulation (see Table 5). Stereotypy comprises a variety of repetitive components which are not necessarily the same for the various psychostimulants. For instance, *d*-amphetamine in mice causes repetitive licking and rapid movements of the head and forelegs whereas the stereotypy induced by methylphenidate consists almost exclusively of compulsive gnawing (PEREL and DAYTON, 1977). Differential pharmacologic effects produced by various agents are presented in Table 5. Although most of the studies were made in rats, several other species respond to *d*-amphetamine with stereotyped behavior, including mice (BERGER et al., 1973; SOUTHGATE et al., 1971; ROSS and RENYI, 1967; ZIEGLER et al., 1972), guinea pigs (GOETZ and KLAWANS, 1974; KLAWANS et al., 1972; SRIMAL and DHAWAN, 1970; RANDRUP and SCHEEL-KRÜGER, 1966), cats (COOLS and ROSSUM, 1970; COOLS, 1971; FUNATOGAWA, 1964), dogs (WILLNER et al., 1970; KLINGENSTEIN et al., 1973; WHITE et al., 1961), monkeys (RANDRUP, MUNKVAD, 1967b), and man (KRAMER et al., 1967). Reviews on stereotyped behavior induced by *d*-amphetamine (MUNKVAD et al., 1968; RANDRUP and MUNKVAD, 1972; LEWANDER, 1977a; IVERSEN, 1977) or other psychostimulants (FOG, 1972; SCHEEL-KRÜGER, 1972b) have been compiled. The mechanism of action underlying the stereotypy induced by *d*-amphetamine has been worked out in a manner similar to that described for locomotor stimulation. Briefly, it appears that release of DA is responsible and, in fact, blocking DA synthesis by α-methyltyrosine abolishes *d*-amphetamine stereotypy (ERNST, 1967a, b; FOG et al., 1967; RANDRUP and MUNKVAD, 1967a). Similarly, antidopaminergic drugs selectively block stereotyped behavior (SAMANIN et al., 1978a, 1979; ELLINWOOD and BALSTER, 1974; JANSSEN et al., 1968; COSTAL et al., 1972a, b, c), but α- or β-adrenergic receptor blockers have no such effect (LEWANDER, 1977a). Selective lesions of the dopaminergic, but not of the noradrenergic terminals (SAMANIN et al., 1978a, 1979), completely block stereotyped behavior (FOG et al., 1970; CREESE and IVERSEN, 1973, 1975; KELLY et al., 1975). The lesion must, however, be made in the striatum; a dopaminergic lesion of the n. accumbens reduces locomotor stimulation induced by amphetamine but has no effect on stereotypy (KELLY et al., 1975) or anorexia (KOOB et al., 1979). It should be remembered that dopaminergic lesions of the striatum did not influence the locomotor stimulant effect (KELLY et al., 1975) or the anorexia (GARATTINI et al., 1978) induced by *d*-amphetamine (for comparison see Table 6). However, not all the literature is in agreement with these findings; for a critical appraisal of this field, the reader is referred to a recent review (COSTAL and NAYLOR, 1977).

The concept of two different mechanisms also applies to stereotypy:

1) One important for *d*-amphetamine which is not inhibited by reserpine (EVERETT et al., 1957; FISHER and HELLER, 1967; HERMAN, 1967; PAPESCHI and RANDRUP, 1973; JANSSEN et al., 1965; LAL and SOURKES, 1972; RANDRUP and JONAS, 1967) but is blocked by α-methyltyrosine (see above) and

2) One unimportant for amphetamine and common to methylphenidate and nomifensine (and probably mazindol and amineptine) which is blocked by reserpine but not by α-methyltyrosine (BRAESTRUP, 1977; BRAESTRUP and SCHEEL-KRÜGER, 1976).

The class of agents described here as producing stereotypy can be distinguished in their mechanism of action from drugs such as apomorphine and piribedil, which are supposed to induce stereotypy by direct agonistic effects on dopaminergic receptors (ANDÉN et al., 1967; CORRODI et al., 1972).

F. Other Effects

It is impossible to summarize all the pharmacologic effects induced by *d*-amphetamine; an attempt has been recently made by LEWANDER (1977a). An incomplete list of such effects includes:

1) Increase of social interactions at low doses (TIKAL and BENESOVA, 1972) but disruption at high doses (TIKAL and BENESOVA, 1972), the latter effect being inhibited by dopaminergic antagonists such as pimozide (SCHIRRING and RANDRUP, 1971);

2) Induction or increase of aggressive behavior in various animal species and under various experimental conditions (LAL et al., 1971; VERGNES and CHAURAND, 1972; ELLINWOOD and ESCALANTE, 1970; TEDESCHI et al., 1969; CONSOLO et al., 1965);

3) An increase of sexual behavior, particularly at low doses of *d*-amphetamine (SOULAIRAC, 1963; BIGNAMI 1966), which may have a serotonergic (ELISASSON et al., 1972) rather than a catecholaminergic origin (MEYERSON, 1968);

4) An increase of the response rate in a number of different conditioned avoidance tasks after low doses (TEITELBAUM and DERKS, 1958; SCHUSTER et al., 1966; NIEMEGEERS et al., 1970) but disruption at higher doses (GUPTA and HOLLAND, 1969); and

5) A change in positively reinforced operant behavior, depending on the baseline response rate, the low rates increasing and the high rates decreasing (DEWS, 1958; RAY and BIVENS, 1966; CAREY at al., 1974);

6) Enhancement of intracerebral self-stimulation both in terms of response rates and current threshold (OLDS, 1958; GERMAN and BOWDEN, 1974; STEIN, 1962, 1964);

7) The onset and persistence of intravenous self-administration (PICKENS et al., 1972; STRETCH et al., 1971; YOKEL and PICKENS, 1974);

8) An increase, under given experimental conditions, of "learning and memory" (LIBERSON et al., 1959; CASTELLANO, 1974; RAHMANN, 1970);

9) Rise in body temperature, reportedly centrally related to catecholaminergic mechanisms (BRODIE et al., 1969; BORBÉLY et al., 1974) and peripherally connected to increase of oxygen consumption (WATERMAN, 1949; ANDRES et al., 1967; WEIS, 1973), glucose metabolism (MOORE et al., 1965; BEWSHER et al., 1966), and mobilization of free fatty acids (HAJOS and GARATTINI, 1973; BIZZI et al., 1970; GESSA et al., 1969);

10) An increase of blood pressure (BIZZI et al., 1970; REINERT, 1958; DAY and RAND, 1962), heart rate (WEIS, 1973; HARVEY et al., 1968; TRENDELENBURG et al., 1963), and peripheral resistance (HARVEY et al., 1968; BURN and RAND, 1958), probably related to a release of catecholamines from peripheral NA neurons and from adrenal medulla (for review see LEWANDER, 1977a).

G. Tolerance

Repeated treatments with psychostimulants result in attenuation of the pharmacologic and biochemical effects present after an acute treatment. However, tolerance develops to a different extent, depending on the animal species, the dose of psychostimulant, the intervals between doses, and the biochemical or pharmacologic parameter considered (for review see KOSMAN and UNNA, 1968).

Table 8. Tolerance to some biochemical effects of amphetamine after repeated administrations[a]

Pretreatment (mg/kg i.p. × no. of days)	Treatment (mg/kg i.p.)	NE in brain stem (ng/g ± SE)	HVA in striatum (ng/g ± SE)	DOPAC in striatum (ng/g ± SE)
Saline	Saline	460 ± 13	245 ± 23	544 ± 30
Saline	d-Amphetamine (15)	265 ± 16	602 ± 21	248 ± 27
d-Amphetamine (5 × 2)	d-Amphetamine (15)	252 ± 8	561 ± 8	–
d-Amphetamine (5 × 3)	d-Amphetamine (15)	362 ± 8[b]	493 ± 16[b]	–
d-Amphetamine (5 × 4)	d-Amphetamine (15)	395 ± 6[b]	300 ± 19[b]	270 ± 16
d-Amphetamine (5 × 8)	d-Amphetamine (15)	401 ± 5[b]	–	400 ± 17[b]

[a] Animals were killed 1 h after treatment
[b] $p < 0.01$ compared with rats given single dose of amphetamine

As previously described, d-amphetamine in rats increases the level of striatal HVA and reduces striatal DOPAC and brainstem NA in a dose-related manner (Jori et al., 1978 b). Doses of d-amphetamine (5 mg/kg), which are only slightly active on these biochemical parameters if given for few days, make a fully active dose of d-amphetamine less effective, as shown in Table 8. Tolerance to the increase of striatal HVA and the reduction of brainstem NA develops more rapidly than to the reduction of DOPAC (Jori et al., 1978 b). Several findings rule out the possibility of this tolerance being related to changes in d-amphetamine kinetics and metabolism, with particular reference to the availability of amphetamine and its metabolites in brain structures (Jori et al., 1978 b; Lewander, 1968; Kuhn and Schanberg, 1977; Lewander, 1971 b; Ellison et al., 1971). In fact, while tolerance developed to the above-mentioned effects on catecholamines, d-amphetamine, p-hydroxyamphetamine, and p-hydroxynorephedrine levels in the striatum and brainstem were comparable when the challenge with d-amphetamine was given to control animals or to rats previously treated with repeated doses of d-amphetamine (Jori et al., 1978 b). If any, the uptake of labeled d-amphetamine in discrete rat brain areas was greater after chronic treatement than in controls (Kuhn and Schanberg, 1977).

Table 9 shows that tolerance develops in respect to the striatal HVA increase not only for d-amphetamine, but also for the l-isomer, as well as for a number of psychostimulant drugs including methylphentermine, mazindol, amineptine, and nomifensine.

It is also interesting to note that cross tolerance arises between different psychostimulants. Short treatment with d-amphetamine induce cross tolerance to mazindol, amineptine, and nomifensine, and short treatments with these three psychostimulants induce cross tolerance to d-amphetamine. When there is tolerance to d-amphetamine, striatal HVA may, however, still be increased by agents such as fenfluramine, a nonstimulant drug inducing anorexia through a mechanism different from that of d-amphetamine (Garattini et al., 1978; Garattini and Samanin, 1976). At present, the intimate mechanism of the onset of tolerance and cross tolerance is not understood. It has been suggested that the hydroxylated metabolites of d-amphetamine may play a role in the onset of resistance by acting as false transmitters (Groppetti and Costa, 1969; Brodie et al., 1970). However, the fact that tolerance to d-amphetamine can be

Table 9. Tolerance to the increase of rat striatal HVA induced by psychostimulant agents[a]

Pretreatment (mg/kg i.p. × 4 days)		Challenge (mg/kg i.p.)		Tolerance (T) or cross tolerance (CT) based on lack of striatal HVA increase	Ref.
d-Amphetamine	5	d-Amphetamine	15	T	Jori and Bernardi (1972)
l-Amphetamine	5	l-Amphetamine	15	T	Jori and Dolfini (1977)
Mazindol	5	Mazindol	15	T	Jori and Dolfini (1977)
Amineptine	7.5	Amineptine	40	T	Samanin et al. (1977c)
Methylphentermine	10	Methylphentermine	30	T	Jori et al. (1978b)
Nomifensine	10	Nomifensine	20	T	Algeri (unpublished)
d-Amphetamine	5	Fenfluramine	15	No effect	Jori and Bernardi (1972)
d-Amphetamine	5	l-Fenfluramine	15	No effect	Jori and Dolfini (1977)
d-Amphetamine	5	Mazindol	15	CT	Jori and Dolfini (1977)
d-Amphetamine	5	Amineptine	40	CT	Samanin et al. (1977c)
d-Amphetamine	5	Nomifensine	10	CT	Algeri (unpublished)
d-Amphetamine	5	l-Amphetamine	15	CT	Jori et al. (1978b)
pOH-Amphetamine	20 × 2	d-Amphetamine	15	CT	Jori and Bernardi (1972)
l-Fenfluramine	5	d-Amphetamine	15	No effect	Jori and Dolfini (1977)
l-Amphetamine	5	d-Amphetamine	15	No effect	Jori et al. (1978b)
Mazindol	5	d-Amphetamine	15	CT	Jori and Dolfini (1977)
Amineptine	7.5	d-Amphetamine	15	CT	Samanin et al. (1977c)
Nomifensine	10	d-Amphetamine	15	CT	Algeri (unpublished)

[a] The interval between pretreatment and challenge was 24 h. There was no residual effect on striatal HVA at the time of challenge. The doses used for the challenge increased striatal HVA in naive rats

induced by other psychostimulants with a completely different chemical structure makes this hypothesis unlikely at least as far as the effect on striatal HVA is concerned.

It is worth stressing again the importance of the length of treatment and the doses involved; high doses of d-amphetamine given for several weeks induce a pronounced decrease of DA in the whole brain (Gunne and Lewander, 1967; Lewander, 1971c) and in the hippocampus, but not in the striatum (Herman et al., 1971). As regards pharmacologic effects during repeated courses of amphetamine, rats develop tolerance to the hyperthermic (Harrison et al., 1952), anorexigenic (Tormey and Lasagna, 1960; Lewander, 1977b), and cardiovascular effects (Burn and Rand, 1958; Day and Rand, 1963), but not to locomotor stimulation (Lewander, 1971d; Kosman and Unna, 1968; Magour et al., 1974b) or stereotyped behavior (Lewander, 1971d; Segal and Mandell, 1974). A review has been compiled (Gunne, 1977) on the development of tolerance in man after repeated treatment with d-amphetamine.

There is no doubt that tolerance develops during the use of d-amphetamine as far as appetite depression is concerned (Modell, 1960; Welsh, 1962; Gallagher and Knight, 1958), although there are no systematic and well-controlled studies. Similarly, tolerance arises to the euphoria-like effects induced by *d*-amphetamine (ROSEN-BERG et al., 1963) and to the awakening effect (KRAMER, 1972; GUNNE, 1977). Relatively little is known about tolerance to other psychostimulants.

H. Toxicology

d-Amphetamine is a fairly toxic compound when given parenterally, the LD_{50} in most animal species lying between 5 and 20 mg/kg (LEWANDER, 1977a). However, it is difficult to give exact figures because many factors (e.g., diurnal rhythms, ambient temperature, illumination, and strain) influence the outcome. Crowding (several animals per cage) is a widely studied factor; the LD_{50} in isolated mice (around 110 mg/kg) may in fact be about 10 times that of grouped animals (14 mg/kg) (CHANCE, 1946). The cause of death is largely unknown; the animals die with convulsions (ALLES, 1933; HÖHN and LASAGNA, 1960) and with elevated body temperatures (ASKEW, 1962; GREENBLATT and OSTERBERG, 1961).

Several studies have investigated how the toxicity of *d*-amphetamine could be prevented. Some of the most active antagonists in rats or mice are neuroleptics (phenothiazines and butyrophenones) (ASKEW, 1962; BURN and HOBBS, 1958; DAVIS, et al., 1974; FROMMEL and CHMOULIOVSKY, 1964), α-adrenoreceptor blocking agents (phenoxybenzamine, Dibenamine, and phentolamine) ASKEW, 1962; GRADOCKI et al., 1966; COHEN and LAL, 1963), β-adrenoreceptor blocking agents (propranolol) (DAVIS et al., 1974; MANTEGAZZA et al., 1968b, 1970; RAEVSKII and GURA, 1970), α-methyl-tyrosine (GOLDBERG and SALAMA, 1969; ALHAVA, 1973), and phenobarbital (FROMMEL and CHMOULIOVSKY, 1964).

In man large doses of *d*-amphetamine, ingested accidentally or for nonmedical use, induce a number of symptoms which have been summarized by GUNNE (1977):

1) Paranoid psychosis was first observed in 1938 (YOUNG and SCOVILLE, 1938); it was carefully described by CONNELL (1958) and subsequently reviewed by several authors (KALANT, 1966; BELL, 1971; GRIFFITH, 1977). "The amphetamine psychosis is an amorphous clinical syndrome characterized by well-systematized paranoid delusions with ideas of reference, with or without altered mood, illusions, and hallucinations of all senses. Usually absent are manifestations of organic delirium such as disorientation, memory impairment, and clouding of consciousness" (GRIFFITH, 1977). This psychosis can be experimentally induced in either short or prolonged *d*-amphetamine treatment;

2) Stereotyped behavior as also described for animals;

3) Choreic syndrome;

4) Excitation syndrome, frequently accompanied by increased blood pressure, tachycardia, hyperthermia, pupillary dilatation, and motor unrest (KRISKO et al., 1969; GINSBERG et al., 1970);

5) Dysautonomic syndrome, characterized by cardiovascular shock with repeated convulsions; and

6) Cerebrovascular accidents which may be related to the sustained high blood pressure (JÖNSSON, 1972).

An onset of psychosis or an intensification of psychotic symptoms has been described after small intravenous doses of methylphenidate (JANOWSKY et al., 1973a, b);

these effects can be counteracted by a cholinesterase inhibitor such as physostigmine (DAVIS et al., 1972; JANOWSKI et al., 1973a).

The most important side-effects of psychostimulants have been described by CONNELL (1978). Cardiovascular effects, including development of malignant hypertension, disruption of sleep organization, and allergy have been described for d-amphetamine. Dryness of the mouth, constipation, and mild adrenergic effects have been reported for mazindol and methylphenidate. For newer psychostimulants, any assessment of side-effects is premature. It should be recalled that the most serious aspect of all psychostimulants is their abuse potential.

A review of the interactions of stimulants with clinically relevant drugs has recently been published (ELLINWOOD et al., 1976).

References

Änggård, E.: General pharmacology of amphetamine-like drugs. A. Pharmacokinetics and metabolism. In: Drug addiction II. Amphetamine, psychotogen, and marihuana dependence. Martin, W.R. (ed.), pp. 3–31. Berlin, Heidelberg, New York: Springer 1977

Änggård, E., Gunne, L.M., Jönsson, L.E., Niklasson, F.: Pharmacokinetic and clinical studies on amphetamine dependent subjects Eur. J. Clin. Pharmacol. *3*, 3–11 (1970a)

Änggård, E., Gunne, L.M., Niklasson, F.: Gas chromatographic determination of amphetamine in blood, tissue, and urine. Scand. J. Clin. Lab. Invest. *26*, 137–143 (1970b)

Ahlskog, J.E., Hoebel, B.G.: Overeating and obesity from damage to noradrenergic system in the brain. Science *182*, 166–169 (1973)

Algeri, S., Brunello, N., Catto, E., Mennini, T., Ponzio, F.: Biochemical effect of some new proposed antidepressant drugs on the monoaminergic systems in the rat brain. In: Depressive disorders. Garattini, S. (ed.), pp. 155–168. Stuttgart: Schattauer 1978

Alhava, E.: Modification by methyltyrosine methylester (H 44/68) of the amphetamine-induced toxicity and brain catecholamine changes in developing mice. Acta Pharmacol. (Kbh.) *32*, 119–128 (1973)

Alles, G.A.: The comparative physiological actions of dl-phenylisopropylamines. I. Pressor effect and toxicity. J. Pharmacol. Exp. Ther. *47*, 339–354 (1933)

Alleva, J.J.: Metabolism of tranylcypromine-C^{14} and dl-amphetamine-C^{14} in the rat. J. Med. Chem. *6*, 621–624 (1963)

Andén, N.-E., Rubenson, A., Fuxe, K., Hökfelt, T.: Evidence for dopamine receptor stimulation by apomorphine. J. Pharm. Pharmacol. *19*, 627–629 (1967)

Andres, F., Ohnesorge, F.K., De Vries, R.: Zum Mechanismus der stoffwechselstimulierenden Wirkung von Weckaminen an isolierten Organen. Naunyn Schmiedebergs Arch. Pharmacol. *257*, 261–262 (1967)

Angrist, B. Sudilovsky, A.: Central nervous system stimulants: Historical aspects and clinical effects. In: Hanbook of psychopharmacology, Vol. 11: Stimulants. Iversen, L.L., Iversen, S.D., Snyder, S.H., (eds.), pp. 99–165. New York: Plenum 1978

Asatoor, A.M., Galman, B.R., Johnson, J.R., Milne, M.D.: The excretion of dexamphetamine and its derivatives. Br.J. Pharmacol. *24*, 293–300 (1965)

Askew, B.M.: Hyperpyrexia as a contributory factor in the toxicity of amphetamine to aggregated mice. Br. J. Pharmacol. *19*, 245–257 (1962)

Axelrod, J.: Enzymatic demethylation of sympathomimetic amines. Fed. Proc. *13*, 332 (1954a)

Axelrod, J.: Studies on sympathomimetic amines. II. The biotransformation and physiological disposition of D-amphetamine, D-P-hydroxamphetamine and D-methamphetamine. J. Pharmacol. Exp. Ther. *110*, 315–326 (1954b)

Axelrod, J.: The enzymatic deamination of amphetamine (Benzedrine). J. Biol. Chem. *214*, 753–763 (1955)

Axelrod, J., Tomchick, R.: Increased rate of metabolism of epinephrine and norepinephrine by sympathomimetic amines. J. Pharmacol. Exp. Ther. *130*, 367–369 (1960)

Azzaro, A.J. Rutledge, C.O.: Selectivity of release of norepinephrine, dopamine and 4-hydroxy-tryptamine by amphetamine in various regions of rat brain. Biochem. Pharmacol. 22, 2801–2813 (1973)

Azzaro, A.J., Ziance, R.J., Rutledge, C.O.: The importance of neuronal uptake of amines for amphetamine-induced release of ^{3}H-norepinephrine from isolated brain tissue. J. Pharmacol. Exp. Ther. 189, 110–118 (1974)

Baggot, J.D., Davis, L.E., A comparative study of the pharmacokinetics of amphetamine. Res. Vet. Sci. 14, 207–215 (1973)

Baggot, J.D., Davis, L.E., Neff, C.A.: Extent of plasma protein binding of amphetamine in different species. Biochem. Pharmacol. 21, 1813–1816 (1972)

Banarjee, U. Lin, G.S.: On the mechanism of central action of amphetamine- the role of catecholamines. Neuropharmacology 12, 917–931 (1973)

Bareggi, S.R., Markey, K., Paoletti, R.: Effects of amphetamine, electrical stimulation and stress on endogenous MOPEG-SO₄ levels in rat brain. Pharmacol. Res. Commun. 10, 65–73 (1978)

Bartlett, M.F., Egger, H.P.: Disposition and metabolism of methylphenidate in dog and man. Fed. Proc. 31, 537 (1972

Beani, L., Bianchi, C., Santinoceto, L., Marchetti, P.: The cerebral acetylcholine release in conscious rabbits with semipermanently implanted epidural cups. Int. J. Neuropharmacol. 7, 469–481 (1968)

Beckett, A.H., Rowland, M.: Urinary excretion kinetics of amphetamine in man. J. Pharm. Pharmacol. 17, 628–639 (1965a)

Beckett, A.H., Rowland, M.: Urinary excretion kinetics of methylamphetamine in man. J. Pharm. Pharmacol. [Suppl.] 17, 109S–114S (1965b)

Beckett, A.H., Rowland, M.: Urinary excretion of methylamphetamine in man. Nature 206, 1260–1261 (1965c)

Beckett, A.H., Rowland, M. Turner, P.: Influence of urinary pH on excretion of amphetamine. Lancet 1965 I, 303

Beckett, A.H., Salmon, M.A., Mitchard, M.: The relation between blood levels and urinary excretion of amphetamine under controlled acidic and under fluctuating urinary pH values using [^{14}]C amphetamine. J. Pharm. Pharmacol. 21, 251–258 (1969)

Beckett, A.H., Coutts, R.T., Ogunbona, F.A.: Metabolism of amphetamines. Identification of N-oxygenated products by gas chromatography and mass spectrometry. J. Pharm. Pharmacol. 25, 708–717 (1973)

Bell, D.S.: The precipitants of amphetamine addiction. Am. J. Psychiatry 119, 171–177 (1971)

Belvedere, G., Caccia, S., Frigerio, A., Jori, A.: A specific gas chromatographic method for the detection of p-hydroxyamphetamine and p-hydroxynorephedrine in brain tissue. J. Chromatogr. 84, 355–360 (1973)

Beregi, L.G., Hugon, P., Le Douarec, J.C., Laubie, M., Duhault, J.: Structure-activity relationships in DF₃ substituted phenethylamines. In: Amphetamines and related compounds. Costa, E., Garattini, S. (eds.), pp. 21–61. New York: Raven 1970

Berger, H.J., Brown, C.C., Krantz, J.C.: Fenfluramine blockade of CNS stimulant effects of amphetamine. J. Pharm. Sci. 62, 788–791 (1973)

Bernhard, K., Bühler, U., Bickel, M.H.: The biochemical action of a psychoanaleptic, the methyl ester of phenylpiperidylacetic acid. Helv. Chim. Acta 42, 802–807 (1959)

Besson, M.J., Cheramy, A., Feltz, P., Glowinski, J.: Release of newly synthesized dopamine from dopamine-containing terminals in the striatum of the rat. Proc. Natl. Acad. Sci. USA 62, 741–748 (1969a)

Besson, M.J., Cheramy, A., Glowinski, J.: Effects of amphetamine and desmethylimipramine on amines synthesis and release in central catecholamine containing neurons. Eur. J. Pharmacol. 7, 111–114

Besson, M.J., Cheramy, A., Feltz, P., Glowinski, J.: Dopamine: spontaneous and drug-induced release from the caudate nucleus in the cat. Brain Res. 32, 407–424 (1971)

Besson, M.J., Cheramy, A., Gauchy, C., Musacchio, J.: Effects of some psychotropic drugs on tyrosine hydroxylase activity in different structures on the rat brain. Eur. J. Pharmacol. 22, 181–186 (1973)

Bewsher, P.D. Hillman, C.C., Ashmore, J.: Studies on the hypoglycemic effect of d-amphetamine in aggregated mice. Biochem. Pharmacol. 15, 2079–2085 (1966)

Biel, J.H.: Structure-activity relationships of amphetamine and derivatives. In: Amphetamines and related compounds. Costa, E., Garattini, S. (eds.), pp. 3–19. New York: Raven 1970

Biel, J.H., Bopp, B.A.: Amphetamines: Structure-activity relationships. In. Handbook of psychopharmacology, Vol. 11: Stimulants. Iversen, L.L., Iversen, S.D., Snyder, S.H. (eds.), pp. 1–38. New York: Plenum 1978

Bignami, G.: Pharmacologic influences on mating behavior in the male rat. Effects of d-amphetamine LSD-25, strychnine, nicotine and various anticholinergic agents. Psychopharmacology 10, 44–58 (1966)

Bizzi, A., Bonaccorsi, A., Jespersen, S., Jori, A., Garattini, S.: Pharmacological studies on amphetamine and fenfluramine. In: amphetamine and related compounds. Costa, E., Garattini, S. (eds.), pp. 577–595. New York: Raven 1970

Blaschko, H.: Amine oxidase and amine metabolism. Pharmacol. Rev. 4, 415–458 (1952)

Blundell, J.E., Latham, C.J.: Pharmacological manipulation of feeding behavior: Possible influence of serotonin and dopamine on food intake. In: Central mechanisms of anorectic drugs. Garattini, S., Samanin, R. (eds.), pp. 83–109. New york: Raven 1978

Blundell, J.E., Leshem, M.B.: Dissociation of the anorexic effects of fenfluramine and amphetamine following intrahypothalamic injection. Br. J. Pharmacol. 47, 183–188 (1973)

Boissier, J.R. Hirtz, J. Dumont, C., Gérardin, A.: Some aspects of the metabolism of anorexic phenylisopropylamines in the rat. In: Amphetamines and related compounds. Costa, E., Garattini, S. (eds.), pp. 141–152. New York: Raven 1970

Booth, D.A.: Amphetamine anorexia by direct action on the adrenergic feeding system of rat hypothalamus. Nature 217, 869–870 (1980)

Borbély, A.A., Baumann, I.R., Waser, P.G.: Amphetamine and thermoregulation: Studies in the unrestrained and curarized rat. Naunyn Schmiedebergs Arch. Pharmacol. 281, 327–340 (1974)

Borella, L., Herr, F., Wojdan, A.: Prolongation of certain effects of amphetamine by chlorpromazine. Cand. J. Physiol. Pharmacol. 47, 7–13 (1969a)

Borella, L.E., Paquette, R., Herr, F.: The effect of some CNS depressants on the hypermotility and anorexia induced by amphetamine in rats. Can. J. Physiol. Pharmacol. 47, 841–847 (1969b)

Borsini, F., Bendotti, C., Carli, M.; Poggesi, E., Samanin, R.: The roles of brain noradrenaline and dopamine in the anorectic activity of diethylpropion in rats. A comparison with d-amphetamine. Res. Commun. Chem. Phathol. Pharmacol. (1979 to be published)

Braestrup, C.: Biochemical differentiation of amphetamine vs. methylphenidate and nomifensine in rats. J. Pharm. Pharmacol. 29, 463–470 (1977)

Braestrup, C., Scheel-Krüger, J.: Methylphenidate-like effects of the new antidepressant drug nimifensine (HOE 984). Eur. J. Pharmacol. 38, 305–312 (1976)

Bridges, J.W., Gorrod, J.W., Parke, D.V. (eds.): Biological oxidation of nitrogen in organic molecules. London: Taylor & Francis 1972

Brodie, B.B., Gilette, J.R., La Du, B.N.: Enzymatic metabolism of drugs and other foreign compounds. Annu. Rev. Biochem. 27, 427–454 (1958)

Brodie, B.B., Cho, A.K., Stefano, F.J.E., Gessa, G.L.: On mechanisms of norepinephrine release by amphetamine and tyramine and tolerance to their effects. Adv. Biochem. Psychopharmacol. 1, 219–238 (1969)

Brodie,, B.B., Cho, A.K., Gessa, G.L., Possible role of p-hydroxynorephedrine in the depletion of norepinephrine induced by d-amphetamine and in tolerance to this drug. In. Amphetamines and related compounds. Costa, E., Garattini, S. (eds.), pp. 217–230. New York: Raven 1970

Brookes, L.G.: Amphetamines. In: Psychotherapeutic drugs, pt. II: Applications. Usdin, E., Forrest, I.S. (eds.), pp. 1267–1286. New York: Dekker 1977

Burn, J.H., Hobbs, R.: A test for tranquilizing drugs. Arch. Int. Pharmacodyn. Ther. 113, 290–295 (1958)

Burn, J.H., Rand, M.J., The action of sympathomimetic amines in animals treated with reserpine. J. Physiol. (Lond.) 144, 314–336 (1958)

Burt, D.R., Creese, I., Snyder, S.H.: Properties of ^{3}H haloperidol dopamine binding associated with dopamine binding associated with dopamine receptors in calf brain membranes. Mol. Pharmacol. 12, 800–812 (1976)

Buus Lassen, J.: The effect of amantadine and (+)-amphetamine on motility in rats after inhibition of monoamine synthesis and storage. Psychopharmacology 29, 55–64 (1973)

Calderini, G., Morselli, P.L., Garattini, S.: Effect of amphetamine and fenfluramine on brain noradrenaline and MOPEG-SO₄. Eur. J. Pharmacol. 34, 345–350 (1975)

Caldwell, J., Dring, L.G., Williams, R.T.: Metabolism of ¹⁴C methamphetamine in man, the guinea pig and the rat. Biochem. J. 129, 11–22 (1972a)

Caldwell, J., Dring, L.G., Williams, R.T.: Norephedrines as metabolites of ¹⁴C amphetamine in urine in man. Biochem. J. 129, 23–24 (1972b)

Caldwell, J., Dring, L.G., Williams, R.T.: Biliary excretion of amphetamine and methamphetamine in the rat. Biochem. J. 129, 25–29 (1972c)

Campbell, B.A., Fibiger, H.C.: Potentiation of amphetamineinduced araousal by starvation. Nature 223, 424–425 (1971)

Carenzi, A., Cheney, D.L., Costa, E., Guidotti, A., Racagni, G.: Action of opiates, antipsychotics, amphetamine and apomorphine on dopamine receptors in rat striatum: In vivo changes of 3',5'-cyclic AMP content and acetylcholine turnover rate. Neuropharmacology 14, 927–939 (1975)

Carey, R.J., Goodall, E.B., Procopio, G.F.: Differential effects of d-amphetamine on fixed ratio 30 performance maintained by food versus brain stimulation reinforcement. Pharmacol. Biochem. Behav. 2, 193–198 (1974)

Carlsson, A.: Pharmacology of synaptic monoamine transmission. Prog. Brain Res. 31, 53–59 (1969)

Carlsson, A.: Amphetamine and brain catecholamines. In: Amphetamines and related compounds. Costa, E., Garattini, S. (eds.), pp. 289–300. New York: Raven 1970

Carlsson, A., Fuxe, K., Hamberger, B., Lindqvist, M.: Biochemical and histochemical studies on the effect of imipramine like drugs and (+)-amphetamine on central and peripheral catecholamine neurons. Acta Physiol. Scand. 67, 481–497 (1966)

Carlsson, A., Corrodi, H., Fuxe, K., Hökfelt, T.: Effects of some antidepressant drugs on the depletion of intraneuronal brain catecholamine stores caused by 4,α-methyl-m-tyramine. Eur. J. Pharmacol. 5, 367–373 (1969)

Carr, L.A., Moore, K.E.: Release of norepinephrine and normetanephrine from cat brain by central nervous system stimulants. Biochem. Pharmacol. 19, 2671–2675 (1970)

Carruba, M.O., Groppetti, A., Mantegazza, P., Vicentini, L., Zambotti, F.: Effects of mazindol, a non-phenylethylamine anorexigenic agent, on biogenic amine levels and turnover rate. Br. J. Pharmacol. 56, 431–436 (1976)

Carruba, M.O., Zambotti, F., Vicentini, L., Picotti, G.B., Mantegazza, P.: Pharmacology and biochemical profile of a new anorectic drug. Mazindol. In: Central mechanisms of anorectic drugs. Garattini, S., Samanin, R. (eds.), pp. 145–164. New York: Raven 1978

Castagnoli, N., Jr.: Drug metabolism: Review of principles and the fate of one-ring psychotomimetics. In: Handbook of psychopharmacology, Vol. 11: Stimulants. Iversen, L.L., Iversen, S.D., Snyder, S.H. (eds.), pp. 335–387. New York: Plenum 1978

Castellano, C.: Cocaine, pemoline and amphetamine on learning and retention of a discrimination test in mice. psychopharmacology 36, 67–76 (1974)

Cattabeni, F., Racagni, G., Groppetti, A.: p-hydroxynorephedrine: Its selective distribution in different rat brain areas. In: Frontiers in catecholamine research. Usdin, E., Snyder, S.H. (eds.), pp. 1035–1037. New York: Pergamon 1973

Cavanaugh, J.H., Griffith, J.D., Oates, J.A.: Effect of amphetamine on the pressor response to tyramine: Formation of p-hydroxynorephedrine from amphetamine in man. Clin. Pharmacol. Ther. 11, 656–664 (1970)

Chance, M.R.A.: Aggregation as a factor influencing the toxicity of sympathomimetic amines in mice. J. Pharmacol. Exp. Ther. 87, 214–219 (1946)

Chiueh, C.C., Moore, K.E.. d-Amphetamine-induced release of "newly synthesized" and "stored" dopamine from the caudate nucleus in vivo. J. Pharmacol. Exp. Ther 192, 642–653 (1975a)

Chiueh, C.C., Moore, K.E.: Blockade by reserpine of methylphenidate-induced release of brain dopamine. J. Pharmacol. Exp. Ther. 193, 559–563 (1975b)

Cho, A.K., Hodshon, B.J., Lindeke, B., Miwa, G.T.: Application of quantitative GC-mass spectrometry to study of pharmacokinetics of amphetamine and phentermine. J. Pharm. Sci. 62, 1491–1494 (1973)

Cho, A.K., Schaeffer, J.C., Fischer, J.F.: Accumulation of 4-hydroxyamphetamine by rat striatal homogenates. Biochem. Pharmacol. *24*, 1540–1542 (1975)

Clineschmidt, B.V., Hanson, H.M., Pflueger, A.B., McGuffin, J.C.: Anorexigenic and ancillary actions of MK-212 (6-chloro-2-[1-piperazinyl]-pyrazine; CPP). Psychopharmacology *55*, 27–33 (1977)

Cohen, M., Lal, H.: A study of the mechanism of amphetamine toxicity in aggregated mice. Pharmacologist *5*, 261 (1963)

Connell, P.H.: Amphetamine psychosis. London: Chapman & Hall 1958

Connell, P.H.: Central nervous system stimulants and anorectic agents. In: Side effects of drugs. Annual 2. Dukes, M.N.G. (ed.), pp. 1–8. Amsterdam: Excerpta Medica 1978

Consolo, S., Garattini, S., Valzelli, L.: Amphetamine toxicity in aggressive mice. J. Pharm. Pharmacol. *17*, 53–54 (1965)

Consolo, S., Dolfini, E., Garattini, S., Valzelli, L.: Desipramine and amphetamine metabolism. J. Pharm. Pharmacol. *19*, 253 (1967)

Consolo, S., Ladinsky, H., Garattini, S.: Effect of several dopaminergic drugs and trihexyphenidyl on cholinergic parameters in the rat striatum. J. Pharm. Pharmacol. *26*, 275–277 (1974)

Consolo, S., Fanelli, R., Garattini, S., Ghezzi, D., Jori, A., Ladinsky, H., Marc, V., Samanin, R.: Dopaminergic-cholinergic interaction in the striatum: Studies with piribedil. In: Advances in neurology, Vol. 9: Dopaminergic mechanisms. Calne, D., Chase, T.N., Barbeau, A. (eds.), pp. 257–272. New York: Raven 1975

Cools, A.R.: The function of dopamine and its antagonism in the caudate nucleus of cats in relation to the stereotyped behavior. Arch. Int. Pharmacodyn. Ther. *194*, 259–269 (1971)

Cools, A.R.: Basic considerations on the role of concertedly working dopaminergic, GABAergic, cholinergic and serotonergic mechanisms within the neostriatum and nucleus accumbens in locomotor activity, stereotyped gnawing, turning and dyskinetic activities. Adv. Behav. Biol. *21*, 97–141 (1977)

Cools, A.R., van Rossum, J.M.: Caudal dopamine and stereotyped behavior of cats. Arch. Int. Phrmacodyn. *187*, 163–173 (1970)

Corrodi, H., Fuxe, K., Ljungdahl, A., Ogren, S.O.: Studies on the action of some psychoactive drugs on central noradrenaline neurones after inhibition of dopamine-β-hydroxylase. Brain Res. *24*, 451–470 (1970)

Corrodi, H., Farnebo, L.-O., Fuxe, K., Hamberger, B., Ungerstedt, U.: ET 495 and brain catecholamine mechanism: Evidence for stimulation of dopamine receptors. Eur. J. Pharmacol. *20*, 195–204 (1972)

Costa, E., Garattini, S. (eds.): Amphetamines and related compounds. New York: Raven 1970

Costa, E., Groppetti, A., Naimzada, M.K.: Effects of amphetamine on the turn-over rate of brain catecholamines and motor activity. Br. J. Pharmacol. *44*, 742–751 (1972)

Costall, B., Naylor, R.J.: Mesolimbic and extrapyramidal sites for the mediation of stereotyped behavior patterns and hyperactivity by amphetamine and apomorphine in the rat. Adv. behav. Biol. *21*, 47–76 (1977)

Costall, B., Naylor, R.J., Olley, J.E.: Stereotypic and anticataleptic activities of amphetamine after intracerebral injections. Eur. J. Pharmacol. *18*, 83–94 (1972a)

Costall, B., Naylor, R.J., Olley, J.E.: The substantia nigra and stereotyped behavior. Eur. J. Pharmacol. *18*, 95–106 (1972b)

Costall, B., Taylor, R.J., Wright, T.: The use of amphetamine induced stereotyped behavior as a model for the experimental evaluation of antiparkinson agents. Arzneim. Forsch *22*, 1178–1183 (1972c)

Creese, I., Iversen, S.D.: Blockage of amphetamine-induced motor stimulation and stereotypy in the adult rat following neonatal treatment with 6-hydrosydopamine. Brain Res. *55*, 369–382 (1973)

Creese, I., Iversen, S.D.: The pharmacological and anatomical substrates of the amphetamine response in the rat. Brain Res. *83*, 419–436 (1975)

Creveling, C.R., Daily, J.W., Witkop, B., Udenfriend, S.: Substrate and inhibitors of dopamine-β-oxidase. Biochim. Biophys. Acta *64*, 125–134 (1962)

Crunelli, V., Bernasconi, S., Samanin, R.: Effects of d- and l-fenfluramine on striatal homovanillic acid concentrations in rats after pharmacological manipulation of brain serotonin: Evidence of a serotonin interaction. Pharmacol. Res. Comm. *12*, 215–223 (1980)

Danielson, T.J., Petrali, E.H., Wishart, T.B.: The effect of acute and chronic injections of d-amphetamine sulfate and substantia nigra lesions on the distribution of amphetamine and *para*-hydroxyamphetamine in the rat brain. Life Sci. *19*, 1265–1270 (1976)

Dankova, J., Boucher, R., Poirier, L.J.: Effects of 1694 and other dopaminergic agents on circling behavior. Eur. J. Pharmacol. *42*, 113–121 (1977)

Davis, J.M., Kopin, I.K., Lemberger, L., Axelrod, J.: Effect of urinary pH on amphetamine metabolism. Ann. N.Y. Acad. Sci. *179*, 493–501 (1971)

Davis, J.M., Janowsky, D.S., El-Yousef, M.K., Sekerke, H.J.: The effects of methylphenidate and physiostigmine in altering psychological behavior in man. Psychopharmacology [Suppl.] *26*, 37 (1972)

Davis, W.M., Logston, D.G., Hickenbottom, J.P.: Antagonism of acute amphetamine intoxication by haloperidol and propanolol. Toxicol. Appl. Pharmacol. *29*, 397–403 (1974)

Day, M.D., Rand, M.J.: Antagonism of guanethidine by dexamphetamine and other related sympathomimetic amines. J. Pharm. Pharmacol. *14*, 541–549 (1962)

Day, M.D., Rand, M.J.: Tachyphylaxis to some sympathomimetic amines in relation to monoamine oxidase. Br. J. Pharmacol. *21*, 84–96 (1963)

Dayton, P.G., Read, J.M., Ong, V.: physiological disposition of methylphenidate C^{14} in man. Fed. Proc. *29*, 345 (1970)

Deffenu, G. Bartolini, A., Pepeu, G.: Effect of amphetamine on cholinergic systems of the cerebral cortex of the cat. In: Amphetamines and related compounds. Costa, E., Garattini, S. (eds.), pp. 357–368. New York: Raven 1970

Dews, P.B.: Studies on behavior. IV. Stimulant actions of methamphetamine. J. Pharmacol. Exp. Ther. *122*, 137–147 (1958)

Di Giulio, A.M., Groppetti, A., Cattabeni, F., Galli, C.L., Maggi, A., Algeri, S., Ponzio, F.: Significance of dopamine metabolites in evaluation of drugs acting on dopaminergic neurons. Eur. J. Pharmacol. *52*, 201–207 (1978)

Dingell, J.V., Bass, A.D.: Inhibition of the hepatic metabolism of amphetamine by desipramine. Biochem. Pharmacol. *18*, 1535–1538 (1969)

Dolfini, E., Tansella, M., Valzelli, L., Garattini, S.: Further studies on the interaction between desipramine and amphetamine. Eur. J. Pharmacol. *5*, 185–190 (1969)

Dominic, J.A., Moore, K.E.: Supersensitivity to the central stimulant actions of adrenergic drugs following discontinuation of a chronic diet of α-methyltyrosine. Psychopharmacology *15*, 96–101 (1969)

Domino, E.F., Olds, M.E.: Effects of d-amphetamine, scopolamine, chlordiazepoxide and diphenylhydantoin on self-stimulation behavior and brain acetylcholine. Psychopharmacology *23*, 1–16 (1972)

Domino, E.F., wilson, A.: Psychotropic drug influences on brain acetylcholine utilization. Psychopharmacology *25*, 291–298 (1972)

Dring, L.G., Smith, R.L., Williams, R.T.: The fate of amphetamine in man and other mammals. J. Pharm. Pharmacol. *18*, 402–405 (1966)

Dring, L.G., Smith, R.L., Williams, R.T.: The metabolic fate of amphetamine in man and ohter species. Biochem. J. *116*, 425–435 (1970)

El Guedri, H., Rapin, J., Jacquot, C., Cohen, Y.: Localisation subcellulaire centrale comparée des dérivés p-hydroxylés de l'éphédrine et de l'amphétamine dans le cervau du rat. C.R. Acad. Sci. [D] (Paris) *281*, 587–589 (1975)

Eliasson, M., Michanek, A., Meyersson, B.J.: A differential inhibitory action of LSD and amphetamine on copulatory behaviour in the female rat. In: Animal Pharm. 1972, p. 22. In: Uppsala University Biomedical Center, Uppsala, 1972

Ellinwood, E., Balster, R.: Rating the behavioral effects of amphetamine. Eur. J. Pharmacol. *28*, 35–41 (1974)

Ellinwood, E.H., Jr., Escalante, O.: Behavior and histopathological findings during chronic methedrine intoxication. Biol. Psychiatry *2*, 27–39 (1970)

Ellinwood, E.H., Jr., Eibergen, R.D., Kilbey, M.M.: Stimulants: Interaction with clinically relevant drugs. Ann. N.Y. Acad. Sci. *281*, 393–408 (1976)

Ellison, T., Gutzait, L., Van Loon, E.J.: The comparative metabolism of d-amphetaime-C^{14} in the rat, dog and monkey. J. Pharmacol. Exp. Ther. *152*, 383–387 (1966)

Ellison, T., Siegel, M., Silverman, A.G., Okun, R.: Comparative metabolism of dl-^{3}H-amphetamine hydrochloride in tolerant and nontolerant cats. Proc. West Pharmacol. Soc. *11*, 75–77 (1968)

Ellison, T., Okun, R., Silverman, A., Siegel, M.: Metabolic fate of amphetamine in the cat during development of tolerance. Arch. Int. Pharmacodyn. *190*, 135–149 (1971)

Engstrom, R.G., Kelly, L.A., Gogerty, J.H.: The effects of 5-hydroxy-5-(4′-chlorophenyl)-2,3-dihydro-5H-imidazo(2,1-a)isoindole(Mazindol,SaH 42–548) on the metabolism of brain norepinephrine. Arch. Int. Pharmacodyn. *214*, 308–321 (1975)

Ernst, A.M.: Mode of action of apomorphine and dexamphetamine on gnawing compulsion in rats. Acta Physiol. Pharmacol. Neerl. *14*, 341 (1967a)

Ernst, A.M.: Mode of action of apomorphine and dexamphetamine on gnawing compulsion in rats. Psychopharmacology *10*, 316–323 (1967b)

ERnst, A.M.: The role of biogenic amines in the extra-pyramidal system. Acta Physiol. Pharmacol. Neerl. *15*, 141–154 (1969)

Estler, C.-J., Ammon, H.P.T., Fickl., W., Fröhlich, H.-N.: Substrate supply and energy metabolism of skeletal muscle of mice trated with methamphetamine and propranolol. Biochem. Pharmacol. *19*, 2957–2962 (1970)

Everett, G.M., Thoman, J.E.P., Smith, A.H.: Central and peripheral effects of reserpine and 11-desmethoxyreserpine (Harmonyl) on the nervous system. Fed. Proc. *16*, 295 (1957)

Faraj, B.A., Israili, Z.H., Perel, J.M., Jenkins, M.L., Holtzman, S.G., Cucinell, S.A., Dayton, P.G.: Metabolism and disposition of methylphenidate-^{14}-C: Studies in man and animals. J. Phrmacol. Exp. Ther. *191*, 535–547 (1974)

Farnebo, L.O.: Effect of d-amphetamine on spontaneous and stimulation-induced release of catecholamines Acta Physiol. Scand. [Suppl.] *371*, 45–52 (1971)

Feller, D.R., Malspeis, L.: Metabolism of D(-)-ephedrine and L(+)-ephedrine in the microsomal and 9,000 × g supernatant fractions of rabbit liver. Fed. Proc. *30*, 225 (1971)

Ferris, R.M., Tang, F.L.M., Maxwell, R.A.: A comparison of the capacities of isomers of amphetamine, deoxypipradrol and methylphenidate to inhibit the uptake of tritiated catecholamines into rat cerebral cortex slices. J. Pharmacol. Exp. Ther. *181*, 407–416 (1972)

Fibiger, H.C.: Behavioural pharmacology of d-amphetamine: Some metabolic and pharmacological considerations: In: Frontiers in catecholamine research. Usdin, E., Snyder, S.H. (eds.), pp. 933–937. New York: Pergamon 1973

Fibiger, H.C., Trimbach, C., Campbell, B.A.: Enhanced stimulant properties (+)-amphetamine after chronic reserpine treatment in the rat: Mediation by hypophagia and weight loss. Neuropharmacology *11*, 57–67 (1972)

Fibiger, H.C., Fibiger, H.P., Zis, A.P.: Attenuation of amphetamine-induced motor stimulation and stereotypy by 6-hydroxydopamine in the rat. Br. J. Pharmacol. *47*, 638–692 (1973)

Fisher, E., Heller, B.: Pharmacology of the mechanism of certain effects of reserpine in the rat. Nature *216*, 1221–1222 (1967)

Fog, R.: On stereotyped and catalepsy: Studies on the effect of amphetamines and neuroleptics in rats. Copenhagen: Munsgaard 1972

Fog, R., Randrup, A., Pakkenberg, H.: Aminergic mechanisms in corpus striatum and amphetamine induced stereotyped behaivor. Psychopharmacology *11*, 179–193 (1967)

Fog, R., Randrup, A., Pakkenberg, H.: Lesions in corpus striatum and cortex of rat brains and the effect on pharmacologically induced stereotyped, aggressive and cataleptic behavior. Psychopharmacology *18*, 346–356 (1970)

Franksson, G. Änggård, E.: The plasma protein binding of amphetamine, catecholamines and related compounds. Acta Pharmacol. Toxicol. (Kbh.) *28*, 209–214 (1970)

Frommel, E., Chemouliovsky, M.: De l'action antidotale de l'haloperidole envers l'amphétamine chez la souris. C.R. Soc. Biol. (Paris) *158*, 48–50 (1964)

Fulginiti, S., Orsingher, O.A.: Effects of learning, amphetamine and nicotine on the level and synthesis of brain noradrenaline in rats. Arch. Int. Pharmacodyn. Ther. *190*, 291–298 (1971)

Fuller, R.W.: Selective inhibition of monoamineoxidase. Adv. Biochem. Psychopharmacology *5*, 339–354 (1972)

Funatogawa, S.: Methamphetamine-induced changes in behavior of cats and in topographical distribution of brain serotonin. Psychiatr. Neurol. Jp. *66*, 743–754 (1964)

Gal, J., Hodshon, B.J., Pintauro, C., Flamm, B.L., Cho, A.K.: Pharmacokinetics of methylphenidate in the rat using single-ion monitoring GLC-mass spectrometry. J. Pharm. Sci. *66*, 866–869 (1977)

Gallagher, N.I., Knight, W.A. : Evaluation of amphetamine as an appetite depressant. J. Chronic Dis. *8*, 244–252 (1958)

Garattini, S.: Similitudes et différences entre la fenfluramine et l'amphétamine. Vie Méd. Can. Fr. *2*, 318–324 (1973)

Garattini, S.: Importance of serotonin for explaining the action of some anorectic agents. Inf. J. Obes. to be published

Garattini, S., Samanin, R.: Anorectic drugs and brain neurotransmitters. In: Dahlem workshop on appetite and food intake. Silvestone, T. (ed.), pp. 83–108, Dahlem Konferenzen, Berlin 1976

Garattini, S., Consolo, S., Chitto, G., Peri, G., Ladinsky, H.: Effect of nomifensine on acetylcholine and choline in the rat striatum and brain stem. Eur. J. Pharmacol. *35*, 199–201 (1976a)

Garattini, S., Jori, A., Samanin, R.: Interactions of various drugs with amphetamine. Ann. N.Y. Acad. Sci. *281*, 409–425 (1976b)

Garattini, S., Pujol, J.F., Samanin, R. (eds.): Interactions between putative neuro-transmitters in the brain, New York: Raven 1977

Garattini, S. Borroni, E., Mennini, T., Samanin, R.: Differences and similarities among anorectic agents. In: Central mechanism of anorectic drugs. Garattini, S., Samanin, R. (eds.), pp. 127–143. New York: Raven 1978

Garattini, S. Caccia, S., Mennini, T., Samanin, R., Consolo, S., Ladinsky, H.: Biochemical pharmacology of the anorectic drug fenfluramine: A review. Curr. Med. Res. Opin. [Suppl. 1] *6*, 15–27 (1979)

Gardocki, J.F., Schuler, M.E., Goldstein, L.: Reconsideration of the central nervous system. Pharmacology of amphetamine. II. Influence of pharmacological agents on cumulative and total lethality in grouped and isolated mice. Toxicol. Appl. Pharmacol. *9*, 536–554 (1966)

Gerhards, H.J., Carenzi, A., Costa, E.: Effect of nomifensine on motor activity, dopamine turnover rate and cyclic 3′,5′-adenosine monophosphate concentrations of rat striatum. Naunyn Schmiedebergs Arch. Pharmacol. *286*, 49–64 (1974)

German, D.C., Bowden, D.M. Catecholamine systems as the neural substrate for intracranial selfstimulation. A hypothesis. Brain Res. *73*, 381–419 (1974)

Gessa, G.L., Clay, G.A., Brodie, B.B.: Evidence that hyperthermia produced by d-amphetamine is caused by a peripheral action of the drug. Life Sci. *8*, 135–141 (1969)

Ginsberg, M.D., Hertzman, M., Schmidt-Nowara, W.W.: Amphetamine intoxication with coagulopathy, hyperthermia, and reversible renal failure. A syndrome resembling heatstroke. Ann. Intern. Med. *73*, 81–85 (1970)Glick, S.D., Jerussi, T.P., Waters, D.H., Green, J.P., Amphetamine induced changes in striatal dopamine and acetylcholine levels and relationship to rotation (circling behavior) in rats. Biochem. Pharmacol. *23*, 3223–3225 (1974)

Glowinski, J.: Release of monoamines in the central nervous system. In: Bayer Symposium II. New aspects of storage and release mechanism of catecholamines. Schüman, H.J., Kroneberg, G. (eds.), pp. 237–247. Berlin, Heidelberg, New York: Springer 1970a

Glowinski, J.: Effects of amphetamine on various aspects of catecholamine metabolism in the central nervous system of the rat. In: Amphetamines and related compounds. Costa, E., Garattini, S. (eds.), pp. 301–316. New York: Raven 1970b

Gluckman, M.I., Baum, T.: The pharmacology of iprindole, a new antidepressant. Psychopharmacology *15*, 169–185 (1969)

Goetz, C., Klawans, H.L.: Studies on the interaction of reserpine, d-amphetamine, apomorphine and 5-hydroxytryptophan. Acta Pharmacol. Toxicol. (Kbh.) *34*, 119–130 (1974)

Goldberg, M.E., Salama, A.I.: Amphetamine toxicity and brain monoamines in three models of stress. Toxicol. Appl. Pharmacol. *14*, 447–456 (1969)

Goldstein, M., Anagnoste, B.: The conversion in vivo of d-amphetamine to (+)-p-hydroxynorephedrine. Biochim. Biophys. Acta *107*, 166–168 (1965)

Goldstein, M., Contrera, J.F.: The substrate specificity of phenylanine-β-hydroxylase. J. Biol. Chem. *237*, 1898–1902 (1962)

Goldstein, M. McKereghan, M.R., Lauber, E.: The stereospecificity of the enzymatic amphetamine β-hydroxylation. Biochim. Biophys. Acta 89, 191–193 (1964)

Gorrod, J.W.: The metabolism and excretion of "amphetamine" in man. In: Frontiers in catecholamines research. Usdin, E., Snyder, S.H. (eds.), pp. 945–950. New York: Pergamon 1973

Greenblatt, E.N., Osterberg, A.C.: Correlations of activating and lethal effects of excitatory drugs in grouped and isolated mice. J. Pharmacol. Exp. Ther. 131, 115–119 (1961)

Griffith, J.D.: Amphetamine dependence. Clinical features. In: Handbook of experimental pharmacology, Vol. 45/II: Drug addiction. Martin, W.R. (ed.), pp. 277–304. Berlin, Heidelberg, New York: Springer 1977

Groppetti, A., Costa, E.: Tissue concentrations of p-hydroxynorephedrine in rats injected with d-amphetamine. Effect of pretreatment with desipramine. Life Sci. 8, 653–665 (1969)

Gunn, J.A., Gurd, M.R.: The action of some amines related to adrenaline. Cyclohexylalkylamines. J. Physiol. (Lond.) 97, 453–470 (1940)

Gunne, L.-M.: Effects of amphetamine in humans. In: Handbook of experimental pharmacology, Vol. 45/II: Drug addiction II. Martin, W.R. (ed.), pp. 247–275. Berlin, Heidelberg, New York: Springer 1977

Gunne, L.-M., Lewander, T.: Long-term effects of some dependence-producing drug on the brain monoamines. In: Molecular basis os some aspects of mental activity, Vol. 2. Otto Walaas, pp. 75–81. London. Academic Press 1967

Gupta, B.D., Holland, H.C.: An examination of the effects of stimulant and depressant drugs on escape/avoidance conditioning in strains of rat selectively bred for emotionality/nonemotionality interarterial activity. Int. J. Neuropharmacol. 8, 227–234 (1969)

Hadler, A.J., Mazindol, a new non-amphetamine anorexigenic agent. J. Clin. Pharmacol. 12, 453–458 (1972)

Hajos, G.J.T., Garattini, S.: A note on the effect of (+) and (−)-amphetamine on lipid metabolism. J. Pharm. Pharmacol. 25, 418–419 (1973)

Harris, J.E., Baldessarini, R.J.: Amphetamine-induced inhibition of tyrosine-hydroxylation in homogenates of rat corpus striatum. J. Pharm. Pharmacol. 25, 755–757 (1973)

Harris, J.E., Baldessarini, R.J., Roth, R.H.: Amphetamine-induced inhibition of tyrosine hydroxylation in homogenates of rat corpus striatum. Neuropharmacology 14, 457–471 (1975)

Harrison, J.W.E., Ambrus, C.M., Ambrus, J.L.: Tolerance of rats towards amphetamine and methamphetamine. J. Am. Pharm. Assoc. 41, 539–541 (1952)

Harvey, S.C., Sulkowski, T.S., Weenig, D.J.: Effect of amphetamines on plasma catecholamines. Arch. Int. Pharmacodyn. Ther. 172, 301–322 (1968)

Heikkila, R.E., Orlansky, H., Cohen, G.: Studies on the distinction between uptake inhibition and release of ³H-dopamine in rat brain tissue slices. Biochem. Pharmacol. 24, 847–852 (1975a)

Heikkila, R.E., Orlansky, H., Mytilinfou, C., Cohen, G.: Amphetamine: Evaluation of d- and l-isomers as releasing agents and uptake inhibitors for ³H-dopamine and ³H-norepinephrine in slices of rat neostriatum and cerebral cortex. J. Pharmacol. Exp. Ther. 194, 47–56 (1975b)

Heikkila, R.E., Cabbat, F.S., Mytilineou, C.: Studies on the capacity of mazindol and dita to act as uptake inhibitors or releasing agents for ³H-biogenic amines in rat brain tissue slices. Eur. J. Pharmacol. 45, 329–333 (1977)

Heimstra, N.W., McDonald, A.: Social influence on the response to drugs. III. Response to amphetamine sulfate as a function of age. Psychopharmacology 3, 212–218 (1962)

Hemsworth, B.A., Neal, M.J.: The effect of stimulant drugs on the release of acetylcholine from the cerebral cortex. Br. J. Pharmacol. 32, 416–417 (1968a)

Hemsworth, B.A., Neal, M.J.: The effect of central stimulant drugs on acetylcholine release from rat cerebral cortex. Br. J. Pharmacol. 34, 543–550 (1968b)

Hendley, E.D., Snyder, S.H., Fauley, J.J., La Pidus, J.B.: Stereoselectivity of catecholamine uptake by brain synaptosomes: Studies with ephedrine, methylphenidate and phenyl-2-piperidyl carbinol. J. Pharmacol. Exp. Ther. 183, 103–116 (1972)

Heptner, W., Hornke, I., Cavagna, F., Fehlhaber, H.W., Rupp, W., Neubauer, H.P.: Metabolism of nomifensine in man and animal species. Arzneim. Forsch. 28, 58–64 (1978)

Herman, Z.S.: Influence of some psychotropic and adrenergic blocking agents upon amphet-amine stereotyped behaviour in white rats. Psychopharmacology *11*, 136–142 (1967)

Herman, Z.S., Kmieciak-Kolada, K., Drybanski, A., Sokola, A., Trzeciak, H., Chrusciel, T.L.: The influence of 1-(o. allylphenoxy)-3-isopropylamino-2-propranolol hydrochloride (al-prenolol) in the central nervous system of the rat. Psychopharmacology *21*, 66–75 (1971)

Ho, A.K.S., Gershon, S.: Drug-induced alterations in the activity of rat brain cholinergic en-zymes. I. In vitro and in vivo effect of amphetamine. Eur. J. Pharmacol. *18*, 195–200 (1972)

Höhn, R., Lasagna, L.: Effects of aggregation and temperature on amphetamine toxicity in mice. Psychopharmacology *1*, 210–220 (1960)

Hoekenga, M.T., Dillon, R.H., Leyland, H.M.: A comprehensive review of diethylpropion hy-drochloride. In: Central mechanisms of anorectic drugs. Garattini, S., Samanin, R. (eds.), pp. 391–404. New York: Raven 1978

Hollister, A.S., Breese, G.R., Cooper,, B.R.: Comparison of tyrosine hydroxylase and dopa-mine-β-hydroxylase inhibition with the effects of various 6-hydroxy-dopamine treatments on d-amphetamine-induced motor acitvity. Psychopharmacology *36*, 1–16 (1974)

Horn, A.S., Snyder, S.H.: Steric requirements for catecholamine uptake by rat brain synapto-somes: Studies with rigid analogs of amphetamine. J. Pharmacol. Exp. Ther. *180*, 523–530 (1972)

Hunt, P., Kannengiesser, M.-H., Raynaud, J.P.: Nomifensine: A new potent inhibitor of dopa-mine uptake into synaptosomes from rat brain corpus striatum. J. Pharm. Pharmacol. *26*, 370–371 (1974)

Irwin, S., Slabok, K., Thomas, G.: Individual differences. I. Correlation between control locomotor activity and sensivtivity to stimulant and depressant drugs. J. Pharmacol. Exp. Ther. *123*, 206–211 (1958)

Isaac, W.: A study of the relationship between the visual system and the effects of d-amphet-amine. Physiol. Behav. *6*, 157–160 (1971)

Iversen, L.L., Horn, A.S., Miller, R.J.: Actions of dopaminergic agonists on cyclic AMP pro-duction in rat brain homogenates. Adv. Neurol. *9*, 197–212 (1975)

Iversen, S.D., Striatal function and stereotyped behaviour. In: Psychobiology of the striatum. Cools, A.R., Lohman, A.H.M., Van den Bercken, J.H.L. (eds.), pp. 99–118. Amsterdam: Elsevier 1977

Janowsky, D.S., El-Yousef, M.K., Davis, J.M., Sekerke, J.H.: Antagonistic effects of physo-stigmine and methylphenidate in man. Am. J. Psychiatr. *130*, 1370–1376 (1973 a)

Janowsky, D.S., El-Yousef, M.K., Davis, J.M., Sekerke, H.J.: Provocation of schizophrenic symptoms by intravenous administration of methylphenidate. Arch. Gen. Psychiatry *28*, 185–191 (1973 b)

Janssen, P.A.J., Niemegeers, C.J.E., Schellekens, K.H.L.: It is possible to predict the clinical effects of neuroleptic drugs (major tranquilizers) from animal data? Part 1: Neuroleptic ac-tivity spectra for rats. Arzneim. Forsch. *15*, 104–117 (1965)

Janssen, P.A.J., Niemegeers, J.E., Schellekens, K.H.L., Dresse, A.D., Lenaerts, F.M., Pin-chard, A., Schaper, W.K.A., von Nueten, M.J., Verbruggen, F.J.: Pimozide, a chemically novel, highly potent orally long-acting neuroleptic drug. Arzneim. Forsch. *18*, 261–287 (1968)

Jenden, D.J., Hinsvark, O.N., Cho, A.K.: Some aspects of the comparative pharmacology of amphetamine and phentermine. In: Central mechanisms of anorectic drugs. Garattini, S., Samanin, R. (eds.), pp. 165–177. New York: Raven 1978

Jönsson, L.E.: Pharmacological blockade of amphetamine effects in amphetamine dependent subjects. Eur. J. Clin. Pharmacol. *4*, 206–211 (1972)

Jonsson, G., Sachs, C.: Subcellular distribution of ^{3}H-noradrenaline in adrenergic nerves of mouse atrium. Effect of reserpine, monoamine oxidase and tyrosine hydroxylase inhibition. Acta Physiol. Scand. *77*, 344–357 (1969)

Jonsson, J., Lewander, T.: Effects of diethyldithiocarbamate and ethanol on the in vivo metab-olism and pharmacokinetics of amphetamine in the rat. J. Pharm. Pharmacol. *25*, 589–591 (1973)

Jonsson, J.A.: Hydroxylation of amphetamine to parahydroxyamphetamine by rat liver micro-somes. Biochem. Pharmacol. *23*, 3191–3197 (1974)

Jori, A., Bernardi, D.: Further studies on the increase of striatal homovanillic acid induced by amphetamine and fenfluramine. Eur. J. Pharmacol. *19*, 276–280 (1972)

Jori, A., Caccia, S.: Distribution of amphetamine and its hydroxylated metabolites in various areas of the rat brain. J. Pharm. Pharmacol. 26, 746–748 (1974)

Jori, A., Dolfini, E.: One the effect of anorectic drugs on striatum homovanillic acid in rats. Pharmacol. Res. Commun. 6, 175–178 (1974)

Jori, A., Dolfini, E.: Tolerance to the increase of striatal homovanillic acid elicited by several anorectic drugs. Eur. J. Pharmacol. 41, 443–445 (1977)

Jori, A., Garattini, S.: Catecholamine metabolism and amphetamine effects on sensitive and insensitive mice. In: Frontiers in catecholamine research. Usdin, E., Snyder, S. (eds.), pp. 939–941. New York: Pergamon 1973

Jori, A., Dolfini, E., Tognoni, G., Garattini, S.: Differential effects of amphetamine, fenfluramine and norfenfluramine stereoisomers on the increase of striatum homovanillic acid in rats. J. Pharm. Pharmacol. 25, 315–318 (1973)

Jori, A., Caccia, S., Garattini, S.: Possible storage of (+)-amphetamine in catecholaminergic terminals of the striatum and brainstem. Eur. J. Pharmacol. 41, 275–279 (1977)

Jori, A., Caccia, S., De Ponte, P.: Differences in the availability of d- and l-enantiomers after administration of racemig amphetamine to rats. Xenobiotica 8, 589–595 (1978a)

Jori, A., Caccia, S., Dolfini, E.: Tolerance to anorectic drugs. In: Central mechanisms of anorectic drugs. Garattini, S., Samanin, R., (eds.), pp. 179–189. New York: Raven 1978b

Jori, A., Caccia, S., Guiso, G. Garattini, S.: Distribution and localization of p-hydroxy-d-amphetamine in rat brain. Eur. J. Pharmacol. 52, 361–365 (1978c)

Jori, A., Caccia, S., Guiso, G., Ballabio, M., Garattini, S.: Selective storage of p-hydroxy-d-amphetamine in the dopaminergic nerve terminals, Biochem. Pharmacol. 28, 1205–1207 (1979)

Kalant, O.J.: The amphetamines toxicity and addiction, Springfield, Ill.: Thomas 1966

Katz, R.I., Chase, T.N.: Neurohumoral mechanisms in the brain slice. Adv. Pharmacol. Chemother. 8, 1–30 (1970)

Kellner, H.-M., Baeder, C., Christ, O., Heptner, W., Hornke, I., Ings, R.M.J.: Kinetics and metabolism of nomifensine in animals. Br. J. Clin. Pharmacol. 4, 109S–116S (1977)

Kelly, P.H., Seviour, P.W., Iversen; S.D.: Amphetamine and apomorphine responses in the rat following 6-OHDA lesions of the nucleus accumbens septi and corpus striatum. Brain Res. 94, 507–522 (1975)

Klawans, H.L., Rubowits, R., Patel, B.C., Weiner, W.J.: Cholinergic and anticholinergic influences on amphetamine-induced stereotyped behavior. J. Neurol. Sci. 17, 303–308 (1972)

Klingenstein, R.J., Wallach, M.B., Gershon, S.: A comparison of pimozide and thioridazine as antagonists of amphetamine-induced stereotyped behaviour in dogs. Arch. Int. Pharmacodyn. Ther. 203, 67–71 (1973)

Koob, G.F., Riley, S.J., Smith, S.C., Robbins, T.W.: Effects of 6-hydroxydopamine lesions of the nucleus accumbens septi and olfactory tubercle on feeding, locomotor activity, and amphetamine anorexia in the rat. J. Comp. Physiol. Psychol. 92, 917–927 (1978)

Kosman, M.E., Unna, K.R.: Effects of chronic administration of the amphetamines and other stimulants on behavior. Clin. Pharmacol. Ther. 9, 240–255 (1968)

Kramer, J.C.: Some observations on and a review of the effects of high-dose use of amphetamines. In: Drug abuse, proceedings of the international conference. Zarafonetis, C.J.D. (ed.), pp. 253–261. Philadelphia, Pa.: Lea & Febiger 1972

Kramer, J.C., Fishman, V.S., Littlefield, D.C.: Amphetamine abuse. Pattern and effects of high doses taken intravenously. J. Am. Med. Assoc. 201, 305–309 (1967)

Krisko, I., Lewis, E., Johnson, J.E.: Severe hyperpyrexia due to tranylcypromine-amphetamine toxicity. Ann. intern. Med. 70, 559–564 (1969)

Krueger, G.L., McGrath, W.R.: 2-Benzylpiperidines and related compounds. In: Psychopharmacological agents, Vol. I, Gordon, M. (ed.), pp. 225–250. New York: Academic 1964

Kruk, Z.L., Zarrindast, M.R.: Mazindol anorexia is mediated by activation of dopaminergic mechanisms. Br. J. Pharmacol. 58, 367–372 (1976)

Kruse, H., Hoffmann, I., Gerhards, H.J., Leven, M., Schacht, U.: Pharmacological and biochemical studies with three metabolites of nomifensine. Psychopharmacology 51, 117–123 (1977)

Kuczenski, R.: Effects of catecholamine releasing agents on synaptosomal dopamine biosynthesis: Multiple pools of dopamine or multiple forms of tyrosine hydroxylase. Neuropharmacology 14, 1–10 (1975)

Kuczenski, R., Segal, D.S.: Differential effects of d- and l-amphetamine and methylphenidate on rat striatal dopamine biosynthesis. Eur. J. Pharmacol. 30, 244–251 (1975)

Kuhn, C.M., Schanberg, S.M.: Distribution and metabolism of amphetamine in tolerant animals. Adv. Behav. Biol. 21, 161–177 (1977)

Ladinsky, H., Consolo, S.: The effect of altered function of dopaminergic neurons on the cholinergic system in the striatum. Progr. Brain Res. (1979 to be published)

Ladinsky, H., Consolo, S., Bianchi, S., Samanin, R., Ghezzi, D.: Cholinergic-dopaminergic interaciton in the striatum: The effect of 6-hydroxydopamine or pimozide treatment on the increased striatal acetylcholine levels induced by apomorphine, piribedil and d-amphetamine. Brain. Res. 84, 221–226 (1975)

La Du, B.N., Mandel, H.G., Way, E.L. (eds.): Fundamentals of drug metabolism and drug disposition. Baltimore: Williams & Wilkins 1971

Lal, H., O'Brien, J., Puri, S.K.: Morphine-withdrawal aggression sentization by amphetamines. Psychopharmacology 22, 217–223 (1971)

Lal, S., Sourkes, T.L.: Protentiation and inhibition of the amphetamine stereotypy in rats by neuroleptics and other agents. Arch. Int. Pharmacodyn. Ther. 199, 289–301 (1972)

Latini, R., Placidi, G.F., Riva, E., Fornaro, P., Guarnieri, M., Morselli, P.L.: Kinetics of distribution of amphetamine in cats. Psychopharmacology 54, 209–215 (1977)

Lawlor, R.B., Trivedi, M.C., Yelnosky, J.: A determination of the anorexigenic potential of dl-amphetamine, d-amphetamine, l-amphetamine and phentermine. Arch. Int. Pharmacodyn. Ther 179, 401–407 (1969)

Le Douarec, J.C., Neveu, C.: Pharmacology and biochemistry of fenfluramine. In: Amphetamines and related compounds. Costa, E., Garattini, S. (eds.), pp. 75–105. New York: Raven 1970

Le Douarec, J.C., Schmitt, H., Laubie, M.: Etude pharmacologique de la fenfluramine et de ses isomers optiques. Arch. Int. Pharmacodyn. Ther. 161, 206–232 (1966)

Leibowitz, S.F.: Hypothalamic beta-adrenergic "satiety" system antagonizes and alpha-adrenergic "hunger" system in the rat. Nature 226, 963–964 (1970a)

Leibowitz, S.F.: Reciprocal hunger-regulating circuits involving alpha- and beta-adrenergic receptors located, respectively, in the ventromedial and lateral hypothalamus. Proc. Natl. Acad. Sci. USA 67, 1063–1070 (1970b)

Lewander, T.: Urinary excretion and tissue levels of catecholamines during amphetamine intoxication. Psychopharmacology 13, 394–407 (1968)

Lewander, T.: On the presence of p-hydroxynorephedrine in the rat brain and heart in relation to changes in catecholamine levels after administration of amphetamine. Acta Pharmacol. Toxicol. (Kbh.) 29, 33–48 (1971a)

Lewander, T.: Effects of acute and chronic amphetamine intoxication on brain catecholamines in the guinea pig. Acta Pharmacol. Toxicol. (Kbh.) 29, 209–225 (1971b)

Lewander, T.: Effects of chronic amphetamine intoxication on the accumulation in the rat brain of labelled catecholamines synthesized from circulating tyrosine-^{14}C and dopa-^{3}H. Naunyn Schmiedebergs Arch. Pharmacol. 271, 211–233 (1971c)

Lewander, T.: A mechanism for the development of tolerance to amphetamine in rats. Psychopharmacology 21, 17–31 (1971d)

Lewander, T.: Effects of amphetamine in animals. In: Drug addiction II. Martin, W.R. (ed.), pp. 33–246. Berlin, Heidelberg, New York: Springer 1977a

Lewander, T.: In food deprivation in relation to amphetamine tolerance. Adv. Behav. Biol. 21, 201–213 (1977b)

L'Hermite, P., Jacquot, C., Goffic, F., Cohen, Y., Valette, G.: Capture et stockage des derivés de la beta-phenylethylamine dans le fibres adrénergiques du système nerveux peripherique retention préferentielle de la noradrénaline. J. Pharmacol. (Paris) 4, 325–340 (1973)

Liberson, W.T., Ellen, P., Feldman, R.S.: Effect of "somatic" vs "guidance" therapies on behaviour rigidity rats. J. Neuropsychiatry 1, 17–19 (1959)

Lindenbaum, A., Marcher, K., Wepierre, J., Cohen, Y.: Barrière hematoencephalique II: Cinetique de distribution de la parahydroxyamphetamine ^{3}H dans les structures du cerveau de rat après administration intraveineuse. Arch. Int. Pharmacodyn. Ther 215, 168–176 (1975)

Magour, S., Coper, H., Fähndrich, C.H.: The effects of chronic treatment with d-amphetamine on food intake, body weight, locomotor activity and suncellular distribution of the drug in rat brain. Psychopharmacology 34, 45–54 (1974)

Maickel, R.P., Cox, R.H., Jr., Miller, F.P., Segal, D.S., Russell, R.W.: Correlation of brain levels of drugs with behavioral effects J. Pharmacol. Exp. Ther. *165*, 216–224 (1969)

Maickel, R.P., Cox, R.H., Jr., Ksir, C.J., Snodgrass, W.R., Miller, F.P.: Some aspects of the behavioral pharmacology of the amphetamine. In: Amphetamines and related compounds, Costa, E., Garattini, S. (eds.), pp. 747–759. New York: Raven: 1970

Maj, J., Sowinska, H., Kapturkiewicz, Z., Sarnek, J.: The effect of l-dopa and (+)-amphetamine on the locomotor activity after pimozide and phenoxybenzamine. J. Pharmacol. *24*, 412–413 (1972)

Maj, J., Sowinksa, H., Barab, L.: Effects of amantadine, amphetamine and apomorphine on the locomotor activity in rats. Life Sci. *12*, 511–518 (1973)

Maj, J., Sowinska, H., Baran, L., Kapturkiewicz, Z.: The effects of clozapine, thioridazine and phenoxybenzamine on the action of drugs stimulating the central catecholamine receptors. Pol. J. Pharmacol. Pharm. *20*, 437–448 (1974)

Malmfors, T.: Studies on adrenergic nerves. The use of rat and mouse iris for direct observations on their physiology and pharmacology at cellular and subcellular levels. Acta Physiol. Scand. [Suppl. 248] *64*, 1–93 (1965)

Mandell, A.J., Knapp, S.: Cholinergic adaptation in the brain to chronic administration of amphetamine. In: Current concepts on amphetamine abuse (DHEW Publ. no. HSM 72-9085). Ellinwood, E.H., Cohen, S. (eds.), pp. 77–86. Washington, D.C.: U.S. G.P.O. 1972

Mantegazza, P., Naimzada, K.M., Riva, M.: Activity of amphetamine in hypothyroid rats. Eur. J. Pharmacol. *5*, 10–16 (1968a)

Mantegazza, P., Naimazada, K.M., Riva, M.: Effects of propranolol on some activities of amphetamine. Eur. J. Pharmacol. *4*, 25–30 (1968b)

Mantegazza, P., Müller, E.E., Naimzada, M.K., Riva, M.: Studies on the lack of correlation between hyperthermia, hyperactivity and anorexia induced by amphetamine. In: Amphetamines and related compounds. Costa, E., Garattini, S. (eds.), pp. 559–575. New York: Raven 1970

Martindale, the extra pharmacopoeia.Central and respiratory stimulants. Wade A. (ed.), pp. 305–318, London: Pharmaceutical Press 1977

McDowell, A.A., Ziller, H.H., Krise, G.M.: Effects of previous radiation exposure on the activity response to d-amphetamine hydrochloride. J. Genet. Psychol. *111*, 241–243 (1967)

McLean, J.R., McCartney, M.: Effect of d-amphetamine on rat brain noradrenaline and serotonin. Proc. Soc. Exp. Biol. Med. *107*, 77–79 (1961)

Meyerson, B.J.: Amphetamine and 5-hydroxytryptamine inhibition of copulatory behaviour in the female rat. Ann. Med. Exp. Biol. Fenn. *46*, 394–398 (1968)

Miller, K.W., Freeman, J.J., Dingell, J.V., Sulser, F.: On the mechanism of amphetamine potentiation by iprindole. Experientia *26*, 863–864 (1970)

Modell, W.: Status and prospect of drugs for overeating. J. Am. Med. Assoc. *173*, 1131–1136 (1960)

Moisset, B., Welch, B.L.: Effects of d-amphetamine upon open field behaviour in two inbred strains of mice. Experientia *29*, 625–626 (1973)

Moore, K.E.: Amphetamines: Biochemical and behavioral actions in animals. In: Handbook of psychopharmacology, Vol. 11, Stimulants, Inversen, L.L., Iversen, S.D., Snyder, S.H. (eds.), pp. 41–98. New York: Plenum 1978

Moore, K.E., Lariviere, E.W.: Effects of d-amphetamine and restraint on the content of norepinephrine and dopamine in rat brain. Biochem. Pharmacol. *12*, 1283–1288 (1963)

Moore, K.E., Sawdy, L.C., Shaul, S.R.: Effects of d-amphetamine on blood glucose and tissue glycogen levels of isolated and aggregated mice. Biochem. Pharmacol. *14*, 197–204 (1965)

Moore, K.E., Carr, L.A., Dominic, J.A.: Functional significance of amphetamine-induced release of brain catecholamines. In: Amphetamines and related compounds. Costa, E., Garattini, S. (eds.), pp. 371–384. New York: Raven 1970

Morpurgo, C., Theobald, W.: Influence of imipramine-like compounds and chlorpromazine on the reserpine-hypothermia in mice and the amphetamine-hyperthermia in rats. Med. Pharm. Ther. *12*, 226–232 (1965)

Munkvad, I., Pakkenberg, H., Randrup, A.: Aminergic systems in basal ganglia associated with stereotyped hyperactive behavior and catalepsy. Brain Behav. Evol. *1*, 89–100 (1968)

Nicholson, P.A., Turner, P. (eds.): Nomifensine. Br. J. Clin. Pharmacol. [Suppl. 2] *4*, 55 (1977)

Niemegeers, C.J.E., Verbruggen, F.J., Janssen, P.A.J.: The influence of various neuroleptic drugs on shock avoidance responding in rats. Psychopharmacology *17*, 151–159 (1970)

Nistri, A., Bartolini, A., Deffenu, G., Pepeu, G.: Investigations into the release of acetylcholine from the cerebral cortex of the cat: Effects of amphetamine of scopolamine and of septal lesions. Neuropharmacology *11*, 665–674 (1972)

Nose, T., Takemoto, H.: The effect of penfluridol and some psychotropic drugs on monoamine metabolism in central nervous system. Eur. J. Pharmacol. *31*, 351–359 (1975)

Nybäck, H., Sedvall, G., Kopin, I.J.: Accelerated synthesis of dopamine-C^{14} from tyrosine-C^{14} in rat brain after chlorpromazine. Life Sci. *6*, 2307–2312 (1967)

Obianwu, H.O., Stitzel, R., Lundborg, P.: Subcellular distribution of (^{3}H)-amphetamine and (^{3}H)-guanethidine and their interaction with adrenergic neurons. J. Pharm. Pharmacol. *20*, 585–594 (1968)

Offermeier, J., Du Prez, H.G.: Effects of anorectics on uptake and release of monoamines in synaptosomes. In: Central mechanisms of anorectic drugs. Garattini, S., Samanin, R. (eds.), pp. 217–231. New York: Raven 1978

Olds, J.: Studies of neuropharmacologicals by electrical and chemical manipulation of the brain in animals with chronically implanted electrodes. Neuropsychopharmacology *1*, 20–32 (1958)

Papeschi, R., Randrup, A.: Catalepsy, sedation and hypothermia induced by alphamethyl-p-tyrosine in the rat. An ideal tool for screening of drugs active on central catecholaminergic receptors. Pharmakopsychiat. Neuropsychopharmacology *6*, 137–157 (1973)

Pepeu, G., Bartolini, A.: Effetto di alcuni psicofarmaci sulla liberazione di acetilcolina dalla corteccia cerebrale di gatto. Boll. Soc. Ital. Biol. Sper. *43*, 1409–1413 (1967)

Pepeu, G., Bartolini, A.: Effect of psychoactive drugs on the output of acetylcholine from the cerebral cortex of the cat. Eur. J. Pharmacol. *4*, 254–263 (1968)

Pepeu, G.C., Bartolini, A., Deffenu, G.: Investigations into the increase of acetylcholine output from the cerebral cortex of the cat caused by amphetamine. In: Drugs and cholinergic mechanisms. Heilbronn, E., Winters, S. (eds.), pp. 387–396. Stockholm: Res. Inst. Natl. Dept. 1970

Perel, J.M., Dayton, P.G.: Methylphenidate. In: Psychotherapeutic drugs, pt. II: Applications. Usdin, E., Forrest, I.S. (eds.), pp. 1287–1316. New York: Dekker 1977

Pfeiffer, A.K., Csaki, L., Fodor, M., György, L., Ökrös, I.: The subcellular distribution of (+)-amphetamine and 8±)-p-chloroamphetamine in the rat brain as influenced by reserpine. J. Pharm. Pharmacol. *21*, 687–689 (1969)

Pickens, R., Thompson, T., Yokel, R.A.: Characteristics of amphetamine self-administration by rats. In: Current concepts on amphetamine abuse (DHEW Publ. no. HSM 72-9085). Ellinwood, E.H., Cohen, S. (eds.), pp. 43–48. Washington, D.C.: U.S. G.P.O. 1972

Poat, J.A., Woodruff, G.N., Watling, K.J.: Direct effect of a nomifensine derivative on dopamine receptors. J. Pharm. Pharmacol. *30*, 495–497 (1978)

Portoghese, P.S., Pazdernik, T.L., Kuhn, W.L., Hite, G., Shafi'ee, A.: Stereochemical studies on medicinal agents. V. Synthesis, configuration, and pharmacological activity of pipradrol enantiomers. J. Med. Chem. *11*, 12–15 (1968)

Quattrone, A., Bendotti, C., Recchia, M., Samanin, R.: Various effects of d-amphetamine in rats with selective lesions of brain noradrenaline-containing neurons or treated with penfluridol. Commun. Psychopharmacol. *1*, 525–531 (1977)

Quinn, G.P., Cohn, M.M., Reid, M.B., Greengard, P., Weiner, M.: The effect of formulation on phenmetrazine plasma levels in man studied by a sensitive analytic method. Clin. Pharmacol. Ther. *8*, 369–373 (1967)

Raevskii, K.S., Gura, S.J.: Effect of adrenergic blocking agents on toxicity of amphetamine in mice kept in groups or in isolation. Boll. Exp. Biol. Med. *69*, 539–541 (1970)

Rahmann, H.: The influence of methamphetamine on learning, longterm memory, and transposition ability in golden hamster. In: Amphetamines and related compounds. Costa, E., Garattini, S. (eds.), pp. 813–817. New York: Raven 1970

Raiteri, M., Bertollini, A., Angelini, F., Levi, G.: d-Amphetamine as a releaser or reuptake inhibitor of biogenic amines in synaptosomes. Eur. J. Pharmacol. *34*, 189–195 (1975)

Randrup, A., Jonas, W.: Brain dopamine and the amphetamine-reserpine interaction. J. Pharm. Pharmacol. *19*, 483–484 (1967)

Randrup, A., Munkvad, I.: Brain dopamine and amphetamine-induced stereotyped behaviour. Acta Pharmacol. Toxicol. (Kbh.) [Suppl. 4] 25, 62 (1967a)

Randrup, A., Munkvad, I.: Stereotype activities produced by amphetamine in several animal species and man. Psychopharmacology 11, 300–310 (1967b)

Randrup, A., Munkvad, I.: Influence of amphetamines on animal behaviour: Stereotypy, functional impairment and possible animal-human correlations. Psychiatr. Neurol. Neurochir. 75, 193–202 (1972)

Randrup, A., Scheel-Krüger, J.: Diethyldithiocarbamate and amphetamine stereotype behavior. J. Pharm. Pharmacol. 18, 752 (1966)

Ray, O.S., Bivens, L.W.: Chlorpromazine and amphetamine effects on three operant and on four discrete trial reinforcement schedules. Psychopharmacology 10, 32–43 (1966)

Rech, R.H., Stolk, J.M.: Amphetamine-drug interactions that relate brain catecholamines to behavior. In: Amphetamines and related compounds. Costa, E., Garattini, S. (eds.), pp. 385–413. New York: Raven 1970

Reinert, H.: The effect of amphetamine on peripheral synaptic structures. Neuropsychopharmacology 1, 399–404 (1958)

Ringoir, S., Lameire, N., Munche, M., Heptner, W., Taeuber, K.: Pharmacokinetics of nomifensine in impaired renal function. Br. J. Clin. Pharmacol. [Suppl.] 4, 129–134 (1977)

Rolinski, Z., Scheel-Krüger, J.: The effect of dopamine and noradrenaline antagonists on amphetamine induced locomotor activity in mice and rats. Acta Pharmacol. Toxicol. (Kbh.) 21, 226–239 (1964)

Rommelspacher, H., Honecker, H., Schulze, G., Strauss, S.M.: The hydroxylation of d-amphetamine by liver microsomes of the male rat. Biochem. Pharmacol. 23, 1065–1071 (1974)

Rosenberg, D.E., Wolbach, A.B., Miner, E.J., Isbell, H.: Observations on direct and cross tolerance with LSD and d-amphetamine in man. Psychopharmacology 5, 1–15 (1963)

Ross, S.B., Renyi, A.L.: Inhibition of the uptake of tritiated catecholamines by antidepressant and related agents. Eur. J. Pharmacol. 2, 181–186 (1967)

Rowland, M.: Amphetamine blood and urine levels in man. J. Pharm. Sci. 58, 508–509 (1969)

Salama, A.I., Goldberg, M.E.: Effect of several models of stress and amphetamine on brain levels of amphetamine and certain monoamines. Arch. Int. Pharmacodyn. Ther. 181, 474–483 (1969)

Samanin, R., Bernasconi, S., Garattini, S.: The effect of nomifensine on the depletion of brain serotonin and catecholamines induced respectively by fenfluramine and 6-hydroxydopamine in rats. Eur. J. Pharmacol. 34, 377–380 (1975)

Samanin, R., Bendotti, C., Bernasconi, S., Borroni, E., Garattini, S.: Role of brain monoamines in the anorectic activity of mazindol and d-amphetamine in the rat. Eur. J. Pharmacol. 43, 117–124 (1977a)

Samanin, R., Bendotti, C., Miranda, F., Garattini, S.: Decrease of food intake by quipazine in the rat: Relation to serotoninergic receptor stimulation. J. Pharm. Pharmacol. 29, 53–54 (1977b)

Samanin, R., Jori, A., Bernasconi, S., Morpurgo, E., Garattini, S.: Biochemical and pharmacological studies on amineptine (S 1694) and (+)-amphetamine in the rat. J. Pharm. Pharmacol. 29, 555–558 (1977c)

Samanin, R., Bendotti, C., Bernasconi, S., Pataccini, R.: Differential role of brain monoamines in the activity of anorectic drugs. In: Central mechanisms of anorectic drugs. Garattini, S., Samanin, R. (eds.), pp. 233–242. New York: Raven 1978a

Samanin, R., Quattrone, A., Peri, G., Ladinsky, H., Consolo, S.: Evidence of an interaction between serotoninergic and cholinergic neurons in the corpus striatum and hippocampus of the rat brain. Brain Res. 151, 73–82 (1978b)

Sbarra, C., Negrini, P., Fanelli, R.: Quantitative analysis of amineptine (S-1694) in biological samples by gas chromatography-mass fragmentography. J. Chromatogr. 162, 31–38 (1979)

Schacht, U., Heptner, W.: Effect of nomifensine (HOE 984), a new antidepressant, on uptake of noradrenaline and serotonin and on release of noradrenaline in rat brain synaptosomes. Biochem. Pharmacol. 23, 3413–3422 (1974)

Scheel-Krüger, J.: Comparative studies of various amphetamine analogues demonstrating different interactions with the metabolism of the catecholamines in the brain. Eur. J. Pharmacol. 14, 47–59 (1971)

Schell-Krüger, J.: Behavioral and biochemical comparison of amphetamine derivatives cocaine, benzotropine and tricyclic antidepressant drugs. Eur. J. Pharmacol. *18*, 63–73 (1972a)

Scheel-Krüger, J.: Some aspects of the mechanism of action of various stimulant amphetamine analogues. Psychiatr. Neurol. Neurochir. *75*, 179–192 (1972b)

Schiørring, E., Randrup, A.: Social isolation and changes in the formation of groups induced by amphetamine in an open-field test with rats. Pharmakopsychiatr. Neuropsychopharmakol. *4*, 2–11 (1971)

Schuster, C.R., Dockens, W.S., Woods, J.H.: Behavioral variables affecting the development of amphetamine tolerance. Psychopharmacology *9*, 170–182 (1966)

Seegal, R.F., Isaac, W.: Sensory influences upon amphetamine tolerance. Physiol. Behav. *7*, 877–879 (1971)

Segal, D.S., Mandell, A.J.: Long-term administration of d-amphetamine-progressive augmentation of locomotor activity and stereotypy. Pharmacol. Biochem. Behav. *2*, 249–255 (1974)

Segal, J.L., Cunningham, R.F., Dayton, P.G., Israili, Z.H.: [^{14}C] methylphenidate hydrochloride. Studies on disposition in rat brain. Drug Metab. Dispos. *4*, 140–146 (1976)

Shafi'ee, A., Hite, G.: The absolute configurations of the pheniramines, methyl phenidates, and pipradols. J. Med. Chem. *12*, 266–270 (1969)

Shafi'ee, A., Marathe, S., Bhatkar, R., Hite, G.: Absolute configurations of the enantiomeric pheniramines, methylphenidates, and pipradols. J. Pharm. Sci. *56*, 1689–1690 (1967)

Sheppard, H., Tsien, W.H., Rodegker, W., Plummer, A.J.: Distribution and elimination of methylphenidate-C^{14}. Toxicol. Appl. Pharmacol. *2*, 353–362 (1960)

Shulgin, A.T.: Psychotomimetic drugs: Structure-activity relationships. In: Handbook of psychopharmacology, Vol. 11: Stimulants. Iversen, L.L., Iversen, S.D., Snyder, S.H. (eds.), pp. 243–333. New York: Plenum 1978

Siegel, M., Ellison, T., Silverman, A.G., Okun, R.: Tissue distribution of dl-^{3}H-amphetamine HCl in tolerant and nontolerant cats. Proc. West. Pharmacol. Soc. *11*, 90–94 (1968)

Simon, P., Tillement, J.P., Larousse, C., Breteau, M., Guernet, M., Boissier, J.R.: Pharmacological and biochemical effects of amphetamine and paracloromethamphetamine. J. Pharmacol. (Paris) *1*, 95–108 (1970)

Smith, R.L., Dring, L.G.: Patterns, of metabolism of β-phenylisopropylamines in man and other species. In: Amphetamines and related compounds. Costa, E., Garattini, S. (eds.), pp. 121–139. New York: Raven 1970

Sofia, R.D.: Effects of chlorpromazine and d-amphetamine in Long Evans rats of different age, body weight and brain weight. Arch. Int. Pharmacodyn. Ther. *182*, 139–146 (1969)

Soulairac, M.L.: Etude experimentale des regulations hormononerveuses du comportement sexuel du rat male. Ann. Endocrinol. (Paris) [Suppl.] *24*, 1–98 (1963)

Southgate, P.J., Mayer, S.R., Boxhall, E., Wilson, A.: Some 5-hydroxytryptamine-like actions of fenfluramine: A comparison with (+)-amphetamine and diethylpropion. J. Pharm. Pharmacol. *23*, 600–605 (1971)

Spengler, J.: Potenzierung der anorexigenen und psychomotorischen Wirkung von d-Amphetaminen durch die Monoaminoxydasehemmer Iproniazid und Pivaloylbenzylhydrazin. Naunyn Schmiedebergs Arch. Pharmacol. *244*, 153–160 (1962)

Srimal, R.C., Dhawan, B.N.: An analysis of methylphenidate induced gnawing in guinea pigs. Psychopharmacology *18*, 99–107 (1970)

Stein, L.: Effects and interactions of imipramine, chlorpromazine, reserpine, and amphetamine on self-stimulation: Possible neurophysiological basis of depression. In: Recent advances in biological psychiatry. Wortis, J. (ed.), Vol. 4, pp. 288–309. New York: Plenum 1962

Stein, L.: Self-stimulation of the brain and the central stimulant action of amphetamine. Fed. Proc. *23*, 836–850 (1964)

Stein, L., Wise, C.D.: Mechanism of the facilitating effects of amphetamine on behavior. In: Psychotomimetic drugs. Efron, D.H. (ed.), pp. 123–145. New York: Raven 1970

Stitzel, R.E., Lundborg, P.: Effect of reserpine and monoamine oxidase inhibition on the uptake and subcellular distribution of ^{3}H-noradrenaline. Br. J. Pharmacol. *29*, 99–104 (1966)

Stolk, J.M., Rech, R.H.: Antagonism of d-amphetamine by alphamethyl-L-tyrosine: Behavioral evidence for the participation of catecholamine, stores and synthesis in the amphetamine stimulant response. Neuropharmacology *9*, 249–263 (1970)

Stretch, S., Gerber, J., Wood, M.: Factors affecting behavior maintained by response-contingent intravenous infusions of amphetamine in squirrel monkeys. Can. J. Physiol. Pharmacol. *49*, 581–589 (1971)

Sugrue, M.F., Charlton, K.G., Mireylees, S.E., McIndewar, I.: Drug-induced anorexia and monoamine reuptake inhibition. In: Central mechanisms of anorectic drugs. Garattini, S., Samanin, R. (eds.), pp. 191–203. New York: Raven 1978

Sulser, F., Sanders-Bush, E.: Effects of drugs on amines in the CNS. Annu. Rev. Pharmacol. Toxicol. *11*, 209–230 (1971)

Sulser, F., Owens, M.L., Norwich, M.R., Dingell, J.V.: The relative role of storage and synthesis of brain norepinephrine in the psychomotor stimulation evoked by amphetamine or by desipramine and tetrabenzamine. Psychopharmacology *12*, 322–332 (1968)

Svensson, T.H.: Functional and biochemical effects of d- and l-amphetamine on central catecholamine neurons. Naunyn Schmiedebergs Arch. Pharmacol. *271*, 170–180 (1971)

Szporny, L., Görög, P.: Investigations into the correlations between monoamine oxidase inhibition and other effects due to methylphenydate and its stereoisomers. Biochem. Pharmacol. *8*, 263–268 (1961)

Taylor, B.: Dopamine-β-hydroxylase-stereochemical course of the reaction. J. Biol. Chem. *249*, 454–458 (1974)

Taylor, K.M., Snyder, S.H.: Differential effects of d- and l- amphetamine on behavior and on catecholamine disposition in dopamine and norepinephrine containing neurons of rat brain. Brain Res. *28*, 205–309 (1971)

Taylor, W.A., Sulser, F.: Effects of amphetamine and its hydroxylated metabolites on central noradrenergic mechanisms. J. Pharmacol. exp. Ther. *185*, 620–632 (1973)

Tedeschi, D.H., Fowler, P.F., Miller, R.B., Macko, E.: Pharmacological analysis of footshock-induced fighting behaviour. In: Aggressive behaviour. Garattini, S., Sigg, E.B. (eds.), pp. 245–252. Amsterdam: Excerpta Medica 1969

Teitelbaum, P., Derks, P.: The effect of amphetamine on forced drinking in the rat. J. Comp. Physiol. Psychol. *51*, 801–810 (1958)

Thoenen, H., Hürlimann, A., Gey, K.F., Haefely, W.: Liberation of p-hydroxynorepinephrine from cat spleen by sympathetic stimulation after pretreatment with amphetamine. Life Sci. *5*, 1715–1722 (1966)

Tikal, K., Benesova, O.: The effect of some psychotropic drugs on contact behavior in a group of rats. Ac. Nerv. Super. (Praha) *14*, 168–169 (1972)

Tilson, H.A., Sparber, S.B.: Studies on the concurrent behavioral and neurochemical effects of psychoactive drugs using the pushfull cannula. J. Pharmacol. Exp. Ther. *181*, 387–398 (1972)

Tormey, J., Lasagna, L.: Relation of thyroid function to acute and chronic effects of amphetamine in the rat. J. Pharmacol. Exp. Ther. *128*, 201–209 (1960)

Trabucchi, M., Cheney, D.L., Racagni, G., Costa, E.: In vivo inhibition of striatal acetylcholine turnover by L-Dopa, apomorphine and (+)-amphetamine. Brain Res. *85*, 130–134 (1975)

Trendelenburg, U., Gomez, B.A.S., Muskus, A.: Modification by reserpine of the response of the atrial pacemaker to sympathomimetic to amines. J. Pharmacol. Exp. Ther. *141*, 301–309 (1963)

Tseng, L.F., Loh, H.H.: Significance of dopamine receptor activity in dl-p-methoxy-amphetamine and d-amphetamine induced locomotor activity. J. Pharmacol. Exp. Ther. *189*, 717–724 (1974)

Valzelli, L., Consolo, S., Morpurgo, G.: Influence of imipraminelike drugs on the metabolism of amphetamine. In: Antidepressant drugs. Garattini, S., Dukes, M.N.G. (eds.), pp. 61–69. Amsterdam: Excerpta Medica 1967

Van Rossum, J.M., Simons, F.: Locomotor activity and anorexigenic action. Psychopharmacology *14*, 248–254 (1969)

Vereczkey, L., Bianchetti, G., Garattini, S., Morselli, P.L.: Pharmacokinetics of nomifensine in man. Psychopharmacology *45*, 225–227 (1975)

Vereczkey, L., Bianchetti, G., Rovei, V., Frigerio, A.: Gas chromatographic method for the determination of nomifensine in human plasma. J. Chromatogr. *116*, 451–456 (1976)

Vergnes, M., Chaurand, J.P.: Activation amphetaminique, rythme hippocampoque et comportement d'aggression interspécifique ratsouris. C.R. Soc. Biol. (Paris) *166*, 936–941 (1972)

Vree, T.B.: Pharmacokinetics and metabolism of amphetamines. Ph. D. Thesis, University of Nijwegen, Netherlands 1973

Waterman, F.A.: Relationship between spontaneous activity and metabolic rate as influenced by certain sympathomimetic compounds. Proc. Soc. Exp. Biol. *71*, 473–475 (1949)

Weiner, N.: Pharmacology of central nervous system stimulants. In: Drug abuse. Zarafonetis, C.J.D. (eds.), pp. 243–251. Philadelphia: Lea & Febiger 1972

Weis, J.: On the hyperthermic response to d-amphetamine in the decapitated rat. Life Sci. *13*, 475–484 (1973)

Welsh, A.L.: Side effects of anti-obesity drugs. Springfield, Ill.: Thomas 1962

Westerink, B.H.C., Korf, J.: Influence of drugs on striatal and limbic homovanillic acid concentration in the rat brain. Eur. J. Pharmacol. *33*, 31–40 (1975)

White, R.P., Nash, C.B., Westerbeke, E.J., Possanza, G.J.: Phylogenetic comparison of central actions produced by different doses of atropine and hyoscine. Arch. Int. Pharmacodyn. Ther. *132*, 349–363 (1961)

Wilkinson, G.R., Beckett, A.H.: Absorption, metabolism and excretion of the ephedrines in man. I. The influence of urinary pH and urine volume output. J. Pharmacol. Exp. Ther. *162*, 139–147 (1968)

Williams, R.T., Caldwell, J., Dring, L.G.: Comparative metabolism of some amphetamines in various species. In: Frontiers in catecholamine research. Usdin, E., Snyder, S.H. (eds.), pp. 927–932. New York: Pergamon 1973

Willner, J.H., Samach, M., Angrist, B.M., Wallach, M.B., Gershon, S.: Drug-induced stereotyped behavior and its antagonism in dogs. Commun. Behav. Biol. *5*, 135–141 (1970)

Wong, D.T., Van Frank, R.M., Horng, J.S., Fuller, R.W.: Accumulation of amphetamine and p-chloroamphetamine into synaptosomes of rat brain. J. Pharm. Pharmacol. *24*, 171–173 (1972)

Yen, T.T., Acton, J.M.: Stimulation of locomotor activity of genitically obese mice by amphetamine. Experientia *29*, 1297–1298 (1973)

Yokel, R.A., Pickens, R.: Drug level of d- and l-amphetamine during intravenous self-administration. Psychopharmacology *34*, 255–264 (1974)

Young, D., Scoville, W.B.: Paranoid psychosis in narcolepsy and the possible danger of benzedrine treatment. Med. Clin. North Am. *22*, 637–645 (1938)

Young, R.L., Gordon, M.W.: The disposition of [^{14}C] amphetamine in rat brain. J. Neurochem. *9*, 161–167 (1962)

Ziegler, H., Del Basso, P., Longo, V.G.: Influence of 6-hydroxydopamine and of α-methyl-p-tyrosine on the effects of some centrally acting agents. Physiol. Behav. *8*, 391–396 (1972)

CHAPTER 15

The Behavioral Pharmacology
of Psychomotor Stimulant Drugs

C. R. SCHUSTER

The purpose of this chapter is to selectively review the behavioral pharmacology of psychomotor stimulant drugs. In this context, psychomotor stimulant drugs are defined as those which produce increased spontaneous motor activity and/or the frequency of occurrence of learned behaviors at doses far below those producing convulsions. An attempt will be made to show the generality of the behavioral effects of this class of compounds. Unfortunately, relatively few behavioral studies have specifically compared more than a few of the psychomotor stimulant drugs. Most studies have used one of the amphetamines with significantly fewer studies investigating and then contrasting the actions of other drugs in this class. For this reason the literature covered in this review will primarily be concerned with amphetamines, but where possible, comparison will be made to other psychomotor stimulant drugs.

A. Unconditioned Behavior

I. Effects of Psychomotor Stimulant Drugs on Motor Activity

1. Acute Effects

Psychomotor stimulant drugs produce a characteristic profile of action in mice and rats; at low doses they produce an alerting effect characterized by increased exploration, locomotion, grooming, and rearing. As the dose is increased, exploration and forward locomotion disappear, and the animals exhibit only stereotyped head bobbing, gnawing, sniffing, and licking. Finally, further increases in dose produce convulsions, coma, and death (LEWANDER, 1977). Although the precise mechanisms underlying these actions may differ for various psychomotor stimulant drugs, all of them presumably have the common effect of increasing activity in catecholaminergic systems in the brain. Present evidence indicates that the increased locomotor activity is mediated by both noradrenergic and dopaminergic systems, whereas the stereotypy is mediated by dopaminergic systems. [For a fuller discussion of the neurochemistry of psychomotor stimulant drugs see LEWANDER (1977)].

Although studied less extensively, the general pattern of motor activity produced by amphetamines in mice and rats is seen in other species. Furthermore, while the topography of the responses exhibited varies from one species to the next, most species show some form of stereotypy (e.g., RANDRUP and MUNKVAD, 1967). The effects of psychomotor stimulant drugs in certain species, however, show some significant differences. In the chicken, for example, amphetamines produce an unexpected spectrum of action composed of sleep-like behavior interrupted by eating, wing drop, postural changes and twittering, foot shuffle, and aggressiveness (LEWANDER, 1977).

Environmental factors as well influence the occurrence of certain motor responses induced by amphetamine administration. For example, rats do not show any rearing response following administration of *d*-amphetamine if tested on an elevated Y-maze, whereas this response is markedly increased in a Y-maze with walls (Mumford et al., 1979).

Methods for studying the effects of psychomotor stimulant drugs on fine motor control in rats (Falk, 1969) and rhesus monkeys (Johanson et al., 1979) have been developed. In both species animals are reinforced for holding a response lever within a narrow force band for a fixed period of time. Rats treated with *d*-amphetamine showed increased phasic activity (tremors) with little effect on tonic activity (Falk, 1969). Similar results were obtained with *d*-methamphetamine in rhesus monkeys (Johanson et al., 1979). These methods are exquisitely sensitive to amphetamines and shoud prove valuable in the investigation of the effects of other psychomotor stimulant drugs on fine motor control.

2. Chronic Effects

It has generally been accepted that tolerance does not develop to increases in general activity produced by psychomotor stimulant drugs (Kosman and Unna, 1968). In a more recent review of this literature, however, Lewander (1977) cites several studies in which tolerance to this effect of amphetamines was found. Therefore, he concluded that a definite statement with regard to tolerance development to amphetamine-induced increases in motor activity cannot yet be made. Since that review, no evidence has been provided which alters that conclusion.

The repeated administration of amphetamines to mice and rats has also been reported to produce increased sensitivity to the drug (Segal and Mandell, 1974). Under certain circumstances part of this increased sensitivity may be attributable to the classical conditioning of activity to stimuli associated with the drug injection procedure (Pickens and Crowder, 1969; Tilson and Rech, 1973). However, increases in sensitivity have been reported as well under conditions where conditioning factors were minimized (Segal, 1975). This issue is complicated by the fact that increased responsiveness to amphetamines may shift the actions of the drug qualitatively. For example, the repetitive administration of low doses of *d*-amphetamine gives rise to increasing activity levels. Repeated administration of intermediate doses, however, results in a gradual decline in drug-induced increments in activity, suggesting tolerance to this action of the drug. Observation of the animals reveals, however, that this decrement in locomotor activity occurs because it is superseded by stereotypy, a response usually seen only at higher doses. Thus, increased sensitivity to successive amphetamine injections may shift the dose-response relationships in such a way that new actions are revealed. [For a full discussion of this issue see Segal (1975).] A recent report suggests a similar interaction between locomotor activity and stereotypy in rats treated with cocaine (Bhattacharyya and Pradhan, 1979). These complications may be responsible for the confusion in the literature regarding the development of tolerance to the gross motor effects of psychomotor stimulant drugs.

II. Effects of Psychomotor Stimulant Drugs on Food and Water Intake

1. Acute Effects

One of the most prominent actions of psychomotor stimulant drugs is the reduction in food intake in most species of animals including humans (VAN ROSSUM, 1970; LE-WANDER, 1977). That this is a specific effect of the drug is suggested by the fact that the ED_{50} of d-amphetamine for its anorexic effect is approximately one-tenth of the LD_{50} (SPENGLER and WASER, 1959; ABDALLAH and WHITE, 1970; ABDALLAH, 1973).

Amphetamines have been reported to cause a decrease in drinking in dogs (AN-DERSSON and LARSSON, 1956) as well as rats (EPSTEIN, 1959; MAICKEL et al., 1970; YEL-NOSKY and LAWLOR, 1970; KNOWLER and UKENA, 1973; WAYNER et al., 1973). STOLERMAN and D'MELLO (1978) have compared the hypodipsic potency of d-, l-, and methamphetamine as well as p-chloromethamphetamine, fenfluramine, chlorphenter-mine, and cocaine in rats. The order of potency for these compounds based upon ED_{50} values obtained with 15 and 60 min of water availability was: d-amphetamine; methamphetamine; CL-methamphetamine; l-amphetamine; fenfluramine; chlorop-hentermine; and cocaine. The halogen-substituted compounds had a longer duration of action. In contrast, cocaine was very short acting and did not produce greater than a 34% decrease in drinking at any subconvulsive dose.

2. Chronic Effects

When given repeatedly, tolerance rapidly develops to the anorexia produced by psy-chomotor stimulant drugs (LEWANDER, 1977). Further, cross tolerance to the anorexi-genic effects has been demonstrated between a number of the members of this class including: d- and l-amphetamine and methamphetamine (TAGLIAMONTE et al., 1969; KANDEL et al., 1975), methylphenidate and d-amphetamine (PEARL and SEIDEN, 1976), and cocaine and d-amphetamine (WOOLVERTON et al., 1978a). Of interest in this regard is that fenfluramine does not show cross tolerance to amphetamine (KANDEL et al., 1975). Fenfluramine is a chemical analog of amphetamine whose anorexic actions are presumably based on a different mechanism of action (LE DOUAREC and NEVEU, 1970). Additionally, fenfluramine has been shown in rats to reduce the rate of eating but not its duration, whereas d-amphetamine has the opposite effects (COOPER and FRANCIS, 1979).

With repeated administration of the amphetamines, tolerance develops to their hy-podipsic effects as well (LAWLOR et al., 1969; YOKEL and PICKENS, 1970).

III. Effects of Psychomotor Stimulant Drugs on Aggression

1. Acute Effects

The effects of amphetamine on the aggressive behavior of a wide variety of species have been investigated (e.g., chickens: DEWHURST and MARLEY, 1965; Siamese fight-ing fish: WEISCHER, 1966; rats: TEDESCHI et al., 1969; cats: ELLINWOOD and ES-CALANTE, 1970; mice: ROLINSKI, 1973; squirrel monkeys: HUTCHINSON et al., 1976).

Further more, a variety of conditions have been used to generate aggression (e.g., isolation, electric shock, competition for food, morphine withdrawal). In general, these studies have found that amphetamines increase aggression at dose levels below those producing stereotypy. There is evidence, however, which suggests that we must interpret this generalization of increased aggression carefully. Hutchinson et al. (1976) reported on an evaluation of several psychomotor stimulant drugs using a method in which noncontingent electric shock generated both aggressive attack behaviors and a lever-pressing response from squirrel monkeys. When amphetamines were administered at low and intermediate doses, aggressive attack frequency increased, as did to a lesser extent, the lever-pressing response. This suggests that at least some portion of the increased aggressiveness found in many experiments may represent a nonspecific increase in all ongoing behaviors. This study demonstrates the necessity of measuring other concurrent behaviors to determine whether drugs have specific actions on aggression. Hutchinson et al. (1976) also reported that nicotine and cocaine produced greater increases in the lever-pressing response than in the aggressive attack behavior, suggesting again that we cannot generalize from amphetamines to other psychomotor stimulant drugs. This has been supported by a recent report by Miczek (1979), who compared cocaine and d-amphetamine using a new method for producing aggressive behavior in rats. At low and intermediate doses, d-amphetamine increased the aggressiveness of dominant rats. On the other hand, at higher doses of d-amphetamine and at all effective doses of cocaine, aggressiveness was decreased. These studies strongly suggest the need for cautiousness in generalizing from the effects of amphetamines on aggression to other psychomotor stimulant drugs. Clearly what is needed is a systematic dose-response study of a variety of psychomotor stimulant drugs, using a single procedure designed to concurrently measure both aggressive and nonaggressive behaviors.

2. Chronic Effects

Repeated administration of methamphetamine has been reported to produce aggression in rats (Randrup and Munkvad, 1967) and in cats (Ellinwood and Escalante, 1970). Whether there is any change in sensitivity to the drug's effect on aggression with repeated administration is not known. Chronic ingestion of cocaine and amphetamine has been reported to produce a toxic psychosis in humans in which aggressive behavior is a prominent feature (Kramer et al., 1967; Ellinwood, 1971).

B. Conditioned Behavior

I. Effects of Psychomotor Stimulant Drugs on Schedule-Controlled Behavior

1. Acute Effects

Since the early work of Skinner and Heron (1937), schedule-controlled operant behavior has been extensively used to generate baselines for the investigation of the effects of psychomotor stimulant drugs. It would be impossible to enumerate (let alone critically review) this vast literature. Fortunately, there has emerged from this research a unifying principle – the rate dependency principle which allows us to make certain general statements about the effects of psychomotor stimulant drugs on operant behavior. This section will include a historical development of the rate dependency principle, a description of critical experiments designed to determine its generality, and a discussion of classes of operant behavior which do not respond to psychomotor stimulant drugs in a rate-dependent manner.

Dews (1955), in a classic study, investigated the effects of methamphetamine on patterns of operant key pecking behavior of pigeons maintained under different schedules of food reinforcement. In the study a short fixed-ratio schedule (FR 50) and a variable-interval 60 s schedule (VI 60 s) were used to generate high rates of key pecking by the pigeon. Fixed ratios requiring 900 responses (FR 900) and a long fixed-interval schedule (FI 15 min) were used to generate relatively low rates. Methamphetamine administration at lower doses produced increased responding during the schedules generating low rates and little or no effect on responding in the schedule components producing high rates. At higher doses of methamphetamine, key pecking rate was decreased under all conditions. Dews (1958) suggested on the basis of these results that an important determinant of the effects of amphetamines was the control rate of responding. This was the first explicit recognition of what later developed into the rate dependency principle which states that the effects of amphetamine (and presumably other psychomotor stimulant drugs) on operant behavior are inversely related to control rates of responding prior to drug administration.

There are a variety of ways in which the rate-dependent effects of psychomotor stimulant drugs can be studied. Basically, any behavioral procedure which generates a range of response rates under nondrug conditions can be used to determine whether drug effects are rate dependent. In many instances differences in response rates are also confounded with other differences in the procedure used to generate the range of control rates. For any single experiment this confounding does not allow a real test of the rate dependency principle. If despite this confounding, rate dependency is found under all conditions, the principle receives even more support, since it would appear that rate is the predominant variable determining the action of the drug. The evidence to date does not justify this blanket endorsement of the rate dependency principle, but it does indicate that rate is a very important but not exclusive determinant of the effects of psychomotor stimulant drugs. The evidence regarding rate-dependent effects of drugs has been critically reviewed by a number of researchers (e.g., Sanger and Blackman, 1976; Dews and Wenger, 1977; McKearney and Barrett, 1978). Therefore, only representative data showing both the generality and the limitations of the rate dependency principle will be reviewed here.

In many experiments using schedule-controlled performance, the baseline rates of responding show wide variance between subjects. Ray and Bivens (1966) utilized this variance to study the rate dependency of dl-amphetamine. Rats selected for high and low rates of responding generated by a fixed ratio schedule of food reinforcement respond to dl-amphetamine in a manner predicted by the rate dependency principle. That is, in animals with low control response rates, there was an increase in lever pressing frequency following drug administration, whereas in high rate responders there was no change or a decrease in rates of responding. At higher doses of dl-amphetamine the rate of responding of both groups declined; however, the low rate group was less sensitive to the drug. On the other hand, high and low rates of responding generated by a variable-interval schedule showed dose-response relations with dl-amphetamine which were not supportive of the rate dependency principle. The range of rates generated by the variable-interval schedule, however, was much smaller than that generated by the fixed-ratio schedule. As these studies indicate, the approach of selecting animals with different rates of responding under control conditions to study the rate-dependent effects of psychomotor stimulants has yielded variable results (SANGER and BLACKMAN, 1976).

A second approach to determining the generality of the rate dependency principle has been to use different schedules. Certain schedules of reinforcement generate very low response rates [e.g., differential reinforcement of low rates (DRL) schedules] and others, very high response rates [e.g., fixed-ratio schedules]. As one would predict on the basis of the rate dependency principle, low rates of responding generated by DRL schedules are increased by psychomotor stimulant drugs using a variety of animals species, including humans (DEWS and MORSE, 1958; SCHUSTER and ZIMMERMAN, 1961; STRETCH and DALRYMPLE, 1968; WEBB and LEVINE, 1978; WOOLVERTON et al., 1978b). In contrast, high rates of responding generated by fixed-ratio schedules are generally decreased by psychomotor stimulant drugs (MCMILLAN, 1969; JOHANSON, 1978; WOOLVERTON et al., 1978b).

It is also possible to generate markedly different response rates in the same animal by using a multiple schedule of reinforcement. A number of investigations have used a multiple fixed-ratio, fixed-interval schedule of food reinforcement. The results of these investigations have shown that in general, low doses of psychomotor stimulant drugs increase the low rates of responding generated by the fixed-interval component while producing no effects or a decrease in the high rates of responding generated by the fixed-ratio schedule. This has been found in pigeons, rats, and monkeys (SMITH, 1964; MCMILLAN, 1969; GONZALEZ and GOLDBERG, 1977).

Under most circumstances, the rate of responding generated by a schedule is correlated with the frequency of reinforcement. To ensure that it is rate of responding rather than reinforcement density that determines the effects of psychomotor stimulant drugs, it is necessary to disentangle these two variables. This has been done in several recent experiments by employing pacing schedules in which responses separated by certain minimal intervals are intermittently reinforced (SANGER and BLACKMAN, 1975, STITZER and MCKEARNEY, 1977). By employing the same interresponse time requirement but varying the frequency of reinforcement, rate and reinforcement density can be independently manipulated. Using such schedules it has been demonstrated that rate of responding, not density of reinforcement, is the primary determinant of the actions of psychomotor stimulant drugs.

Another method commonly used to study the rate-dependent effects of psychomotor stimulant drugs is to take advantage of the different rates of responding generated over time by a fixed-interval schedule of reinforcement. Fixed-interval schedules of reinforcement characteristically produce a low rate of responding following the delivery of a reinforcer with a gradual acceleration in responding until the next reinforcer is delivered. By dividing the fixed-interval into time segments, it is possible to generate baselines covering a wide range of response rates to investigate the rate-dependent effects of drugs. Using this method it has been established that psychomotor stimulant drugs generally increase low rates of responding generated in the initial segment of the fixed interval and decrease the high rates of responding generated in the later segments (e.g., MCMILLAN, 1968; HEFFNER et al., 1974; MCKEARNEY, 1974; GONZALEZ and GOLDBERG, 1977).

Most studies using fixed-interval schedules in this manner have used food as the reinforcer. It is also possible, however, to generate the same temporal pattern of responding by having the first response after a preset interval terminate a stimulus periodically paired with shocks. KELLEHER and MORSE (1964, 1968) compared the effects of d-amphetamine using multiple fixed-ratio, fixed-interval schedules in which the reinforcer was either food or escape from a shock-associated stimulus. The effects of d-amphetamine were rate dependent regardless of the nature of the reinforcer generating responding, i.e., high rates generated by the fixed-ratio schedule were unaffected or decreased at doses causing an increase in responding generated by the fixed-interval schedule.

Under certain conditions it is possible to maintain fixed-interval responding by the presentation (rather than the avoidance) of electric shock. Using a fixed-interval schedule of shock presentation it has been demonstrated that amphetamine produces a rate-dependent change in responding (MCKEARNEY, 1974). It would thus appear that rate-dependent effects of amphetamines (and possibly all other psychomotor stimulant drugs) are independent of the nature of the reinforcer being used to maintain behavior. This obviates any explanation of the effects of psychomotor stimulant drugs on operant behavior being mediated by the anorexigenic action of these drugs. There are conditions, however, in which the nature of the reinforcer has been found to be of importance. In one well-controlled study, JOHANSON (1978) demonstrated that behaviors maintained under fixed-ratio schedules of food reinforcement were suppressed by intravenous doses of cocaine, diethylpropion, and d-amphetamine at doses which had minimal effects on behavior maintained by fixed-ratio shock avoidance. Of critical importance in this study is that the baseline control response rates generated by food presentation and shock avoidance were similar. The rate dependency principle would predict that psychomotor stimulant drugs should produce comparable changes in response rate regardless of the reinforcer; such was not the case in this study. In addition, there are other circumstances in which behaviors are generated which do not show rate-dependent effects when psychomotor stimulant drugs are administered (SANGER and BLACKMAN, 1976; DEWS and WENGER, 1977; MCKEARNEY and BARRETT, 1978). These include behaviors occurring at a very low frequency, low rates of responding which are under strong stimulus control, and behavior suppressed by punishment. Such low rate behaviors are not increased by psychomotor stimulant drugs. Thus, certain conditions appear to generate behaviors which are not subject to the rate-dependent actions of psychomotor stimulant drugs. Only further research will delineate the range of the limiting conditions for the rate dependency principle. At present, however, it represents the single most unifying principle relating psychomotor stimulant drugs to schedule-controlled operant behavior. Recently, DEWS and WENGER (1977) have extended the rate dependency analysis of the actions of psychomotor stimulant drugs to behaviors other than schedule-controlled operants. Their analysis demonstrated that this principle has utility in the prediction of the effects of psychomotor stimulant drugs on behaviors such as general activity. More research is needed to collect data on a broad range of behaviors (e.g., fighting) in a manner allowing measures of behavior necessary for rate dependency analysis.

It has been suggested that the rate dependency principle may apply to the effects of psychomotor stimulant drugs on human behavior (WEISS and LATIES, 1970). It is well established that psychomotor stimulant drugs are able to improve human performance which has deteriorated because of fatigue or boredom (e.g., Kornetsky et al., 1959, Fischman and Schuster, 1980). In contrast, performance under normal conditions shows little if any improvement with the administration of psychomotor stimulant drugs. Weiss and Laties (1970) argue that the differential sensitivity of behaviors disrupted by fatigue or boredom to psychomotor stimulant drugs is based upon the same mechanisms as their rate-dependent effects. In both instances behaviors sensitive to the rate-increasing effects of psychomotor stimulant drugs occur at a low rate because of inadequate reinforcement. Low rates generated in the initial portions of a fixed-interval schedule, for example, occur because the probability of reinforcement at that time in zero. Thus, responding early in the fixed interval has been extinguished. Similarly, when we state that a subject's performance has deteriorated because of boredom with a task, we also may be dealing with behavior weakened by extinction. This analysis would predict that performance enhancement should be obtainable not only by the administration of psychomotor stimulant drugs, but by increasing the magnitude of reinforcement as well. Clearly, research of this type is needed to determine whether the deterioration in human performance generally attributed to fatigue and/or boredom can best be understood as behavior that is not being maintained because of inadequate reinforcement.

There have been several recent studies of the effects of psychomotor stimulant drugs on human operant behavior (Griffiths et al., 1977; Stitzer et al., 1978; Fischman and Schuster, 1980). In all these studies, response rates were increased by drug in some subjects but not in others. Unfortunately an analysis was not done to determine whether this variance was predictable on the basis of the rate dependency hypothesis. It remains for future research to be specifically designed to determine the importance of this principle to the effects of drugs on human behavior.

2. Chronic Effects

Sensitivity to a drug which is repeatedly administered may decrease (tolerance), increase (sensitization), or remain the same, depending on both pharmacologic and behavioral variables. Not surprisingly, therefore, all three effects have been reported with the chronic administration of psychomotor stimulant drugs. The most common finding for schedule-controlled operant behavior, however, is for tolerance to develop to the actions of psychomotor stimulant drugs. It has been suggested that tolerance development may in part be based upon the animal's relearning under the drug condition to meet the environmental requirement for reinforcement. Schuster et al. (1966) stated that tolerance would develop to those actions of a drug which disrupted an animal's behavior so that reinforcement density decreased. Conversely, where reinforcement frequency was increased or unchanged, behavioral tolerance would not develop to the drug. This suggestion was put forth on the basis of several studies of amphetamines using rats lever pressing for food reinforcement or to avoid electric shock. In their first studies (Schuster and Zimmerman, 1961; Zimmerman and Schuster, 1962), rats were trained to lever press for food under a DRL schedule of reinforcement. A low or moderate dose of *dl*-amphetamine increased the animal's response rate and decreased the frequency of reinforcement. With repeated administration of the drug, however, response rates were progressively less affected and reinforcement frequency increased. Measures of locomotor activity taken in these same rats did not systematically change over the course of the repeated drug regimen. Since there was differential development of tolerance to one effect but not to the other, metabolic tolerance was ruled out. In a subsequent experiment, rats were trained under a multiple fixed-interval 30 sec DRL 30 sec schedule of food reinforcement (SCHUSTER et al., 1966). Under this schedule, increases in lever pressing response rate would decrease reinforcement frequency in the DRL component but not in the fixed-interval component. When d-amphetamine was repeatedly administered, tolerance developed to the rate increases produced by d-amphetamine in the DRL component but not in the fixed-interval. Of particular interest were the results for one rat where d-amphetamine initially produced a large rate decrease in the fixed-interval component sufficient to decrease the frequency of reinforcement. In this animal, tolerance developed to the rate-decreasing actions of the drug in the fixed-interval component and the rate-increasing actions in the DRL component. In a further experiment in this study, d-amphetamine was repeatedly administered to rats lever pressing to avoid electric shock. In these animals, d-amphetamine increased rate of lever pressing and significantly decreased the frequency with which they received electric shocks. No tolerance was observed under these conditions to the rate increases produced by d-amphetamine. These studies were interpreted as supporting the hypothesis that tolerance represented an adaptation to the reinforcement contingencies under the drug condition.

Another type of experiment suggesting the critical role of adaptation to the reinforcement contingencies is illustrated in a study by CAMPBELL and SEIDEN (1973). In this study, rats were trained under a DRL schedule of reinforcement, and the previous findings of SCHUSTER and ZIMMERMAN (1961) on tolerance development to d-amphetamine were replicated. In addition, however, these investigators demonstrated that rats given the same dose of the drug after the DRL session did not develop tolerance. Similar findings have been reported for milk consumption by rats by CARLTON and WOLGIN (1971) with amphetamine and by WOOLVERTON et al. (1978a) using cocaine. In this latter study, animals receiving cocaine after the session developed supersensitivity to the drug's anorexic properties. It would thus appear that animals must be exposed to the reinforcement contingencies while under the influence of the drug for behavioral tolerance to develop.

Not all tolerance which develops to the behavioral actions of amphetamines is based upon an adaptation to reinforcement contingencies. This is demonstrated by a series of studies using rhesus monkeys. In these studies, tolerance to the disrupting effects of d-methamphetamine on food-reinforced operant performance has been reported to occur at dosage levels well above the acutely lethal dose (FISCHMAN and SCHUSTER, 1974, 1977). It seems probable that this phenomenal tolerance development is based primarily on the irreversible depletion of brain dopamine found in these animals to have been produced by the repeated administration of d-methamphetamine (SEIDEN et al., 1975). That the tolerance to the behavioral disruption was not based upon a behavioral adaptation is demonstrated by a recent finding that monkeys not in contact with the reinforcement contingencies during the chronic methamphetamine regimen showed comparable tolerance to that of animals which were so exposed (FINNEGAN, personal communication). It would thus appear that tolerance to amphetamines can be based both upon behavioral and neurochemical mechanisms. Recent evidence demonstrating that in rats an irreversible depletion of brain dopamine can be produced by d-methamphetamine and d-amphetamine, but not methylphenidate, suggests that we must be cautious in generalizing results from amphetamines to other psychomotor stimulant drugs (Wagner et al., 1980). More research is needed to determine the conditions under which behavioral variables will determine the direction of change in sensitivity to psychomotor stimulant drugs and how these behavioral variables interact with pharmacologic variables.

II. Stimulus Properties of Psychomotor Stimulant Drugs

Psychomotor stimulant drugs have been shown to serve a variety of stimulus functions. In this section, we will describe and illustrate three of these: (1) as an unconditioned stimulus in a respondent conditioning paradigm; (2) as a discriminative stimulus for operant responding; and (3) as a reinforcing stimulus for operant behavior.

1. Psychomotor Stimulant Drugs as Unconditioned Stimuli

As previously stated, the administration of low to moderate doses of most psychomotor stimulant drugs causes an increase in locomotor activity in rats. It has been demonstrated (Pickens and Crowder, 1969; Tilsen and Rech, 1973) that stimuli associated with the administration of d-amphetamine can acquire this ability to increase locomotor activity. This has been interpreted as an instance of respondent conditioning in which the drug serves as the unconditioned stimulus (UCS) and the stimulus acquiring the ability to elicit the effects originally produced by the UCS is termed the conditioned stimulus (CS).

Psychomotor stimulant drugs have as well been shown to serve as unconditioned stimuli in the formation in rats of conditioned taste aversions. In 1955, Garcia and his colleagues reported that rats given a saccharin solution to drink and subsequently exposed to gamma radiation developed an aversion to saccharin (Garcia et al., 1955). This report has been followed by a number of studies demonstrating that a variety of drugs including the amphetamines (d, l, and methyl) can produce an aversion to comestibles (Martin and Ellinwood, 1973; Carey and Goodall, 1974; Gamzu, 1977; Cappell and Leblanc, 1977). Relatively low doses of the amphetamine will serve this UCS function, raising the question of the action of the drug responsible for the "aversion." As will be discussed in a subsequent section, it is possible to demonstrate that rats will self-administer amphetamines at the same dose levels used as the UCS to produce conditioned taste aversion. For many theorists who would like to believe that the hedonic value of a stimulus event is an inherent property, the finding that amphetamine will both be self administered (i.e., has positive properties) and serve to produce aversions (i.e., has negative properties) presents a paradox. It should be remembered, however, that we have already referred to experiments in which electric shocks would be administered by squirrel monkeys at intensity levels normally used in avoidance schedules (McKearney, 1974). These data strongly suggest that under certain circumstances, factors other than the inherent properties of the stimulus event imbue it with its functional significance. (For a discussion of this issue, see Morse and Kelleher, 1977.)

It has been suggested that the conditioned taste aversion using amphetamines as the UCS might be an instance of conditioned anorexia and/or adipsia (Carey and Goodall, 1974). This is certainly possible in the case of amphetamines; however, conditioned taste aversion has also been established with drugs which do not produce decreases in food intake (CAPPELL and LEBLANC, 1977). Further more, STOLERMAN and D'MELLO (1978) have established conditioned taste aversion using doses of fenfluramine well below those necessary to produce adipsia. It is also important to note that it has been difficult to establish cocaine as a UCS in the conditioned taste aversion paradigm (CAPPELL and LEBLANC, 1978; GOUDIE et al., 1977), despite the fact that it is a potent anorexigenic drug (WOOLVERTON et al., 1978a).

BOOTH et al. (1977) conducted one of the few studies designed to compare the potencies of a range of compounds in their ability to serve as a UCS in a conditioned taste aversion paradigm. This study confirmed the previous work showing that at best, cocaine produced only moderate taste aversions. This study also demonstrated that (1) d- and l-amphetamine were similar in potency (in contrast CAREY and GOODALL [1974] found a 4 to 1 potency difference); (2) p-chloromethamphetamine was more potent than methamphetamine; and (3) the rank order of potency for amphetamine congeners was fenfluramine > chlorphentermine > p-hydroxyamphetamine. It would thus appear that with the possible exception of cocaine the ability to serve as a UCS in the conditioned taste aversion paradigm is a general property of psychomotor stimulant drugs.

2. Psychomotor Stimulant Drugs as Discriminative Stimuli

Stimuli which are uniquely associated with the availability of a reinforcer are called discriminative stimuli when they acquire the ability to increase the frequency of the response reinforced in their presence. A variety of drugs have been shown to serve as discriminative stimuli, including many of those in the psychomotor stimulant class (SCHUSTER and BALSTER, 1977; LAL, 1977). In most experiments using drugs as discriminative stimuli, animals are trained to make one response when given drug and another response when given the drug vehicle, which is generally saline. Stimulus control is considered established when the animal makes the appropriate response when given drug or saline. There are a variety of problems in the use of drugs as discriminative stimuli, most all of which are related to the inability of the experimenter to have precise control over the intensity and duration of the stimulus. Nevertheless, a variety of psychomotor stimulant drugs have been successfully used as discriminative stimuli.

For many years drugs have been classified, at least in part, on the basis of their subjective effects in humans. Until recently, it was felt that this approach was only possible with humans because of their unique verbal abilities. It has been suggested that the development of the methods for establishing drugs as discriminative stimuli allows us to study similar processes in animals. For example, HARRIS and BALSTER (1971) established a discrimination between dl-amphetamine and saline injections in rats. Subsequently, they determined with drugs would substitute for dl-amphetamine, i.e., to which drugs would the animals generalize. Generalization was obtained with methylphenidate, but not with atropine. Similarly, SCHECHTER and ROSECRANS (1973) established d-amphetamine as a discriminative stimulus and found a generalization to l-amphetamine, but not to nicotine, mescaline, fenfluramine, or LSD. Furthermore, specificity was demonstrated by the fact that animals brought under the stimulus control of sedative-hypnotic agents responded to amphetamine injections as if they were saline (OVERTON, 1966; OVERTON and LEBMAN, 1973). Generalization was also found between *d*-amphetamine and cocaine (ANDO and YANAGITA, 1978). A recent review by SILVERMAN and HO (1977) summarizes the generalization studies conducted with psychomotor stimulant drugs. Although most studies have employed one of the amphetamines, sufficient work has been done with other psychomotor stimulant drugs to warrant the conclusion that this class of drugs possesses unique stimulus properties.

3. Psychomotor Stimulant Drugs as Reinforcing Stimuli

Many investigators have demonstrated that behavior leading to the injection of psychomotor stimulant drugs can be established and maintained (JOHANSON and BALSTER, 1978). Psychomotor stimulant drugs serve as reinforcers, for example, in rats (PICKENS, 1968), cats (BALSTER et al., 1976), squirrel monkeys (GOLDBERG, 1973), rhesus monkeys (DENEAU et al., 1969; WILSON et al., 1971), baboons (GRIFFITHS et al., 1979), and humans (JOHANSON and UHLENHUTH, 1978). It would thus appear that this is a general property of all psychomotor stimulant drugs occurring in a broad variety of mammalian species.

In most studies drugs have been given intravenously, usually through chronically implanted catheters. However, other studies have demonstrated that amphetamine and cocaine can serve as reinforcers by intramuscular and oral routes of administration (GOLDBERG et al., 1976; JOHANSON and UHLENHUTH, 1978).

The most extensive comparative studies of psychomotor stimulant drugs have been carried out in the rhesus monkey, using drugs delivered through chronic venous catheters contingent upon a lever pressing response. Using this general procedure, it has been established that naive rhesus monkeys can be conditioned to press a lever for *d*-, *l*-, and *d*-methamphetamine as well as diethylpropion and cocaine (JOHANSON et al., 1976). When given 23-h day access to these drugs under conditions where each lever press resulted in a drug injection (FR 1), rates of responding varied markedly from hour to hour and day to day. This variability was correlated with signs of CNS toxicity ending in many instances with the death of the animal. If access to psychomotor stimulant drugs under a fixed-ratio schedule is limited to 3–4 h daily, intake is remarkably stable within and between daily sessions (WILSON et al., 1971). Using this limited access procedure, dose-response relationships for cocaine, pipradrol, methylphenidate, and phenmetrazine (WILSON et al., 1971), *d*-, *l*-, and *d*-methamphetamine (BALSTER and SCHUSTER, 1973), mazindol (WILSON and SCHUSTER, 1976), and diethylpropion (JOHANSON and SCHUSTER, 1977) have been obtained. Three general relations have emerged from these studies: (1) All these drugs at certain dose levels maintain rates of responding greater than that generated by saline injections; (2) There is an inverse function relating dose to response rate; and (3) The total daily dose of drug received is relatively independent of dose per injection. This latter feature is a unique characteristic of drugs in the psychomotor stimulant class.

There has been a great deal of speculation concerning the interpretation of the relationship between response rate and reinforcement efficacy (JOHANSON, 1975). Dose-response functions relating rate of responding under a fixed-ratio schedule to dose per injection would suggest that higher doses are less reinforcing than lower doses. It seems likely that this result is due to the fact that psychomotor stimulant drugs can not only reinforce behavior preceding their injection but can have behavioral effects after their injection, as well.

On the basis of studies of the effects of psychomotor stimulant drugs on behaviors maintained by food, water, etc., we would expect that higher doses would decrease response rates for any reinforcer, including the drug maintaining the response (for a full discussion of this issue see JOHANSON, 1975). Thus, response rate is determined by both a drug's reinforcing actions and rate-modifying actions. For a variety of reasons, investigators have been interested in obtaining less confounded measures of the reinforcing efficacy of psychomotor stimulant drugs. First, such procedures would allow the determination of the relationship between dose and reinforcement magnitude. Second, such procedures might also be useful for predicting the relative "abuse potential" of new agents in this class (THOMPSON and UNNA, 1977). Measures which would allow the ranking of psychomotor stimulant drugs according to their reinforcing efficacy might show a good correlation with their actual abuse. It this were the case, then such measures might be useful in predicting the relative abuse potential of new agents.

A variety of procedures have been developed to compare the reinforcing actions of psychomotor stimulant drugs. These include preference procedures (IGLAUER and WOODS, 1974; JOHANSON and SCHUSTER, 1975), progressive ratio procedures (YANAGITA, 1973; GRIFFITHS et al., 1979), and response rate measures during extinction (BALSTER and SCHUSTER, 1977). In contrast to the results obtained using response rate under fixed-ratio schedules, a direct relationship between dose and reinforcement magnitude has been found using these procedures.

Furthermore, it has been found that members of the class of psychomotor stimulant drugs vary in their reinforcing efficacy. In a choice study, for example, JOHANSON and SCHUSTER (1977) found that cocaine was generally preferred to diethylpropion, regardless of the doses in the comparison. On the other hand, preference between cocaine and methylphenidate was determined by whichever drug was available at a higher dose (JOHANSON and SCHUSTER, 1975). Similarly, GRIFFITHS et al. (1979), using a progressive ratio procedure, have found that the highest ratios are maintained by cocaine with lower ratios being reached with diethylpropion and chlorphentermine, in that order. It would thus appear that the reinforcing efficacy of members of the psychomotor stimulant drug class does vary. It remains for more drugs in this class to be investigated before it is possible to say that the rank ordering of drugs according to their reinforcing efficacy will be correlated with their actual abuse.

Procedures allowing the unconfounded measurement of reinforcing efficacy are also essential for the investigation of the pharmacologic basis of drug reinforcement. For example, WILSON and SCHUSTER (1972, 1973) used a FR1 schedule of cocaine reinforcement to study the effects of drugs used to modify various neurochemical systems. The most striking finding was that chlorpromazine and atropine were the only agents producing an increase in rate of cocaine self-administration. Unfortunately, it is impossible to determine from these data whether these drugs were modifying the reinforcing actions or the direct rate-decreasing property of cocaine.

In this section we have been dealing with the reinforcing effects of psychomotor stimulant drugs as an inherent property. It is possible to do this when comparing drugs under similar environmental conditions. It must be recognized, however, that the rank ordering of drugs in terms of their reinforcing efficacy will not be the same under all environmental circumstances. As stated previously, there is a wealth of evidence demonstrating that under certain circumstances, environmental conditions may be the predominant determinant of a reinforcer's efficacy or even valence (MORSE and Kelleher, 1977). Wise et al. (1976) have demonstrated that at the same time apomorphine was serving as a positive reinforcer in rats, it was also serving as an unconditioned stimulus for producing aversion to a saccharin solution. Furthermore, many studies have used amphetamines as the UCS for the establishment of conditioned taste aversion at the same dose levels that other investigators have used as a reinforcer. A recent study by Spealman (1979) has demonstrated that cocaine can serve as a positive reinforcer for one response in a concurrent schedule where responses on the second lever terminates its availability. These findings lead one to seriously question the importance of the inherent properties of the event as a determinant of its reinforcing actions. Clearly, more research is necessary to delineate the manner in which environmental factors interact with the pharmacologic properties of events to determine their reinforcing actions.

C. General Comments

This review has discussed only certain aspects of the immense literature on the behavioral actions of psychomotor stimulant drugs. Even with this brief and selective review it is apparent that most of our generalizations about the actions of psychomotor stimulant drugs derive from experiments using amphetamines. In several areas it has become apparent that certain actions of amphetamine may not be shared by other psychomotor stimulant drugs. Clearly what is needed are parametric studies in which a number of psychomotor stimulant drugs are investigated using a wide variety of behavioral tasks. It is already apparent that this class of drugs will share a variety of behavioral actions. On the other hand, it is equally likely that certain psychomotor stimulant drugs will have some unique properties. This research should offer behavioral pharmacologists an exciting challenge.

References

Abdallah, A.H.: Comparative study of the anorexigenic activity of 5-(3,4-dichlorophenoxy-methyl)-2-amino-2-oxazoline HCl and d-amphetamine in different species. Toxicol. Appl. Pharmacol. 25, 344–353 (1973)

Abdallah, A.H., White, H.D.: Comparative study of the anorectic activity of phenindamine d-amphetamine and fenfluramine in different species. Arch. Int. Pharmacodyn. 188, 271–283 (1970)

Andersson, B., Larsson, S.: Water and food intake and the inhibitory effect of amphetamine on drinking and eating before and after "Prefrontal lobotomy" in dogs. Acta Physiol. Scand. 38, 22–30 (1956)

Ando, K., Yanagita, T.: The discriminative stimulus properties of intravenously administered cocaine in rhesus monkeys. In: Colpaert, F.C., Rosecrans, J.A. (eds.): Stimulus properties of drugs: Ten years of progress. Amsterdam: Elsevier/North Holland Press 1978

Balster, R.L., Schuster, C.R.: A comparison of d-amphetamine, l-amphetamine and methamphetamine self-administration in rhesus monkeys. Pharm. Biochem Behav. 1, 67–71 (1973)

Balster, R.L., Schuster, C.R.: A preference procedure that compares the efficacy of different intravenous drug reinforcers in the rhesus monkey. In: Ellinwood, E.H., Kilbey, M.M. (eds.): Cocaine and other stimulants. New York: Plenum Press 1977

Balster, R.L., Kilbey, M., Ellinwood, E.H.: Methamphetamine self-administration in the cat Psychopharmacologia 46, 229–233 (1976)

Bhattacharyya, A.K., Pradhan, S.N.: Interactions between motor activity and stereotypy in cocaine-treated rats. Psychopharmacology 63, 311–312 (1979)

Booth, D.A., Pilcher, C.W.T., D'Mello, G.D., Stolerman, I.P.: Comparative potencies of amphetamine, fenfluramine and related compounds in taste aversion experiments in rats. Br. J. Pharmacology. 668–677 (1977)

Campbell, J.C., Seiden, L.S.: Performance influence on the development of tolerance to amphetamine. Pharmacol. Biochem. Behav. *1*, 703–708 (1973)

Cappell, H., Le Blanc, A.E.: Parametric investigations of the effects of prior exposure to amphetamine and morphine on conditional gustatory aversion. Psychopharmacology *51*, 265–271 (1977)

Cappell, H., Le Blanc, A.E.: Gustatory avoidance conditioning by drugs of abuse. In: Food aversion learning. Milgram, N.W., Krane, K., Alloway, T.M. (eds.) New York: Plenum Press 1978

Carey, R.J., Goodall, E.B.: Amphetamine-induced taste aversion: A comparison of *d*- versus *l*-amphetamine. Pharmacol. Biochem. Behav. *2*, 325–330 (1974)

Carlton, P., Wolgin, D.: Contingent tolerance to the anorexigenic effects of amphetamine. Physiol. Behav. *7*, 221–223 (1971)

Cooper, S.J., Francis, R.L.: Feeding parameters with two food textures after chlordiazepoxide administration, alone or in combination with *d*-amphetamine or fenfluramine. Psychopharmacology *62*, 253–259 (1979)

Deneau, G., Yanagita, T., Seevers, M.H.: Self-administration of psychoactive substances by the monkey: A measure of psychological dependence. Psychopharmacologia *16*, 30–48 (1969)

Dewhurst, W.G., Marley, E.: Action of sympathomimetic and allied amines on the central nervous system of the chicken. Brit. J. Pharmacol. *25*, 705–727 (1965)

Dews, P.B.: Studies on behavior. II. The effects of pentobarbital, methamphetamine and scopolamine on performances in pigeons involving discriminations. J. Pharmacol. Exp. Ther. *115*, 380–389 (1955)

Dews, P.B.: Studies on behavior. IV. Stimulant actions of methamphetamine. J. Pharmacol. Exp. Ther. *122*, 137–147 (1958)

Dews, P.B., Morse, W.H.: Some observations on an operant in human subjects and its modification by dextroamphetamine. J. Exp. Anal. Behav. *4*, 359–364 (1958)

Dews, P.B., Wenger, G.R.: Rate-dependency of the behavioral effects of amphetamine. In: Thompson, T.I., Dews, P.B. (eds.): Advances in behavioral pharmacology, Vol. 1, New York: Academic Press Inc. 1977

Ellinwood, E.H., Jr.: Assault and homicide associated with amphetamine abuse. Am. J. Psychiat. *127*, 1170–1175 (1971)

Ellinwood, E.H., Jr., Escalante, O.: Behavior and histopathological findings during chronic methedrine intoxication. Biol. Psychiatry *2*, 27–39 (1970)

Epstein, A.H.: Suppression of eating and drinking by amphetamine and other drugs in normal and hyperphagic rats. J. Comp. Physiol. Psychol. *52*, 37–45 (1959)

Falk, J.L.: Drug effects on discriminative motor control. Physiol. Behav. *4*, 421–427 (1969)

Fischman, M.W., Schuster, C.R.: Tolerance development to chronic methamphetamine intoxication in the rhesus monkey. Pharm. Biochem. Behav. *2*, 503–508 (1974)

Fischman, M.W., Schuster, C.R.: Long-term behavioral changes in the rhesus monkey after multiple daily injections of *d*-methylamphetamine. J. Pharm. Exp. Ther. *201*, 593–605 (1977)

Fischman, M.W., Schuster, C.R.: Cocaine effects in sleepdeprived humans. Psychopharmacology (in press)

Gamzu, E.: The multifaceted nature of taste-aversion-inducing agents: Is there a single common factor? In: Learning mechanisms in food selection. Barker, L.M., Best, M.R., Domjan, M. Houston: Baylor University Press 1977

Garcia, J., Kimeldorf, D.J., Koelling, R.A.: A conditioned aversion towards saccharin resulting from exposure to gamma radiation. Science *122*, 157–159 (1955)

Goldberg, S.R.: Comparable behavior maintained under fixed ratio and second order schedules of food presentation, cocaine injection or *d*-amphetamine injection in the squirrel monkey. J. Pharm. Exp. Ther. *186*, 18–31 (1973)

Goldberg, S.R., Morse, W.H., Goldberg, D.M.: Behavior maintained under a second-order schedule by intramuscular injection of morphine or cocaine in rhesus monkeys. J. Pharmacol. Exp. Ther. *199*, 278–286 (1976)

Gonzalez, F.A., Goldberg, S.R.: Effects of cocaine and d-amphetamine on behavior maintained under various schedules of food presentation in squirrel monkeys. J. Pharm. Exp. Ther. 201, 33–43 (1977)

Goudie, A.J., Dickins, D.W., Thornton, E.W.: Cocaine-induced conditioned taste aversions in rats. Pharmacol. Biochem. Behav. 8, 757–761 (1977)

Griffiths, R., Stitzer, M., Corker, K., Bigelow, G., Liebson, I.: Drug-produced changes in human social behavior: Facilitation by d-amphetamine. Pharmacol. Biochem. Behav. 7, 365–372 (1977)

Griffiths, R.R., Brady, J.V., Bradford, L.D.: Predicting the abuse liability of drugs with animal drug self-administration procedures: Psychomotor stimulants and hallucinogens. In: Advances in Behavioral Pharmacology. Thompson, T.I., Dews, P.B. (eds.), Vol. 2. New York: Academic Press 1979

Harris, R.T., Balster, R.L.: Discriminative control by dl-amphetamine and saline of lever choice and response patterning. Psychon. Sci. 10, 105–106 (1968)

Harris, R.T., Balster, R.L.: An analysis of the function of drugs in the stimulus control of operant behavior. In: Stimulus properties of drugs. Thompson, T.I., Pickens, R. (eds.). New York: Appleton-Century-Crofts 1971

Heffner, T.G., Drawbaugh, R.B., Zigmond, M.J.: Amphetamine and operant behavior in rats: Relationship between drug effect and control response rate. J. Comp. Physiol. Psychol. 86, 1031–1043 (1974)

Hutchinson, R.R., Emley, G.S., Krasnegor, N.W.: The effects of cocaine on aggressive behavior. In: Mule, S.J. (ed.): Cocaine: Chemical, biological, clinical, social and treatment aspects. CRC Press 1976

Iglauer, C., Woods, J.H.: Concurrent performances: Reinforcement by different doses of intravenous cocaine in rhesus monkeys. J. Exp. Anal. Behav. 22, 179–196 (1974)

Johanson, C.E.: Pharmacological and environmental variables affecting drug preference in rhesus monkeys. Pharmacol. Rev., 27, 343–355 (1975)

Johanson, C.E.: The effects of electric shock on responding maintained by cocaine injections in a choice procedure in the rhesus monkey. Psychopharmacology 53, 277–282 (1977)

Johanson, C.E.: Effects of intravenous cocaine, diethylpropion, d-amphetamine, and perphenazine on responding maintained by food delivery and shock avoidance in rhesus monkeys. J. Pharm. Exp. Ther. 204, 118–129 (1978)

Johanson, C.E., Balster, R.L.: A summary of the results of a drug self-administration study using substitution procedures in rhesus monkeys. Bull. Narcotics 30, 43–54 (1978)

Johanson, C.E., Schuster, C.R.: A choice procedure for drug reinforcers: cocaine and methylphenidate in the rhesus monkey. J. Pharm. Exp. Ther. 193, 676–688 (1975)

Johanson, C.E., Schuster, C.R.: Procedures for the preclinical assessment of abuse potential of psychotropic drugs in animals. In: Predicting dependence liability of stimulant and depressant drugs. Thompson, T., Unna, K. Baltimore: University Park Press 1977

Johanson, C.E., Uhlenhuth, E.H.: Drug self-administration in humans. In: Krasnegor, N. (ed.): Self-Administration of abused substances: Methods for study. National Institute on Drug Abuse. Research Monograph Series 20, 68–85 (1978)

Johanson, C.E., Aigner, T., Seiden, L., Schuster, C.R.: The effects of methamphetamine on fine motor control in rhesus monkeys. Pharmacol. Biochem. Behav. 11, 273–278 (1979)

Johanson, C.E., Balster, R.L., Bonese, K.: Self-administration of psychomotor stimulant drugs: the effects of unlimited access. Pharmacol. Biochem. Behav. 4, 45–51 (1976)

Kandel, D.A., Doyle, D., Fischman, M.W.: Tolerance and cross tolerance to the effect of amphetamine, methamphetamine and fenfluramine on milk consumption in the rat. Pharmacol. Biochem. Behav. 3, 705–707 (1975)

Kelleher, R.T.: Psychomotor stimulants. In: Drug abuse. Pradhan, S.N., Sutta, N.S. (eds.). St. Louis: Mosby 1977

Kelleher, R.T., Morse, W.H.: Escape behavior and punished behavior. Fed. Proc. 23, 808–817 (1964)

Kelleher, R.T., Morse, W.: Determinants of the specificity of the behavioral effects of drugs. Ergeb. Physiol. Biol. Chem. Exp. Pharmakol. 60, 1–56 (1968)

Knowler, W.C., Ukena, T.E.: The effects of chlorpromazine, pentobarbital, chlordiazepoxide and d-amphetamine on rates of licking in the rat. J. Pharmacol. Exp. Ther. 185, 385–397 (1973)

Kornetsky, C., Mirsky, A., Kessler, E.K., Dorff, J.E.: The effect of dextroamphetamine on behavioral deficits produced by sleep loss in humans. J. Pharmacol. Exp. Ther. *127*, 46–59 (1959)

Kosman, J., Unna, K.: Effects of chronic administration of the amphetamines and other stimulants on behavior. J. Clin. Pharmacol. Ther. *9*, 240–254 (1968)

Kramer, J., Fischman, V., Littlefield, D.: Amphetamine abuse: pattern and effects of high doses taken intravenously. J. Am. Med. Assoc. *201*, 305–309 (1967)

Lal, H. (ed.): Discriminative stimulus properties of drugs: Advances in behavioral biology, Vol. 22. New York, London: Plenum Press 1977

Lawlor, R.B., Trivedi, M.C., Yelnosky, J.: A determination of the anorexigenic potential of *dl*-amphetamine, *d*-amphetamine, *l*-amphetamine and phentermine. Arch. Int. Pharmacodyn. *179*, 401–407 (1969)

Le Douarec, J.C., Neveu, C.E.: Pharmacology and biochemistry of fenfluramine. In: International Symposium on amphetamines and related compounds. Costa, E., Garattini, S. (eds.). New York: Raven Press 1970

Lewander, T.: Effects of amphetamines in animals. In: Drug Addiction II. Martin, W.R. (ed.). Berlin, Heidelberg, New York: Springer 1977

Maickel, R.P., Cox, Jr., R.H., Ksir, C.J., Snodgrass, W.R., Miller, F.P.: Some aspects of the behavioral pharmacology of the amphetamines. In: International symposium on amphetamines and related compounds. Costa, E., Garattini, S. (eds.): New York: Raven Press 1970

Martin, J.C., Ellinwood, Jr., E.H.: Conditioned aversion to a preferred solution following methamphetamine injections. Psychopharmacologia *29*, 253–261 (1973)

McKearney, J.W.: Effects of *d*-amphetamine, morphine, and chlorpromazine on responding under fixed-interval schedules of food presentation or electric shock presentation. J. Pharmacol. Exp. Ther. *190*, 141–153 (1974)

McKearney, J.W., Barrett, J.E.: Schedule-controlled behavior and the effects of drugs. In: Blackman, D.E., Sanger, D.J. (eds.): Contemporary research in behavioral pharmacology. New York: Plenum Press 1978

McMillan, D.E.: The effects of sympathomimetic amines on schedule controlled behavior in the pigeon. J. Pharmacol. Exp. Ther. *160*, 315–325 (1968)

McMillan, D.E.: Effects of *d*-amphetamine on performance under several parameters of multiple fixed-ratio, fixed-interval schedules. J. Pharmacol. Exp. Ther. *167*, 26–33 (1969)

Miczek, K.A.: A new test for aggression in rats without aversive stimulation, differential effects of *d*-amphetamine and cocaine. Psychopharmacology *60*, 253–259 (1979)

Morse, W.H., Kelleher, R.T.: Determinants of reinforcement and punishment. In: Handbook of operant behavior. Honig, W.K., Staddon, J.E.R. (eds.). Englewood Cliffs, New Jersey: Prentice-Hall Inc. 1977

Mumford, L., Teixeira, A.R., Kumar, R.: Sources of variation in locomotor activity and stereotypy in rats treated with *d*-amphetamine. Psychopharmacology *62*, 241–245 (1979)

Overton, D.A.: State-dependent learning produced by depressant and atropine-like drugs. Psychopharmacologia *10*, 6–31 (1966)

Overton, D.A., Lebman, R.I.: Rapid drug discrimination produced by ketamine, a dissociative anesthetic. Proc. Am. Psychol. Assoc. (1973)

Pearl, R., Seiden, L.: The existence of tolerance to and cross tolerance between *d*-amphetamine and methylphenidate for their effects on milk consumption and DRL performance. J. Pharmacol. Exp. Ther. *198*, 635–647 (1976)

Pickens, R.: Self-administration of stimulants by rats. Int. J. Addict. *3*, 215–221 (1968)

Pickens, R.W., Crowder, W.F.: Effects of CS-UCS interval on conditioning of drug response with assessment of speed of conditioning. Psychopharmacologia *11*, 88–94 (1969)

Randrup, A., Munkvad, I.: Special antagonism of amphetamineinduced abnormal behavior. Psychopharmacologia *7*, 416–422 (1965)

Randrup, A., Munkvad, I.: Stereotyped activity produced by amphetamine in several animal species and man. Psychopharmacologia *11*, 300–310 (1967)

Randrup, A., Munkvad, I.: Various forms of stereotype activity produced by amphetamine in certain animal species and man. Neuropsychopharmacology *127*, 1224–1225 (1967)

Ray, O.S., Bivens, L.W.: Chlorpromazine and amphetamine effects on three operant and on four discrete trial reinforcement schedules. Psychopharmacologia *10*, 32–43 (1966)

Rolinski, Z.: Analysis of aggressiveness-stereotypy complex induced in mice by amphetamine or nialamide and *l*-dopa. Pol. J. Pharmacol. Pharm. *25*, 551–558 (1973)

Sanger, D.J., Blackman, D.E.: Rate dependent effects of drugs on the variable-interval behavior of rats. J. Pharmacol. Exp. Ther. *194*, 343–350 (1975)

Sanger, D.J., Blackman, D.: Rate dependent effects of drugs: A review of the literature. Pharmacol. Biochem. Behav. *4*, 73–83 (1976)

Schechter, M.D., Rosecrans, J.A.: *d*-Amphetamine as a discriminative cue: Drugs with similar stimulus properties. Eur. J. Pharmacol. *21*, 212–216 (1973)

Schuster, C.R., Balster, R.: The discriminative stimulus properties of drugs. In: Advances in behavioral pharmacology. Thompson, T.I., Dews, P.B. (eds.) New York, San Francisco, London: Academic Press 1977

Schuster, C.R., Zimmerman, J.: Timing behavior during prolonged treatment with *dl*-amphetamine. J. Exp. Anal. Behav. *4*, 327–350 (1961)

Schuster, C.R., Dockens, W.S., Woods, J.H.: Behavioral variables affecting the development of amphetamine tolerance. Psychopharmacologia *9*, 170–182 (1966)

Segal, D.S.: Behavioral and neurochemical correlates of repeated *d*-amphetamine administration. In: Neurobiological mechanisms of adaptations and behavior. Mandell, A.J. (ed.) New York: Raven Press 1975

Segal, D.S., Mandell, A.J.: Long-term administration of *d*-amphetamine: progressive augmentation of motor activity and stereotypy. Pharm. Biochem. Behav. *2*, 249–255 (1974)

Seiden, L.S., Fischman, M.W., Schuster, C.R.: Long-term methamphetamine induced changes in brain catecholamines in tolerant rhesus monkeys. Drug Alcohol Depend. *1*, 215–219 (1975)

Silverman, P.B., Ho, B.T.: Psychomotor stimulant discrimination. In: Discriminative stimulus properties of drugs: Advances in behavioral biology. Lal, H. (ed.), Vol. 22. New York: Plenum Press 1977

Skinner, B.F., Heron, W.T.: Effects of caffeine and benzedrine upon conditioning and extinction. Psychol. Rep. *1*, 340–346 (1937)

Smith, C.B.: Effects of *d*-amphetamine upon operant behavior of pigeons: Enhancement by reserpine. J. Pharmacol. Exp. Ther. *146*, 167–174 (1964)

Spealman, R.D.: Behavior maintained by termination of a schedule of self-administered cocaine. Science *204*, 1231–1233 (1979)

Spengler, J., Waser, P.: Der Einfluß verschiedener Pharmaka auf den Futterkonsum von Albino Ratten im akuten Versuch. Naunyn-Schmiedebergs Arch. Exp. Path. Pharmak. *237*, 171–185 (1959)

Stitzer, M., McKearney, J.W.: Modifications of drug effects by pause requirements. J. Exp. Anal. Behav. *27*, 51–59 (1977)

Stitzer, M.L., Griffiths, R.R., Liebson, I.: Effects of *d*-amphetamine on speaking in isolated humans. Pharmacol. Biochem. Behav. *9*, 57–63 (1978)

Stolerman, I.P., D'Mello, G.D.: Amphetamine-induced hypodipsia and its implications for conditioned taste aversion in rats. Pharmacol. Biochem. Behav. *8*, 333–338 (1978)

Stretch, R.G., Dalrymple, D.: Effects of methylphenidate, pentobarbital and reserpine on behavior controlled by a schedule of inter-response time reinforcement. Psychopharmacologia *13*, 49–64 (1968)

Tagliamonte, A., Tagliamonte, P., Gessa, G.L.: Cross tolerance to the anorexigenic effect of *d*-amphetamine, *l*-amphetamine, fenfluramine and desmethylimipramine in rats. Pharmacologist *11*, 264 (1969)

Tedeschi, D.J., Fowler, P.F., Miller, R.B., Macko, E.: Pharmacological analysis of foot shock-induced fighting behavior. In: Aggressive behavior. Garrattini, S., Sigg, E.B. (eds.) Amsterdam: Excerpta Medica Foundation 1969

Thompson, T., Unna, K.: Predicting dependence liability of stimulant and depressant drugs. Baltimore, Md: University Park Press 1977

Tilson, H.A., Rech, R.H.: Conditioned drug effects and absence of tolerance to *d*-amphetamine induced motor activity. Pharmacol. Biochem. Behav. *1*, 149–153 (1973)

Van Rossum, J.M.: Mode of action of psychomotor stimulant drugs. Int. Rev. Neurobiol. *12*, 307–383 (1970)

Wagner, G.C., Ricaurte, G.A., Johanson, C.E., Schuster, C.R., Seiden, L.S.: Amphetamine induces depletion and loss of dopamine uptake sites. Neurology *30*, 547–550 (1980)

Wayner, M.J., Greenberg, I., Trowbridge, J.: Effects of d-amphetamine on schedule induced polydipsia. Pharmacol. Biochem. Behav. *1*, 109–111 (1973)

Webb, D., Levine, T.E.: Effects of caffeine on DRL performance in the mouse. Pharmacol. Biochem. Behav. *9*, 7–10 (1978)

Weischer, M.L.: Einfluß von Anorektica der Amphetamine-Reihe auf das Verhalten des Siamesischen Kampffisches Betta splenden. Arzneim. Forsch. *16*, 1310–1311 (1966)

Weiss, B., Laties, V.G.: Reconciling the effects of amphetamine on human and animal behavior. Excerpta Medica International Congress series No. 220, 1970

Wilson, M.C., Schuster, C.R.: The effect of various pharmacological agents on cocaine self-administration by rhesus monkeys. In: Current concepts on amphetamine abuse. Ellinwood, E.H., Cohen, S. (eds.): DHEW Publ. No. (HSM) 72-9085 Washington, D.C.: U.S. Government Printing Office 1972

Wilson, M.C., Schuster, C.R.: The effects of stimulants and depressants on cocaine self-administration behavior in the rhesus monkey. Psychopharmacologia *31*, 291–304 (1973)

Wilson, M., Schuster, C.R.: Mazindol self-administration in the rhesus monkey. Pharmacol. Biochem. Behav. *4*, 207–210 (1976)

Wilson, M.C., Hitomi, M., Schuster, C.R.: Psychomotor stimulant self-administration as a function of dosage per injection in the rhesus monkey. Psychopharmacologia *22*, 271–281 (1971)

Wise, R.A., Yokel, R.A., De Wit, H.: Both positive reinforcement and conditioned aversion from amphetamine and from apomorphine in rats. Science *191*, 1273–1275 (1976)

Woolverton, W.L., Kandel, D., Schuster, C.R.: Tolerance and cross-tolerance to cocaine and d-amphetamine. J. Pharmacol. Exp. Ther. *205*, 525–535 (1978a)

Woolverton, W., Kandel, D., Schuster, C.: Effects of repeated administration of cocaine on schedule-controlled behavior of rats. Pharmacol. Biochem. Behav. *9*, 327–337 (1978b)

Yanagita, T.: An experimental framework for evaluation of dependence liability of various types of drug in monkeys. Pharmacology and the future of man. Proc. 5th Int. Congr. Pharmacology *1*, 7–17 (1973)

Yelnosky, J., Lawlor, R.G.: A comparative study of the pharmacologic actions of amphetamine and fenfluramine. Arch. Int. Pharmacodyn. *184*, 374–388 (1970)

Yokel, R.A., Pickens, R.: Chronic methamphetamine self-administration by rats. Pharmacologist *12*, 226 (1970)

Zimmerman, J., Schuster, C.R.: Spaced responding in multiple DRL schedules. Investigation of several behavioral and pharmacologic variables. J. Exp. Anal. Behav. *5*, 497–504 (1962)

CHAPTER 16

The Dependence-Producing Properties of Psychomotor Stimulants

J. E. VILLARREAL and L. A. SALAZAR

A. Introduction

This review deals with a singular form of pathology induced by certain drugs, including some of the group that are currently classified as psychomotor stimulants. For historical reasons, this form of pathology is now generically called drug dependence, with subclasses defined in terms of the type of pharmacologic agent that generates or maintains the disorder. Other terms such as toxicomania, habituation, or addiction have been employed for the disease. It is possible that its name will change again in the future as the new, growing knowledge about its nature develops more fully. The main objective of this chapter is to review the disease of dependence to psychomotor stimulants as well as the results of experimental work aimed at understanding and measuring the dependence-producing properties that these drugs possess. Simultaneous attention to these two levels of study – analysis of dependence as a disease and experimental analysis of drug actions related to dependence production – has been deemed necessary to maintain the complete perspective that the subject requires.

In the not too distant past many human diseases were classified as "fevers," and some prominent physicians regarded cardiac acceleration as a sort of pathognomonic indicator of the generic family of the fever diseases; high body temperature, chills, and other signs were also part of the picture. These remarks about an outdated concept for a semiologic variable (sign or symptom) thought to be primary in febrile diseases, are not meant to be disparaging; their purpose is to provide a perspective of analogy pertinent to the subject of this paper. Modern medicine, in fact, had its origins in the first series of systematic efforts to describe, classify, and define diseases as nosologic entities (see SYDENHAM 1666–1686; BOISSIER DE SAUVAGES 1762). Such empirical taxonomic approach had a profound value for medicine and promoted the incorporation of the advances in other sciences.

The nosologic approach was also applied, especially in this century, to the class of diseases of drug dependence. Until recently, however, with limited knowledge and with clinical pictures of protean and shifting semiologic variables, quite different features of the behavior, psychology, etc., of human subjects suffering from drug dependence, and/or features of drug action, were variously regarded as of primary or defining significance by different authors.

With the opioids, prototypal drugs of dependence, it became progressively apparent that chronic intoxication with these compounds produced marked pharmacologic changes that strongly suggested themselves as mechanisms for the continued tenacious consumption of these drugs. Yet, it is worthy of note that, even in the case of opioids, studies in human addicts carried out in the late 1920s could not determine whether the disturbances after drug withdrawal were physiologic, psychological, or even a form of malingering (see review by Schuster and Villarreal 1968). Nevertheless, studies on the pharmacology of opioids, both in animals and humans, produced a body of evidence which clearly indicated that pharmacologic factors were strong enough to account for a major part of the fully developed picture of addition. It should be pointed out, however, that some of the prominent features of opioid dependence were well suited to study by approaches that were part, or extensions, of conventional physiologic pharmacology, e.g., features such as tolerance, physiologic dependence, and relief of the abstinence syndrome. Here, what is meant by conventional physiologic pharmacology is the linear approach in which the investigator administers a compound to an organism and then records the consequent changes produced.

The issue of dependence to psychomotor stimulants acquired prominence 2–3 decades ago, at a time when the biomedical community was without the specific conceptual and methodologic tools necessary to handle it. On this issue, the approaches of conventional pharmacology would simply not do. The nosologic approach had a difficult struggle. The development of clinical nosologic concepts can be appreciated in an excellent review on amphetamine dependence by Kallant (1966). At such a late date, this author had to go to great lengths to defend the proposition that addiction to amphetamine-like drugs does indeed exist.

A statement by one of the authors quoted by Kallant (1966) illustrates one type of problem raised for clinical nosology by amphetamine dependence. The quoted author considered that most so-called amphetamine addicts are instances of "symptomatic addiction," that is, a nonspecific type of addiction where the patient uses a substitute when his favorite drug is not available. He says: "It appears, . . . that addiction or habituation to amphetamine is caused by a factor in the individual's psychologic make-up which leads him to abuse the drugs rather than by any pharmacologic action of the drugs themselves."

The idea that "factors in the individual's psychological make-up" *cause* habituation or addiction is a persistent, though now qualified, theme in the literature. It probably arises from an understandable, but fallacious, type of logic. In an exaggerated form, this type of reasoning seems to go as follows: a person who takes drugs does something that does not make sense; therefore, that person is mad or, at least, there is something wrong with his "make-up."

A new type of pharmacologic experiment on animals quickly led to a major reformulation of the concept of dependence, including dependence on psychomotor stimulants. For the latter, this new approach provided a focus of clarity and a means to study their dependence-producing properties. When animals of different species are put under conditions that make it likely that they will accidentally operate a device (e.g., a lever or a button) that will activate a system that in turn will inject into their bloodstream a dose of an amphetamine-like drug, the behavior that at first occurred accidentally will be repeated again and again. The animal will self-administer large amounts of the drug with temporal patterns of high and low intake similar to those seen in human addicts to this class of drugs. Since this phenomenon occurs in all animals, of at least seven different species, the above-mentioned logic of psychological make-up causing amphetamine consumption does not hold. It is not sensible to infer that all animals are psychopathologic, if all of them, when put in the proper conditions for making a special kind of contact with CNS stimulants, do in fact acquire the disease of dependence. We now know that the disease requires the availability of drugs with certain pharmacologic properties and that the contact of the drug with the organism must be produced by self-administration, or a very close equivalent of it.

Important misunderstandings still persist. In the latest edition of a textbook of psychiatry with widespread use, we found the following statement about cocaine: "Taken daily in fairly large amounts it can disrupt eating and sleeping habits; ... and create a serious psychologic dependence." Dependence starts with the first self-administration of the drug. Dependence can be terminated, of course, but if an individual is taking cocaine "daily in fairly large amounts" the subject is already under some degree of dependence and need not wait for it to be "created."

As with infectious diseases, laboratory experimentation on drug dependence is revealing key layers of pathogenesis that do not seem easy to dissect in clinical observation. However, we find it quite fitting that a perceptive clinician should furnish us with the words to state what the nodal feature of dependence appears to be. Talking about psychomotor stimulants, BEJEROT (1969) says: "... the state of addiction is mainly a biological phenomenon ... forces of the strength of natural instincts, and often even stronger ... have been artificially induced by chemical means." Such induced forces are behavioral impulses for the self-administration of the drug.

Even if the above notion is a great step forward, it is also only a point of departure. Strong evidence, epidemiologic, clinical, and from the experimental laboratory, indicates that environmental variables play a determining role in the risk, severity, time course of dependence, and its reversibility. The present chapter discusses the role of such environmental variables not only because of their pertinence to dependence as a human disease but also because the dependence-producing effects of drugs can only exist in the context of the dynamic interaction of the behavior of organisms with the "anatomy and physiology" of their environments. The kind of environmental basis for interaction with the organism, whether man or experimental animal, will determine whether self-administration of stimulants takes on a pattern of consumption that leads to severe toxicity and even death. An outstanding case will be discussed later on where a major dependence-producing drug of widespread use is so controlled by environmental variables that the drug has come to be generally regarded as of low danger and low dependence capacity.

The purposes of the present chapter are twofold: (1) to assemble key concepts, methodologies, and findings into a coherent whole, with emphasis on concepts that may orient and stimulate interest in the subject; and (2) to draw attention to the new dimensions that compulsive drug-seeking behavior presents to science. Dependence differs in a fundamental way from other drug-induced phenomena. The scientific study of dependence implies the need not only for new methodologies and forms of analysis, but also for new forms of thought. We have to face it as it demands to be faced and not try to force it improperly into more familiar but inadequate molds.

The present task is somewhat difficult because crucial concepts emerge from and cut across different disciplines with very different styles of thought and different languages. Certain important concepts are not easy to convey in abstract form or in succinct statements as are conventional in physiologic pharmacology. Experience has led us to conclude that some of these concepts, to be effectively transmitted, have to be presented in a more vivid way, with examples, analogies, and selected descriptions of experimental procedure.

B. Evolution of the Concepts of Dependence

Concepts from the experimental study of dependence have pushed some early, simplified notions aside. One type of such simplified notion assigned to the character or personality of the addict the main role in dependence. Another notion appeared to explain the craving for drugs in the case of opioids: physiologic dependence as a sort of biologic "hunger." Physiologic dependence does not appear to play a determining role in the case of self-administration of psychomotor stimulants. Villarreal (1970) gives a brief account of the changing concepts:

> The stories of drug addicts, alcoholics, gamblers, and others who compulsively engage in behavior which predictably brings about life tragedy have always been a source of great puzzlement for more fortunate mortals. ...Not surprisingly, many have agreed with John Johnes, who, at the turn of the XVIII century concluded that the source of mischief (in opium dependence) is not in the drug but in the people (the addicts). However, attempts to define the nature of this mischief through studies of the personality or character of drug addicts have been far from revealing factors which are either *necessary* and/or *sufficient conditions* for the generation of compulsive tendencies to self-administer certain drugs.

Such conditions can only be identified by experiment, as with the postulates of Koch for infectious diseases.

> Against a background in which self-administration of drugs appeared to be unaccountable except by the postulation of a psychological disorder in the addict, the emergence of the concept of physical dependence (to opioids) had a profound (explanatory) impact. ...Physical dependence was established as a strong biological need ... which could be represented as a physiological hunger to a large extent responsible for the strong craving of the addict. ...However, it was acknowledged that factors other than physical dependence play a very important role... Human addicts to opiates continued to crave for these drugs even after prolonged drug-free periods, when they were no longer physically dependent. Furthermore, stabilizing schedules of drug administration which met the physical requirements of opiate addicts did not always satisfy their "emotional" needs for drug.
>
> The findings of laboratory studies have now made it clear that physical dependence is neither a necessary nor a sufficient condition for the initiation or the maintenance of self-administration (although opioid physical dependence can markedly enhance the strength of self-administration behavior).
>
> ... there have been two major contributions of laboratory work to our understanding of human drug dependence. First, the fact that simpleminded organisms behave like man when they are given access to drugs of dependence indicates that compulsive self-administration is a relatively simple form of reflex action (operant reflex), eliminating the necessity to postulate needs ... peculiar to the mind of man. Second, the fact that for practical purposes all animals that are given the opportunity to take the major drugs of dependence will develop steady self-administration behavior indicates that any individual differences in susceptibility that may exist in this regard are of secondary import when these drugs are freely available to subjects who do not have other strong competing behaviors.

Describing the epidemic of intravenous amphetamine dependence that took place in San Francisco in the late 1960s, Smith (1972) states that:

> Although the number (of subjects) that progress from experimental or occasional use of *speed* (amphetamine) is not known, our observations suggest that it is probably *much higher* than is the case with other substances. ...*The individual variables* which antedate involvement in the drug scene (drug-using group or subculture) *appear to be less important* in determining the direction drug use will take than such immediate factors as prevailing community attitudes, peer sanctions imposed on certain kinds of social behavior, *drug availability*, subjective interpretations of the drug experience, the quality of social interactions in the speed drug scene, and, finally, the structure of the illicit marketplace to which the user must relate.

Thus, laboratory and clinical evidence indicates that necessary and sufficient conditions for the production of dependence as strong self-administration behavior lie with the properties of certain drugs and the immediate environmental base on which the organism functions.

Decades of experimental laboratory analysis of behavior have profited from the use of a concept that applies with remarkable fitness to drug self-administration behavior. Such a concept is *reinforcement of operant behavior*. "The term reinforcement refers neither to a theory nor an explanation for behavior. It is, instead, a name for a particular relation between behavior and environmental events" (CATANIA 1976). When an item of behavior produces a stimulus and such behavior increases because it produces such stimuli, it is appropriate to apply the term "operant reinforcement" to the process. A *primary reinforcer* is a stimulus which, if presented closely after a given behavior is emitted, will increase the probability that such behavior will occur again. If the stimulus once more occurs after the new emission of the behavior in question, the behavior will be further reinforced. The behavior is called operant because it is defined in terms of what it does to the environment (what it operates) and not in terms of its anatomic description; any behavior will do, as long as it operates the same change in the environment.

Those drugs that when injected by laboratory devices into animals following an operant behavior (e.g., pressing a lever) generate further emissions of the operant behavior are, therefore, said to have primary reinforcing properties.

In casual language and in some instances in the literature there is sometimes a misuse of the concept of reinforcement. For example, it is sometimes said that an event has been very reinforcing when what is meant is that the event has caused a subjective sensation of pleasantness, i.e., that the event is liked. Pleasure and reinforcement are not necessarily associated and it has been amply demonstrated that it can be very misleading to make them synonymous.

Very extensive laboratory research has shown that drugs that produce dependence in man also function as primary reinforcers of self-administration behavior in a wide variety of animal species (rats, cats, dogs, various primate species). Also, drugs that do not produce drug-seeking behavior in man – phenothiazines, tricyclic antidepressants – do not generate self-administration in animals, i.e., they do not function as primary reinforcers (WIKLER et al. 1963; YANAGITA et al. 1965; SCHUSTER and VILLARREAL 1968; DENEAU et al. 1969; SCHUSTER and THOMPSON 1969; HOFFMEISTER and GOLDBERG 1973; WOODS and TESSEL, 1974; HOFFMEISTER and WUTTKE 1975; HOFFMEISTER 1975; World Health Organization 1975; DE V. COTTEN 1976; JOHANSON and SCHUSTER 1976; YANAGITA 1977; WOODS 1977; SPEALMAN and GOLDBERG 1978; GRIFFITHS et al. 1978a, b).

These findings in animals indicate not only that the laboratory preparations that have produced them represent strong animal models of dependence, but also that reinforcement of operant behavior by the drugs that we call dependence producing occurs through mechanisms that have wide biologic generality and, therefore, that laboratory findings in such animal preparations are in principle highly extrapolative to man. This contribution of laboratory work is especially significant since experimentation in humans in the field of dependence is severely limited for ethical reasons.

It is clear that two conditions are necessary to generate the predisposition of organisms to engage in drug-seeking behavior: the availability of drugs with operant reinforcing properties, and acts of self-administration. Students of drug-taking behavior, both at the clinical and experimental level, place great emphasis on environmental circumstances and the schedules of reinforcement in determining the pattern and severity of drug-taking behavior. Very severe forms of drug dependence with psychomotor stimulants have been observed in humans. The evidence available makes it clear that the joint presence of drugs with primary reinforcing properties and a "facilitating" schedule of reinforcement jointly constitute the *necessary and sufficient* conditions for the development of severe cases of dependence on stimulants.

Drug dependence is a disorder of behavior, even if one of its consequences is the toxic disturbance of nonbehavioral functions. The proper level of analysis for understanding this pathology and its possible forms of therapy is the behavioral level. Now, behavior is not simply the flow in time of what an organism does. The central nervous system is, in large part, the system of the life of relation with the environment. Many of the important variables in this system are, therefore, located outside, in the environment. These variables encompass the current environment and all the rules of interchange with outside entities and stimuli (what investigators of behavior call by the technical term *schedules of reinforcement*). Drug dependence needs to be analyzed in this context in order to be productively understood.

Another quote from C. R. SMITH (1972) about the epidemic of amphetamine dependence in San Francisco provides details of a schedule of reinforcement that brings out the susceptibility for severe forms of dependence to stimulants.

Given the receptive attitudes toward drug experimentation which most young transients brought to the neighborhood with them, it was predictable that a large percentage would experiment with speed (amphetamine) at one time or another ... Progression depended on several factors. ...Fears were dissipated and the first "fix" (injection) was often administered by a friend. ...Other factors which seem to facilitate progression into compulsive use include: living in an area which either overtly condones drug use or applies no moral sanctions on users; estrangement from meaningful family or social relationships. ...For most individuals, the turn ing point comes when they totally abandon their former life styles and assume the daily routine of the compulsive drug user (falling into a schedule in which drug reinforcement is the major controlling component); developing an identity as a speed freak (addict); forming alliances, both social and business, with other freaks; developing a "hustle" which will support the drug habit; and adopting the rhetoric, values, and attitudes of the speed culture which allow one to justify his way of life to himself. The most important function of the speed culture is to teach participants the art of survival.

The notion of schedule of reinforcement obviously has a strong bearing on the pathogenesis of human dependence on psychomotor stimulants. At times, such as in epidemics of intravenous use of stimulants, the drugs seem to generate a new social form of living, a new schedule of reinforcement for all concerned. The wide diversity of possible schedules of reinforcement under which drugs are self administered may account for the diversity of pictures of drug use presented by reinforcing drugs in the midst of societies during the course of history. There has been a major disproportion between massive availability of stimulants, some of which have been available for centuries or millenia, and the relatively small number of cases of severe dependence on stimulants. It is not yet clear what exactly it is that paves the way for catastrophe. The risk is there, however. Investigators who have personally witnessed monkeys having their first experiences with cocaine self-administration and have seen how their behavior is dramatically "taken over" by the drug, are appalled at the current casual attitudes, reflected in portions of the medical literature, about the "safety" of cocaine.

There are strong reasons to assume that the current schedules of reinforcement under which it is possible for humans to self-administer cocaine do not easily allow the deleterious effects of such drug use to emerge. However, from the knowledge gained through laboratory investigation, it is quite legitimate to be concerned. The barriers to loss of control and damage probably present in certain privileged circles of cocaine users may easily disappear for those belonging to those circles, or such protective schedules may not exist for other social groups and we may again have to face epidemics of damaging use as we had with the amphetamines – epidemics that occurred after decades of widespread availability when everybody, including experts, regarded such compounds as rather safe.

In a recent book about cocaine, its author states that "observations on users and their own comments indicate no true craving or addiction." The content of this quote represents a sample of a widespread opinion about the safety of cocaine. It is at present natural, but regrettable, that the drug itself gets the qualification of "safe" or "dangerous," as if the compound were the only major determinant of dependence. Also, much of our current estimations of risk and dependence severity come from impressions of instances of human drug use, as if dependence were only the result of the contact between the drug and the organism and nothing else mattered much.

Cocaine can produce fierce forms of dependence in animals, resulting in death, under conditions of unlimited availability and low cost. Then, an outstanding question is why severe forms of dependence on cocaine occur so infrequently in humans (at least under current social conditions). The answer can be found in the experimental laboratory itself, but not in the observation of the behavior of animals with access to self-administration; the answer lies in observation of the behavior of laboratory investigators. Inspection of the literature on self-administration of psychomotor stimulants shows that a majority of research papers deal with studies where animals are only allowed restricted access to the drugs. When access is unlimited, animals behave erratically and die quickly. Not much research can be done and published from experiments of unlimited access. Laboratory investigators need their subjects alive, productive, and well behaved. So do sellers of cocaine to humans; sellers need users that are alive and productive. The behavior of the seller is reinforced by earnings he gets from the behavior of users. The schedule of reinforcement in human dependence involves not only the addict but also the seller and other human or economic interactions. From this, it is easy to conceive further factors that may determine the schedule of drug reinforcement of addicts: production costs, local and world supply, etc. Of course, neither the laboratory investigator nor the cocaine seller need be conscious of the determinants of his behavior or explicit about it.

There is no way to account for the facts that give the impression of the safety of cocaine except by factors in the marketplace. This is not an idle speculation. The case of cocaine is probably the best current piece of evidence that schedule factors in the marketplace and not the drug alone determine the pharmacologic effects observed. Another important point is that the pharmacologic properties of the drug in turn contribute to determine the structure of the marketplace; cocaine and heroin generate two different types of marketplace.

It is now possible to make contact between pharmacologic experimentation and notions about the dynamics of the marketplace.

A recent publication by ELSMORE et al. (1980) challenges the validity of another widespread notion about dependence. These authors, together with HURSH (1980), open new research pathways for the understanding and possible control of dependence with incisive concepts that enrich the range of laboratory analysis of behavior with notions borrowed from the field of economics. We shall touch here only the notion of "elasticity of demand." HURSH (1980) makes a strong case for the view that "reinforcers can be distinguished by their demand elasticity apart from differences in value." For the purposes of this paper, demand can be considered as equivalent to the quantity of a reinforcer that is consumed under varying circumstances. An item (or a reinforcer) whose demand (consumption) drops when its price increases or when resources for its purchase decrease is said to be a "luxury." An item whose consumption resists change when its price increases or when resources decrease is said to be a "necessity." The demand for a luxury is said to be elastic whereas the demand for a necessity is said to be inelastic. Thus, in these concepts there is a means of determining in a quantitative fashion whether a dependence-producing drug generates a demand that makes it more a luxury than a necessity, or vice versa. For decades, there has been a solid consensus that heroin dependence constitutes a "need" for this drug. Yet, ELSMORE et al. (1980) have shown in heroin-dependent baboons that the demand for heroin is quite elastic compared with the demand for food. These authors tested the elasticity of the demand for heroin by systematically reducing the "purchasing resources" of the animals. Throughout the day, the baboons were given choice trials with the opportunity to purchase either 3.0 g of food or a 0.1 mg/kg intravenous infusion of heroin. Choice trials were presented at intervals that varied from 2 to 12 min. Therefore, the number of purchasing options during 24 h varied from 720 to 120. The daily number of purchasing options represents the economic resources of the animals. Reduction in economic resources led to a small decrease (23%) in the demand for food (total amount consumed) and to a large decrease (83%) in the demand for heroin. In another study, ELSMORE (quoted in HURSH, 1980) increased the price of food and heroin by increasing the number of lever presses required for the delivery of either reinforcer. Again, the demand for heroin was found to be more elastic than the demand for food. Increasing the price from one required lever press to about 250 produced only a small decrease in the daily amount of food consumed and a large decrease (about 95%) in the number of injections of heroin taken.

For pharmacologists with firsthand experience with opioid dependence, the above results about the elasticity of demand for heroin appear, at first sight, incredible. In fact, careful examination of the data shows that during test conditions involving high resources or low prices, the daily number of heroin self-injections is between 80 and 100. When resources are reduced or prices increased, the daily number of self-injections decreases to a level of about ten. Ten daily injections of 0.1 mg/kg per injection of heroin correspond to daily dose levels at which physical dependence should be expected to be maintained and abstinence prevented. This consideration suggests that Elsmore's experiments should be extended to test whether there might be a region further down, in terms of numbers of daily injections, where demand for heroin becomes inelastic.

Fortunately, we were able to find in the literature data about heroin-reinforced behavior that allowed us to construct demand elasticity curves for heroin at dose levels and daily number of injections below those tested in Elsmore's experiments. HOFF-

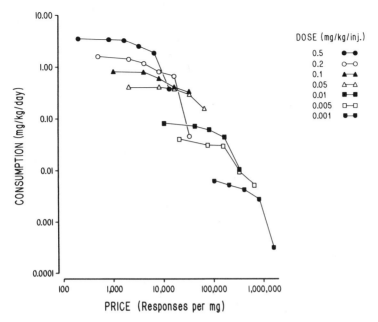

Fig. 1. Curves of elasticity of demand for intravenous heroin in rhesus monkeys. Prices (lever presses required for each injection) were progressively increased until the monkeys no longer paid for the injection. The graph depicts consumption changes as a function of the price per milligram. Each set of points joined by a line represents behaviors maintained by a single dose level. The figure was constructed with data published by HOFFMEISTER (1979)

MEISTER (1979) studied progressive-ratio performances in rhesus monkeys maintained by infusions of several opioids. Procedural details are different from those employed by Elsmore, and the two studies are not strictly comparable on a quantitative basis. For example, Hoffmeister's procedure only allowed for a maximum of eight daily injections; furthermore, heroin was not in competition with food. Data published in tabular form by HOFFMEISTER (1979) were used to construct the demand elasticity curves presented in Fig. 1 and 2 for heroin and pentazocine, respectively.

The curves presented in the figures are families of individual curves, each corresponding to a different unit dose per injection. "Prices" (responses required) for each injection were progressively increased until the animals no longer paid for them. The two families of curves for the two different drugs seem to constitute overall demand elasticity curves for each compound. As behavioral price per milligram increases, consumption decreases. However, every point in the figures indicates the outcome of conditions where self-administration behavior was maintained by the drug for at least some monkeys. Thus, at the extreme point on the right of Fig. 1, prices paid for this drug were computed to reach 1,600,000 responses per milligram. All the monkeys tested at the lowest dose per injection of heroin (0.001 mg/kg) paid prices ranging from 100,000 to 800,000 responses per milligram.

The demand elasticity curves for pentazocine (Fig. 2) are far to the left of those for heroin. The extreme point on the right represents the maximum price paid of 32,000 responses per milligram, 50 times less than the maximum prices paid for her-

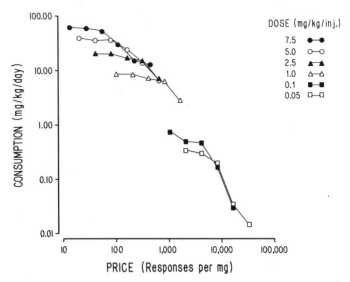

Fig. 2. Curves of elasticity of demand for intravenous pentazocine in rhesus monkeys. Prices (lever presses required for each injection) were progressively increased until the monkeys no longer paid for the injection. The graph depicts consumption changes as a function of the price per milligram. Each set of points joined by a line represents behaviors maintained by a single dose level. The figure was constructed with data published by HOFFMEISTER (1979)

oin. All the monkeys tested at the lowest dose paid prices for pentazocine ranging from 2,000 to 8,000 responses per milligram of the drug, 50–80 times less than the prices paid for the lowest dose of heroin.

A great deal more could be said about the demand elasticity curves in Figs. 1 and 2. However, the main purpose for including them in this paper is to demonstrate that quantitative determinations can be made in the laboratory of the tenacity of drug-seeking behavior generated by dependence-producing drugs. We do not have to rely on visual impressions of the behavior of human or animal addicts or on verbal reports. Unfortunately, we could not find published data in the literature of self-administration of psychomotor stimulants that would allow us to construct wide demand elasticity curves for these drugs.

A few more points deserve attention. Behavior (self-administration or other) can be excessive, but as such it is not necessarily strong. We tend to regard the predisposition to take drugs in dependence as very strong. The fact is that we do not really know much about this. Rats made obese by hypothalamic lesions overeat, but their overeating is very easily disrupted; such behavior is weak. With regard to drug dependence, research on the issue of tenacity has obviously just begun. Excessiveness had not been separated from tenacity. It is now necessary to consider at least these two aspects of reinforcement: the generation of demand and demand elasticity.

The curves in Figs. 1 and 2 for heroin and pentazocine might be misleading if elasticity of demand were to be considered as a single entity. They represent demand elasticities when the amount of drug is regarded as an economic good where price paid per unit weight has uniform significance in commerce. The figures indicate why sellers are a lot more interested in heroin than in pentazocine. The behavioral tenacity of behavior generated by heroin or pentazocine needs to be more precisely determined in a new experiment. HOFFMEISTER (1979) was not attempting to determine behavioral demand elasticities. At the highest prices he required for drug injections, the animals were also under conditions where their resources may be said to have been limited. Time available for lever pressing was 2 h and 45 min (9,900 s) for each injection. The highest price demanded was 12,800 responses per injection, This price was not paid by any animal for any dose of opioids. To pay that price monkeys would have to maintain a rate of lever-pressing of 1.29 responses per second for 2 h and 45 min for each injection. They would have had no time to sleep if they worked for eight injections in a day.

In view of all the above, we may now propose a definition of dependence, in objective terms, that may lead to more quantitative questions about its characteristics and also to sharper questions about the properties of drugs.

C. The Nature of Dependence and Pertinent Aspects of the Properties of Dependence-Producing Drugs

A definition of dependence as a disease, considering its semiologic variables as susceptible to objective quantitation, at least in idealized form, is likely to clarify the experimental questions that may be asked about drugs that are thought or known to be dependence producing.

A wide consensus about the characteristics of dependence may perhaps be formulated explicitly in the following manner. In extreme forms drug dependence consists of

(1) Excessive behavior maintained and centered on drug self-administration (excessive drug-seeking and drug-consuming behavior); (2) Drug-reinforced behavior that is resistant, relative to other behaviors reinforced by other reinforcers necessary to personal and social health, to increases in price requirements or decreases in economic or behavioral resources; (3) Drug-reinforced behavior that assumes a monopoly of all behavior, either because of the prepotency of the reinforcing effects of the drug, or its inelasticity of demand, or direct drug effects that weaken behavioral channels maintained by other reinforcers (this notion should be extended to the weakening of human and moral values); (4) Neurobehavioral toxicity for the individual; (5) Undesirable consequences for family and community.

The above characteristics overlap somewhat, but it seems convenient to state them separately. Also, some terms cut across the different characteristics. For example, excessive behavior may mean behavior that occurs at high frequency, behavior that occurs in a sustained manner, behavior that is inelastic, and behavior that looks excessive because of its toxic or undesirable consequences. Idealized definitions serve only a general purpose. The intention here is to open the way for concrete quantitative assessments.

In the past, definitions of dependence have been made in terms of the type of drug that generates or maintains the disorder. Therefore, the question of pharmacologic specificity deserves discussion. Many kinds of behavior can be nonspecifically reinforced by dependence-producing drugs such as psychomotor stimulants, for example, establishing associations with members of the drug subculture. However, there is one behavior that is always specifically reinforced because it is the necessary terminal point in the chain of events of drug reinforcement. This is the behavior of self-administration. In the case of dependence on stimulants, drug self-administration is also likely to be reinforced by central depressants, barbiturates, or opioids that the individual often takes to avoid or terminate the aversive effects of either excessive dosage or the comedown following episodes of repeated stimulant injections. After a while, a person addicted to central stimulants may come under the control of multiple types of drugs with operant reinforcing properties. Heroin addiction seems to be a common end result of dependence initiated by psychomotor stimulants.

From an epidemiologic point of view, drug dependence behaves as an infectious disease. It requires an etiologic agent, vectors for the distribution of the agent, and a population in a receptive condition. Dependence can spread like infectious epidemics or it can be endemic.

Concerning the "etiologic" agents, i.e., the drugs, it should be emphasized again that the end result of contagion depends not only on pharmacologic characteristics but also on the other determining factors as well. However, sufficient knowledge has been acquired about the entire phenomenon of dependence to make possible the assessment of pharmacologic characteristics that could predict what would happen if contagion occurred under different conditions of receptivity.

First, risk may be regarded as related to high values of primary operant reinforcing characteristics determined in a wide variety of circumstances. Drugs with these wide reinforcing characteristics pose a generalized risk. Second, high values of primary reinforcing efficacy indicate that drug-seeking behavior can be rapidly induced and that such behavior can be excessive in frequency and in amount. Third, the tenacity of dependence can be assessed in appropriate tests where drug-reinforced behavior is made to compete with behaviors maintained by other reinforcers. Fourth, some characteristics of the drug marketplace may be inferred from certain pharmacologic properties. Drugs that have steep dose-response curves or that have a narrow range of doses with reinforcing properties are likely to maintain a market where users cannot cut down or adulterate and resell a portion of their purchased doses. Drugs that induce paranoid ideation may restrict the range of criminal activities aimed at obtaining money to purchase the drug. SMITH (1972) states:

> In the heroin community, the brunt of the hustling activities is borne by the non-using population. In the speed scene, most of the criminality is directed toward other members of the drug scene. The speed scene differs from other drug scenes in that the money needed to sustain the marketplace is not generated with any regularity by the individual user who is committed to the life style centering around speed use. Unable to generate money outside the community, the culture has turned on itself, creating a climate of fear, suspicion, and violence which shows litte sign of abating.

D. Epidemiologic and Clinical Aspects of Dependence on Psychomotor Stimulants

GRIFFITH (1977) has published an interesting and comprehensive review of human dependence to psychomotor stimulants, including a detailed relation of historical developments. MASAKI (1956) and KATO (1972) discuss the Japanese experience of epidemic amphetamine dependence. The proceedings of a symposium on abuse of central stimulants (SJÖQVIST and TOTTIE, 1969) contain contributions describing medical and social aspects of the abuse of central stimulants in the Scandinavian peninsula. KALLANT (1966, 1973) reviewed the world literature on human amphetamine addiction.

Isolated instances of dependence on psychomotor stimulants self-administered by the oral route are well documented. Cases are reported that last years with consumption levels that are not too high. However, most reports of dependence refer to individuals who take large doses, up to daily levels about 100 times the unit available dose, and who develop profound somatic behavioral and psychiatric alterations that require hospitalization.

The most severe forms of psychostimulant dependence occur with intravenous self-administration. Vivid accounts of amphetamine intravenous dependence are given by GRIFFITH (1966), KRAMER et al. (1967), CAREY and MANDEL (1968), HAWKS et al. (1969), and SMITH (1972). Early intravenous use is intermittent and doses on the order of 20–40 mg per injection may be taken once or a very few times over a day or two. Then the drug is taken in sprees. Weeks may intervene between the sprees. Gradually, the sprees become longer, the doses larger, and the intervals between sprees shorter. A final pattern is reached where subjects self-inject the drug many times a day, reaching dose levels that may be as high as 1,000 mg; they remain awake for 3–6 days, becoming anxious, tense, tremulous, and paranoid. Spree runs are interrupted by periods where self-administration is "spontaneously" interrupted and a complex called "crashing" occurs, where subjects fall into profound sleep. Amphetamine users uniformly lose weight and after the crash ravenous hunger ensues.

A paranoid psychosis is an almost inevitable consequence of stimulant overconsumption. Clearly, this effect has been observed in persons who are psychiatrically normal, and the available evidence overwhelmingly indicates that the psychosis is a drug-induced phenomenon. Termination of drug use leads to quick and complete recovery of the thought disorder.

It is worthy of note that severe dependence on psychomotor stimulants appears unstable on the whole. Drug-taking occurs in irregular cycles. In contrast with opioids, complete remissions occur.

Stimulant dependence is also unstable as a social group phenomenon. SMITH (1972), in discussing the San Francisco epidemic of amphetamine dependence, refers to three types of career patterns for amphetamine users: (1) continued marginal adjustment, usually terminated by arrest, hospitalization, voluntary treatment, or death; (2) elevation to the upper levels of the marketplace; and (3) progression to barbiturates or heroin.

E. Methods for the Laboratory Study of Drug Self-Administration

Techniques and procedures have been developed to allow experimental animals the self-administration of drugs by the intravenous route. Intravenous self-administration is the most sensitive way of assessing the dependence-producing properties of drugs. First, a great deal of laboratory work has shown that positive reinforcers of operant behavior are much more effective in generating behavior when the reinforcer makes contact with the organism at the shortest time interval after the emission of the operant. Second, clinical observation has produced a wide consensus that intravenous self-administration of dependence-producing drugs presents the highest risk of acquiring dependence and causes its most tenacious forms. Third, intravenous injection is likely to produce the severest kinds of toxicity for the majority of drugs. Details of the techniques, equipment, and procedures used with different animal species can be found elsewhere (e.g., Weeks, 1962; Thompson and Schuster, 1964; Stretch and Gerber, 1970; Findley et al., 1971, 1972; Jones and Prada, 1973; Balster et al., 1976). The following is a brief summary of the general procedure. One of the major veins (e.g., external or internal jugulars, femorals) is surgically exposed under general anesthesia. A plastic catheter is fixed in place and its opposite end is passed under the skin to a place of exit the animal will find it difficult to reach, the middle of the back, for example. Usually, the animal is previously trained to carry a harness that will further protect the catheter from being reached at its exit and provide a final point of attachment for a more or less flexible arm through which the catheter passes to an infusion machinery located in the outside of the cage. The flexible arm is fixed to the cage and must be flexible enough to permit relative freedom of movement to the experimental animal, but it must be sturdy enough to withstand the stresses imposed by the movements of the sometimes hyperactive animal and prevent damage to the catheter. The infusion system can be a peristaltic, a rotary, or a syringe pump that can deliver a few mililiters per minute, depending on the size of the experimental animal. The infusion pump is controlled by electronic programming equipment that makes possible the administration of drugs under a wide variety of rules called programs or schedules.

The levels and patterns of drug intake and the amounts and patterns of the operant and associated behavior maintained or produced by central stimulants depend on a number of factors: (a) the reinforcing properties of the drug, (b) the schedule of drug delivery and availability, (c) the dosage per injection, (d) the half-life of the drug, and (e) the state variables. This last class of variables are those describing manipulations other than those strictly described by the schedule of drug delivery, e.g., food and water deprivation or satiation and pharmacologic pretreatment.

For studies of self-administration, the control equipment is set up to deliver a drug infusion whenever a behavioral requirement is met, e.g., pressing a lever with a given force.

When drug delivery is made dependent on the animal's behavior, it can be made dependent on a required number of responses or on a time requirement, or on some combination of both. When an animal has to repeat a certain behavior a fixed or variable number of times in order to produce an infusion of a drug, it is said to be in a ratio schedule (a number schedule). Ratio schedules can be fixed (FR), variable (VR), or progressive (PR). When the first response after a time interval is followed by a drug infusion, it is said to be in an interval schedule. Interval schedules can be fixed (FI) or variable (VI).

Combinations of these elementary schedules are possible. Manipulations of schedules are experimental probes into different aspects of behavior and direct pharmacologic actions. The purposes of their experimental use and the significance of results obtained will be discussed further on in appropriate sections.

F. Self-Administration of Psychomotor Stimulants by Laboratory Animals

When one of a wide variety of central stimulants is made available to an animal from one of several laboratory species at a cost of one or a few responses per injection, the animal rapidly acquires a predisposition to respond for drug injections. The number of self-injected doses of the drug increases rapidly, faster than with narcotics or barbiturates. The species tested for self-administration of psychomotor stimulants, all with positive results, include rats (e.g., PICKENS and THOMPSON, 1967), rhesus monkeys (e.g., DENEAU et al., 1969), baboons (e.g., GRIFFITHS et al., 1975), cats (e.g., BALSTER et al., 1976), squirrel monkeys (e.g., KELLEHER and GOLDBERG, 1977), dogs (e.g., JASINSKI et al., 1978), and pig-tailed macaques (e.g., YOUNG and WOODS, 1980).

A number of central stimulants have been tested and proven capable of starting and maintaining varying levels and patterns of drug-taking behavior in several laboratory species. The following is a list of compounds which are psychomotor stimulants or substances related to them either in chemistry or pharmacology. The list includes names of the compounds, a notation of whether positive or negative results were obtained with regard to their positive reinforcing properties, and a reference number to published papers also listed further below. The list of referenced papers includes the range of doses tested in milligram per kilogram per injection, the species, and the author(s) and date of the study.

List of Compounds

D-Amphetamine (+) [5, 7, 9, 13, 18, 20, 22, 24, 26, 27, 28, 32, 36, 38, 39]

L-Amphetamine (+) [18, 20, 26]

Apomorphine (+) [38]

Caffeine (+) [7]

DL-Cathinone (+) [30]

L-Cathinone (+) [30, 40]

Chlorphentermine (+) [13, 14]

Chlortermine (+) [13]

Cocaine (+) [1, 2, 3, 4, 7, 8, 11, 12, 13, 14, 15, 16, 17, 18, 19, 20, 21, 23, 24, 25, 28, 29, 31, 33, 34, 35, 36, 37, 41]

Diethylpropion (+) [13, 14, 20]

DITA (+) [9]

DMA (−) [13]

N-Ethylamphetamine (+) [33, 34]

N-Ethylamphetamine, m-fluoro (+) [34]

N-Ethylamphetamine, m-bromo (+) [34]

N-Ethylamphetamine, m-methyl (+) [34]

N-Ethylamphetamine, m-iodo (−) [34]

N-Ethylamphetamine, m-t-butyl (−) [34]

Fencamfamin (+) [10]

Fenfluramine (−) [13, 14, 33]

Mazindol (+) [37]

MK-212 (−) [5]

Mescaline (−) [7]

Metamphetamine (+) [2, 7, 18]

D-Metamphetamine (+) [20]

Methylphenidate (+) [12, 18, 19, 27, 35, 36]

L-Noradrenaline (+) [6]

Norcocaine (+) [3, 28]

β-Phenethylamine (+) [18]

Phenmetrazine (+) [13, 18, 27, 35, 36]

Phentermine (+) [13]

Pipradrol (+) [35, 36]

SPA (+) [10].

List of Referenced Papers

1. Cocaine (+), 0.025–0.8, rhesus monkeys, BALSTER and SCHUSTER (1973); 2. Methamphetamine (+), 0.005–0.16; cocaine (+), 0.05, cats, BALSTER et al. (1976); 3. Cocaine (+), 0.025–0.8, rhesus monkeys, BEDFORD et al. (1978); 4. Cocaine (+), 0.2, norcocaine (+), 0.05–0.8, rhesus monkeys, BEDFORD et al. (1980); 5. MK-212[6-chloro-2-(1-piperazinyl)-pyrazine] (−), 0.1–0.5, D-amphetamine, (+), 0.1–0.3, rats, CLINESCHMIDT et al. (1977); 6. L-Noradrenaline (+), 0.021 [in the lateral hypothalamus], rats, CYTAWA et al. (1980); 7. Cocaine (+), 0.25–1.0, D-amphetamine (+), 0.1, methamphetamine (+), 0.1, caffeine (+), 1.0–5.0, mescaline (−), 1.0–10.0, rhesus monkeys, DENEAU et al. (1969); 8. Cocaine (+), 0.32–0.64, rats, DOUGHERTY and PICKENS (1973); 9. DITA[3′,4′-dichloro-2-(2-imidazolin-2-yl-thio)-, acetophenone hydrobromide] (+), 0.01–0.1, D-amphetamine (+), 0.01–0.03, rhesus monkeys, DOWNS and WOODS (1975); 10. Fencamfamine [2-phenyl-3-ethylaminobicyclo-(2,2,1)-heptane] (+), 0.1–2.0, SPA [(L)-1-2-diphenyl-1-dimethyl-aminoethane] (+), 0.1–2.0, rhesus monkeys, ESTRADA et al. (1967); 11. Cocaine (+), 0.75–3.0, rhesus monkeys, GOLDBERG et al. (1976); 12. Cocaine (+), 0.4–1.6, methylphenidate (+), 0.1–0.8, baboons, GRIFFITHS et al. (1975); 13. Cocaine (+), 0.4, D-amphetamine (+), 0.01–0.5, phenmetrazine (+), 0.1–2.0, phentermine (+), 0.1–1.0, diethylpropion (+), 0.1–10.0, chlorphentermine (+), 0.1–5.0, chlortermine (+), 0.1–5.0, fenfluramine (−), 0.02–5.0, DMA [methylenedioxy-amphetamine] (−), 0.1–5.0, baboons, GRIFFITHS et al. (1976); 14. Cocaine (+), 0.01–3.0, chlorphentermine (+), 0.03–10.0, diethylpropion (+), 0.1–10.0, fenfluramine (−), 0.02–5.0, baboons, GRIFFITHS et al. (1978a); 15. Cocaine (+), 0.01–4.0, baboons, GRIFFITHS et al. (1979); 16. Cocaine (+), 0.03, rhesus monkeys, HERLING et al. (1979); 17. Cocaine (+), 0.013–0.8, rhesus monkeys, IGLAUER and WOODS (1974); 18. Cocaine (+), 0.15–0.6, D-amphetamine (+), 0.025–0.2, L-amphetamine (+), 0.2–0.8, methamphetamine (+), 0.03–0.12, methylphenidate (+), 0.05–0.4, phenmetrazine (+), 0.2–1.6, β-phenethylamine (+), 1.5–6.0, dogs, JASINSKI et al. (1978); 19. Cocaine (+), 0.05–1.5, methylphenidate (+), 0.075–0.7, rhesus monkeys, JOHANSON and SCHUSTER (1975); 20. Cocaine (+), 0.2, D-amphetamine (+), 0.05, L-amphetamine (+), 0.05, D-methamphetamine (+), 0.025, diethylpropion (+), 0.5, rhesus monkeys, JOHANSON et al. (1976a); 21. Cocaine (+), 0.1–0.2, rhesus monkeys, JOHANSON et al. (1976b); 22. D-Amphetamine (+), 0.05, dogs, JONES and PRADA (1973); 23. Cocaine (+), 0.03–0.6, squirrel monkeys, KELLEHER and GOLDBERG (1977); 24. Cocaine (+), 0.25–3.0, D-amphetamine (+), 0.25–1.0, rats, PICKENS and THOMPSON (1967); 25. Cocaine (+), 0.25–3.0, rats, PICKENS and THOMPSON (1968); 26. D-Amphetamine (+), 0.05–0.1, L-amphetamine (+), 0.2–0.8, dogs, RISNER (1975); 27. D-Amphetamine (+), 0.025–0.2, phenmetrazine (+), 0.2–1.6, methylphenidate (+), 0.05–0.4, dogs, RISNER and JONES (1975); 28. Cocaine (+), 0.15–0.6, norcocaine (+), 0.15, D-amphetamine (+), 0.05–0.1, dogs, RISNER and JONES (1980); 29. Cocaine (+), SÁNCHEZ-RAMOS and SCHUSTER (1977); 30. DL-Cathinone [α-aminopropiophenone] (+), unknown doses, L-cathinone (+), unknown doses, rhesus monkeys, SCHUSTER and JOHANSON (1979); 31. Cocaine (+), 0.01–0.1, squirrel monkeys, SPEALMAN (1979); 32. D-Amphetamine (+), 0.05–0.8, rats, TAKAHASHI et al. (1978); 33. Cocaine (+), 0.03, N-ethylamphetamine (+), 0.01–0.1, fenfluramine (−), 0.01–0.3, rhesus monkeys, TESSEL and WOODS (1975); 34. Cocaine (+), 0.03, N-ethylamphetamine (+), 0.01–0.1, *meta*-fluoro N-ethylamphetamine (+), 0.01–0.1, m-bromo N-ethylamphetamine (+), 0.03–0.3, m-methyl N-ethylampheta-

mine (+), 0.03–0.3, m-iodo N-ethylamphetamine (−), 0.01–0.3, m-t-butyl N-ethyl-lamphetamine (−), 0.01–0.3, rhesus monkeys, TESSEL and WOODS (1978); 35. Cocaine (+), 0.025–1.2, pipradrol (+), 0.025–0.4, methylphenidate (+), 0.025–0.4, phenmetrazine (+), 0.025–0.8, rhesus monkeys, WILSON et al. (1971); 36. Cocaine (+), 0.1–0.2, phenmetrazine (+), 0.1, methylphenidate (+), 0.05, pipradrol (+), 0.1, D-amphetamine (+), 0.025, rhesus monkeys, WILSON and SCHUSTER (1972); 37. Mazindol [5-p-chloro-phenyl-5-hydroxy-2,3-dihydro-5H-imidazo (2,1-a) isoindol] (+), 0.05–0.2, cocaine (+), 0.2, rhesus monkeys, WILSON and SCHUSTER (1976); 38. D-Amphetamine (+), 0.25, apomorphine (+), 0.5, rats, WISE et al. (1976); 39. D-Amphetamine (+), 0.25, rats, WISE et al. (1977); 40. L-Cathinone (+), 0.06–0.25, rhesus monkeys, YANAGITA (1979); 41. Cocaine (+), 0.01–1.0, rhesus macaques *(M. mulatta)* and pig-tailed macaques *(M. nemestrina)*, YOUNG and WOODS (1980).

I. Self-Administration Under Unlimited Drug Access

Two main types of experiment of drug self-administration with psychomotor stimulants have been employed. In one the drug is made continuously available, 24 h a day, at low cost, and in the absence of other strong behaviors that may compete with self-administration. The purpose of this type of experiment is to allow the emergence of the overall picture of self-administration and its possible accompanying behavioral and somatic toxicities under conditions of minimal restriction; risk and maximum severity of consequences are thus amply facilitated. In the second main type of experiment, the drug is made available either during sessions of limited length, and/or with schedule manipulations, with the purpose of seeking answers to more specific behavioral or pharmacologic questions.

Under continuous drug availability at low cost, animals self-administer stimulants at high rates, easily reaching 1,000 injections per day when the unit dose per injection is not high. However, the pattern of intake over successive days is very irregular, with peaks and valleys of high and low rates of self-administration of disorderly duration (e.g., ESTRADA et al., 1967; PICKENS and THOMPSON, 1967, 1968; DENEAU et al., 1969; BALSTER et al., 1976; JOHANSON et al., 1976a; JASINSKI et al., 1978).

Most of the reports coincide in that animals engage in sprees of rapid intake for a few days during which the animal does not eat and does not sleep, and severe toxic effects develop. Usually, after these episodes of frantic activity and very high rates of drug intake, the animal spontaneously ceases self-injecting and overeats and oversleeps. After 1 or a few days, the animal starts another spree of high drug intake. Monkeys usually die after a short exposure to this schedule of drug availability (DENEAU et al., 1969; JOHANSON et al., 1976a). Lower mortalities seem to occur in other animal species. However, studies of this kind in other species are fewer. Despite wide variations in the daily and even in the hourly rate of drug intake, within the effective range of doses an inverse relationship has been observed between the maximum number of self-administrations per day and the unit dose per injection (ESTRADA et al., 1967).

The following is the description given by DENEAU et al., (1969) of the toxic effects seen in the rhesus monkey self-administering cocaine under continuous availability:

> During self-administration of cocaine the monkeys became apprehensive and restless, showed almost constant choreiform movements, stereotypy, dysmetria, tremors, mydriasis, pilo-erection and gross ataxia during the first several days. As the dosage increased in daily

amount and duration, signs of somatic and psychotoxicity increased. The monkeys showed an extremely rapid loss of muscle mass and grand mal convulsions became frequent. Behavior consistent with visual hallucinations (staring and grasping at the wall) and tactile hallucinations (continued scratching and biting of the skin of the extremities, to the point of producing extensive wounds and even amputation of the digits) was consistently observed. The monkeys also appeared to become unaware of their surroundings in that they ignored raisins and candy which were proffered by the experimenters. These manifestations of toxicity were rapidly reversible when cocaine administration was discontinued.

The same authors state that with D-amphetamine and methamphetamine the picture of the toxic syndrome was similar except that it was slightly less severe.

The effects of unlimited access to cocaine, D- and L-amphetamine, D-methamphetamine, and diethylpropion were studied comparatively in rhesus monkeys by JOHANSON et al. (1976a). Doses tested per injection were in the upper middle range of reinforcing effectiveness. The monkeys took from 400 to 1,200 injections per day at the peak rates observed in the irregular cycles of self-administration. The monkeys on cocaine died within 5 days. With amphetamine and methamphetamine, the animals also died but survived a little longer than with cocaine. Severe overall toxicity also occurred with diethylpropion, but three of five animals on this drug survived for the 30 days that the experiment lasted.

II. Self-Administration Under Restricted Drug Access

Since unlimited access to stimulants leads to irregular behavior, severe toxicity, and early death, studies with limited availability were initiated with the objective of achieving longer lives for the animals and behavioral performances better suited to experimental analysis. When access to stimulants is restricted to daily sessions of a few hours' duration, even if the costs per injection are low and there are no competing behaviors, behavioral and organic toxicity is reduced and several orderly relationships appear (ESTRADA et al., 1967; PICKENS and THOMPSON, 1967, 1968; WILSON et al., 1971; RISNER, 1975; RISNER and JONES, 1975, 1980; DOUGHERTY and PICKENS, 1976) (1) Drug intake per session becomes very stable from day to day; (2) For all stimulants studied, there is a threshold unit dose per injection that generally gives the highest number of self-administrations per session; (3) Beyond the threshold dose, frequencies of self-administration decrease as the unit dose per injection increases; (4) As a consequence of this inverse relationship between unit dose and frequency of infusions, total drug intake per session varies little over a wide range of unit doses.

The factors responsible for the contrast between the irregular patterns of drug intake observed under unlimited access to stimulants and the regularity obtained with limited access have not been formally identified. However, the excessive neurobehavioral toxicity produced by sustained high drug concentrations during several days of spree use is likely to play a role in the irregularity of intake. Possible contributing factors may include total disorganization of sleep and other biologic rhythms. Whatever the mechanisms, there seems to be a disruption of processes related to reinforcement and/or inhibition of behavior by aversive consequences. It is attractive to think of the extended drug-free periods imposed by restricted access as necessary for the consolidation of behavioral controls. Nevertheless, this idea must be tested against the notion that high concentrations of stimulants directly disrupt such controls.

Another point that deserves attention is that with restricted access to stimulants there is no long-term tendency to increase the dose consumed per session. High doses are taken from the start. This fact raises questions about the meaning of tolerance in human addicts, when tolerance is considered in the sense of a progressive increase in dose self administered.

A good review of the finer features of self-administration behavior under limited availability and low costs was made by DOUGHERTY and PICKENS (1976) with regard to intravenous cocaine self-injection by rats. The principal findings they review are: (1) There is an initial burst of shortly spaced self-injections at the start of each session; (2) After the initial burst, the animals develop a very regular spacing of drug injections; (3) After the initial burst, a slight (7% per hour) positive trend in the mean interinjection interval is observed along the session, across the effective dose range; (4) The regular spacing of drug injections does not appear in the first contact of the animal with the drug, but it is developed within the first several days of exposure to sessions of limited drug access, indicating the necessity of time for the acquisition of controls; (5) Short-term oscillations in interinjection interval length occur along the session around the mean interval; (6) The mean interinjection interval is directly and linearly related to unit dose, not to its logarithm; (7) Enzymatic induction with phenobarbital (40 mg/kg per day) reduced the mean interinjection interval; (8) Enzymatic inhibition with SKF 525 A (5, 20, 20, and 40 mg/kg) produced a dose-related increase in the mean interinjection interval; (9) Cocaine injected via a chronically implanted catheter, while a rat is responding for food, makes the animal stop responding totally for dose-related periods. The size of these pauses in food-maintained responding is similar to that seen between injections of self-administered cocaine when a rat is responding for that drug.

DOUGHERTY and PICKENS (1976) also review the pharmacokinetics of cocaine and suggest that in the self-administration of this drug under restricted access, the intensity of effect may be close to 100% and that the regularity of intervals between injections may be due to the regular decline in intensity of effect because of drug disposition. For example, the decline of effect to a particular level may be a stimulus condition for the initiation of a new self-administration response. Likewise, the increase in the intensity of some effect to a certain level may be a discriminating stimulus for the cessation of responding.

Pharmacokinetic dynamics are likely to be involved in the determination of the regularities of self-administration under limited access. However, the question remains as to how the dynamics of blood and tissue levels of a drug or its metabolites could determine behavior.

Three general possible explanations have been or could be offered for the regularity in frequency of self-administration with any given unit dose as well as for the relatively small variation in total session intake over a broad range of unit doses: (1) that progressively higher drug doses exert progressively longer direct disruptive effects on behavior that correspond to the intervals between responses of self-administration; (2) that at high blood levels, there occur aversive effects that counterbalance the process of reinforcement and, thus, lead to a suppression of self-administration until enough of the drug has been metabolized or excreted; (3) that there may be some regulatory mechanism that tends to maintain a sort of "optimum" blood or tissue level of the drug.

This last mechanism is most unlikely, but it deserves discussion. Properly formulated, the mechanism of feedback regulation, to be different from the first two mentioned, must be formulated as a mechanism with a regulatory "set point." The initial rapid responding at the start of the self-administration session could appear as behavior leading to an optimum level. Once that level is reached, a quite regular and dose-related spacing appears. Within this relatively stable phase, the observed short-term oscillations could be interpreted as the amount of deviation from the optimum drug level that is permitted before the feedback systems sends a "correction" signal of feedback control. However, the existence of a set-point mechanism for the self-administration of stimulants, similar to that participating in processes such as body temperature regulation, must be regarded as highly unlikely. Therefore, the weight of evidence for its existence should be proportionate to the a priori degree of its improbability. The attainment of an "equilibrium" dose level, as well as oscillations around that level, occurs in systems without regulatory set-points. Further, if there were any regulation, the set-point would seem far off any reasonably expected level; in spite of the appearance of regulation, the total drug intake per session is very high. More importantly, there is a great deal of evidence indicating that direct actions of stimulants, and other self-administered drugs, suppress behavior at high doses for a length of time proportional to their presence in the body (see review by KELLEHER, 1976). PICKENS and THOMPSON (1967, 1968) have shown that cocaine, injected by the experimenter into animals whose lever-pressing behavior is maintained by food, produces dose-dependent pauses which are almost identical in duration to the intervals found between self-injections of the drug.

There is experimental and clinical evidence for the presence of aversive properties in psychomotor stimulants, especially at high doses. Therefore, it would seem that the apparent regulation observed in sessions of restricted access to psychomotor stimulants merely represents equilibrium points reached between the opposing tendencies of the process of reinforcement, the direct suppressant drug effects, and the punishing effects of aversive drug properties.

G. Chains of Behavior Maintained by Psychomotor Stimulants

Since one of the aims of laboratory research on drug self-administration is to investigate the quantitative characteristics of drugs as reinforcers, "an important perspective can be gained by considering behavior that is engendered and maintained by drug injections in the context of what is known about behavior maintained by other events" (KELLEHER, 1976).

The proceedings of a symposium on the control of drug-taking behavior by schedules of reinforcement (DE V. COTTEN, 1976) give a comprehensive review of research work where the reinforcing effects of drugs are compared with those of other reinforcers under schedules of reinforcement that have been in widespread use for the experimental analysis of behavior. The reader interested in the behavioral characteristics and mechanisms of drug dependence is referred to the papers presented in that symposium. There is ample evidence that psychomotor stimulants maintain orderly chains of behavior with performances that match quantitatively and qualitatively the performances maintained by food or other well-known reinforcing stimuli.

Because drug dependence is not just self-administration behavior, but all of the behavior that is engendered by the reinforcing effects of drugs, the laboratory study of the chains of behavior that lead to drug injection is of special interest and offers great promise for an understanding of the whole phenomenon of dependence. One type of schedule that generates long chains of behavior, second-order schedules, will be discussed here. Later sections will examine how schedules of reinforcement can be utilized to assess in a quantitative fashion the reinforcing potencies and efficacies of psychomotor stimulants as well as the strength of the drug-seeking behavior that these drugs produce.

Second-order schedules (KELLEHER, 1966) take advantage of a process by which a primary or unconditioned reinforcer confers reinforcing properties to previously neutral stimuli. In the laboratory such neutral stimuli can be colored lights, sounds, or poker chips; in real life, one may think of pieces of paper called money, or others.

A second-order schedule of drug reinforcement can be arranged in the following manner. Initially, the reinforcing drug is given in the presence of some salient neutral stimulus such as a light. This paired presentation of the primary reinforcer with the neutral stimulus is made to follow the emission of the response to be reinforced. After a number of pairings of the two stimuli, the schedule is changed in such a way that some responses produce as their only consequence the light previously associated with the administration of the reinforcing drug. After a sequence, at first short, of responses producing only the light, this is presented together with an injection of the reinforcing drug. By gradually lengthening the sequence of responses reinforced by the secondary reinforcer (the light), very large amounts of behavior can be generated and maintained by a few injections of the reinforcing drug. In its final form, a performance under a second-order schedule is usually formed by sequences of responses reinforced by the secondary reinforcer; then a succession of these sequences is in turn reinforced by the primary reinforcer. GOLDBERG (1973), GOLDBERG et al. (1976, KELLEHER and GOLDBERG (1977), and SÁNCHEZ-RAMOS and SCHUSTER (1977) have published on the characteristics of behavior generated by second-order schedules, with psychomotor stimulants as primary reinforcers.

Besides their contribution to understanding behavior in drug dependence, second-order schedules have practical applications. One such application permits the study of drug-seeking behavior with intramuscular instead of intravenous injections of psychomotor stimulants (GOLDBERG, 1973, GOLDBERG et al., 1976). Intramuscular injections eliminate the technical necessities associated with long-term intravenous catheters and the problems of infectious disease these preparations carry.

H. Quantitative Assessment of Reinforcing Properties

Different experimental paradigms have been employed and adapted to assess the magnitude of the reinforcing properties of drugs. Some of these deal with important aspects of self-administration behavior but are not directly aimed at estimating the reinforcing actions of drugs. An example of the latter is the determination of frequencies of drug injections, given at low cost, that are maintained by different dose levels per injection. Other experimental paradigms deal with aspects of behavior more precisely related to the operational definition of reinforcement and reinforcer. As stated previously, reinforcement of operant behavior consists primarily in the increase in the probability of its occurrence (rate and amount) by a consequent stimulus. There are two general types of these paradigms that have been most widely used in the study of self-administration of psychomotor stimulants. One is the measurement of preference by the experimental subject for one of two simultaneously available stimuli. Preference of one stimulus over another indicates that the behavior maintained by the former stimulus is preportent over the behavior maintained by the latter. Another paradigm consists in the systematic determination of the maximum behavioral output that is consistently sustained by a drug (progressive ratio schedules). Both general methods comprise a diversity of procedural alternatives.

JASINSKI et al. (1978), RISNER (1975), and RISNER and JONES (1975, 1980) using dogs as experimental subjects have made bioassays of the self-administration of a number of central stimulants. The variable they use is the number of self-injections that the animal takes during 4-h sessions on an FR-1 schedule (under an FR-1, one response produces one self-injection). The bioassay is based on dose-response curves of frequencies of self-injection. These bioassays compare the relative potencies of drugs that maintain equivalent levels of self-administration behavior. However, these investigations, as well as a number of other studies (e.g., DOUGHERTY and PICKENS, 1976; ESTRADA et al., 1967; JOHANSON and SCHUSTER, 1975; PICKENS and THOMPSON, 1967, 1968; WILSON et al., 1971), have shown that with psychomotor stimulants, for a broad range of doses, the frequency of injections decreases as the dose per injection increases (the interval between injections grows in proportion to the dose injected). In the previous section, evidence was presented that intervals between self-injections, under low-cost schedules of restricted access, are more a reflection of drug duration and of other drug actions than of reinforcing properties. In fact, when the experimental preparation is focused primarily on reinforcing properties, it has been shown that within a broad range of doses, reinforcing efficacy of psychomotor stimulants increases with increments in dosage (see below). The bioassay of self-administration of psychomotor stimulants that measures frequency of injections at different dose levels and that determines equivalent levels of self-injection behavior provides useful pharmacologic information. Yet, as with other dose-response curves for drugs that simultaneously exert actions that tend to move the biologic system in opposite directions, the dose-response curves of self-administration in terms of frequency of injections are the end result of the mixture of reinforcing properties with other behavioral actions of the drugs.

In order to dissect experimentally the reinforcing actions proper of psychomotor stimulants, the choice and the progressive ratio procedures have been used with success. A brief description of these and a discussion of the information thus far obtained follow.

I. Evaluation of Preference

In this field there are two general instances in which preference procedures can be applied: one, to ascertain whether a drug is a positive reinforcer; another, to assess the relative potency of two or more known reinforcers. In either case, a set of options is presented to the experimental subject. In the first case, the options must be, on one hand, a solution of the test drug, or, on the other hand, just the inert drug vehicle. In the second case, the options can be solutions with different concentrations (different doses) of the same drug, or solutions of equal or different concentrations of different drugs. In the first case, if the animal chooses the drug over the vehicle option, the drug can be regarded as a positive reinforcer under the test conditions.

Drug choice behavior can be assessed by means of two types of general procedures: One type consists of discrete trials in which the options are presented at the beginning of the trial in order to let the animal choose, and once the choice is made, the other alternatives are no longer available until the next trial (e.g., FINDLEY et al., 1972; JOHANSON and SCHUSTER, 1975). The second type of procedure arranges for the continuous and simultaneous availability of the alternatives. One particular case of this kind of procedures is that of concurrent schedules (e.g., IGLAUER and WOODS, 1974).

FINDLEY et al., (1972) gave the first detailed description of a choice procedure employing intravenous self-administration of psychoactive drugs (secobarbital and chlordiazepoxide).

The following methodologic points have been included in drug choice tests with psychomotor stimulants: (1) The experimental subjects must make enough contacts with each of the options so that they get to "know" them well. (2) Some external stimulus must be paired with each of the alternatives being presented in a trial; this allows the animal to choose the alternatives by its associated external stimulus and it also permits one to test whether the preference is based on the pharmacologic properties of the alternatives, or if it is based on the external stimuli (this test is made by reversing the stimuli associated with each of the alternatives after a clear and stable preference is developed for the first association). (3) The choice must be permitted enough times to establish a clear, consistent preference. (4) Choice trials must not be closely spaced in time to avoid the interaction of some of the pharmacologic effects of the drugs with all the subject's behavior, i.e., there must be time-outs after drug injections.

JOHANSON and SCHUSTER (1975) first compared the psychomotor stimulants cocaine and methylphenidate in choice tests. Each session began with two "sampling" periods during which the experimental subject was faced five times with each of two options at the start of the session. After that, the choice trials were started, each followed by a time-out of 15 min. At the start of each trial the exteroceptive stimuli associated with each of the options were presented. The first response on one of the two levers served as a choice response; four more responses on the same lever produced the chosen option. They found that no preference was shown for either cocaine or methylphenidate when these drugs were given in equal doses. When different doses were presented, the higher was always preferred, for both drugs. These authors also found that during the sampling periods, when the options were presented separately without time-outs between injections, the rate of self-injection was inversely related to the dose of the drug in turn. For all doses, the frequency of self-injections was always two to three times higher for cocaine than for methylphenidate. The higher rate of cocaine self-injections during the sampling periods of the sessions was regarded as the consequence of the shorter disruption of self-administration behavior produced by this drug because of its shorter half-life. Thus, cocaine and methylphenidate were preferred about equally, and higher doses of either drug were preferred to low doses.

This indicates that the reinforcing actions of these two drugs are about equal in this test, and that higher doses are more reinforcing than the lower ones. This conclusion would not have been borne out if rates of self-injection (during the sampling periods) had been taken as measures of reinforcing action; such rates are lower for the higher doses of either drug and higher for cocaine than for methylphenidate at all doses tested.

In another study of drug choices, JOHANSON and SCHUSTER (1976) found that diethylpropion is about one-tenth as potent as cocaine and is generally less efficacious in terms of drug preference.

The fact that high doses of cocaine are more reinforcing than lower ones was documented in a different procedure designed to evaluate preferences through a concurrent schedule (IGLAUER and WOODS, 1974; IGLAUER et al., 1976). In concurrent schedules, the two optional reinforcements are simultaneously and continuously available, but to reach either option the experimental subject must perform a task. In this particular case, the task was lever-pressing on a variable interval schedule of cocaine reinforcement on two levers, each associated with injections of different doses of drug. Timeouts followed each injection. Higher rates of lever pressing were obtained on the lever option associated with higher doses of drug.

J. Progressive Ratios: Evaluation of the Maximum Behavioral Output Sustained by Self-Administration

Another experimental procedure conceptually related to the operational definition of reinforcement is one in which the amount of behavior (lever presses) required from the experimental animal, for a given amount of a reinforcer, is systematically increased until the animal no longer pays the behavioral price of the increased requirement. Since some behavior continues to be emitted, practical decisions about failure of completion of the requirement need a criterion cutoff point, for example, failure to complete at least two ratios within a period of 24 h. The response requirement at which the reinforcer no longer maintains behavior above the cutoff point is called the "breaking point."

A number of studies have shown that progressive ratio tests provide a measure that is sensitive to changes in the amount as well as in the quality of the reinforcer (e.g., HODOS, 1961; HODOS and KALMAN, 1963; KEESEY and GOLDSTEIN, 1968; YANAGITA, 1973; GRIFFITHS et al., 1975, 1978, 1979; BEDFORD et al., 1978; HOFFMEISTER, 1979).

The particular form in which the procedure is arranged can vary depending on the kind of reinforcer to be tested. For example, with small amounts of food or with electric brain stimulation, successive ratios can follow one after another without serious disturbance because of stimulus aftereffects. However, with reinforcers such as psychomotor stimulants, their disruptive effects must be allowed to dissipate before presenting the animal with the opportunity to respond for one more reinforcer. Thus, each ratio must be presented as a single trial separated from the others by time-out periods. Another important feature that can be varied in the progressive ratio procedures is the rule for the numeric progression of the ratios. Some authors have used increments of equal size while others have used increments of varying sizes.

The following is a summary of the main general steps of the progressive ratio procedures used to assess the reinforcing efficacy of drugs administered intravenously: (1) Establishment of the behavior of self-administration with a drug such as cocaine until a stable performance is reached at a relatively low fixed ratio; (2) Substitution of the standard dose of the reference drug for the dose of the drug to be tested and progressive increase of the ratio until reaching the breaking point according to the chosen criterion; (3) Return to the dose and drug of reference to reassess the baseline performance; (4) Repetition of steps 4 and 5 for each dose and drug tested; (5) Sometimes performance under saline baseline periods is also obtained.

YANAGITA (1973 and GRIFFITHS et al. (1975, 1978a, 1979) have studied a number of psychomotor stimulants on progressive ratio tests. Maximum prices paid for a single dose of cocaine have reached 6000–6400 responses.

The function relating the drug dose to the breaking points, for various psychomotor stimulants, has an ascending limb in the lower dose range. The ascending limb leads to a more or less extended plateau in some intermediate range, and afterward, a descending limb starts. Cocaine has maintained the highest ratios among the psychomotor stimulants tested. The rank ordering of different psychomotor stimulants according to their dose-response curves on progressive ratios put diethylpropion, methylphenidate, and chlorphentermine as drugs with less potency and less efficacy as reinforcers than cocaine.

Compared with the opioids (HOFFMEISTER, 1979), the psychomotor stimulants maintain high behavioral prices only over a narrow dose range.

Early on we proposed that drug dependence is characterized by excessive drug-seeking and drug-consuming behavior. Progressive ratio tests yield information about the maximal behavioral output that can be commanded by a given dose of a drug. Therefore, results in this test appear to give a measure of how much behavior could be generated by a reinforcing drug under conditions where there is no competition with behaviors reinforced by other reinforcers.

Previous considerations about the elasticity of demand generated by a reinforcer suggested that this aspect of the strength of behavior is a very important semiologic variable to characterize dependence. Results obtained in progressive ratio tests may be used to estimate the elasticity of demand generated by a drug, but the design of the procedure must be different. The elasticity of demand of a reinforcer cannot a priori be considered as a single unmovable function. It is sure to vary depending on the nature of other reinforcers that may compete with drug self-administration.

In real life, it is very important to know how drug reinforcement and elasticity of drug demand interact in competition with other reinforcers. Information on this point might enrich even more the great insight that has been gained about what is possibly the best understood disorder of human behavior.

References

Balster, R.L., Schuster, C.R.: Fixed-interval schedule of cocaine reinforcement: effect of dose and infusion duration. J. Exp. Anal. Behav. *20*, 119–129 (1973)

Balster, R.L., Kilbey, M.M., Ellinwood, jr., E.H.: Methamphetamine self-administration in the cat. Psychopharmacologia (Berl.) *46*, 229–233 (1976)

Bedford, J.A., Bailey, L.P., Wilson, M.C.: Cocaine reinforced progressive-ratio performance in the rhesus monkey. Pharmacol. Biochem. Behav. *9*, 631–638 (1978)

Bedford, J.A., Borne, R.F., Wilson, M.C.: Comparative behavioral profile of cocaine and nor-cocaine in rats and monkeys. Pharmacol. Biochem. Behav. *13*, 69–75 (1980)

Bejerot, N.: In: Sjöqvist, F., Tottie, M. (eds.): Abuse of central stimulants, p. 298. Stockholm: Almqvist & Wiksell 1969

Boissier de Sauvages, F.: Nosologie methodique. French translation by Nicolas, M. (1771) of the original Latin version of 1762. Facsimile at the National Library of Medicine, Washington, D.C.

Carey, J.T., Mandel, J.: A San Francisco bay area "speed" scene. J. Hlth. Soc. Behav. *9*, 164–174 (1968)

Catania, A.C.: Drug effects and concurrent performances. Pharmacol. Rev. *27*, 385–394 (1976)

Clineschmidt, B.V., Hanson, H.M., Pflueger, A.B., McGuffin, J.C.: Anorexigenic and ancillary actions of MK-212 (6-chloro-2-[1-piperazinyl]-pyrazine; CPP). Psychopharmacology *55*, 27–33 (1977)

Cytawa, J., Jurkowlaniec, E., Biatowas, J.: Positive reinforcement produced by noradrenergic stimulation of the hypothalamus in rats. Physiol. Behav. *25*, 615–619 (1980)

Deneau, G.A., Yanagita, T., Seevers, M.H.: Self-administration of psychoactive substances by the monkey: a measure of psychological dependence. Psychopharmacologia (Berl.) *16*, 30–48 (1969)

De V. Cotten, M. (ed): Symposium on control of drug taking behavior by schedules of reinforcement. Pharmacol. Rev. *27*, 291–548 (1976)

Dougherty, J., Pickens, R.: Fixed-interval schedules of intravenous cocaine presentation in rats. J. Exp. Anal. Behav. *20*, 111–118 (1973)

Dougherty, J., Pickens, R.: Pharmacokinetics of intravenous cocaine selfinjection. In: Mulé, S.J. (ed.) Cocaine: chemical, biological, clinical, social, and treatment aspects. Cleveland, Ohio: CRC Press 1976

Down, D.A., Woods, J.H.: Food- and drug-reinforced responding: effects of DITA and d-amphetamine. Psychopharmacologia (Berl) *43*, 13–17 (1975)

Elsmore, T.F., Fletcher, G.V., Conrad, D.G., Sodetz, F.J.: Reduction of heroin intake in baboons by an economic constraint. Pharmacol. Biochem. Behav. *13*, 729–731 (1980)

Estrada, U., Villarreal, J.E., Schuster, C.R.: Self-administration of stimulant drugs as a function of the dose per injection. Minutes of the twentyseventh meeting of the CPDD. pp. 5056–5059. National Academy of Sciences, Washington, D.C. 1967

Findley, J.D., Robinson, W.W., Gilliam, W.: A restraint system for chronic study of the baboon. J. Exp. Anal. Behav. *15*, 69–71 (1971)

Findley, J.D., Robinson, W.W., Peregrino, L.: Addiction to secobarbital and chlordiazepoxide in the rhesus monkey by means of self-infusion preference procedure. Psychopharmacologia (Berl.) *26*, 93–114 (1972)

Goldberg, S.R.: Comparable behavior maintained under fixed-ratio and second-order schedules of food presentation, cocaine injection or d-amphetamine injection in the squirrel monkey. J. Pharmacol. Exp. Ther. *186*, 18–30 (1973)

Goldberg, S.R., Morse, W.H., Goldberg, D.M.: Behavior maintained under a second-order schedule by intramuscular injection of morphine or cocaine in rhesus monkeys. J. Pharmacol. Exp. Ther. *199*, 278–286 (1976)

Griffith, J.D.: A study of illicit amphetamine drug traffic in Oklahoma City. Amer. J. Psychiat. *123*, 560–569 (1966)

Griffith, J.D.: Amphetamine dependence; clinical features. In: Martin, W.R. (ed.): Drug addiction II. pp. 277–304. Handb. exp. pharm. Vol. 45/II. Berlin Heidelberg New York: Springer-Verlag 1977

Griffiths, R.R., Findley, J.D., Brady, J.V., Dolan-Gutcher, K., Robinson, W.: Comparison of progressive-ratio performance maintained by cocaine, methylphenidate, and secobarbital. Psychopharmacologia (Berl.) *43*, 81–83 (1975)

Griffiths, R.R., Winger, G., Brady, J.V., Snell, J.D.: Comparison of behavior maintained by infusions of eight phenylethylamines in baboons. Psychopharmacology *50*, 251–258 (1976)

Griffiths, R.R., Brady, J.V., Snell, J.D.: Progressive-ratio performance maintained by drug infusions: comparison of cocaine, diethylpropion, chlorphentermine, and fenfluramine. Psychopharmacology (Berl.) *56*, 5–13 (1978a)

Griffiths, R.R., Brady, J.V., Snell, J.D.: Relationship between anoretic and reinforcing properties of appetite suppressant drugs: implications for assessment of abuse liability. Biol. Psychiat. *13*, 283–290 (1978 b)

Griffiths, R.R., Bradford, L. DiAnne, Brady, J.V.: Progressive ratio and fixed ratio schedules of cocaine-maintained responding in baboons. Psychopharmacology *65*, 125–136 (1979)

Hawks, D., Mitcheson, M., Ogborne, A., Edwards, G.: Abuse of methylamphetamine. Brit. Med. J. 1969 II, 715–721

Herling, S., Downs, D.A., Woods, J.H.: Cocaine, d-amphetamine, and pentobarbital effects on responding maintained by food or cocaine in rhesus monkey. Psychopharmacology *64*, 261–269 (1979)

Hodos, W.: Progressive ratio as a measure of reward strength. Science *134*, 943–944 (1961)

Hodos, W., Kalman, G.: Effects of increment size and reinforcer volume on progressive ratio performance. J. Exp. Anal. Behav. *6*, 387–392 (1963)

Hoffmeister, F.: Negative reinforcing properties of some psychotropic drugs in drug-naive rhesus monkeys. J. Pharmacol. Exp. Ther. *192*, 468–477 (1975)

Hoffmeister, F.: Progressive ratio performance in the rhesus monkey maintained by opiate infusions. Psychopharmacology *62*, 181–186 (1979)

Hoffmeister, F., Goldberg, S.R.: A comparison of chlorpromazine, imipramine, morphine, and d-amphetamine self-administration in cocaine-dependent rhesus monkeys. J. Pharmacol. Exp. Ther. *187*, 8–14 (1973)

Hoffmeister, F., Wuttke, W.: Further studies on self-administration of antipyretic analgesics with codeine in rhesus monkeys. J. Pharmacol. Exp. Ther. *193*, 870–875 (1975)

Hursh, S.R.: Economic concepts for the analysis of behavior. J. Exp. Anal. Behav. *34*, 219–238 (1980)

Iglauer, C., Woods, J.H.: Concurrent performances: reinforcement by different doses of intravenous cocaine in rhesus monkeys. J. Exp. Anal. Behav. *22*, 179–196 (1974)

Iglauer, C., Llewellyn, M.E., Woods, J.H.: Concurrent schedules of cocaine injection in rhesus monkeys: dose variations under independent and non-independent variable-interval procedures. Pharmacol. Rev. *27*, 367–383 (1976)

Jasinski, D.R., Gilbert, P.E., Vaupel, B., Risner, M.E., Cone, E.J.: Stimulant self-administration studies in dog. Progress Report from the NIDA addiction research center. Proceedings of the fortieth annual scientific meeting of the CPDD, pp. 171–177. National Academy of Sciences, Washington, D.C. 1978

Johanson, C.E., Schuster, C.R.: A choice procedure for drug reinforcers: cocaine and methylphenidate in the rhesus monkey. J. Pharmacol. Exp. Ther. *193*, 676–688 (1975)

Johanson, C.E., Schuster, C.R.: A comparison of cocaine and diethylpropion under the different schedules of drug presentation. In: Ellinwood, E.H., Kilbey, M.M. (eds.): Cocaine and other stimulants, pp. 545–570. New York: Plenum 1976

Johanson, C.E., Balster, R.L., Bonese, K.: Self-administration of psychomotor stimulant drugs: the effects of unlimited access. Pharmacol. Biochem. Behav. *4*, 45–51 (1976a)

Johanson, C.E., Kandel, D.A., Bonese, K.: The effects of perphenazine on self-administration behavior. Pharmacol. Biochem. Behav. *4*, 427–433 (1976b)

Jones, B.E., Prada, J.A.: Relapse to morphine use in dog. Psychopharmacologia (Berl.) *30*, 1–12 (1973)

Kallant, O.J.: The amphetamines: toxicity and addiction. Toronto: University of Toronto Press, 1966

Kallant, O.J.: The amphetamines: toxicity and addiction, 2nd ed. Springfield, Ill.: Thomas 1973

Kato, M.: Epidemiology of drug dependence in Japan. In: Zarafonetis, C.J.D. (ed.): Drug abuse, pp. 67–70. Philadelphia: Lea & Febiger 1972

Keesey, R.E., Goldstein, M.D.: Use of progressive fixed ratio procedures in the assessment of intracranial reinforcement. J. Exp. Anal. Behav. *11*, 293–301 (1968)

Kelleher, R.T.: Conditioned reinforcement in second-order schedules. J. Exp. Anal. Behav. *9*, 475–485 (1966)

Kelleher, R.T.: Characteristics of behavior controlled by scheduled injections of drugs. Pharmacol. Rev. *27*, 307–323 (1976)

Kelleher, R.T., Goldberg, S.R.: Fixed-interval responding under second order schedules of food presentation or cocaine injection. J. Exp. Anal. Behav. *28*, 221–231 (1977)

Kramer, J.C., Fishman, V.S., Littlefield, D.C.: Amphetamine abuse. Pattern and effects of high doses taken intravenously. J. Amer. Med. Ass. *201*, 305–309 (1967)

Masaki, T.: The amphetamine problem in Japan. Wld. Hlth. Org. Techn. Rep. Ser. *102*, 14–21 (1956)

Pickens, R., Thompson, T.: Self-administration of amphetamine and cocaine by rats. Minutes of the twenty-seventh meeting of the CPDD, pp. 5049–5055. National Academy of Sciences, Washington, D.C. 1967

Pickens, R., Thompson, T.: Cocaine-reinforced behavior in rats: effects of reinforcement magnitude and fixed ratio size. J. Pharmacol. Exp. Ther. *161*, 122–129 (1968)

Risner, M.E.: Intravenous self-administration of D- and L-amphetamine by dog. Eur. J. Pharmacol. *32*, 344–348 (1975)

Risner, M.E., Jones, B.E.: Self-administration of CNS stimulants by dog. Psychopharmacologia (Berl.) *43*, 207–213 (1975)

Risner, M.E., Jones, B.E.: Intravenous self-administration of cocaine and norcocaine by dogs. Psychopharmacology *71*, 83–89 (1980)

Sánchez-Ramos, J.R., Schuster, C.R.: Second-order schedules of intravenous drug self-administration in rhesus monkeys. Pharmacol. Biochem. Behav. *7*, 443–450 (1977)

Schuster, C.R., Johanson, C.E.: Behavioral studies of cathinone in monkeys and rats. In: Harris, L.S. (ed.): Problems of drug dependence, 1979. NIDA research monograph 27, pp. 324–325

Schuster, C.R., Thompson, T.: Self-administration of and behavioral dependence on drugs. Ann. Rev. Pharmacol. *9*, 483–502 (1969)

Schuster, C.R., Villarreal, J.E.: Experimental analysis of opioid dependence. In: Efron, D.H. (ed.): Psychopharmacology – a review of progress 1957–1967, pp. 811–828. Washington, D.C.: U.S. Government Printing Office 1968

Sjöqvist, F., Tottie, M. (eds.): Abuse of central stimulants. Stockholm: Almqvist & Wiksell 1969

Smith, R.C.: Speed and violence: compulsive methamphetamine abuse and criminality in the Haight-Ashbury District. In: Zarefonetis, C.J.D. (ed.): Drug abuse, pp. 435–448. Philadelphia: Lea & Febiger 1972

Spealman, R.D.: Behavior maintained by termination of a schedule of self-administered cocaine. Science *204*, 1231–1233 (1979)

Spealman, R.D., Goldberg, S.R.: Drug self-administration by laboratory animals: control by schedules of reinforcement. Ann. Rev. Pharmacol. Toxicol. *18*, 313–339 (1978)

Stretch, R., Gerber, G.J.: A method for chronic intravenous drug administration in squirrel monkeys. Canad. J. Physiol. Pharmacol. *48*, 575–581 (1970)

Sydenham, T.: The works, on acute and chronic diseases (1666–1686). Version published in English by Rush, B. in 1815. Facsimile at National Library of Medicine, Washington, D.C.

Takahashi, R.N., Singer, G., Oei, T.P.S.: Schedule induced self-injection of D-amphetamine by naive animals. Pharmacol. Biochem. Behav. *9*, 857–861 (1978)

Tessel, R.E., Woods, J.H.: Fenfluramine and N-ethylamphetamine: comparison of the reinforcing and rate-decreasing actions in the rhesus monkey. Psychopharmacologia (Berl.) *43*, 239–244 (1975)

Tessel, R.E., Woods, J.H.: Meta substituted N-ethylamphetamine selfinjection responding in the rhesus monkey: estructive-activity relationships. J. Pharmacol. Exp. Ther. *205*, 274–281 (1978)

Thompson, T., Schuster, C.R.: Morphine self-administration, food-reinforced, and avoidance behaviors in rhesus monkeys. Psychopharmacologia (Berl.) *5*, 87–94 (1964)

Villarreal, J.E.: Contributions of laboratory work to the analysis and control of drug dependence. In: Bachly, P.H. (ed.): Drug abuse, data, and debate, pp. 82–103. Springfield, Ill.: Thomas 1970

Weeks, J.R.: Experimental morphine addiction: method for automatic intravenous injections in unrestrained rats. Science *138*, 143–144 (1962)

Wikler, A., Martin, W.R., Pescor, F.T., Eades, C.G.: Factors regulating oral consumption of an opioid (Etonitazine) by morphine-addicted rats. Psychopharmacologia (Berl.) *5*, 55–76 (1963)

Wilson, M.C., Schuster, C.R.: The effects of chlorpromazine on psychomotor stimulant self-administration in the rhesus monkey. Psychopharmacologia *26*, 115–126 (1972)

Wilson, M.C., Schuster, C.R.: Mazindol self-administration in the rhesus monkey. Pharmacol. Biochem. Behav. *4*, 207–210 (1976)

Wilson, M.C., Hitomi, M., Schuster, C.R.: Psychomotor stimulant self-administration as a function of dosage per injection in the rhesus monkey. Psychopharmacologia *22*, 271–281 (1971)

Wise, R.A., Yokel, R.A., DeWitt, H.: Both positive reinforcement and conditioned aversion from amphetamine and from apomorphine in rats. Science *191*, 1273–1275 (1976)

Wise, R.A., Yokel, R.A., Hansson, P.A., Gerber, G.J.: Concurrent intracranial self-stimulation and amphetamine self-administration in rats. Pharmacol. Biochem. Behav. *7*, 459–461 (1977)

Woods, J.H.: Behavioral effects of cocaine in animals. In: Petersen, R.C., Stillman, R.C. (eds.): Cocaine. 1977. NIDA Research monograph 13, pp. 63–95.

Woods, J.H., Tessel, R.E.: Fenfluramine: amphetamine congener that fails to maintain drug-taking behavior in the rhesus monkey. Science *185*, 1067–1069 (1974)

World Health Organization, Techn. Rep. Ser., No. 577, Evaluation of dependence liability and dependence potential of drugs 1975

Yanagita, T.: An experimental framework for evaluation of dependence liability in various types of drugs in monkeys. Bull. Narc. *1*, 25–57 (1973)

Yanagita, T.: Brief review on the use of self-administration techniques for predicting drug abuse potential. In: Thompson, T., Unna, K. (eds.): Predicting dependence liability of stimulant and depressant drugs, pp. 231–242. Baltimore: University Park 1977

Yanagita, T.: Studies on cathinones: cardiovascular and behavioral effects in rats and self-administration experiment in rhesus monkeys. In: Harris, L.S. (ed.): Problems of drug dependence, 1979. NIDA Research monograph 27, pp. 326–327

Yanagita, T., Deneau, G.A., Seevers, M.H.: Evaluation of pharmacological agents in the monkey by long-term intravenous self- or programmed-adminiseration. Excerpta Med. Int. Congr. Ser. *87*, 453–457 (1965)

Young, A.M., Woods, J.H.: Behavior maintained by intravenous injection of codeine, cocaine, and etorphine in the rhesus macaque and the pigtail macaque. Psychopharmacology *70*, 263–271 (1980)

Author Index

Subject Index

Handbook of Experimental Pharmacology

Continuation of "Handbuch der experimentellen Pharmakologie"

Editorial Board:
G. V. R. Born, A. Farah,
H. Herken, A. D. Welch

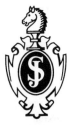

Springer-Verlag
Berlin
Heidelberg
New York

Handbook of Experimental Pharmacology

Continuation of "Handbuch der experimentellen Pharmakologie"

Editorial Board:
G. V. R. Born, A. Farah,
H. Herken, A. D. Welch

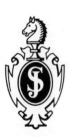

Springer-Verlag
Berlin
Heidelberg
New York